Pocket Guide to the Operating Room

Pocket Guide to the Operating Room

THIRD EDITION

Maxine A. Goldman, BS, RN
Clinical Nurse IV
Formerly, Operating Room Clinical Education Instructor
Medical Center of Tarzana
Tarzana, California

JAYPEE BROTHERS
MEDICAL PUBLISHERS (P) LTD.
New Delhi

F.A. DAVIS COMPANY • Philadelphia

FIRST INDIAN EDITION 2009

As new scientific information becomes available through basic and clinical research, recommended treatments and drug therapies undergo changes. The authors and publisher have done everything possible to make this book accurate, up to date, and in accord with accepted standards at the time of publication. The authors, editors, and publisher are not responsible for errors or omissions or for consequences from application of the book, and make no warranty, expressed or implied, in regard to the contents of the book. Any practice described in this book should be applied by the reader in accordance with professional standards of care used in regard to the unique circumstances that may apply in each situation. The reader is advised always to check product information (package inserts) for changes and new information regarding dose and contraindications before administering any drug. Caution is especially urged when using new or infrequently ordered drugs.

Printed in India

Published by

Jitendar P Vij
Jaypee Brothers Medical Publishers (P) Ltd
B-3 EMCA House, 23/23B Ansari Road, Daryaganj
New Delhi 110 002, India
Phones: +91-11-23272143, +91-11-23272703, +91-11-23282021, +91-11-23245672
Rel: 32558559, Fax: +91-11-23276490, +91-11-23245683
e-mail: jaypee@jaypeebrothers.com
Visit our website: www.jaypeebrothers.com

Branches

- 2/B, Akruti Society, Jodhpur Gam Road Satellite
  Ahmedabad 380 015, Phones: +91-079-26926233 Rel: +91-079-32988717
  Fax: +91-079-26927094 e-mail: ahmedabad@jaypeebrother.com
- 202 Batavia Chambers, 8 Kumara Krupa Road, Kumara Park East,
  Bengaluru 560 001, Phones: +91-80-22285971, +91-80-22382956,
  Rel: +91-80-32714073, Fax: +91-80-22281761 e-mail: bangalore@jaypeebrothers.com
- 282 IIIrd Floor, Khaleel Shirazi Estate, Fountain Plaza, Pantheon Road,
  Chennai 600 008, Phones: +91-44-28193265, +91-44-28194897,
  Rel: +91-44-32972089, Fax: +91-44-28193231 e-mail: chennai@jaypeebrothers.com
- B-2, Sector - 4, Lekhraj Market, Faizabad Road, Indira Nagar
  Lucknow 226 016, Phones: +91-0522-3040553, +91-0522-3040554
  e-mail: lucknow@jaypeebrothers.com
- 4-2-1067/1-3, 1st Floor, Balaji Building, Ramkote Cross Road
  Hyderabad 500 095, Phones: +91-40-66610020, +91-40-24758498
  Rel:+91-40-32940929, Fax:+91-40-24758499 e-mail: hyderabad@jaypeebrother.com
- No. 41/3098, B & B1, Kuruvi Building, St. Vincent Road
  Kochi 682 018, Kerala, Phones: 0484-4036109, +91-0484-2395739, +91-0484-2395740
  e-mail: kochi@jaypeebrothers.com
- 1-A Indian Mirror Street, Wellington Square
  Kolkata 700 013, Phones: +91-33-22451926, +91-33-22276404, +91-33-22276415
  Rel: +91-33-32901926, Fax: +91-33-22456075 e-mail: kolkata@jaypeebrothers.com
- 106 Amit Industrial Estate, 61 Dr SS Rao Road, Near MGM Hospital, Parel
  Mumbai 400 012, Phones: +91-22-24124863, +91-22-24104532, Rel: +91-22-32926896
  Fax: +91-22-24160828 e-mail: mumbai@jaypeebrothers.com
- "KAMALPUSHPA" 38, Reshimbag, Opp. Mohota Science College, Umred Road
  Nagpur 440 009 (MS), Phones: Rel: 3245220, Fax: 0712-2704275
  e-mail: nagpur@jaypeebrothers.com

ISBN 978-81-8448-463-2

Printed by Rajkamal Electric Press, B-35/9, G.T.Karnal Road, Delhi-33

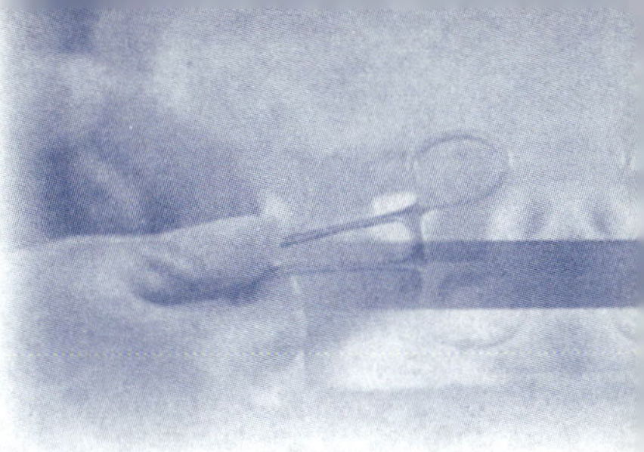

I dedicate this work to those special registered nurses and surgical technologists who are entrusted daily with the responsibility of the care and safety of patients in the perioperative environment.

M.A.G.

Preface

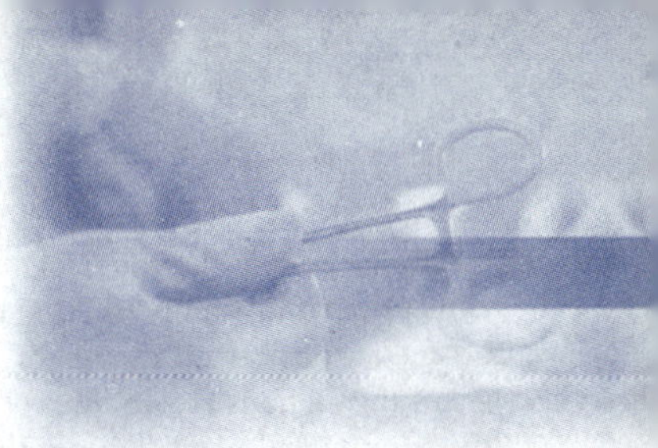

Although the format appears the same as in previous editions, this third edition of *Pocket Guide to the Operating Room* reflects completely revised and thoroughly researched "state of the art" material that will enable the practitioner to elevate his/her level of perioperative patient care to new standards of excellence. The reader will find approximately 100 new procedures or their modifications in this third edition; previously included procedures have been updated to reflect current knowledge of evolving technology and perioperative patient care measures. Chapters containing the latest information on advanced surgical modalities employing lasers, endoscopy, robotics, microsurgical techniques and instrumentation, the Harmonic® and Plasma® scalpels, the Argon beam coagulator®, and radiofrequency ablation are included and cited throughout the work. New chapters on various dental and orthognathic procedures and intraoperative radiotherapy are presented. New surgical entries and/or approaches to previously described surgeries include total joint replacement surgeries; microneuroendoscopy; prosthetic disc replacement; micro, percutaneous, and endoscopic discectomy; percutaneous vertebroplasty and kyphoplasty; and multiple approaches to correct scoliosis. The chapter on pediatric surgery provides comprehensive measures with explanations particularly designed for the care of the child in surgery. My intent is to continue to limit the text's physical size for convenience while maintaining the concise format of previous editions and describing perioperative care with an emphasis on the intraoperative phase. The most recent principles, standards, recommendations, and/or mandates set forth by the Association of periOperative Registered Nurses (AORN), the Joint Commission (JC) [formerly the Joint Commission on Accreditation of Healthcare Organizations (JCAHO)], the Centers for Disease Control and Prevention (CDC), the Occupational Safety and Health Administration (OSHA), and the North American Nursing Diagnoses Association (NANDA) International have been incorporated into the text.

Measures for providing psychological support and physical safety of the patient in the perioperative environment are emphasized in this edition, particularly in the expanded Special Notes section at the end of each surgical entry. The Special Notes also serve to alert the circulator and the scrub person to important information that may not necessarily be found elsewhere. This information assists the practitioner with anticipating and predicting the perioperative needs of the patient and the surgical team members. The reader is encouraged in Chapter 1, and throughout conduction of the surgical procedures in Part 4, to assess individual needs unique to the surgical patient by developing a plan of care and by implementing that plan of care according to currently established safe standards. Perioperative practitioners are also encouraged to evaluate the effectiveness of implemented care by examining patient outcomes to maintain a level of excellence. The discussion section for each surgery includes information on the application of "state of the art" technologic modalities and updated surgical techniques. More than 500 surgical procedures are presented in a preestablished, standardized format. Each includes a definition, a discussion, and a description of each procedure, as well as notes on preparation of the patient and safe positioning practices, skin preparation, draping techniques, equipment, instrumentation, supplies, and Special Notes pertinent to patient care for each procedure. In the Special Notes section, the perioperative practitioner is alerted to care measures of particular importance that are preceded by the notation **N.B.**

The conduction of a surgical procedure may appear to differ from institution to institution, between different sections of the country, and according to the preferences of individual surgeons, but the common goal regarding the best outcome for the patient remains the same. As noted in the previous editions, the particular equipment, instruments, and supplies suggested for use are not to be regarded as exclusive. Rather, the suggested surgical items represent those that are basic and commonly used; items can be added or deleted according to preference. Draping techniques, instrument nomenclature, equipment, supplies, etc. will also vary accordingly. Precise details regarding certain items such as suture material have been omitted due to the ever-increasing availability of products and brands.

In this edition, the bibliography lists references that include pertinent Internet sites. As in previous editions, the text is reflective of the most current drug information with reference to safety precautions and includes anesthetic agents and their administration in their respective chapters. An encyclopedic reference to every surgical procedure has not been attempted. Infrequently performed procedures or those procedures performed only at select surgical facilities, such as organ transplantation surgery, complex cardiac procedures, etc. have been omitted.

Incumbent upon the perioperative practitioner is the need to ever expand knowledge on a daily basis, to provide a continuum of safe patient care in the perioperative environment, and to adapt the latest surgical modalities to established basic concepts. I hope the information presented herein will serve as a generally applicable foundation upon which to build.

M.A.G.

Acknowledgments

In writing this third edition, I am indeed indebted to many surgeons, anesthesia providers, perioperative nurses, and surgical technologists for sharing their knowledge with me. They offered highly informative insights gained through years of diligent observation and active participation in the conduction of their respective specialties. I wish to thank the many providers of surgical instruments, equipment, prostheses, and pharmaceuticals who have generously supplied detailed product information and resources.

I wish to acknowledge and thank my long-term friend and colleague, Patricia Gautreau, RN, BSN, CNOR, director of perioperative services at West Hills Hospital and Medical Center, West Hills, California, who suggested that I write the first edition of this text over twenty years ago. She continues to be a great source of professional encouragement, support, and enlightenment, unsparing in her assistance in obtaining technical information.

I also wish to thank Chris Keegan, CST, MS, FAST Professor/Chair Surgical Technology and Surgical Assisting, Vicennces University, Evansville, Indiana, who advised me on the role of the surgical technologist. She initially reviewed and proposed a number of suggestions regarding surgical entries for the text and lent her expertise to the writing of the chapter on dental surgery.

I appreciate the considered critique of the 2nd edition of this Pocket Guide by the following Reviewers:

- Janet Cadorette, Instructor, Surgical Technology, Tennessee Technical Center at Knoxville, Knoxville, TN
- Tracy L. Ray, RNFA, CNOR, ST, Coordinator and Instructor, Surgical Technology, Ozarks Technical Community College, Springfield, MO
- Jane Roman, RN, MEd, Chair, Surgical Technology, Bunker Hill Community College, Chelsea, MA, and
- Elizabeth Slagle, MS, RN, CST, Director and Associate Professor, Surgical Technology, University of Saint Francis, Fort Wayne, IN.

These highly qualified professionals provided encouragement and certain insights to write a future 3rd edition.

I very much appreciate the patience and understanding of my editor, Christa Fratantoro, regarding the nature of delays inherent in compiling the text and the support and encouragement I received from her and the staff at F. A. Davis Company, especially Elizabeth Zygarewicz, Editorial Assistant. I also thank Robert H. Craven, Jr., President, who encouraged me to proceed with the writing of the third edition of this text. I again thank Francine Kubrin, former medical librarian, Valley Presbyterian Hospital, Van Nuys, California, for obtaining many valuable references. I thank Colleen Ward, Marla Sussman, and Linda Kern and her staff at Progressive Publishing Alternatives for their efforts in preparing the manuscript for production.

I am also pleased to acknowledge the love, kind encouragement, and unwavering support of my adult children Laurie, Emily, Judith, and David, and that of my dear friends during the preparation of this work. And finally, as always, I wish to thank my husband Harris, my partner in all endeavors, whose knowledge and love sustained me through the completion of this work.

Contents

PART 1 PERIOPERATIVE CONSIDERATIONS: Preoperative, Intraoperative, and Postoperative Care Including Psychological Support of the Surgical Patient

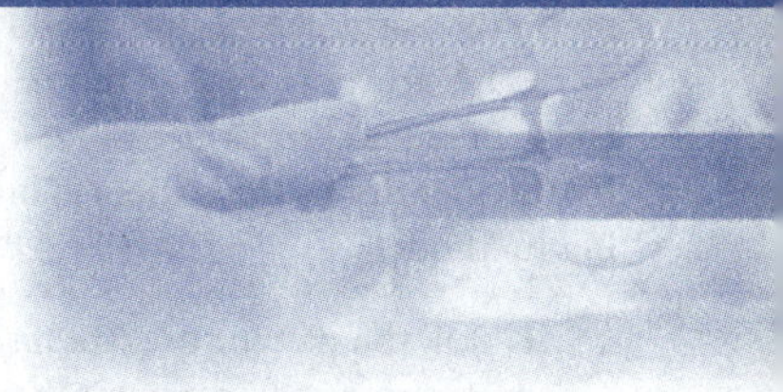

CHAPTER 1

Perioperative Care of the Patient

Psychological Support of the Patient in Surgery

When surgery is recommended to an individual, the proposed operation, regardless of its extent, is perceived by the patient to be a "major" procedure. The patient's emotional support begins with the referring physician who recommends a surgeon qualified to perform the surgery. The surgeon explains the indications for surgery, the course of events prior to and following the surgical procedure, and the medical terminology used. During the discussion, the surgeon, in a supportive manner, will outline a favorable course of events, but will not make any guarantees regarding the outcome of the surgical procedure. In addition, the surgeon must inform the patient of the possibility of poor results and the potential complications or injuries related to the procedure or the anesthetic, including death, even though the likelihood may be remote. The surgeon then clarifies any information pertaining to the surgery until the patient (or legal representative) indicates that he/she understands and is satisfied with the explanation. If there are alternative treatments or therapies, these must be disclosed prior to asking the patient to sign the "informed consent." The surgeon may comfort the patient by stating that the chosen hospital or surgicenter is an accredited facility that has a capable and dedicated staff and that every measure will be taken to assure a successful outcome.

In some facilities, when time permits, a perioperative nurse telephones the patient prior to the day of surgery to verify the patient's name, date of birth, height and weight, and other personal data, as necessary. He/she answers the patient's questions and tries to help the patient feel more comfortable about the impending surgical procedure. This initial patient contact optimally is made prior to the date of surgery, but may not take place until immediately before the surgical procedure.

The patient usually arrives at the hospital or surgicenter the day before or the day of the scheduled surgery, according to the surgeon's orders. Following admission to a unit, as time permits, the patient may be offered a perioperative teaching session and/or a teaching video. Whenever possible, the patient is afforded an opportunity to express anxieties and/or ask questions. The nurse preparing the patient for surgery completes the Surgical Assessment and Preoperative Checklist (**Form 1-1**).

Prior to transporting the patient to the surgical suite, operating room personnel must use at least two sources of identification to verify the identity of the patient. This may include any two of the following methods:

1. ask the patient to state his/her name
2. compare the name on the chart to the patient's stated name
3. compare the name on the patient's armband to the name on the chart
4. compare the name on the addressograph plate to the name on the chart.

In addition, as a safety measure, personnel should check the front of the chart to obtain a list of the patient's allergies and current medications.

Once the patient arrives in the surgical holding area preoperatively, the circulator, a perioperative practitioner, will implement the Joint Commission (JC) (formerly the Joint Commission on Accreditation of Healthcare Organizations) 2004 *Universal Protocol* to identify the patient by asking the patient to state his/her name and by using another identifier from the list above. (Note that by asking for the patient's name, rather than by asking directly, "Are you Mary Jones," one minimizes the possibility of misidentification.) The patient's name, date of birth, the name of the admitting doctor or surgeon, and other identifiers on the patient's hospital armband must match those identifiers on the chart. The patient is asked to state the proposed procedure; the perioperative practitioner records the patient's response in the patient's *own* words on the record. Obtaining and confirming important information from the patient and the patient's chart helps to ensure the patient's safety in the operating room. For patients who are unable to communicate effectively (e.g., a young or shy child, a patient with a language barrier, or a patient who is physically or emotionally impaired or otherwise unable to speak coherently or obtunded), the above information is verified with the patient's legal representative.

In the surgical suite, the circulator again asks the patient to state his/her name. (Note that the patient's name and identifiers are verified a number of times by different personnel.) The circulator compares the patient's name and identification number with the armband, chart, and addressograph plate. The procedure to be performed, the appropriately marked site/side (or laterality) of the body as applicable, and the name of the surgeon are reconfirmed with the patient or the patient's representative.

FORM 1-1 Surgical Assessment and Preoperative Checklist

Patient Identification Verification for Patient Safety

Use at least two identifiers

☐ Ask the patient to state his/her name
☐ Compare stated name to the name on chart
☐ Compare the name on chart to the name on armband.
☐ Compare armband information to addressograph plate

Name of anticipated surgical procedure
(*write in patient's own words*)
"____"

Surgical procedure ______________________

Consent signed
☐ yes ☐ no Comment ______________

Special consent signed
☐ yes ☐ no ☐ N/A Comment ______________

Prep by ______________________
Skin condition before prep ______________
after prep ______________

History and physical examination charted
☐ yes ☐ no Comment ______________

Medications on front of chart *(include OTC, herbal products)*
☐ yes ☐ no Comment ______________

Sensitivities on front of chart
☐ yes ☐ no Comment ______________

ALLERGIES on front of chart
☐ yes ☐ no Comment ______________

Blood or blood products ordered ☐ refuses transfusions
☐ yes ☐ no Time available Initials

Preoperative instructions given by ______________

Skin preparation by ______________ Site ______________ Solution ______________

Skin condition
before prep ______________ After prep ______________

NPO since *(time)* ______________ Height ______________ Weight ______________
B/P ______________ TPR ______________

Old charts in OR
☐ yes ☐ no Comment ______________

continued on following page

FORM 1-1 Surgical Assessment and Preoperative Checklist (continued).

☐ Drains type
site N/A
Comment

☐ Catheter(s) type
(1) site
(2) site
Comment

☐ Intravenous line started: solution type
by
Comment

Prostheses:

☐ Dental (*dentures, bridges, retainers*)
retained by
removed by
disposition by

☐ Limb type/location
retained by
removed by
disposition by

☐ Eye: ☐ R ☐ L
retained by
removed by
disposition by

Implanted Electronic Devices (IED):

☐ Hearing devices: *implantable hearing aids, cochlear implant bone conduction aids*
type signature

☐ Cardiac: *defibrillator, pacemaker, or ventricular assist devices (VAD)*
type signature

☐ Bone growth stimulator
type signature

☐ Medication infusion pump
type signature

☐ Neurologic devices: *ventricular shunts, nerve stimulators, brain stimulators*
type signature

VALUABLES:

☐ Eyeglasses
removed/disposition by

☐ Contact lenses ☐ R ☐ L
removed/disposition by

☐ Hearing aids ☐ R ☐ L
retained/removed/disposition by

☐ Jewelry type
retained/removed/disposition by

☐ Shaver/radio type
removed/disposition by

☐ Wallet/money
removed/disposition by

Entries on the Surgical Assessment and Preoperative Checklist (pp. 3–4) are begun on the nursing unit as the information is reviewed with the patient. The circulator is also required to verify the information with the patient and initial each item on the checklist. (Note that every facility has its own policy and procedure.) The patient's fasting status, prosthetic devices, special physical needs, and drug and substance intolerances, including sensitivities and ALLERGIES, are reviewed by the circulator with the patient or his/her representative and noted in the chart. The patient's allergies and current medications should be listed on the front of the chart, although this requirement is not mandated in every health-care institution. Documentation of this information is valuable for preventing errors in patient care; it provides an extra measure of patient safety. Laboratory data are reviewed; a current record of the patient's history and physical examination (dated according to institution policy) are confirmed. Any deviations from the norm, omissions, or discrepancies are to be reported immediately to the anesthesia provider and surgeon. Any valuables or personal property items not previously collected are secured, and their destination is noted on the chart.

When the patient enters the operating room, the circulator may offer a warm blanket and/or touch the patient's hand or shoulder to indicate concern for the individual. When the circulator answers the patient's questions or directs the questions to the surgeon as appropriate, the patient may feel more secure. Adding to that security, the circulator should inform the patient that he/she acts as the patient's advocate during surgery, particularly when the patient is anesthetized or otherwise unable to respond. A simple explanation of "patient's advocate" may contribute significantly to the patient's confidence in the course of events to follow. Incidentally, operating room personnel must know and implement patient care safety measures when interacting with patients (e.g., protecting the patient's fingers from injury when the foot of the table is dropped and later raised).

The chart is checked once again by the circulator with respect to the Authorization for and Consent to Surgery (**Form 1-2**), p. 6. This document may include authorization for the administration of blood, blood products, and/or blood transfusions. Additional special consents may be required, i.e., Authorization for and Special Consent to Surgical Sterilization Procedure (**Form 1-3**), p. 7. This document indicates that the patient will become sterile. The circulator must verify and document in the Perioperative Record that the surgeon has informed the patient and the patient has stated that he/she understands that he/she will no longer be able to procreate.

Once the patient data requirements are verified by the circulator, everyone on the surgical team must agree that the patient on the operating table is the correctly named patient, of the named surgeon present,

FORM 1-2 Authorization for and Consent to Surgery

I, ____,
do hereby authorize Dr. ______________________
and his/her assistant ________________________
(certified to assist in surgery) to perform the
following procedure(s) ________________________
at this hospital (name) ______________________
on (date) ____________________________________.

I have been informed of the risks, benefits, and alternative treatments to this surgery.

I do/do not authorize permission for a blood or blood products transfusion, if necessary, as deemed advisable by my surgeon and/or anesthesia provider. (If consent is withheld, as for religious reasons, document refusal in (Form 1-1) Surgical Assessment and Perioperative Checklist.)

I have been informed and understand the purpose of the procedure and the possible complications.

I have received no guarantee regarding the consequences or outcome of the aforementioned procedure, including risk of death.

I agree to photography (in which I cannot be identified). The photographer and others may be in the operating room for educational purposes.

I leave to the discretion of the pathologist the disposition of any specimen(s).

I understand that I am responsible for the fees for any specialized services I receive while in surgery, independent from hospital fees.

I acknowledge that I read this document, that I fully understand it, and that I am not under the influence of any preoperative or other sedating medication.

Patient (or legal representative)
Signature ______________________________
date ______________________________

Relationship to patient, if patient is a minor or if patient requires a legal representative ______________________________
Signature ______________________________
date ______________________________
Signature of witness ______________________________
date ______________________________

FORM 1-3 Authorization for and Consent to Surgical Sterilization Procedure

I, ____ ,
do hereby authorize Dr. ______________________
and his/her assistant ________________________
(certified to assist in surgery) to perform the
following procedure(s) ______________________
at this hospital (name) ______________________
on (date) ________________________________

My physician has fully explained the hysterectomy/tubal ligation/vasectomy (or other) surgical procedure and appropriate alternatives to me. I was offered the opportunity to ask questions and to refuse to have the procedure. I understand that following the hysterectomy/tubal ligation/vasectomy I will be sterile, that is, not able to have children. I understand that the procedure is to be regarded as ***irreversible***. If I change my mind after the sterilization procedure (e.g., tubal ligation or vasectomy) has been performed, a reversal procedure, if available, may not be successful in restoring my fertility. Following a hysterectomy procedure there is no possibility that I will be able to become pregnant.

Signature ______________________________
date ______________________________
Witness ______________________________
date ______________________________

AFFIRMATION OF INFORMED CONSENT BY PHYSICIAN

I, in agreement with the Health and Safety Code of the (state), have given the above named patient (or legal representative) information explaining the nature of the procedure: purpose, alternative methods, risks and potential complications, and limitations. After receiving the foregoing information, the patient consents to the treatment and/or procedure described.

Signature ______________________________
date ______________________________
Witness ______________________________
date ______________________________

with the correct site and side marked for the particular surgery, and that the patient's position on the table is correct for the procedure to be performed. Should any member of the team notice something amiss, it is his/her obligation to bring it to the attention of the team. Any special equipment, instrumentation, and/or implants must be available in the operating room, ready for use prior to starting the surgery. If blood or blood products have been ordered, their availability should be determined prior to surgery by the circulator. The information above needs to be corroborated by all members of the surgical team during the obligatory "time out" mandated by the JC before the surgery may proceed. Any unresolved discrepancies must be reported to the surgeon, the anesthesia provider, and the surgery supervisor, documented in the Perioperative Record, and reported in an Incident Report. The surgery may not proceed until all discrepancies are resolved. All pertinent issues and events during the patient's surgery must be documented on the Perioperative Record, p. 12. Documentation on this record provides the legal accounting of the surgery in detail. Any incident that occurs while the patient is in the operating room that has not been documented cannot be considered "fact" in a court of law. Documentation of all that occurs intraoperatively during the patient's perioperative experience is recorded for medicolegal purposes as well as to provide information.

During the induction of anesthesia, the circulator may hold the patient's hand and/or make eye contact with the patient until the patient is anesthetized; these measures may be continued intermittently throughout the surgical procedure when the patient experiences varying degrees of awareness (e.g., when sedation and analgesia/conscious sedation are employed). Be aware that the patient may be able to perceive, in varying degrees, what is said during the induction of general anesthesia, and even subsequently, as hearing is the last sense to be lost. It is imperative that all who are in the operating room maintain silence during the induction of anesthesia to prevent distraction. Talking is best kept to a minimum throughout the surgical procedure. The number of people in the operating room should be kept to a minimum to avoid distractions and to avoid the possibility of inadvertent contamination of the sterile field.

Postoperatively, the anesthesia provider and the circulator safely transport the patient to the Post Anesthesia Care Unit (PACU), alert to any untoward events. The perioperative RN in the PACU is given orders from the anesthesia provider upon the patient's arrival. Similarly, the circulator from the operating room gives report to the PACU RN regarding the patient's condition, pertinent surgery details, and the patient's immediate needs. The patient's care is transferred at that time to the perioperative RN in the PACU, who now assumes the role of the patient's advocate.

PERIOPERATIVE CARE PLAN

NURSING FOCUS I:

PATIENT APPEARS ANXIOUS DUE TO ANTICIPATED SURGERY/PROCEDURE AND UNFAMILIAR ENVIRONMENT

ASSESSMENT — Cognitive Status

☐ Awake ☐ Alert ☐ Oriented
☐ Asleep ☐ Drowsy ☐ Responsive
☐ Obtunded ☐ Lethargic ☐ Disoriented/confused
☐ Unresponsive/comatose Comment ____________

PAIN 1–10 ________ Other Factors: ☐ Alcohol abuse history ☐ Drug abuse history
Language: Speaks English ☐ yes ☐ no Patient speaks another language ________
Deficits: ☐ Hearing ☐ Sensory ☐ Mobility ☐ Visual ☐ Memory
Discuss impairment(s): ____________

CARE PLAN

☐ Greet patient by name (with titles), as necessary
☐ Encourage patient to express concerns and questions; incorporate them into the care plan
☐ Respond to concerns or questions with calm reassurance and accurate facts; defer to surgeon/anesthesia provider when appropriate
☐ Orient patients to surroundings and advise them of events as they occur
☐ Consider using touch to enhance communication
☐ Consider special needs of pediatric and geriatric patients

DESIRED OUTCOME Patient is able to speak calmly, cooperate, and follow directions.
Outcome met ☐ yes ☐ no
Comment ____________

NURSING FOCUS II:

PATIENT MAY PERCEIVE BODY IMAGE AS ALTERED/IMPAIRED SELF ESTEEM

CARE PLAN

☐ Consider developmental age of all patients, especially pediatric or geriatric patients
☐ Answer patient's questions and explain procedures before doing them
☐ Avoid unnecessary exposure of patient's body
☐ Adhere to policy regarding visitors and photography; keep number of people in the room to a minimum

DESIRED OUTCOME Patient refers to the surgery with positive attitude, acceptance, and understanding.
Outcome met ☐ yes ☐ no
Comment ____________

NURSING FOCUS III:

PREVENT INJURY TO NERVES, JOINTS, AND SKIN INTEGRITY WHEN POSITIONING PATIENT

CARE PLAN

☐ Smooth sheets under the patient, remove knots on gown ties to maintain smooth surfaces for skin integrity
☐ Consider pediatric patient's size and adjust table, accessories, equipment, and instrumentation accordingly
☐ Pad all bony prominences, e.g., the sacrum, particularly in elderly patients with fragile skin; use adequate padding also on elbows and heels to prevent pressure sores; use positioning aides for support, as necessary
☐ Use rolls and/or pillows to ease pressure on skin and nerves, to allow for adequate lung expansion, to relieve pressure between breasts and under scrotum, to support the patient in the desired position, and for comfort, as a pillow placed under the knees to minimize back strain or a small pillow under the head
☐ Use safety belt across the thighs, taking care to be sure it is not so tight that venous return is impaired
☐ Position patient so that the body is in good alignment and symmetry; avoid extreme flexion or extension of joints to prevent pain and injury
☐ Use supports above and below joints when moving an extremity; the surgeon is responsible for moving or lifting broken extremities
☐ Avoid placing patient's hands at the break in the table, use arm boards as procedure permits; check position of the fingers, especially when raising the foot of the table

Patient position ____________
Positioning aids ____________
Padding used ________ Type ________ Site ________
Grounding pad used ☐ yes ☐ no Type ________
Control lot number # ________ Location ________
Skin condition before surgery ________ After surgery ________

DESIRED OUTCOME:
Patient shows no signs or symptoms of injury to nerves, joints and skin integrity.
Outcome met ☐ yes ☐ no
Comment ____________

(**NOTE**: When patient arrives in PACU or on the floor unit, patient should be examined and asked about **PAIN 1–10** ________ or paresthesiae,and the ability to move, i.e., to rule out paralysis)

continued on following page

PERIOPERATIVE CARE PLAN (continued)

NURSING FOCUS IV:

PREVENT PATIENT'S DISCOMFORT ON THE TABLE AND LOSS OF BODY HEAT

CARE PLAN

- ☐ Provide comfort measures as appropriate with pillows, pads, and specially warmed blankets as necessary
- ☐ Confer with anesthesia provider and surgeon regarding application of forced-air warming blanket or MUL-T blanket (hypo/hyperthermia blanket or mattress pad)
- ☐ Observe that skin temperature feels warm and that color appears normal
- ☐ Ask patient if room temperature is comfortable; check room temperature and adjust if necessary. Monitor patient's body temperature
- ☐ Use warm irrigation solutions (noting also that cold or iced solutions may be employed, e.g., for active bleeding)
- ☐ Avoid over-warming patients with fever
- ☐ Increase room temperature, use radiant heat lamps, thermal blankets, and fluid warmers for pediatric patients according to weight
- ☐ Adjust room temperatures for geriatric patients as necessary
- ☐ Incorporate temperature control measures into procedures, e.g., keep patient well covered when inserting Foley catheter

DESIRED OUTCOME Patient has warm, dry skin with normal color.

Outcome met ☐ yes ☐ no

Comment ____________________

NURSING FOCUS V:

PREVENT IMPAIRMENT OF SKIN INTEGRITY DURING SKIN PREPARATION

CARE PLAN

- ☐ Document condition of skin before beginning skin preparation and following completion of preparation
- ☐ Work carefully to prevent nicks in skin when shaving or using clippers; work carefully to avoid moles, papillomata, and skin tags
- ☐ Assess skin for reaction to prep solution; observe for rash or hives; discontinue using solution as necessary, ask surgeon for further directions and document the finding if reaction occurs
- ☐ Work carefully to prevent skin preparation solutions from pooling under patient as they may cause skin irritation and excoriation and the solution could support combustion

DESIRED OUTCOME Patient's skin will remain intact and in good condition.

Outcome met ☐ yes ☐ no

Comment ____________________

NURSING FOCUS VI:

ASSIST ANESTHESIA PROVIDER DURING INDUCTION AND ASSIST HIM/HER TO CORRECT PATIENT'S FLUID VOLUME LOSS DURING SURGICAL PROCEDURE

CARE PLAN

- ☐ Monitor blood loss in suction canisters and in sponges
- ☐ Monitor urine output
- ☐ Communicate with anesthesia provider and/or surgeon regarding total fluid losses and assist with fluid replacement to maintain fluid and electrolyte balances
- ☐ Consider special needs of the pediatric patient by weighing sponges as soon as possible to prevent evaporation of blood or fluid in sponges
- ☐ Utilize blood warmers to prevent shock from cold transfusion and infusion pumps to speed fluid correction. Use warm saline irrigation unless contraindicated

DESIRED OUTCOME Alterations in patient's fluid volume losses due to NPO and intraoperative losses are restored.

Outcome met ☐ yes ☐ no

Comment ____________________

NURSING FOCUS VII:

PREVENT INJURY AND RISK TO PATIENT WITH IMPLANTED ELECTRONIC DEVICE WITH SPECIAL PRECAUTIONS TO PREVENT ELECTROMAGNETIC INTERFERENCE (e.g., interference with implanted pacemaker by ESU)

CARE PLAN

- ☐ If IED is to be inserted or replaced, check that IED and instrumentation for implantation are in OR
- ☐ Know details regarding IED (by attending in-service education); circulator is notified in advance about the patient with IED
- ☐ Check that appropriate industry representatives are present in OR
- ☐ Verify representative's credentials; that rep. has taken AORN OR course (or similar course) for understanding and knowledge of asepsis and the sterile field
- ☐ Assure patient you know about IED; that you will take all safety precautions necessary for patient safety
- ☐ Prevent inherent electromagnetic interference and risk to the patient with a pacemaker or similar device
- ☐ Take special care to see that device is not damaged
- ☐ Complete Special Log if IED is inserted

DESIRED OUTCOME Patient will leave OR with IED without injury to patient or damage to device.

Outcome met ☐ yes ☐ no

Comment ____________________

PERIOPERATIVE CARE PLAN (continued)

NURSING FOCUS VIII:

PREVENT PATIENT DISCOMFORT OR INJURY DURING TRANSFER TO GURNEY AND TRANSPORT TO PACU

CARE PLAN

- ☐ Cover patient with warmed blankets following procedure
- ☐ Ensure adequate assistance for transfer from table to gurney, lock wheels, check side rails are up
- ☐ Observe safety measures by using good body mechanics, bend knees, lift with strength from legs
- ☐ Consider size and weight of the pediatric patient to determine if isolette, crib, or gurney is needed following procedure
- ☐ Circulator accompanies patient to PACU; assisting anesthesia provider, as necessary
- ☐ Circulator will give verbal report to PACU RN to provide continuity of care

DESIRED OUTCOME Patient is safely transferred to PACU.

Outcome met ☐ yes ☐ no

Comment ____________________

PERIOPERATIVE RECORD

PREOPERATIVE, INTRAOPERATIVE, AND PACU RECORD

[STAMP PATIENT ADDRESSOGRAPH PLATE]

PREOPERATIVE RECORD :

IMPLEMENT JCAHO *UNIVERSAL PROTOCOL CORRECT SITE/SIDE SURGERY*

Patient speaks English ________ If not, other language ____________

IDENTIFICATION:

Preoperative Assessment and Checklist

ASK PATIENT/PARENT/GUARDIAN

☐ Patient's name ______________________________

☐ DOB ________________

☐ Age ________________

☐ Sex ________________

VERIFY

☐ I.D. band, chart, and hospital patient numbers match

☐ Surgeon(s) names correct

☐ Scheduled surgical procedure correct

Comment ______________________________

Patient states (in his/her own words) the proposed surgery is

" ______________________________

______________________________ "

☐ Signed consent(s) in chart ☐ Correct site/side marked

Limitations ______________________________

Comment ______________________________

☐ Implanted Electronic Device ______________________________

Specify ________ OR notified ______________________________

Comment ______________________________

☐ Prosthesis or implant in OR as ordered

☐ (Industry representative in OR, if requested)

☐ Blood/blood products ordered

\# units available ______________________________

type ______________________________

☐ Radiology exams (X-rays, MRI, CT scan) in OR

☐ Endoscopy reports in OR

☐ Old records/previous charts in OR

☐ Radiology notified in advance, if anticipated

SENSITIVE to: (*including foods, contrast media, medications, dose related problems with medications, OTCs, herbal, and LATEX*)

____

ALLERGIC to: *(including contrast media, foods, medications, dose related problems with medications, OTCs, herbal, and LATEX)*

____

PATIENT RESPONSES MUST CORRESPOND TO THE CHART DATA. ACCURATE RESPONSES ARE REQUIRED FOR *UNIVERSAL PROTOCOL*. DO **NOT** PROCEED UNTIL ANY DISCREPANCY IS RESOLVED. DOCUMENT DISCREPANCY AND ITS RESOLUTION. NOTIFY THE OR SUPERVISOR OR PERSON IN CHARGE.

Comment ______________________________

Signature ______________________________

PERIOPERATIVE RECORD (continued)

INTRAOPERATIVE RECORD

OR # ____________ Time IN ______ Time OUT ______

STAMP PATIENT IDENTIFICATION
NAME PLATE HERE

PREOPERATIVE DIAGNOSIS ____________ ☐ major ☐ minor

SURGEON ____________
ASSISTANT ____________
ANESTHESIA PROVIDER ____________

CIRCULATOR ____________
SCRUB PERSON ____________
Relief ____________
Relief ____________

TYPE OF ANESTHESIA USED ____________
time started ______ time ended ______
Oxygen saturation ____________
IV/lines/CVP/arterial/other ______ (include location)
B/P cuff location ____________

"TIME OUT" OBSERVED ______ Initials ______
Comment ____________
SURGERY ______ time started ______ time ended ______

PATIENT'S POSITION ______ supports used ______
POSTOPERATIVE DIAGNOSIS ____________
SURGICAL PROCEDURE PERFORMED ____________
Prep solution ____________
Skin intact before starting prep ______ Comment ______
Skin intact after starting prep ______ Comment ______

ESU grounding pad site ______ applied by ______ ESU serial # ______
Coagulation setting ______ cutting setting ______ blend/pure setting ______
Skin area before pad ______ after ______
Plume evacuator type ____________

Laser type ____________
Key obtained by ______ Signature ______
Type of handpiece ____________
Laser operation checked by ______ initials ______
Laser test fired by ______ initials ______
- Room warning signs • windows covered • Limit number of people in room
- Eye protection for staff and patient • Non-reflective instrumentation and supplies
- Operative area surrounded with water or saline dampened sponges, towels or drapes
- Special Halon fire extinguisher in room
- Laser plume evacuator type ______ filter type ______
- "Standby" mode on and foot pedal to surgeon ______

☐ Room safety protocol observed
Comment ____________
Signature ____________

continued on following page

PERIOPERATIVE RECORD (continued)

INTRAOPERATIVE RECORD (continued)

Type of Lithotripsy:

ESWL with portable lithotripter ____ ☐ Delta II ☐ Compact S

☐ Ultrasonic lithotripsy ☐ Laser lithotripsy ☐ Electrohydraulic lithotripsy

Patient warned before shockwaves start ____ by ____

☐ Stent or catheter in place on patient's arrival Type ____ Size ____

☐ Stent or catheter inserted Type ____ Size ____ Location ____

☐ IV urography performed ☐ Retrograde urography performed

Fluoroscopy total time ____

X-ray precautions taken ____

Appearance of patient's skin at lithotripsy site

preprocedure ____ postprocedure ____

Equipment problem encountered ____

Intervention ____

Incident report filed ____

Outcome ____

Heating devices/warming mattress/lamps type ____ setting ____

Comment ____

TED hose ____ Sequential hose ____

Catheters/drains/devices

1) Foley catheter ____ size ____

2) Nasogastric tube ____

3) Hemovac ____

4) Other type drain ____

Tourniquet

site ____ pressure ____

time inflated ____ time deflated ____

Skin condition before tourniquet ____ after ____

MEDICATIONS/DOSE/ROUTE ____ Time ____ Given by ____

1) ____

2) ____

INTRAVENOUS FLUIDS

type ____ 1) ____ amount ____

2) ____ amount ____

INTAKE IV ____ Other ____

TOTAL INTAKE ____

OUTPUT Urine ____ Nasogastric tube ____ Other ____

TOTAL OUTPUT ____

☐ **TRANSFUSIONS** type ____ *(whole, packed RBCs, autologous, cell saver, washed WBC, FFP, Other)*

☐ **Blood ID checked with patient ID** Signatures ____ and ____

Bag # ____ type ____ Signatures ____ and ____

Bag # ____ type ____ Signatures ____ and ____

Albumin ____ Plasmanate ____

Blood pump type ____ warmer ____

Comment ____

PROTHESIS/IMPLANT/GRAFT

Type ____ Manufacturer ____ Serial/lot # ____

Implanted Electronic Device (IED)

Type ____ Manufacturer ____ Serial/lot # ____

External Cardiac Pacemaker (temporary)

____ Manufacturer ____ Serial/lot # ____

SPECIMENS Source ____ 1) ____

2) ____

Frozen section source ____

TOTAL # SPECIMENS ____

CULTURES Aerobic Anaerobic

1) ____ 1) ____

2) ____ 2) ____

PERIOPERATIVE RECORD (continued)

INTRAOPERATIVE RECORD (continued)

COUNTS

SPONGE	first	second
NEEDLES/SHARPS	first	second
INSTRUMENTS	first	second
Other type	first	second

ALL COUNTS CORRECT ☐ yes ☐ no

Comment

If the count is incorrect, TAKE ANOTHER COUNT

COUNT CORRECT ☐ yes ☐ no

INCIDENT REPORT filed ☐

Comment

OPERATIVE NURSING NOTES

Integrity and sterility of packaging and indicators have been confirmed. The standards set by AORN for perioperative clinical practice were applied appropriately for this patient throughout the procedure and were within the scope of my practice. I have met the patient's needs and charted the outcomes in accordance with those as proposed in the patient's care plan. I verify that there have been no changes in the patient's condition (other than those inherent in the surgical procedure) during the preceding interval since my preoperative assessments.

Other comments

Signatures

Circulator

Scrub person

Relief

Circulator

Scrub person

PERIOPERATIVE RECORD (continued)
POSTOPERATIVE RECORD

Time admitted to Postanesthesia Care Unit (PACU) ____________
IDENTIFICATION checked by ____________ transported by ____________
Report given to ____________ PACU RN by ____________ OR RN ____________

INTRAOPERATIVE TRANSFER DATA
Surgery Preop Diagnosis ____________
Postop Diagnosis ____________
Surgeon ____________ Assistant ____________
Scrub person ____________ Circulator ____________
Anesthesia provider ____________ Type Anesthesia ____________

Nasal or oral airway ____________
Comment ____________
Oxygen set at ____________ l/m ____________
Dressings intact ____________
Comment ____________
Surgical site dry ____________
Comment ____________
Respirator ____________
settings ____________
color normal ____________
Comment ____________
Monitor in sinus rhythm ____________
Comment ____________
IV in progress from OR ____________
site ____________
solution ____________
Comment, if redness or swelling ____________
IV in PACU ____________
solution ____________
site ____________
Comment ____________
CVP catheter/intraartial ____________
Swan Ganz type/site ____________ pressure ____________
Comment ____________
Skin color normal, warm, dry ____________
Comment ____________
Foley catheter draining ____________
Comment ____________
Nasogastric tube draining ____________
Comment ____________
Other drains type ____________
Comment ____________
Position on gurney ____________
side rails up ____________ restraints ____________ type/location ____________

Level of consciousness ____________
Patient able to move lower extremities with
Spinal, Epidural, or Caudal L ____________ R ____________
Transfusions from OR in progress
type ____________ checked bag # with chart # initials ____________

PERIOPERATIVE RECORD (continued)
POSTOPERATIVE RECORD (continued)

Vital signs on arrival

(*record or graph all the following vital signs on graph*)

Pulse oximeter Oxygen saturation %

• Pulse o Respiration X B/P

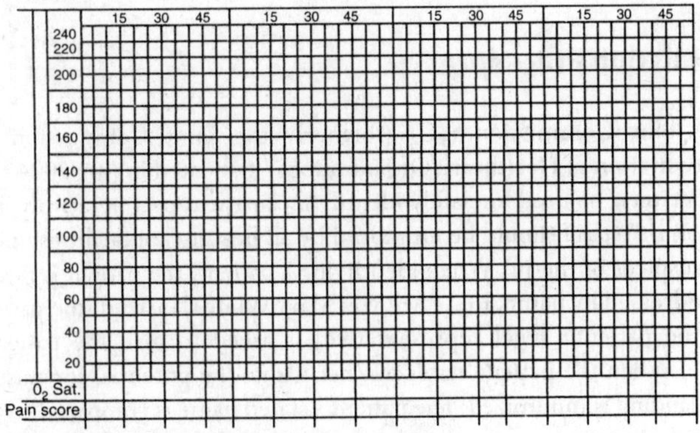

MEDICATIONS/DOSE/ROUTE

time ______ given by ______

1) ______

2) ______

INTRAVENOUS FLUIDS

type 1) ______

2) ______

INTAKE IV ______ Other ______ TOTAL INTAKE ______

OUTPUT Urine ______ Nasogastric tube ______ Other ______

TOTAL OUTPUT ______

TRANSFUSIONS

Type (whole, packed RBCs, autogous, cell saver washed WBC, FFP, Other)

Blood ID checked with patient ID Signatures ______ and ______

Bag # ______ type ______ Signatures ______ and ______

Bag # ______ type ______ Signatures ______ and ______

Albumin ______ Plasmanate ______

PAIN on departure from PACU 1–10 ______

NURSING NOTES:

OBSERVATIONS, INTERVENTIONS, DESIRED OUTCOMES MET

______

______

______

Time out of PACU ______

Transferred to ______ Transport via ______

by ______

Signature(s) ______

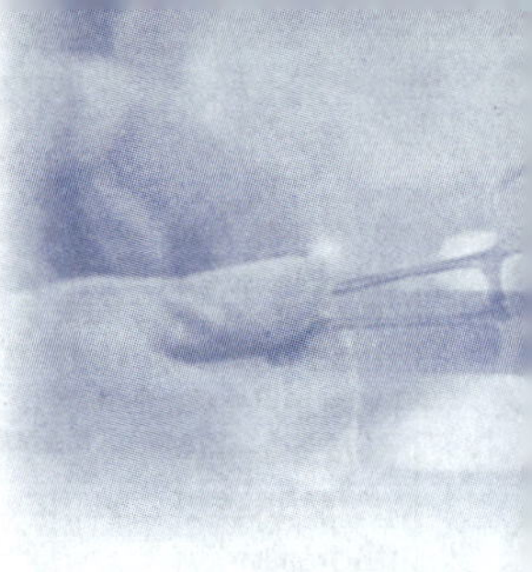

CHAPTER 2
Protection of the Patient in Surgery/ Patient Safety

Admission Procedure

The Joint Commission (JC) (formerly the Joint Commission on Accreditation of Healthcare Organizations) mandated in July 2004 that new criteria be used for safely identifying a patient preoperatively. The *Universal Protocol* should be employed by all health-care facilities under the auspices of the JC. When identifying a patient, the patient is not to be addressed by name, i.e., "Are you Mary White?" Instead, the patient (or the patient's legal representative) is asked to give the patient's name. When the patient states his/her name, the potential for misunderstanding is minimized. The patient's stated name is compared to the name and patient number on the armband, the chart, and the addressograph plate. The patient is asked the name of the surgeon, the type of surgical procedure that he or she anticipates having, the location (site on the body), and the laterality (side) where the procedure will be performed. The location is identified by the patient and corroborated by the perioperative nurse and/or the surgeon. The site is marked with indelible ink. Even when the procedure will be performed on both sides of the body (either left or right but not both sides on the same day), the site for the procedure is marked (boldly), the designated site/side stated on the consent for surgery. Before the surgery begins, before the scalpel is passed to the surgeon, everyone on the surgical team observes a "time out" during which all must verbally agree to the identity of the patient, the surgery to be performed, and the operative site (correctly marked) according to laterality.

The following year, in March 2005, the Association of periOperative Registered Nurses (AORN) recommended adding to the "time out" that everyone on the surgical team must agree that the patient is in the "correct position" on the table before the surgery begins. This "time out" requires the active participation of every member of the surgical team. Should any member find something amiss, he/she is obligated to bring it to the attention of the surgical team. The JC, AORN, American Medical Association (AMA), and other professional organizations consider the mandatory protocol for "wrong site/side, wrong procedure, and wrong patient" in addition to noting that the patient is correctly positioned on the operating table necessary to preventing tragic errors.

Every health-care facility has a policy regarding the procedure to be followed when preparing a patient for surgery (ascribing to the recommendations by the JC). (Please note that any facility where surgery is performed may be referred to as a hospital, surgicenter, or health-care facility, and these names are used interchangeably in this text.) Authorization for and Consent to Surgery, p. 6, and any other special consent form, as necessary, i.e., Authorization for and Special Consent to Surgical Sterilization Procedure, p. 7, or any similar record, must be contained in the chart prior to admitting the patient to the surgical suite preoperatively.

Other requirements may include a recent history and physical examination report, hematology and blood chemistry reports, urinalysis report, chest x-ray report, EKG, and any other reports that may be required depending on the patient's age, diagnosis, and medical condition, and the hospital's policy.

Procedure for Safely Transferring the Patient to the Operating Table

The patient should be transferred to the operating table by at least two persons to prevent injury to the patient and personnel. One or more persons is necessary to stabilize the gurney (stretcher) as close as possible to the operating table, taking care to lock the wheels. Similarly, at least one person must stand on the opposite side of the operating table (bed) to receive the patient and prevent him/her from falling. When the patient is alert and physically able, he/she is given directions for moving onto the table; however, if the patient is unable to move without assistance, adequate help should be summoned before the transfer is made.

Using proper body mechanics is imperative when lifting patients to prevent injury to the musculoskeletal system of the employee(s). Back injuries, in particular, can be avoided when there is adequate help to move the patient safely. Personnel need to lift the patient in unison, bending their knees and using their leg muscles to provide strength during the lifting. Special devices, such as the Davis roller or the Hoyer pad, serve to reduce the weight being lifted, thereby facilitating the lifting and/or moving of a patient. During the transfer, care is taken to protect all catheters and tubings (e.g., Foley catheter, intravenous lines, Swan Gans lines, etc.) from becoming tangled or pulled out. Following the transfer, the restraint (safety) strap is fastened securely across the patient's thighs (about three inches above the knees). <u>Do not</u> apply the restraint too tightly to avoid tissue ischemia and nerve damage.

Once the patient is on the table, correct alignment is required to prevent injuries to the patient's musculoskeletal system. All bony prominences and the extremities must be adequately padded to prevent tissue damage (e.g., to nerves and skin). Some hospitals provide a specially trained staff, a *lift team,* who can be deployed to any area within the facility to assist in moving patients or heavy objects. The cost/benefit of employing individuals to accomplish heavy lifting safely far outweighs the cost of sick days taken by personnel with back injuries.

Preventing Patient Injuries from Falls

Appropriate application of the safety belt (restraint) firmly fastened across the patient's mid-thighs is the single most important measure taken to prevent falls from the OR table. It is fastened firmly, but not excessively as to interfere with the patient's circulation. The patient is ***never*** left unattended in the operating room (OR). The upper extremities may be protected with softly padded restraints that are secured to padded armboards or the table to ensure stabilization of that extremity, but not too tightly as to compromise local circulation.

Positioning/Surgical Positions

The surgeon determines the position of the patient by considering the particular surgical approach, the physical condition of the patient, the technique used for anesthesia administration, and his/her preference in consultation with the anesthesia provider. Factors such as height, weight, body habitus, age, coexisting disease limitations, and cardiopulmonary status are taken into consideration. The desired patient outcome at the conclusion of the surgery is the avoidance of integumentary, nervous, vascular, and musculoskeletal injuries related to positioning or the change of position.

NOTE: Once the anesthesia provider assumes care of the patient, the patient must ***never*** be moved without the anesthesia provider's permission and direction. In all instances, proper body alignment is to be maintained; adequate assistance should be obtained prior to moving or lifting the patient. Positioning aids (devices), when used, must be brought into the OR prior to the admission of the patient to avoid prolonging OR and anesthesia time (for which the patient is charged) while these devices are located. For patients with fractures, severe injuries, significant deformities, or applied devices, it is the surgeon's responsibility to protect the area involved when the patient is moved.

The ultimate position employed may begin with a basic position, appropriately modified to ensure the patient's safety and to obtain the best exposure of the surgical site. The patient's physical mobility is assessed to prevent pain and injury by avoiding excessive flexion or extension of the joints, especially in the patient with arthritis, paralysis, or other physically limiting preexisting conditions. An (oscillating) air mattress may be placed on the table (OR bed) for selected patients (with fragile skin) to protect the skin integrity from injury caused by pressure ischemia. The patient's body should not hang over the table in any direction; if necessary, a padded extension can be added to the table. The skin must not be in contact with any metal surface, as the exposed area would become a potential grounding site when electrosurgery is employed. Disregard of this measure may result in serious burns (see electrosurgery safety precautions, p. 38). When using unipolar electrosurgery, the pencil must be replaced in the holster when not in use.

As previously noted, when positioning the patient, the circulator protects bony areas with padding, pillows, donuts, towel or blanket rolls, etc. Blanket rolls are utilized under the chest to facilitate adequate lung expansion when the patient is prone. In the prone position, extra padding is placed to protect genitalia and breasts. Table accessories, such as shoulder braces, kidney rests, stirrups, and footboards must be well padded to avoid nerve damage and/or tissue ischemia. Care is taken to prevent strain on lower back muscles (e.g., a pillow is placed under the knees) and hyperextension injuries are avoided with proper support of the arms, hands, fingers, neck, and lower extremities, including feet and toes. The circulator and scrub person must ascertain, when applicable, that neither drape sheets nor the Mayo stand are causing undue pressure on the common peroneal nerve (resulting in foot drop) and/or direct pressure on the feet and toes.

The following descriptions include the most common patient positions employed in surgery (See Fig. 2-1 A–J, pp. 27–30). Please note that the protective measures as noted above apply to all standard positions and their modifications.

Supine/Dorsal Recumbent (see Figure 2-1A, p. 27)

In the supine position, the patient lies face up on the padded table with arms tucked in at the sides (using the lift sheet), or extended on (padded) armboards. The body is maintained in proper alignment to prevent straining muscles. The legs may not be crossed to avoid local presure ischemia. When the upper extremities are extended on padded armboards, they are placed at the level of the table to prevent injury to the brachial plexus with padding under the elbows and wrists to prevent pressure injury to soft tissues, for example, the ulnar nerve; the hands are placed with the palms up (in supination). The head may be positioned on a donut or a small pillow; a pillow may also be placed under the knees, and an additional small pillow may be placed at the sacral area to prevent pressure injury to the soft tissue. The elbows and heels are protected with padding (and protective plastic cups, if necessary), as are other bony prominences. The supine position is the most frequently used. It may be employed for procedures on the face (the head may be stabilized on a donut), the neck (with a small pillow under the neck to provide increased extension, improving access), the abdomen, the upper extremities (a hand table may be needed), and the lower extremities.

Trendelenburg (see Figure 2-1B, p. 27)

Trendelenburg is a variation of the supine position. The head and the torso are tilted downward (to a 30°- to 45°-angle), permitting gravity to pull the abdominal contents toward the head (cephalad); this allows for better visualization of the pelvic contents during surgery. Softly padded shoulder braces placed over the supraclavicular area may be used to prevent the patient from sliding off the table. This position should be maintained no longer than absolutely necessary. (In Trendelenburg, blood pools in the torso and the head, increasing blood pressure and intracranial pressure.) The knees are positioned over the lower break in the table to permit flexion. The feet are supported on a padded footboard. Trendelenburg may be employed to minimize hypotension produced by acute blood loss or resulting from the effects of an epidural or spinal anesthetic. Trendelenburg increases venous emptying of the lower extremities to reverse hypotension; additional measures are necessary to treat this condition. Trendelenburg is employed for abdominal hysterectomy and other procedures in the pelvic area.

Reverse Trendelenburg (see Figure 2-1C, p. 28)

Reverse Trendelenburg is a variation of the supine position. The entire table is tilted upward so that the head is higher than the feet. A padded footboard is placed at the end of the table to prevent the patient from sliding off the table. The arms may be secured on a pillow placed on the patient's lap, extended on padded armboards, or tucked in at the patient's sides. Do not allow the fingers to be trapped and injured as the foot of the table is dropped and subsequently raised. Neither the drape sheets nor the Mayo stand should place undue pressure on the feet, toes, and common peronal nerve. A sequential compression device with the application of antiembolitic hose or leg wraps is recommended to avoid venous stasis. This position is employed for neck procedures as thyroidectomy, parathyroidectomy, and scalene node biopsy. It is also used to perform laparoscopic procedures as cholecystectomy.

Fowler's/Sitting (see Figure 2-1D, p. 28)

Fowler's position is also a modification of the supine position; the patient appears to be sitting on a chair. The buttocks are positioned over the middle bend (kidney rest) at the table's edge, and the knees are positioned over the lower break in the table. The head of the table is tilted (angled) upward to as much as a 90° angle; this position supports the head and torso. The knees are flexed slightly as the legs are placed on a pillow over the lower section of the table, angled downward. The feet are placed on a padded footrest (horizontal to the table). A small pillow may be placed at the patient's sacrum to prevent back strain; another pillow may be placed under the knees for comfort. The elbows and heels are protected with padding (and protective plastic cups, if necessary). The arms are frequently placed on a pillow on the patient's lap, secured with softly padded restraints, tucked in at the patient's sides, or extended on padded armboards. This position is employed for posterior craniotomy, selected shoulder, and ear, nose, and throat (ENT) procedures. A traction device (e.g., Crutchfield tongs) is used to immobilize the head during procedures on the brain and cervical spine. All bony prominences must be protected with padding, donuts, or pillows, etc. A variation of this position is known as semi-Fowler's position, in which the degree of elevation of the head and torso is less; the patient appears to be sitting on a lounge chair. In the past, this position was used to permit postoperative intraabdominal secretions or septic exudates to pool in the pelvis to facilitate subsequent surgical drainage. This position may be employed for posterior craniotomy.

Dorsal Lithotomy (see Figure 2-1E, p. 28)

Dorsal lithotomy position is also a modification of the supine position. Stirrup or strap attachments, adjusted to equal height are secured on the table at the middle break. The buttocks are positioned at the edge of the middle break in the table and the sacrum is padded. The lower extremities are simultaneously elevated (preferably by two persons) and the hips and knees are flexed as the feet are placed in one of the many types of padded stirrups or padded straps looped above and below the ankle. After the feet are secured in stirrups or strap attachments, the lower mattress section is removed and the foot of the table is lowered completely. Extreme abduction of the hips is to be avoided; extra care must be used when positioning elderly or arthritic patients (some of whom cannot tolerate this position at all). When the foot of the table is subsequently raised, care is taken to prevent injury to the fingers. This position is employed for obstetric, gynecologic, perineal, anorectal, and urologic procedures. The term "lithotomy" originally referred to the extraction of bladder stones transperineally. A modification of this position employs leg and foot supports (e.g,. Allen stirrups) that permit a less exaggerated elevation of the lower extremities while giving access to both the abdomen and the perineum. Therefore, this position may be employed for low rectal resections without having to change the patient's position during the procedure. Another variation of this position is Edebohl's or Simon's position, in which the knees and hips are somewhat less flexed for some vaginal surgeries. At the completion of the procedure, after dressings are placed, both lower extremities are disengaged from the stirrups and slowly lowered simultaneously to prevent a dramatic drop in blood pressure, as the foot of the table is raised.

Sims' (Semi-Prone) (see Figure 2-1F, p. 29)

In the Sims' position, the patient is placed on his/her left side with the left thigh and leg extended. The right knee and hip are flexed and supported by a padded table restraint with a pillow placed between the legs to prevent undue pressure. The patient's body is rotated to lie more prone than supine (pillows or other supports may be employed). The left arm is protected and secured at the patient's side and the right arm, supported by a pillow-padded Mayo stand, is placed over the patient's body. The skin of the right buttocks is protected with tincture of benzoin, distracted by wide (e.g., four inch) adhesive tape, and secured to the underside of the table. Care is taken to keep the pillow between the legs out of the operative field. Having the left side dependent is preferred, especially if sigmoidoscopy, colonoscopy, or enemas may be performed; minimizes the angulation of the distal colon. A variation of this position is utilized for a combined abdominosacral resection of a low rectal lesion. In this situation, the patient's torso is rotated to provide access to the lower abdomen and the sacral area (with appropriate tissue protection using tincture of benzoin applied to sites prior to the application of tape to achieve distraction of the buttocks and pillows to pad and maintain the position). Draping is done to permit access to both sites without having to reposition the patient during the procedure. Sims' position is employed for procedures requiring access to the vagina, anorectum, and perineum.

Fracture Table (see Figure 2-1G, p. 29)

Patients who arrive in the surgical suite in discomfort and/or in a traction device (e.g., with an acute fracture) may first be anesthetized in the hospital bed in which he/she arrives. Following the administration of anesthesia, the surgeon, with adequate assistance, protectively transfers the patient to the fracture table. The patient is placed supine with both arms extended on padded armboards, or the arm on the unaffected side may be extended on a padded armboard and the arm on the affected side may be flexed over the chest, supported by a pillow-padded Mayo stand, and secured with tape or a double armboard may be used. The sacral area and genitalia are well padded (as most of these patients are elderly with fragile skin) and supported by a specially designed saddle with a perineal post (that is padded for comfort and covered for hygienic reasons). The lower extremities are secured in padded stirrups or padded leg supports. Care is taken not to permit the legs to be in contact with the metal part of the stirrups (when positioning) to prevent the skin from being burned inadvertently when electrosurgery is employed. Separate leg extensions can be moved independently in a variety of positions to permit optimal access to the surgical site. Orthopedic procedures on the lower extremities are performed; x-rays are taken intraoperatively to ensure proper positioning of a prosthesis, plate, or rod. The unaffected extremity may be raised and abducted from the field by adjusting the stirrup height and positioning the leg extension. This position is most often employed for insertion of a hip prosthesis and total hip replacement.

Prone (see Figure 2-1H, p. 29)

The patient, depending on the selected anesthetic, is placed face down in the prone position, with a padded donut to protect the face, or the head is turned to either side with a donut or pillow to protect the face and ear from undue pressure. The hips are positioned over the middle table break to permit flexion, as required. In this position, caudal or hypobaric spinal anesthesia can be induced without having to turn the patient. Epidural anesthetics are usually administered with the patient in a modified lateral mode. When general anesthesia is employed, the patient is supine. Following induction, the airway (including the endotracheal tube) is secured with adhesive tape (the skin is protected with tincture of benzoin) and the patient is turned over to the prone position (at the direction of the anesthesia provider). The head is turned to the side and placed on a well-padded donut that protects the ear and the face. In this position, blanket rolls are placed bilaterally under the chest to facilitate respiratory excursion. Female breasts and male genitalia are well padded to prevent pressure injury. The arms may be tucked in at the sides or extended on padded armboards. If anorectal or sacrococcygeal surgery is performed, the buttocks are distracted with tape secured to the ipsilateral sides of the table, after the skin is protected with tincture of benzoin. A pillow may be placed under the pelvic region to elevate the buttocks and to prevent pressure on the pubis and genitalia. The table is flexed at the hips (more so for procedures requiring the Kraske approach, a modification of the prone position to expose the sacral area; the "jackknife" approach is employed for anorectal and coccygeal surgeries). Adrenalectomy (unilateral or bilateral) and various spinal surgeries may employ the prone position. For some spinal surgeries, a convex curvilinear padded frame is placed anterior to the prone patient to provide additional flexion. Another modification of this position has the patient flexed at the waist over the middle bend of the table; the patient is kneeling with the thighs perpendicular to the floor, the legs horizontal (both areas protected by a pillow), and the feet angled downward. A pillow may also be placed in front of and under the knees, and a rolled towel is placed in front of the ankles to prevent undue pressure. When the lower table section is raised subsequently during the procedure, protect the patient's fingers. This position may be employed for anorectal procedures.

Lateral Kidney (see Figure 2-1I, p. 30)

After anesthesia is established, the patient is placed in the lateral position (with the affected side up) and the iliac crest positioned over the "kidney" elevator (rest, bend, bar). The head is placed on a padded donut, protecting the face and ear on the unaffected side from undue pressure. Bony prominences, including the shoulder, knee, hip, and ankle are well padded. On the unaffected side, the lower extremity is flexed on the table and the leg on the affected side is extended straight over the leg below secured with wide adhesive tape to the underside of the table (with a pillow padding between the legs); the feet and ankles are well-padded, supported, and held in position secured by softly padded restraints or adhesive tape. The position is maintained by adhesive tape applied to the chest and the legs, secured to the underside of the table. All areas of skin that are taped are protected by an application of tincture of benzoin. Care is taken to avoid compromising circulation with all tape restraints. The arms may be placed on padded double armboards or the dependent arm may be extended on a padded armboard with the upper arm brought over the chest onto a pillow-padded Mayo stand and secured. The head and neck are aligned without tension, under the care of the anesthesia provider to avoid airway problems or undue stress on the brachial plexus. After the kidney elevator is raised and the table flexed, the patient is observed for respiratory and cardiodynamic changes. Potential compromise of venous return from the lower extremities may occur and pulmonary function in the dependent lung may be compromised, as well. Following the completion of the definitive procedure, the elevated kidney rest may be lowered and the table flexion reduced to facilitate wound closure Postoperatively, the patient may experience muscle pain related to the "unnatural" position employed during surgery. This position is primarily employed for procedures on the upper urinary tract (e.g., kidney), and structures in the retroperitoneal space.

Lateral Chest/Posterolateral Thoracotomy (see Figure 2-1J, p. 30)

After anesthesia is established, the patient is placed on the unaffected side with the head on a padded donut (to protect the face and dependent ear). The arm on the unaffected side is extended on a padded armboard while the superior arm on the affected side is bent over the chest, supported by a pillow-padded Mayo stand, and secured. The arm is pulled slightly forward and downward to provide some traction on the scapula. The lower extremity on the unaffected side is flexed on the table, and the extremity on the affected side is extended straight over the dependent leg (with pillow padding between the legs to prevent undue pressure). A padded restraint (e.g., the table strap) is secured over the hips, or the patient's position may be secured by wide tape (four inch) to the underside of the table, following the application of tincture of benzoin to protect the skin. A small roll is placed under the shoulder and thorax at the posterior axillary line; female breasts and genitalia are protected with padding, as are the feet and ankles and any other pressure points. The shoulders are padded and tincture of benzoin is applied to the skin under the adhesive tape that is secured to the underside of the table. A soft pad may be placed under the unaffected hip to prevent undue strain on the lumbar region and to relieve pressure on the skin. A modification of this is the anterior chest position; the patient position is more supine than lateral. This position is employed for procedures requiring thoracoabdominal access. Padding and support are altered accordingly. The lateral chest position is employed for thoracotomy procedures.

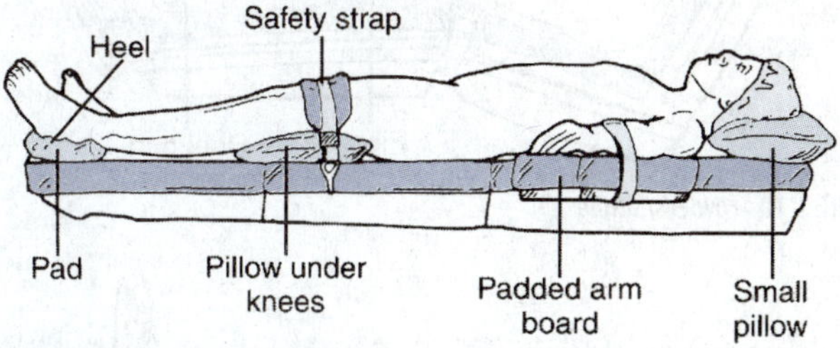

FIGURE 2-1A.

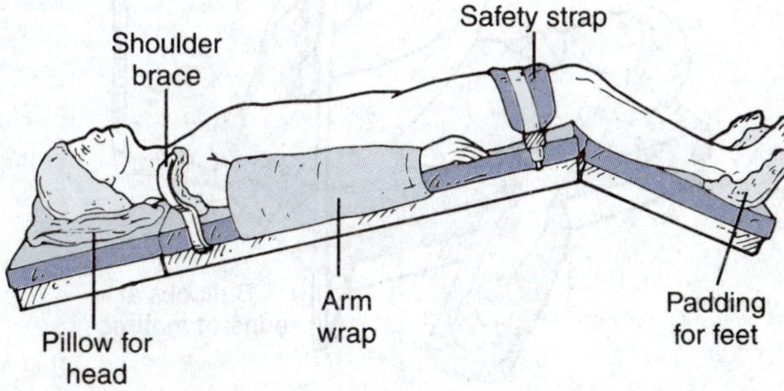

FIGURE 2-1B. Trendelenburg

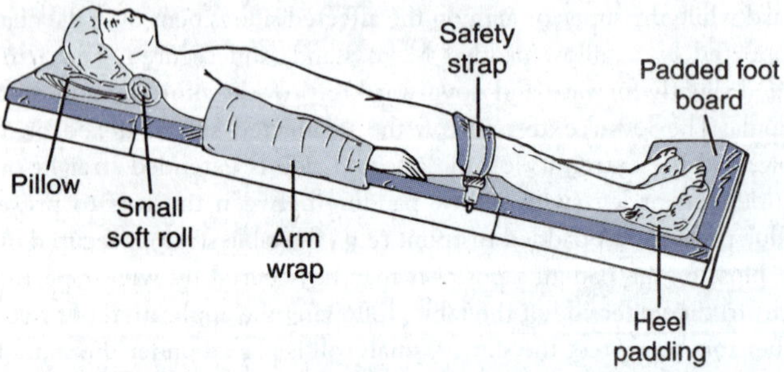

FIGURE 2-1C. Reverse Trendelenburg

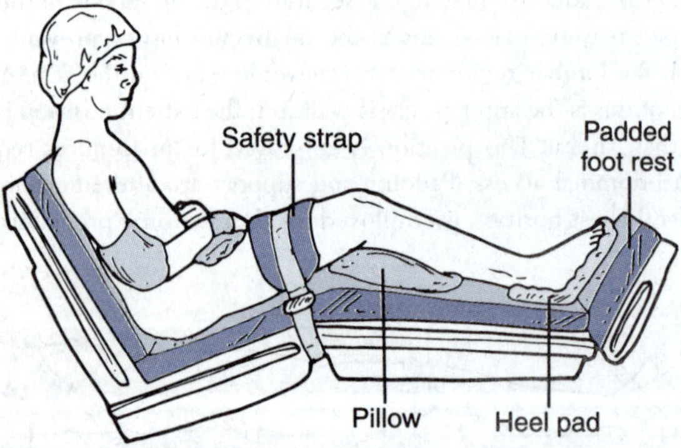

FIGURE 2-1D. Fowler's/Sitting

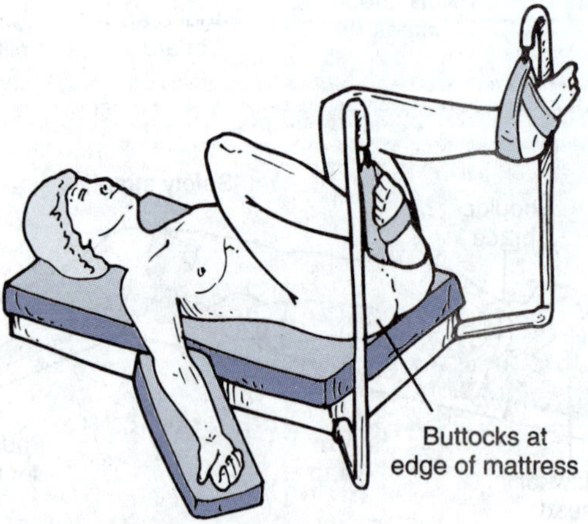

FIGURE 2-1E. Dorsal Lithotomy

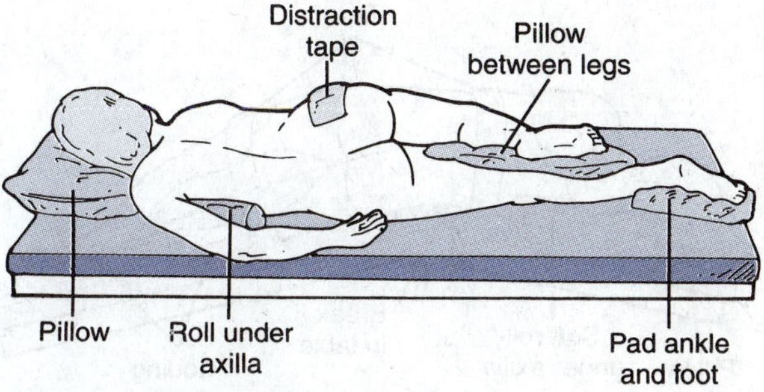

FIGURE 2-1F. Sims' (Semi-Prone)

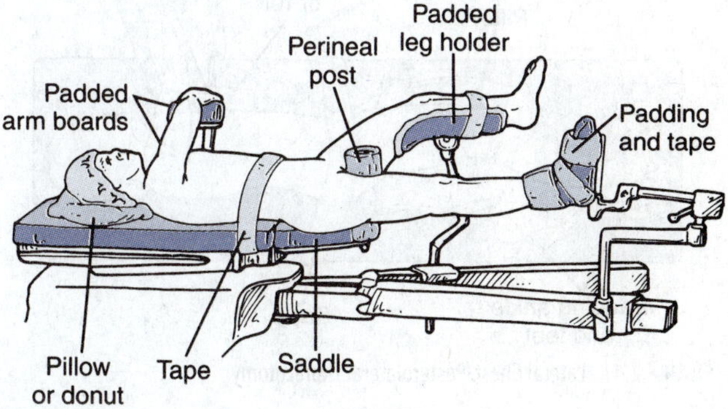

FIGURE 2-1G. Fracture Table

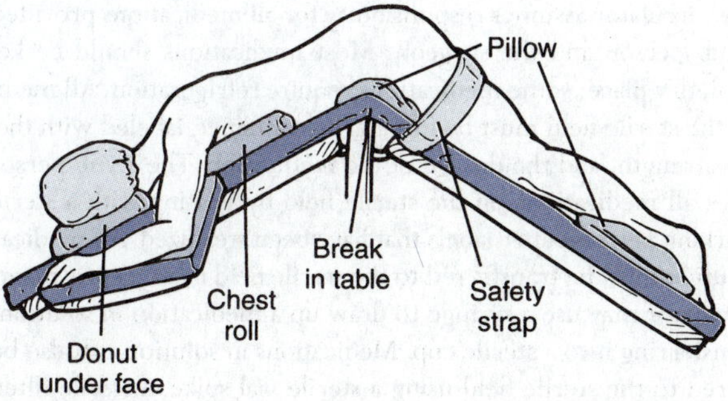

FIGURE 2-1H. Prone

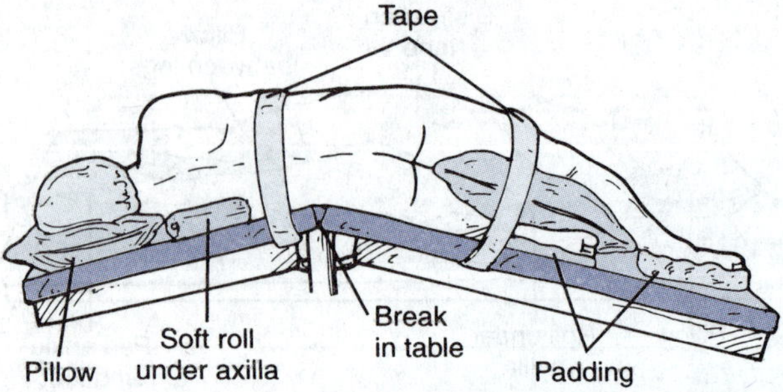

FIGURE 2-1I.

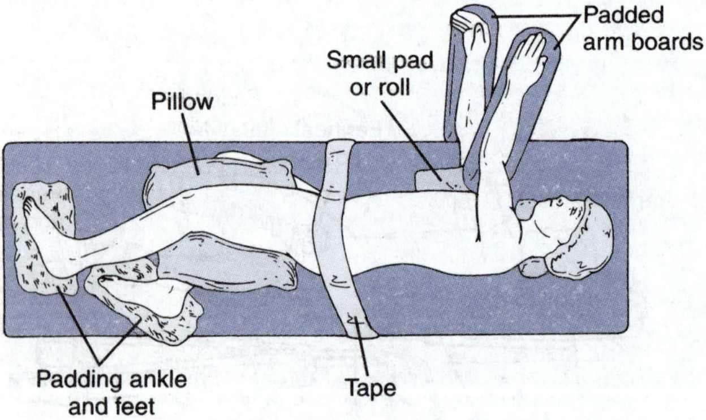

FIGURE 2-1J. Lateral Chest/Posterolateral Thoracotomy

Medication Practices and Guidelines to Avoid Medication Errors

The circulator assumes responsibility for all medications provided to the scrub person and the surgeon. Most medications should be kept in a cool, dry place; some medications require refrigeration. All medications on the sterile field must be in a sterile container, labeled with the name, the strength, and the dosage of the medication. The scrub person identifies all medications on the sterile field by writing with a sterile skin-marking pen on paper labels that have been sterilized. All medications in solution must be transferred to the sterile field in an aseptic manner. The circulator may use a syringe to draw up a medication in solution before transferring it to a sterile cup. Medications in solution can also be transferred to the sterile field using a sterile vial spike, a sterile filter straw, or a sterile catheter; they may not be poured from bottles with stoppers.

A current, reliable medication reference book should always be available in the OR department for use by personnel. Medication errors must be reported and corrected immediately; an Incident Report form should be available for reporting medication errors. Periodic reviews of medication errors should be made to analyze how and why a particular medication error was made and how it can be prevented in the future. "Constraints," as recommended by AORN, are approaches that should be used to avoid errors when administering medications; examples include minimizing the number of medication calculations required and stocking dose-related bottles of medication whenever possible. In addition, the competency of perioperative personnel who administer medications should be evaluated on a regular basis.

To ascertain if a patient is allergic to a requested medication, the patient is asked directly (if possible), and the front of the chart and the preoperative assessment checklist are consulted. Adequate time must be taken to verify that the correct medication is being given, by the correct route, in the correct dosage, and, to the correct patient, as ordered by the surgeon. The protocol for the administration of medication should be checked and rechecked.

When a medication is dispensed to the scrub person, the circulator should state the name of the medication, the strength, and its dosage aloud, while showing the labeled bottle to the scrub person for verification. When a medication must be prepared (in solution), calculations should be checked and rechecked by the person dispensing the medication and the calculations should be verified by another licensed professional. Any unused portions of a used (i.e., opened) medication should be discarded at the completion of the procedure. Any unlabeled medications found in the OR are ***always*** discarded. When the scrub person and the circulator are relieved, all labeled medications being used are shown to the relief person(s). The relief person(s) is/are required to take note of specific medications and their locations on the sterile field. Medication containers or vials and the items used for medication preparation and delivery during a surgical procedure must remain in the room until the completion of the procedure. During a procedure, the trash is ***never*** to be removed from the room before the conclusion of the procedure.

AORN guidance statement suggests using the five "rights" when administering medication: 1) the right patient, 2) the right medication, 3) the right dose, 4) the right time, and 5) the right route.

Allergies

The circulator should speak directly to the patient about any allergic reactions to medications, foods, herbal preparations, and other substances. Check the front of the chart for the list of the patient's allergies;

listing the patient's allergies on the front of the chart can be an invaluable safety measure. The patient allergies most frequently encountered in the OR are those to adhesive tape, latex, and iodine (often contained in some skin preparations and contrast dye agents). Patients who are allergic to certain foods are often allergic to certain types of medications.

NOTE: Allergic reactions can be serious; they may lead to anaphylactic shock and possibly even death. Be prepared for this emergency situation by knowing the location of the cardiac arrest "crashcart" prior to bringing the patient into the room.

Latex Sensitivity and Allergy

When identifying patients before surgery, it is imperative that perioperative personnel question the patient regarding all sensitivities and allergic responses to foods, substances, and medications. Individuals who have a food allergy to bananas, avocados, chestnuts, and kiwi fruit are frequently sensitive or allergic to latex. Patients need to be asked specifically about being sensitive or allergic to those fruits listed, in addition to *latex,* or any product that may contain latex. Knowing in advance that a patient is allergic to latex may literally save that patient's life.

Latex sensitivity and latex allergic reaction vary in intensity from causing an "irritant dermatitis" that results in dry, red and cracked, itching skin to causing a true (delayed) allergic reaction, an "allergic contact dermatitis" within 48 hours of exposure that exhibits similar symptoms, but may not be limited to the point of contact. The most serious reaction is a "true allergic response" (anaphylaxis) that occurs almost immediately and may be characterized by rapidly developing urticaria, facial edema, and a generalized swelling of body tissues (i.e., the larynx and bronchi), followed by respiratory distress secondary to bronchospasm and laryngospasm and hypotensive shock that may result in death.

When an "at-risk" person simply touches a balloon or has cutaneous or mucous membrane contact with latex proteins, an allergic response may result. In surgery, the allergic response may be far greater if the patient or the staff member has had repeated contact with products made of latex, as gloves, nasogastric tubes, anesthesia and respiratory support equipment, urinary catheters, enema equipment, etc. Patients, particularly pediatric patients, who have had multiple surgeries (e.g., procedures for spina bifida, staged hypospadias and epispadias, etc.) and have been exposed to latex proteins during previous operative experiences are at the greatest risk for developing an allergic response. Individuals who frequently don latex gloves or work with latex products may also be at great risk for developing an allergic response. Latex allergy may not be evident until the individual has been exposed to latex proteins numerous times.

The best method for treating a latex reaction is to prevent it by creating an environment that is "latex safe" or "latex-free." Corticosteroids, antihistamines, and other appropriate medications are used to lessen the severity of an allergic reaction. Medications (including epinephrine, diphenhydramine, steroids, H-2 blockers, inhalants such as albuterol, glucagon, etc.), a variety of latex free airways and tubings, and all equipment necessary to treat anaphalactic shock should be kept on a well-stocked "latex-free crash cart" in the surgical suite. Health care facilities should develop a protocol for treating latex reactions.

The Food and Drug Administration (FDA) requires the manufacturers of products and devices containing latex (proteins) to have a warning label stating that use of the product may cause an allergic response. Decision makers in hospitals and health-care facilities need to adopt a policy requiring latex-safe environments for both patients and health-care workers by selecting alternate products for use in the OR, and throughout the facility, making the environment safer for personnel and patients

Environmental Controls

Preventing Infections

In 1996, the Center for Disease Control and Prevention (CDC) issued *Standard Precautions* directed to health-care facilities and personnel for the purpose of prevention of and transmission of infectious diseases. These guidelines were initially prompted by the HIV/AIDS emergence, but are applicable to all infectious diseases encountered in the health care system. *Universal Precautions,* previously established, listing measures to safely deal with blood products, bodily fluids (including vaginal secretions and seminal fluid), was incorporated into *Standard Precautions*. Patients and health-care givers are presumed to be potentially infectious or susceptible to infection. The practice of hand washing, utilization of gloves, masks, facial shields, gowns, cleansing of patient care equipment, environmental control, linen processing, occupational health and bloodborne pathogens, and patient placement considerations are addressed. By observing these measures, the spread of pathogenic microorganisms can be controlled or limited. The discussions that follow are the practice of these measures, as applied to the OR environment.

Each OR, including furnishings and equipment, should be cleaned with a germicidal cleaning agent after every procedure. Numerous studies have shown that selected "ritual cleaning" that was done in the past following "contaminated" or "dirty" cases is an obsolete practice as all cases are known to be potentially infectious. Each OR needs to be cleaned in the same manner every time using a germicide. In addition, the entire surgical department, including its corridors, storage rooms, and other auxiliary areas, is cleaned according to an established schedule.

Traffic patterns are developed to minimize intrusion into restricted areas. Airborne contaminants are reduced by air conditioning (utilizing high-efficiency particulate air filters) and laminar airflow systems. The barriers created in and around special areas in the department must be observed.

Specially laundered or disposable clothing (scrub attire) is worn. Disposable head coverings, masks, protective facial shields, and waterproof fire-retardant gowns and shoe coverings are utilized and replaced (changed) between cases and removed when leaving the department.

Probably the greatest single factor in preventing the nosocomial infections is frequent hand washing with an antimicrobial agent. Nosocomial infections are those infections acquired while in the hospital. Hand washing should be performed upon entering the surgical suite before starting work, and it should be the last thing done by each member of the staff when leaving the department. Hand washing is just as important for the circulator as for the scrub person (following a case even if gloves were worn). Hands should be washed after caring for each individual patient, and gloves should be changed after performing each task (even when on the same patient) while working as a circulator (as in handling of soiled sponges and instruments, tissues, or fluids). Gloves are always changed between patients.

Following their initial hand washing, individuals who are not working within the sterile field may use a waterless cleansing agent (antimicrobial gel) following their initial scrub upon entering the department. Personnel with cuts and abrasions of the hands or forearms should not scrub.

Jewelry such as rings and bracelets is to be removed. Artificial fingernails (which may harbor bacteria and fungi) may not be worn in surgery according to AORN. An appropriate cap (containing all of one's hair) and a mask (to cover facial hair) should be adjusted before scrubbing, as should eyeglasses. Disposable masks of synthetic materials are preferable to cloth masks that are permeable to the passage of pathogens. Similarly, the mask protects the wearer from inhaling contaminants or particulate matter generated in the operative field. Additionally, facial shields prevent splashing or spattering of blood and other fluids into the eyes, nose, or mouth. Laser-related eye protective measures are addressed in the chapter on lasers, p. 95.

Surgical Scrubbing Technique

"Scrubbing" refers to a specified length of time (and number of brush strokes) needed to cleanse all anatomical aspects of the nails, fingers, hands, and forearms and the order in which each zone is washed and rinsed prior to donning gown and gloves. Each institution selects a variety of disposable brushes and cleansing agents approved by the Occupational Safety and Health Administration (OSHA). Strict attention to "scrubbing" technique by those working in the sterile field, in addition to proper skin preparation of the surgical site, and the constant vigilance and attention paid to the implementation of aseptic technique by the entire surgical team will help to reduce the number of contaminants present about the surgical field.

Aseptic Technique

Careful attention must be given to the controlled sterilization of instrumentation, instrument trays, and supplies by specifically noting the time and the condition of the sterility indicators and wrappers. The careful, proper opening of individually packaged sterile instruments, instrument trays, and supplies must be observed. All wrapped items are to be unwrapped by holding the package away from one's body and unwrapping the item starting with the corner that is farthest away and ending with the corner closest to the body. Disposal of waste material and the removal of laundry into specially colored or marked and labeled plastic bags or containers is mandatory to prevent contamination of the environment inside and outside the hospital/health-care facility.

Utilizing an enzymatic foaming agent that can be sprayed on instruments following a surgery before removing trays from the OR aids in preventing blood and other contaminants from drying on the instruments. This debris is sometimes overlooked, and it dries inside the lumen of an instrument as well as in other areas (e.g., crevices, joints of instruments, etc.). Enzymatic foaming agents also prevent contaminated spilled liquids from becoming a biohazard. When this foam is not available, instruments should be covered with a sheet and carefully transported to the decontamination area. Spills are to be mopped up using a germicidal agent.

Implanted Electrical Devices

It is not unusual to encounter patients with an implanted electrical device (IED). The devices include implantable hearing devices, cardiac devices, infusion pumps, neurological devices, brain stimulators, bone stimulators, and gastric devices. Perioperative personnel should be aware that some IEDs are susceptible to electromagnetic interference, causing them to malfunction in the OR when other electrical equipment (e.g., electrosurgical unit) is used. In 2005, AORN stated that perioperative personnel must possess current knowledge regarding the many types of IEDs; this information is often provided by the surgical department through in-service education. When scheduling a patient for surgery, the surgeon must notify the OR if a patient requires insertion or replacement of an IED. The patient's status regarding an IED should be noted on the patient's chart in the nursing surgical assessment preoperatively.

If an IED is initially being implanted or replaced, the appropriate industry representative may be present during the surgery. He/she must take the AORN special OR instruction course (or its equivalent) in order to be present in the OR. The industry representative is in the OR to lend his/her expertise and support to the OR team. Documentation should be made in the Intraoperative Record that the industry representative is present in the OR (with the permission of the patient, surgeon, and OR supervisor).

Documentation of all the special care measures and precautions taken by the circulator and the team members must be recorded in the Intraoperative Record, as well as the IED ownership log. Before the patient arrives, the circulator needs to review all necessary information regarding the IED. Often a separate log for a particular type of device is kept in the OR; the circulator is responsible for maintaining current information, as the name of the device, type, manufacturer, serial number, and other applicable information to help identify the device.

Electrical and Fire Hazards

Electrical and fire safety precautions are set forth in hospital policy and are carried out by members of the OR staff. The National Fire Protection Association (NFPA) provides health-care facilities with standards for fire prevention and safety. NFPA recommends that specific types of portable fire extinguishers (labeled according to the source of the fire to be extinguished) should be accessible and in close proximity to the ORs. Health-care facilities provide in-service programs and fire drills for personnel. These programs should address the potential causes of surgical fires, their prevention, and methods for extinguishing a fire in the department. Most facilities request that members of the local fire department teach a fire prevention class; they may also be requested to teach methods for rescue and evacuation of patients.

The engineering department determines the safety of equipment before permitting its use in the OR. Inspection of the equipment prior to each use is the responsibility of the person(s) who will participate in using said equipment. Personnel are required to receive instruction for the safe operation of all electrical equipment and then demonstrate their ability to use the equipment safely before putting it to use. All electrical equipment used in the OR must be grounded. A three-pronged plug on equipment cords indicates that it is grounded. Electrical cords should be inspected for damage; any electrical equipment in the OR must not be used if it has a damaged cord. When a surgeon asks the circulator to increase the current of an ESU several times, eventually above normal limits, this indicates a malfunction of the unit. It is imperative for the perioperative RN to investigate whenever a red light suddenly appears on a piece of electrical equipment as it is a warning sign that indicates a problem. That particular ESU or other piece of electrical equipment should be unplugged. If the source of the defect or malfunction cannot readily be determined and corrected, the unit should be replaced and referred to the engineering department. The model number of the replacement equipment should be noted on the intraoperative record along with the reason why the previous unit was replaced, e.g., red warning light remained on.

Fires result from a combination of HEAT plus OXYGEN plus FUEL; an inciting source of ignition (e.g., electrical spark) sets off the fire. These three elements create the fire triangle and are replete in an OR. Personnel must be instructed how to prevent fires in the OR, as well as what action is required of each individual should a fire occur. The location of fire extinguishers, the fire alarm, and the code name (e.g., CODE RED) to alert personnel are to be known by everyone in the surgical department and the entire facility. All personnel should receive special instruction regarding their responsibilities in case of fire and may be asked during fire drills to perform those duties. Fire drills are not scheduled; they should be called at least twice a year. Fire drills are to be taken seriously.

Flammable anesthetic agents are infrequently employed today; however, there are flammable materials and liquids that may be in use at any time in an OR (e.g., alcohol-based skin preparation solutions). Paper or fabric items, such as gowns, head and shoe coverings, and drapes used in the OR, are made as fire retardant as possible, but they are not *fireproof*. Flammable liquids should be avoided, but when absolutely necessary, are to be used with great caution when preparing the skin. These solutions must not be permitted to pool under the patient or in the drapes, as they can ignite from a spark when using the electrosurgical unit (ESU) or the laser. Note that the pooling of any solution under the patient or in the drapes is also to be avoided to prevent injury to the skin by excoriation, and to prevent the solution from becoming the fuel for a fire.

Neither the ESU nor the laser should be used in the mouth or oropharynx concurrent with the administration of high concentrations of oxygen. When the administration of oxygen is absolutely necessary, the oxygen should be halted transiently when the ESU or laser is employed in these locations to avoid local, tracheal, and pulmonary burn injury. Rapport between surgeon and anesthesia provider is to be maintained in these circumstances. Insulated nonflammable endotracheal tubes or modified metal endotracheal tubes that have been covered with a nonflammable, nonreflective material are employed during laser applications. Towels, drapes, and sponges placed about the surgical site during laser applications are to be premoistened to prevent combustion. For laser safety precautions, see p. 94.

When all factors are considered, careful forethought and vigilance regarding the use of flammable materials in the OR are the best defense in preventing surgical fires that could result in an injury or the death of patients and personnel.

Electrosurgery

The ESU is commonly employed in the OR for the coagulating or cutting of tissue. In a bipolar ESU, the current flows from the generator (ESU) to an active electrode, one side of the forceps, through the tissue, and returns to the ESU through an inactive electrode, i.e., the other side of the forceps. In the monopolar ESU, the active electrode is usually an electrosurgical "pencil," and the inactive electrode is the dispersive (grounding) pad. In the monopolar system, when using an adhesive dispersive pad, the pad is placed on the patient's skin, as close as possible to the surgical site to minimize the pathway of the current through the body. The pad must make direct contact with the skin; shaving the area may be necessary for good contact. It must also be placed as far as possible from ECG leads to prevent interference. All connections must be secure.

A variety of ESU dispersal pad (return electrode or ground), *Megadyne 2000,* utilizes a nonadhesive pad that is large enough to cover an adult torso. It is placed on the operating table under the patient. This reusable pad, covered by a sheath and a linen sheet, does not make direct contact with the patient's skin; no shaving of the area is required.

Safety precautions must always be taken when employing an ESU to prevent burn injury to the patient. These include the following:

1. All connections must be secure.
2. The disposable adhesive pad (the inactive electrode) of the ESU should cover a sufficiently large area of skin, relatively free of hair (which acts as an insulator).
3. The patient's body should *never* make direct contact with any metal surfaces when an ESU is being used during the procedure. If the return circuit is faulty, the ground circuit could be completed through the contact area, causing an inadvertent burn injury.
4. Keep the electrosurgical pencil in its holster when not in use to prevent direct skin burns.
5. Although the electrosurgical pad should be placed as close as possible to the operative site, it should be placed as far away as possible from ECG leads to avoid interference with the heart's electrical field forces.

As noted in the section above, repeated requests to increase the current on an ESU should be thoroughly investigated by the circulator.

All connections and the dispersive pad should be checked. If no problem is found, e.g., a frayed cord, the unit may be faulty. Turn off and unplug the ESU. Label the faulty unit, request repair, and obtain another ESU. Be certain that this occurrence and the serial number of the units involved are documented in the patient's operative record.

Special Notes

- Drapes, gowns, shoe coverings, head coverings, etc. must be fire retardant. ***NOTE:*** These items are *not* fireproof.
- If the patient has an implanted pacemaker, the ESU could cause malfunctioning of the pacemaker. The patient needs to be continuously monitored and observed closely.
- When the ESU is in use, the cardiac arrest cart or the "crash" cart, complete with defibrillator and paddles, should be in close proximity to the particular OR. This is of extra concern when the patient being operated on has a pacemaker. The unit should be brought close to that OR before the surgery begins. Documenting that this has been done before surgery began is imperative for medicolegal reasons.
- During surgery, the electrosurgical pencil should be kept in a holster when not in use to avoid inadvertently burning the patient with the tip.

Counting Procedures

Each institution has its own written policy and procedure regarding the counting of sponges (varying types), sharps, and instruments. The following guidelines should be observed when counting all objects potentially subject to inadvertent inclusion within a wound:

1. The scrub person and the circulator count together (aloud) all items on the sterile field as the scrub person touches to each item.
2. The circulator immediately records the number (count) of each type of item. Keeping a record of the count is the legal responsibility of the circulator.
3. If there is any uncertainty regarding any count, it is repeated.
4. As additional items (e.g., sponges or needles) are introduced to the sterile field during the procedure, the scrub person counts the item(s) with the circulator, who adds the item to the count in the record and initials it.
5. *Nothing* (including laundry, trash, instruments, or sponges) may be removed from an OR while a procedure is in progress

until the final count is acknowledged to be correct. The only exception to this is when a specimen is sent to the laboratory for immediate inspection (e.g., frozen section) and the specimen remains attached to a "counted" item (as by sutures to maintain its orientation); this must be noted and initialed on the intraoperative record.

6. Whenever there is a change of team members, a count is taken. The name of the replacement person(s) is documented on the intraoperative record.
7. When a package containing an incorrect number of items is opened, the items should be passed off the table, bagged, and labeled accordingly. The bag with the incorrect number of sponges is labeled, set aside, and not included in the count. The bag may not be removed from the room.
8. Counts are taken before the procedure begins, before wound closure begins, and when skin closure is initiated.
9. An additional count is taken prior to the closure of an organ with a cavity (e.g., uterus, bladder, or bowel).

Incorrect closure counts must be repeated immediately. If the count remains incorrect, the circulator alerts the surgeon, who will inspect the patient's wound for the missing item. If the item is not located, hospital policy must be followed, i.e., usually to include immediate x-ray examination. Notification of the OR supervisor and an incident report must be filed as part of the chart, the permanent record. Any item inadvertently left in a wound may become a source of infection and result in subsequent litigation.

Sponge Counts

All sponges, including neurosurgical sponges (cottonoids and patties), soft goods (e.g., umbilical tapes), and loose items are counted. Each type of sponge according to size is counted together and kept separate from all other types or sizes. All sponges used within the wound must be x-ray detectable. X-ray-detectable sponges are never used for dressings, and dressing sponges are never used to dry the wound or surgical field as undetectable sponges could be inadvertently left in the wound (if placed on the sterile field before the final count). Soiled sponges are counted by the scrub person and the circulator together and then bagged in impervious plastic bags according to a predetermined number (usually in sets of 5 or 10). When the counts are taken, the scrub person counts the sponges according to type, beginning with the sponges on the sterile field, proceeding to the sponges on the back table, and following with those off the field. The circulator wears gloves when separating or counting soiled items. The circulator informs the surgeon of the results of the counts. As noted above, if the sponge count is *not correct*, the surgeon examines the wound and the count is repeated immediately. If it is still *incorrect*, hospital policy is to be followed (i.e., usually policy states the incident must be reported to the OR supervisor and an x-ray must be taken). An incident report must be filed in the chart as a part of the permanent record.

Sharps Counts

All needles, knife blades, electrosurgical tips and all other sharp or edged items ("sharps") are counted. Needles in multiple-suture packs may be counted according to the number on the package; some hospitals require each package to be opened and each needle counted individually. Used needles, blades, and other sharps should be retained on a magnetic pad to prevent inadvertent loss and to facilitate counting. Dispose of the sharps on the magnetic pad (usually encased in a compact). This compact can be closed and discarded in a specially marked container designated for sharps disposal only following the final count. All parts of any needle (or other sharp item) broken during a procedure must be accounted for in its entirety. If a minor fragment of a broken needle cannot be retrieved without undue trauma to the patient and the surgeon concurs, the fragment is left in situ. The surgeon will describe this event in the operative report. Follow hospital policy regarding the filing of an incident report when a sharps item is broken (e.g., a needle or knife blade) or when all of its parts are not recovered. Closure counts for sharps follow the same protocol as that for sponges.

Instrument Counts

Instruments are counted before the surgery begins and subsequently following, using the protocol for sponges and sharps. All parts of disassembled or broken instruments must be accounted for in their entirety. Follow the policy noted above if an instrument (or part of an instrument) is lost.

Sterilization Modalities

All items (e.g., instruments, supplies, and equipment) that come in contact with the sterile field and the wound must be sterile. As soon as possible, following the completion of a surgical procedure, soiled instruments are cleaned in the washer-sterilizer. After terminal decontamination in the washer-sterilizer has been completed, the instruments are cleaned in an ultrasonic cleaner to remove any remaining soilage. When available, an enzymatic foaming agent may be sprayed on the instruments initially in the OR before they are taken to the decontamination area.

The most commonly used methods of sterilization employed in the OR (or central supply) include:

1. Saturated steam under pressure
2. Gas chemical sterilization
3. Liquid chemical sterilization
4. Low-temperature hydrogen peroxide gas plasma sterilization

Saturated Steam Under Pressure Sterilization

The *flash sterilizer* is utilized in the OR for urgently needed equipment, unwrapped instruments, and trays. Customarily, the temperature is set at 270°F (132°C) for a 3- or 10-minute cycle. The length of the cycle is determined according to the density of the item(s) to be sterilized. The manufacturer of any item used in the sterile field must provide directions for its sterilization; the recommended temperature and length of exposure time for the sterilization of that particular item must be given. The recording device on the sterilizer should be checked to confirm that the instrument(s) to be sterilized has (have) been exposed to the proper temperature for the desired length of time. Heat-sensitive indicators should accompany the instrument(s). Trays with mesh bottoms are recommended for complete exposure to the steam.

Wrapped instruments, trays, basins, and other items are usually sterilized in a prevacuum, high-temperature steam sterilizer. Proper packing and wrapping of instruments and trays is mandatory, as is the proper loading of the sterilizer; the *Bowie-Dick* test is used to verify that there were no air pockets in the sterilizer that would negate the sterilizing process. A heat-sensitive indicator is placed within each wrapped tray (or package), and each package is secured with heat-sensitive tape.

The packaging of instruments and trays must be unwrapped by holding the item away from the body using aseptic technique when opening. The corner of the wrapper farthest away from the body is unwrapped first, then either of the sides is unwrapped, and lastly the corner closest to the body is unwrapped. By utilizing this technique, one will not contaminate the item by reaching over the sterile field.

Gas Chemical Sterilization

Ethylene oxide gas is used to sterilize items that are vulnerable to heat and/or moisture. Any item that can withstand sterilization by steam under pressure should not be gas-sterilized. Ethylene oxide sterilization depends on concentration of gas, temperature, humidity, and exposure time. The ethylene oxide sterilizer must be operated exactly according to the manufacturer's instructions to ensure that the requirements for sterilization are met. The type of item, arrangement of the load, and rate of penetration of the gas influence the amount of exposure time required. A vacuum that is created within the sterilizer aids gas penetration. Usually cycles of 3 to 7 hours are employed. An ethylene oxide chemically sensitive indicator that is placed inside the wrapped package indicates that the item was exposed to ethylene oxide, but it does not necessarily indicate that sterilization has occurred. Therefore, for sterilization to have occurred, the process must conform completely to manufacturer's specifications.

Inhalation of ethylene oxide is to be avoided, as is direct contact with the sterilized items prior to aeration. The length of aeration time required depends on the composition of the items, the type of wrapper used, the concentration of the ethylene oxide used, the airflow rate, and the temperature during the aeration process. When items are aerated in a mechanical aerator, the air is automatically changed a minimum of four times an hour, depending on the size and composition of the load. The temperature is controlled at 122°F (50°C) to 140°F (60°C) for 8 to 12 hours. If a mechanical aerator is unavailable, items should be aerated in a well-ventilated room at a controlled temperature of 65°F (18°C) to 72°F (22°C) for 7 days.

Liquid Chemical Sterilization

When items cannot tolerate sterilization by saturated steam under pressure and when the time required for gas sterilization is impractical, liquid chemical sterilization is employed. A 2% activated aqueous glutaraldehyde solution (e.g., Cidex) is the agent often employed when liquid disinfection is desired. Instruments must be completely immersed in the solution for 10 hours to achieve sterilization. High-level disinfection is effected if the instrument is submerged for 10 minutes. All items must be thoroughly rinsed in sterile distilled water before use to prevent irritation of the skin and mucous membranes.

The glutaraldehyde solution may be reused after testing it for potency, noting that the solution soon loses its potency after it is activated. Frequent testing with a test strip or a kit of reagents (obtained from the manufacturer) is recommended to be certain of its effectiveness. Polyethylene gloves or doubled latex gloves should be worn for skin protection. Directly breathing the fumes is to be avoided; OSHA recommends wearing a monitor for those individuals at risk. Following use, Cidex may be disposed of into most sewer systems.

Steris 20™ is a single-use sterilant that employs peracetic acid as the active sterilizing agent. Peracetic acid, a highly biocidal oxidizer, maintains its efficiency even when high levels of organic soil are present. Steris 20 has a low surface tension, which makes it very effective at reaching all instrument surfaces. To sterilize items, they must be completely immersed in Steris 20 for 12 minutes at 50°C. The sterilant is prepackaged in single-use containers where dilution is automatically prepared within the environmental processing chamber. The sterilized items are rinsed in microfiltered tap water in the processor. The used solution is disposed of in an ordinary drain during the processing cycle, eliminating exposure to chemicals to the operator. After use, the peracetic acid decomposes into acetic acid (vinegar) and oxygen.

Low-Temperature Hydrogen Peroxide Gas Plasma Sterilization

A hydrogen peroxide gas plasma sterilization system employs 1.8 ml of 58% hydrogen peroxide that is vaporized in a sterilization chamber after a vacuum is created; the vapor is converted into a plasma by means of radio-frequency energy. The resulting plasma consists of highly charged particles and free radicals that sterilize instruments at low temperature in one hour without producing toxic emissions or residues. Its by-products are simply water vapor and oxygen. The plasma particles destroy a wide variety of microorganisms, including bacteria, fungi, viruses, and spores. An indicator of bacterial spores is used to monitor the sterilization process.

An FDA-approved commercially available self-contained system, STERRAD®, using cassettes or cartridges of hydrogen peroxide, can be used to sterilize metallic and nonmetallic instruments, fiber-optic cables, endoscopes, microsurgical equipment, glass, ceramic, and electrical equipment in a low-temperature (50°C, 122°F) and low-moisture environment. As there are no toxic by-products, aeration and cooling post cycle are not necessary, in contrast to ethylene oxide, which is toxic, explosive, carcinogenic, and takes up to 12 hours for effect, and packs must be thoroughly aerated prior to use. However, the hydrogen peroxide gas plasma system is not appropriate for sterilization of cellulose products, as towels, paper, cotton, dressings, organic matter, and similar items that absorb the sterilant, making it incompletely effective. A standard electrical outlet is the only connection for the contained system. The initial cost of these units is high, but its safety features, effectiveness, shorter turn around, and lower operating cost will lead to increasing utilization of the modality.

Reuse of "Single-Use" Instruments

The reuse of instrument(s) or device(s) intended for "single use" (by the manufacturer) that have been opened but <u>unused</u> remains controversial. The issue regarding the reprocessing and resterilization of instrument(s) or device(s) that have been <u>used</u> is very highly controversial. The FDA has set up rules to regulate the reuse of "single-use" instruments in an effort to help to control rising hospital costs. The manufacturer of "single-use" or disposable instrumentation must follow the FDA's guidelines precisely. Validation of the process used by the company should be enclosed in the packaging of the resterilized item. The FDA has a published list of instruments that may be resterilized if the instrument has been opened but *not used*. They also have a list of instruments that may be resterilized and reused in addition to a list of those instruments or devices that may not be resterilized and reused once they have been used. If there is doubt regarding the sterility of a "reprocessed instrument," consult the website www.FDA.com and follow the prompts for instrument resterilization or reuse of "single-use" instruments. A hospital may resterilize an item (opened and unused or a used item), or it may be sent out to a third party to be resterilized if it is resterilized according to the guidelines established by the FDA. The FDA mandated in August of 2000 the requirements for resterilization of "single-use" items. AORN's guidance statement requires the patient's safety to be of utmost consideration in the acceptance of a reprocessing procedure. Even with the FDA's ruling, the acceptance of the reprocessing and the resterilization of "single-use" items remains somewhat controversial. This topic is discussed further in the chapter on Endoscopy, p. 102.

Safe Use of Pneumatic Tourniquet

A pneumatic tourniquet is often employed for surgical procedures on the extremities, particularly during orthopedic procedures. For perioperative personnel unfamiliar with the use of tourniquets, return demonstration is recommended (before permission to apply tourniquets is granted). The tourniquet used in most operating rooms today is comprised of a cuff with pressure sensor, tubing, and an inflation device equipped with a pressure gauge (microprocessor) that is used to regulate pressure and time settings in addition to providing audible and visual feedback (a micro pressure and time settings regulator). The surgeon wraps Webril (or other soft material) around the extremity at the level of tourniquet placement, and the cuff applied. Following skin preparation and draping, the extremity is elevated and abducted, and a sterile rubber bandage (e.g., Esmarch, Ace, or self-adherent Coban) is applied from the tips of the fingers or toes to the level of the tourniquet, proximally, to achieve exsanguination after which the tourniquet is inflated by the circulator or anesthesia provider at the direction of the surgeon. The time of inflation and the pressure employed is recorded (including on the anesthesia record). The tourniquet is inflated for the least amount of time possible.

Guidelines for Safe Use of the Pneumatic Tourniquet. An appropriately sized tourniquet should be used. The ends of the tourniquet must overlap by about 3 inches but not more than 6 inches. Do not apply the tourniquet at or near the elbow. For the average adult, tourniquet use should not exceed 1 hour on the upper extremity and $1\frac{1}{2}$ hours on the lower extremity. Pressure setting is approximately 250 to 300 mm Hg (up to 6 pounds) on the upper extremity and 350 mm Hg on the lower extremity. Thin adults and children may require less pressure. When tourniquet use is anticipated to exceed these time limits, the tourniquet is deflated at intervals at the discretion of the surgeon to avoid tissue ischemia. The location, placement of, and use of the tourniquet, the pressure setting, and the times at which the tourniquet is inflated and deflated are recorded on the Perioperative Record and initialed by the circulator. In addition, the anesthesia provider records use of the tourniquet.

Safe Use of Pulsed Lavage

This suction-irrigator for single-patient use pulsed lavage (with cojoined suction and irrigation tubing) is used for controlled, high powered irrigation with or without suction; 1 or 2 irrigation bags may be used. The scrub person attaches tubing with spike adaptor to the pistol grip handle (contains batteries) and passes off the single- or dual-spike tubing to the circulator; one channel of the cojoined tubing (either straight or a "Y") is connected to the irrigation bag(s), and the other channel of the cojoined tubing is connected to suction (if used).

The scrub person inserts the tip of choice (e.g., soft splash shield tip) into the pistol grip handle and primes the unit by squeezing the trigger until irrigation solution exits the tip. The circulator may squeeze the irrigation bag(s) to facilitate priming.

Safety Measure Guidelines for Pulsed Lavage Usage. Read manufacturer's instructions prior to use. Do not use if packaging has been damaged. All persons scrubbed are advised to wear a face shield for protection from splashed irrigation fluid. The pulsed lavage is a "single use" unit and may not be resterilized or reused. Do not submerge handle of the unit. Do not use it close to an oxygen-enriched area. Do not use in presence of flammable anesthetics. Following use, the unit and/or its batteries is disposed of according to hospital regulations regarding the disposal of a *biohazard*.

Safe Use of Powered Saws and Drills

Powered saws and drills are employed in various surgical specialties to save intraoperative time, resulting in many tangible and intangible benefits to the patient. The hospital engineering department must be consulted before any new piece of powered equipment may be permitted or used in the OR. Reading the manufacturer's recommendations for the safe operation of this powered equipment in the operating room is mandatory. Power equipment should be tested prior to use whenever possible. All attachments must be appropriately secured; attachments previously used must be tested for their sharpness. Size discrepancy of the jigs and templates used with powered equipment must be determined prior to their use and if found, adjustment or use of properly fitting accessories must be employed (before the surgery is begun). Immediately following its use, the rotary section of the instrument must come to complete standstill before it is set aside. When not in use for a substantial interval, the power source (electrical, battery, or air compressor) should be deactivated and the instrument secured.

Emergency and Disaster Considerations

Operating rooms are required to be equipped with a special emergency signal (usually a flashing red light) to alert others to an emergency; the signal can be operated from within each separate OR.

In the event that a patient suffers a cardiopulmonary arrest, the anesthesia provider and surgeon administer cardiopulmonary resuscitation (CPR). In the absence of the anesthesia provider, the surgeon, assisted by nursing personnel, must administer CPR. Health-care providers must be knowledgeable regarding CPR and be prepared to perform it. An emergency cardiopulmonary arrest cart/"crash" cart should be available in the surgery department at all times. Included on this well-stocked cart are in-date emergency drugs, needles and syringes, infusion equipment, a defibrillator with paddles, ventilation devices (e.g., bag-valve-mask/"Ambu"), and monitoring equipment. Nursing personnel responding to the emergency signal should bring the "crash" cart into the room. Documentation of all medications administered to the patient, according to the strength and dosage, and route of administration; the treatments and procedures performed, including the time and the name of the person giving each type of care. Perioperative personnel who care for pediatric patients are required to have pediatric advanced life systems (PALS) skills to assess and assist in the treatment of "at risk" pediatric patients.

Hospitals are required to be equipped with an alternative power source, usually an independent generator that is triggered when a power failure occurs. During the time lapse, or should the independent generator not function, high-intensity flashlights (kept in the department) should be located by members of the surgery staff and brought into the individual OR. All team members are required to know the location of these high-intensity flashlights kept in the department for use during the time lapse following a loss of power until the alternate power source begins functioning and during any emergency where the lights are needed.

Malignant Hyperthermia

Malignant hyperthermia (MH) is a rare, potentially lethal condition triggered by the use of inhalation anesthetics and depolarizing muscle relaxants (e.g., succinylcholine chloride). This condition requires proper treatment to be initiated immediately; documentation of treatment for MH must be recorded. As soon as MH is suspected, one should call for assistance. Immediate treatment is begun, usually by the anesthesia provider, who administers dantrolene (Dantrium), steroids, and iced intravenous (IV) solutions, the gavage of all open cavities with iced saline, and the cooling of the patient with ice packs. These treatments can significantly reduce mortality. In preparation to meet this emergency situation, OR personnel are required to be informed of the protocol set up by their anesthesia department.

Setting up a Malignant Hyperthermia (MH) Protocol and Emergency Treatment Cart in the OR department is highly recommended by the American Association of Anesthesiologists (AAA). Again, documentation must be made of all medications given, IV and pressure lines established, and treatments performed. Additional discussion of this entity is presented in Chapter 4, General Anesthesia, p. 68.

Legal Rights

The patient's legal rights and the rights of OR personnel are significantly protected by the documentation recorded in the patient's Intraoperative Record. The JC requires the Intraoperative Record to include the name of the surgeon, the preoperative diagnosis, the procedure performed, the postoperative diagnosis, the type and number of specimens obtained, and the names of the surgical team members providing intraoperative care. The documentation of important intraoperative information, such as the skin preparation (noting the condition of the skin prior to and following the skin preparation), the results of the counts (e.g., sponges, sharps, and instruments), the placement of catheters, intravenous lines, and wound packing, and the use of equipment (e.g., ESU, the pneumatic tourniquet, etc.), in addition to other notations, is an invaluable tool for verification of actions, observances, and the delivery of specific treatments, and/or medications administered. An example of the suggested format for the Intraoperative Record is on p. 12. Documentation is of major importance, as it is the *legal* record of the surgical procedure. The circulator should remember that in a court of law, only information that was documented is accepted as a legal fact.

Legal Records

In addition to the Intraoperative Record that is maintained by the circulator, the JC mandates that an Anesthesia Record must be maintained for every patient during a surgical procedure. The anesthesia provider documents his/her care in the Anesthesia Record, but in his/her absence, a perioperative RN (in addition to the circulator) assumes this role and is responsible for the Conscious Sedation and Analgesia Record. According to the policy of the hospital, when an anesthesia provider is not present during a surgical procedure, a perioperative RN (specially trained) may provide the patient care to include the monitoring of the patient's vital signs, administering of treatments, medications, etc. (as directed by the surgeon). Documentation should provide the name of any person giving medications or treatments, including all pertinent times, dosages, and routes of administration, in addition to his/her observations of the patient throughout the surgical procedure. *Everything* that takes place must be documented. This nursing anesthesia record, complete with full documentation of the events as they occurred in the OR, will legally protect the RN providing conscious sedation and analgesia. The Analgesia and Conscious Sedation Record is on p. 76.

Death in the OR

Should the death of a patient occur in the OR, individual state law and hospital policy must be adhered to regarding the handling and disposition of the deceased patient. Most often, the scrub person and the circulator prepare the body for departure from the OR by removing all lines, tubings, and devices and by washing the body until it is free of all visible blood and body secretions and excretions. An Incident Report must be recorded by the circulator, and the death must be recorded in the Intraoperative Record, detailing the times, the interventions, and the outcome of events leading to the patient's death. These documents are part of the patient's permanent medicolegal record.

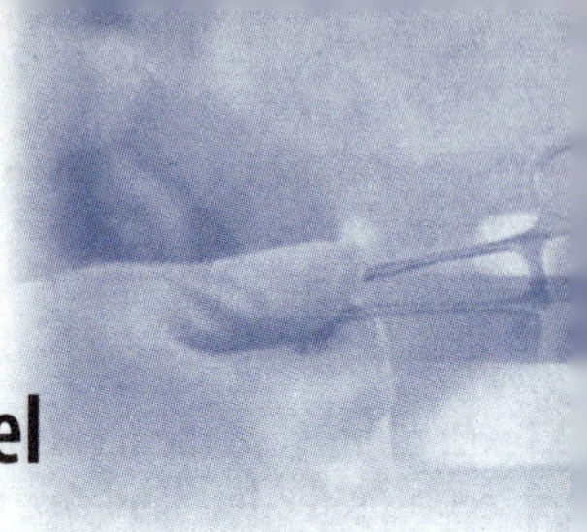

CHAPTER 3

Safety Measures for Operating Room Personnel

Perioperative personnel are directly involved in patient care. They must become aware of the many potential risks and hazards that exist in today's surgical environment, not only for the benefit of the patients, but for their own safety as well. Their opportunity and the obligation to observe safe practices in the performance of their roles as health-care providers in an environment in which potentially lethal drugs, noxious gases, and life-threatening diseases may be encountered is a continuous process.

Orientation

The orientation programs for the new employees of a health-care facility are designed to familiarize them with the policies and procedures of the facility. Working in a health-care facility is very different from working in any other environment. Housekeeping, engineering, maintenance, security, and other health-care personnel are exposed to potential health hazards. These hazards should be identified by the facility, and procedures to prevent or minimize their transmission of disease and other risks must be learned by the employees.

Hospitals are required to inform new employees about numerous other safety measures advised by the facility, e.g., the prevention of fires, the prevention of falls from spilled liquids, and the prevention of creating a biohazard when body fluids are present, in addition to many other important factors that serve to create a hazard for the health-care worker and the environment inside and outside the facility. *Fire drills* are held at least twice each year in hospitals; other safety drills, including disaster training, are mandatory.

Perioperative employment necessitates a special type of orientation and knowledge for those who work in the OR.

Orientation to the OR prepares the employee to deliver safe care to the patient and familiarizes him/her with the techniques and procedures specific to the OR. During this period, AORN recommends that new employees have a mentor or that they work on the buddy system with more experienced personnel.

Surgery Department In-Service Education

Hospital perioperative departments are required to have in-service education programs for their employees. Most perioperative departments schedule monthly in-service education meetings to provide their staff with information regarding the safest methods to use for delivering care to the surgical patient, information regarding new procedures and the latest techniques, equipment, and instrumentation for use in the department, as well as other matters of concern, including patient safety.

Body Mechanics/Ergonomic Safety

Personnel must employ good body mechanics, particularly when lifting or moving (unconscious) patients, heavy instrument trays, or equipment, to prevent strains and other injuries to their musculoskeletal systems. Lifting should be done by bending the knees, positioning one's body under the load, and then straightening the legs, allowing the lower-extremity muscles to do the lifting.

A roller (e.g., Davis) can be of significant value in preventing strains when moving unconscious or obese patients; see Procedure for Safely Transferring the Patient to the Operating Table, p. 19. Another moving device that can be of significant value is the Hoyer pad, which is placed on the operating table preoperatively. Following the surgical procedure, a crane-like machine directed by an employee is attached to the Hoyer pad and lifts the patient. In 2002, the Occupational Safety and Health Administration (OSHA) required hospitals and other health-care facilities to reduce the number of ergonomic injuries to health-care personnel. Suggestions enumerated by OSHA can be found on the Web at www.OSHA.gov.

Lift teams may be hired by health-care facilities to assist personnel in lifting obese patients or heavy objects. They are very effective in helping to prevent injuries to employees.

Fatigue Factors

Fatigue is one of the most important factors influencing job performance. Although becoming fatigued can be minimized through working quickly and efficiently, the underlying reason for frequently feeling fatigued must be investigated. In our fast-paced world, one may feel pressured to perform more tasks than he/she can reasonably handle. Often employees with this problem are sleep-deprived because they attempt to perform too many tasks at home as well. Sleep deprivation prevents the body from being restored. It takes longer for someone who is sleep-deprived to complete a task correctly than the individual who has had 7 or 8 hours of sleep.

AORN's statement on safe practices in the OR recommends that an RN should not work in direct patient care for more than 12 consecutive hours. The association further recommends 8 hours of uninterrupted sleep per night and a workweek (including on-call time) of no longer than 60 hours. The time away from the OR allows the individual adequate time to recuperate.

Fatigued staff members are more prone to errors than others who have had adequate rest. Errors in the health-care field, in particular, can result in harm to or death of a patient and/or employee. Sleep deprivation can greatly influence one's efficiency, job performance (including patient care), and endurance. It would be unethical to work in the OR when one's judgment is affected.

Radiation Safety

Operating room personnel may be exposed to radiation during intraoperative x-rays and when radioactive implant procedures are performed. To reduce the deleterious effects of radiation exposure, hospital policy must be strictly followed. Radiation exposure (received by an individual) depends on the amount of radiation, the proximity of the radiation source, the length of time of the exposure, and the frequency of exposure. Personnel should stand as far away from the radiation source as possible when x-ray equipment is in use. Additional protective measures should include, but are not limited to, the following:

1. All nonsterile team members should leave the room (whenever possible) or wear a lead apron.
2. Sterile team members should either stand behind a lead screen or wall or wear a lead apron donned before scrubbing, i.e., in cases using fluoroscopy.
3. Monitoring devices or badges (e.g., dosimeters) should be worn by personnel who may be exposed to radiation; readings should be computed weekly.
4. Pregnant personnel or those who may be pregnant should avoid all cases involving exposure to radiation, as radiation may harm the unborn fetus and possibly the mother's reproductive capabilities.

Personnel holding x-ray cassettes during radiography should wear lead gloves. In addition to wearing a lead apron, special eyewear and thyroid shields were once frequently worn when older equipment was employed; today this is infrequently done.

Modern x-ray machines have a direct beam that limits the size of the area exposed. When the beam of the x-ray machine cannot be limited, the patient's reproductive organs and thyroid gland must be shielded. Female patients must be asked if they *are* or *could be* pregnant to prevent x-ray exposure to the fetus.

Infection Control and Prevention

The Centers for Disease Control and Prevention (CDC) mandates that one should consider body secretions and excretions of all individuals as contaminated. It is impossible to determine whether a patient or health-care worker has a contagious disease due to the latency (conversion time period) of serological tests for various communicable diseases, such as human immunodeficiency virus (HIV), acquired immunodeficiency syndrome (AIDS), strains of hepatitis, and many other diseases; therefore, *standard precautions* must be observed at all times during patient care.

AIDS, hepatitis (several strains), pyogenic infections, and numerous other blood-borne infections can be transmitted via puncture wounds. Hospital procedure must be followed regarding the disposal of "sharps" (needles and edged implements) to help to control the transmission of blood-borne diseases. In the OR (in the sterile field) a needle magnet is available encased in a flat plastic compact, the lid of which can be used for counting needles and sharps and for containing them. Following a surgical procedure, the compact is closed for its safe disposal (including its contents). A designated rigid plastic container is used for the disposal of sharps (knife blades and needles) and for plastic syringes; an attached device separates the hub and shaft of the needle while breaking the syringe tip prior to its disposal. Some syringes are made for use specifically without needles (in particular situations/setups).

Biologically engineered sharps or needleless systems offer the safety protection recommended by OSHA. Some of these devices include:

1. Syringes with a sliding sheath that shields needles after use.
2. Needles that retract back into the syringe after use.
3. A jet injection system without needles.
4. An intravenous delivery system that uses a catheter port to house the needle in a protective covering.
5. A delivery system that uses plastic capillary tubes.

Sharps must be handled responsibly in all situations. The scrub person must always pass the handle of the knife to the surgeon while holding the knife by the shaft. It is safest if suture is mounted just before use, again, passing the handle to the surgeon.

A "no-passing" technique can be employed. It requires both the scrub person and the surgeon to agree on a neutral zone where the sharps will be placed. A magnetic pad may be used to prevent the sharps (and all instruments) in the neutral zone from falling. The scrub person places the sharps object on the pad in the same direction it would be passed. The sharps object is used and returned to the same place by the surgeon. In this way, the "no-passing" technique limits the potential for either person being stuck by sharps. All personnel should wear gloves when performing patient-care tasks, i.e., when catheterizing a patient, when starting intravenous fluids, and when handling potentially contaminated articles, such as soiled sponges, instruments, intravenous lines, blood transfusion sets and blood pouches, and any other items soiled by body secretions or excretions that might provide the source of infection through a break in the skin. Some authorities advocate double gloving when virulent infections are present or suspect.

Similarly, during endoscopy procedures or procedures in which drills or saws are employed, and when one is involved in any surgery where he or she may be spattered or sprayed by potentially contaminated tissue fragments, saliva, or irrigation fluids, it is necessary for scrubbed personnel to wear a protective facial shield.

Latex Allergy Precautions

In the surgical suite, health-care personnel and patients who are sensitive to latex are not only sensitive to the latex in latex gloves, but they may also be sensitive to the powder found in various types of latex gloves. The powder containing latex proteins is released into the air when latex gloves are handled. A "sensitivity" response has the appearance of varying degrees of irritant dermatitis, i.e., red, itchy, irritated, and/or broken skin. Most often, mild reactions merely require the individual to change into gloves that do not contain latex.

Latex allergy and its serious systemic effects, the prevention of an allergic response to latex products, the medications and equipment needed for a latex allergy cart, and the precautions necessary for a latex safe environment are discussed on p. 32.

Chemical Waste Hazards

The National Institute of Occupational Safety and Health (NIOSH) has established guidelines regarding the unsafe levels of waste (anesthetic) gases in the operating room. The harmful effects of these gases are leaked to health-care personnel during surgery and may cause harmful effects as a decrease in mental performance, audiovisual ability, and manual dexterity. Exposure to anesthetic chemicals may result in an increased risk of abortion in female employees and developmental defects in an unborn fetus. Fire, explosion, and the toxicity of compressed gases are additional potential hazards of these chemical wastes.

The control of waste gases in the OR is accomplished with an efficient scavenger system, a well-designed anesthetic system that includes securely fitting patient masks, tubings, and connectors, and an efficient room air-dilution ventilation conditioning system. A similar ventilation air conditioning system should also be provided for the PACU, due to the unit's close proximity to the surgical suite. Well-maintained scavenging systems, air-conditioning systems using high-efficiency particulate air filters that do not recirculate the air, and anesthetic gas leak detectors help to minimize the exposure of personnel and patients to hazardous waste gases in the operating room.

Fires, explosions, and the toxicity of compressed gases are sources of potential chemical hazards. Cylinders containing compressed gases must be secured. Care must be taken to *never* drop a canister or allow one cylinder to forcefully strike another.

The skin may be exposed to harmful chemical liquids that are used in the OR; they include methyl methacrylate (an acrylic "cement" molded to replace sections of bone or used to secure some types of prostheses) and paracetic acid (used as a cold sterilant). OSHA recommends that hospitals advise surgical personnel to mix the cement in a closed unit and to follow manufacturers' recommendations for safe handling, storage, and disposal of chemical wastes.

Noxious Smoke Hazards

A plume of noxious smoke results from the burning of patient tissues (and vaporization of potentially infectious lesions such as papilloma virus lesions and various secretions) when the electrosurgical unit or the laser is used during surgical procedures to cut, or coagulate tissue. The plume pollutes the air in the immediate vicinity unless a plume evacuator is employed to suck up the smoke into a suction apparatus or the wall suction unit. The masks made of man-made materials worn by personnel function to filter the air are more efficient than cotton cloth masks that are easily made damp (from the wearer).

The high-particulate air-filtering action of the air conditioning systems found in modern ORs can be very effective in removing smoke from the air. The concern regarding plume smoke is that it may be carcinogenic or contain infectious particles.

Fire Hazards

Obviously, the best way to deal with fires in the OR is to prevent them. All employees need to be responsible for learning about how fires occur in the OR and how, in the delivery of care to patients, steps can be taken to minimize the risk of fire. Employees in the department are responsible for attending fire drills and learning fire evacuation plans.

In 2005, the Joint Commission (JC) (formerly the Joint Commission on Accreditation of Healthcare Organizations) issued a "Sentinel

Alert" on fires in surgical facilities to alert the health-care worker to the ever-present danger fires pose to patients and employees.

Innumerable items found in the OR are flammable; they support combustion. A fire requires fuel (which includes anything flammable), oxygen, heat, and a source of ignition. The fuel might be the paper drapes, clothing, or paper from packaging, all of which have been treated to become "nonflammable" (i.e., less flammable) but not truly fireproof. Chemical agents, preparation fluids, and substances like methyl methacrylate glue are found in the OR; these substances all support combustion. Some anesthetic gases and liquids also support combustion. The OR is an "oxygen–rich" environment because oxygen escapes from the anesthesia delivery tubing system. Gases arrive via this route as well. Liquids, particularly solutions used to prepare the skin, are often highly flammable. Manufactured preparation solutions that are flammable are not recommended for use in the OR. However, there are times when a surgeon will request that a combustible solution be used, even though he/she is aware of its dangerous properties, because the particular solution does the best preparation (in a particular situation).

Never allow flammable solutions to pool under a patient. To prevent skin excoriation and a flammable reaction, dry all prep solution puddles.

One should know the location of all fire-fighting equipment in the OR.

Knowledge of the methods for rescue and evacuation of patients should be practiced so that the execution of those skills will be automatic should they ever be needed.

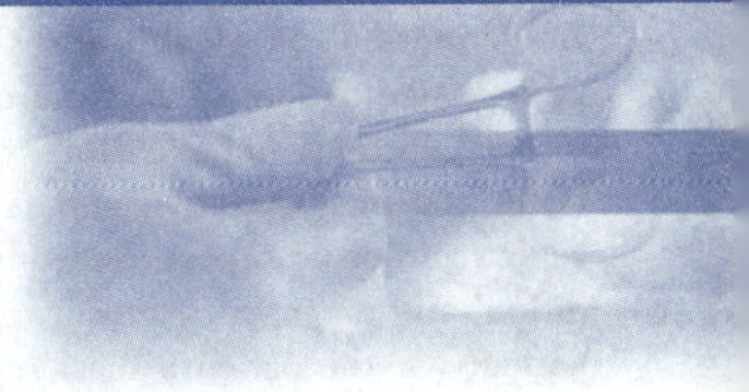

CHAPTER 4
Anesthesia Modalities

General Information

Anesthesia is defined as the absence of sensation. A physician (anesthesiologist), or certified registered nurse anesthetist (CRNA), administers anesthesia in the operating room (OR). Surgeons also may administer local or regional anesthesia to their own patients. In this guide, the term *anesthesia provider* refers to the anesthesiologist or CRNA.

Using an anesthesia preoperative evaluation form, the anesthesia provider interviews the surgical patient prior to his/her arrival in the OR. He/she identifies the patient and discusses the patient's medical, surgical, and anesthesia history as well as a drug/medication history. He/she reviews the patient's lab work and diagnostic studies and the history and physical examination report made by the surgeon, and then the anesthesia provider performs a pertinent physical examination of the patient. If the patient has had previous surgery, the anesthesia provider asks the patient if he/she had an unusual response to anesthesia or if there has been any familial history of unusual responses to anesthesia. The anesthesia provider explains a "plan of anesthesia," including risks, benefits, and alternatives to the particular type of anesthesia modality (if any alternative methods are permissible), to the patient. The patient is given the opportunity to ask relevant questions about alternative methods of anesthesia. The anesthesia provider follows through with the agreed plan for anesthesia. The anesthesia provider then verifies the site and side of the procedure with the patient and with the chart, as well as the position on the table that the patient will assume for the administration of the anesthetic.

After the patient is brought to the surgical suite, the circulator, identifies and admits the surgical patient to the OR by using at least two identifiers, e.g., the patient's chart and hospital armband. The circulator must implement the *Universal Protocol for Preventing Wrong Site, Wrong Side, Wrong Procedure, and Wrong Person Surgery* mandated by the Joint Commission (JC) (formerly the Joint Commission on

Accreditation of Healthcare Organizations). In addition, he/she reviews the patient's chart thoroughly, noting that there is a current written history and physical examination, a complete blood count (CBC), urinalysis (UA), and possibly an electrocardiogram (EKG) report and other reports depending on the patient's age, physical condition, and diagnosis. He/she verifies the chart information with the patient (or the patient's legal representative) and ascertains whether the patient has any sensitivities or allergies to foods, medications, latex, or other allergens. The importance of documenting and relaying information (to the surgeon and anesthesia provider) regarding patient allergies and current medications is vital; for latex allergy safety, see Chapter 2, p. 32.

When an anesthesia provider is not present during a patient's surgery, a perioperative RN, in addition to the circulator, will start intravenous fluids (IV) and monitor the patient's vital signs, blood pressure (B/P), and EKG (ECG); and apply a pulse oximeter to the patient's finger to monitor the patient's pulse and oxygen saturation. He/she monitors all aspects of the patient's physical condition and also oversees the care of the anesthesia equipment used for the patient during the surgical procedure (such as a mask and anesthesia circuit delivery system for oxygen). The perioperative RN, who stands in for the anesthesia provider, must document an initial assessment and medications given (with the route, dose, time, and response); monitor and chart the vital signs, including temperature, pulse, and respirations (TPR), oxygen saturation, and method of oxygen administered (e.g., nasal catheter, mask, etc and flow rate in liters per minute); and record nursing observations and interventions, and whether the desired or expected outcomes were met. Remember, documentation of nursing interventions is the proof necessary for medicolegal consideration in a court of law. The importance of documenting *all* that transpires during a surgical procedure cannot be exaggerated.

The techniques of anesthesia administration utilized in the OR include:

1. *General anesthesia*. The patient is made unconscious.
2. *Conduction anesthesia*. Anatomical sites are anesthetized by infiltration or topical application of various anesthetic agents. A peripheral nerve block may be produced by injecting an agent about nerve(s) supplying sensation to the operative site, or a block may be placed at a central level. *Local anesthesia* and *topical anesthesia* are established by employing anesthetic agents immediately about the area to be treated. Conduction anesthesia may be supplemented by varying degrees of general anesthesia or sedation.

The American Society of Anesthesiologists (ASA) recommends the following standards for basic intraoperative monitoring:

1. An *anesthesia* provider must be present throughout the administration of all general and most conduction anesthetics.
2. During the administration of the anesthetic, vital signs and EKG are to be continually monitored and evaluated.
3. Oxygen saturation is determined by use of an oxygen analyzer, pulse oximeter, and observing skin and nailbed color.
4. The patient's temperature can be evaluated with a forehead tape strip or transesophageal or urinary bladder temperature probe.

Breathing efficiency may be evaluated by observing chest excursions and by using respirometry. During general anesthesia the monitoring of the carbon dioxide content of expired gas is accomplished by use of tidal carbon dioxide monitors ($ETCO_2$). A "disconnect" alarm; indicators for various volatile agents; and monitors and gauges for measuring invasive arterial pressure, pulmonary artery (PA) pressure, and central venous pressure (CVP) are immediately available. *Bispectral Index System (BIS)* can be employed to monitor the effect of general anesthesia via electroencephalogram (EEG) patterns to better titrate the amount and level of anesthesia with respect to awareness, but it is not universally utilized for this purpose. BIS also can be used during neurosurgery to detect early signs of brain ischemia. The choice of an anesthetic technique is influenced by the feasibility of the particular modality of anesthesia, position to be assumed, extent of the surgical procedure, medical status, prior history of exposure to anesthetics, surgeon's preference, patient's preference (when not contraindicated), and anticipated need for particular postoperative analgesia (e.g., with an indwelling epidural catheter). The anesthesia provider will classify the patient's physical status according to the guidelines of the ASA into six categories (P1–6, 1–6, I–VI), where P1 is a healthy patient and P6 describes a brain-dead patient maintained on life support to permit harvesting of donor organs according to accepted ethical protocols.

Prior to the administration of anesthesia, premedication, as a single drug or a combination of various drugs, is often given. The purpose of the premedication is to allay anxiety, to help the patient relax, and to diminish secretions. Premedication is administered by intramuscular injection about 30 to 60 minutes before surgery, prior to the patient's arrival in the OR suite, or by the anesthesia provider, intravenously, immediately prior to induction of anesthesia, or not at all. Similarly, when surgery must be performed in an emergent situation, premedication may be given intravenously or may be omitted. These drugs are selected according to the patient's general condition and the extent and nature of the surgery to be performed. Outpatients or surgicenter patients are given less premedication or none at all.

Specialized equipment is required to deliver anesthesia. For general inhalation anesthesia, an anesthesia machine delivers an anesthetic gas mixture to the patient at a specific rate and concentration as determined by the anesthesia provider. The most simplistic machine consists of a cart with attached key-coded tanks of nitrous oxide (or other agents) and oxygen with flow meters and pressure gauges. Usually, expired "air" from the patient passes through a carbon dioxide absorbing tank or cartridge.

Currently, a sophisticated machine that is able to store and deliver several compressed gaseous and highly volatile liquid anesthetic agents is employed in the OR. In addition, the compact anesthesia cart contains a variety of monitoring devices, an oxygen depletion alarm, and special equipment that includes masks, laryngoscopes with interchangeable blades, McGill forceps, endotracheal tubes, and obturators, as well as a source of suction and anesthesia circuits. An additional cart of drawers is required for drugs and supplies. Equipment and prepackaged kits for various procedures (e.g., insertion of arterial and central venous pressure catheters) must be stored nearby. A variety of intravenous fluids, administration sets, and stands for these items should be located nearby in the surgical suite.

One role of the circulator with respect to the administration of anesthesia is to provide an "extra hand" for the anesthesia provider, particularly during the induction of anesthesia. In some institutions, an anesthesia technician may perform this role. The circulator is responsible for maintaining the patient's immediate safety, helping to allay the patient's anxiety, and being attentive to the special needs of the patient. Some patients' fear can elicit psychological distress; the circulator may extend a caring gesture, such as holding the patient's hand during induction. Even after the patient is anesthetized, the circulator assumes the role of the patient's advocate, as a diligent observer and administrator of the total care of the patient in surgery. As a perioperative practitioner, he/she identifies the needs of the patient in a preoperative care plan that is written for the individual patient and that is implemented preoperatively, intraoperatively, and postoperatively.

The information gathered is used to implement a plan of care that is "tailor made" to address the needs of the individual patient while taking into consideration the potential problems that might be incurred, their possible solutions, and desired patient outcomes. Special consideration is made for the patient who cannot move by himself/herself, for the patient with a "bad" back or "stiff" joints, for one who is hearing impaired, or for one with any other physical or mental impairment.

Following surgery, the circulator accompanies the anesthesia provider to transport the patient to the postanesthesia care unit (PACU). The anesthesia provider reports the patient's immediate needs and condition and gives orders to the PACU practitioner. The circulator gives additional information according to his/her observations of the patient during the course of the surgery performed. This documented report is vital for providing for the patient's safety and continuity of care.

General Anesthesia, Overview

For the administration of general anesthesia, the patient is initially in the supine position. An intravenous line is inserted, if not already present, an automatic B/P cuff is applied, and the oxygen sensor (pulse oximeter) and EKG monitoring electrodes are placed. Oxygen may be administered by mask for a few minutes. A minimal test dose of intravenous agent or muscle relaxant may be given to observe any untoward reaction.

Induction is usually begun by injecting a rapidly acting intravenous agent, e.g., thiopental (Pentothal), propofol (Diprovan), or methohexital (Brevital). (For children, a nonmalodorous inhalation agent, such as sevoflurane [Ultane], can be given by mask, and as consciousness is lost, intravenous lines are placed and other anesthetic measures are introduced.) As the patient loses consciousness, oxygen and gaseous agents are gradually introduced by mask. For cases of lesser duration or when profound muscle relaxation is not required, maintenance can be achieved with an intravenous agent alone or with an inhalation agent administered by facemask and oral airway or by utilizing a laryngeal mask airway.

If an endotracheal tube is to be inserted (transnasally, transorally, or via tracheostomy), a fast-acting muscle relaxant, e.g., succinylcholine chloride (Anectine), may be used in adults, or an intermediately fast-acting curare-like drug, e.g., rocuronium (Zemuron), atracurium (Tracrium), or vecuronium (Norcuron), is used in children. In adults and some children, following the administration of the muscle relaxant, the endotracheal tube is inserted under direct vision with the aid of a laryngoscope (and McGill forceps, as needed). Several milliliters of a 4% lidocaine solution may be instilled into the larynx prior to placing the endotracheal tube that has been lubricated with anesthetic ointment. The tube cuff is inflated, except in infants and small children, and the tube is secured with tape (hypoallergenic tape for children and adults who are sensitive to adhesives). For the duration of the procedure, muscle relaxation is maintained with any of the several curare-like drugs.

Additional monitoring devices may be applied, and the patient's position changed as necessary, with the permission of the anesthesia provider. (In situations such as clinical emergency or when gastric emptying is not assured [trauma, intestinal obstruction, obstetrical labor, etc.], a "crash" insertion of an endotracheal tube may be required, even in the conscious patient, by employing rapid-acting muscle relaxants and by pressure exerted transiently on the cricoid cartilage to avoid pulmonary aspiration of potentially regurgitated gastric contents.) A working suctioning device that must be checked before starting anesthesia should be immediately available; suction apparatus should be checked on the anesthesia equipment, and the circulator is responsible for checking the room suction.

Changes in the position of the patient as directed by the anesthesia provider may also be made to permit the anesthetic to "settle" in the desired area following a central block. The circulator assists the anesthesia provider in any way necessary, such as by helping the patient to maintain a position, displaying easy access to the equipment, giving additional premeasured drugs as directed by the anesthesia provider, and manipulating the cricoid cartilage, at the instruction of the anesthesia provider. A wide variety of drugs and inhalation agents is described in **Table 4-1**, p. 63.

To supplement the anesthetic agents, numerous additional drugs may be administered intravenously to "balance" the anesthesia. These drugs include various narcotics (e.g., morphine, meperidine, fentanyl, remifentanil, alfentanil, and sufentanil), amnestics (e.g., midazolam), and neuroleptics (e.g., haloperidol). Muscle relaxants, as referred to above, are regarded as depolarizing agents (e.g., succinylcholine) or nondepolarizing agents (e.g., the curare-like drugs). Succinylcholine (Anectine) and mivacurium (Mivacron) are short-acting with rapid onset and recovery; intermediate-acting muscle relaxants include vecuronium (Norcuron), atracurium (Tracrium), cisatracurium (Nimbex), and rocuronium (Zemuron). The longer-acting muscle relaxants include pancuronium (Pavulon) and lesser used d-tubocuarine, doxacurium, pipecuronium, metocurine, and gallamine.

Shorter-acting agents often need not be reversed; however, neostigmine (Prostigmin) or edrophonium (Enlon and Enlon Plus containing atropine) can be used to effect reversal of the longer-acting agents as necessitated by the patient's response, dosage, postoperative respiratory status, etc. If cholinesterase deficiency is encountered, prolonged respiratory support (hours to days) will be needed. The anesthesia provider must be familiar with all of these agents (and others), although frequently utilizing only a select few in daily practice.

Antiemetics in common use include chlorpromazine (Compazine), promethazine (Phenergan), metochlopramide (Reglan), hydroxyzine

TABLE 4-1 General Anesthetics

Agent	Route of Administration	Form	Comments
Thiopental (Pentothal)	intravenous	stable liquid	rapid induction; short duration; respiratory depressant; can cause laryngospasm and hypotension (opiate or additional agent required for adequate pain control) induction: 3–4 mg/kg maintenance: 50–100 mg/q 10–12 min
Methohexital (Brevital)	intravenous	stable liquid	ultra-short-acting; rapid induction; rapid recovery; may cause hiccoughs; can be administered rectally (pediatrics) induction: 1–1.5 mg/kg maintenance: 20–40 mg/q 4–7 min pediatric rectal induction via 14Fr catheter 7 cm into rectum as 10% solution 20–25 mg/kg
Propofol (Diprovan)	intravenous	stable liquid	rapid induction; short duration; can be used for continuous infusion with clear-headed rapid recovery; used for endoscopy; may cause respiratory depression, transient hypotension; some pain on injection; some anti-emetic effect; common usage induction: 1–2.5 mg/kg maintenance: 50–150 mcg/kg/min (with nitrous oxide or opiate) sedation: 25–75 mcg/kg/min
Ketamine (Ketaject, Ketalar)	intravenous; intramuscular	stable liquid	short-acting anesthetic, long-acting analgesic; used for pediatric and burn wound procedures; trauma cases; may cause emergence hallucinations if given in larger dosages (especially in adults)

continued on following page

TABLE 4-1 General Anesthetics (continued)

Agent	Route of Administration	Form	Comments
			induction: 0.5–2.0 mg/kg; 4–6 mg/kg IM maintenance: 0.5–1.0 mg/min (with nitrous oxide) sedation: 0.2–0.8 mg/kg q 3 min; 2–4 mg/kg IM (pediatric usage)
Etomidate (Amidate, Hypnomidate)	intravenous	stable liquid	induction used for unstable cardiac patients; some nausea; local pain on injection; debatable cause of steroid depression; may be used for sedation in critically ill patients and with fentanyl for percutaneous angioplasty induction: 0.2–0.6 mg/kg maintenance: 0.010 mg/kg/min sedation: 0.005–0.010 mg/kg/min
Nitrous oxide	inhalation	compressed gas	commonly used; employed with other agents to potentiate their action to produce deeper anesthesia
Halothane (Fluothane)	inhalation	volatile liquid	slow, smooth induction; maintenance; for pediatric and burn patients as well as adults; bradycardia; may cause ventricular arrhythmia if epinephrine given; hepatotoxic in some recipients (check prior history); nonmalodorous
Enflurane (Ethrane)	inhalation	volatile liquid	rapid induction; maintenance; rapid recovery; may cause hypotension; associated with seizures in children; less often used
Desflurane (Suprane)	inhalation	volatile liquid	maintenance; good relaxation; rapid recovery; malodorous; increased postoperative nausea

TABLE 4-1 General Anesthetics (continued)

Agent	Route of Administration	Form	Comments
Isoflurane (Forane)	inhalation	volatile liquid	maintenance; good relaxation; cardiovascular stability; useful for cardiac patients
Sevoflurane (Ultane)	inhalation	volatile liquid	rapid induction (useful for mask induction in children); rapid recovery; good relaxation; may cause emergence delirium in children

(Vistaril), ondansetron (Zofran), dolasetron (Anzemet), and granisetron (Kytril). These agents can be used for premedication as well as for antiemetics. (Droperidol, employed commonly until recently, has limited use due to an incidence of ventricular arrhythmias.)

Malignant Hyperthermia

Malignant hyperthermia (MH) is a rare hypermetabolic, highly lethal state triggered by exposure to halogenated inhalation anesthetics (e.g., halothane, enflourane, desflurane, and isoflurane) and depolarizing muscle relaxants (e.g., succinylcholine). There is a predisposition to this syndrome; various myopathies (e.g., muscular dystrophy) present a high risk.

MH usually develops during the administration of an anesthetic, not necessarily on the first exposure, and it can also present in the postoperative period. The major pathophysiological event is the release of an abnormally large amount of an intracellular calcium ion that leads to inordinate muscle contraction (often manifested initially in the masseter muscle).

There is tachycardia with dysrhythmias, increased end-tidal carbon dioxide levels, and muscle cell breakdown (rhabdomyolysis) with production of myoglobinemia. Myoglobinuria can lead to renal failure, and there is respiratory and metabolic acidosis.

Hyperkalemia results, with an increased creatine phosphokinase (CPK) and a progressive rise in core body temperature (even to over 110°F [43°C]). Untreated or suboptimally treated MH results in cardiac and renal failure. Intravascular coagulopathy, muscle necrosis due to hypoxia, and neurologic sequelae also related to hypoxia result in coma and death (occurring in 80% to 90% of the cases).

Suspicion of and prompt recognition of MH when any of the clinical findings occur must be treated well before actual temperature elevation presents. Immediate institution of treatment can significantly reduce mortality.

A protocol for treatment has been proposed and promulgated by the Malignant Hyperthermia Association of the United States (MHAUS). MHAUS is a nonprofit entity with a 24-hour hotline; it also provides educational material. The MHAUS chart (Figure 4-1, p. 68–69) is clear for establishing guidelines for treatment of MH.

As soon as this syndrome is suspect, the anesthetic and/or depolarizing relaxant should be discontinued and positive pressure oxygenation begun.

If the surgical procedure has been started and cannot be aborted, safe "nontriggering" agents can be used, such as nitrous oxide, opiates, and various intravenous anesthetics (e.g., thiopental, propofol, and ketamine), and most local anesthetics can be used to complete the surgery expeditiously.

Treatment is begun as soon as this entity is suspected. The surgeon is notified. Succinylcholine and volatile agents are discontinued. The circulator should obtain Dantrolene and immediately call for assistance. Hyperventilate patient with 100% oxygen at 10 l/min.

Dantrolene sodium (Dantrium) 2 to 3 mg/kg reconstituted with 60 ml of sterile (nonpreservative) water (containing 3 g of mannitol) is given as an IV bolus and repeated every 5–10 minutes to a limit of 10 mg/kg (up to 30 mg/kg) or until the manifestations subside, and it is then administered 1mg/kg every 4 to 6 hours for 24 to 72 hours. This agent is effective (within minutes) due to its prevention of the calcium ions from being released into the muscle cells, thus interfering with the excessive contractions.

Simultaneously, multiple laboratory parameters related to the entities noted above must be checked serially, as well as blood gases. Dysrhythmias are treated (e.g., by procainamide or other antiarrhythmia drugs, noting that calcium channel blocking agents are not to be used). Sodium bicarbonate is given; hyperkalemia is treated with insulin and calcium.

Additional mannitol and furosemide are administered to prevent an accumulation of myoglobin in the renal tubules and to maintain adequate urine flow. A CVP line should be established. Cooling measures are begun with an intravenous infusion of iced saline 15 ml/kg every 15 minutes × 3. Gastric and/or transrectal iced lavage must be initiated; external ice packs and/or a hypothermia blanket are indicated (while monitoring the core body temperature so as not to produce hypothermia).

Any electrolyte, blood gas, coagulation factor, or other abnormality is corrected. On occasion, partial cardiopulmonary bypass may be required as a life-saving measure (to assist with cooling and providing adequate oxygenation). Patients are kept in the intensive care unit (ICU) and are closely monitored using the numerous parameters noted above that are necessary for survival.

Anesthesia providers must be familiar with all of the aspects of MH and must establish a protocol to be followed in the surgical department. The OR staff should be instructed regarding the protocol that requires a coordinated effort to assure the patient's survival. An MH treatment cart stocked with the various agents listed above, including additional IV fluids and fluid administration equipment, defibrillators, and other items, must be available in the department.

Whereas MH can occur *de novo*, all candidates for anesthesia should be questioned regarding any family history of this problem. Elevation of CPK should trigger further investigation. When there is any increased likelihood of MH, prophylaxis with dantrolene may be begun preoperatively and avoidance of the "triggering" types of anesthetic agents should be observed.

It is to be noted that each patient who suffers this problem will present with an individual spectrum of what has been described. The discussion above by no means addresses the entire subject of MH. Please refer to the Emergency Therapy for Malignant Hyperthermia chart on pages 68–69.

Conduction Anesthesia, Overview

Nerve Blocks

The term *central block* refers to spinal, epidural, or caudal anesthesia. Appropriate supplies for their administration are available in most hospitals in disposable prepackaged trays. Additional drugs may be requested. If a longer procedure is contemplated or postoperative central analgesia is to be utilized, the anesthesia provider places a catheter to deliver increments of an anesthetic agent, as in continuous epidural or continuous caudal anesthesia. Postoperatively, morphine (Duramorph) specially prepared for this purpose may be similarly injected for pain relief. For these blocks, the anesthesia provider positions the patient with an established intravenous line; the circulator helps the patient maintain this position while the block is administered. When an anesthetic catheter is placed, it must be secured with tape. The patient may then be placed in a temporary position to allow the block to take effect or moved to the position of surgery at the direction of the anesthesia provider. When the patient is positioned prone (and slightly flexed), a *hypobaric spinal anesthetic* can be accomplished; sterile water is added to the anesthetic mixture, causing the anesthetic to rise to the site of the injection (as employed sterile water is for anorectal surgery).

MHAUS — Malignant Hyperthermia Association of the United States

Emergency Therapy for Malignant Hyperthermia

MH Hotline
1-800-MH-HYPER
(1-800-644-9737)
Outside the US:
1-315-464-7079

DIAGNOSIS

Signs of MH:

- Increased $ETCO_2$
- Trunk or total body rigidity
- Masseter spasm or trismus
- Tachycardia/tachypnea
- Acidosis
- Increased temperature (may be late sign)

Sudden/Unexpected Cardiac Arrest in Young Patients

- Presume hyperkalemia and initiate treatment (see #6)
- Measure CK, myoglobin, ABGs, until normalized
- Consider dantrolene
- Usually secondary to occult myopathy (e.g., muscular dystrophy)
- Resuscitation may be difficult and prolonged

Trismus or Masseter Spasm with Succinylcholine

- Early sign of MH in many patients
- If limb muscle rigidity, begin treatment with dantrolene
- For emergent procedures, continue with nontriggering agents; consider dantrolene
- Follow CK and urine myoglobin for 36 hours at least. Check CK immediately and at 6-hour intervals until returning to normal. Observe for cola-colored urine. If present, test for myoglobin.
- Observe in PACU or ICU for at least 12 hours

ACUTE PHASE TREATMENT

GET HELP. GET DANTROLENE —

1. **Notify Surgeon**
   - Discontinue volatile agents and succinylcholine.
   - Hyperventilate with 100% oxygen at flows of 10 L/min or more.
   - Halt the procedure as soon as possible; if emergent, use nontriggers.

   (The circle system and CO_2 absorbent need not be changed.)

5. **Dysrhythmias** usually respond to treatment of acidosis and hyperkalemia.
   - Use standard drug therapy **except calcium channel blockers, which may cause hyperkalemia or cardiac arrest in the presence of dantrolene.**

2. Dantrolene 2.5 mg/kg rapidly IV through large-bore IV, if possible
To convert kg to lbs for amt of dantrolene, give patients 1 mg/lb (2.5 mg/kg approximates 1 mg/lb).

- Repeat until there is control of the signs of MH.
- Sometimes more than 10 mg/kg (up to 30 mg/kg) is necessary.
- Dissolve the 20 mg in each vial with at least 60 ml **sterile preservative-free water** for injection. Prewarming (not to exceed 38°C) the sterile water will speed solublization of dantrolene.
- The crystals also contain NaOH for a pH of 9; each 20 mg bottle has 3 gm mannitol for isotonicity.

3. Bicarbonate for metabolic acidosis.

- 1-2 mEq/kg if blood gas values are not yet available.

4. Cool the patient with core temperature > 39°C. Lavage open body cavities, stomach, bladder, or rectum. Apply ice to surface. Infuse cold saline intravenously. Stop cooling if temp < 38°C and falling to prevent drift < 36°C.

6. Hyperkalemia - Treat with hyperventilation, bicarbonate, glucose/insulin, calcium.

- Bicarbonate 1-2 mEq/kg IV.
- For **pediatric**, 0.1 units insulin/kg and 1 ml/kg 50% glucose **or** for **adult**, 10 units regular insulin IV and 50 ml 50% glucose.
- Calcium chloride 10 mg/kg or calcium gluconate 10-50 mg/kg for life-threatening hyperkalemia.
- Check glucose levels hourly.

7. Follow $ETCO_2$, electrolytes, blood gases, CK, core temperature, urine output and color, coagulation studies. If CK and/or K+ rise more than transiently or urine output falls to less than 0.5 ml/kg/hr, induce diuresis to >1 ml/kg/hr urine to avoid myoglobinuria-induced renal failure.

- Venous blood gas (e.g., femoral vein) values may document hypermetabolism better than arterial values.
- Central venous or PA monitoring as needed and record minute ventilation.
- Place Foley catheter and monitor urine output.

POST ACUTE PHASE

A. Observe the patient in an ICU for at least 24 hours, due to the risk of recrudescence.

B. Dantrolene 1 mg/kg q4-6 hours or .25 mg/kg/hr by infusion for at least 24 hours. Further doses may be indicated.

C. Follow vitals and labs as above (see #7)

- Frequent ABG
- CK every 6 hours

D. Follow urine myoglobin and institute therapy to prevent myoglobin precipitation in renal tubules and the subsequent development of Acute Renal Failure. Follow standard intensive care therapy for acute rhabdomyolysis and myoglobinuria (urine output > 200 ml/h, alkalinization of urine with Na-bicarbonate infusion with careful attention to both urine and serum pH values, etc.).

E. Counsel the patient and family regarding MH and further precautions; refer them to MHAUS. Fill out and send in the Adverse Metabolic Reaction to Anesthesia (AMRA) form (www.mhreg.org) and send a letter to the patient and her/his physician. Refer patient to the nearest Biopsy Center for follow up.

Non-Emergency Information
MHAUS
11 East State Street, PO Box 1069
Sherburne, NY 13460-1069
Phone
1-800-986-4287 (607-674-7901)
Fax
607-674-7910
E-mail
info@mhaus.org
Website
www.mhaus.org

CAUTION: This protocol may not apply to all patients; alter for specific needs.

FIGURE 4-1. Wall chart distributed by the Malignant Hyperthermia Association of the United States (MHAUS), which describes the protocol for managing hyperthermia crisis. (Reprinted with permission from the Malignant Hyperthermia Association of the United States, Sherburne, NY.)

In an *isobaric spinal block*, spinal fluid is mixed with the agent(s), with minimal migration of the anesthetic within the intrathecal space. Similarly, for *hyperbaric spinal*, 10% dextrose is added so that by positioning the patient, the anesthetic will (being heavier than spinal fluid) gravitate accordingly (i.e., in sitting position, a "saddle" block for pelvic procedures or on the dependant side, such as for a unilateral inguinal herniorrhaphy). A vasoconstrictor (e.g., ephedrine) can be added to the anesthetic mix to provide a longer effect.

A *central block* can be supplemented by a variety of narcotics, amnestics, and intravenous anesthetic agents; oxygen and inhalation anesthetics may be administered by mask as well.

To control postoperative pain, a catheter may be left (or newly placed) in the epidural space (or at caudal, thoracic, and, less often, cervical levels) for continuous or intermittent bolus infusion of narcotic and/or low-dosage local anesthetic. Similarly, a single dose of a narcotic (e.g., morphine) may be given and the catheter removed. When these modalities are employed, most hospitals require the concurrent use of an apnea monitor in addition to a postoperative protocol regarding the use of additional analgesics, antiemetics, and certain other medications prescribed by an attending anesthesia provider until 8 to 24 hours after the catheter is removed.

There are numerous types of *regional blocks* and agents used to affect anesthesia (**Table 4-2** p. 72). Often, the surgeon will administer these anesthetics. Examples include *brachial plexus blocks*, *retrograde intravenous blocks* (e.g., Bier for surgery upon the extremities, most often for upper extremity or ankle level in the lower extremity), *pudendal blocks* (for gynecologic surgery), *perianal blocks* (for anorectal surgery), *inter-costal nerve blocks* (for segmental thoracic pain), and *"field" blocks* (for inguinal hernia repair). These blocks may be supplemented with various systemic agents, as described under central nerve blocks earlier.

Etidocaine (Duranest), benzocaine (Americaine), chloroprocaine (Nesacaine), and procaine (Novocaine) currently have minimal usage in the OR. Alternative dosages of these agents are employed for pediatric surgeries. Numerous ancillary drugs, including tranquilizers, narcotics, and amnestic agents, likewise, have not been specifically listed, as use of these agents varies widely between anesthesia providers, surgeons, and institutions.

Local Anesthesia

Local anesthesia is frequently used for lesser procedures, e.g., plastic, ophthalmic, and anorectal procedures. The surgeon administers the anesthetic by the infiltration of the agent or the diluted agent (and by utilizing a "tumescent" degree of dilution, such as for liposuction).

With few exceptions, an intravenous line is inserted. When "anesthesia standby" is requested, the anesthesia provider will monitor the patient and administer supplemental sedation or even general anesthesia, should it be required.

When an anesthesia provider is not present, a perioperative RN, in addition to the circulator, will insert an intravenous line (in accordance with hospital policy); place EKG electrodes and pulse oximeter; and monitor the patient's vital signs, B/P, and other parameters, as applicable. At the direction of the surgeon, the perioperative RN may administer various drugs parenterally, including narcotics (e.g., morphine, meperidine, fentanyl [Sublimaze], or sufentanil [Sufenta]), sedatives (e.g., diazepam [Valium] or hydroxyzine [Vistaril]), and agents that have an amnestic effect (e.g., midazolam [Versed]).

Upon completion of the procedure, drugs to reverse the effects of the aforementioned agents may be required, such as naloxone (Narcan) or flumazenil (Mazicon). The perioperative RN completes the Conscious Sedation and Analgesia Record (p. 76), which includes the documentation of the time at the beginning and at the termination of the procedure, the patient's vital signs and B/P at appropriate intervals, and the times and dosage of anesthetic agents or any other drugs administered.

Topical Anesthesia

Topical anesthesia is the direct application of an anesthetic agent such as a liquid solution, eye drops, jelly, ointment, and/or spray to the site of the surgery; see Table 4-2, p. 72. Local or general anesthesia may be required to supplement these anesthetics.

Table 4-2 lists only several of the more commonly employed agents for adult patients. Again, numerous other agents can be utilized, and stated dosages must be altered for pediatric patients. In addition, a wide array of ancillary agents, including tranquilizers, narcotics, and amnestic agents, have not been listed because their use varies widely among anesthesia providers and institutions. Special considerations in the administration of pediatric anesthesia can be found on p. 984.

Conscious Sedation and Analgesia

The perioperative RN is not intended to take the place of an anesthesia provider. The American Association of Nurse Anesthetists (AANA) suggests that health care facilities consider professional nursing standards and scope of practice of the RN, not in the capacity of an anesthesia provider who is qualified to administer conscious sedation and analgesia.

"Sedation and analgesia" describes a modality that allows patients to tolerate unpleasant procedures while maintaining adequate cardiorespiratory function and the ability to respond purposefully to verbal commands and tactile stimulation, states the American Society of Anesthesiologists (ASA) Task Force. The Task Force believes that "conscious sedation," a term in common usage, is imprecise terminology and that "sedation and analgesia" more accurately describes this state. When a patient is able to respond only to painful stimulation, a greater degree of sedation exists. Procedures in which sedation and analgesia are employed include those in which regional or local anesthetics are used.

TABLE 4-2 Commonly Used Conduction Anesthetics*

Agent	Route of Administration	Concentration/ Dose	Comments
Lidocaine (Xylocaine)	spinal**	5%/100 mg	rapid onset; shorter acting
Bupivacaine (Marcaine, Sensorcaine)	spinal**	0.75%/15–22.5 mg	longer acting; longer analgesia after return of sensation
Tetracaine (Pontocaine)	spinal**	0.5%–1.0%/ 5–12 mg	rapid onset; longer acting with higher dosage and/or added ephedrine or epinephrine**
Lidocaine (Xylocaine)	epidural/** caudal	1.0%–2.0%/ 500 mg	rapid onset; shorter duration
Bupivacaine (Marcaine, Sensorcaine)	epidural/** caudal	0.25–0.7.5%/ 150 mg	longer acting; obstetrics; postoperative analgesia (including obstetrics) as infusion via catheter; cardiac arrest in higher dosage reported
Ropivacaine (Naropin)	epidural/** caudal	0.5%–0.75%/ 75–200 mg	as per bupivacaine but less toxic
Mepivacaine (Polocaine)	epidural/** caudal	1.5%–2.0%/ 150–400 mg	as per bupivacaine
Lidocaine (Xylocaine)	regional nerve block/ retrograde (Bier) intravenous block	1.0%–2.0%/ 500 mg; 5%/40–60 ml (200–300 mg)	rapid onset; double-cuffed tourniquet required

TABLE 4-2 Commonly Used Conduction Anesthetics* (continued)

Agent	Route of Administration	Concentration/ Dose	Comments
Bupivacaine (Marcaine, Sensorcaine)	regional nerve block	0.25%–0.5%	long acting
Ropivacaine (Naropin)	regional nerve block	0.5%–0.75%/ 75–300 mg	long acting
Mepivacaine (Polocaine)	regional nerve block	1%–2%/50–400 mg	long acting
Lidocaine (Xylocaine)	local	0.5%–2%/ 500 mg	commonly used
Bupivacaine (Marcaine, Sensorcaine)	local	0.25%–0.5%/ 225 mg	long acting
Ropivacaine (Naropin)	local	0.5%/5–200 mg	long acting
Mepivacaine (Polocaine)	local	1.0%/400 mg	long acting
Lidocaine (Xylocaine)	topical liquid ointment; gel	2% or 4% 2%/15–30 ml; 4%/15 ml	low toxicity; short acting; intra-tracheally cystoscopy; other endoscopies
Lidocaine (LMX 4; LMX 5)	topical cream	4% or 5%	on intact skin or mucous membranes; not for open wounds or ophthalmic use; superficial skin procedures; to lessen pain of subsequent puncture (children); may take 5–40 min to be effective; occlusive dressing for skin use
Lidocaine/ Prilocaine	topical cream dressing use for skin (up 1–2 hr) before procedure	2.5%/2.5% (25 mg/ 25 mg/g) 1–2 g/10 cm²	as per lidocaine 4%–5% cream; occlusive (EMLA)

continued on following page

TABLE 4-2 Commonly Used Conduction Anesthetics* (continued)

Agent	Route of Administration	Concentration/ Dose	Comments
Cocaine	topical liquid	2%-10% (4% common)/ 200 mg	high potency; rapid absorption through mucous membranes; ENT procedures
Tetracaine (Pontocaine)	topical liquid ointment; cream	0.5%–1.0% 0.5%–1.0%	rapid onset; ophthalmic use mucous membranes (anorectal)

*All conduction anesthetic agents, when administered in greater than recommended dosages or if accidentally given intravenously (or by idiosyncratic reaction), may cause extreme agitation, convulsions, cardiac arrest, and death. Resuscitative equipment and drugs must be immediately available whenever these agents are employed. The dosages of agents listed in this table are approximate, modified by the patient's weight, height, duration of the procedure (with incremental doses), and cardiac arrhythmias.
** Vasoconstrictors such as ephedrine and epinephrine can be added to an anesthetic agent to prolong the effect of the block. A diffusing agent such as hyaluronidase (Wydase) may be added to local anesthetics to hasten the onset of the anesthetic effect.
This table lists only several of the most commonly used anesthetic agents in the dosages used primarily for adult patients.

There are four levels of sedation and analgesia described by the JC. They are:

1. minimal sedation and analgesia (the patient responds normally)
2. moderate sedation (conscious sedation)
3. deep sedation (the patient is not easily aroused but maintains respiration), and
4. anesthesia in which the patient requires assisted ventilation.

Patients can easily slip from moderate sedation to deeper levels of sedation, the deeper levels necessitating the assistance of a skilled anesthesia provider.

The JC (last revised, 2003), has set forth qualifications for the nonanesthesia provider, the perioperative RN who administers conscious sedation and analgesia in a health-care facility. The competency of the perioperative RN should be periodically evaluated and documented. The RN must have knowledge of anatomy and physiology, pharmacology, EKG arrhythmias, and complications related to sedation and analgesia. See Analgesia and Conscious Sedation Record, p. 76.

The perioperative RN who administers conscious sedation and analgesia must continually assess the patient's physical status and behavioral changes. He/she is required to know about oxygen saturation and the use of the pulse oximeter and to understand the indications for oxygen supplementation and its administration. He/she must be able to recognize signs and symptoms of drug toxicity and hypersensitivity to medications and anesthetic agents resulting in anxiety, sweating, pallor, nausea, vomiting, urticaria, tachycardia, laryngeal swelling, severe hypotension, convulsions, and shock.

It is mandatory that he/she be familiar with the treatment for these conditions and know when to request assistance in an urgent manner. Similarly, he/she must be able to assess, diagnose, and intervene during the procedure to manage the airway and to request the intervention of an anesthesia provider.

The perioperative RN administers agents, e.g., meperidine (Demerol) and midazolam (Versed), as ordered by the anesthesia provider or surgeon for sedation and analgesia *only*; anesthetics are not to be given by the perioperative RN who is not a qualified anesthesia provider. He/she who provides conscious sedation and analgesia is to have no other responsibilities during the procedure. Frequent monitoring and documentation of the patient's physiologic status (vital signs, B/P, and oxygen saturation) and the charting of medications according to the time administered are required.

An emergency cart or "crash cart" must be readily available, and an anesthesia provider is required to be present (in the facility) to handle emergencies and complications and, in some facilities, to discharge the patient.

Postoperative Transfer of the Patient to the PACU

Upon completion of the surgical procedure and placement of dressings, the circulator accompanies the anesthesia provider or RN provider of conscious sedation and the patient to the recovery room. The patient is repositioned (as necessary) for movement onto the gurney (or special bed or frame); intravascular lines, urinary catheter, and splinted extremities are protected. The security of the airway is the responsibility of the anesthesia provider. The patient may *never* be moved until the anesthesia provider is ready.

When the patient has been expeditiously transported to the recovery room, the anesthesia and perioperative records, special appliances, and equipment are given to the PACU provider. The circulator also reports to the PACU provider any significant intraoperative events, as a severe fluctuation in cardiovascular or pulmonary functions, any untoward reaction to drugs, or the need for multiple transfusions or special medications.

The patient's chart may be temporarily retained by the surgeon to complete the operative note, postoperative orders, or dictation. If the chart is not immediately available, the circulator will advise the PACU

ANALGESIA AND CONSCIOUS SEDATION RECORD

PROCEDURE ______________________________

SURGEON ______________________ **DATE** __________

TIME CONSCIOUS SEDATION STARTED __________

PROCEDURE STARTED __________

PROCEDURE ENDED __________

CONSCIOUS SEDATION ENDED __________

ANALGESIA AND CONSCIOUS SEDATION ADMINISTERED BY:

____

RN signature

PREOPERATIVE PHYSIOLOGICAL ASSESSMENT

Respiration:	Preprocedure	Postprocedure
Deep breathes and coughs freely		
Dyspnic or limited		
Cyanotic		

Skin color:	☐ normal	☐ pale	☐ flushed	☐ jaundiced
Skin moisture:	☐ normal	☐ dry	☐ moist	☐ diaphoretic
Skin temperature:	☐ normal	☐ warm	☐ cool	☐ cold

PREOPERATIVE

Behavior, mental status		**Speech**
☐ Conscious	☐ Cooperative	☐ Coherent
☐ Drowsy	☐ Uncooperative	☐ Incoherent
☐ Confused	☐ Combative	☐ Silent
☐ Unconscious	☐ Anxious	☐ Slurred
☐ Oriented x __	☐ Other	☐ Crying
☐ Agitated		

POSTOPERATIVE

Behavior ______________________________

Speech ______________________________

VITAL SIGNS RECORD

Time	**Temp.**	**B/P**	**Pulse**	**Respirations**	**O2 Sat.**

POSITION

Aids for positioning (e.g., pillows, rolls, donut) __________

Skin condition: ______________________ preprocedure

Does patient's skin appear free from injury postprocedure?

____

ANALGESIA AND CONSCIOUS SEDATION RECORD

IV INSERTED (site) ______ ANGIOCATHETER # ______

BY ______

SOLUTION #1 ______ #2 ______ #3 ______

B/P CUFF PLACED (site) ______ PULSE OXIMETER yes ☐ no ☐

OXYGEN BY MASK ______ BY CANNULA ______ l/m ______

NURSING FOCUS:
OBSERVATIONS/INTERVENTIONS/OUTCOME

Continuous Assessment is made of the patient's condition PRE, INTRA, AND POSTPROCEDURE: Note anxiety, degree of alertness during procedure, ability to follow commands while receiving conscious sedation, etc.

Use the suggested PERIOPERATIVE PATIENT CARE PLAN, p ______, as applicable.

DOCUMENT ALL OBSERVATIONS AND CARE INTERVENTIONS for continuity of care and for medicolegal purposes.

NURSING FOCUS I: PATIENT APPEARS ANXIOUS DUE TO ANTICIPATED SURGERY/ PROCEDURE AND UNFAMILIAR ENVIRONMENT

List nursing interventions e.g., Orient patients to surroundings and advise them of perioperative events as they occur

Explain to the patient that you will act as his/her advocate. Presence near patient during anesthetic injections suggests you want to provide comfort and emotional support. Explain the sequence of perioperative events before starting a procedure, as insertion of an IV.

DESIRED OUTCOME: Patient is able to speak calmly, cooperates, and follows directions.

Outcome met ☐ yes ☐ no

Comment *Outcome met; patient stated he/she felt minimal discomfort and did not appear to be in distress.*

MEDICATION ROUTE DOSE TIME RESPONSE

Midazolam IV ______

Fentanyl IV ______

Demerol IV ______

Romazicon IV ______

Narcan IV ______

______

______

Signature ______

provider of any postoperative orders made to him/her requiring immediate attention, as the application of an ice pack or the connection of drainage systems to a suction source. If significant nausea occurs, the anesthesia provider may administer an antiemetic, e.g., ondansetron (Zofran) or dolasetron (Anzamet). The circulator will remain with the patient until the transfer to the PACU is completed.

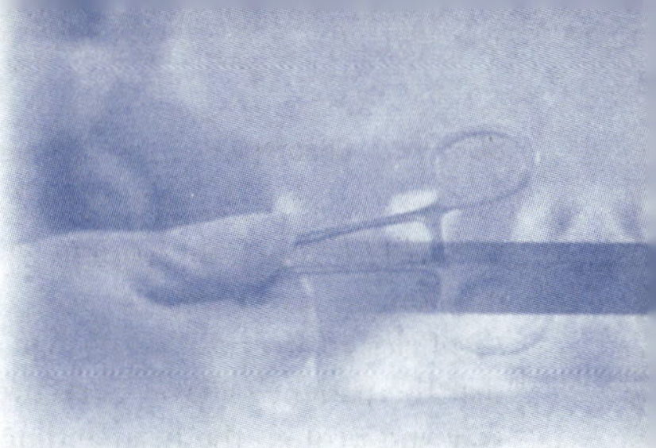

CHAPTER 5
General Anesthesia

Perioperative Considerations

Definition

General anesthesia is the administration of agents by intravenous injection or inhalation that renders the patient unconscious or obtunded.

Discussion

This anesthetic method is commonly employed. The depth and duration of anesthesia are regulated according to the type of anesthetic employed and the amount of the agent(s) administered. In addition to numerous intravenous and inhalation anesthetics, a large number of other agents, including muscle relaxants, tranquilizers, and narcotics, are employed. Rarely is a single drug used, although for limited procedures, a single agent (e.g., ketamine) may be employed. Intramuscular injection and rectal instillation of a primary agent are rarely used. During all general anesthetics, the patient must be well oxygenated and the patency of the airway maintained. The anesthesia provider must also maintain the patient's cardiovascular system and other vital functions. For more information on general anesthesia, see Chapter 4.

Preparation of the Patient

The patient is supine, with the safety strap in place across the thighs (about 3 inches above the knees). Care is taken not to compromise circulation by securing the restraint too tightly. The head support, a donut, pillow, or headframe is adjusted or removed at the discretion of the anesthesia provider. For procedures performed in the supine or lithotomy position that are of short duration, i.e., those in which profound muscle relaxation is not usually required, patency of the airway is managed with a mask and oral (or nasal) airway or by means of a laryngeal mask airway (LMA).

Following induction, the insertion of an endotracheal tube will be required if the patient's position is to be other than supine or lithotomy, for a prolonged procedure in the supine position, for surgeries that affect respiration, or when profound muscular relaxation is needed. A variety of types and sizes of endotracheal tubes is available. Most often the endotracheal tube is placed transorally, but it may also be inserted transnasally or via an established tracheostomy.

NEVER move the patient without the anesthesia provider's permission.

Prior to any position change, the anesthesia provider must indicate that the patient's airway is secure and that he/she will control the airway and protect the head and neck as the patient is repositioned. The patient's eyes are protected by the instillation of ophthalmic ointment and/or by taping the lids closed. For details on positions, see pp. 20–27; the position diagrams are on pp. 27–30, or refer to the specific surgical procedure.

Draping

No draping is required.

Equipment and Supplies

The anesthesia equipment and supplies necessary to care for and monitor the patient in surgery are selected by the anesthesia provider to meet the needs of the individual patient. Factors considered include whether the patient is a child or an adult, the patient's age, stature (physical size), physical condition, and state of health.

The following should be available for general anesthesia and maintenance:

- Suction sou e, preferably a separate unit (in addition to the one on anesthesia cart)
- Laryngoscope and blades
- Suction catheters and suction tips, e.g., Yankauer (disposable, as requested)
- McGill forceps (or similar) to facilitate endotracheal tube or nasogastric tube (and other transesophageal probe) insertion
- Face mask, head strap, variety of endotracheal tubes (with obturators), oral and nasal airways, connectors for masks or endotracheal tubes, sterile anesthetic lubricant (for the endotracheal tube and obturator), syringe (to inflate the tube cuff), tongue blades, topical anesthetic for instillation into the larynx, e.g., local tracheal anesthesia (LTA) kit
- Anesthesia breathing circuit (disposable)
- Stethoscopes, standard and esophageal
- Monitoring devices for blood pressure and pulse, electrocardiogram (EKG), oxygen and carbon dioxide monitors, oxygen alarm, pulse oximeter, and EEG (as appropriate)
- Intravenous (IV) line(s), central venous pressure line (CVP), intraarterial line and the specific tray containing the items needed for insertion of the line and appropriate gauges
- Ether screen, IV standards, and drape clips

Padded armboards and shoulder supports, pillows, headrest or headframe, and chest rolls
Nasogastric tube (NG tube), if requested
BIS (bispectral index system) attachments and monitor (if requested)

Special Notes

These **Special Notes** are in regard to the administration of a general anesthetic. Prior to the surgical procedure, the circulator must use the Universal Protocol mandated by the Joint Commission (JC) (formerly the Joint Commission on Accreditation of Healthcare Organizations) to identify the patient, "time out" must be observed by the OR team, etc. Apply **Special Notes** from ***Abdominal Extraintestinal Surgery***, p. 151, as applicable.

- The circulator should be familiar with the anesthesia equipment (the name, function, and assembly of each piece of equipment) and know its location. This is invaluable in saving time and is potentially lifesaving as well.
- The circulator should check the working order of the room suctions prior to bringing the patient into the room. In the event that the suction on the anesthesia cart does not function properly, the room suctions must be substituted immediately.
- The circulator should confirm that the compressed oxygen cylinder contains more than 250 psi of oxygen to avoid needing to replace the oxygen tank before the surgery is completed. When cylinder pressure is below 250 psi or if a long procedure is anticipated, the cylinder should be replaced before the patient is brought into the room.
- The circulator is required to know the location of the emergency "crash" cart (supplied with medications, syringes, supplies, defibrillator paddles, etc.); if the patient suffers a *cardiac or respiratory arrest* additional assistance should be summoned immediately.
- Prior to bringing the patient into the room, the circulator should obtain pillows, pads, rolls, etc. necessary for positioning the patient for the correct surgical procedure.
- Positioning aids may be needed during endotracheal intubation (e.g., shoulder roll to support the scapulae, shoulders, and posterior neck of an obese patient); the circulator should bring the necessary aids into the room prior to the patient's arrival to save time.

- The circulator must know the location of the anesthesia "Emergency Airway Cart"; it should be positioned immediately outside the room whenever a difficult intubation is anticipated or when there is concern regarding the patient's medical status.
- The circulator must know what emergency equipment (by name) is on the Emergency Airway Cart; knowing the names, parts, and assembly of each piece of equipment is vital.
- When the circulator brings the patient into the OR, he/she can help to allay or minimize the patient's anxiety by directly addressing the patient's concerns and questions with knowledgeable information when appropriate and by referring questions to the surgeon as necessary.
- The circulator may want to explain to the patient that he/she will act as the patient's advocate (i.e., that he/she will act or speak on the patient's behalf), particularly while the patient is anesthetized.
- Conversation and movement in the room should be kept to a minimum during the induction of anesthesia, particularly endotracheal intubation. The induction and administration of anesthesia is facilitated by a quiet atmosphere. Remember that hearing is the last sense to be lost and that movement can be distracting.
- The circulator needs to be prepared to assist the anesthesia provider at all times during the surgery, particularly prior to, and during, induction.
- The circulator should stand at or near the head of the table during endotracheal intubation to assist the anesthesia provider by manipulating the cricoid cartilage (thereby providing better visualization of the glottis) and by injecting premeasured intravenous drugs, as directed by the anesthesia provider.
- Following the induction of anesthesia (and placement and securing of an endotracheal tube when utilized), the circulator reaffirms with the surgeon and the anesthesia provider regarding the patient's position for the anticipated surgical procedure. Perioperative personnel should ***never*** move or reposition the patient until directed to do so by the anesthesia provider.
- Care must be taken to protect the patient to avoid injuries as the result of burns, neurological damage, pressure sores, or other traumas that cannot be perceived by the anesthetized

patient. Use adequate cushioning for all bony prominences to prevent excessive pressure injuries to the skin, nerves, and soft tissues that would eventually lead to tissue necrosis.

- When the patient's medical status is compromised and minimizing anesthesia time is desirable, the surgical area may be prepared and draped prior to the induction of the anesthetic.

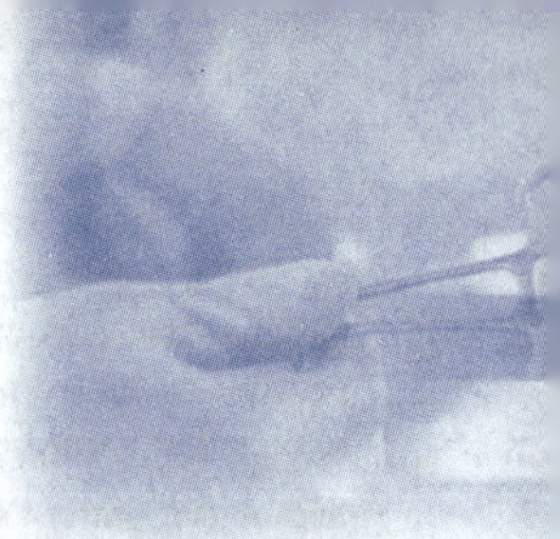

CHAPTER 6
Conduction Anesthesia

Central Nerve Blocks: Spinal, Epidural, and Caudal

Definition

Central nerve blocks are achieved by injecting anesthetic solutions intrathecally into the subarachnoid space, into the epidural space, or into the caudal canal (an extension of the epidural space).

Discussion

Conduction anesthetics are often employed when surgical procedures are performed on the lower abdomen and lower extremities. The composition and concentration of the anesthetic solution used determines the duration of the block. The patient's position immediately after the injection of the anesthetic solution influences the level and distribution of the block. These anesthetics may be supplemented by varying depths of general anesthesia and/or sedation.

Preparation of the Patient

The patient's position during the administration of the anesthetic is determined by the type of anesthetic block being administered, the surgical procedure to be performed, the patient's physical condition, the preference and ability of the anesthesia provider to administer the particular block, and the preference of the surgeon. The physician selects the type of anesthesia that he/she considers safest for the patient. During the administration of the anesthetic block, the patient may be placed in a sitting, lateral, or prone position.

Sitting: with the back arched and feet supported on a stool (spinal or epidural)

Lateral: with the knees, hips, back, and neck flexed (spinal or epidural)

Prone: with the body flexed at the waist (caudal or hypobaric spinal)

Following the injection of the anesthetic agent (after an interval determined by anesthesia provider), the patient is placed in the selected operative position or the patient remains in the same position, as appropriate (e.g., patient remains in the prone position after caudal or hypobaric spinal is administered for anorectal surgery). The circulator or other available personnel helps to support the patient in the required position necessary to administer the block.

For prolonged procedures and/or postoperative analgesia, "continuous epidural" or "caudal" anesthesia is established at the time of the initial needle placement by inserting a catheter into the appropriate space (epidural space or caudal canal) for the nerve block. Increments of anesthetic solution may then be administered via the catheter.

Skin Preparation and Draping

Prior to administering the anesthetic, the anesthesia provider usually preps the skin and drapes the patient. The supplies for the skin prep and draping are often included in a prepackaged disposable tray. When the circulator preps the skin, the prep begins at the site of injection, extending for an appropriately wide margin circumferentially. The anesthesia provider then drapes the patient.

Equipment

Stool/lift (for patient's feet, sitting position)
Sitting stool (for anesthesia provider)

Supplies

Appropriate sterile disposable prepackaged tray, according to type of block to be administered (e.g., spinal, epidural, or caudal)
Additional anesthetic agents, needles, catheters, tubing, etc. (as requested)

Special Notes

These **Special Notes** are in regard to the administration of the anesthetic, not a surgical procedure. For a surgical procedure, the circulator must use the Universal Protocol mandated by the Joint Commission (JC) (formerly the Joint Commission on Accreditation of Healthcare Organizations) to identify the patient, "time out" must be observed by the OR team, etc. Apply **Special Notes** from ***Abdominal Extraintestinal Surgery***, p. 151, as applicable.

- The circulator may want to explain to the patient that he/she will act as the patient's advocate (i.e., that he/she will act or speak on the patient's behalf) particularly while the patient is anesthetized.
- The circulator should be familiar with the anesthetic agents, supplies, equipment, and trays required to perform each type of anesthetic block.
- The circulator should know the location of necessary additional anesthesia supplies not included in the prepackaged anesthetic

tray to save valuable time. The patient is charged for all time spent in the OR.

- The circulator may be requested to make preparations for starting an intravenous line (the anesthesia provider usually inserts the line) or the circulator may be asked to insert the intravenous line.
- The circulator or scrub person assists the anesthesia provider by helping the patient to assume and maintain the position required during administration of the block.
- The circulator (in addition to the anesthesia provider) must closely observe the patient for signs of respiratory distress caused by the sedation or by the inadvertent administration of a "high" spinal resulting in the depression or paralysis of the respiratory muscles. In this situation, the patient would require immediate endotracheal intubation and ventilatory assistance, as he or she would be paralysed (physically unable to breathe).
- The circulator must know the location of the anesthesia "Emergency Airway Cart"; it should be positioned immediately outside the room in case of respiratory distress or when there is concern regarding the patient's medical status.
- The circulator must know what emergency equipment (by name) is on the Emergency Airway Cart; knowing the names, parts, and assembly of each piece of equipment is vital to patient safety during an emergency.
- The circulator should check the working order of the room suctions prior to bringing the patient into the room. Room suctions must be ready for use at all times. In the event that the suction on the anesthesia cart does not function properly, the room suctions must be substituted immediately.
- The circulator is required to know the location of the emergency "crash" cart supplied with medications, syringes, supplies, defibrillator paddles, etc. in case of *cardiac or respiratory arrest*, assistance must be obtained immediately.
- Special care must be taken to protect the patient to avoid injuries as the result of burns, neurological damage, pressure sores, or other traumas that cannot be perceived by the "unfeeling" anesthetized patient. Use adequate cushioning for all bony prominences to prevent excessive pressure injuries to the skin, nerves, and soft tissues that would eventually lead to tissue necrosis.
- The circulator should determine what equipment is needed to administer the nerve block and to perform the surgery before

bringing the patient into the OR; the electrical equipment must be in working order before it is brought into the room.

- In order to avoid postspinal headache, patients must be instructed preoperatively and reminded postoperatively to remain on bedrest without raising their heads for 24 to 48 hours. A good deal of fluids via an appropriate route (oral, intravenous, or both), as ordered, should be given until the possibility of headache has passed.
- Special needles with a trocar tip and side port are available for intrathecal injection (e.g., Whitacre needle) to minimize the leakage of spinal fluid. For persistent leakage, an epidural puncture is made at approximately the level of the prior spinal puncture and a "patch" of autologous blood is injected to facilitate closure of the leak.
- Adhesive, hypoallergenic plastic, or paper tape is used to secure intravenous and pressure lines, the anesthetic catheter, and all other tubes or lines. The circulator should ask the patient about and check the patient's chart regarding tape allergies.
- **Do not** dispose of any items on the disposable anesthetic tray until the anesthesia provider indicates that the appropriate information needed for the anesthetic record has been obtained. The tray may be disposed of *in* the room ***only***. The room trash is ***not*** removed until the surgical procedure is completed.
- The patient, although often sedated, may be alert enough to hear, as hearing is the last sense to be lost. Therefore, discussion of the diagnosis, other medical information, and idle conversation should be limited accordingly.
- Perioperative personnel should employ all measures necessary to ensure the patient's privacy.

Regional, Local, Topical Anesthesia Modalities

Definition

An anesthetic agent may be applied by injection about the peripheral nerve trunk, by injection adjacent to or directly into the surgical site, or by application directly to the surface to be treated.

Discussion

Regional nerve block (e.g., brachial plexus block or ankle block) is achieved by depositing an anesthetic agent immediately adjacent to a larger peripheral nerve(s). This anesthetic is used primarily for surgery on the extremities. Intercostal nerve block is administered for local pain control, such as for a patient with a fractured rib or herpes zoster. A field block is used for limited abdominal surgery (e.g., gastrostomy or inguinal herniorrhaphy).

Local anesthesia refers to the injection of the anesthetic agent into, or immediately adjacent, to the site of surgery, anesthetizing smaller nerves directly.

In *topical anesthesia*, the anesthetic agent (cream, gel, or liquid) is absorbed through the tissues (usually mucous membrane) to anesthetize the area immediately beneath where it is being applied (i.e., ophthalmic or gingival) or the agent is applied to the tissue overlying a larger nerve trunk that courses close to the surface (e.g., glossopharyngeal nerve block). These anesthetic modalities (local or topical) may be administered by the surgeon (without the presence of an anesthesia provider); however, when the patient is medically fragile, or when general anesthesia or deep sedation is employed, an anesthesia provider is required. When the patient receives "conscious sedation," a perioperative registered nurse (RN), in addition to the circulator, is required to monitor the patient.

Hyaluronidase (Wydase™) may be added to an injectable agent to promote more rapid spread and resolution of the local edema related to the injection. Epinephrine (adrenalin) added to the anesthetic solution will prolong the effect of the anesthetic solution.

Preparation of the Patient

The patient is positioned to expose the site of the proposed injection or application. In local or topical anesthesia, this site is often identical to the site of the surgery; whereas in regional anesthesia, the site of injection may be remote from that of surgery.

Skin Preparation

Regional: Skin preparation is done before the block is established, most often by the person performing the block (anesthesia provider or surgeon). The circulator may be requested to prep the skin; the prep begins at the site of injection, extending for an appropriately wide margin circumferentially.

Local: Skin preparation for the injection and the surgery are usually the same.

Topical: Usually none is required, but an occlusive dressing is recommended for the transdermal application of EMLA™ or LMX™ (anesthetic agents in a cream formula).

Supplies

Skin preparation tray, often located inside the regional or local tray
Needles and syringes (regional or local)
Medicine cup (for anesthetic agent)
Sponges
Anesthetic agent(s)

Special Notes

- See **Special Notes** from Central nerve blocks above and apply, as applicable.
- When the surgical site is anesthetized using a regional, local, or topical anesthetic agent, equipment for administration of general anesthesia and performing resuscitative measures must be immediately available.
- A perioperative RN may insert an intravenous line, according to hospital policy.
- In the absence of an anesthesia provider, a perioperative RN (in addition to the circulator) is needed to monitor and record the patient's vital signs and blood pressure, monitor the intravenous line, and record any other important information on the ***Analgesia and Conscious Sedation Record***.
- Determine the type of anesthesia chosen for the patient and the supplies that will be needed; the items should be in the operating room prior to bringing the patient into the room.
- Be aware of special items needed to administer selected anesthetic blocks (e.g., Bier block [retrograde intravenous], requires two tourniquets [or a double-cuff tourniquet]), in addition to the medication cup, anesthetic agent (as requested), paper labels, sterile marking pen, needles, and syringes.
- Although the patient receiving regional, local, or topical anesthetic is often sedated, he/she may be alert enough to hear; discussion of the diagnosis, other medical information, and idle conversation should be limited accordingly.
- Perioperative personnel must ***always*** observe measures necessary to maintain the patient's privacy.

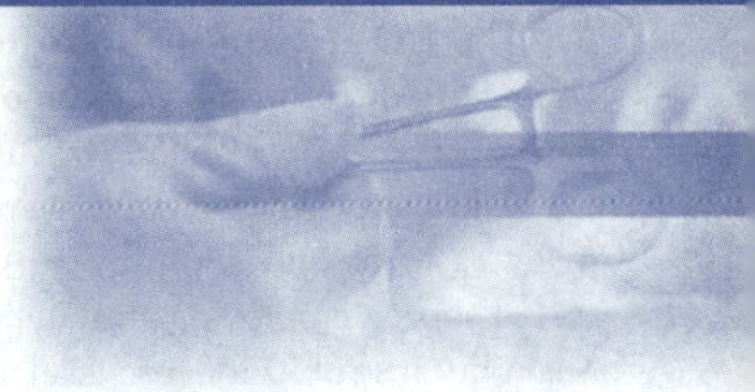

CHAPTER 7
Laser Technology

Types of Lasers

Definition

The ***laser*** (an acronym for *light amplification by stimulated emission of radiation*) is an energy source derived from light.

Discussion

The laser emits light energy produced by stimulating the electrons of various media (solid, liquid, tunable dye, or gas) with electricity (or xenon flash lamp or another laser) to reach a high-energy (excitement) state, releasing this energy in the form of photons. The photons collide within the laser chamber between mirrors, creating more energy that then escapes in a controlled manner as the *laser beam*. This beam is ***collimated*** (parallel), maintaining a constant diameter for great distances (unlike an ordinary light beam, which expands). This beam is monochromatic and of a single optical frequency, and the energy particles, ***photons***, travel in a coordinated fashion with the light waves in phase with each other, i.e., ***coherently***. These properties allow the laser light beam to travel over great distances with extremely concentrated energy that focuses the light into a tiny spot, the ***focal point***. Each individually stimulated substance emits energy of a different wavelength, which influences the absorption of this energy in a selective manner. The laser does not produce ionizing radiation and is not hazardous in that sense, as are radioactive substances or x-rays.

Body tissues are affected by the laser beam as the light energy is converted to heat (or acoustical energy). The result is the vaporization, fragmentation, cutting, or coagulation (or "welding") of these tissues. The level of the laser power setting, the ***wattage,*** the duration of the contact time with the target tissues, the use of continuous or pulsed mode, the cooling action of the local blood flow pigmentation, translucency of the target, and adjacent tissues determine the effect of the laser beam on tissues.

Several lasers of different wavelengths measured in nanometers (nm) and with different clinical capabilities are commonly used in the operating room.

The **CO_2 (carbon dioxide)** 10,600-nm laser is used in a noncontact mode for cutting and vaporization of tissues (and welding of certain tissues, for example, vascular anastamoses). This laser may be excited by electricity or radiowaves. The source of CO_2 (and accompanying gases helium and nitrogen) can be from a replaceable tank or a sealed source employing a catalytic reaction to reclaim the gases. Previously, because of its longer wavelength, the CO_2 laser beam could not be transmitted through lengthy fiber delivery systems. However, a hollow tubular articulated arm within which are specially positioned mirrors that permit adaptation of the laser beam via a microscope or handpiece with a lens system to focus the beam is in use. Another variant is a flexible hollow wave guide lined with reflective metal ribbons and a dielectric (electrically nonconducting) coating that extends the CO_2 laser's ability to treat previously inaccessible areas, but with loss of laser energy.

The **Nd:YAG (neodymium yttrium aluminum garnet)** 1064-nm laser can pass through clear fluid, targeting darker tissues beyond, or it can be transmitted by a flexible probe (fiber) through an endoscope for the destruction of gastrointestinal, urinary, and respiratory tract lesions. With the use of a sapphire tip, the Nd:YAG laser can be used in a contact mode.

The **argon** 488-nm (blue) to 515-nm (green) laser composes blue-green laser energy that is absorbed by melanin and hemoglobin and is used in ophthalmology (e.g., photo coagulation of retinal vessels and bleeding points), in plastic surgery to ablate hemangiomata, and in various dermatologic applications.

The **KTP (potassium titanyl phosphate)** 532-nm laser is a variant of the Nd:YAG wherein the beam is passed through a potassium titanyl phosphate crystal, doubling its frequency (halving its wavelength), giving this laser properties similar to the argon laser but with increased tissue-destructive capability.

The **Ho:YAG (holmium)** 2100-nm laser with penetration to 0.4 to 0.6 mm is absorbed by water (as is CO_2 laser energy) and can be applied directly or via a fiber. It can be used for acoustical effect to shatter biliary or urinary tract calculi.

The **Er:YAG (erbium)** 2940-nm laser is absorbed by water with shallow tissue penetration, making it useful for local ablation and skin resurfacing.

Tunable dye lasers refer to laser energy derived from various dyes exposed to intense light (e.g., the argon laser), the wavelength (400 to 1000 nm) modified by a tuning crystal. Included in this modality are pulsed dye lasers of various frequencies, depending on the particular liquid dye medium and a pulsed light source. For example, this laser (with a frequency of 504 nm), as conducted through a fine (0.2-mm) quartz fiber, can be passed through a ureteroscope immediately adjacent to or in direct application to a calculus, causing it to shatter. A 530-nm wavelength yellow dye laser will also disrupt urinary tract calculi.

A **flashlamp pumped pulse dye (FLPPD) laser** depends on a dye activated by a flashlamp and tuned to 400 to 1000 nm by changing the dye and the use of prisms to treat dermatologic conditions involving specific pigments.

Candela lasers (585 nm and 510 nm) are used for urologic purposes or can be used to ablate colored skin lesions as hemangiomata and are often used in outpatient settings for a variety of cosmetic purposes as pigmented lesion ablation, reduction of fine varicose veins, and tattoo removal.

An additional application is **photodynamic therapy**, which involves the systemic injection of a photosensitive dye (e.g., modified porphyrin as 5-aminolaevulinic acid [5ALA], porfirmer sodium [Photofrin], meso tetra hydroxyphenyl chlorin [m-THPC, Foscan]), which are selectively retained by malignant (and other) tissues. These tissues (e.g., urinary bladder, breast, retina, and maxillary sinus) are exposed to a laser light of appropriate wavelength (range, 400 to 1000 nm) to produce a photochemical reaction, resulting in tumor destruction. Thus, a tunable dye laser adjusted (tuned) by prism to emit, for example, red light (argon laser energy source for rhodamine B laser 630 nm) produces the photochemical effect in conjunction with the administration of hematoporphyrin to ablate certain superficial lesions, as carcinoma in situ, pigmented skin lesions, and transitional cell bladder tumors, and to restore a lumen in cases of obstructive esophageal and lung malignancies.

Via image guidance technique, a needle through which a laser fiber is introduced interstitially can be used to destroy liver metastases, pancreatic tumors, and breast tumors, benign and malignant. Photodynamic therapy is also employed to reopen arterial stenosis after angioplasty. Pulsation and wattage can be adjusted to minimize adjacent tissue damage (e.g., Q-switched lasers with which very brief but frequent pulses attain a high level of target destruction, sparing surrounding tissues).

The **ruby laser** (694 nm) is used for tattoo removal.

The **excimer** (excited dimeric medium) **laser** utilizes an inert gas-halide system (including argon-fluoride 193 nm, krypton-fluoride 248 nm, xenon-chloride 308 nm, and xenon-fluoride 351 nm), which can be incorporated in a fine catheter that includes a video system and irrigating mechanism used to open occluded coronary arteries (pulsed 308 nm) by direct contact destruction of intimal plaque. An additional excimer laser use is in optical contouring of the cornea. These gases are toxic so that appropriate apparatus housing structures and exhaust systems are inherent in their use.

The **Diode** laser, 750 to 950 nm (or gallium arsenide, 840 to 910 nm), has been introduced in a compact system for photocoagulation in ophthalmologic use, delivered directly by fiber or introduced through a slit lamp. The diode laser also may be used for urological applications. Delivery fibers with a rotary mirror (metallic) to orient the beam are available, as are units that can deliver a selection of lasers of different wavelengths.

As CO_2 and Nd:YAG laser beams are colorless, an accompanying neon-helium beam that emits a red light is used for "aiming."

Adapted to use with the operating microscope, the laser is invaluable in microlaryngeal and ophthalmologic procedures. Many laser procedures can be performed in outpatient surgery or special-procedure units (e.g., eye laboratories) with reduced operating room and anesthesia time.

There are many advantages to using any one of the many types of lasers. In general, they include the following:

Less blood loss, as most small blood vessels are sealed
Working in a relatively dry field, which facilitates visibility
Minimal tissue trauma, with reduced injury to adjacent structures
Faster wound healing, with less pain and edema (due to sealing of nerve endings and lymphatics)
Decreased chance of malignant cells being spread through the lymphatics
Decreased scarring due to precision
Decreased stenosis due to decreased scarring in the lumen of structures
Faster recovery time in most cases
Treatment of areas otherwise inaccessible via catheters and endoscopes

Safety Precautions

Any time a laser procedure is performed, a scrub person, a circulator, and a laser safety officer should be present. The laser safety officer may be a registered nurse or a surgical technologist (ST). All laser team members need continuing in-service education regarding their expanded responsibilities.

Strict safety precautions must be enforced. Signs posted on all of the entrance doors must warn of laser use with the words **"DANGER, Laser in use; Special Eyewear Required."**

Windows must be appropriately covered.

All equipment must be checked prior to the procedure, including but not limited to testing the beam focus, electrical connections, and suction apparatus.

Only personnel trained in laser safety and technique should participate. A master key enabling operation of the laser must be obtained and then returned at the completion of the procedure; the key should be kept in a locked box. A "sign-out" log is suggested for the key.

The pedal (when used) is identified as it is placed in front of the operating surgeon to avoid accidental activation.

The laser is set at "*standby*" or "*stop*" mode during significant interruptions in its use.

Eye protection for patients and all personnel in the room is mandatory for most lasers, except when the conditions of minimum permissible exposure exist (i.e., when optical injury from "scatter" is not a danger).

Flammable prep solutions and other flammable liquids should not be used in the area where the laser is used.

A large amount of water or saline, a Halon fire extinguisher, and a fire blanket must be in the room in case of fire.

All dry materials in or near the operative field must be dampened with saline or water.

Nonflammable endotracheal tubes must be used, or traditional tubes should be wrapped with commercially available tape prepared specifically for this purpose. The cuff should be inflated with saline; the tube is wrapped in wet sponges around the lips.

All instrumentation should be ebonized, or in the case of large retractors being used, covered with wet towels.

Everything around the impact site, excluding the target site, must be moistened; the sterile field must be monitored for strike-through wetness contamination.

Special surgical masks should be worn when the laser is in use to filter out microscopic particulate matter that has hazardous potential concerning the respiratory tract.

A smoke evacuator must be used, held close to the target to evacuate the plume with its toxic by-products and odor.

Small amounts of plume can be evacuated with the in-line room suction.

An individual smoke evacuator with charcoal and ultra-low penetration air filters is recommended when there is a large amount of plume.

Smoke evacuation filters must be changed according to manufacturer's instructions.

Disposal of "used" evacuation filters is controversial regarding whether they should be considered general waste or medical waste. Treating the used filter as a "biohazard" will eliminate the possibility of its contamination of the environment.

According to standards set by the American National Standards Institute (ANSI), maximal permissible exposure, as determined by wavelength, power, exposure time, and pulsed versus continuous laser energy, must be observed to avoid skin injury. A nominal hazard zone can be calculated regarding wherein the operating room laser hazard to eye, skin, and fire considerations exists. For practical considerations, appropriate maximal protection should be employed for all procedures. Ordinary eyeglasses and contact lenses are inadequate for protection. Lens filters for endoscopes are necessary to avoid scatter. When using the CO_2 laser, clear glasses with side wings are worn by everyone in the room, including the patient, if he or she is awake. Under general anesthesia, the patient's eyes are taped shut and covered with wet pads and the face is covered with a wet towel. If the area to be operated is on the face, wet towels are placed about the site. All flammable materials near the area of laser use should be covered with wet towels. The Nd:YAG laser requires blue-green safety goggles, and the argon laser requires orange goggles.

Fire is a realistic potential hazard, particularly when the CO_2 laser is used in or near the airway (as in laryngeal procedures). Only nonflammable anesthetics are permitted. Conventional endotracheal tubes must be wrapped with a specific laser-retardant protective (wrap) tape. A polyvinyl chloride (PVC) tube is highly flammable and should never be employed when the laser is used in the oropharanyx or in procedures about the head.

Insulated silicone endotracheal tubes are available. The cuff of the endotracheal tube should be filled with saline. The protocol for an endotracheal tube fire must be rehearsed to minimize fire's untoward effects. The first thing to do in cases where the endotracheal tube has caught fire is to remove the endotracheal tube and turn off the flow of oxygen from the tank. Water or saline should always be available in abundance. Having fire extinguishers readily available is a must. A technique of jet ventilation, employing a rigid laryngoscope through which a thin needle-like metal catheter delivers calibrated amounts of anesthetic agent into the trachea, can be used in microlaryngoscopy as a means to avoid fire hazard. (see Box 7–1).

All employees in the surgical suite must receive safety education regarding laser use to prevent injuries. A variety of instruments to protect the tissue surrounding the laser target have been devised (e.g., Donnez "backstop"), some with plume suction incorporated. Similarly, nonreflective instruments (with anodized or ebonized finishes) that defocus and disperse the laser energy are used. Larger instruments and

BOX 7-1 In Case of Laser-Induced Fire Involving the Endotracheal Tube

1) Remove the endotracheal tube
2) Pinch or shut off the supply of oxygen
3) Assist the anesthesia provider in the reintubation of the patient
4) Open the oxygen supply

NOTE: As the mucous membranes will become edematous very rapidly, reintubation of the patient is of great importance.

retractors are covered with wet towels or pads during laser use to protect against scatter of laser energy if a beam is accidentally misdirected. If mirrors are needed to reflect a laser beam to an otherwise directly inaccessible site, the reflecting surface is to be stainless steel or rhodium rather than glass, which may shatter.

Wet towels or sponges must be used to surround the operating field, but precautions are taken to prevent strike-through contamination. A saline-filled irrigating syringe should be available to cool local tissues or extinguish a flash fire around the operative field. Special fire extinguishers, e.g., Halon (halogenated hydrocarbon), can be used for a flash fire in any portion of the laser system apparatus without significant damage to the expensive and delicate components. The solution used for skin preparation must not contain combustible agents (i.e., no alcohol or ether).

As noted previously, the laser should be in the "standby" mode when not in use. Only the operating surgeon should control the laser activation switch or pedal. Other controls (such as for the electrosurgical unit [ESU]) may be delegated to the assistant. When a laser fiber is passed through a scope or tube (catheter), the laser must not be activated until the laser tip is beyond the tip of the scope or tube to avoid heating the tube and inadvertently burning the patient. A satisfactory smoke evacuator to remove noxious smoke (plume) is necessary. Plume smoke evacuate filters should be changed as recommended by the manufacturer with appropriate "hazardous waste" technique (as some viable microorganisms may be contained in the plume). Laser masks filter out particles of a finer size (1–2 microns) than do ordinary masks (5 microns). During endoscopic procedures, smoke evacuation is important to eliminate the noxious plume and also to maintain visibility. The plume may contain carbonized microscopic particulate matter that, when inhaled on repetitive exposure, may lead to respiratory distress, hyperplasia of bronchial tissue, bacterial or viral diseases, and possibly even cancer.

The smoke evacuator should have an in-line filter when room suction is used. When large amounts of plume are to be evacuated, an individual smoke evacuator that has a charcoal filtration system and ultra-low penetration air (ULPA) filter is required.

In the presence of pneumoperitoneum during laparoscopy, smoke evacuation done too rapidly is to be avoided. Special suction devices with high-flow CO_2 insufflators are available to counter the loss of intraabdominal pressure during the evacuation of the plume.

When lasers are employed, movement by the patient is limited by restraints, if the patient is awake; for delicate microscopic surgery, general anesthesia with muscle paralysis is necessary.

The circulator assists the laser officer to enforce all precautions, to support the patient, to explain the need for wetting sponges and drapes, and to explain the need for protective eyewear. He/she documents use of the laser in the Intraoperative Record, the medicolegal record of the procedure. The scrub person keeps the immediate field surrounded by wet sponges, towels, and drapes while guarding against strike-through contamination, assists in suctioning the plume, and anticipates the need for special instruments or supplies. The laser officer, working in conjunction with the surgeon, tests the laser equipment to assure that it is functioning properly. The laser officer also maintains all rules, regulations, and precautions regarding the use of the laser by all personnel. He/she maintains an individual patient record in the laser log book for each patient.

Care and Competency Standards for Use of Lasers

Care and competency standards for use of the lasers (various types) have been established, with ongoing revisions by several agencies, including the Food and Drug Administration (FDA), National Institute of Occupational Safety and Health (NIOSH), Occupational Safety and Health Administration (OSHA), American Society for Laser Medicine and Surgery (ASLMS), Association of periOperative Registered Nurses (AORN), and the American National Standards Institute (ANSI).

The Joint Commission (JC) (formerly the Joint Commission on Accreditation of Healthcare Organizations) mandates that physicians employing the laser must be credentialed and that all operating room personnel (including orderlies and housekeepers, as applicable) must be instructed in laser safety. All employees involved in laser use must receive hands-on training. Quality maintenance of the expensive equipment is essential. Documentation of laser procedures becomes part of the patient's intraoperative record. The data must include type of procedure, type of laser, duration of use, wattage settings, and verification that the safety protocol was observed.

[A significant proportion of laser equipment is not owned by the hospital or surgicenter, but is rented; a certified technician may accompany the equipment and assist in its use.]

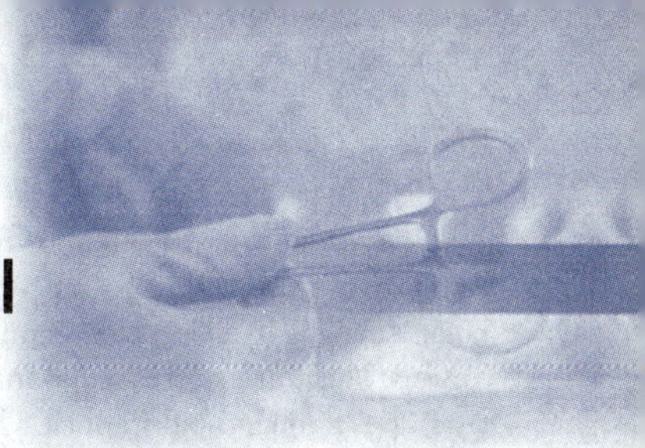

CHAPTER 8
Endoscopy: A Minimal Access Approach

Endoscopy refers to the direct visualization of a body cavity or tissue space through an illuminated tubular instrument inserted via a natural body orifice or a minimal incision to view, diagnose, or treat a wide variety of conditions.

When appropriate, the surgeon chooses an endoscopic approach for a given surgical procedure. In making this determination, the surgeon must consider his/her clinical judgment and endoscopic experience.

Advantages of the endoscopic approach versus open surgery may include:

- out-patient treatment versus a hospital stay
- smaller incision; less-invasive, less-traumatic procedure
- precise control of a laser beam (via instrument channel)
- unobstructed view of the operative site
- minimal trauma to tissues as retraction is obviated or lessened
- less postoperative pain
- faster healing, shorter recovery, and faster return to usual activities
- potential for a decrease in overall cost of treatment

Diagnostic capabilities, including assessment of metastatic disease, infertility, endometriosis, sepsis, extent of trauma, etc. may be achieved. Biopsies, fluid samples, and cultures may be taken.

Disadvantages include expensive instrumentation and equipment, need for special training with updating for the surgeon and surgical team, possible equipment failure, and potential complications requiring that an open procedure be performed.

The basic tenet of endoscopy is that the definitive portions of the procedure be accomplished in identical fashion to that of an "open" procedure. If, for any reason, the inability to safely expose and visualize structures due to hemorrhage, inflammation and sepsis, dense adhesions, obesity, or excessive anesthesia time ensues, or consequent surgical injury is sustained, the urgency of the situation dictates, or there is equipment failure, the procedure must promptly be converted to the traditional approach. In certain instances, endoscopic surgery may be performed in conjunction with an additional lesser formal incision (e.g., "laparoscopic-assisted" colon resection).

Endoscopes may be rigid or flexible and all perform a similar task, i.e., provide the ability to see within a body cavity (or tissue space). Their shape and size is determined by the part of the body to be viewed. There are some scopes made of plastic that are disposable, e.g., otoscopes and sigmoidoscopes. The rigid endoscopes are usually metal and permit the surgeon a straight-ahead or angulated view, e.g., otoscope, nasal sinus scope, laryngoscope, thorascope, mediastinoscope, esophagogastroscope, laparoscope, arthroscope, hysteroscope, cystoscope, anoscope, proctosigmoidoscope, and trans-anal microsurgical scope. Flexible endoscopes provide the ability to survey the entire operative field. Advantages such as intense illumination, magnification, and the ability to see "around" corners gives the surgeon better visualization of the operative field. A fiber-optic light source is used with a direct lens-viewing system or a video camera that displays the images on a television monitor. In many surgical specialties, flexible endoscopes have supplanted rigid endoscopes in many applications (or by the surgeon's preference). Some of these flexible endoscopes include the mediastinascope, bronchoscope, angioscope, choledochoscope, cystonephrostoscope, ureteroscope, hysteroscope, esophagogastroduodenoscope, and colonoscope.

Incandescent bulbs have been replaced by fiber-optic bundles that produce an evenly distributed, nonglaring, high-intensity, "cool" light that remains cool inside the patient's body. Electricity furnishes the power for the lighting systems. The scrub person attaches one end of the power cable to the instrument with the light, and the other end of the power cable is handed to the circulator, who inserts it into the light source. The drape sheet covering the patient's body should be very carefully wrapped around the power cable and secured so that the cable does not hang down or slide off the sterile field and become contaminated. The fibers in the power cable are extremely fragile and must be handled with extreme care. The cable should never be bent, folded, or handled roughly, as the fibers in this very expensive component will break.

The lamps are 175 to 300 watts and have a use life of 250 to 700 hours. They require changing the bulb at a moment's notice. Care should be taken when replacing a lamp (bulb) in use, as it will be "hot." Lamp-life status monitors are often incorporated into the light source units to anticipate the need to change the lamp.

Imaging is by lens systems or by a miniaturized video camera chip charged-coupled device (CCD) that is transmitted to a video monitor displayed near the operating table. Other recording modalities, such as videotape, distant broadcasting, and still image photos, are also available. Use of the additional modalities should be readily available, preferably with the necessary equipment placed compactly on multileveled carts. Angulated viewing (e.g., 0°, 25°, 30°, 50°, 70°, 90°, and 120°) may be employed accordingly to provide optimal visualization of a particular site. Dual cameras are available so that two images can be seen on separate monitors (or split screen).

The light source needs to be "balanced" so that white light is achieved in most instances. The current technologies provide a variety of settings for light and monitor adjustment. The light cable must be of sufficient length to go from the sterile field (if present) to the visualization system. Numerous connectors (couplers) are available, permitting various viewing permutations. The monitors must exceed camera specifications and also must be compatible to receive the three varieties of camera signal: composite, S-video comprised of Y (brightness) and C (chroma/color) components, and RGB (red, green, blue) color components. To prevent fogging, commercial solutions and pads (e.g., FRED®, ELVIS®) are made; special lenses, scope warmers, CO_2 insufflator warmers, and simply "touching" the scope end to adjacent tissues are effective.

Instrumentation for endoscopic surgery is generally similar to that used for traditional surgery but is smaller with respect to the working end and often controlled by pistol grip or palm grip activation, with capability of locking, rotating, and angle changing. Dissectors, graspers, various shaped scissors, needle holders and suture passers, clip applicators, staplers, sponging devices, irrigator/aspirator/coagulator devices, specimen bags, expandable fans or balloon retractors, and a host of specialty-oriented products are available. Many of these implements have insulated shafts so that electrosurgical modalities (cutting or coagulation) can safely be performed with the primary function (e.g., graspers and scissors). Adapted laser devices, argon beam coagulator, harmonic scalpel, and other sophisticated dissectors (e.g., hydrodissectors), cutting, and coagulating modalities can be employed.

The ability to use multiple instruments depends on the placement of additional access ports when the site permits. Numerous trocars with cannula devices used in abdominal surgery must have pneumatic sealing valves and lumen reducers (permitting the passage of smaller-diameter instruments) in order to prevent deflation of the induced pneumoperitoneum. Cannulae may have expandable tips to effect larger bore access; some have "grippers" (screw-like coarse threads) to avoid dislodgement. Many of the cannulae are radiolucent to permit radiographic studies (e.g., cholangiogram) without undue interference. Cannulae for use other than in the abdomen usually do not require valves.

Various suture-tying and knot-passage techniques have been devised to minimize the tedious effort to tie knots with instruments alone; special kits and suture passers, some with pretied knots, are available, such as the Laparomed® applier, Surgitie®, and Surgiwhip®.

There also are techniques where the actual knot is tied extracorporeally and placed with the suture-passer device.

To facilitate some procedures, both laparoscopic and open (but through a smaller incision than would ordinarily be used) techniques are employed. This is referred to as laparoscopic-*assisted* surgery. After initial evaluation and dissection is performed laparoscopically, the secondary incision is made. The wound is protected, and by using a modified sleeve device, through which a hand can be inserted ("handport"), larger specimens are retrieved and anastomoses and suture tying are performed.

Pneumoperitoneum, required for laparoscopic procedures, will be discussed in the laparoscopic procedures, pp. 136-138.

Instrument processing for endoscopic surgical devices is similar to processing for devices used in standard procedures; however, as many of the instruments are miniaturized and more fragile, meticulous care must be exercised to carefully remove all debris (e.g., enzymatic and ultrasound cleaning); light cables must be handled with great care so as to not shorten their use life by fracturing delicate fibers. The usual "cold" sterilization techniques using glutaraldehyde and peracetic acid solutions, ethylene oxide, or hydrogen peroxide gas plasma are used for instruments containing heat-sensitive elements (e.g., lenses and fibers). Cutting instruments such as scissors and trocar tips, when reused, require sharpening.

There is a huge inventory of "single-use" or disposable instrumentation available; however, many of these expensive items are well made and can be reused if Food and Drug Administration-approved commercial reprocessing is performed, certifying the reuse of single-use instruments. Some hospitals are certified to perform reprocessing. Stapling devices are not recycled. In addition to the special care given to the instrumentation, the electronic equipment, CO_2 insufflator, monitors, and other related devices, equipment, and supplies must be cared for by specially trained personnel.

Innovative techniques and the introduction of new instrumentation are ongoing. Robotics (see Chapter 9) are used to control the light/camera in certain applications and also have been adapted (some highly miniaturized) to the performance of intricate surgical maneuvers, controlled when applicable from sites remote to the procedure, by means of televised connections.

Virtually every surgical specialty employs endoscopic procedures. Special training courses (often included in surgical residency programs) for physicians and in-service programs for the perioperative RN and surgical technologist (ST) accredited for credentialing have accompanied the new technology. Surgical discretion, experience, and availability of all aspects necessary for the success of the procedure must dictate the propriety of the endoscopic modality for each individual patient.

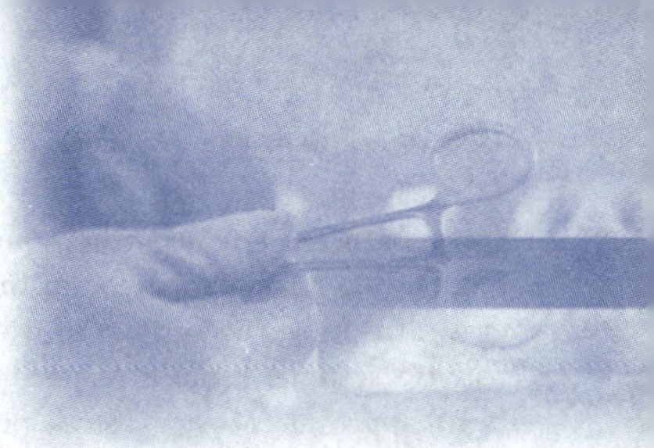

CHAPTER 9
Robotics

Robotics is an emerging modality in the surgical armamentarium. Robots have been developed to perform relatively simple tasks, such as controlling an endoscopic camera, but also to perform intricate surgical maneuvers, even beyond the capability of a surgeon's hand.

Robotic systems respond to manual or voice-activated commands to maneuver mechanical arms or an endoscopic camera. As manual manipulation of endoscopic instruments can be affected by fatigue-induced tremor of the surgeon, some delicate procedures such as endoscopic anastomosis may be difficult, and in other situations, visualization may be suboptimal or positional application of instruments may be limited. The master/slave robotic application can improve dexterity with large control movements translated into micromotions that enhance manipulation and decrease any tremor effect, allowing the surgeon to be more comfortable (ergonomic improvement). In regard to surgeon fatigue and reproducibility, robots work (i.e., with the ability to perform technically precise maneuvers repetitively) with no discernable difference between the first or last time the maneuver is performed. Visualization and hand-eye coordination perception have been improved in current robotics over former systems, and the "fulcrum"effect (i.e., the need to move an instrument in the opposite direction as on the monitor image) has been eliminated. The surgeon can now view the field in 3D using natural hand-eye coordination with the adaptation of "all-around"vision. He/she can zoom in and out of the surgical field as well. There has been an improved feeling of dexterity, resulting in the surgeon feeling as though the manipulations done during laparoscopic procedures are being performed in "open" surgery. There has been improved access using smaller incisions for many procedures, such as laparoscopic cholecystectomy, laparoscopic radical prostatectomy and other pelvic procedures, thoracoscopic-assisted cardiotomy, and others. Clinical trials are being performed for coronary artery bypass graft (CABG) surgery and repair of atrial-septal defects, as well as many other surgeries. Heart surgeries that once could only be performed via sternal splitting incision are being done through mini-incisions. It has been predicted that soon many surgeries will be performed utilizing as few as three 1-cm incisions. Pain and bleeding are reduced, and the patient has a faster recovery when procedures are performed using this technology.

The robotic modality can permit the surgeon to operate in comfort from workstations (with video display, utilizing a control panel) about 5 feet from the operating table. The robot may be operated by controls that are moved synchronously with the surgeon's hand movements; other robots may be in the form of mechanical arms or cameras that move according to voice activation. Procedures utilizing robotic systems require governmental (Food and Drug Administration) approval. Most systems permit the surgeon to perceive that he/she is closer to the operative field than human vision would allow, resulting in the extremely precise excision of malignancies and other lesions, thus, perhaps, affording a better potential for cure.

With respect to the **EndoWrist®** (da Vinci System), surgeons have 7° of freedom and 90° articulation. Surgical maneuvers can be performed by a miniaturized robotic "hand" inserted into the depth of a wound that can perform minimally invasive heart valve (e.g., mitral valve) and CABG procedures. Other procedures being performed include the Nissen fundoplication for gastroesophageal reflux disease, gastric bypass surgery for obesity, esophageal surgery, thymectomy for myasthenia gravis, and insertion of endocardial pacemaker leads for biventricular resynchronization, to name just a few. Surgery can be performed from a remote site. (In 2001, a procedure in Strasbourg, France was controlled by a surgeon in New York City.)

There are some negatives regarding the use of robotics, including evolving technology requiring the constant upgrading of equipment and the high cost of the electronics and compatible instruments. As the systems are cumbersome in an already crowded operating room, increasing the size of suites and/or downsizing robotic systems will be required; newly built facilities suspend the necessary equipment from the ceiling (or conceal it in ceiling compartments).

A problem with long-distance operations is the time delay. In these cases of remote-control surgery, there is about a 1-second "real-time" delay in current application (to which the surgeon must adapt). A telerobotic remote surgical facility has been set up to service hospitals in rural Canada (controlled by surgeons in Hamilton). Remote control battlefield surgery can be done, but it is not yet a practical measure. Complex transmission and reception video networking is required for remote-control application.

Historically, in 1985, the **Puma 560™** system was capable of performing neurological surgical biopsies, and in 1988, it could perform transurethral resection of the prostate (TURP). The **Probot™** system also could perform TURP, and a **Robodoc™** system was used to machine the femur in hip arthroplasty. Updated systems such as **AESOP™** (automated endoscopic system for optimal positioning, Computer Motion, Inc.) respond to voice commands to manipulate an endoscopic camera. **ARTEMIS™** provides two arms to be controlled by the surgeon from a console. The **da Vinci™** system (Stanford Research Institute/Green Telepresence Surgery is mounted on a cart and has dual light sources and computer chip telecameras that can produce a 3D image, a master remote control console for the surgeon, and four instrument arms (one of which controls the camera and light source) attended directly on the operative field by the assistant surgeon, who passes the instrumentation manipulated by the robotic wrist, and provides exposure, foot pedals for electrosurgical unit control and camera focus, and grips to control the arms. The **Zeus**™ system (Computer Motion, Inc.) is mounted on the operating table with three arms, using straight and jointed instruments, and includes the **AESOP** camera control. The **Socrates**™ "telestrator," a remote site control of **AESOP**, has been introduced. A system for colonoscopy has been used that applies "inch-worm" advancement of the scope with suction.

Current applications include endoscopic camera control and femoral preparation in hip arthroplasty, as noted. Multiple procedures have been performed in general surgery utilizing robotics, including cholecystectomy, Nissen fundoplication, right hemicolectomy, sigmoid colectomy, gastroplasty and bypass in bariatric surgery, Heller myotomy, esophagectomy, intrarectal procedures, inguinal herniorrhaphy, and adrenalectomy. In urology, radical prostatectomy with superior potency outcomes is being performed in many centers; nephrectomy, ureteral repair, varicocelectomy, and renal transplantation are being performed robotically. In gynecology, robotics has greatly enhanced tubal reanastomosis. In orthopedics, total hip arthroplasty (femoral preparation and acetabular cup replacement), total knee arthroplasty, and spinal surgery can be performed with robotics enhancement. Robotics are also used in neurological surgery image-guided procedures and in lumbar sympathectomy and in ENT for laryngeal surgery. Cardiac surgery, internal mammary artery harvest, CABG, total endoscopic coronary artery bypass (TECAB), mitral valve repair, and closed chest off-pump procedures are all enhanced by robotics. In pediatrics, microanastomoses, as for biliary and esophageal atresia, are being performed with increasing frequency employing robotic technology.

At present, the practicality and availability of the modality is not a reality for many hospital centers. Research is ongoing. Issues regarding malpractice insurance, credentialing and training, and interstate licensing (for telesurgery) are being addressed. Magnetic resonance imaging (MRI) and 3D models created prior to performing robotic neurosurgical procedures are in practice. Increasing tactile perception between surgeon and robot has been further improved.

Economic constraints and improved patient care must be balanced. Potentially, robotics could lower the cost of health care some time in the future. When that happens, in addition to cost efficiency over conventional surgery, the benefits of the enhanced precision afforded by robotics that cause minimal trauma to the patient will be undeniable.

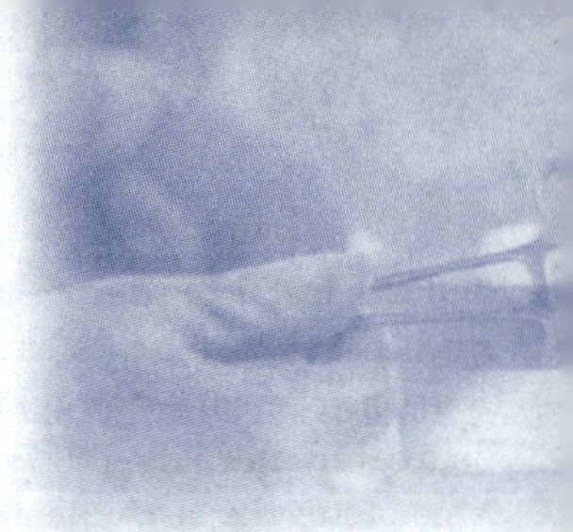

CHAPTER 10
Microsurgery

Microsurgery employs magnification, fine instrumentation, fine suture material, and minimal tissue manipulation for precision procedures on diminutive structures. These techniques are applicable in many surgical fields as procedures to enhance fertility, fertilization, microlaryngeal and otoscopic surgery, intracranial neurological surgery, construction of musculocutaneous flaps, and anastomoses of small-caliber arteries, veins, nerves, and tendons.

In ophthalmology, procedures performed with a slit lamp are regarded as a modality of microsurgery. Although these procedures are otherwise similar to most surgical procedures, intense practice sessions for the surgeon and training for the perioperative personnel are required. The procedures are often tedious, with special attention required of the anesthesia provider (e.g., to prevent sudden patient movement, especially when anesthesia other than general is employed).

More than the usual care of the delicate instruments is necessary. The technique for handling microsurgical instruments, tissue, and suture material requires that meticulous attention be paid to detail; working in the microsurgical field requires techniques that are often precise, time consuming, and complex. Both the circulator and, particularly, the scrub person need to know what their responsibilities are (which varies according to the type of procedure) during a microsurgical procedure. The scrub person needs to develop skills to assure his/her movements are smooth and not at all jerky; the slightest movements are exaggerated under magnification. It is important that the surgeon, the assistant surgeon, and the scrub person refrain from drinking caffeinated beverages the day of surgery. Care must also be employed to avoid obstructing the operative field in the exchange of instruments.

For the circulator, being prepared for dealing with problems involving the operating microscope (e.g., having extra lamps available) and knowing how to solve them is a valuable asset. Surgeons and support personnel must be familiar with all aspects of use of the operating microscope, including special drapes, foot controls, beam splitters, laser adapters, eyepiece protectors, and filters. The surgeon's and assistant surgeon's chairs must be stable, as must be the support of the patient's operative site. Attention to padding, e.g., donut, pillow, foam, gel, an egg-crate mattress, and well-padded armboards, is vital. When used, a hand table must be padded as well. Paying attention during the long procedures by the scrub person is mandatory; this is more easily accomplished when the operative field is displayed on a television monitor.

The operating microscope is composed of two or more lens systems in a compound binocular instrument of magnifying equipment that provides stereoscopic viewing. There are a variety of objective lenses and interchangeable eyepieces that combine to present different magnifications according to the working distance required. Both the scrub person and the circulator need to know and understand how the parts of the microscope work. As the scrub person drapes the microscope, the circulator often needs to assist with pulling the distal ends of the drape cover over the scope. The microscope is electrically powered (as light waves provide the illumination); the cord requires a grounded three-prong plug.

When lesser magnification (e.g., up to five times) is needed, loupes may be used; most often the microscope is set for 16- to 40-times power with a working focal length of 40 cm. Commonly used fine instruments employ spring-locking mechanisms rather than ratchets (to minimize jarring) and include jeweler's forceps (straight and curved), microscissors, microirrigators, microvascular clamps and needle holders, probes, microbipolar coagulation forceps, and sutures of varying composition (9–0, 10–0, 11–0, 12–0). Blue tinged titanium steel instruments are lightweight and produce less glare in the microscopic operative field and are preferable to antiglare-finished stainless steel. Micro power drills and small lint-free sponges are used. During surgery, the scrub person protects instrument tips and keeps the instruments free of tissue debris and secretions.

Microsurgery in the field of orthopedic trauma includes *reimplantation/replantation* of amputated digits and more proximal levels of the extremities. Accidental amputation involving varying levels of the extremities may be associated with more significant life-threatening injuries, which take precedence over digital or limb salvage.

Multiple factors influence the reattachment of severed portions of the extremities, including:

- interval from time of injury
- age of patient
- severity of injury
- additional injuries to the amputated part
- site, level, multiplicity of amputations, and bilaterality (if present)
- general medical status and associated injuries

A reattached member should be expected to regain at least 30% of normal function. Rehabilitation potential, occupation, intelligence, and the patient's economic situation must be considered prior to performing these extensive surgical undertakings. Larger amputations require reimplantation/replantation within 4 to 6 hours after injury; smaller members (such as digits) can be preserved longer in iced saline solution.

When surgery is completed, the concept of tension-free repairs of soft-tissue structures may require shortening of the involved bone after complete inspection. Debridement of nonviable tissues and cleansing of the wound are also performed. K (Kirshner) wires are employed for smaller bones (e.g., digits), and other rods or pins are used for larger bones.

Nerve and tendon repair may be done initially, if time, with respect to the patient's general condition, permits and the local tissues are not severely crushed or questionably viable. Arterial and venous repair must be done at the initial procedure. Common to all reimplantations, including, for example, transfer of a great toe to replace a thumb, are techniques of vascular and nerve repair. These will be described in their respective chapters; see individual procedures for further information.

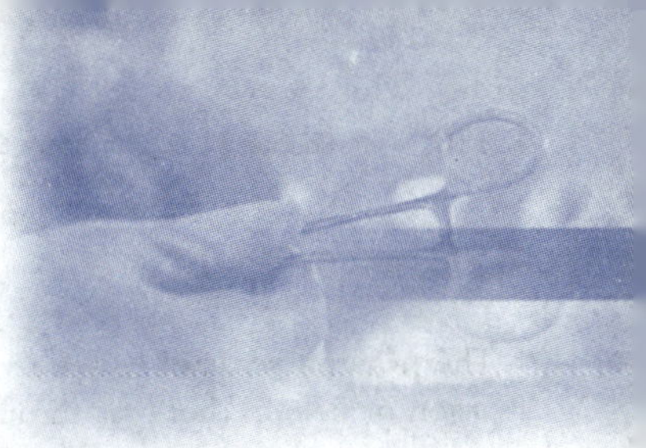

CHAPTER 11 Harmonic Scalpel and Plasma Scalpel

Harmonic Scalpel

The **Harmonic Scalpel®** and **LaparoSonic Cutting Shears (LCS)** employ ultrasonic energy to affect cutting and coagulation of tissues. Using the piezoelectric principle, mechanical effect, e.g., vibration, is produced by stimulating a reactive substance (certain crystals or discs) with electricity (and vice versa in that mechanical energy imparted to an appropriate crystal will generate an electrical force).

A single-use titanium blade or cutting forceps is made to vibrate (at its working end) at 55,500 Hz (cycles per second), which produces heat in the local tissues. This causes a cutting effect by denaturing the proteins into a coagulum that also provides hemostasis, but without smoke and at a lower temperature, usually 176°F (80°C) [with range of 122°F to 212°F (50°C to 100°C)], than an electrosurgical unit, which vaporizes water and other tissue substances at 302° to 752°F (150°C to 400°C) resulting in smoke and eschar formation.

There is less lateral thermal injury to surrounding tissue with the ultrasound energy, making it safer to use closer to vital structures than using electrosurgery. The surgeon controls precision cutting and coagulation by adjusting the power level, blade edge, tissue traction, and blade pressure. As there is no electrical effect on tissue, no electrodispersive pad is necessary for its use. The harmonic scalpel unit consists of a hand piece (blade or shears), cable, generator, and footswitch.

Advantages for using the harmonic scalpel over electrosurgery are:

- no noxious smoke plume is produced
- greater precision near vital structures
- minimal, if any, lateral thermal tissue damage
- minimal charring and desiccation
- reduces the need for ligatures
- fewer instrument changes during procedure
- does not produce the eschar of electrosurgery (bleeding can reoccur if an eschar is disrupted)

This modality has many applications in traditional surgery, such as for tonsillectomy, hemorrhoidectomy, and a wide variety of laparoscopic and thoracoscopic procedures, etc.

Plasma Scalpel

The **plasma scalpel** passes a visible stream of inert noncombustible argon or helium (hot) gas through an electric arc that ionizes the gas into a high thermal state. The single-use applicator, acting like a tiny "blowtorch," lightly cauterizes as it cuts through tissue.

The plasma scalpel is a large surgical pencil that simultaneously cuts and coagulates tissue, effecting hemostasis of blood vessels up to 4 mm, making it is especially useful in areas of greater vascularity.

A smaller amount of inflammatory response is generated with the plasma scalpel than with an electrosurgical blade. It can be used with the same efficacy and low complication rate as the CO_2 laser. The visible beam permits control, and unlike the argon beam coagulator (p. 111), there is no electrical effect to the tissues so that an electrodispersive pad is not needed.

Advantages of the plasma scalpel over electrosurgery are thought to be:

- better precision
- less scarring
- faster healing
- reduced operating room time

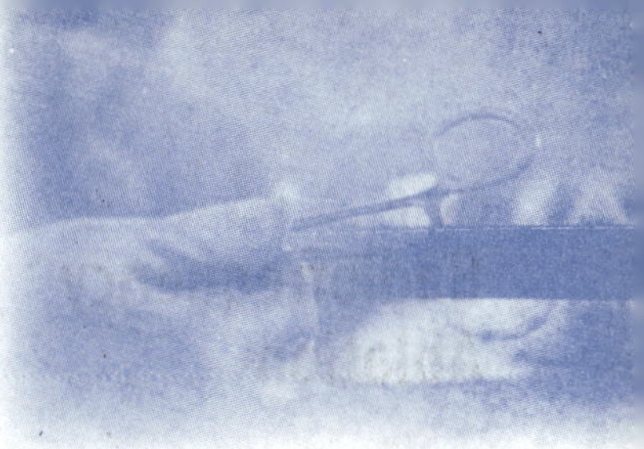

CHAPTER 12
Argon Beam Coagulator

The **argon beam coagulator** allows a jet of argon gas to carry electrons from a unipolar electrode through space to impact on tissue in a grounded patient, delivering electrosurgical energy in a way similar to a standard unipolar electrosurgical unit (ESU). However, inherent in the argon beam coagulator is a no-touch technique, and the stream of argon gas, as it conducts the electrical energy, simultaneously has a "blast" effect on the target tissues, momentarily blowing away blood, fluid, and debris for more efficient coagulation. The flow of gas (i.e., 4 l/min), power (40 to 50 W), and spot diameter of the beam can be adjusted. The coagulation effect is good on solid organ surfaces such as the spleen, liver, and myometrium and broad oozing surfaces such as in enterolysis. Smoke is minimal as argon gas surrounds the target site.

In a laparoscopic adaptation, 5- and 10-mm diameter (disposable) probes are employed. Excess gas must be evacuated to prevent it from creating an increase in intraperitoneal pressure (rare cases of fatal gas embolism have been reported). A suction irrigation probe, therefore, is placed near the argon beam coagulator probe when it is activated.

Additional safety precautions include:

- purging the electrode and argon tank gas line of air
- limiting the flow of gas to 4 l/min
- placing the electrode tip no more than several millimeters from the target tissue
- being certain that the laparoscopic insufflator has functioning audible and visual over-pressurization alarms
- following manufacturer's recommendations and other established procedures to prevent gas embolism during laparoscopic surgery

[Doppler ultrasonography, awareness of decreasing end-tidal carbon dioxide, and electrocardiographic signs of gas embolism can detect these changes (i.e., indicating gas embolism) early on to permit therapeutic measures in due time.]

The argon beam coagulator has been used to obliterate endometrial implants and ovarian cancer metastatic implants and to perform presacral neurectomy through laparotomy or laparoscopy.

Whereas the electrical generator is less costly than a laser, the electrode tips are relatively expensive, requiring frequent replacement; however, the efficacy of the argon beam coagulator, with its potential for a reduction of operating room time and its efficient achievement of (otherwise tedious) hemostasis, may negate these expenses.

CHAPTER 13

Radiofrequency Ablation

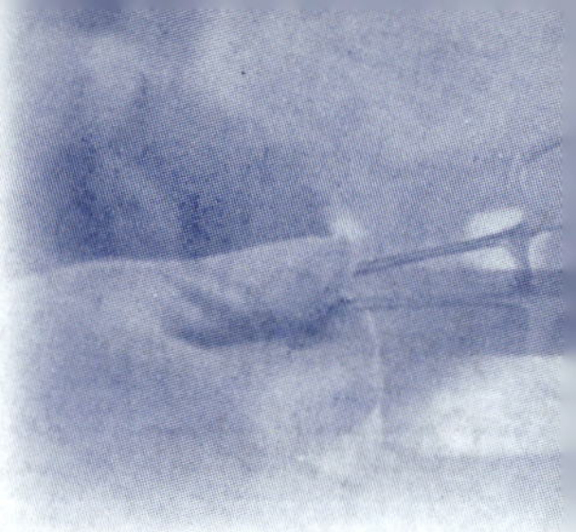

Radiofrequency (RF) energy is a form of electromagnetic wave energy occurring in nature, but in medical usage, directed from a generator. The energy is transformed to heat at the target tissue level, causing local cell death. RF energy is "nonionizing," as opposed to x-ray or gamma-ray emission. It is applied via a catheter inserted in approximation to the target area via guided needle technique.

Local anesthesia is administered to the patient in a radiology suite to ablate liver and lung metastases (without the need for the procedure to be performed in an operating room). RF may be employed to destroy local nerve endings, such as for (painful) facet syndrome, and by cardiologists to ablate cardiac foci causing arrhythmias.

Intraoperative uses include treatment for benign prostatic hypertrophy, varicose veins, osteoid osteoma, sleep apnea, endometrial ablation for dysfunctional uterine bleeding, and prevention of pregnancy.

When used in the uterus, the goal of therapy is to create endometrial fibrosis or stenosis of the uterine cavity. The system does not depend upon a distensive medium (as for hysteroscopy) and is less expensive than laser equipment. The endometrial tissues are heated to 144°F to 149°F (62°C to 65°C) for approximately 15 minutes. Uterine blood flow, thermal nonconductivity of the myometrium, and geometrically proportional "fall-off" of the heating effect combine to protect surrounding organs. The cervix is dilated to Hegar size 10, and the uterus is sounded. A probe (the length appropriate to avoid heating the endocervical canal) is selected. The probe is then passed into the uterine cavity through an insulated vaginal sleeve (which also affords protection to the bladder). Thermal monitoring probes and a special grounding belt are employed. Care is taken to be certain that the patient is not in contact with any metal surfaces (to avoid an accidental burn). During the procedure, the thermal probe may be rotated to achieve more uniform tissue destruction.

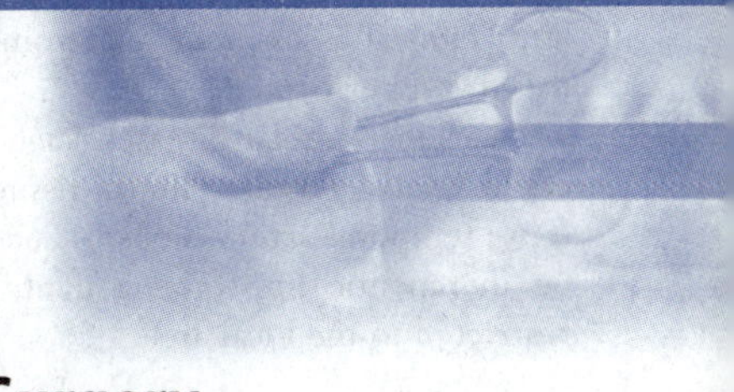

CHAPTER 14
Integumentary and Minimally Invasive Surgery

Excision (or Destruction) of Skin Lesions

Definition

Excision or ablation of epidermal, dermal, and subcutaneous lesions.

Discussion

Numerous small benign skin lesions, including nevi, papillomata, cysts, warts, indolent ulcers, and unsightly scars, and minimally invasive malignant skin lesions, such as squamous cell carcinoma, basal cell carcinoma, and malignant melanoma, can be excised, often employing local anesthetics. Usually, these patients are treated in same-day surgery or outpatient surgery facilities.

Procedure

Following the skin prep, the outline of the lesion is marked prior to infiltrating the area with a local anesthetic. An elliptical incision is made about the lesion oriented to the skin lines (Langer's lines). Primary closure is achieved by undermining the wound edges to facilitate tension-free approximation. After hemostasis is achieved, the wound is closed. When there are numerous lesions, after excisions of representative specimens, e.g., condylomata, and the remaining lesions do not require histological examination, the electrosurgery unit (ESU) or laser of choice (e.g., CO_2 laser) may be used.

Muscle Biopsy

Definition

Excision of a representative section of muscle tissue for histological study.

Discussion

Various neuromuscular diseases, such as muscular dystrophies, myotonia, and myositis, may require a muscle biopsy for definitive diagnosis after clinical assessment, electromyography, and biochemical studies have been performed.

Various vascular diseases, such as inflammatory arteritis and giant cell arteritis, require similar tissue sampling for definitive diagnosis (e.g., temporal artery biopsy). Sectioning of the temporal artery may be therapeutic for some patients when the symptoms related are restricted to the local area.

Procedure

Following skin preparation, a local anesthetic is administered. An incision is made at the selected site (e.g., forearm, calf, or temporal artery) and continued through the muscle tissue layers (epimysium and perimysium) or other investing connective tissue to expose the tissue to be sampled. After an appropriate specimen is excised and hemostasis is achieved, the wound is closed.

Excision of Subcutaneous Lipoma

Definition

The surgical removal of a fatty tumor.

Discussion

A lipoma is usually a benign fatty tumor presenting subcutaneously, most often over the trunk, neck, and extremities. Superficial lipomata are primarily removed for cosmetic or nuisance tactile symptoms. A lipoma may be encapsulated with attached nutrient vessels or amorphous with fibrous tissue of increased vascularity, which can cause discomfort. Lipomata occur singly, multiply, or as part of a condition called lipomatosis. The excised tissue should be submitted for histological study to ensure that no malignant component (such as liposarcoma) is present.

Procedure

Following skin preparation, depending on the size and number of lesions, appropriate anesthesia is instituted. An incision is made following the skin lines over the prominence of the lesion. The incision can be smaller than the lesion in many instances; after the superficial fascia is incised and local enveloping tissues are dissected about the lipoma (and if the lesion is mobile and discrete), manual pressure can cause this soft lesion to protrude so that its vascular attachment can easily be cross clamped and divided, facilitating the removal of the lesion. Hemostasis is assured and the wound closed. When the lipoma is amorphous, i.e., without discrete margins, dissection is more tedious and a wound drain may be needed.

Incision and Drainage of an Abscess

Definition

Surgical release of septic fluid from a confined tissue space (compartment) in the body.

Discussion

An abscess is a collection of fluid and inflamed or necrotic tissue, usually related to a bacterial infection in a confined tissue space. The fluid is comprised of leukocytes, serum, and local tissue exudates that cannot be locally absorbed, accumulating under pressure and spreading towards the tissue planes of least resistance. In superficial or even those presentations of deeper origin, the abscess "points" to the skin producing the classical signs of inflammation, swelling, heat, redness, and tenderness. Once an abscess develops, prompt drainage is required. This may occur spontaneously when pressure necrosis destroys the overlying skin, releasing the septic fluid, to relieve the symptoms and avoid dissection of additional areas. On occasion, the abscess contents are "sterile."

Any abscess, whether from a deep (e.g., ruptured viscus) or a superficial (e.g., puncture wound) source, must be drained. Rarely will antibiotics alone reverse the process without accompanying drainage. Abscesses affecting certain structures must be treated according to special anatomical considerations (e.g., acute tenosynovitis).

Procedure

After skin preparation, choice of anesthetic is influenced by the local consideration and the patient's tolerance to pain. The prominence of the inflammatory swelling is incised, obviously necrotic tissue is excised, and, often, an ellipse of skin about the incision is excised to prevent premature closure of the wound. The depth of the wound is cleansed (may be irrigated with antibiotic agent of choice), and the wound is packed loosely with gauze stripping to facilitate drainage. If the origin of the abscess is deep, a drain may be inserted. These wounds are not closed; dressings or a fluid-collecting pouch is applied.

Percutaneous Insertion of Catheters

Definition

Introduction of a cannula into a deeper structure via the skin.

Discussion

Vascular access via internal jugular or subclavian vein or radial, brachial, or femoral artery is achieved by means of a catheter introduced through a needle puncture (guided by anatomical landmarks). A "cut-down" (small incision) may be used to facilitate catheter placement.

In addition to vascular cannulation, hollow organs or ducts (e.g., biliary system) or an abscessed cavity may be accessed. A needle threaded with a guidewire is introduced under fluoroscopy or scan (CT, ultrasound, etc.) to provide passageway for dilators that enlarge the tract. An endoscope, cannula, or tube (e.g., feeding tube) may then be safely placed in the channel leading to the targeted structure. These latter procedures are often performed in the radiology suite; for examples of this type of cannulazation, see percutaneous gastrostomy (p. 212), jejunostomy (p. 226), and nephrostomy (p. 420).

Procedure

After skin preparation, local anesthesia is injected at the puncture site to ease the passage of a larger bore-introducing needle through which the catheter will be passed. Following verification of the position of the catheter by evidence of blood return or presence of specific fluids, the catheter is attached to an intravenous line, arterial strain gauge, fluid collecting apparatus, etc. The catheter is anchored to the skin by means of suture or tape (check the chart for patient sensitivities and allergies when choosing tape).

The following directions for **Skin Preparation, Equipment, Draping**, etc., are to be modified according to the location of the operative site for any of the aforementioned procedures. Some suggestions are offered here as guidelines.

Preparation of the Patient

The patient is positioned to permit optimal access to the operative site, as determined by the surgeon (and the anesthesia provider, when necessary); see pp. 20–27 for position descriptions. Bony prominences and all areas vulnerable to skin and neurovascular trauma or pressure are padded. The patient's physical limitations (e.g., arthritis) must be taken into consideration when positioning the patient. The patient's circulation should not be compromised by placing the restraints too tightly or by crossed legs. An electrosurgical dispersive pad is applied to a skin area relatively free of hair (the area may need to be shaved). The pad should be placed on the body as close as possible to location of the procedure.

Skin Preparation

Begin at the intended site of incision, cleansing the skin outwardly for an adequate margin (or as directed by the surgeon). If the site is a draining abscess, leave a sponge **saturated** with prep solution on the abscess while cleansing outwardly with another sponge. Cleanse immediately around the abscess last, working inward. Remove the sponge covering the abscess when the prep has been completed.

Draping

The operative field is draped with folded towels around the perimeter of the intended incision. An optional sterile adhesive plastic drape may be placed. For a single operative site, a fenestrated sheet may be used, e.g., a laparotomy sheet; when multiple incision sites are anticipated, use individual drape sheets.

Equipment

Electrosurgical unit
Suction

Instrumentation

Limited procedures tray
Small sharp self-retaining retractor, e.g., Weitlaner

Supplies

Small basin
Steridrape (plastic skin drape), optional
Local anesthetic and medicine cup
Needles, #22 and #25 and Luer-lok syringes
Sterile marking pen and labels
Blades, (1) #10 and (1) #15; #11 blade, optional
Suction tubing, as needed
Electrosurgical pencil
Culture tubes, two for abscess, one aerobic and one anerobic
Cannula for percutaneous insertion; cannula may be contained in a prepackaged kit
Small drain, e.g., 1/4-inch Penrose (with sterile safety pin), optional
Gauze (plain or iodoform) for packing the wound, as needed
Bulb syringe, optional

General Special Notes

- These detailed General Special Notes will not be restated following every surgery, as they were presented previously in Chapter 1, but they are included here (in this first chapter of surgical procedures) as a reminder. These reminders should be taken into consideration for all surgical procedures, e.g., always follow ***Universal Protocol*** as mandated by the Joint Commission (JC) (formerly the Joint Commission on Accreditation of Healthcare Organizations) for identifying the correct patient, the correct procedure, and the correct site and side (laterality).

- *Always* ascertain that a signed **Authorization and Consent for Surgery** is contained in the chart before bringing the patient into the room.
- Before every surgery begins, an official "time out" must be taken. It is a safety measure to ensure the correct patient is on the table to have the correct surgery (site and laterality); all members of the team must participate.
- *Time out* is required and must be documented on the Perioperative Record for medicolegal reasons.

Special Notes

- See the suggested Patient Care Plan, p. 9. The circulator adapts care to meet the patient's needs in order to implement nursing interventions that result in optimal desired outcomes for the patient. Adjust the plan of care with the Special Notes to ensure that all reasonable considerations have been taken into account.
- Advise the patient that you will act as his/her advocate.
- Provide emotional support by maintaining eye contact when conversing with the patient and by holding the patient's hand during the injection of the (local) anesthetic.
- Prevent musculoskeletal injuries to personnel and the patient by employing ergodynamic measures when positioning or moving the patient, as necessary.
- Ascertain that accessory equipment (when used) has been properly secured onto the table to ensure patient safety.
- Provide emotional support to the patient regarding feelings of altered body image and allow the patient the opportunity to express his/her feelings.
- Regarding physical exposure of the patient, keep the patient well covered; exposing only the immediate area for the procedure.
- Employ reassuring measures to help the patient cope with fears and anxiety of the unfamiliar environment (e.g., answer questions in a knowledgeable manner).
- Take appropriate measures to maintain patient's body temperature (e.g., offer a warm blanket, raise room temperature, apply forced-air warming blanket for long procedures).

- Assess hemodynamic factors, e.g., keep patient's legs uncrossed, apply antiembolitic hose before positioning patient, if requested.
- Check chart for patient sensitivities and allergies, including to latex products (e.g., gloves, drains, or elasticized dressings).
- These procedures are usually performed using a local anesthetic. Medication safety precautions are always observed; see Medication Guidelines and Practices to Avoid Medication Errors, pp. 30–31.
- The circulator confirms selection of the local anesthetic agent and its strength with the scrub person and surgeon aloud.
- All medicine containers in use must be labeled according to agent and strength and remain in the room until the conclusion of the procedure.
- In integumentary and minimally invasive procedures, Wydase™ (hyaluronidase) may be requested by the surgeon to facilitate dispersion of the anesthetic agent and to minimize related localized associated swelling.
- For **muscle biopsy**, an elastic bandage (e.g., Elastoplast™ tape) may be used to create a pressure dressing.
- When an **abscess is drained**, culture tubes are needed for *aerobic* and *anaerobic* cultures; requisitions for culture and sensitivity are prepared in advance by the circulator. Cultures are dispatched to the laboratory as soon as possible (to prevent their drying out).
- Antimicrobial agents may be requested for wound irrigation (such as in drainage of abscess).
- A Penrose drain with a gauze wick (for fluid absorption) may be referred to as a "cigarette drain."
- A Penrose drain, if used, should be moistened with saline before passing it to the surgeon.
- If a drain is placed, it is usually sutured to the skin; a sterile safety pin also may be attached to the exposed portion. (A cut rubber band may be used in a smaller wound.)
- Gauze strips may be used to drain the wound.
- Electrosurgery is often employed; see safety precautions, p. 38.
- A laser may be employed; see safety precautions, p. 94.
- When the surgeon closes the skin, he may use one of the following methods to minimize scarring:
  1. interrupted or continuous subcuticular nonabsorbable sutures (e.g., nylon) on a cutting needle,
  2. continuous subcuticular absorbable suture (e.g., plain gut, Vicryl™) placed just under the epithelium,

3. liquid skin sealant that forms a clear, plastic-like protective barrier when it dries, or
4. semipermeable, microporous closure tapes (e.g., Steristrips™). Apply tapes to dry skin or skin prepared with tincture of benzoin or Mastisol®; remove half of the backing on the tape strips along perforations to facilitate their application.

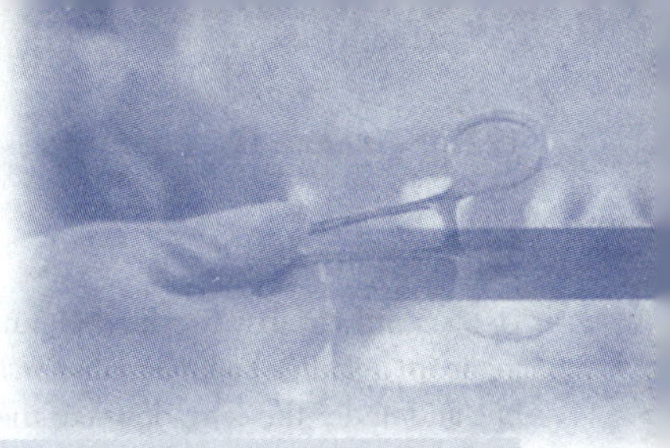

CHAPTER 15
Breast Surgery

Breast Biopsy

Definition

Removal of tissue from the breast to determine the nature of a breast lesion.

Discussion

When the lesion is not palpable, prior to the biopsy procedure, the patient is taken to the radiology department, where needles are inserted into the breast under imaging techniques to localize the lesion. Alternatively, a specimen can be obtained for examination utilizing a stereotactic-guided needle; this biopsy may obviate the need for open surgical biopsy.

A frozen section can be performed on the specimen immediately, if indicated.

Procedure

The incision may be made over the lesion; however, most often the incision is made circumareolar, if it is at all possible to reach the lesion. The lesion is grasped and dissected free. The specimen may be sent for a frozen section. After hemostasis is obtained, a drain may be inserted. Subcuticular tissue is approximated. Skin is closed with fine subcuticular suture or fine interrupted skin stitches. A stitch secures the saline-moistened drain; a safety pin is attached to the drain to prevent its retraction into the wound.

Preparation of the Patient

Patient is supine with the arm on the affected side extended on a padded armboard; the other arm may be padded and tucked in at the patient's side using the draw sheet. Antiembolitic hose may be put on the legs, particularly if a long procedure is anticipated. A pillow may be placed under the head, as well as an additional small pad placed under the lumbar spine and/or a pillow placed under the knees to avoid straining back muscles, to prevent pressure damage to tissue, and for comfort. Apply electrosurgical dispersive pad.

When local anesthesia is to be administered by the surgeon and the presence of an anesthesia provider is not required, a perioperative registered nurse (RN), in addition to the circulator, will monitor the patient's vital signs, etc.; for the perioperative RN's monitoring duties, see p. 58, and for the Analgesia and Conscious Sedation Record, see p. 76.

Skin Preparation

Use a *gentle* circular motion beginning at the site of incision and extending from neckline to lower ribs, including a wide margin beyond the midline and under the arm, down to the table on the affected side. For lesions in the upper outer quadrant, include the axilla. The scrub is performed with a "gentle touch," as cancer cells could (theoretically) be dislodged from the specimen into the bloodstream if vigorous scrubbing were done.

Draping

Four folded towels and a laparotomy sheet

Equipment

Electrosurgical unit (ESU)

Instrumentation

Basic/minor procedures tray

Supplies

Antiembolitic hose, as requested
Basin set
Local anesthetic, as requested, and medicine cup
Disposable needles and syringe (to administer local anesthesia)
Paper labels and marking pen (to label local medication)
Blades, (2) #15 and (1) #10, if specimen is likely to be "large"
Electrosurgical pencil and cord
Abrasive electrosurgical cleaner (adhesive-backed)
Needle magnet or counter
Small drain (e.g., ¼-inch Penrose) and safety pin

Special Notes

- The circulator, using *Universal Protocol*, must confirm the side and site of the lesion with the patient and the chart. (The site should have been marked preoperatively with an indelible pen.)
- See the suggested Patient Care Plan, p. 9. The circulator adapts care to meet the individual patient's needs by implementing the nursing interventions that result in optimal desired outcomes. Use the Special Notes to augment the plan of care to ensure that all reasonable considerations have been taken into account.
- Before every surgery begins, an official "time out" must be taken. This safety measure ensures the correct patient will have the correct surgery (site and laterality); all members of the team

must participate. *Time out* must be documented on the Perioperative Record for patient safety and medicolegal reasons.

- The circulator should provide measures of emotional support to the patient, e.g., maintain eye contact with the patient and hold the patient's hand during the administration of anesthesia, etc.
- The circulator conveys to the patient that he/she will act as the patient's advocate.
- The patient may have fear and anxiety regarding the surgery and the unfamiliar environment; answer questions in a knowledgeable manner whenever possible or refer questions to the surgeon.
- The circulator can provide emotional support regarding feelings of altered body image by allowing the patient an opportunity to express his/her feelings.
- Take appropriate measures to maintain patient's body temperature (e.g., offer warm blanket, raise room temperature, or apply forced-air warming blanket when a long procedure is anticipated).
- In regard to local anesthetic, label all medications according to name and strength, and keep all containers in room until procedure ends; use precautions to avoid medication errors (see pp. 30–31).
- Keep the patient adequately covered to avoid overexposure of areas not involved in the procedure.
- Check chart for patient sensitivities and allergies, including to latex products, e.g., gloves, drains (such as Penrose), or elasticized dressings (such as pressure bandages).
- Assess hemodynamic factors, e.g., keep the patient's legs uncrossed and apply antiembolitic hose before positioning the patient, if requested.
- Exercise all precautions in handling excised tissue to avoid misidentification of biopsies when multiple specimens are taken. Each specimen must have the exact location (from which the specimen was taken) indicated on the request form.
- The surgeon may indicate the orientation of the specimen with a suture; the circulator needs to indicate this on the request form along with the surgeon's explanation.
- The circulator is responsible for sending the specimen to the laboratory immediately for "frozen section." **Do not** put the specimen in formalin or other fixative.
- ***The circulator* must *notify the pathologist if the patient is awake; this should be indicated in an obvious area on the request form in large letters, e.g., PATIENT AWAKE.***

Mastectomy

Definition

The removal of breast tissue; the amount of tissue excised is determined by the extent, type, and size of the malignancy and the elected procedure.

Partial Mastectomy (Lumpectomy). Excision of a breast tumor with appropriate tumor-free margins.

Subcutaneous Mastectomy. Removal of all breast tissue; overlying skin and nipple are left intact.

Simple Mastectomy. Removal of the entire breast (subcutaneous tissue, skin, and nipple).

Radical Mastectomy. Removal of the breast and axillary lymph nodes; the most frequently performed "radical" procedure.

Modified Radical Mastectomy.

Classic Radical Mastectomy. Includes the removal of the entire breast, pectoralis muscles, axillary lymph nodes, fat, fascia, and adjacent tissues. A skin graft may be necessary for skin closure. Radical mastectomy is less frequently employed unless there is an invasion of deeper structures.

Extended Radical Mastectomy. En bloc removal of the breast, axillary contents (total axillary dissection), pectoralis muscles, and internal mammary lymph nodes. Resection of the ribs and sternum may also be included. The surgeon would choose this procedure for patients who have invasive or infiltrating tumors that have spread beyond the breast tissue. A skin graft may be required for closure of the wound.

Sentinel Node Biopsy. Procedure in which the axillary lymph node(s), into which tumor cells metastasize, are excised and sent for "frozen section."

Discussion

Patients, over 95% of whom are female, are particularly emotionally affected by any of these procedures. Prior to bringing the patient to the operating room (OR), the surgeon must (by law) discuss the risks and benefits of each type of procedure with the patient. In the past, most breast cancers were treated very aggressively, but today, studies have shown that some patients will benefit as much from a lesser procedure, depending on the type, extent, and size of the malignancy. Having a *lumpectomy* is not an option for every patient. Ultimately, the surgeon presents his/her (educated and experienced) opinion, and the patient decides from the choices offered. In some states, the surgeon must explain the different types of breast surgery alternatives, as mandated by law, before the surgeon may operate. Every effort must be made on the part of the surgical team, particularly the perioperative practitioner, to be understanding of and sensitive to the patient's feelings, vulnerability, and needs.

Ductal or *lobular* cancers may be confined to the breast; however, they may metastasize to other parts of the body. An infrequently occurring, rapidly growing carcinoma is *inflammatory breast carcinoma* that spreads aggressively to the lymph glands and blocks them. The breast with this type of carcinoma generally appears red and swollen.

Partial mastectomy (lumpectomy) followed by radiation treatments and/or chemotherapy is widely employed for those patients for whom this is an option.

A *subcutaneous mastectomy* is recommended for patients with small, centrally located, noninvasive lesions, including chronic cystic mastitis and gynecomastia (excessive growth of male breast tissue), and patients with a strong family history of breast cancer (who have the BRCA2 gene) who require prophylactic mastectomy. **Gynecomastia** is not usually cancerous; it may subside in the young male and will not necessarily require surgery.

A *simple mastectomy* is usually reserved for patients with no lymph node involvement (as per biopsy and/or other diagnostic modalities, patients who are elderly, or poor surgical risk patients who cannot tolerate a more extensive procedure).

A *radical mastectomy* is performed on patients with malignant lesions in which axillary fat and lymphatic tissues are excised and pectoral muscles may be removed to more widely encompass any potential tumor and its spread.

Sentinel node biopsy is performed to obviate the need for axillary dissection (and its potential morbidity) when metastatic spread is not identified; conversely, if the nodes are tumor positive, complete axillary dissection would be indicated. One to four hours before surgery (or immediately after induction of anesthesia), radioactive technetium-labeled sulfur colloid (0.3 to 1.96 mCi) is injected about the lesion or subareolarly. At surgery, a handheld Geiger counter (gamma detecting probe [GDP]) is employed to determine if any axillary lymph nodes are radioactive (to twice the background level). Suspect nodes are excised.

Alternatively, or as suggested by recent studies, concomitantly, 5 ml of a blue dye, isosulfan blue 1% (Lymphazurin™) is injected about the lesion. After several minutes, blue dyed nodes are displayed. When the tissues are obese, the GDP will help to find the dyed nodes. The combination of dyed and radioactive nodes is most accurate.

Nevertheless, palpation of the axillary contents is done as well, as infrequently, the lymphatic channels are blocked so that the dye and/or tracer do not extend to tumor-containing nodes. These identified nodes are excised and submitted as a *sentinel node biopsy.* The pathologist examines a "frozen section" of the lymph nodes in the OR. The histological findings provide the determining factors regarding the removal of additional lymph nodes and axillary contents. Thus, when the cancer is metastatic, the surgeon may remove all of the axillary nodes (*total axillary dissection).* If the axillary nodes are "clean," no further dissection need be done. This is a great advantage to the patient who could potentially develop lymphedema and restrictive arm movements when total axillary dissection is done.

In current practice, when discussed with the patient preoperatively, immediate breast reconstruction may be performed at the time of mastectomy. A breast prosthesis, a myocutaneous flap, or a combination of both may be employed. When the prosthesis is employed, a muscular pocket is created into which a tissue expander balloon is inserted (to be incrementally inflated postoperatively) to attain appropriate size for insertion of a permanent prosthesis subsequently placed as an outpatient procedure. The pocket created will vary with the patient's breast size and availability of adjacent musculature. When necessary, a latissimus dorsi myocutaneous (LDM) flap may be used to enhance the symmetry. An alternative to the use of a breast prosthesis is a transverse rectus abdominus myocutaneous (TRAM) flap, in which case a mesh prosthesis may be necessary to reconstruct the abdominal wall donor-site defect as well as additional sites of adjacent tissue mobilization. A greater omentum pedicle graft and free gluteal flap requiring *microvascular anastomotic techniques* have been used. For breast reconstruction in appropriate candidates, microvascular technique may also be employed for the autologous transfer of subcutaneous tissue and skin (e.g., from the buttocks).

Procedure

In *partial mastectomy (lumpectomy)*, the incision may be made over the lesion, or if centrally located on the breast, a circumareolar incision is made. The skin is elevated and the breast mass is excised. Hemostasis is obtained. The wound may be irrigated, and a drain may be inserted. Skin is closed with interrupted stitches. A skin stitch secures the drain, or it may be pinned with a safety pin to prevent retraction of the drain into the wound. When elected, prior to wound closure, ***APBI (accelerated partial breast irradiation)*** technique is used in the OR in conjunction with ***"lumpectomy,"*** see p. 124 and p. 969.

In *subcutaneous mastectomy*, the incision is generally made in the inframammary fold. If the breast is small (or in male patients with gynecomastia), a circumareolar incision may be employed. The skin is elevated, and all subcutaneous and connective tissues are removed, with the nipple and the skin left intact. Hemostasis is obtained. The wound may be irrigated, a suction drain may be placed; alternatively, a prosthesis may be inserted at this time. The skin is closed.

In *modified radical mastectomy,* usually a transverse or longitudinal incision is used. Skin flaps are developed, and often pectoralis fascia is dissected free from underlying structures. The axillary contents are dissected free from vascular and nervous structures and are removed. Care is taken to avoid injury to the nerve supply to various muscles. After hemostasis is achieved, the skin flaps are approximated over drains or suction catheters (e.g., Hemovac™). A skin graft may be required for skin closure.

In *classic radical mastectomy*, (performed less frequently because patients and physicians are finding breast lesions earlier), additional structures, including the pectoralis major and minor muscles and the intervening lymphatic and fatty tissues, are excised.

Preparation of the Patient

Antiembolitic hose may be put on the lower extremities, as requested. The patient is supine with arms extended on padded armboards. A folded sheet is placed under the shoulder on the affected side to facilitate exposure of the operative site. All bony prominences and areas prone to skin and neurovascular pressure or trauma are padded, e.g., elbows and heels. A small pillow may be placed under the lumbosacral spine, and/or a pillow may be placed under the knees to avoid muscle strain. Apply electrosurgical dispersive pad.

Skin Preparation

Using a ***gentle*** circular motion, begin at the intended site of the incision, extending upward to the neckline and downward to the umbilicus, with a wide margin beyond the midline. Prep the area around the shoulder, under the arm, and down to the table on the affected side. Gentle motions used while performing the prep may prevent malignant cells from being dislodged and entering the bloodstream. ***Do not*** allow solution to pool under the patient; a potential fire hazard exists when a flammable prep solution is used.

Draping

The patient's arm on the affected side is held up in a tube, or impervious stockinette as a drape sheet is placed under the axilla. The field around the breast is draped with folded towels. The arm is brought through the fenestration of a laparotomy sheet.

Equipment

Sequential compression device with leg wraps, as requested
Forced-air warming blanket, if ordered

ESU
Plume evacuator unit
Suction
Scales (2) to weigh sponges, optional

Instrumentation

Major procedures tray
Additional curved Crile clamps and large towel clips
Hemoclips™ appliers (small, medium, large)
Rake retractors (four-or six-prong)

Supplies

Antiembolitic hose
Tube (or impervious) stockinette
Basin set
Blades, several #10 for a large breast
Electrosurgical pencil and cord with holder and scratch pad
Suction tubing
Needle magnet or counter
Hemoclips (small, medium, large)
Dermatome (e.g., Brown), for skin graft and necessary supplies, including mineral oil, saline, tongue blades, and petrolatum-impregnated gauze, as requested
Drainage unit (e.g., Hemovac)
Pressure dressing
Marlex™ mesh, optional
Breast prothesis, optional

Special Notes

- The circulator must confirm with the patient, using the ***Universal Protocol***, the site/side of the lesion, as well as verifying that the patient understands the Consent to Surgery (when lumpectomy or mastectomy will be performed following the frozen section, should the results confirm a malignancy). The circulator should ask the patient to state in her own words what surgery will be performed; her quote must be documented in the Perioperative Record, p. 12, for patient safety and medicolegal reasons. The site should be marked and its location confirmed preoperatively before the patient is brought into the OR.
- Before every surgery begins, an official "***time out***" must be taken. It is a safety measure to ensure the correct patient is on the table to have the correct surgery (site and laterality); all members of the team must participate.

- ***Time out*** is required and must be documented on the Perioperative Record for patient safety and medicolegal reasons.
- A biopsy may have been done in the radiology department. The radiologist identifies the location from which the specimen was taken with a marker, such as a ligating clip, e.g., Hemoclip. The circulator must ascertain that the films are in the room before bringing the patient into the room.
- When a biopsy is taken in the operating room, the laboratory request for "frozen section" should be prepared and sent as soon as possible to facilitate a "speedy" reply from the pathologist. More than one biopsy may be taken; the biopsy request forms must be accurate, i.e., indicate the exact location of each specimen (and possibly its orientation as designated by a suture). Indicate on the pathology requisition, in big letters "PATIENT IS AWAKE," when applicable.
- See the suggested Patient Care Plan, p. 9. The circulator adapts a plan of care to meet the individual patient's needs by implementing the nursing interventions that result in optimal desired outcomes. Use the Special Notes (at the end of each procedure) to augment the plan of care, ensuring that all reasonable considerations have been taken into account.
- The circulator conveys to the patient that he/she will act as the patient's advocate while the patient is in surgery.
- It is especially important for the circulator to provide measures of emotional support to the patient, e.g., maintain eye contact with the patient and hold the patient's hand during the administration of anesthesia.
- The patient may receive general anesthesia when surgery for the biopsy begins if the surgeon strongly suspects the lesion is malignant.
- If the biopsy specimen is malignant and the patient has had local anesthesia, accordingly, the anesthesia provider will immediately begin to administer general anesthesia, as had been discussed with the patient preoperatively and the definitive surgery performed. The circulator stands at the head of the table to lend support to the patient and to assist the anesthesia provider, e.g., by pressing on the cricoid cartilage to facilitate endotracheal intubation.
- The patient may have fear and anxiety regarding the serious nature of the surgery and the unfamiliar environment; answer her questions in a knowledgeable manner whenever possible or refer them to the surgeon, as necessary.

- Provide emotional support regarding feelings of altered body image for the mastectomy patient in particular, considering the emotional nature of this surgery. Give the patient an opportunity to express his or her feelings.
- Take appropriate measures to maintain the patient's body temperature (e.g., offer warm blanket, raise room temperature, apply forced-air warming blanket).
- Keep patient adequately covered to avoid overexposure of areas not involved in the procedure.
- Prior to bringing the patient into the room, check the chart for the patient's sensitivities and allergies, including latex products, e.g., gloves, drains, and elasticized dressings.
- The circulator must continually assess and evaluate the patient's physiological status throughout the procedure and consult with the anesthesia provider and/or the surgeon, as necessary.
- Assess hemodynamic factors, e.g., keep patient's legs uncrossed and place antiembolitic hose on the patient's legs before positioning, if requested.
- Disposable leg wraps (may be applied over the hose); they are attached to the sequential compression device (pump), if requested.
- Check that blood and/or blood products have been ordered and that the correct number of units is available.
- When "lumpectomy" or "mastectomy" is to follow a breast biopsy, the skin is *reprepped* and *redraped*, the team is *regowned* and *regloved*, and the instruments are changed for a "fresh" set. This is done in an effort to prevent inadvertent contamination with cells from the malignant specimen.
- Prepare the skin with *gentle* motions to avoid the (potential) dislodging of tumor cells.
- Following the skin prep, the circulator will hold out the prepped arm to receive the double (or impervious) stockinette, the arm is supported and held by scrubbed personnel.
- The circulator needs to check "coagulation" and "cutting" settings on the ESU. Often a great deal of the dissection is performed with the electrosurgical pencil. If repeated requests are made to increase the settings on the ESU, suspect a malfunction. Check the unit and replace if necessary.
- The scrub person should keep the electrosurgical pencil tip clean by removing eschar using a scratch pad (an abrasive electrosurgical pencil cleaner with an adhesive backing). The use of

two electrosurgical pencils may be requested so that a clean tip will always be available.

- Large amounts of noxious smoke and odor resulting from the thermal destruction from the ESU or the laser should be evacuated with an in-line filter attached to the room suction or by a smoke evacuation system. The tip of the suction should be placed within 1 cm of the tissue interaction site.
- Avoid an inadvertent burn injury to the patient by keeping the electrosurgical pencil (when not in use) in a holder.
- Several knife blade changes may be required (especially if the breast is large) due to the fibrous nature of the tissues incised; *always* notify the surgeon when a blade is ***"new."***
- Weigh sponges for accurate fluid replacement assessment.
- Keep an accurate record of irrigation fluid used to assess need for fluid replacement. Irrigation fluid is usually ***water***, not saline, to lessen the survival of tumor cells.
- When a skin graft is necessary, one thigh must be prepared and draped (for obtaining the graft, at the time the main operative site is prepared). An additional prep set is necessary. The surgical site of the graft (e.g., thigh) is generally covered with a drape sheet until the graft is needed.
- Estrogen and progesterone receptor assays may be requested on the specimen; be prepared with laboratory request forms.
- With breast reconstruction, intravenous fluorescein dye may be employed to determine viability of the flap. The scrub person attaches a name label to the basin containing the dye, indicating its strength.

CHAPTER 16
Abdominal Extraintestinal Surgery

Abdominal Laparotomy

Definition

An incision made through the abdominal wall into the peritoneal cavity, preperitoneal space, or retroperitoneal space for the purpose of exploration, diagnosis, and treatment.

Discussion

Literally, laparotomy refers to an incision through the flank; however, laparotomy usually refers to an incision through the anterior abdominal wall into the peritoneal cavity. Laparotomy is performed for diagnostic and/or therapeutic purposes.

Procedure

The skin is incised with the "skin" knife. Subcutaneous tissue and deeper structures are incised with the "deep" knife or electrosurgical unit (ESU). Blood vessels may be clamped and ligated or cauterized with electrosurgery. Fascia is incised, and the underlying muscles are retracted or transected. The surgeon grasps the peritoneum (usually with a smooth forceps) and incises it with the "deep" knife. The incision is completed with a scissors (Metzenbaum or curved Mayo) or electrosurgical pencil. Wound edges are retracted accordingly by Deaver and/or Richardson retractors or by a self-retaining retractor (e.g., Balfour). The abdomen is explored. The surgery is performed. The wound/peritoneal cavity may be irrigated; the irrigation fluid is removed by suction. Drains may be brought out through stab wound incisions and sutured to the skin. A safety pin is often placed on the exposed portion of a simple drain. The peritoneum is closed with a continuous suture. Two toothed forceps or several Pean or Kocher clamps may be used to grasp the peritoneum to assist in its exposure for closing. The musculofascial tissues are closed in layers or, less often, in a single layer. The skin is approximated with suture mounted on a small cutting needle, skin strips/tapes, or skin staples. The skin may also be closed using Dermabond™, a skin sealant. For infected cases (e.g., peritonitis), skin and subcutaneous tissues may be left open to drain using appropriate wound packing and dressings. If a stoma is created or a fluid-collecting catheter is placed, a collection device is applied to the surrounding skin following the application of tincture of benzoin or Mastisol® to protect the skin.

Preparation of the Patient

Antiembolitic hose are put on the legs, as requested. The patient is supine; arms may be extended on padded armboards. A pillow may be placed under the lumbar spine and/or knees (to avoid straining back muscles). Pad all bony prominences and areas vulnerable to skin and neurovascular pressure or trauma. A Foley catheter is not routinely placed. An electrosurgical dispersive pad is applied.

Skin Preparation

Determine the intended site of incision; begin at this "clean" site, working outward. ***Never*** use the same used sponge to go back over an area; instead, take a new sponge. Include skin surface area from nipples to mid-thigh level and down to the table at the sides. For women, a vaginal prep may be indicated; check with surgeon.

Draping

4 folded towels and a laparotomy sheet

Equipment

Sequential compression device with leg wraps, as requested
Forced-air warming blanket, if ordered
Suction
ESU

Instrumentation

Major procedures tray
Large self-retaining retractor (e.g., Balfour)
Ligating clip appliers, e.g., Hemoclip® appliers (various sizes and lengths)

Supplies

Antiembolitic hose
Basin set
Blades, (2) #10 and (1) #15
Needle magnet or counter
Suction tubing
Electrosurgical pencil and cord with holder and scratch pad
Ligating clips, e.g., Hemoclips, variety of sizes

Special Notes

- The circulator must always use the Joint Commission (JC) (formerly the Joint Commission on Accreditation of Healthcare Organizations) *Universal Protocol* to identify that the patient is the correct patient, anticipating the correct surgery on the correctly marked side (laterality) and site. See the JC's *Universal Protocol,* p. 18.
- Before every surgery begins, an official **"time out"** must be taken; it is a safety measure. A *time out* is required and must be documented on the **Perioperative Record** for patient safety in continuity of care and for medicolegal reasons
- See the suggested **Patient Care Plan,** p. 9, for the care of the patient. The circulator adapts care to meet the individual patient's needs by implementing the nursing interventions that result in the optimal desired outcomes. Use the **Special Notes** to augment the plan of care to ensure that all reasonable considerations have been taken into account.
- The circulator assists the anesthesia provider during the induction of anesthesia, e.g., during endotracheal intubation (by applying pressure to the cricoid cartilage), during the administration of a block (e.g., by holding the patient in position for an epidural anesthetic), or by injecting medications the anesthesia provider has prepared (at his/her direction). For a description of the circulator's role during the administration of anesthesia, see Chapter 5, pp. 81 to 83.
- All patient care must be documented in the **Perioperative Record** for continuity of care and for medicolegal reasons.
- The circulator conveys to the patient that he/she will act as the patient's advocate by speaking for him/her while the patient is in surgery.
- It is important for the circulator to provide measures of emotional support to the patient, e.g., maintain eye contact and hold the patient's hand during the administration of anesthesia.
- The patient may have fear and anxiety regarding the surgical procedure and the unfamiliar environment; answer questions in a knowledgeable manner.
- Provide emotional support regarding the patient's feelings of altered body image and permit an opportunity to express his/her feelings.

- Provide emotional support to the patient by keeping the patient adequately covered and exposing only those areas that are involved in the procedure.
- Check chart for patient sensitivities and allergies, including to latex products, e.g., gloves, drains, elasticized tape, etc. Note that simple drains (e.g., Penrose) and pressure bandages (e.g., containing Elastoplast® tape) contain latex, as do many other items in general use. Also, check for patient allergy to iodine found in many prep solutions.
- The circulator should assess hemodynamic factors; he/she should keep the patient's legs uncrossed and apply antiembolitic hose before positioning the patient for the procedure, (when the hose have been requested by the surgeon).
- The surgeon may order a sequential compression device with leg wraps (disposable) to be applied over the antiembolitic hose (to prevent deep vein thrombosis).
- The circulator should take appropriate measures to maintain the patient's body temperature; when the patient is cold, he/she should offer a warmed blanket and/or adjust the room temperature accordingly. When ordered, a forced-air warming blanket may be placed over legs and/or chest.
- The electrosurgical pad should be applied to skin that is relatively hair-free (to obtain good contact); it may be necessary to shave the area. The pad should be placed as close to the surgical site as possible.
- The electrosurgical pencil tip should be kept free of debris and eschar (by using the scratch pad) and kept in its holder when not in use.
- Large amounts of noxious smoke and fumes resulting from thermal destruction are a health hazard; smoke should be suctioned away by the room suction with an in-line filter or with a smoke evacuation system (e.g., Clear View® smoke evacuator).
- Masks with a filtering capacity of between 2 and 5 microns should be worn by all personnel in the operating room (OR) during an operative procedure to prevent inhalation of toxic matter.
- Only laparotomy pads (lap pads) are used once the abdminal cavity has been entered. All lap pads must have a radio-opaque strip incorporated in the fabric (making them x-ray detectable).
- After the abdominal cavity has been entered, "free" raytec sponges (4″ × 4″ sponges with a visible blue radio-opaque

thread) are ***never*** placed on the sterile field, except when mounted on a sponge forceps (or other clamp).

- A raytec sponge, when mounted on a sponge forceps, is frequently referred to as a "*spongestick*."
- Most surgeons prefer that the lap pads be lightly moistened with warm saline once the peritoneal cavity has been entered.
- The peritoneal cavity may be irrigated with copious amounts of normal saline that may be suctioned with a Poole suction.
- A protective face shield is suggested for those scrubbed to avoid inadvertent splashing of contaminated fluids onto mucous membranes and eyes.
- Prior to leaving the OR, the circulator assures that the patient is properly positioned on the gurney, that all tubings and lines are not kinked, and that measures necessary to maintain the patient's body temperature have been taken.
- The circulator accompanies the anesthesia provider taking the patient to the Post Anesthesia Care Unit (PACU); he/she gives the PACU perioperative practitioner a detailed intraoperative report regarding the course of events when the patient was in surgery.
- In the PACU, the perioperative practitioner observes that the patient's breathing is unobstructed, monitors the patient's blood pressure and vital signs, and documents all pertinent information in the Perioperative Record in the Postoperative Record. Documentation is vital for patient safety regarding continuity of care and for medicolegal reasons.
- In the PACU, the perioperative practitioner assumes the role as the patient's advocate.

Abdominal Laparoscopy

Definition

The introduction of an endoscope through the abdominal wall to directly visualize the peritoneal cavity and the preperitoneal and retroperitoneal spaces for diagnosis and treatment.

Discussion

Inherent in intraperitoneal laparoscopic procedures is the need to distend or distract the parietal wall, most often by establishing pneumoperitoneum or by the less frequently employed gasless technique.

Both laparoscopic techniques are described below. Laparoscopy is not advisable in patients who have had multiple surgeries due to adhesion formation. Laparoscopic procedures, when performed, should have the same outcome as those performed by "open" laparotomy. For further details regarding endoscopic surgery, see Chapter 8, pp. 99 to 102.

Procedure

A minimal infraumbilical incision is made after the table is moved into Trendelenburg position. An insufflator needle, e.g., Verres needle (with sheath), is inserted, angled towards the pelvis, and gently pushed until it penetrates the peritoneum. The surgeon ascertains that the position of the needle is correct; the needle is removed, leaving the sheath in place. The surgeon attaches the Silastic® tubing to the sheath. (The scrub person passed off the other end of the tubing earlier to the circulator who attached it to the CO_2 source following draping.) Pneumoperitoneum is established.

The sheath is removed and the initial incision is made larger to accommodate a 10- or 11-mm trocar. This disposable trocar (with its sharp siliconized tip and sheath) is introduced; the tip automatically retracts as the peritoneum is pierced. The trocar is removed; the sheath (now an established port) is secured to the abdominal wall with incorporated screw threads. Stay sutures may be used to further secure the port. A laparoscope is inserted through the port; the CO_2 line is attached to the sheath. The laparoscope contains a (computer chip at its distal end) camera that provides an image directly to the monitors. Additional ports are placed under visual control using the telescopic property of the laparoscope.

In the alternative Hasson technique to establish pneumoperitoneum, a mini skin incision is made; the deeper tissues are incised. An Hasson trocar is inserted into the peritoneal cavity under direct vision through this 1- to 2-cm incision. Interchangeable adaptors, i.e., pneumatic seals or reducers, prevent leakage of CO_2. Initial insufflation pressure begins at a low level between 5 and 7 mm Hg; pressure may be increased to 12 to 15 mm Hg during the definitive procedure.

Following either technique to perform laparoscopy, appropriate intraabdominal maneuvers are made and the surgery is completed. Pneumoperitoneum is released. The instruments and ports are removed. The incisions are sutured closed. On occasion, a port may be removed and its insertion defect enlarged to effect the extraction of a large specimen or via a specialized port; e.g., LAP DISC™ or HAND-PORT™ placed to accommodate the surgeon's hand while maintaining the pneumoperitoneum. The procedure is then referred to as ***laparoscopically assisted.*** The wound is closed by standard techniques.

Complications that may arise (usually related to CO_2 pneumoperitoneum) include:

- Respiratory compromise and decreased venous return due to the elevated intraabdominal pressure
- Subcutaneous emphysema
- Hypercarbia with ensuing acidosis in patients with respiratory compromise.

In trauma patients with lacerated vessels, gas emboli are a potential risk, and if the diaphragm is injured, pneumothorax can be induced. The effects of CO_2 on the fetus in pregnant patients are not completely understood.

A gasless technique for laparoscopy employs a mechanical lifting device to establish a working cavity. The advantages of this modality are the following:

- avoids any potential physiologic ill effects of CO_2
- may cost less
- avoids the need to maintain pneumatic seals
- permits the use of large instruments
- may reduce the formation of adhesions

Laparolift®, a special mechanized fan retractor with arms closed, is introduced through a port under visualization. The retractor is usually placed intraperitoneally, or when significant adhesions are anticipated, into the immediate preperitoneal space. The retractor is attached to a mechanical lifting arm previously secured to the table. The fan arms are spread, and the retractor is mechanically elevated. A second fan retractor may be employed, if necessary, particularly in obese patients or to expose the paracolic gutters. However, exposure may be limited to a single area or quadrant, necessitating the repositioning of the fan retractors. Retraction of adjacent structures requires additional manual effort or the gravity effects of Trendelenburg position (rather than the gaseous pressure effect of pneumoperitoneum). Another retractor system has been introduced employing one or two rods with shape memory alloy (SMA) inserted through deep subcutaneous tissue singly or crisscrossed and fixed to side table mounts. As indicated, this device does not preclude the use of pneumoperitoneum. Accordingly, when advantageous, the two techniques can be combined for alternate phases of a procedure. In some approaches to inguinal herniorrhaphy, *extra*peritoneal insufflation may be employed as well.

Preparation of the Patient

Antiembolitic hose are put on the legs, as requested. The patient is supine with arms extended on padded armboards, or both arms may be padded and tucked in at the patient's sides using the draw sheet. During the procedure, the patient is placed in Trendelenburg position to facilitate establishment of the pneumoperitoneum. Padded shoulder braces are utilized. A small pillow may be placed at the lumbosacral area, and another pillow may be placed under the knees to avoid straining the back muscles. All areas vulnerable to skin and neurovascular pressure or trauma are padded. A Foley catheter may be requested. An electrosurgical dispersive pad is applied.

Skin Preparation

Begin cleansing at the umbilicus. Include area from the nipples to mid-thighs and down to the table at the sides. For women, a vaginal prep may be indicated and the bladder is drained with a straight catheter (e.g., Robinson).

Draping

4 folded towels and a laparotomy sheet

Equipment

Padded shoulder braces
Sequential compression device with leg wraps, if requested
Forced-air warming blanket, if ordered
Monitors (1 or 2)
Insufflation device (CO_2)
Fiberoptic light source, e.g., Xenon™ 300 W
VCR
ESU
Suction
Pressure bag to facilitate irrigation (when done), optional
Laser, see safety precautions, p. 94 (optional)
CD burner
Printer
Camera console

Instrumentation

Limited procedures tray
Major procedures tray, available (used if procedure converted to open procedure)
Verres needle
Trocars (5 mm, 10 or 11 mm, 12 mm, or Hasson)
Fiberoptic laparoscopes, with camera and cord, 30° and 0°
Reducers
Endoscopic instruments: dissectors, graspers, scissors (blunt and sharp), electrosurgical suction-irrigator

Multifire ligating clip applier, if requested
Loop sutures (e.g., Endoloop®) , if requested
Intracorporeal suturing device with introducer sleeve, e.g., Endostitch®, if requested

Supplies

Antiembolitic hose
Small basin
Blades, (1) #10, (1) #15, (1) #11
Needle magnet or counter
Suction tubing
Electrosurgical cord
Silastic tubing (for insufflation)
Cystoscopy or similar straight tubing, e.g., K50; add 1000-ml bag normal saline and three-way stopcock for irrigation
Loop ligation sutures, e.g., Endoloop and/or Endostitch (with introducer sleeve), if requested
Multifire ligating clip applier, if requested
Fog reduction agent, e.g., FRED®, ELVIS™ (optional)
Endoscopic specimen retrieval bag, e.g., Endo Pouch™, ENDOBAG™, LAP-BAG™, LapSac®, GRABAG ™ (optional)
Hand port, e.g., LAP DISC, HANDPORT, Intromit™, Omniport™, Dexterity Device™ for hand-assisted procedures, if requested

Special Notes

- Apply **Special Notes** from ***Abdominal Laparotomy***, p. 134, as indicated.
- Well-padded shoulder braces are secured to the table (to prevent the patient from sliding off) when table is in Trendelenburg. The table is positioned this way to encourage organs to slide cephalad; in this way, the danger of inadvertently puncturing an organ or vital structure is reduced.
- Prevent musculoskeletal injuries to personnel and the patient by employing ergodynamic measures (see p. 51) when positioning the patient, as necessary.
- Ascertain that accessory equipment has been properly secured onto the table to ensure patient safety.
- **REMINDER:** The circulator will assist the anesthesia provider during the induction of anesthesia, e.g., during endotracheal intubation (by applying pressure to the cricoid cartilage), or by

injecting medications the anesthesia provider has prepared (at his/her direction). For a description of the circulator's role during the administration of anesthesia, see p. 81.

- The circulator connects and turns on the light source.
- Circulator will turn on the VCR, if requested.
- Circulator needs to recheck position of monitors to ensure that they can be viewed easily.
- Circulator connects remaining items (irrigation tubing, suction tubing, and electrosurgical cord) after the team is in position (to avoid tripping over the cords).
- Check that equipment is appropriately plugged in before investigating that it (or one of its parts) is not working.
- The circulator and the scrub person must familiarize themselves with the instrumentation used in laparoscopy and the equipment on the laparoscopy cart. This should be done before the patient is brought into the room.
- The gas cylinder (tank) used for abdominal insufflation is verified to be CO_2.
- The circulator is responsible for having adequate levels of CO_2 in the tank (cylinder) prior to bringing the patient into the room. There should be at least 250 psi of CO_2 pressure in the tank before starting the procedure. If CO_2 is below that level, the cylinder should be changed before the procedure begins.
- All equipment (in working order) should be checked prior to bringing the patient into the OR.
- The circulator positions the two monitors after the patient is on the table, as the gurney will have been removed (and located out of the way).
- Following the draping, the scrub person will pass off the end of the CO_2 Silastic insufflation tubing, fiberoptic light cord (cable), suction tubing, and electrosurgical cord to the circulator.
- *When the scrub person is unsure which end of the tubing, cords, and cables to pass off to the circulator, he/she will resolve any doubt by connecting the cords, etc., to their respective instruments ahead of time and then dismantling the same before passing the item to the surgeon.*
- The circulator connects the CO_2 insufflator tubing and adjusts the insufflator pressure level. The beginning flow rate of CO_2

should be low (1 to 1.5 l/min) to effect a pressure of between 5 and 7 mm Hg; later, the flow rate is adjusted higher, as directed by the surgeon.

- Scrub person keeps the lens of the laparoscope clean as necessary, as well as the tips of the instruments.
- All fiber-optic instruments and light cables must be handled with great care to avoid breaking the fragile light fibers.
- Most scopes cannot be autoclaved; they may be sterilized using ethylene oxide, peracetic acid, or low temperature hydrogen peroxide gas plasma; see pp. 42–44.
- **NOTE:** Nondisposable instruments may be flash-sterilized, except the scopes; very few scopes are autoclaveable.
- Steris 20™ (peracetic acid) solution system (most frequently employed) may be used to sterilize instruments; the instrument must be completely submerged for 12 minutes at 122°F to 131°F (50°C to 55°C) for specifications to be met; see p. 43.
- An endoscopic specimen pouch may be employed to obtain the specimen, e.g., Endopouch, Endosac, ENDOBAG, LAP-BAG, LapSac, GRABAG (optional).
- **REMINDER:** Prior to leaving the OR, the circulator assures that the patient is properly positioned on the gurney, that all tubings and lines are not kinked, and that measures necessary to maintain the patient's body temperature have been taken.
- **REMINDER:** The circulator accompanies the anesthesia provider taking the patient to the PACU; he/she gives the PACU perioperative practitioner a detailed intraoperative report regarding the course of events of the patient in surgery.

Abdominal Herniorrhaphy

Definition

Repair of a musculofascial defect, through which various organs or tissues may present.

Classification

Inguinal (Direct and Indirect) and Femoral. The musculofascial defect is in the groin, the herniated tissues presenting through the abdominal wall medial to the deep inferior epigastric vessels (direct); or through the deep inguinal ring and inguinal canal, emerging at the superficial inguinal ring (indirect); or through the femoral canal (femoral).

Umbilical. Within the umbilicus (or about the umbilicus: paraumbilical); most often seen in children, pregnant women, or obese adults.

Epigastric. Defect in the abdominal wall between the xiphoid process and the umbilicus through which fat protrudes.

Incisional (Ventral). A defect underlying the scar of a previous surgical site in the abdomen through which viscera or fat may protrude.

Discussion

Hernias are either reducible or irreducible, i.e., incarcerated. When the contents of an incarcerated hernia become strangulated, compromising the viability of entrapped tissue (leading to gangrenous changes), resection of the involved tissue or organ must be performed on an emergent basis, in addition to the herniorrhaphy. If significant local sepsis is present, the definitive hernia repair is delayed.

Herniorrhaphy may be done laparoscopically.

Procedures

There are several techniques that may be employed for each of these hernia types. Usually an incision is made over the site of the defect. Both blunt and sharp dissection are employed to expose the hernia sac and the surrounding musculofascial defect. With incisional hernias, the peritoneal cavity may be entered. The hernia sac may be allowed to retract; it is sutured over (imbricated) or excised. The musculofascial defect may be closed, employing a wide variety of techniques (including mobilization of fascial flaps and anchoring tissue to adjacent ligaments, e.g., Cooper's ligament), suture materials, and, often, a mesh-type prosthesis. A fibrin sealant (e.g., Tisseel VH™ or Tissicol™) may be employed to prevent mesh migration. Staples (ProTack™) may also be used for this purpose. The employment of mesh potentially allows for a tension-free repair. The subcutaneous tissue and skin are approximated.

Preparation of the Patient

Antiembolitic hose may be put on the legs, as requested. The patient is supine with the arm on the affected side extended on a padded armboard. The opposite arm is padded and tucked in at the patient's side with the draw sheet. A pillow may be placed under the sacrum and/or under the knees to reduce muscle strain on the back and pressure on tissues. Pad all bony prominences and areas vulnerable to skin and neurovascular pressure or trauma. Apply electrosurgical dispersive pad. When local anesthesia is administered and an anesthesia provider is not required, a perioperative RN, in addition to the circulator, must be present to monitor the patient

Skin Preparation

Inguinal and Femoral. Begin at the inguinal region on the affected side, extending from just below the nipples to mid-thighs (including a wide margin beyond the midline) and down to the table on the affected side; external genitalia are prepped last; check with surgeon regarding a vaginal prep for a female.

Umbilical. Begin at the umbilicus, extending from the nipples to upper thighs and down to the table at the sides.

Epigastric. Begin at the midline, extending from the nipples to the upper thighs and down to the table at the sides.

Incisional. Begin at the site of previous incision; prep widely enough to allow for a generous operative field; ask surgeon for parameters (when in doubt).

Draping

4 folded towels and a laparotomy or transverse sheet

Equipment

Sequential compression device with leg wraps, if requested
Forced-air warming blanket, if requested
ESU

Instrumentation

Basic/Minor procedures tray
Self-retaining retractor (e.g., Adson)
Ligating clip appliers, e.g., Hemoclip appliers, assorted sizes

Supplies

Antiembolitic hose
Basin set
Blades, (2) #10 and (1) #15
Needle magnet or counter
Penrose drain, small, ¼″ for retraction, optional
Dissectors (e.g., peanut, Kittner sponges)
Electrosurgical pencil and cord with holder and scrape pad
Ligating clips, e.g., Hemoclips, assorted sizes
Mesh, e.g., Marlex™, Gor-Tex™, Surgipro™, or PreFix Plug™, as requested
Fibrin sealant/tissue glue to secure mesh, e.g., Tisseel VH, Tissicol, optional
Stapler with staples (e.g., ProTack), if requested

Special Notes

- Apply **Special Notes** from ***Abdominal Laparotomy,*** p. 134, as indicated.
- A small Penrose drain (used to isolate the spermatic cord) is moistened in saline and passed on a Pean clamp.
- Synthetic meshes, secured with and without staples, e.g., Mersilene, Marlex, Gor-Tex, or Surgipro Prolene Hernia System, are often used to repair hernia defects, recurrent hernias, or large ventral defects.
- A fibrin sealant, acting as a tissue glue, e.g., Tisseel VH or Tissicol, may also be used for the purpose of stabilizing the mesh. Do not open package until it is requested by the surgeon as these items are expensive.
- When an anesthesia provider is not required, see the perioperative RN's responsibilities in monitoring the patient, p. 58.
- Keeping a medicolegal record of the patient's vital signs and blood pressure is mandatory for the perioperative RN monitoring the patient; see responsibilities for the RN administering analgesia and conscious sedation, p. 74; see the Analgesia and Conscious Sedation Record, p. 76.
- Dissectors (peanut sponges, Kittner sponges) are included in the sponge count.

Laparoscopic Groin Herniorrhaphy

Definition

Repair of an inguinofemoral musculofascial defect employing laparoscopic technique.

Discussion

The techniques of "open" hernia repair are performed without violation of the abdominal cavity, often under local anesthesia. However, ***Laparoscopic Herniorrhaphy*** is frequently employed, usually as an outpatient procedure.

The advantages of a laparoscopic hernia repair over "open" hernia repair are:

- Reduction of pain
- Smaller incisions with less tissue manipulation and dissection
- A more rapid return to normal activity
- May result in fewer recurrences

The disadvantages of the laparoscopic approach include:

- Need for general anesthesia
- A lack of long-term follow-up data
- The cost of instrumentation must be weighed against other economic factors

Procedure

The table is positioned in Trendelenburg. Following the establishment of a pneumoperitoneum, a 10- or 11-mm laparoscope is inserted through the umbilical port and the abdomen is inspected. Second and third 10- or 11-mm ports are created, lateral to the rectus sheath at the level of the umbilicus on the side of the defect. Both inguinal rings are examined for hernias. Commonly employed is the transabdominal approach to the preperitoneal space (TAPP). A discrete hernia sac, if present, is retracted out of the inguinal canal, and a segment is excised. Peritoneal flaps are developed by blunt dissection. Care is taken to avoid injury to the spermatic vessels and vas deferens in the male. Mesh (e.g., Marlex, Gor-Tex Surgipro, etc.) may be secured with staples (e.g., ProTack) or tissue glue to cover the hernia defect. The Gor-Tex patch although expensive, is impregnated with an antimicrobial agent, resulting in a decreased rate of infection). Slits are made in the mesh for the epigastric vessels and the spermatic cord. Some surgeons staple mesh into the surrounding rim of the abdominal wall as a reinforcement to the repair. Care is again taken to avoid injury to the spermatic vessels, vas deferens, and the epigastric and iliac vessels. The pneumoperitoneum is relaxed. The peritoneal flaps are then stapled together to cover the mesh (and, also, as an attempt to prevent adhesion formation to the bowel). The employment of mesh potentially allows for a tension-free repair. Some authorities advocate a contralateral repair despite the absence of a frank hernia.

The peritoneal cavity may be flushed with copious amounts of Ringer's Lactate or normal saline to aid in the prevention of adhesion formation. Hemostasis is verified. The peritoneum is completely deflated. Others may repair indirect, direct, and recurrent inguinal hernias extraperitoneally with insufflation of CO_2 into the preperitoneal space, or by employing a lubricated inflatable balloon to provide exposure. The ports are removed, and the incisions are closed.

Preparation of the Patient

Antiembolitic hose may be put on the legs, as requested. The patient is supine; the arms may be extended on padded armboards. A pillow may be placed under the sacrum and/or under the knees to avoid straining the back muscles. Pad all bony prominences and areas vulnerable to skin and neurovascular pressure or trauma. The table will be placed in Trendelenburg to facilitate the establishment of pneumoperitoneum. An electrosurgical dispersive pad is applied. A Foley catheter is not routinely inserted.

Skin Preparation

Begin at the groin on the affected side, extending from just below the nipple to mid thigh (on the affected side), well beyond the midline on the unaffected side and down to the table on the affected side.

Draping

Folded towels and a laparotomy sheet

Equipment

Padded shoulder braces
Forced-air warming blanket, if requested
ESU
Suction, optional (infrequently used)
Fiberoptic light source, e.g., Xenon 300 W
Video monitor
VCR
CO_2 insufflator
Pressure bag, optional
Hydraulic dissector generator, when requested
CD burner
Printer
Camera console

Instrumentation

Limited procedures tray
Basic/minor procedures tray (available, in case procedure converted to open)
Verres needle
Trocars, 5 mm, 10 or 11 mm, and 12 mm
Fiberoptic laparoscopes, 30° and 0°, with camera and power cord
Reducers
Endosurgical instruments: dissectors, graspers (Babcock, Allis clamps), scissors (blunt), sharp scissors (straight, micro), double-action shears, and electrosurgical dissector
Multifire ligating clip applier, optional
Loop sutures (e.g., Endoloop), optional
Suturing device (with introducer sleeve) e.g. Endostitch, optional, for

Stapler (endostapler with self-contained staples), e.g., ProTack, as requested
Hydraulic dissector handpiece (laparoscopic) and cord with a variety of tungsten blades and scissors, optional

Supplies

Antiembolitic hose
Small basin set
Blades, (1) #10, (1) #15, (1) #11
Needle magnet or counter
Fog reduction agent, e.g., FRED, ELVIS
Suction tubing
Electrosurgical cord
Silastic tubing (for insufflation)
Cystoscopy or similar straight tubing, e.g., K50; add 1000-ml bag normal saline and three-way stopcock (for irrigation)
Mesh, Marlex, Gor-Tex, or Surgipro, or PreFix
Plug (prosthesis made of Marlex mesh), as requested
Fibrin sealant/tissue glue to secure mesh, e.g., Tisseel VH, Tissicol, optional
Stapler with self-contained staples, e.g. EndoTack®, optional

Special Notes

- Apply **Special Notes** from ***Abdominal Laparoscopy***, p. 140, as indicated.

Cholecystectomy

Definition

Excision (removal) of the gallbladder.

Discussion

Cholecystectomy may be performed to treat chronic or acute cholecystitis, with or without cholelithiasis, or to resect a malignancy.

Related Procedures Include:

Cholecystotomy. The establishment of an opening into the gallbladder to allow for drainage of bile from the organ (gallbladder) and removal of stones. A catheter (e.g., Foley, Pezzer, or Malecot) is placed in the gallbladder to establish external drainage **(cholecystostomy)**. This is performed when the patient cannot tolerate cholecystectomy.

Choledochoscopy. The insertion of a choledochoscope into the common bile duct to directly visualize the duct or to facilitate stone extraction.

Choledochotomy. The opening of the common bile duct to remove choledocholiths (gallstones). It is performed to relieve choledocholithiasis or otherwise drain an obstructed common bile duct. Drainage is usually established by placing a T-tube in the common bile duct **(choledochostomy)**.

Procedure

The incision is right subcostal, right paramedian, or midline. The abdominal cavity is entered in the usual manner. The gallbladder is grasped (generally with a Pean clamp). The cystic duct, cystic artery, and common bile duct are exposed. The surgeon must be aware of anomalies of these structures. The cystic artery is clamped (using two right-angle clamps) and ligated with a suture passed on a long instrument or by clips (e.g., Hemoclips), as is the cystic duct. The gallbladder is mobilized by incising the overlying peritoneum and after local dissection is removed. The underlying liver bed may be reperitonealized. A drain (e.g., Jackson-Pratt™) may be employed exiting a stab wound and secured to the skin with a stitch. The wound is closed in layers. The skin is closed with interrupted stitches, tapes, or skin staples.

For cholangiogram, the x-ray performed to demonstrate the anatomy and any abnormalties of the extrahepatic bilary tract prior to the ligation of the cystic duct. A catheter is passed through the stump of the cystic duct into the common bile duct. A suture or special cystic duct clamp secures the catheter. Prior to taking x-ray films, all extraneous metal clamps and retractors are removed from the field. The catheter is tested with saline for leakage, and then radiopaque dye is injected. X-rays are taken. The catheter is removed, and the cystic duct is ligated.

For choledochotomy and choledochoscopy, the common bile duct is exposed, and traction sutures are placed. A longitudinal incision is made in the duct, and a variety of stone-removing forceps, scoops, and irrigation and balloon or mushroom catheters may be employed to explore for and extract stones either proximally (hepatic bile ducts) or distally (common bile duct). A choledochoscope may also be employed. Further cholangiograms may then be taken. The duct is usually closed over a T-tube drain.

Ultrasonography is a technique that utilizes a hollow ultrasound probe that is inserted into the common bile duct to transmit high-frequency sound waves that fragment the stones. The abdominal cavity may be irrigated with warm saline to enhance the sound waves.

An Nd:YAG laser fiber or pulsed dye laser may also be used via choledochoscope to fragment the stones and to facilitate their removal.

Cholelithotripsy, performed in the lithotripsy suite, is a noninvasive technique that utilizes high-energy shock waves to fragment the stones. The pulverized stones are then passed through the common bile duct. Ursodiol (deoxycholic acid), taken by mouth, may be prescribed for the patient following lithotripsy to help dissolve the stone fragments. For an explanation of extracorporeal shock wave lithotripsy (ESWL), see p. 430.

Preparation of the Patient

Antiembolitic hose may be put on the legs, as requested. The patient is supine; both arms may be extended on padded armboards. A pillow may be placed under the sacrum and/or under the knees to avoid straining back muscles. Some surgeons position the patient with a roll under the right upper flank, which facilitates visualization for the cholangiogram, by "separating" the biliary tree from the spine. Pad all bony prominences and areas vulnerable to skin and neurovascular pressure or trauma. A preliminary x-ray ("scout") film may be taken to ensure correct placement of the cassette. A nasogastric tube may be inserted by the anesthesia provider. A Foley catheter is not routinely placed. An electrosurgical dispersive pad is applied.

Skin Preparation

Begin at the intended site of incision, either right subcostal (most frequently used), right paramedian, or midline, extending from the axilla to the pubic symphysis and down to the table on the sides.

Draping

4 folded towels and a laparotomy sheet

Equipment

Folded blanket or pad (for positioning)
Sequential compression device with disposable leg wraps, if ordered
Suction
ESU
Ultrasound generator, if requested
Laser (e.g., **Nd:YAG laser fiber or pulsed dye)** when requested; see mandatory safety precautions, pp. 94–98.

Instrumentation

Major procedures tray
Long Metzenbaum scissors
Hemoclip or other ligating clip appliers (various sizes and lengths)
Biliary tract tray (for common duct exploration)
Choledochoscope when requested; if unavailable, a ureteroscope or small cystoscope may be substituted

Supplies

Antiembolitic hose
Basin set
Blades, (2) #10, (1) #15, or (1) #11
Suction tubing
Hemoclips or similar ligating clips (various sizes)
Electrosurgical pencil and cord with holder and scrape pad
Needle magnet or counter
Dissectors (e.g., peanut or Kittner sponges)
Drains, e.g., Penrose 1″ or suction drain (e.g., Jackson-Pratt or Hemovac™), optional
T-tubes (if choledochotomy is done)
Mushroom-tipped (retention) catheters, e.g., Pezzer or Malecot, available
Culture tubes, one aerobic and one anaerobic
Hemostatic agent, e.g., Surgicel™, Helistat™, Thrombostat™, Avitene™, available

For Cholangiogram, Add

Catheter (surgeon's preference)
Radiopaque dye, e.g., Hypaque™ or Renografin 60™ diluted to half strength (labeled as such)
Small basins, one for saline and one for dye
Biliary tract tray
Sterile marking pen and labels
Syringes, 2 35–50 ml conical tipped or Luer lok to connect to dye catheter
K50 polyethylene cystoscopy tubing or surgeon's preference and three-way stopcock

For Choledochoscopy, Add

Flexible fiber optic choledochoscope (when unavailable, use rigid ureteroscope or small cystoscope) and cord with accompanying instrumentation such as suction, stone retrieval basket, etc. and equipment such as light source

Special Notes

- Apply **Special Notes** from ***Abdominal Laparotomy***, p. 134, as indicated.
- When the circulator reviews patient allergies with the patient, he/she ascertains that the patient has no history of allergy to radiopaque dye.
- If the patient is cold, offer a warmed blanket. **Do not** use a forced-air blanket, as a forced-air warming blanket or

hyper/hypothermia blanket or mattress pad interferes with the x-ray image.

- Circulator must advise x-ray department in advance that x-rays will be taken.
- A "scout" film will be taken before surgery begins to ensure correct positioning.
- It is imperative that the patient be positioned over the correct area on the table to ensure accurate visualization of the biliary tract when the x-ray is taken.
- All medications, dyes, etc., on the operating field must be labeled. Scrub person should use a marking pen on labels to identify all solutions. All medication containers should be kept in the room until the completion of the procedure. Follow all safety precautions to avoid medication errors; see pp. 30–31.
- Instruments used on the gallbladder are isolated in a basin (considered contaminated).
- Use a small basin to accept the specimen.
- Aerobic and anaerobic cultures may be taken of the bile or gallbladder bed.
- Scrub person needs to have a right angle clamp (Mixter) available throughout the dissection of the biliary tree.
- When cholangiogram is anticipated, the scrub nurse should prepare the necessary supplies in advance.
- Usually a stab wound is made in the cystic duct using a #11 blade. The incision is extended with Potts' scissors.
- Anticipate a common duct exploration if stones are seen (on x-ray). Stones are removed with Randall stone forceps, malleable scoops, dilators, baskets, Fogarty catheters, etc.
- Have T-tubes available following common duct exploration.
- One syringe is filled with saline, and a second syringe is filled with radiopaque dye diluted to half strength (labeled accordingly).
- Scrub person takes care to make certain that the saline or dye filled cholangiogram catheters are devoid of air bubbles (which can be confused for calculi).
- Both basins and syringes must be labeled to avoid confusion and to ensure successful x-ray exposures.
- Observe x-ray precautions when films are taken; see p. 52.
- Cover (to protect) the surgical field with a sterile towel when x-rays are taken.

- If surgical team members are to remain in the room during x-ray exposure, they should don a chest/abdominal protective shield before scrubbing.
- A protective facial shield is suggested for those scrubbed to avoid inadvertent splashing of contaminated fluids onto mucous membranes and eyes.

Laparoscopic Cholecystectomy

Definition

Endoscopic excision of the gallbladder.

Discussion

Cholecystectomy, performed laparoscopically, is the preferred treatment for symptomatic gallstones unless the patient is extremely obese, there are excessive adhesions (related to a previous surgery, recurrent attacks of cholecystitis, etc.), or ductal or vascular anomalies exist. If unexpected pathology is encountered, if acute inflammation distorts normal tissue planes, or if there is excessive bleeding or surgical injury, the laparoscopic procedure is promptly converted to "open" laparotomy.

Procedure

Pneumoperitoneum is achieved. A 10- or 11-mm trocar (with sheath) is inserted infraumbilically and removed after the sheath is secured. A laparoscope is introduced; it may be removed and reinserted via a subsequently placed port. The abdomen is explored. A subxiphoid trocar is inserted and port established. The patient's right side is rotated anteriorly 15 to 20°. A third trocar is inserted and a port established in the right anterior axillary line halfway between the iliac crest and the twelfth rib. A locking grasping forceps is introduced through this port, seizing the fundus of the gallbladder and distracting it until the hilum can be seen; local dissection of fat or adhesions may be necessary to achieve visualization of the gallbladder prior to this maneuver. A fourth trocar may be inserted and port established 2 to 3 cm below the right costal margin just medial to the shaft of the grasper (holding the gallbladder). Following appropriate dissection, the hilum of the gallbladder is visualized, including the cystic duct and the cystic artery. The cystic artery is divided between clips. A clip is placed on the proximal portion of the cystic duct and just proximal the junction of the cystic duct and common bile duct and the cystic duct divided unless a cholangiogram is to be performed, after which the distal cystic duct is clipped close to the junction with the common bile duct.

Cholangiogram. The cystic duct is incised as close to the gallbladder as possible. A cholangiogram catheter is inserted (with or without prior placement of a guide wire) and clipped or held in place with a cholangiogram clamp. Saline may be injected into the catheter to verify patency. Radiopaque dye (diluted to half strength and labeled accordingly) is injected after the patient is repositioned, as necessary. X-rays are obtained or fluoroscopy or ultrasonography is performed. The cholangiogram catheter is then withdrawn and the distal cystic duct clipped.

Choledochoscopy. The cystic duct is pneumatically dilated, through which the common bile duct is cannulated with a choledochoscope or ureteroscope. A guide wire is passed via the cystic duct, and the choledochoscope is advanced over the wire. An endoscopic stone basket may be used to retrieve calculi. If the stone is too large to have been removed via the cystic duct, lithotripsy of the stone may be employed using a mechanical, electrical, or laser energy source (crushing forceps, electrohydraulic lithotripter, or pulse-dye laser). The distal portion of the cystic duct is clipped after the instrumentation is withdrawn. Limitations of choledochoscopy exist due to the size of the instruments. Postoperatively, extraction of remnants of calculi may be facilitated by endoscopic retrograde cholangiopancreaticography (ERCP), including duodenal papillary sphincterotomy.

Some surgeons may perform "duct" choledochotomy, i.e., by direct incision into the common bile duct. (As indicated, the procedure may require conversion to open laparotomy to correct the common duct pathology.) The cystic duct is then ligated and divided. The neck and the fundus of the gallbladder are freed from the liver bed using either monopolar electrosurgery or laser dissection. (Before the gallbladder is completely detached, the area may be irrigated to expose and cauterize sites of bleeding in the liver bed.) A closed suction drain may be passed through the lateral port in an appropriate position and secured to the skin. When the gallbladder is freed of its attachments, bile and small stones may be aspirated to facilitate its extraction. If very large stones are encountered, the umbilical incision is extended and the gallbladder is removed directly through a large (18-mm) port. Hemostasis is achieved, and the incisions are closed following the release of the pneumoperitoneum.

Preparation of the Patient

Antiembolitic hose may be put on the legs, as requested. The patient is positioned supine with both arms extended on padded armboards. A standard table with an x-ray cassette in place or an image intensifier in conjunction with a C-arm or fluoroscopy may be used for film taking. A padded footboard and shoulder braces are secured to the table. An electrosurgical dispersive pad is placed. A pillow may be placed under the sacrum and/or the knees to prevent strain on back muscles. Pad all bony prominences and areas vulnerable to skin and neurovascular pressure or trauma. Neither a nasogastric tube nor a Foley catheter is routinely requested. The table is placed in Trendelenburg at 5 to 10° to establish pneumoperitoneum and then in reverse Trendelenburg at 10° to 20° to allow the abdominal viscera to gravitate inferiorly, away from the gallbladder. The table may also be rotated slightly to the left to increase exposure of the gallbladder and cystic duct.

Skin Preparation

Begin at the midline and extend from level of the axilla to the pubic symphysis and down to the table at the sides.

Draping

Folded towels and a laparotomy sheet

Equipment

Padded shoulder braces
Padded footboard
Sequential compression device with leg wraps, as requested
Suction
ESU
Fiber optic light source (e.g., Xenon 300 W)
Video monitors (2)
VCR
CO_2 insufflator
Nd:YAG or other laser, as requested
Pressure bag to facilitate irrigation
Cavitron™ or other lithotripter (infrequently used)
CD burner
Printer
Camera console

Instrumentation

Basic/Minor procedures tray
Major tray (available)
Biliary tract tray (available)
Choledochoscopy tray (available)
Verres needle
Hasson trocar (available)
Reducer caps
Fiber optic laparoscopes (2), 0° and 30°, with camera and cord

Endoscopic instruments: electrosurgical suction-irrigator; dissector clamps (two); electrosurgical right-angle hook suction (L shaped); electrosurgical J-hook with spatula tip; Babcock clamps, (two) 5 mm, (two) 10 mm; Allis clamps (two); scissors (micro, straight); Metzenbaum double-action shears; cholangiography clamp (with nipple for guide wire), several types available; Maryland clamp (almost right angle); stone basket or three-prong grasper; stone-crushing forceps; and fan retractors (two), optional

Multifire ligating clip applier (with self-contained clips)

Loop sutures, e.g., Endoloop (for ties)

Supplies

Antiembolitic hose

Basin set

Blades, (2) #10, (1) #15, (1) #11

Needle magnet or counter

Electrosurgical cord

Suction tubing

Silastic tubing for insufflation

Cystoscopy or similar straight tubing, e.g., K50; add 1000-ml bag normal saline and three-way stopcock for irrigation

Guide wire (e.g., 0.035 mm)

Fog reduction agent, e.g., FRED, ELVIS

Loop sutures (for ties), e.g., Endoloop

Catheter, e.g., Taut®, #5 ureteral

Catheter, open-ended, e.g., Karlan™

Culture tubes (aerobic, anaerobic)

Luer lok syringes, 35 ml (2), for cholangiogram

Radiopaque dye (e.g., Renographin 60 mixed half strength with normal saline)

Labels and sterile marking pen to label medications, dyes, etc.

Endoscopic specimen retrieval bag, Endo Pouch, ENDOBAG, LAP-BAG, LapSac, GRABAG (optional)

Hemostatic agent, e.g., Thrombin, Surgicel, Avitene, cryoprecipitate

Ductal dilating balloon catheter (e.g., 7 Fr. available)

Special Notes

- Apply **Special Notes** from ***Abdominal Laparoscopy***, p. 140, and ***Cholecystectomy***, p. 151, as indicated.
- When the circulator reviews patient allergies with the patient, he/she ascertains that the patient has no history of allergy to radiopaque dye.

- When patient is cold, offer warmed blanket. As x-rays may be taken, **do not** use a forced-air blanket or hyper/hypothermia blanket or mattress pad (may interfere with x-ray visualization).
- Whenever possible, fluoroscopy is used, as the image is immediately available to view findings. An image intensifier-compatible OR table may be used; however, if unavailable, place x-ray cassette in a standard table (ahead of time) to be used with a C-arm.
- A lithotripter, e.g., Cavitron, is infrequently requested for stone crushing; it must be planned for and set up in advance.
- When a laser (e.g., Nd:YAG or pulsed dye) is used, laser safety precautions must be observed; see pp. 94–98.
- Some surgeons use 5000 U Heparin in 1 liter of 0.9% (normal) saline for irrigation.
- Circulator will notify x-ray department when cholangiogram is anticipated.
- Scrub person takes care to make certain that the saline or dye filled cholangiogram catheters are devoid of air bubbles (which can be confused for calculi).
- The scrub person needs to drape the C-arm, when used. A drape may also be used to cover the x-ray screen to block the light.
- Circulator will turn off the power source to the laparoscopic camera during the cholangiogram.
- Following the cholangiogram, the circulator reconnects the ESU and other necessary equipment.

Drainage of Pancreatic Cyst (Pseudocyst)

Definition

Internal drainage of a pseudocyst is performed by anastomosing the cyst wall to an adjacent hollow viscus (stomach, duodenum, jejunum) or, less frequently, by external drainage or marsupialization.

Discussion

A pseudocyst of the pancreas is so named because this "cyst" does not have an epithelial lining, as does a true cyst. These cysts develop secondary to pancreatic trauma or acute pancreatitis in which pancreatic fluid and/or blood have been encased in adhesions that later form the cyst wall. As the cyst often contains pancreatic enzymes, internal drainage is preferable to external drainage to avoid external fistula formation and excoriation of the skin. Laparoscopic approach is usually preferred. These pseudocysts may be drained into a Roux-en-Y jejunal loop, the duodenum, or the stomach.

Procedure

A vertical or transverse incision is made. The cyst is identified and anastomosed to an adjacent abdominal viscus (organ). An incision is made into the anterior wall of a hollow viscus (e.g., stomach) to gain access to the posterior wall to which the anastomosis is made. Prior to suturing the cyst, the contents are aspirated to facilitate the anastomosis and to avoid spillage of pancreatic fluid into the operative field. After the anastomosis is completed, the anterior gastric wall is closed. If biliary tract disease is responsible for the pancreatitis, a concomitant biliary tract procedure is performed (e.g., cholecystectomy with common bile duct exploration (see p. 148). A drain may be placed and secured to the skin. The abdomen is closed in layers.

Preparation of the Patient

Apply antiembolitic hose, as requested. The patient is supine; arms may be extended on padded armboards. A pillow maybe placed under the sacrum and/or the knees to avoid straining back muscles. All bony prominences and areas prone to skin and neurovascular pressure or trauma are padded. An electrosurgical dispersive pad is applied.

Skin Preparation

Begin at the intended site of incision (vertical or transverse) extending from nipples to upper thighs and down to the table at the sides.

Draping

Folded towels and a laparotomy or transverse sheet (depending on incision)

Equipment

Sequential compression device with leg wraps, as requested
Forced-air warming blanket, as requested
ESU
Suction

Instrumentation

Major procedures tray
Biliary tract tray (available)
Hemoclip or other ligating clip appliers (variety of sizes and lengths)

Supplies

Antiembolitic hose
Basin set
Electrosurgical pencil and cord with holder and scratch pad
Suction tubing
Foley catheter, if requested
Antibiotic irrigation, optional
Blades, (2) #10 and (1) #15
Ligating clips, e.g., Hemoclips (small, medium, large)
Umbilical tapes
Dissectors (e.g., peanut or Kittner sponges)

Special Notes

- Apply **Special Notes** from ***Cholecystectomy***, p. 151, as indicated.
- The trocar (on the biliary tract tray) can be used to attach the suction tubing to aspirate the cyst.
- The Poole suction may be employed to suction out the antibiotic irrigation.
- Umbilical tapes and dissector sponges are included in the sponge count.

Pancreaticoduodenectomy (Whipple Procedure)

Definition

Removal of the head of the pancreas, the entire duodenum, the very proximal portion of the jejunum, the distal third of the stomach, and the distal half of the common bile duct, with the reestablishment of continuity of the biliary, pancreatic, and gastrointestinal tracts.

Discussion

Pancreaticoduodenectomy (Whipple Procedure) is usually performed for regional malignancy or benign obstructive chronic pancreatitis.

Pancreaticoduodenectomy can be performed laparoscopically.

Procedure

Approach is through a transverse, midline, or paramedian incision. The operability of the findings is assessed. The distal stomach, extra-hepatic biliary tract, head of the pancreas, and duodenum are mobilized. The distal stomach, the distal common bile duct, and the neck of the pancreas are resected. A total pancreatectomy, splenectomy, cholecystectomy, and vagotomy may be included. If the tumor has invaded the base of the mesocolon, portal vein, aorta, vena cava, or superior mesenteric vessels, this procedure is abandoned and a lesser procedure, usually a bypass (of the biliary tree and/or stomach), will be performed. Palliative double bypass may also be performed for unresectable pancreatic tumors. The proximal end of the jejunum is anastomosed to the distal pancreas (when proximal pancreatectomy, only, is performed). The common bile duct is anastomosed to the jejunum in end-to-side fashion. The distal stomach is anastomosed to the jejunum, also in end-to-side fashion. Stapling devices may be utilized in mobilizing and transecting multiple blood vessels and in the transection of the stomach and the gastrojejunal anastomoses. Various plastic stents may be placed in the biliary or pancreatic anastomosis. A fibrin sealant may be applied to suture lines. The wound is drained. The drain is secured with a stitch, and the abdomen is closed in layers.

Preparation of the Patient

Apply antiembolitic hose, as requested. The patient is supine; arms may be extended on padded armboards. A pad or pillow may be placed under the sacrum and/or the knees to avoid strain on back muscles. All bony prominences and areas prone to skin and neurovascular pressure or trauma are padded. The anesthesia provider inserts a nasogastric tube. A Foley catheter is inserted. An electrosurgical dispersive pad is applied.

Skin Preparation

Begin at the intended site of the incision (transverse, midline, or paramedian), extending from nipples to upper thighs and down to the table at the sides.

Draping

Folded towels and a laparotomy or transverse sheet (depending upon incision)

Equipment

Sequential compression device with leg wraps (disposable), as requested
Forced-air warming blanket, as requested
ESU
Suction
Scales (2) for weighing sponges
Blood pump and blood warmer, available

Instrumentation

Major procedures tray
Biliary tract tray
Gastrointestinal procedures tray
Long instruments tray (available)
Balfour or other large self-retaining retractor (e.g., Bookwalter)
Harrington retractors
Hemoclip, or other ligating appliers (variety of sizes and lengths)

Supplies

Antiembolitic hose
N/G tube to the anesthesia provider, as requested
Foley catheter with urimeter and continuous drainage unit, as requested
Basin set
Electrosurgical pencil and cord with holder and scratch pad
Suction tubing
Blades, (2) #10 and (1) #15
Hemoclips or similar ligating clips, variety of sizes and lengths
Dissectors (e.g., peanut or Kittner sponges)
Needle magnet or counter
Drains, for retraction (e.g., 1″ Penrose) and suction drain for wound drainage (e.g., Jackson-Pratt or Hemovac)
Umbilical tapes
Disposable automatic stapler (for closure of gastric pouch), e.g., TA™
Disposable linear stapler with cutter, e.g., GIA™ and staple cartridges (note various sizes, parameters, etc.) for gastrotomy, as requested
Stent, e.g., Gianturco Z™ or Wallstent™
Fibrin sealant/glue, e.g., Tissucol or Tisseel VH (optional)
Disposable skin and fascia stapler, e.g., DFS™, or skin stapler, e.g., DSS™, or skin suture, as requested

Special Notes

- Apply **Special Notes** from ***Abdominal Laparotomy***, p. 134, as indicated.
- The circulator must verify with blood bank that the correct number of units (of blood or blood products) are ready and available as ordered.
- The circulator assists the anesthesia provider in verifying the numbers on the units (of blood or blood products), comparing them to the patient identification number.

- The circulator prepares intravenous (IV) tubing, blood warmer, and blood pump, as requested by the anesthesia provider.
- The circulator may insert an intravenous (IV) line as requested by the anesthesia provider (according to hospital policy).
- **REMINDER:** After the peritoneal cavity has been entered, warm, moist lap sponges are used.
- Do not open any disposable stapling devices, etc., until surgeon requests exact size and type, as they are expensive.
- Weigh sponges to determine fluid loss replacement. To weigh sponges, two scales are used: one for raytec sponges and one for lap pads. To weigh sponges, calculate the weight of the dry sponge and set the scale to 0 after weight adjustment.
- An accurate record of the amount of irrigation used also helps to determine fluid loss replacement.
- The scrub person may want to receive the large specimen in a basin.
- Keep all soiled instruments isolated in a basin.
- Umbilical tapes and dissector sponges (e.g., peanuts, Kittner) are included in the sponge count.
- Record the insertion of a stent (name and type), in the **Perioperative Record** in the **Intraoperative Record** section.
- The stent information may be recorded in the hospital log book, according to hospital policy.
- **REMINDER:** A protective face shield is suggested for those scrubbed to avoid inadvertent splashing of contaminated fluids onto mucous membranes and eyes.
- **REMINDER:** The circulator accompanies the anesthesia provider to the PACU and gives the PACU perioperative practitioner a detailed report regarding the course of intraoperative events during the patient's surgery.
- The PACU perioperative practitioner monitors the patient, taking extra care to monitor vital signs and blood pressure, to observe the appearance of dressing sponges and blood loss, and to observe the patient for signs of hemorrhage.

Pancreatectomy

Definition

Removal or excision of a portion of or the entire pancreas.

Discussion

Partial pancreatectomy usually refers to the removal of the tail portion of the pancreas. The extent of the procedure performed depends on the site and nature of the lesion. Indications for pancreatectomy include ductal obstruction, pancreatic stones, pancreatic cysts, trauma, benign or malignant tumors, and endocrine tumors. If total pancreatectomy is performed for benign disease or a malignancy restricted to a very distal portion of the pancreas, a small portion at the head of the pancreas may remain attached to the duodenum along with the common bile duct. When the entire pancreas including the head is to be removed, see ***Pancreaticoduodenectomy***, p. 159. In cases where the distal pancreatic duct is obstructed by calculi, a longitudinal incision into the distal duct is made, the calculi removed, and the jejunum anastomosed to the distal pancreas (***Peustow procedure***).

Pancreatectomy may be performed laparoscopically.

Procedure

A transverse, midline, or right paramedian incision is made. The abdomen is explored. If total pancreatectomy is to be performed, see Pancreaticoduodenectomy, p. 159. If only the distal portion of the pancreas is removed, the pancreas is mobilized by dissecting it from its numerous vascular attachments. The gland is transected at the appropriate level and the distal end of the proximal portion of the pancreas is oversewn; an omental patch may be employed. The operative site is usually drained. The drain is secured with a stitch, and the wound is closed in layers.

For **Preparation of the Patient, Skin Preparation, Draping, Equipment, Instrumentation, Supplies,** and **Special Notes,** *see* ***Pancreaticoduodenectomy (Whipple Procedure)***, pp. 160–162.

Drainage of Abscess(es) in the Region of the Liver

Definition

Evacuation of purulent material within a confined space in or about the liver.

Discussion

The location of the abscess is determined by the surgeon using sonogram, computed tomography (CT) scan, or other x-ray study. A radiologist may aspirate and drain the abscess percutaneously. If percutaneous drainage is inadequate, open surgical drainage is performed. The abscesses are classified as left and right subdiaphragmatic, subhepatic, and intrahepatic. Multiple abscesses may be present

Procedure

An incision is made posteriorly along the twelfth rib extraperitoneally or anteriorly, either extraperitoneally or transperitoneally. The abscess is identified, and cultures are taken. The abscess is evacuated, and the area is irrigated with an antibiotic solution. Drains are placed and secured with a skin stitch. The wound is closed in layers.

Preparation of Patient

For a **subcostal approach**, the patient may be in supine position with arms extended on padded armboards. A pillow may be placed under the sacrum and/or the knees to avoid straining back muscles.

For **a posterolateral approach**, the patient is in the lateral position with the right side uppermost. The left arm is extended on a padded armboard; the right arm is supported by a Mayo stand (padded with a pillow), or a padded double armboard may be used. The left leg is flexed, and the right leg is extended with a pillow between the knees, or both legs may be flexed. Padding is placed around the feet and ankles. Female breasts and male genitalia are protected with padding. Following the application of tincture of benzoin, the position is secured by wide adhesive tape (check chart for patient allergies) from the shoulders, hips, and legs to the underside of the table.

For either position, antiembolitic hose may be applied. All bony prominences and areas vulnerable to skin and neurovascular pressure or trauma are padded. Neither a nasogastric tube nor a Foley catheter is routinely inserted. An electrosurgical dispersive pad is applied.

Skin Preparation

For a ***subcostal approach***, begin at the bottom of the ribcage, extending from axilla to just above the pubic symphysis and down to the table at the sides.

For a ***posterolateral approach***, begin at the eighth interspace, extending from the shoulder to the iliac crest and down to the table, anteriorly and posteriorly.

Draping

Folded towels and a laparotomy or transverse sheet (depending on incision)

Equipment

Sequential compression device with disposable leg wraps, as requested
Forced-air warming blanket, if requested
ESU
Suction

Instrumentation

Major procedures tray
Long instruments tray
Biliary tract tray (available)
Balfour or other large self-retaining retractor
Harrington retractor
Ligating clip applier, e.g., Hemoclip applier

Supplies

Antiembolitic hose
Basin set
Electrosurgical pencil and cord with holder and scratch pad
Suction tubing
Blades, (2) #10 and (1) #15
Needle magnet or counter
Culture tubes, one aerobic and one anaerobic
Antibiotic irrigation, as requested
Drains, e.g., Hemovac or as requested
Ligating clips, e.g., Hemoclips
Disposable fascia and skin stapler, e.g., DFS or DSS, or skin closure as requested

Special Notes

- See Special Notes for *Pancreaticoduodenectomy (Whipple Procedure)*, p. 161, as indicated.
- The circulator should consult the surgeon and the anesthesia provider to determine the position of the patient during the procedure to obtain all padding, supports, etc., for positioning available before bringing the patient into the room.
- Protect skin under adhesive tape with tincture of benzoin after checking chart regarding patient's allergies.
- Scrub person should anticipate culture and sensitivity (aerobic and anaerobic) will be taken; he/she should have culture tubes, etc., on the back table in advance.
- The circulator must accurately identify area from which cultures are taken on the lab requisitions.
- Those scrubbed should wear face shields to protect them from inadvertent splashing or spraying of contaminated material.
- All instruments that come in contact with the abscess are isolated in a basin.

- The peritoneal cavity may be irrigated with an antibiotic solution, a Poole suction may be used.
- **REMINDER:** The PACU perioperative practitioner monitors the patient, taking extra care to monitor and record vital signs and blood pressure, to observe the appearance of dressing sponges and blood loss, and to observe the patient for signs of hemorrhage.

Hepatic Resection

Definition

Refers to a small wedge biopsy, the local excision of tumors, or a major segmentectomy of the liver.

Discussion

Indications for hepatic resection include trauma, cysts, or tumors, benign (e.g., hemangioma) and malignant (e.g., primary or secondary, i.e., metastatic). A preoperative CT scan or angiogram delineates the pathology. Major resections follow the liver segments as defined by the vascular and biliary channels rather than the traditional lobar pattern. As significant blood loss is inherent in major resections, use of the cell saver with auto transfusion should be available.

Procedure

The location of the incision is determined by the section of the liver to be resected. Feasibility of resection is determined. When a thoracoabdominal incision is employed, the abdominal portion is incised first. The thoracic portion of the incision is made next, incising the diaphragm. Hepatic artery, portal vein, and major biliary ducts are controlled by vascular forceps or vessel loops at the porta hepatis (the Pringle maneuver) to avoid excessive bleeding or bile leakage until more peripheral control is established. Similarly, special bow-shaped clamps have been devised to compress large segments of the liver until local hemostasis is effected. The liver parenchyma is divided, pausing to ligate major vascular and biliary channels. Tissue finger fracture, cavitational ultrasonic surgical aspirator CUSA™, Harmonic Scalpel®, Plasma Scalpel™, jet-cutter (high frequency jet beam employing hypertonic NaCl cutting solution), argon beam coagulator, and/or electrosurgical unit may be employed. Careful technique is necessary when approaching the posterior surface where the hepatic veins enter the inferior vena cava. If bleeding is excessive, the vena cava may be controlled by the insertion of balloon catheters, intracavally. After hemostasis is obtained and the bile ducts are ligated, the exposed parenchyma may be covered by greater omentum or absorbable hemostatic agents. A fibrin sealant may be employed to control bleeding, seal tissue planes, or "glue" tissues. The area is drained. The drains are secured with a skin stitch, and the abdomen is closed in layers.

Hepatic resection may be performed laparoscopically.

Preparation of Patient

A hyper/hypothermia blanket or mattress pad (e.g., MUL-T-Blanket®) may be placed on the table before the patient is brought into the room (consult with surgeon and anesthesia provider). Apply antiembolitic hose as requested. Pad all bony prominences and areas vulnerable to skin and neurovascular pressure or trauma. The anesthesia provider inserts a nasogastric tube. A Foley catheter is inserted. Apply electrosurgical dispersive pad.

For a partial left lobe excision, employing a subcostal approach, the patient is supine with arms extended on padded armboards. A pillow is placed under the sacrum and/or under the knees to avoid straining back muscles.

For a major resection, the approach is thoracoabdominal; the patient is in a modified (45°) lateral position with right side uppermost. The left arm is extended on a padded armboard; the right arm is supported by a Mayo stand (padded with a pillow) or placed on a padded double armboard. The right leg is extended, and the left leg is flexed (or both legs may be flexed) with a pillow between the knees. Areas around the feet and ankles are well padded. Following the application of tincture of benzoin, the position is secured by wide adhesive tape (after checking chart for patient allergies) from the shoulders, hips, and thighs to the underside of the table. Pad female breasts and male genitalia, as necessary.

Skin Preparation

For a subcostal approach, begin at the bottom of the ribcage, extending from axilla to just above the pubic symphysis and down to the table at the sides.

For a posterolateral approach, begin at eighth interspace, extending from the shoulder to the iliac crest and down to the table anteriorly and posteriorly.

Draping

Folded towels and a transverse or laparotomy sheet

Equipment

MUL-T-Blanket (hyper/hypothermia blanket or mattress pad), optional
Sequential compression device with leg wraps, as requested
ESU

Suctions (2)
Scales (2) for weighing sponges
Manometer (for measuring portal pressure), optional
Cell-saver (optional, check with surgeon)
Blood pump
Blood warmer
Cavitron, Cavitational Ultrasonic Surgical Aspirator (CUSA), Harmonic scalpel, Plasma scalpel, Jet-cutter with hypertonic NaCl or Argon beam coagulator, as requested

Instrumentation

Major procedures tray
Long instruments tray
Vascular procedures tray
Thoracotomy tray (for thoracoabdominal approach)
Gastrointestinal procedures tray
Biliary tract tray, available
Large self-retaining retractor, e.g., Balfour, Finochietto
Hemoclip or similar ligating clip appliers (various sizes and lengths)
Bow-shaped liver compression clamp, e.g., Lin (available)
Liver compression clamp curved on both sides, e.g., Masters-Schwartz (available)
Handpiece for CUSA, Harmonic scalpel, Jet-cutter, Argon beam coagulator, optional

Supplies

Antiembolitic hose, as requested
N/G tube to anesthesia provider, as requested
Foley catheter with urimeter and continuous drainage unit,
Basin set
Blades, (3) #10
Electrosurgical pencil and cord with holder and scrape pad
Suction tubing
Hemoclips or similar ligating clips (various sizes)
Dissectors (e.g., peanut)
Needle magnet or counter
Hemostatic agent, e.g., Gelfoam, Surgicel, Helistat, Hemostat, Thrombostat, Avitene, or cryoprecipitate
Fibrin glue/sealant, e.g., Tissucol or Tisseel VH (optional)
Vessel loops, optional

For Thoracoabdominal Approach, Add

Chest tubes, e.g., 2 Argyle

Intrapleural sealed drainage unit, e.g., Pleurevac™
Y-connector
Bulb syringe

Special Notes

- Apply Special Notes from *Pancreaticoduodenectomy (Whipple Procedure),* p. 161, as indicated.
- **REMINDER:** A hyper/hypothermia blanket or mattress pad (e.g., MUL-T-Blanket) may be placed on the table before the patient is brought into the room (consult with surgeon and anesthesia provider).
- The circulator should bring the patient's x-rays and scan reports into the room before bringing the patient into the room.
- The circulator should consult the surgeon regarding whether the cell-saver will be used; if so, it should be set up in the room before the patient is brought in.
- Additional personnel needed to operate the cell-saver must be notified. The policy regarding capabilities or special training of personnel to run the cell-saver varies according to the institution.
- Blood collected in the cell-saver for autotransfusion must be free of contamination. Blood contaminated by foreign body intraabdominal contents (as in perforation of the bowel) or by medications administered (as in antibiotic irrigation) cannot be used.
- In addition to the blood that is collected by suctioning the abdomen, blood saturated sponges "wrung out" by the scrub person before they are discarded into the kick basin.
- The circulator must confirm with blood bank that the number of units of blood (or blood products) ordered by the surgeon are ready and immediately available.
- The circulator assists the anesthesia provider in verifying the numbers on the units (of blood and/or blood products) and comparing the numbers to the patient's identification numbers prior to administering the units.
- The circulator must be sure at least two suction units in the room (besides the one on the anesthesia cart) are operational.
- The OR team must be prepared for a potentially significant amount of blood loss; extra lap sponges should be available on back table (already counted) so that there is no delay.

- Keep strict accounting of lap sponges, as a saturated sponge can be overlooked.
- **REMINDER:** Use warm moist lap sponges after entering abdominal cavity; "free" raytec sponges should **not** be on the sterile field.
- Special liver sutures (2-0 chromic on a large blunt needle) are available and may be requested; do not open the packages until they are requested, for cost-control reasons.
- Cavitron (or cavitational ultrasonic surgical aspirator [CUSA]), plasma scalpel, or argon beam coagulator may be employed; have this equipment available and ready for use, if requested.
- A fibrin glue/tissue sealant may be employed along suture lines, (e.g., Tissucol or Tisseel VH); do not open the packages until they are requested, for cost-control reasons.
- Keep an accurate record of the amount of irrigation used to determine replacement of fluid loss.
- **REMINDER:** Weigh sponges accurately for determining fluid loss replacement. To weigh sponges, two scales are used, one for raytec sponges and one for lap pads. Calculate the weight of the dry sponge and set the scale to 0 after weight adjustment.
- Dissector sponges (peanuts or Kittner), umbilical tapes, and vessel loops are included in the count.
- A basin is necessary to receive the large specimen.
- **REMINDER:** The PACU perioperative practitioner monitors and records the patient, taking extra care to monitor vital signs and blood pressure, to observe the appearance of dressing sponges and blood loss, and to observe the patient for signs of hemorrhage.

Splenectomy

Definition

Removal or partial removal of the spleen.

Discussion

The most common indication for splenectomy is accidental injury. Other indications include hematological disorders, tumors, cysts, or splenomegaly and in the staging of Hodgkin's disease. Splenectomy may also be indicated as the result of trauma during surgery, as in gastrectomy or mobilization of the splenic flexure of the colon; an attempt is made to preserve the traumatized spleen with suture techniques and hemostatic agents. A portion of the spleen may be preserved when feasible. Total splenectomy is avoided whenever possible to obviate the necessity for indefinite protection against pneumococcal pneumonia. Accessory spleens may be present in perisplenic tissues; rarely they are found in more remote sites. In cases of trauma, transfusion or autotransfusion (with use of the cell-saver) may be required.

Procedure

A midline or left subcostal incision is made. Entry into peritoneal cavity is achieved. The spleen is identified and the splenic hilum is isolated, taking care not to injure the tail of the pancreas. The splenic vessels (may be multiple) are divided and ligated. The enlarged spleen may be adherent to surrounding structures, including the parietal peritoneum and diaphragm. The spleen is removed. The wound may be irrigated. Hemostasis is achieved, and the wound is closed in layers. If optimal hemostasis cannot be achieved or there is a question of pancreatic injury, a closed suction unit may be employed, e.g., Hemovac.

Splenectomy may be performed laparoscopically.

Preparation of the Patient

A hyper/hypothermia blanket or mattress pad (e.g. MUL-T-Blanket) may be placed on the table before the patient is brought into the room (consult with surgeon and anesthesia provider). Apply antiembolitic hose, as requested. The patient is supine **for an abdominal approach**, with arms extended on padded armboards. Pad all bony prominences and areas vulnerable to skin and neurovascular pressure or trauma. Foley catheter is inserted. The anesthesia provider may insert a nasogastric tube. Apply electrosurgical dispersive pad.

A **thoracoabdominal approach** may be employed for massive splenomegaly.

Apply antiembolitic hose as requested.

For thoracoabdominal approach, the patient is in lateral position with left side up at a 45° angle; the right arm is extended on a padded armboard. The left arm is supported on a pillow-padded Mayo stand, or a padded double armboard may be used. The right leg is flexed and the left leg is extended, or both legs may be flexed with a pillow between the knees. The feet and ankles are padded. Following the application of tincture of benzoin, wide adhesive tape secures the position (after checking chart for allergies and sensitivities) at the shoulders, hips, and thighs to the underside of the table. The breasts of women and the genitalia of men are padded. Pad all bony prominences and areas vulnerable to skin and neurovascular pressure or trauma. The anesthesia provider may insert a nasogastric tube. A Foley catheter is inserted. Apply electrosurgical dispersive pad.

Skin Preparation

For abdominal approach, begin at the midline, extending from the axilla to just above the pubic symphysis and down to the table at the sides.

For subcostal approach, begin at the bottom of the ribcage (left side up), extending from axilla to just above the pubic symphysis and down to the table, anteriorly and posteriorly.

Draping

Folded towels and a laparotomy or transverse sheet (depending on incision)

Equipment

Sequential compression device with leg wraps, as requested
Hyper/hypothermia blanket or mattress pad (e.g. MUL-T-Blanket), optional
ESU
Suctions (2)
Cell-saver (optional, check with surgeon)
Blood pump
Blood warmer
Scales (2) for weighing sponges

Instrumentation

Major procedures tray
Gastrointestinal procedures tray
Long instruments tray (available)
Harrington retractor
Ligating clip applier e.g., Hemoclip appliers (various sizes and lengths)

Supplies

Antiembolitic hose, as requested
N/G tube to anesthesia provider, as requested
Foley catheter and urimeter (with continuous drainage unit), as requested
Basin set
Electrosurgical pencil and cord with holder and scraper pad
Suction tubing
Blades, (2) #10 and (1) #15

Needle magnet or counter
Ligating clips, e.g., Hemoclips (various sizes)
Dissectors (e.g., peanut, Kittner sponges)
Hemostatic agents (e.g., Thrombostat, Avitene, Helistat, Surgicel, etc.)
Fibrin glue/tissue sealant, e.g., Tissucol or Tisseel VH (optional)
Drains, for retraction (e.g., 1″ Penrose) and for wound drainage, suction drain (e.g., Jackson-Pratt or Hemovac)
Umbilical tapes

Special Notes

- Apply Special Notes from *Pancreaticoduodenectomy (Whipple Procedure)*, p. 161, as indicated.
- A hyper/hypothermia blanket or mattress pad (e.g. MUL-T-Blanket) may be placed on the table before the patient is brought into the room (consult with surgeon and anesthesia provider).
- Have patient's x-rays and scan reports in the room.
- Inquire if the cell-saver will be used; if so, bring it into the room before the patient. **See *Hepatic Resection,*** p. 166 for use of the cell-saver.
- Confirm with blood bank that the correct number of units of blood (or blood products) have been ordered and are ready and available.
- Assist in verifying identification for administering blood and blood products. Prepare IV tubing, blood warmer, and blood pump, as needed.
- Be sure at least two suction units in the room are operational.
- Be prepared for the possibility of significant amount of blood loss; have extra lap sponges on back table (already counted) so that there is no delay.
- Keep strict accounting of lap sponges, as a saturated sponge could be overlooked.
- Use warm moist lap sponges after entering abdominal cavity.
- A fibrin glue/sealant may be employed at suture lines, e.g., Tissucol™ or Tisseel VH (optional).
- Include vessel loops in the sponge count.
- Keep an accurate record of the amount of irrigation used to determine replacement of fluid loss.

- Weigh sponges accurately for determining fluid loss replacement.
- Initially, dry lap sponges are used, followed by warm moist lap sponges.
- The scrub person may want to receive the large specimen in a basin.

Laparoscopic Splenectomy

Definition

Endoscopic removal of the spleen.

Discussion

Laparoscopic splenectomy has been performed in patients with ***idiopathic thrombocytopenic purpura (ITP)*** or as part of a staging procedure (such as for Hodgkin's disease). For ITP, the splenic tissue should be entirely removed (including possible accessory spleens) to avoid the occurrence of postoperative splenosis. When the procedure is part of a staging laparoscopy, it is performed with bilobar superficial and deep hepatic biopsies; peri-aortic/para-aortic and pelvic lymph node sampling is taken. Large or adherent spleens are often difficult to remove laparoscopically, necessitating an "open" procedure.

Procedure

Pneumoperitoneum is created, and a 10- or 11-mm trocar (with sleeve) is inserted in the midline 2 to 3 cm above the umbilicus. A laparoscope is inserted, and additional ports are established. The abdomen is explored, with emphasis placed on identifying any accessory spleen(s). This is critical in the treatment of patients with ITP. A window into the lesser sac is created adjacent to the greater curvature of the stomach. The vessels are clipped and cut to create an appropriate-sized window. The laparoscope is then introduced into the lesser sac. The splenic artery is meticulously dissected and clipped, but not yet transected. The splenic vein is also clipped. The scope is withdrawn from the lesser sac, and dissection of the spleen is initiated. Retraction is required on both sides of the spleen. Through the most lateral port on the right, an endoscopic Babcock is used to grasp the greater curvature of the stomach (opposite the hilum of the spleen), retracting it medially. An endoscopic extrudable fan retractor is inserted via the most lateral port on the left side to retract the spleen upward and laterally. Any additional vascular supply to the spleen (which can be variable) is identified, clipped, and divided. Electrosurgery should be avoided in controlling these large vessels. Care is taken to avoid injury to the tail of the pancreas. The peripheral attachments or perisplenic adhesions are then severed, the previously controlled hilar vessels are transected, and the spleen is removed through an ancillary incision, or in ITP, when the anatomy of the specimen is not a factor, the spleen may be morcellated within a specimen bag and removed via a port. If visualization of the surgical field is inadequate and/or if bleeding is excessive, the procedure must be promptly converted to an open approach. After hemostasis is assured, the pneumoperitoneum is released. The incisions are closed in the usual manner.

Preparation of the Patient

Antiembolitic hose are applied, as requested. The patient is supine, and the padded arms are tucked in at the patient's sides using the draw sheet, unless the patient is obese; then the right arm may be placed on a padded armboard. A pillow may be placed under the sacrum and under the knees to avoid straining back muscles. A nasogastric tube is usually placed by the anesthesia provider. Bony prominences and all areas vulnerable to skin and neurovascular pressure or trauma are padded. Initially, the patient is placed in Trendelenburg, 5° to 10°, to allow the viscera to gravitate cephalad, thereby assisting in the establishment of pneumoperitoneum. Following this, the table is placed in (slightly) reverse Trendelenburg and rotated to the right to allow organs to fall away from the spleen to increase exposure.

A Foley catheter may be inserted. Apply an electrosurgical dispersive pad.

Skin Preparation

Begin cleansing at the umbilicus. Include area from the nipples to midthighs and down to the table at the sides.

Draping

Folded towels and a laparotomy sheet

Equipment

Sequential compression device with leg wraps, as requested
Hyper/hypothermia blanket or mattress pad (e.g., MUL-T-Blanket), if requested
Suction
ESU
Fiber optic light source, e.g., Xenon 300 W
Video monitors (2)
VCR

CO_2 insufflator
Pressure bag
CD burner
Printer
Camera console

Instrumentation

Major procedures tray (opened)
Verres needle
Hasson trocar
Trocars (2), 10 or 11 mm
Trocars (2), 5 mm
Reducer caps
Laparoscopes with cameras and power cords (2), 0° and 30°
Endoscopic instruments: electrosurgical suction-irrigator-dissector, graspers, scissors (blunt, micro) (3) hook, straight, micro; Metzenbaum double-action shears, extrudable fan retractor, Cushieri liver retractor, and morcellator
Multifire ligating clip applier
Suturing device (with introducer sleeve), Endostitch
Loop sutures (e.g., Endoloop)

Supplies

Antiembolitic hose
Foley catheter (with continuous urinary drainage unit), as requested
N/G tube, e.g., 16 Fr to anesthesia provider, as requested
Blades, (1) #10, (1) #15, (1) #11
Needle magnet or counter
Suction tubing
Fog reduction agent, e.g., FRED, ELVIS
Silastic tubing for CO_2 insufflation
Electrosurgical cord
Cystoscopy or similar straight tubing, e.g., K50; add 1000-ml bag normal saline and three-way stopcock, for irrigation
Hemostatic agent, e.g., Thrombin, Surgicel, Avitene, cryoprecipitate, as requested
Hand port, e.g., LAP DISC, HANDPORT, Intromit, Omniport Dexterity Device for hand-assisted procedures, if requested
Extra large endoscopic impermeable specimen retrievable bag, Endo Pouch II, ENDOBAG, LAP-BAG, LapSac, GRABAG (optional)

Special Notes

- Apply **Special Notes** from ***Abdominal Laparoscopy***, p. 140 and ***Splenectomy***, p. 173, as indicated.
- Generally, when the laparoscopic approach for splenectomy is chosen, significant blood loss is not anticipated. When significant blood loss occurs, the procedure is converted to an "open" procedure; see ***Splenectomy***, p. 171.
- Ascertain that blood is available, as ordered; in case of excessive blood loss, the laparoscopic procedure may be converted to an "open" procedure.

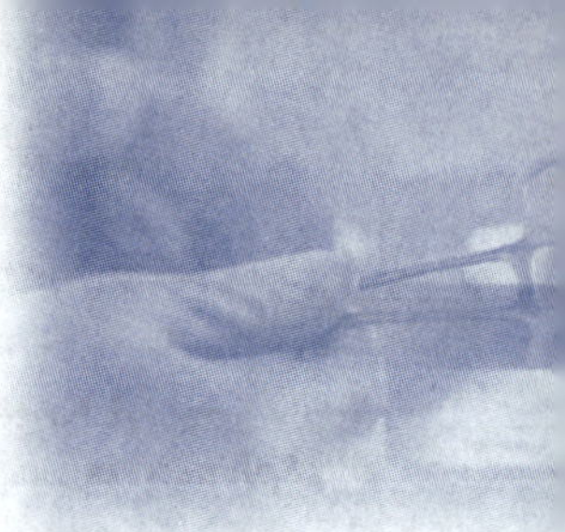

CHAPTER 17
Gastrointestinal Surgery

Esophagoscopy

Definition
Endoscopic inspection of the esophagus.

Discussion
Esophagoscopy is performed to diagnose malignancies, esophagitis (noting reflux), hiatal hernia, strictures, and varices; to remove tissues (biopsy) or secretions for study; for direct therapeutic manipulations such as removal of a foreign body or tumor, injection or coagulation of varices, or insertion of a plastic prosthesis (e.g., stent) to relieve strictures (or relieve obstruction due to a nonresctable tumor), etc. Fiber-optic esophagoscopes are rigid or flexible and are available in a variety of sizes. Scope choice depends on the procedure and the patient's level of discomfort and ability to tolerate the procedure. Rigid scopes are employed when the esophagus is obstructed by a bolus of food or bone or when an object (e.g., dental work) becomes lodged. Esophageal swelling may result from these entrapped objects, creating an emergency (as the airway may become occluded by the ensuing local pressure). A calm and reassuring manner will help to prevent the patient's anxiety from escalating during this uncomfortable procedure.

Care must be taken by the endoscopist or surgeon to prevent perforation of the esophagus during the procedure. Flexible fiber-optic esophagoscopes are the instrument of choice for diagnostic procedures. **Esophagoscopy** is most often performed in the gastrointestinal (GI) lab but may also be done in the operating room (OR) and, occasionally, as necessitated, at the patient's bedside. Bougies may be required to dilate the esophagus.

Using either type of scope requires the patient's full cooperation; the patient may receive *conscious sedation* in addition to the anesthetic spray (used to eliminate the gag reflex). Studies have demonstrated that patients instructed in relaxation techniques pre-procedure (when esophagoscopy is performed for diagnosis) have significantly less anxiety. Playing music also has a calming effect on the patient.

Procedure
The surgeon applies a topical anesthetic spray to the posterior oropharynx to control the gag reflex; some patients may receive intravenous (IV) *conscious sedation*. At least a three-minute wait is required for the spray to take

effect. The patient is encouraged to take deep breaths. In select patients for whom the flexible scope is employed, topical anesthesia may be omitted

For rigid esophagoscopy, the surgeon applies a topical anesthetic spray to the posterior oropharynx to control the gag reflex. During the three-minute wait necessary for the spray to take effect and throughout the procedure, the patient receives intravenous (IV) *conscious sedation* to reduce discomfort and feelings of anxiety or panic. The top section of the table is removed; the patient's head is held (supported) by an assistant, (usually the scrub person, but may also be the circulator), who raises or lowers the head in the direction of the endoscopist or surgeon as the lubricated esophagoscope is passed transorally (with the neck fully extended). Manipulations are performed as indicated.

For flexible esophagoscopy, the lubricated esophagoscope is passed transorally. A bite block is placed. Air and water may be instilled through the scope (for distention and to provide better visualization). Various instruments take biopsies, obtain specimens for brush cytology, and suction secretions for diagnoses and treatment. Bleeding may be controlled with a sclerosing agent, electrosurgery, or laser beam. However, the small diameter of the instrument channel limits the ability to take biopsies larger than 3 mm and to perform certain therapeutic or diagnostic measures. The flexible esophagoscope may also be passed transnasally.

Longer endoscopes may also be passed transorally or transnasally, past the ligament of Treitz into the jejunum to perform ***esophagogastroduodenoscopy***. When ***endoscopy*** includes ***nasopharyngoscopy, laryngoscopy, bronchoscopy,*** and **esophagoscopy,** the procedure is referred to as ***panendoscopy***.

A newly developed two-sided camera, contained in a capsule, provides an alternate option, referred to as ***capsule endoscopy***. The patient swallows the disposable miniature video camera-contained in a capsule, and images are produced at the rate of two per second from both ends of the camera. ***The PillCam™ capsule endoscopy*** is an ambulatory procedure. A disadvantage to this approach is that although the surgeon or endoscopist is able to inspect the mucous membranes of the esophagus and a photographic record can be made; no specimens or biopsies may be obtained. Another disadvantage is that the capsule is expensive. The capsule is similar to that used for small bowel visualization, which requires the patient to wear a belt-supported recording device.

Preparation of the Patient

A Mayo stand is prepared with a tray for administering the topical anesthetic.

Topical Anesthetic Tray

Laryngeal mirrors, lingual spatula, anesthetic spray, laryngeal syringe with straight and curved cannulas, medicine cups for the agent(s) of choice, emesis basin, syringe (e.g., Luer lok, 10 cc), dressing sponges, and tissues.

The patient is sitting (with feet on a stool) during application of the topical anesthetic. Either the circulator or the scrub person stands behind the patient to lend support, as necessary, and to the assist surgeon. During the three-minute wait that is observed to allow time for the anesthetic to work, the surgeon is consulted regarding the need for electrosurgery. Apply the electrosurgical dispersive pad, as necessary.

For rigid esophagoscopy, the patient is positioned supine with the shoulders slightly over the top break in the table.

For flexible esophagoscopy, the patient (usually) is in the ***left lateral position*** (i.e., left side down).

Draping

Patient may be covered with a drape sheet. A drape sheet is used to cover the back table.

Skin Preparation

None required.

Equipment

Suction
Stool for patient's feet (during anesthesia spraying of the oropharynx)

Rigid

Fiber-optic light source for cable
Electrosurgical unit (ESU), monopolar

Flexible

Endoscopy Cart:
Fiber-optic light source, e.g., Xenon™ 300 W
Air insufflation/Irrigation device
Suction unit
Monitor
VCR and printer
CD burner
Printer
Camera console
ESU, monopolar
Laser (e.g., Nd:YAG fiber or as requested), optional; see p. 94 for mandatory laser safety precautions

Instrumentation

Dilators, e.g., bougies (may be passed prior to passing either scope to dilate the esophagus) and stents, available for both types

Rigid

Rigid fiber-optic esophagoscope with camera and cord for light, grasping forceps, suction, electrosurgical suction, biopsy forceps, electrosurgical snare, sponge carrier, and cytology brush

Flexible

Flexible fiber-optic esophagoscope with camera and power cable, forceps, electrosurgical snare, mini grasping forceps, suction, electrosurgical suction, cytology brush, and disposable irrigation tube

N.B. *If laser is employed, all instruments must be treated or coated (e.g., ebonized) and mandatory laser safety precautions, p. 94 must be observed.*

N.B. *If the patient is receiving general anesthesia and a laser is employed, special laser-retardant endotracheal tubes must be used or the endotracheal tube should be wrapped with tape made especially for this purpose. The manufacturer's specifications must be followed precisely when using the protective tape.*

Supplies

- Bite block to protect scope (flexible)
- Small basin (with saline)
- Leur lok syringe (1) on prep table (1) on back table for sclerosing agent, if used (e.g., for treatment of esophageal varices)
- Topical anesthetic spray
- Water-soluble lubricant (to lightly lubricate scopes)
- Bronchoscopy sponges (rigid)
- Specimen containers and slides
- Needle, e.g., 25 gauge (to remove biopsy specimen from biopsy forceps)
- Electrosurgical cord
- Suction tubing
- Sclerosing agent (e.g., ethanolamine oleate or sodium tetradecyl sulfate/Sotradecol® 1% or 3%)

Special Notes

- Apply **Special Notes** from ***Abdominal Laparoscopy,*** p. 140 as indicated.
- These **Special Notes** for ***Esophagoscopy*** in general, apply to most other gastrointestinal endoscopic procedures, as well.

- The circulator must always use the **Joint Commission's (JC) (formerly the Joint Commission on Accreditation of Healthcare Organizations)** *Universal Protocol* to identify that the patient is the correct patient, anticipating the correct surgery. See the **JC**'s *Universal Protocol*, p. 18, as necessary.
- Before every surgery begins, an official "*time out*" is required and must be documented on the **Perioperative Record** for patient safety regarding continuity of care and for medicolegal reasons.
- See the suggested **Patient Care Plan**, p. 9 for care of the patient in surgery. The circulator adapts care to meet the individual patient's needs by implementing the nursing interventions that result in optimal desired outcomes for the patient. Use the **Special Notes** to augment the plan of care to ensure that all reasonable considerations have been taken into account.
- All care given must be documented in the **Perioperative Record,** (p. 12) for patient safety regarding continuity of care and for medicolegal reasons.
- To provide a measure of emotional support to the patient, the circulator may convey to the patient that he/she will act as the patient's advocate.
- It is important for the circulator to provide measures of emotional support to the patient, e.g., by maintaining eye contact when speaking to the patient and holding the patient's hand during the administration of anesthesia.
- The patient may have fear and anxiety regarding the surgery and the unfamiliar environment; the circulator should answer questions in a knowledgeable manner whenever possible and refer questions to the surgeon as necessary.
- Provide emotional support with a nonjudgmental attitude regarding the patient's feelings of an altered body image by providing the patient an opportunity to express his/her feelings.
- The circulator can provide a feeling of physical security to the patient (particularly during local and topical anesthesia when the patient is awake) by limiting exposure of the part of the body involved in the procedure and by keeping the patient well-covered otherwise.
- The circulator takes appropriate measures to maintain patient's body temperature by offering a warmed blanket (from blanket warmer), by raising the room temperature, and by assuring that the patient is adequately covered). When ordered, a forced-air warming blanket may be placed over legs and/or chest.

- Check with surgeon regarding the topical anesthetic spray to be used.
- A bite block should be included with the instruments (for sterilization) to protect the scope from damage.
- All fiber-optic telescopes must be handled carefully, as the fibers that make up the fiber optics are fragile and easily broken.
- High-level disinfection (versus sterilization), see p. 43, is the minimal requirement for instrumentation utilized for procedures on mucous membranes. See sterilization, p. 41; regarding care and disinfection of the endoscopic instruments, see p. 102.
- When an anesthesia provider is not required, a perioperative RN, in addition to the circulator, must monitor the patient and record patient data to promote patient safety and to create a medicolegal record. For RN monitoring guidelines, see p. 58. For the **Analgesia and Conscious Sedation Record,** see p. 76.
- If the monitoring perioperative RN is relieved during the procedure, report of patient data is reviewed with the relief RN and the record maintained to provide continuity of care. As in all nursing interventions, documentation is vital.
- Supportive measures and caring reassurances, etc., in addition to those given by the circulator, are provided by the perioperative RN monitoring the patient.
- The perioperative RN monitoring the patient and the circulator must continually assess and evaluate the patient's physiologic status throughout the procedure. The initial plan of care outlined is adjusted according to the individual's needs and is used to implement nursing interventions resulting in optimal desired outcomes for the patient.
- **N.B.** ***The precautions in endoscopic laser surgery are mandatory for the safety of both the patient and personnel. Select measures are listed below; to see all laser safety precautions, see p. 94.***

Select Laser Safety Precaution Reminders

- Any time a laser procedure is performed, a scrub person, a circulator, and a laser safety officer should be present.
- All equipment must be checked prior to the procedure, including but not limited to testing the beam focus, electrical connections, and suction apparatus.
- The pedal is identified (aloud) as it is placed in front of the operating surgeon to avoid accidental activation.

- The laser is set at "standby" or "stop" mode during significant interruptions in its use.

- When a laser is used to ablate a lesion, e.g., a tumor, the tumor may evaporate (into plume); there will be no specimen to send to the lab.
- A protective face shield should be worn by those scrubbed to prevent the patient's secretions from spraying into the eyes and mucous membranes of team members.
- Scrub person must pass forceps to the surgeon with the tips of the forceps in the closed position.
- Scrub person should help to guide the instruments into the scope, as necessary, to permit the surgeon to keep his/her eyes on the surgical field.
- Scrub person may remove specimens from biopsy forceps without damaging the specimen by using a 25-gauge needle to facilitate tissue removal.
- Careful labeling and handling of specimens is essential for safe patient diagnosis and treatment. (The circulator should prepare several labels and requisitions providing specific information regarding the site of origin.)
- Care is taken to place specimens in the appropriate solutions or on slides (using alcohol) or to save as directed by the surgeon.
- Specimens not placed in fixative should be labeled and delivered promptly to the lab (to avoid their drying out).
- Prior to leaving the OR, the circulator assures that the patient is properly positioned on the gurney, that lines are not kinked, and that measures necessary to maintain the patient's body temperature have been taken.
- The circulator accompanies the anesthesia provider who takes the patient to the Post Anesthesia Care Unit (PACU); he/she gives the PACU perioperative practitioner a detailed intraoperative patient report regarding the course of events as they apply to the individual.
- In the PACU, the perioperative practitioner observes that the patient's breathing is unobstructed, monitors the patient's blood pressure and vital signs, and documents all pertinent information in the **Perioperative Record** in the **Postoperative Record**. Documentation is vital for patient safety regarding continuity of care and for medicolegal reasons.
- In PACU, the perioperative practitioner assumes the role as the patient's advocate.

Gastroscopy

Definition

Endoscopic visualization of the stomach and proximal duodenum.

Discussion

Gastroscopy is performed for diagnosis, aspiration of gastric contents, removal of a foreign body, or tissue biopsy. **Flexible fiberoptic gastroscopy** is usually performed in the GI lab or at the patient's bedside (for critically ill patients); gastroscopy is rarely performed in the OR. By employing the ultra-slim flexible fiber-optic gastroscope, the procedure is more easily done. **Gastroscopy** is employed concomitant with the creation of a **percutaneous gastrostomy (PEG)**, see p. 212.

Often, the esophagus is inspected during the course of the procedure.

Procedure

The patient receives topical anesthesia (applied to the oropharynx) and ***conscious sedation***. The surgeon inserts the lubricated gastroscope, traversing the gastroesophageal sphincter into the stomach. If the scope is further advanced beyond the pylorus, into the duodenum (or proximal jejunum), the term *esophagogastroduodenoscopy* may be used. Inspection is performed with "turn around maneuver" to visualize the cardia (flexible scope), biopsy, destruction of lesions (chemical, electrosurgical, laser, etc.), sphincter dilatation, foreign body retrieval, assistance with **percutaneous gastrostomy**, etc., are performed.

For **Preparation of the Patient, Skin Preparation, Draping, Equipment, Instrumentation, Supplies,** and **Special Notes,** see *Esophagoscopy*, pp. 179–184.

Colonoscopy

Definition

Endoscopic visualization of the large intestine from rectum to cecum (and occasionally the very terminal ileum).

Discussion

Total colonoscopy is almost always performed in the GI lab or the radiology department. Exceptions to this include colonoscopy performed during open laparotomy to positively identify the location of a nonpalpable lesion, or certain pediatric examinations when general anesthesia is required. **Colonoscopy**, limited to the distal colon, may be performed in the OR (for the reasons just stated) by inserting only a portion of a lubricated colonoscope or by employing a flexible fiberoptic sigmoidoscope; see ***Sigmoidoscopy***, p. 186.

Procedure

The lubricated colonoscope is advanced transanally into the distal rectum (usually with the assistance of personnel from the GI lab). By manipulating the controls, torquing, advancing, and withdrawing the scope, the surgeon or endoscopist inspects the entire or limited portions of the colon, as indicated. If the abdomen is open, the surgeon in the operating field may manually facilitate passage of the scope. Depending on the clinical circumstances, biopsy and destruction of lesions, etc. may be performed. Generally, careful inspection is performed as the scope is withdrawn. If a larger lesion is treated with sequential excision by electrosurgical biopsy loop, the scope may have to be withdrawn and reinserted to retrieve the specimens. Hemostasis is achieved electrosurgically.

For **Preparation of the Patient, Skin Preparation, Draping, Equipment, Instrumentation, Supplies,** and **Special Notes,** see ***Sigmoidoscopy***, p. 186, to follow.

Sigmoidoscopy

Definition

Endoscopic inspection of the anal canal, rectum, and sigmoid colon

Discussion

This procedure may be performed for diagnosis, excision of polyps, biopsy of lesions, fulguration of bleeding points, and relief of sigmoid volvulus, etc.

Sigmoidoscopy is often performed in the surgeon's office; usually, no anesthetic of any type is necessary. Sigmoidoscopy is performed in the OR when the patient is unable to tolerate the procedure due to pain and tenderness or when the procedure is too risky to perform outside the OR environment; conscious sedation and/or conduction anesthesia (a block) or general anesthesia may be employed. Modalities as electrosurgery or laser may be employed.

Rigid fiber-optic sigmoidoscopy or flexible fiber-optic sigmoidoscopy is performed as independent procedures, often in conjunction with an anorectal surgery to follow.

Procedure

Rigid Sigmoidoscopy is described. The anus is digitally lubricated and examined. ***Anoscopy*** may be performed. The rigid fiber-optic sigmoidoscope is inserted and advanced under direct visualization until obstructed by an unyielding angulation of the lumen or obstructed by an occlusive lesion or advanced to the full length of the scope. Definitive inspection of the mucous membrane is done as the scope is withdrawn. Air may be insufflated to distend the lumen for better visualization. Biopsy or destruction of a lesion, reduction of a sigmoid colon volvulus, etc. may be performed.

Sigmoidoscopes (rigid) are usually 18 to 19 mm in diameter; larger diameters to 30 mm may be employed when anesthesia is given. An 11-mm sigmoidoscope can be employed to traverse a stricture; also see ***Transanal Endoscopic Microsurgery***, p. 262.

Flexible Sigmoidoscopy. Digital examination and anoscopy are performed after the anus is lubricated. The tip of the sigmoidoscope is inserted, and under direct visualization, the scope is advanced by various torquing and advancement motions to the length of the scope (30 or 65 cm) or until resistance is met, patient discomfort, or inability to see the lumen ahead is reached. Definitive examination is done on withdrawal. Biopsy or destruction of lesions may be performed employing elctrosurgical biopsy forceps, or loop, or laser fiber.

N.B. ***A laser may be employed using either type of scope; see laser safety precautions, p. 94.***

Preparation of the Patient

Positions for **rigid sigmoidoscopy** include jackknife, modified lateral/Sims', or lithotomy; see surgical positions, p. 24. The modified left lateral/Sims' position is generally preferred for **flexible sigmoidoscopy**, although the jackknife position may be employed. For all of the positions, apply antiembolitic hose before positioning patient, as requested.

Jackknife position. The table is flexed, and the patient is prone with arms extended on padded armboards angled toward the head of the table with the forearms pronated. A pillow may be placed under the head and chest for comfort; if the patient is obese, chest rolls may be placed to facilitate respiration. A pillow is placed in front of the legs, and a roll is placed in front of the ankles. Care is taken to pad female breasts or male genitalia, as necessary. When anorectal surgery is to follow, tincture of benzoin is applied to the buttocks. Buttocks are distracted by 3- or 4-inch adhesive tapes (after checking chart for patient's allergies) anchored to the underside of the table (pull tapes toward patient's head before anchoring them for maximal exposure) when surgery, e.g., ***hemorrhoidectomy***, is performed to follow. When general anesthesia is employed, chest rolls are required to facilitate the patient's breathing. Pad all bony prominences and areas vulnerable to skin and neurovascular pressure or trauma. Apply electrosurgical dispersive pad.

Lithotomy position. The patient's legs are placed in padded stirrups, and a folded towel is placed under the sacral area for elevation of the buttocks (permitting better exposure of the surgical field). Arms may be extended on padded armboards. All bony prominences and areas vulnerable to skin and neurovascular pressure or trauma are padded. Tincture of benzoin is applied to the buttocks area. Buttocks may be distracted by 3- or 4-inch adhesive tapes (after checking chart for patient's allergies) that are anchored to the stirrup posts. Apply electrosurgical dispersive pad.

Modified Lateral/Sims' position. The patient lies on the left side with left arm extended on a padded armboard and the right arm flexed over the left, with a pillow placed between the arms (or a padded double armboard may be used). The back is angled so that the anus extends just over the table's edge. The left leg is straight and the right leg is flexed, or both legs may be flexed with a pillow between the knees; additional padding is required at feet and ankles. Pad all bony prominences and areas vulnerable to skin and neurovascular pressure or trauma. Tincture of benzoin is applied to the right buttocks. After checking chart for patient's allergies, the buttocks are distracted by 3- or 4-inch adhesive tape (placed on the right buttock [uppermost]) and anchored to the underside of the table. Apply electrosurgical dispersive pad.

Skin Preparation

None required.

Draping

Drapes for draping the patient depend upon the position. A drape sheet covers the back table.

Equipment

Padded stirrups for *lithotomy* position
Padded stirrups for *modified lithotomy* position, e.g., Allen or Lloyd-Davies usually in conjunction with extensive procedures involving the colon or rectum.
Pillow, pad, and rolls for positioning for Sims' position

Rigid

Suction
ESU
Laser, if requested; see p. 94, mandatory laser safety precautions
Flexible Endoscopy Cart:
Suction unit
Insufflation-Irrigation console
Fiber-optic light source, e.g., Xenon 300 W
Monitor
VCR
Printer
CD Burner

Camera console (control unit)
ESU (monopolar)

Instrumentation

Flexible sigmoidoscope with camera (disposable plastic, 18mm or stainless steel 11, 15, 19, or 30mm), as requested
Sigmoidoscopy (specific) light cord
Sigmoidoscopy tray with suction-electrosurgical (cautery) instrument with cord, bulb insufflator, biopsy forceps, snare (loop), ligating clip appliers, polyp-grasping forceps

Flexible Fiber-optic Sigmoidoscope

Flexible fiber-optic sigmoidoscope with built-in camera, and cable
Endoscopic instruments:
electrosurgical biopsy forceps, snare, polyp grasper, irrigating cannula, and cytology brush

Supplies

Antiembolitic hose, if requested
Lubricant, water-soluble
Suction tubing
Long cotton swabs (rigid)

For Flexible Scope, Add

Cord for electrosurgery

Special Notes

- Apply **Special Notes** from ***Esophagoscopy***, p. 181, as indicated.
- **Reminder:** The circulator must always use the JC's *Universal Protocol* to identify that the patient is the correct patient, anticipating the correct surgery on the correctly marked side (laterality) and site. See the JC's *Universal Protocol*, p. 18, as necessary.
- **Reminder:** Before every surgery begins, an official "time out" must be taken as a patient safety measure. A *time out* is required and must be documented on the **Perioperative Record** for medicolegal reasons.
- **Reminder:** See the suggested **Patient Care Plan**, p. 9, for care of the patient in surgery. The circulator adapts care to meet the individual patient's needs by implementing the nursing interventions that result in the optimal desired outcomes. Use the **Special Notes** to augment the plan of care to ensure that all considerations have been taken into account.

- All care that is given must be documented in the **Perioperative Record** for medicolegal reasons and patient safety related to continuity of care.
- **Reminder:** The circulator will assist the anesthesia provider during the induction of anesthesia, e.g., during endotracheal intubation (by applying pressure to the cricoid cartilage), during the administration of a block (e.g., by holding the patient in position for an epidural anesthetic), or by injecting medications the anesthesia provider has prepared (at his/her direction). For a description of the circulator's role during the administration of anesthesia, see p. 81.
- Check chart for patient sensitivities and allergies, particularly to latex products, e.g., gloves, elasticized dressings. Note that a simple pressure bandage contains latex, as do many other items in general use.
- Follow Medication Guidelines and Practices, p. 30–33, to avoid errors. Remember that trash and linen should not be discarded until the procedure has concluded.
- Apply antiembolitic hose, if requested, before positioning patient.
- The electrosurgical pad should be applied to skin that is relatively hair-free (to obtain good contact) and as close to the surgical site as possible. It may be necessary to shave the area.
- Large amounts of noxious smoke and fumes resulting from thermal destruction are a health hazard; smoke should be suctioned away by the room suction with an in-line filter or with a smoke-evacuation system.
- Masks (with a filtering capacity of between 2 and 5 microns) should be worn by all personnel and the patient in the room during an operative procedure to prevent inhalation of toxic matter.
- The electrosurgical coagulator tip should be free from debris and eschar (use scratch pad) and kept in its holder (fashioned from folded towel) when not in use.
- Prevent musculoskeletal injuries by employing ergodynamic measures when positioning patient, as necessary.
- Adequate padding is required for female breasts and male genitalia when patient's position is prone.
- For ***modified lithotomy position***, prevent risk of positioning injury with stirrups that are padded and positioned correctly to avoid skin and neurovascular pressure or trauma.

- Prevent trauma to patient's fingers when lithotomy position is employed, i.e., when the lower section of the table is returned to level position.
- Protect skin under adhesive tape (after checking chart for patient allergies) with tincture of benzoin.
- **N.B.** *If tapes are to be applied for anorectal surgery to follow, this is done prior to the scope procedure, as the presence of a lubricant will interfere with the adherence of the tape.*
- When **sigmoidoscopy** is performed before an anorectal surgery, a separate back table is set up for the sigmoidoscopy
- A protective face shield should be worn to protect those persons scrubbed to avoid inadvertent splashing of contaminated fluids onto mucous membranes and eyes.
- Extreme care must be taken when handling fiber-optic endoscopic scopes, instruments, and cords, as all are fragile. Do not bend cords, as the fibers within break easily.
- Lubricate the scope with a water-soluble agent to facilitate its passage.
- Clean scope immediately following use to prevent debris from drying and becoming hard and too difficult to remove.
- **N.B.** *Specimens may be removed from biopsy forceps with a 25-gauge needle to avoid crushing the specimen.*
- **Rigid.** The scrub person should assist surgeon by guiding suction, forceps, electrosurgical instruments, etc., guiding instruments into scope, and by removing biopsies from forceps, as necessary.
- **Flexible.** The scrub person should be prepared to help stabilize the flexible scope. Assist surgeon by passing biopsy forceps, endoscopic snare, polyp grasper, etc., as necessary.
- The surgeon may direct the scrub person to open and close the endoscopy snare or biopsy forceps to obtain specimens.

Laparoscopic Esosphagomyotomy for Achalasia (Heller Procedure)

Definition

Incision of the muscular layers of the distal esophagus and proximal stomach to correct esophagogastric sphincter spasm, permitting normal swallowing.

Discussion

Due to degeneration of the ganglion cells in the esophageal neuromuscular plexus (cause unknown) and possibly in vagus nerve fibers, the gastroesophageal sphincter does not relax, with ensuing dysphagia and dilatation of the esophagus. Medical treatment with smooth muscle relaxants (including nitrates and calcium channel blocking agents) is not usually successful, nor does the injection of botulinum toxin through an esophagoscope provide relief for more than a few months.

Pneumatic dilatation, which fractures esophageal muscle fibers, may give relief but is often inadequate or may result in perforation. **Esophagogastric myotomy** provides lasting results in more than 90% of patients. The procedure may be performed by laparotomy, laparoscopically, transthoracically, or thoracoscopically. A partial fundoplication may be done at the same time to prevent gastroesophageal regurgitation. ***Esophagectomy*** is reserved for the rare intractable cases of unsuccessful lesser treatments.

Procedure

The laparoscopic approach for *Esophagomyotomy* is described. Five laparoscopic ports are placed following the establishment of pneumoperitoneum. The short gastric vessels are divided and the distal esophagus mobilized, protecting the anterior vagal nerve trunk. A bougie (50Fr) is illuminated and passed into the esophagus by the anesthesia provider, aiding in the dissection. Using an L-shaped dissector (with or without electrosurgical modality), a longitudinal incision is made down to the submucosal layer 2 to 3 cm distal to the gastroesophageal junction and then proximally onto the esophagus for 6 to 8 cm. The esophageal incision may be longer. If elected, a partial posterior fundoplication (e.g., Toupet) may be performed to prevent gastroesophageal reflux. The port incisions are closed.

Preparation of the Patient

Antiembolitic hose are put on the legs, as requested. The patient is supine with the arms on padded armboards. Padded shoulder braces and a padded footboard are secured to the table. The anesthesia provider passes a lubricated nasogastric tube. All bony prominences and areas vulnerable to skin and neurovascular pressure or trauma are padded, e.g., the heels. Apply electrosurgical dispersive pad. A Foley catheter may be inserted. The table is placed in Trendelenburg 5° to 10° to establish pneumoperitoneum, and then in reverse Trendelenburg 10° to 20° to allow the viscera to gravitate inferiorly. The table may be rotated slightly to the right to facilitate exposure.

Skin Preparation

Begin at the midline (for an abdominal approach), extending from the axilla to the pubic symphysis and down to the table at the sides.

Draping

Folded towels and a laparotomy sheet

Equipment

Sequential compression device with disposable leg wraps, if requested
Padded shoulder braces
Padded footboard
Suction
ESU
Fiber-optic light source, e.g., Xenon 300 W
Video monitors (2)
VCR
Printer
CD burner
Camera console
CO_2 insufflator
Pressure bag to facilitate irrigation

Instrumentation

Limited procedures tray (open)
Major procedures tray (for possible conversion to "open" procedure), available
Esophageal dilator set, e.g., Maloney or Hurst
Verres needle
Hasson trocar
Trocars, (5), e.g., (2) or (3) 10 or 11 mm and (2) or (3) 5 mm
Reducer caps
Fiber-optic laparoscope with camera charged-coupled device (CCD) and power (light) cord
Endoscopic instruments:
electrosurgical suction irrigator/dissector with J hook tip or right angle tip, scissors (hook, straight, and micro), grasping clamps, such as (2) Babcock (atraumatic) 5 mm and (2) 10 mm, and (2) Allis, fan or Nathanson retractor
Suturing device, e.g., EndoStitch®
Multifire ligating clip applier

Supplies

Antiembolitic hose
Foley catheter (with continuous drainage unit), as requested
N/G tube (e.g., 16Fr) to anesthesia provider
Methylene blue dye, if requested
Basin set
Blades, (1) #15 and (1) #11
Fog reduction agent, e.g., FRED®, ELVIS™
Silastic™ tubing for CO_2 insufflation
Suction tubing
Cystoscopy or similar straight tubing, e.g., K50; add 1000-ml bag normal saline and Stopcock 3-way, for irrigation
Electrosurgical cord

Special Notes

- Apply **Special Notes** from ***Abdominal Laparoscopy***, p. 140, and ***Esophagoscopy***, p. 181, as indicated.
- When there is a question regarding penetration of the esophageal mucosa, methylene blue dye may be instilled into the distal esophagus by the anesthesia provider to identify the site of the perforation.

Esophagectomy

Definition

Removal of the esophagus or a portion of the esophagus with reestablishment of the continuity of the gastrointestinal tract.

Discussion

Esophagectomy (in the adult) is performed for stricture, trauma, achalasia not responsive to lesser procedures, Barrett's esophagus, etc., but most often for malignancy. Approximately half of esophageal cancers occur in the proximal two thirds of the esophagus (squamous cell carcinoma) and half in the distal third (adenocarcinoma). Metastasis to adjacent structures as multiple lymph node regions and blood vessels ensues. Most lesions are discovered late; survival rate is poor despite treatment.

Diagnostic evaluation, in addition to routine examination, includes endoscopy and barium studies, computed tomography (CT), magnetic resonance imaging (MRI), positron emission tomography (PET), and ultrasound scans, immunologic studies, and thoracoscopy and laparoscopy (for staging and planning of therapy). For Barrett's esophagus, transendoscopic laser treatment may suffice in early presentations.

When the patient is too debilitated to undergo resectional surgery, the constricting lesion may be cored, employing electrosurgery or laser (with endoscopic placement of an expandable stent, e.g., Song™, Ultraflex™, Gianturco-Z™) to permit the patient to swallow saliva and take liquid nutrition. When a chance of cure is possible, extensive procedures are undertaken.

For tumors of the hypopharyngeal or cervical esophagus, reconstruction requires the use of skin flaps (deltopectoral, etc.), and for more distal lesions, radical en bloc dissection may involve partial ***gastrectomy, splenectomy,*** and excision of multiple lymph node regions, azygous vein, thoracic duct, and adjacent diaphragm. Radiation therapy alone or a combination of surgery and radiation with adjuvant chemotherapy are treatment considerations.

When the lesion is amenable to surgery, a wide variety of procedures may be performed. Surgical resection may be via left or right thoracotomy, with a thoracoabdominal incision or a combination of separate cervical, thoracic, and abdominal incisions. Reconstruction most often utilizes the stomach configured into a variety of tubes after resection of the cardioesophageal junction. When the patient has previously undergone upper gastrointestinal procedures, or, electively for mechanical reasons or to avoid later acid reflux, isolated segments of the right, transverse, or left colon may be used with a colocolostomy to restore colonic integrity. Similarly, a jejunal segment may be used in a Roux-en-Y configuration. The interposed segment is placed transpleurally, or for palliation, endoesophageally. Endoscopic stapling techniques are employed.

Esophagectomy is formidable, with high morbidity and mortality. A combined thoracoscopic and laparoscopic approach, although tedious, is often undertaken; however, it may compromise the dissection. There is controversy regarding the most appropriate procedure.

Procedure

Esophagectomy via left transpleural transdiaphragmatic approach for a lesion inferior to the aortic arch is described. Via left ***thoracotomy***, a portion of the seventh rib (and lesser resection of the sixth and eighth ribs) is resected. The pleural space is entered, and an incision is made into the mediastinal pleura. The esophagus, superior and inferior to the aortic arch (including the tumor-bearing segment), is mobilized. Branches of the esophageal artery from the thoracic aorta are ligated. The azygos vein is either protected or excised, accordingly. Major lymphatic channels and the thoracic duct, likewise, are protected or excised in a more radical procedure. The left recurrent laryngeal nerve is protected. The diaphragm is incised and the stomach mobilized. The esophagocardiac junction is transected, and the esophagus and mobilized stomach are brought up (i.e., superiorly). The proximal esophagus is divided, removing the specimen.

An anastomosis is fashioned between the esophagus and the (now) intrathoracic stomach, anterior to (or posterior to) the aortic arch. Combinations of endoscopic stapling and/or suture techniques are utilized throughout. The stomach is anchored to the mediastinal pleura, and the diaphragm is closed about the distal stomach. (Some surgeons advocate concomitant ***pyloroplasty,*** p. 205, to prevent a gastric outlet obstruction due to spasm created by a vagus nerve branch division inherent to the procedure.) A thoracostomy tube is placed and secured with a stitch. The incision is closed.

Preparation of the Patient

Antiembolitic hose are put on the legs. Following the administration of general anesthesia, the patient is placed in a **modified right lateral position** (left side up). The patient's right arm is extended on a padded armboard, and the left arm is bent and brought over the right (supported by a pillow-padded Mayo stand). The right leg is flexed, and the left leg is straight (or both legs may be flexed) with a pillow placed between the knees. Padding is placed around the feet and ankles. The position is maintained with wide adhesive tape (after checking chart for patient's allergies), following the application of tincture of benzoin, at the shoulders, hips, and legs and secured to the underside of the table. All bony prominences and areas vulnerable to skin and neurovascular pressure or trauma are well padded. A Foley catheter is placed. An electrosurgical dispersive pad is applied.

Skin Preparation

Begin at the intended site of incision (mid-thorax to the abdomen), extending from the shoulders to the iliac crest and to the table, anteriorly and posteriorly.

Draping

Folded towels and a laparotomy sheet

Equipment

Sequential compression device with disposable leg wraps, as requested
MUL-T-Blanket® (hyper/hypothermia blanket or mattress pad), optional
ESU
Suction
Scales for weighing sponges (2)
Blood pump and blood warmer, available
Laser, if requested; see p. 94 for mandatory laser safety precautions

Instrumentation

Major procedures tray
Vascular procedures tray
GI tray
Thoracotomy tray
Long instruments tray, available
Hemoclip® appliers, or similar ligating clip appliers, variety of sizes and lengths
Disposable multi-fire automatic stapling devices, e.g., LDS™ for ligation and division of omentum and vagus nerves, TA 90™ for closure of gastric fundus, GIA™ (available), TA 55™ for closure of gastrotomy, EEA™ for anastomosis

Supplies

Antiembolitic hose
N/G tube to the anesthesia provider
Foley catheter with urimeter and continuous drainage unit
Basin set
Blades, (2) #10 and (1) #15
Needle magnet or counter
Suction tubing
Electrosurgical pencil and cord with holder and scraper
Hemoclips or similar ligating clips, assorted sizes
Small dissectors, e.g., peanut, Kittners

Special Notes

- Apply **Special Notes** from ***Abdominal Laparotomy,*** p. 134, and ***Esophagoscopy***, p. 181, as indicated.
- **Reminder:** The circulator must always use the ***JC Universal Protocol*** to identify that the patient is the correct patient, anticipating the correct surgery on the correctly marked side (laterality) and site. See the **JC**'s *Universal Protocol,* p. 18, as necessary.
- **Reminder:** Before every surgery begins, an official "*time out*" must be taken; it is a safety measure. A "*time out*" is required and must be documented on the **Perioperative Record** for medicolegal reasons.
- **Reminder:** See the suggested **Patient Care Plan,** p. 9. The circulator adapts care to meet the individual patient's needs by implementing the nursing interventions that result in the optimal desired outcomes. Use the **Special Notes** to augment the plan of care to ensure that all considerations have been taken into account.

- All care that is given must be documented in the **Perioperative Record** for medicolegal reasons.
- **Reminder:** The circulator will assist the anesthesia provider during the induction of anesthesia, e.g., during endotracheal intubation (by applying pressure to the cricoid cartilage) or by injecting medications the anesthesia provider has prepared (at his/her direction). For a description of the circulator's role during the administration of anesthesia, see p. 81.
- **Reminder:** Check chart for patient sensitivities and allergies, including to latex products, e.g., gloves, drains, or elasticized dressings. Note that simple drains (e.g., Penrose) and pressure bandages contain latex, among many other items in general use. Also note that some patients may be allergic to the iodine in some prep solutions.
- The circulator must verify with the blood bank that the correct number of units (of blood or blood products) are ready and available as ordered.
- The circulator assists the anesthesia provider in verifying the numbers on the units (of blood or blood products) and comparing them to the patient identification number.
- The circulator prepares intravenous (IV) tubing, blood warmer, and blood pump, as requested by the anesthesia provider.
- The circulator may insert an intravenous (IV) line, as requested by the anesthesia provider (according to hospital policy).
- **Reminder:** After the chest cavity has been entered, warm moist lap sponges are used; free raytec sponges are not used in the open thorax or abdomen. A raytec sponge mounted on a sponge forceps (e.g., Forrester) may be requested. This is referred to as a "spongestick."
- Do not open any disposable stapling devices, etc., until surgeon requests exact size and type, noting that these items are expensive.
- Weigh sponges to determine fluid loss replacement. To weigh sponges, two scales are used, one for raytec sponges and one for lap pads. To weigh sponges, calculate the weight of the dry sponge and set the scale to 0 after weight adjustment.
- An accurate record of the amount of irrigation used also helps to determine fluid replacement.

- Once the chest cavity is opened, lap pads moistened with warm normal saline are placed, and the rib spreader (a self-retaining retractor, e.g., Finocietto) is needed.
- A small sponge for dissection, e.g., peanut or Kittner, is mounted on a tonsil forceps; using a long-tonsil forceps may be requested.
- A protective face shield should be worn by those scrubbed to prevent tbe patient's secretions from sprayng into the eyes and mucous membranes of team members.
- If a ligature is requested, it should be passed mounted on a tonsil (or on long-tonsil) forceps.
- The skin knife used to make the initial incision is used to make the stab wound for the chest tube, e.g., Argyle. A hemostat (e.g., Pean) is inserted into the stab wound to grasp the tube. The chest tube is secured with a skin stitch of heavy material, e.g., #2 silk on a cutting needle.
- Following wound closure, the chest tube may be additionally secured to the adjacent skin with tape; check the chart for patient allergies if adhesive tape is to be used and apply tincture of benzoin or Mastisol® before placing the tape.
- The chest tube is attached to an under water seal drainage, e.g., Pleurevac™ and hung at a level below the patient's chest.

Esophageal Hiatal Herniorrhaphy

Definition

Repair of the esophageal diaphragmatic aperture (hiatus) to prevent herniation of the stomach into the thorax.

Discussion

Esophageal hiatal hernia is often detected on routinc chest x-ray; the patients frequently are asymptomatic.

Indications for surgical repair include severe clinical symptoms as gastroesophageal reflux (GERD) and chest pain with radiographic, endoscopic, and intestinal physiologic and manometric findings. On occasion, the apparent herniation of the stomach into the thoracic cavity is due to a foreshortened esophagus. Numerous procedures have been devised to correct this condition by transabdominal, transthoracic, or endoscopic approach.

The recurrence rate is relatively high. No single procedure has been determined to be the best.

Procedure

A transabdominal approach for Esophageal Hiatal Herniorrhaphy is described.

The upper abdomen is approached through a midline, paramedian, or high-transverse incision. The esophagocardiac region is exposed by either retraction or mobilization of the left lobe of the liver. The herniated stomach is reduced, and the posterior mediastinal space is entered, exposing the distal esophagus. The crural fibers of the diaphragm at the esophageal hiatus are exposed, with the stomach distracted inferiorly and approximated (with nonabsorbable suture) posterior to the distal esophagus. The distal esophagus may be sutured to reflected portions of the peritoneum and the phrenicoesophageal (phrenoesophageal) ligament and to the gastric cardia, maintaining an acute esophagogastric angle. Care must be taken to avoid making the repair too tight and to injuring the vagus nerves. The anesthesia provider may be asked to pass a lubricated large-diameter esophageal bougie (e.g., Maloney or Hurst) to determine that the hiatus is not unduly compromised.

Preparation of the Patient

Antiembolitic hose are put on the legs. The patient is supine with the arms extended on padded armboards, or a modified lateral position may be employed. A pillow may be placed under the knees to avoid strain on the back muscles. Bony prominences and all areas vulnerable to skin and neurovascular pressure or trauma are padded. A lubricated nasogastric tube is passed by the anesthesia provider. A Foley catheter may be inserted. Electrosurgical dispersive pad is applied.

Skin Preparation

Abdominal approach: Begin at the midline, extending from nipples to knees and down to the table at the sides.

Draping

Folded towels and a laparotomy sheet

Equipment

Sequential compression device with disposable leg wraps, if requested
ESU
Suction

Instrumentation

Major procedures tray
GI tray
Vascular procedures tray
Thoracotomy tray, available
Large self-retaining retractor, e.g., Balfour

Hemoclip or similar ligating clip appliers (variety of lengths and sizes)
Bougies, e.g., Maloney or Hurst, to anesthesia provider

Supplies

Antiembolitic hose
Foley catheter with continuous drainage unit, as requested
N/G tube to the anesthesia provider
Basin set
Blades, (2) #10 and (1) #15
Needle magnet or counter
Suction tubing
Electrosurgical pencil and cord with holder and scraper
Hemoclips or similar ligating clips, variety of sizes
Small dissector sponges (e.g., peanut or Kittner)

Special Notes

- Apply **Special Notes** from ***Abdominal Laparotomy***, p. 134, as indicated.
- When the circulator checks the chart for patient sensitivities and allergies, he/she should note an allergy to latex products, as many products used in surgery contain latex, (e.g., gloves, drains [Penrose], adhesive tape, and elasticized bandages). The circulator documents he/she noted the latex allergy; the products substituted must be "latex-free." Document when an allergy to iodine is noted, as most skin prep solutions contain providone iodine; an alternate prep solution should be used. The substitute products used should be documented.
- Take appropriate measures to maintain patient's body temperature, e.g., offer warmed blanket, raise room temperature, apply forced-air warming blanket, when ordered.
- A small sponge used for dissection (e.g., peanut or Kittner) may be requested. Dissector sponges are included in the sponge count; see p. 40.
- The circulator accompanies the anesthesia provider taking the patient to the PACU; he/she gives the PACU perioperative practitioner a detailed intraoperative report regarding the course of events as they apply to the individual.
- Prior to leaving the OR, the circulator assures that the patient is properly positioned on the gurney, that lines are not kinked, and that measures necessary to maintain the patient's body temperature have been taken.

- In the PACU, the perioperative practitioner observes that the patient's breathing is unobstructed, monitors the patient's blood pressure and vital signs, and documents all pertinent information in the **Perioperative Record** in the **Postoperative Record**. Documentation is vital for patient safety regarding continuity of care and for medicolegal reasons.
- In the PACU, the perioperative practitioner assumes the role of the patient's advocate.

Laparoscopic Fundoplication (Nissen Procedure)

Definition

Endoscopic wrapping of the gastric fundus about the cardia to correct gastroesophageal reflux and/or hiatal hernia.

Discussion

In the adult, this procedure is used to treat gastroesophageal reflux disease (GERD) and certain presentations of an esophageal hiatal hernia by physically reestablishing the gastroesophageal angle and a barrier to intrathoracic gastric displacement.

For children, see Pediatric **Laparoscopic Fundoplication (Nissen),** p. 1070.

Procedure

Laparoscopic Fundoplication (Nissen) is described. Five ports are placed following establishment of pneumoperitoneum (as for ***Laparoscopic Vagotomy,*** p. 207). The left lobe of the liver is retracted, and the triangular ligament is incised, as necessary. The esophageal hiatus is visualized.

The gastric cardia is distracted, with reduction of the hiatal hernia, if present, and the phrenicoesophageal ligament is incised. The left gastric artery and vagal nerve branches are displaced. A window is dissected posterior to the distal esophagus, through which a drain or soft catheter (e.g., 12Fr or 14Fr) is placed to provide traction on the esophagus. The stomach is mobilized by dividing the short gastric vessels on the greater curvature.

If the esophageal hiatus is enlarged, several sutures may be placed to minimize the crural defect. The anesthesia provider may pass an esophageal dilator (50Fr to 60Fr), lubricated with water-soluble lubricant, transorally. The gastric fundus is seized with an atraumatic grasping forceps and passed posterior to the esophagus. An adjacent portion of the fundus is seized anterior to the esophagus (apposed to the posteriorly seized segment) and sutured or stapled (incorporating the esophagocardiac wall), completing the fundoplication.

By wrapping the proximal stomach around the gastroesophageal junction and "fixing" it to itself, the fundoplication prevents recurrent herniation. The drain or catheter and esophageal dilators are removed. After the surgical field is inspected for hemostasis and irrigated as necessary, pneumoperitoneum is released. The incisions are closed in the usual manner.

Preparation of the Patient

Apply antiembolitic hose, as requested. The patient is **supine** with arms extended on padded armboards, or the arms may be padded and tucked in at the patient's sides using the draw sheet. Padded shoulder braces and a padded footboard are secured to the table. All bony prominences and areas vulnerable to skin and neurovascular pressure or trauma are padded. A lubricated nasogastric tube is passed by the anesthesia provider. An electrosurgical dispersive pad is applied. A Foley catheter is inserted. The table is placed in Trendelenburg 5° to 10° to establish pneumoperitoneum and then in reverse Trendelenburg 10° to 20° to allow the viscera to gravitate inferiorly. The table may be rotated slightly to the right to increase exposure.

Skin Preparation

Begin at the midline extending from the axilla to the pubic symphysis and down to the table at the sides.

Draping

Folded towels and a laparotomy sheet

Equipment

Sequential compression device with disposable leg wraps, if requested
Padded shoulder braces
Padded footboard
Suction
ESU
Fiber-optic light source, e.g., Xenon 300 W
Video monitors (2)
VCR
CD burner
Printer
CO_2 insufflator
Camera console
Pressure bag to facilitate irrigation

Instrumentation

Limited procedures tray
Major procedures tray (available for conversion to "open" procedure)

Verres needle
Hasson trocar
Trocars, (2) or (3) 10 or 11 mm and (2) or (3) 5 mm
Reducer caps
Fiber-optic laparoscope with camera charged-coupled devices (CCD) and power (light) cord
Endoscopic instruments:
electrosurgical suction-irrigator/dissector with J hook tip or right angle tip, scissors (hook, straight, and micro), grasping clamps, e.g., Babcock (atraumatic) (2) 5 mm, (2) 10 mm, (2) Allis, fan retractor or Nathanson retractor (to retract the liver)
Multifire ligating clip applier, optional
Intracorporeal suturing device with introducer sleeve, e.g., EndoStitch

Supplies

Antiembolitic hose
N/G tube (e.g., 16Fr) to anesthesia provider
Bougies (e.g., Maloney or Hurst) to anesthesia provider, if requested
Foley catheter with continuous drainage unit
Soft catheter for retraction, e.g., Robinson 12Fr or 14Fr
Basin set
Blades, (1) #15 and (1) #11
Fog reduction agent, e.g., FRED, ELVIS
Suction tubing
Silastic tubing for CO_2
Cystoscopy or similar straight tubing, e.g., K50, a 1000-ml bag normal saline and three-way stopcock, for irrigation
Electrosurgical cord

Special Notes

- Apply **Special Notes** from ***Abdominal Laparoscopy,*** p. 140, as indicated.

Vagotomy and Pyloroplasty

Definition

Vagotomy. The transection of the vagus nerves (or peripheral divisions of the vagus nerves) performed at the level of the distal esophagus or at the gastric cardia to reduce gastric secretion (of hydrochloric acid) in patients with peptic ulcers.

Pyloroplasty. Enlargement of the gastric outlet (the pylorus) to enhance emptying of the stomach into the duodenum.

Discussion

Vagotomy is a conservative surgical therapy compared to ***gastrectomy*** regarding controlling gastric acid secretion. Vagotomy may be either truncal or selective.

In **truncal vagotomy,** the main trunks of the vagus nerve are interrupted, including branches to the stomach and other abdominal viscera.

Selective vagotomy (of which there are several modifications) is performed about the gastric cardia, so that only the gastric branches of the vagus nerves are interrupted.

Pyloroplasty is performed in conjunction with *truncal* vagotomy to enhance gastric emptying, which is otherwise delayed when the vagus nerves have been transected. When feasible, highly *selective* vagotomy can be performed, which includes transection of the posterior vagal trunk and seromyotomy along the lesser curvature interrupting the acid production innervation (i.e., selective branches of the anterior trunk). This spares the ability of the antrum to contract, obviating the need for pyloroplasty.

In recent years, the medical regimen for peptic ulcer disease by treatment of *Helicobacter pylori* with antibiotics and acid-reducing agents has greatly decreased the need for peptic ulcer surgery.

For **Discussion** and **Procedure** for **Laparoscopic Vagotomy,** see p. 207.).

Procedure

The upper abdomen is exposed through a midline, paramedian, or high-transverse incision. Physical findings are assessed, and either **truncal** or **selective vagotomy** is performed. Ligating clips (e.g., Hemoclips) are applied to the severed vagus nerve trunks.

Small sections of the vagus nerve are sent to pathology to confirm that neural tissue was actually divided. ***Pyloroplasty*** is then performed. The most common pyloroplasty procedure is the *Heinieke-Mikulicz;* the pyloroduodenal junction is incised longitudinally and closed transversely to facilitate gastric emptying.

In patients with severe bleeding, a gastrotomy or duodenotomy may be necessary to identify and control the bleeding site.

Preparation of the Patient

Antiembolitic hose are applied. The patient is supine; arms may be extended on padded armboards. A pillow may be placed under the sacrum and/or under the knees to relieve strain on back muscles. All bony prominences and areas vulnerable to skin and neurovascular trauma or pressure are padded. A Foley catheter may be inserted. The anesthesia provider places a lubricated nasogastric tube. An electrosurgical dispersive pad is applied.

Skin Preparation

Begin at the midline, extending from axilla to the pubic symphysis and down to the table at the sides.

Draping

Folded towels and a laparotomy or transverse sheet

Equipment

Sequential compression device with disposable leg wraps, as requested
ESU
Suction

Instrumentation

Major procedures tray
Long instruments tray
Gastrointestinal procedures tray
Blunt nerve hook (e.g., Smithwick)
Hemoclip or similar ligating clip appliers (various sizes and lengths, especially long)
Large self-retaining retractor, e.g., Balfour

Supplies

Antiembolitic hose
Foley catheter (with continuous drainage unit), as requested
N/G tube to the anesthesia provider
Basin set
Blades (3) #10 and (1) #15
Needle magnet or counter
Suction tubing
Electrosurgical pencil and cord with holder and scraper
Penrose drains (2), long, 1″ for traction on esophagus
Hemoclips or similar ligating clips, assorted sizes
Hemostatic agents, e.g., Gelfoam®, Surgicel™
Disposable stapler, e.g., TA 55™ for closure of longitudinal incision across pylorus, as requested

Special Notes

- Apply **Special Notes** from ***Abdominal Laparotomy***, p. 134, as indicated.

- Wet the Penrose drain with saline before passing it on clamp (e.g., Pean forceps) to the surgeon; the drain is used for traction.
- **N.B.** *Specimens of the vagus nerve must be correctly identified as "neural" tissue; therefore, the specimens are placed on pieces of Telfa™ (or other nonsticking type pad), labeled, and sent to the lab for a frozen section.*
- If ***Gastrotomy*** or ***Duodenotomy*** is performed, instruments used intraluminally are isolated in a basin.

Laparoscopic Vagotomy

Definition

The endoscopic transection of the vagus nerves (or peripheral divisions) at the level of the distal esophagus or gastric cardia.

Discussion

There are numerous procedures and modifications to diminish gastric acid secretion related to peptic ulcer disease. Many of these modifications can be performed laparoscopically. Most often, interruption of the vagus nerves is performed. **Selective vagotomy** versus **truncal (complete) vagotomy** permits gastric emptying without the need for an accompanying drainage procedure (***pyloroplasty, gastrojejunostomy, partial gastrectomy,*** etc.) unless advanced peptic ulcer disease with fibrosis or stricture is present, in which case the latter may be necessary.

In some instances within several hours of perforation of a peptic ulcer, **vagotomy** may be combined with the application of an omental patch to the site of the perforation.

Procedure

Pneumoperitoneum is established. Additional ports are established inferior to the left and right costal margins, in the mid-axillary line, the subxiphoid, and the mid-left upper quadrant. Through a right subcostal port, an extrudable fan-shaped retractor (e.g., Laparolift™) or Nathanson retractor is inserted to displace the left lobe of the liver (dividing the triangular ligament if necessary). A laparoscope (30°) is preferred for this procedure by most surgeons. A lubricated large-bore nasogastric tube or an esophageal dilator, e.g., Maloney or Hurst's, may be passed to facilitate traction on the stomach. As indicated, an endoscope may be passed to dilate the pylorus.

The lesser sac is entered, and the tissues along the lesser curvature of the stomach to the esophageal hiatus are dissected. The left gastric vein may be divided between sutures or ligating clips. The left margin of the right crus of the diaphragm and the stomach are retracted to the left. The paraesophageal tissues are dissected to expose the esophagus, which is retracted to the left. The posterior vagus nerve is identified, divided, and ligated with clips. A section of the specimen (neural tissue) is sent for histological confirmation.

The anterior vagus nerve is now exposed. Most often a **selective vagotomy** is elected (*versus* **truncal**). Branches to the other viscera (including the nerve of Laterget) are preserved. Gastric branches are identified (employing dissection of the gastric serosa as necessary), clipped, and divided. A tissue specimen is sent for histological examination. Hemostasis is assured. The abdomen is irrigated; an antibiotic solution may be used. Pneumoperitoneum is released, and the incisions are closed.

An alternative procedure is the ***Posterior Truncal Vagotomy with Anterior Seromyotomy (Taylor's Procedure).*** This procedure is identical to the one described up to the division of the posterior vagal trunk. As branches of the anterior vagus nerve are often imbedded within the seromuscular layer of the stomach, preventing division of the individual branches, a seromyotomy 1.5 cm from the lesser curvature from the cardia to a point proximal to the pylorus (5 to 7 cm) is made. Care is taken to avoid penetration of the mucosa. The seromyotomy is then repaired with staples or a running suture. (A variation of the procedure is to distract a seromuscular strip [in lieu of seromyotomy], excising it using a multifire linear stapler, thus interrupting the intramural vagal branches.) Methylene blue dye may be instilled in the stomach via nasogastric tube to verify integrity of the gastric repair. A fibrin sealant (e.g., Tissucol™ or Tisseel VH™) may be applied to the suture line.

After the vagotomy is complete, a ***Congo red test*** may be performed. In addition to histological confirmation that the nervous tissue was removed, testing for gastric acidity may be done intraoperatively. (*Pentagastrin* [to stimulate gastric acid production] 6 μg/kg is given subcutaneously by the anesthesia provider.)

Hemostasis is assured. The pneumoperitoneum is released. Incisions are closed in the usual manner.

Congo Red Test. Twenty minutes prior to the testing, the stomach is lavaged through a gastroscope with sodium bicarbonate solution to remove residual acid. *Congo red dye* is instilled into the stomach to coat the gastric mucosa. If **vagotomy** is complete, the red dye remains unchanged. If even partial innervation remains, the affected area will turn black (as seen via the scope) and additional nerve transection may be done.

Preparation of the Patient

Apply antiembolitic hose to the legs, as requested. The patient is supine; arms may be extended on padded armboards, or arms may be padded and tucked in at the patient's sides using the draw sheet. A pad under the sacral area and/or a pillow may be placed under the knees to relieve strain on back muscles. Padded shoulder braces and a padded footboard are secured to the table. Bony prominences and all areas vulnerable to skin and neurovascular trauma or pressure are padded. The anesthesia provider passes a lubricated nasogastric tube. A Foley catheter may be inserted. Electrosurgical dispersive pad is applied.

The table is placed in Trendelenburg 5° to 10° to establish pneumoperitoneum and then in reverse Trendelenburg 10° to 20° to allow the abdominal viscera to gravitate inferiorly. The table may be rotated slightly to the right to increase exposure of the stomach intraoperatively.

Skin Preparation

Begin at the midline extending from axilla to the pubic symphysis and down to the table at the sides.

Draping

Folded towels and a laparotomy sheet

Equipment

Sequential compression device with disposable leg wraps, if requested
Suction
ESU
Fiber-optic light source (e.g., Xenon 300 W)
Video monitor
VCR
Printer
CD burner
CO_2 insufflator
Camera console
Pressure bag to facilitate irrigation

Instrumentation

Limited procedures tray, open
Major procedures tray, available
Verres needle
Hasson trocar
Trocars, 10 or 11 mm (2 or 3)
Trocars, 5 mm (2 or 3)
Reducer caps
Fiber-optic laparoscope with camera and power (light) cord
Endoscopic instruments:
Electrosurgical suction-irrigator/dissector with J hook tip or right angle tip and cord, scissors (hook, straight, and micro), grasping clamps, e.g., (2) atraumatic Babcock 5 mm, (2) 10 mm,

and (2) Allis, fan retractor, and Nathanson retractor
Multifire ligating clip appliers
Suturing device, e.g., EndoStitch
Flexible fiber-optic gastroscope and associated equipment and instruments, see *Gastroscopy*, p. 185.

Supplies

Antiembolitic hose
Foley catheter with continuous drainage unit, as requested
N/G tube (e.g., 16Fr) to anesthesia provider
Dilators to the anesthesia provider (e.g., Maloney or Hurst), if requested
Basin set
Blades, (1) #15 and (1) #11
Electrosurgical cord
Suction tubing
Fog reduction agent, FRED, ELVIS
Silastic tubing
Cystoscopy or similar straight tubing, e.g., K50, a 1000-ml bag normal saline, and three-way stopcock for irrigation
Methylene blue dye and Luer lok syringe, if requested
Fibrin tissue sealant, e.g., Tissucol or Tisseel VH
Antibiotic irrigation, if requested

Special Notes

- Apply **Special Notes** from ***Abdominal Laparoscopy***, p. 140, as indicated.
- If an endoscopist other than the surgeon is to perform gastroscopy (when included in procedure), ample notification must be given, i.e., the gastroenterologist must be notified regarding the time he/she will be needed (according to the OR schedule).
- The ***Endoscopy Cart*** (with necessary consoles, equipment, etc.) should be brought into the room before the patient when gastroscopy is performed.

Closure of a Perforated Peptic Ulcer

Definition

Repair of a full thickness of gastric or duodenal ulcer that has penetrated into the peritoneal cavity.

Discussion

A complication of *peptic ulcer disease* is spontaneous perforation with the escape of gastroduodenal secretions and contents into the peritoneal cavity, resulting in peritonitis. The presentation may be mild with a spontaneous closure of the perforation treated by nonsurgical means, or it may result in an extensive *life-threatening* peritonitis. Less often, a gastric malignancy may present in similar fashion. Numerous surgical procedures are described for this condition.

When preexisting peptic ulcer disease has been present and the peritoneal irritation is limited, a vagotomy and drainage procedure may be performed; see ***Vagotomy and Pyloroplasty***, p. 204.

Procedure

An upper abdominal incision (midline, right paramedian) is made. The site of perforation is identified. Fluid and debris are aspirated. If not already partially adherent to the perforation, a portion of adjacent greater omentum (or gastrocolic ligament, etc.) is sutured or stapled to the stomach or the duodenum surrounding the perforation. If malignancy is suspected, appropriate biopsies may be taken. Concomitant ***vagotomy and pyloroplasty*** (p. 204) may then be performed. The peritoneal cavity is irrigated with an antibiotic solution. After hemostasis is assured and the drains are placed (and secured with a stitch), the wound is closed in the usual manner.

For Preparation of the Patient, Skin Preparation, Draping, Equipment, Instruments, Supplies, and **Special Notes,** see *Vagotomy and Pyloroplasty*, p. 205.

Special Notes

- Apply **Special Notes** from **Vagotomy and Pyloroplasty**, p. 206, as indicated.
- The scrub person should be prepared to aspirate fluid from the peritoneal cavity, following irrigation of the abdomen (e.g., with Poole suction).
- Instruments used intraluminally for bowel surgeries are isolated in a basin.
- Consult the surgeon regarding the type of antibiotic irrigation he/she plans to use, if any.
- Surgical team members should wear face shields to prevent contaminated gastric and peritoneal contents from splashing or spraying into their eyes, or onto mucous membranes.

Laparoscopic Closure of a Perforated Ulcer (With Vagotomy)

Definition

Closure of a perforated stomach or duodenal ulcer and excision of the vagus nerve and its branches; laparoscopically.

Discussion

Limitations to this approach include advanced peritonitis, dense adhesions, etc.

Procedure

Pneumoperitoneum and ports are established as for ***Laparoscopic Vagotomy***; see p. 207. The pathology is assessed, and fluid is aspirated and sent for culture. The peritoneal cavity may be irrigated. The site of the perforation is closed with endoscopic sutures, if feasible. An omental patch is then stapled or sutured over the site of the perforation.

An alternative technique, less frequently employed, is intralumenal endoscopic. An endoscope is passed transorally, through which a grasping forceps is placed from within the stomach or duodenum into the peritoneal cavity, seizing (with laparoscopic guidance) a portion of omentum. The omentum is retracted onto the perforation. The patch is secured with endoscopic suture or staples, and the endoscope is withdrawn.

Vagotomy (with drainage procedure) may then be performed, as described in ***Laparoscopic Vagotomy,*** p. 207. A closed suction drain may be placed (e.g., Hemovac™) and secured with a stitch. After release of pneumoperitoneum, the incisions are closed in the usual manner.

For **Preparation of the Patient, Skin Preparation, Draping, Equipment, Instruments, Supplies,** and **Special Notes,** see *Laparoscopic Vagotomy*, p. 208.

Gastrostomy

Definition

Establishment of an artificial opening into the stomach exiting onto the skin of the abdominal wall.

Discussion

A **gastrostomy,** either temporary or permanent, is used to drain the stomach when there is an obstruction or to allow for liquid feedings (on long-term or permanent basis) for patients with esophageal stricture or tumor, or for general feeding for the patient unable to take oral nourishment on a long-term basis. A catheter (e.g., Foley) maintains the patency of the gastrostomy tract.

As an alternative to an open surgical procedure, **percutaneous endoscopic gastrostomy (PEG)** may be performed in the radiology department special procedure suite or, if necessary, for critically ill patients at the patient's bedside or in the operating room.

Percutaneous endoscopic gastrostomy (PEG) is described. A well-lubricated flexible fiber-optic gastroscope is passed into the stomach;

the stomach is distended with air. The lighted tip of the scope is impacted on the gastric wall, which is then positioned to be directly under the parietal peritoneum, displacing the liver edge and colon. X-ray or ultrasound may be employed to confirm the position of the gastric wall onto the parietal abdominal wall. If the patient is awake, local anesthesia is injected at the site of the intended gastrostomy. A second operator passes a catheter through a percutaneous stab wound, aiming at the transilluminated gastroscope tip. The catheter passes through the abdominal wall (following a guide wire and dilators, which enlarge the puncture tract) and into the stomach, where it is seized via the scope and its intragastric position confirmed. Various catheters are used, including balloon and loop tips to prevent dislodgement. Tissue anchors may be placed percutaneously to secure the gastric wall to the parietal abdominal wall about the catheter entry site. The catheter is secured to the skin about the stab wound. An alternative method is to pass the catheter transorally, seizing same from within the stomach with a percutaneously inserted grasper.

N.B. *PEG (and tissue anchor) kits are available.*

Gastrostomy is often performed as an adjunct to a more extensive procedure. In the debilitated patient, gastrostomy may be performed under local anesthesia.

Procedure

A gastrostomy (e.g., feeding) as an isolated procedure is described. A limited transverse left upper abdominal incision is employed. The peritoneal cavity is entered, the gastric wall is identified, and concentric purse-string sutures are placed. A small incision is made into the stomach, within the innermost purse-string suture, through which a catheter is passed. The purse-string sutures are secured. The catheter can exit through the incision or preferably through a separate stab wound and secured. The gastric wall is sutured intra-abdominally at a few points to the peritoneal surface about the stab wound. The peritoneal cavity may be irrigated, usually with an antibiotic solution. The abdomen is closed in layers.

Preparation of the Patient

When **gastrostomy** is performed in the OR, the patient is supine; arms may be extended on padded armboards. A pillow may be placed under the sacral area and/or under the knees to relieve strain on back muscles. Antiembolitic hose may be put on the legs, if requested. All bony prominences and areas vulnerable to skin and neurovascular pressure or trauma are padded. Apply electrosurgical dispersive pad.

Skin Preparation

Begin at the intended site of incision (usually transverse left upper abdominal), extending from nipples to upper thighs and down to the table at the sides.

Draping

Folded towels and a transverse sheet

Equipment

Suction
ESU
Fiber-optic light source, e.g., Xenon 300 W
Air insufflation unit

Instrumentation

Flexible fiber-optic gastroscope (for both "open" and percutaneous approach)

"Open" Procedure

Major procedures tray
GI tray, available
Ligating clip appliers, e.g., Hemoclip

Percutaneous Procedure

Limited procedures tray
PEG kit (e.g., Moss, which includes a T-Anchor™ gun and anchors), available

Supplies

Bite block (to protect scope), as necessary
Antiembolitic hose, if requested
N/G tube to anesthesia provider
Electrosurgical pencil and cord
Suction tubing
Basin set
Blades, (2) #10 and (1) #15
Needle magnet or counter
Hemoclips or similar ligating clips, various sizes
Antibiotic irrigation, if requested
Silastic tubing for air insufflator
Gastrostomy catheter (e.g., Foley, Pezzer)
Catheter plug

Special Notes

- Apply **Special Notes** from ***Abdominal Laparotomy***, p. 134, as indicated.
- In **gastrostomy**, instruments used intraluminally are isolated in a basin.

- Surgical team members should wear face shields to prevent contaminated gastric contents from splashing or spraying into their eyes or onto mucous membranes.
- The stab wound made for the catheter is made with a #11 or #15 blade; the catheter is grasped with a Pean clamp. The catheter is secured with a skin stitch.
- A catheter plug is placed at the conclusion of procedure.

Gastrectomy

Definition

Removal of the entire stomach or a portion of the stomach and the reestablishment of the continuity of the gastrointestinal tract.

Discussion

Subtotal (partial) gastrectomy refers to the excision of a portion of the stomach performed primarily for peptic ulcer disease or tumor of the distal stomach. A *vagotomy* (see p. 204) may be included. Gastrointestinal continuity is reestablished by anastomosing of the gastric remnant to the proximal duodenum **(Billroth I)** or to the proximal jejunum (**Billroth II**, or a modification of it). When treating malignancies, the greater omentum, lymph nodes, and adjacent organs (e.g., spleen) are removed.

Total gastrectomy is performed because of malignancy or uncontrollable bleeding. Continuity of the gastrointestinal tract is established by anastomosing distal esophagus to the proximal jejunum, usually with the creation of a pouch or reservoir. (The duodenum or an isolated segment of colon can also replace the resected stomach.) The lymph nodes, adjacent organs (such as spleen), and greater omentum are removed when treating malignancies.

A laparoscopic approach or laparoscopically assisted technique may be employed.

Procedure

The incision may be upper midline or bilateral subcostal. For **total gastrectomy**, a thoracoabdominal incision may be necessary. The pathology is identified, and its operability assessed. The stomach is mobilized by clamping and dividing the vascular attachments.

The greater omentum and sometimes the spleen are resected in continuity with the stomach en bloc when malignancy is present. According to the extent of the resection and the type of anastomosis to be fashioned, the duodenum or jejunum is mobilized and anastomosed to the gastric remnant or the distal esophagus anterior to (or posterior to) the transverse colon.

A retrocolic anastomosis requires an incision to be made in a relatively avascular portion of the transverse mesocolon. The anastomosis is facilitated by the use of automatic stapling devices, or clamps and a wide variety of sutures and suturing techniques may be employed. A side-to-side jejunal pouch may be required when total gastrectomy is performed. A drain (e.g., Jackson-Pratt™ or Hemovac) is inserted. If the pleural space has been entered, an intrapleural sealed drainage unit (e.g., Pleurevac) is necessary. The wound is closed in layers. Drains are anchored with a skin suture.

Preparation of the Patient

For an upper midline or bilateral subcostal approach, antiembolitic hose are applied. The patient is supine with arms extended on padded armboards. A pillow may be placed under the sacrum and/or under the knees to relieve strain on back muscles. All bony prominences and areas vulnerable to skin and neurovascular pressure or trauma are padded. An electrosurgical dispersive pad is applied. A Foley catheter is inserted.

For a thoracoabdominal approach, antiembolitic hose are put on the legs. The patient is in a modified (45° -) right lateral position with the left side uppermost. The right arm is extended on a padded armboard; the left arm is supported by a Mayo stand (padded with a pillow), or a double armboard may be used. The left leg is extended and the right leg is flexed, or both legs may be flexed with a pillow between the knees. Pad areas around the feet and ankles. A pillow folded longitudinally may be necessary to support the back. Pad all bony prominences and areas vulnerable to neurovascular pressure or trauma. The position is secured by wide adhesive tape (after checking chart for patient allergies), following the application of tincture of benzoin, from the shoulders, hips, and legs to the underside of the table. An electrosurgical dispersive pad is applied. A Foley catheter is inserted.

Skin Preparation

For an upper midline or bilateral subcostal approach, begin at intended site of incision, extending from the axilla to just above the pubic symphysis and down to the table at the sides.

For a thoracoabdominal approach, begin at the intended site of incision, extending from the shoulder to the iliac crest and down to the table, anteriorly and posteriorly.

Draping

Four folded towels and a laparotomy sheet

Equipment

Sequential pressure device with disposable leg wraps, as requested
Suction

Electrosurgical unit
Pillows, pads for positioning (for thoracoabdominal approach)
Scales for weighing sponges (2)

Instrumentation

Major procedures tray
Long instruments tray
GI procedures tray
Hemoclip or similar clip appliers (various sizes and lengths)
Long blunt nerve hooks (2), e.g., Smithwick)
Vascular procedures tray (available)
Disposable automatic stapling devices, e.g., LDS™ and TA 55 or 30™ and TA 90™ or GIA™ and EEA™, optional
Large self-retaining retractor (e.g., Balfour, Bookwalter system, Martin arm)

Supplies

Antiembolitic hose
Foley catheter with urimeter and continuous drainage unit
N/G tube to anesthesia provider
Blades, (2) #10 and (1) #15
Basin set
Needle magnet or counter
Suction tubing
Electrosurgical pencil and cord with holder and scraper
Hemoclips or similar ligating clips (variety of sizes)
Drain (e.g., Jackson-Pratt, Hemovac)

For Thoracoabdominal Approach, Add

Chest tubes (e.g., Argyle)
Intrapleural sealed drainage unit (e.g., Pleurevac)
Y-connector
Bulb syringe

Special Notes

- Apply **Special Notes** from ***Abdominal Laparotomy,*** p. 134, as indicated.
- The circulator should check that the correct number of blood (and/or blood product) units that were ordered are ready and available.
- The circulator assists the anesthesia provider in verifying identification for administering blood and blood products. Prepare IV tubing, blood warmer, and blood pump, as needed.

- Weigh sponges to accurately determine fluid loss replacement. Two scales are used, one for raytec sponges and one for lap pads. Calculate the weight of the dry sponge and set the scale to 0 after weight adjustment.
- Keep an accurate record of irrigation used to accurately determine replacement of fluid loss.
- The scrub person should be prepared with large atraumatic vascular clamps ready (prevents tissue damage to bowel).
- Keep all soiled instruments (e.g., those that are used intraluminally) isolated in a basin.
- The scrub person should be prepared with long, free ties mounted on a tonsil (or long tonsil) clamp.
- Frozen section may be requested.
- The specimen is received in a large basin.
- Surgeon may request a "clean" closure of the abdomen; this may include any or all of the following: regowning, regloving, redraping, and a Basic/Minor procedures tray. "Clean" closure is at the discretion of the surgeon, as it is not required in upper GI procedures.

Bariatric Surgery

Definition

Procedures to treat morbid obesity that alter the gastrointestinal tract to effect weight loss by reducing the capacity of the stomach.

Discussion

Persons who are morbidly obese, weighing at least 100 pounds more than their ideal weight, may be candidates for ***bariatric surgery***. Surgery to induce weight loss is performed only after nonsurgical means have failed and the patient has undergone medical and psychological evaluation. While individualized, weight in excess of 100 pounds of "ideal" weight or body mass index (BMI) greater than 40 (35 to 40 in diabetics and hypertensives) are criteria for this surgery with its significant risks, acute and long term.

The physiologic considerations in performing ***bariatric surgery*** are:

1. Anatomical restriction of the ability to comfortably contain ingested food.
2. Metabolic restriction, in which absorptive capacity of the intestinal tract is altered by short circuiting the small intestine and/or diverting biliopancreatic secretions. Some procedures combine both aspects to achieve results.

There are numerous procedures, some of which have been abandoned due to long-term metabolic consequences (such as ***jejuno-ileal bypass***). Other procedures may have to be reversed, revised, or converted to an alternative configuration. Gastroscopic placement of an intragastric balloon has largely been abandoned because of erosive side effects and its ineffectiveness.

A "gastric pacemaker" with electrodes applied to the proximal stomach to produce feelings of satiety with rapid emptying has not been applied for routine use. ***Panniculectomy*** (see p. 762) and/or ***liposuction***, (see p. 765) which directly removes redundant skin and adipose tissues, can be performed in conjunction with or after the procedures that physiologically effect weight loss. The most commonly performed procedures include laparoscopic **adjustable gastric banding** that restricts ingested food volume capacity and **vertical gastric banding** may be performed "open" or laparoscopically; the band (e.g., LAP-BAND®) partitions the stomach and restricts ingested food volume capacity. In **proximal gastric bypass** performed "open" or laparoscopically, a small proximal gastric pouch is anastomosed to the mid-jejunum, and biliopancreatic diversion is achieved with partial gastrectomy and gastric pouch to distal small bowel anastomosis or biliopancreatic diversion with duodenal switch (in which ***partial gastrectomy*** decreases the size of the stomach but preserves the pyloric channel, which is anastomosed to the distal small bowel).

In these procedures, a thorough medical assessment, including history and physical examination, nutritional assessment, and psychiatric evaluation must be performed preoperatively. Anesthesia precautions must be strictly considered and observed in the morbidly obese. These patients must be closely observed for signs of shock and respiratory distress.

Laparoscopic Adjustable Gastric Banding and Proximal Gastric Bypass

Procedure

Laparoscopic Gastric Banding: Laparoscopic entry to the upper abdomen is achieved; ports are placed. Retraction of the liver is often necessary for exposure. A tunnel is created circumferentially by dissection around the proximal stomach. A grasper is used to pass an encircling silicone band (LAP-BAND®) around the proximal stomach and is "locked." Sutures fix the band in place to prevent slippage. The band tubing is brought into a deep subcutaneous position and connected to its reservoir, implanted into the abdominal wall, allowing percutaneous access to inject or withdraw saline to alter the constrictive degree of the band. The wounds are closed.

Proximal Gastric Bypass Roux-en-Y Configuration (open technique): The abdomen is entered through an upper midline incision. If gallstones are noted (or documented on preoperative x-ray), ***cholecystectomy*** (p. 148) may be performed. The distal esophagus and proximal stomach are mobilized, and the gastrohepatic ligament is incised. A drain or catheter may be used for traction. Between the first and second branches of the left gastric artery, the stomach is stapled (three rows) or stapled and transected after being certain that tubes (e.g., nasogastric or esophageal stethoscope) are first withdrawn. The drain or catheter can help to guide placement of the stapler. The proximal pouch created should have 30 ml capacity.

At 45 cm distal to the ligament of Treitz, the jejunum is divided. An 8- to 12-cm segment may be excised to allow more mobility for the ensuing gastric pouch anastomosis (without undue tension in these obese structures). The proximal limb is anastomosed to the distal jejunum (45 to 150 cm from the site of division, depending on the desired weight loss assessment) employing a linear stapler. The distal limb is anastomosed to the gastric pouch, usually retrocolic, via an incision in the transverse mesocolon. Hand-sewn or staple technique can be employed. The anesthesia provider passes a Maloney or Hurst dilator (e.g., 30Fr) down the esophagus before the anterior anastomotic layer is completed to assure a stoma of this diameter. A nasogastric tube is inserted, and methylene blue dye (diluted) is instilled to test for anastomotic leakage. The tube is left in the jejunal limb. A ***gastrostomy*** (p. 212) may be performed to decompress the excluded gastric remnant. All mesenteric defects are closed. Antibiotic irrigation of the subcutaneous tissues may be done. The wound is closed.

This procedure may be performed laparoscopically, employing a disposable endoscopic circular stapler, the anvil of which is passed perorally into the esophagus (when possible) in conjunction with a percutaneously passed snare wire that is used retrogradely to seize the anvil for the pouch-jejunal anastomosis. Using a linear stapler, e.g., GIA™, may be preferable. Also, hand-assisted technique using a hand port, e.g., LAP-PORT™ may be employed.

Preparation of the Patient

Perioperative personnel must be aware of the many surgical and anesthesia risk factors inherent in the extremely obese patient to develop a **Perioperative Care Plan** with interventions that will result in optimal outcomes for the patient. Hemodynamic factors must be assessed in positioning the patient. Also, emotional support is extremely important, the patient's feelings must be considered, as he/she may be sensitive about his/her physical condition. Treating the patient with dignity will go a long way in helping the patient cope and maintain self-esteem while in this vulnerable position (as surgical patient).

The morbidly obese patient may require an extension be placed on the table or two operating tables placed side by side. In some facilities, a specially sized bed is available that is taken into the OR. Safety belts made of Velcro® may be attached to each other, or extenders may be needed, or a specially sized belt may be used. When the patient is moved from the bed to the table, and postoperatively, from table to bed, an automatic lift (e.g., Hoyer or Invacare) can be employed; the lift should be in the room before bringing patient into the room.

In addition, the patient may have difficulty breathing in the supine position when the table is flat. The head of the table is elevated as directed by the anesthesia provider, or extra pillows can be used to ease respiration until anesthesia is induced. Arms are extended on specially sized padded armboards, or two padded armboards may be required for each arm. A padded headboard and padded footboard are secured onto the table. The anesthesia provider may require assistance when inserting the IV, as finding a vein may be difficult. A pillow may be placed under the knees to avoid strain on back muscles. All areas prone to skin and neurovascular pressure or injury (e.g., the heels) are padded. Regarding the use of antiembolitic hose the correct size may not be available; the disposable leg wraps may be put directly onto the legs. The wraps are connected to a sequential compression device (to avoid thrombus formation). Apply an electrosurgical dispersive pad.

Laparoscopic or "open" approach procedures with general anesthesia are employed. Intubation may require bronchofiberscopic assistance perorally or nasally; the fiber-optic bronchoscope should be available at the anesthesia provider's side. The circulator must be ready to stand at the head of the table to render assistance as needed by the anesthesia provider and to provide emotional support to the patient as anesthesia is induced. Following intubation, the anesthesia provider inserts a lubricated nasogastric tube. An indwelling catheter, e.g., Foley, is inserted (prior to the abdominal prep) and attached to continuous drainage.

Skin Preparation

Two prep sets or additional sponges and solution may be necessary. Begin at the midline, extending from the axilla to mid-thighs and down to the table at the sides. If the patient has a large panniculus, the surgeon usually devises a method of support for the panniculus that enables the circulator to prep the skin area under it adequately.

Draping

Folded towels and a laparotomy sheet

Equipment

Automatic lift for moving the patient (e.g., Hoyer or Invacare)
Pillows, pads for positioning

Sequential pressure device with disposable leg wraps
Suction
ESU
Scales (2) for weighing sponges
Padded shoulder braces
Padded footboard
Padded table extension, as necessary

For Laparoscopic Procedure, Add
Endoscopy Cart: (where available)
Fiber-optic light source, e.g., Xenon 300 W
Video monitors (2)
VCR
CO_2 insufflator and irrigator
Suction
Camera console
Pressure bag to facilitate irrigation
CD burner
VCR
Printer

Instrumentation

Major procedures tray (open)
Esophageal dilator set, e.g., Maloney or Hurst (to anesthesia provider)
Long instruments tray
Gastrointestinal (GI) procedures tray
Cholecystectomy tray (available)
Bilary tract procedures tray (available)
Vascular tray (available)
Hemoclip or similar clip appliers (various sizes and lengths)
Vascular procedures tray (available)
Automatic stapling devices, e.g., GIA, EEA (optional)
Self-retaining retractor, extra-large (e.g., Bookwalter retractor system)

For Laparoscopy, Add
Verres needle
Hasson trocar
Trocars, five total, e.g., 2 or 3 10 or 11 mm and 2 or 3 5 mm
Reducer caps
Fiber-optic laparoscope with camera and power (light) cord
Endoscopic instruments:
electrosurgical suction irrigator/dissector with J hook tip or right-angle tip and cord, scissors (hook, straight, and micro,

grasping clamps (total of (6): (2) atraumatic Babcock 5 mm, (2) 10 mm, and (2) Allis), suturing device, fan retractor, Nathanson retractor

Disposable automatic endoscopic stapler/multifire ligating clip appliers, e.g., EEA©, GIA©

Supplies

Foley catheter with urimeter to continuous drainage unit
N/G tube to anesthesia provider
Methylene blue dye to anesthesia provider
Blades, (2) #10 and (1) #11
Basin set
Needle magnet or counter
Suction tubing
Electrosurgical pencil and cord with holder and scraper
Hemoclips or other ligating clips (various sizes and lengths)
Fibrin tissue sealant, e.g., Tisseel VH, Tissucol

For Laparoscopy, Add

Silastic™ tubing (for CO_2 insufflation)
Fog reduction agent, FRED, ELVIS
Suction tubing
Cystoscopy or similar straight tubing, e.g., K50, add 1000-ml bag normal saline and three-way stopcock for irrigation
Hand port (e.g., LAP DISC™, HANDPORT™, LAP-PORT™, Intromit™, Omniport™ Dexterity Device™) for hand-assisted procedures, if requested

Special Notes

- Apply **Special Notes** from ***Pancreaticoduodenectomy (Whipple Procedure)***, p. , as indicated. For endoscopic approaches apply **Special Notes** from *Abdominal Laparoscopy*, p. 140, as indicated.
- The circulator should try to meet the patient in advance (at least the day before whenever possible) to assess the perioperative nursing care requirements of this individual.
- The surgical team should make an ongoing effort to gather information, including research methods others have devised to meet the special perioperative needs of the extremely obese patient. One suggestion made is for antiembolitic hose to not be worn by the patient when a sequential compression device is employed. The disposable leg wraps are used without hose; they are applied directly onto the legs. Another suggestion is using an automatic lift to move the patient (e.g., Hoyer or Invacare).

- Members of the surgical team at some hospitals consult with personnel from the involved hospital departments to develop a coordinated overview of care that will meet the bariatric patient's perioperative needs.
- Consult with surgeon and anesthesia provider to prepare the room in advance (prior to bringing the patient into the OR).
- The circulator must always use the **JC** *Universal Protocol* to identify that the patient is the correct patient, anticipating the correct surgery on the correctly marked side (laterality) and site. See the **JC**'s *Universal Protocol*, p. 18, as necessary.
- Before every surgery begins, an official *"time out"* must be taken as a safety measure. "*Time out*" is required and must be documented on the **Perioperative Record** for patient safety and for medicolegal reasons.
- Perioperative personnel should review the suggested **Patient Care Plan,** p. 9, for care of the bariatric surgical patient, p. 218, and adjust it accordingly. The circulator adapts care to meet the individual patient's needs by implementing nursing interventions that result in optimal desired outcomes for the patient.
- The circulator must continually assess and evaluate the patient's physiological status throughout the procedure to choose and implement nursing interventions that will best result in desired outcomes for the patient.
- All care must be documented in the **Perioperative Record** for continuity of care and medicolegal reasons.
- Assist the anesthesia provider during the administration of general anesthesia. Intubation of the obese patient may be difficult. Obtain additional equipment before the patient is brought into the room (e.g., fiber-optic bronchoscope to the anesthesia provider) as necessary.
- The circulator should have the *Emergency Airway Cart* in the room and be prepared to help anesthesia provider during the induction phase of general anesthesia.
- The circulator should be certain the "*Crash Cart*" is nearby to avoid delay should an emergency situation occur, such as cardiac arrest.
- The circulator should immediately summon help should an emergency situation occur.
- **Reminder:** The circulator conveys to the patient that he/she will act as the patient's advocate while the patient is in surgery.

- **Reminder:** It is important for the circulator to provide measures of emotional support to the patient, e.g., maintain eye contact and hold the patient's hand during the administration of anesthesia.
- Ascertain that equipment has been properly secured onto the table to ensure patient safety. Prevent injuries by checking the strength and functioning of all equipment that will be used or added to the table.
- Prevent musculoskeletal strains to personnel and the patient by employing ergodynamic measures whenever necessary; see Body Mechanics/Ergonomic Safety, p. 51. Use aids such as lifts, rollers, slides, etc. for moving the patient, as necessary.
- Assess hemodynamic factors in positioning the patient and take appropriate measures, such as applying leg wraps directly to the patient's legs for sequential compression, do not cross legs, etc.
- Provide pillows to elevate the head to aid the patient's respiration and to and make positioning more comfortable.
- Take appropriate measures to maintain patient's body temperature by offering a blanket from the warmer, raising room temperature, and/or applying forced-air warming blanket, when ordered.
- Avoid patient feelings of embarrassment by exposing only the area involved in the surgery, while all other areas are adequately covered.
- Provide emotional support to the patient regarding feelings of altered body image by providing the patient an opportunity to express his/her feelings.
- Provide measures of reassurance to help patient cope with fear and anxiety regarding the serious nature of the surgery and the unfamiliar environment by answering questions in a knowledgeable manner whenever possible and referring questions to the surgeon, as necessary.
- The circulator should check that blood and/or blood product units that were ordered are ready and that the correct number of units is available.
- Weigh sponges accurately to help to determine fluid loss replacement. Two scales are necessary to weigh each type of sponges (raytec and lap) separately.
- Keep an accurate record of irrigation fluid used to determine fluid replacement.
- Large atraumatic vascular clamps and Glassman (GI) clamps (that prevent tissue damage to the bowel) are employed for the bowel anastomoses or disposable automatic staplers may be used.

- Do not open disposable staplers, etc., until they are specifically requested and the exact size has been determined, as they are expensive; this is a price control measure.
- Keep all soiled instruments (those used intraluminally) isolated in a basin.
- Prepare long free ties mounted on an extra-long tonsil forceps.
- Check that anesthesia provider has the desired esophageal dilators or obtain same, as necessary.

Jejunostomy

Definition

Creation of an opening between the jejunum and the abdominal wall.

Discussion

The jejunum can be affected by a variety of primary and secondary conditions, including benign, malignant, and metastatic malignant tumors, obstruction due to tumor, inflammatory process or adhesions, diverticula, and congenital anomalies, including atresia. These conditions often require excision of the involved bowel segment with reconstitution of the bowel as jejunojejunostomy (see ***Small Bowel Resection***, p. 230).

The jejunum is also employed surgically as an internal conduit or to bypass a lesion involving other portions of the gastrointestinal tract. Examples include substitution of a jejunal segment in esophageal resection (see ***Esophagectomy***, p. 194), gastrojejunostomy (see ***Gastrectomy***, p. 215), ***choledochojejunostomy*** (see ***Cholecystectomy***, p. 148), pancreaticojejunostomy (see ***Pancreaticoduodenectomy***, p. 159), etc., and in the formation of an externalized segment or tube fistula for alimentation. A feeding jejunostomy is preferred to a feeding gastrostomy when there is obstruction, trauma, fistula, or other compromise of the upper intestinal tract.

Percutaneous placement of a jejunostomy tube (under radiographic control) is most often performed in the radiology suite rather than in the operating room. The use of CT fluoroscopy minimizes the chance of injuring or traversing structures adjacent to the chosen jejunal segment.

In another variation of the percutaneous technique, if an endoscope can be advanced into the proximal jejunum, (PEJ), a procedure similar to the more commonly employed percutaneous endoscopic gastrostomy (PEG) (p. 212) can be done; a kit made for this purpose is Direct PEJ kit using the Endovive™ or the MIC™ jejunostomy tube.

Procedure

Tube jejunostomy (open approach): An incision is made in the left upper abdomen; approximately 30 cm distal to the ligament of Treitz, a pursestring suture is placed on the antimesenteric aspect of the jejunum, within which a 7-18Fr catheter (Silastic™, polyethylene, rubber, etc.) is introduced into the jejunal lumen for several centimeters via a small stab wound. The pursestring suture is tied, and a seromuscular tunnel is made longitudinally by a series of sutures placed in side-to-side fashion for 3 cm proximal to the insertion site (*Witzel technique*). The jejunum is sutured to the abdominal wall adjacent to a stab wound, through which the tube exits to the exterior; the tube is secured to the skin with a suture, and the primary incision is closed. This procedure may be done independently or as part of a more involved procedure that requires a jejunostomy for considerations as stated above.

Laparoscopic jejunostomy. Pneumoperitoneum is established, and three trocars are placed. The appropriate jejunal segment is mobilized as necessary under direct vision, in the left upper abdomen. A grasper is passed from within through the abdominal wall under direct vision and then retracted intraperitoneally holding the tip of a jejunostomy tube. A limited jejunotomy is made (again under direct vision), and the tube is placed intraluminally. Sutures secure the site of entry into the jejunum, and sutures are placed to attach that segment of jejunum to the parietal peritoneal surface at several points.

Alternatively, T- fasteners™ (usually a total of four) are placed percutaneously to fasten a percutaneous endoscopic jejunostomy *(PEJ) tube* using a T-Anchor Introducer Gun™ that fastens the tube into the jejunal lumen. The long limb of these inert anchors (similar to toggle bolts) is fastened to the skin and released 3 weeks later to allow the T-Anchors™ to pass peristaltically. A percutaneously passed needle establishes entry into the lumen (by aspiration of jejunal contents); a guide wire is passed via the needle, and the needle is removed. Serial tubular dilators are passed into the jejunal lumen, removing the dilator after a jejunostomy tube is placed via the final dilator. The trocars are removed, incisions are closed, and the jejunostomy tube is sutured to the abdominal skin with a skin stitch.

Jejunostomy conduit. A left upper-abdominal incision is made when performed as an independent procedure (or otherwise as part of a more extensive procedure). In this procedure, a formal jejunal stoma is made, following Roux-en-Y configuration of the jejunum. The jejunum is divided 30 cm distal to the ligament of Treitz; the proximal end is anastomosed to the more distal jejunum (end to side) employing sutures or staples. The distal end of the divided segment is exited to the abdominal surface via an adequate tunnel or excision of a full-thickness disc of the abdominal wall and secured to the skin (as a stoma) with sutures. The primary incision is closed. This procedure is employed when the need for jejunal feeding will be *permanent* or for an extended period.

Preparation of the Patient

Antiembolitic hose are applied to the legs, as requested. The patient is supine with arms extended on padded armboards. A pillow may be placed under the sacral area and/or under the knees to avoid strain on back muscles. Padded shoulder braces and a padded footboard are secured to the table. Pad all bony prominences and areas vulnerable to skin and neurovascular trauma or pressure. A Foley catheter may be inserted. Apply electrosurgical dispersive pad. The anesthesia provider may pass a lubricated nasogastric tube. The table is placed in Trendelenburg 5° to 10° to establish pneumoperitoneum and then in reverse Trendelenburg 10° to 20° to allow the abdominal viscera to gravitate inferiorly. The table may be rotated slightly to the right to increase exposure of the stomach intraoperatively.

Skin Preparation

Begin at the midline, extending from axilla to the pubic symphysis and down to the table at the sides.

Draping

Folded towels and a laparotomy sheet

Equipment

Sequential compression device with disposable leg wraps, if requested
Suction
ESU

For Laparoscopic Approach, Add
Monitor(s), 1 or 2
Endoscopy Cart:
Fiber-optic light source (e.g., Xenon 300 W)
Suction device
VCR, as requested
Printer
CD burner
CO_2 insufflator and Irrigator
Pressure bag for irrigation
Camera console

Instrumentation

"Open" procedure
Major procedures tray
GI tray

Laparoscopic Approach
Limited procedures tray

Verres needle
Hasson trocar
Trocars 10 or 11 mm (2 or 3)
Trocars 5 mm (2 or 3)
Reducer caps
Fiber-optic laparoscope with camera and power cord
Endoscopic instruments:
Electrosurgical suction-irrigator/dissector with J hook tip or right angle tip, scissors (hook, straight, and micro), grasping clamps, e.g., at (2) Babcock 5mm, (2) 10 mm, and (2) Allis
Multifire ligating clip appliers
Suturing device, e.g., EndoStitch

Supplies

Antiembolitic hose
Foley catheter with continuous drainage unit
N/G tube, e.g., #16Fr (to anesthesia provider)
Small basin
Blades, (1) #10, (1) #15, (1) #11
Suction tubing
Electrosurgical pencil and cord
Jejunostomy kit, e.g., PEJ Kit: Jejunostomy tube, e.g., 7Fr to 18Fr Silastic, polyethene, or rubber, T- Anchor fasteners and introducer gun (if requested)
Catheter plug

Laparoscopic Approach, Add
Electrosurgical cord
Fog reduction agent, FRED, ELVIS
Silastic™ tubing (1) for insufflator (1) for irrigation, as Cystoscopy or similar straight tubing, e.g., K50, a 1000-ml bag normal saline, and 3- way stopcock for irrigation

Special Notes

- **For the "open" approach** to **Jejunostomy,** apply **Special Notes** from *Gastrostomy,* p. 214, as indicated.
- **For laparoscopic approach** to **Jejunostomy,** apply **Special Notes** from *Abdominal Laparoscopy,* p. 140, as indicated.
- **For Percutaneous endoscopic jejunostomy,** a kit, made for this purpose, e.g., "Direct PEJ" kit using the Endovive™ or the MIC™ jejunostomy tube. The kit is similar to the one for gastrostomy, PEG kit.

- Check with surgeon for type of jejunostomy tube preference as procedure progresses however, well before the tube is needed.
- Have available, but do not open, individual items (e.g., tubes, T-Anchors, etc.) or a kit, until the specific item or kit is requested for price control.
- Anticipate need for collection pouch or catheter plug for tube jejunostomy or ostomy pouch for conduit.
- When a pouch is used, protect skin with tincture of benzoin applied to the skin before applying pouch.
- The skin knife is used to make the exit wound for the tube; the tube is secured with a skin stitch.

Small-Bowel Resection

Definition

Excision of a segment of the small intestine to remove an obstruction, a gangrenous portion of the bowel, a perforation, or a source of hemorrhage, etc. with the remaining small bowel proximally anastomosed to a segment of more distal small bowel or colon.

Discussion

Small-bowel resection is infrequently performed as an isolated procedure, as for inflammatory bowel disease, rare primary tumors, and mesenteric infarctions. In addition, whether a *Meckel's diverticulum* is diagnosed preoperatively or discovered intraoperatively, it is similarly excised. More often, the small bowel is resected in the course of other procedures as adhesive obstructive bowel disease, tumors of adjacent organs, and inflammatory processes, e.g., diverticulitis or tubo-ovarian abscess.

Laparoscopic approach may be employed, but may not be applicable in certain circumstances, as when extensive adhesions are encountered due to inflammation.

Procedure

Small Bowel Resection as an isolated procedure is described. An incision is made so that the entire small bowel is accessible, especially if the patient has had previous surgery and there are adhesions. The mesentery is divided, ligating vascular structures; the affected segment is excised, and the continuity of the bowel is restored by anastomosis of the proximal and distal ends of the remaining small bowel. An automatic stapling device (e.g., GIA or TA) may be employed, or one- or two-layered anastomoses may be performed. The abdomen is closed in layers.

Small bowel resection as part of another procedure is described. Similar steps are taken, leaving the resected segment of small intestine attached to the adherent organ (e.g., colon, ovary) also to be resected.

Preparation of the Patient

Antiembolitic hose are applied to the legs. The patient is supine; arms may be extended on padded armboards. A pad may be placed under the sacrum, or a pillow may be placed under the knees to avoid back strain. Pad all bony prominences and areas vulnerable to skin and neurovascular trauma or pressure. The anesthesia provider may pass a lubricated nasogastric tube. Foley catheter is inserted. Apply electrosurgical dispersive pad.

Skin Preparation

Begin at the intended site of the incision (often right paramedian), extending from nipples to upper thighs and down to the table at the sides.

Draping

Folded towels and a laparotomy sheet

Equipment

Sequential pressure device with disposable leg wraps, if requested
Suction
ESU

Instrumentation

Major procedures tray
Long instruments tray (available)
Gastrointestinal procedures tray
Hemoclip or similar ligating clip appliers (variety of sizes and lengths)
Self-retaining retractor, large (e.g., Balfour)
Automatic (disposable) stapling devices, GIA, TA, optional

Supplies

Antiembolitic hose
N/G tube to the anesthesia provider
Foley catheter with continuous drainage unit
Basin set
Blades (2) #10 and (1) #15
Ligating clips, e.g., Hemoclips (assorted sizes)
Electrosurgical pencil and cord with holder and scraper
Needle magnet or counter

Special Notes

- Apply **Special Notes** from ***Abdominal Laparotomy,*** p. 134, as indicated.
- Keep instruments that come in contact with the interior of the small bowel isolated in a basin.
- "Clean" closure of the abdomen may be requested. This may include any or all of the following: clean change of gloves, gown, drapes, and a Basic/Minor procedures instrument tray. "Clean" closure is not mandatory for small bowel procedures and is left to the discretion of the surgeon.

Cutaneous Ileostomy

Definition

Formation of temporary or permanent opening of the ileum, brought out onto the abdomen as a stoma.

Discussion

Cutaneous ileostomy is performed to divert the fecal stream in resection of the colon and rectum (permanent end ileostomy); to protect a distal anastomosis, such as, ileo-anal (temporary loop ileostomy); or to relieve inflammatory bowel disease of the colon with or without distal resection. A continent ileostomy (Kock pouch) consists of a stoma in continuity with a pouch of folded and sutured ileum that serves as a reservoir. The patient will catheterize the stoma to empty the pouch, as necessary.

A laparoscopic approach may be employed.

Procedure

Cutaneous ileostomy is described. The abdomen is entered, usually through a right paramedian or midline incision. A disc of skin and subcutaneous fat is excised at the preoperatively selected ileostomy site; the anterior rectus sheath is incised and a small fragment removed. The incision is deepened into the peritoneum. The ileum is cleared of its mesentery for several centimeters and divided, and the proximal end is passed through the stoma site onto the abdominal wall. The distal end of the ileum, unless resected, is sutured or stapled closed. The proximal end is reverted back on itself and sutured circumferentially to the skin of the stoma site. The mesentery of the terminal ileum is sutured to the parietal peritoneum to prevent internal hernia. (Alternatively, a loop ileostomy may be performed, most often as a temporary stoma.) The abdomen is closed. An ileostomy pouch (appliance) is placed over the stoma following protection of the skin is protected with any of a variety of products (Duradhesive wafer, Stomadhesive™ paste, etc.).

Preparation of the Patient

Antiembolitic hose are applied to the legs, as requested. The patient is supine; arms may be extended on padded armboards. A pad may be placed under the sacrum and/or under the knees to avoid back strain. Pad all bony prominences and areas vulnerable to skin and neurovascular trauma or pressure. Apply electrosurgical dispersive pad. The anesthesia provider passes a lubricated nasogastric tube. Foley catheter is inserted.

Skin Preparation

Begin at midline, extending from above nipples to the upper thighs and down to the table on the sides.

Draping

Folded towels and a laparotomy sheet

Equipment

Sequential pressure device with disposable leg wraps, if requested
Suction
ESU

Instrumentation

Major procedures tray
Long instruments tray
Gastrointestinal procedures tray
Hemoclip or similar ligating clip appliers (various sizes and lengths)
Automatic disposable stapling device, optional

Supplies

Antiembolitic hose
N/G tube to the anesthesia provider
Foley catheter with continuous drainage unit, as requested
Basin set
Blades, (3) #10 and (1) #15
Needle magnet or counter
Electrosurgical pencil and cord with holder and scraper
Suction tubing
Hemoclips or similar ligating clips (various sizes)
Marking pen (to mark stoma site), optional
Ileostomy appliance (e.g., Karaya Seal)
Stoma skin protective wafer or paste (e.g., Stomadhesive)

Special Notes

- Apply **Special Notes** from ***Abdominal Laparotomy***, p. 134, as indicated.
- Keep instruments that come in contact with the interior of the small bowel isolated in a basin.
- "Clean" closure of the abdomen may be requested. This may include clean change of gloves, gown, drapes, and a basic/minor procedures instrument tray. Change is not mandatory for small bowel procedures and is left to the discretion of the surgeon.
- An ileostomy stoma is covered with an ileostomy appliance after the site is protected with a wafer to which the appliance is attached or with a skin protective paste. Ask for the surgeon's preference as the case progresses to have same available when the stoma is placed.

Appendectomy

Definition

Excision of the appendix, usually performed to remove the acutely inflamed organ.

Discussion

When the appendix is acutely inflamed, it may rupture, spilling the contents of the bowel into the peritoneal cavity; peritonitis and abscess formation ensues. Earlier diagnosis and appendectomy can prevent this potentially serious complication. **Incidental appendectomy** may be performed in conjunction with other abdominal surgery.

A laparoscopic approach may be employed (p. 236).

Procedure

Appendetomy is described. An incision is made in the right lower abdomen either transversely, obliquely with a McBurney or a vertical incision for primary appendectomy. The appendix is identified and its vascular supply ligated. The appendix is ligated at its base, i.e., the stump is tied off with absorbable suture. The appendix is removed, and the stump may be inverted in the cecum within a placed pursestring suture, cauterized with chemicals or ESU, or simply left alone after ligation.

Another technique to effect **appendectomy** is to devascularize the appendix and invert the entire appendix into the cecum. The wound is closed in layers, except when an abscess has occurred, as with acute appendicitis. In that case, the skin and subcutaneous tissues may be left open. A drain is placed into the abscess cavity, exiting through the incision or a stab wound. Antibiotic irrigation may be used.

Preparation of the Patient

Antiembolitic hose may be applied to the legs. The patient is supine; arms may be extended on padded armboards. A pad may be placed under the sacrum or under the knees to avoid back strain. Apply electrosurgical dispersive pad. Pad all bony prominences and areas vulnerable to skin and neurovascular trauma or pressure. A Foley catheter is not routinely placed.

Skin Preparation

Begin in lower right quadrant (McBurney incision is most frequently used), extending from nipples to upper thighs and down to the table at the sides.

Draping

Folded towels and a laparotomy sheet

Equipment

ESU

Instrumentation

Basic/Minor procedures tray

Supplies

Antiembolitic hose, if requested
Ice packs, if patient has an elevated temperature, optional
Basin set
Blades, (3) #10
Needle magnet or counter
Electrosurgical pencil and cord with holder and scraper
Culture tubes (aerobic and anaerobic)
Drain (e.g., Penrose, ¼″, optional)
Antibiotic irrigation (optional)

Special Notes

- Apply *Special Notes* from *Abdominal Laparotomy,* p. 134, as indicated.
- Take appropriate measures to maintain patient's body temperature. Consider that the patient may be febrile; infrequently, measures to decrease body temperature may be requested, e.g., with ice packs placed under the arms, at the groin area, etc.
- Instruments used for amputation of the appendix are to be isolated in a basin.

Laparoscopic Appendectomy

Definition

Endoscopic excision of the appendix.

Discussion

Indications for **laparoscopic appendectomy** are the same as for the traditional procedure. An advantage to this approach in addition to the usual considerations of a minimal access procedure is that if the diagnosis of appendicitis is incorrect [e.g., pelvic inflammatory disease (P.I.D.) is encountered], the procedure can either be aborted with limited trauma to the patient, or "incidental" appendectomy may be performed, as appropriate. When an abscess or significant adhesions are encountered and the definitive operative area cannot be exposed expeditiously, or if a mucocele or neoplasm is discovered, the laparoscopic procedure is converted to an "open" procedure.

Incidental appendectomy may be performed in conjunction with other laparoscopic procedures.

Procedure

Laparoscopic appendectomy is described. Pneumoperitoneum is established. Abdominal exploration is performed through a 10-/11-mm or 12-mm port. If appendicitis is confirmed, additional ports in the suprapubic area (5 mm) and right subcostal at the anterior axillary line (12 mm) are established. Additional right or left lower quadrant ports may be required. The cecum is retracted superiorly, employing an atraumatic instrument (e.g., endoscopic Babcock). After appropriate dissection, the appendiceal tip is distracted by grasping forceps (or by endoscopic loop ligature if edematous). The mesoappendix is exposed and a "window" made in an avascular site. Using an endoscopic gastrointestinal stapler or between serial clips, the mesoappendix (including the appendiceal artery) is divided. An endoscopic loop ligature of chromic catgut may be secured around the appendiceal base, and with an endoscopic gastrointestinal stapler placed just distal to the same, the appendix is amputated.

Alternatively, an additional suture loop can be employed and the appendix divided by endolaser fiber or electrosurgery or scissors. The appendiceal stump may be cauterized. During the procedure, the port functions can be alternated. The specimen is withdrawn into the trocar sleeve (of the selected port) or an endoscopic specimen pouch may be employed, particularly if the appendix is inflamed and edematous. Hemostasis is assured. A drain may be placed, as indicated. Pneumoperitoneum is released and the wounds closed in the usual manner.

Preparation of Patient

Antiembolitic hose may be applied to the legs. The patient is supine; arms may be padded and tucked in at the patient's sides. Bony prominences and all areas vulnerable to skin and neurovascular trauma or pressure are padded. An electrosurgical dispersive pad is applied. A Foley catheter is not routinely placed.

Skin Preparation

Begin at the midline, extending from the nipples to the upper thighs and down to the table at the sides.

Draping

Folded towels and a laparotomy sheet

Equipment

ESU
Suction
Video monitor
Printer
CD burner
Insufflation-irrigation device
Fiber-optic light source, e.g., Xenon 300 W
Pressure bag for irrigation
VCR, as requested
Camera console
Laser, if requested (see p. 94 for mandatory laser safety precautions)

Instrumentation

Basic/Minor tray
Verres needles
Trocars (5 mm, 10 mm, 12 mm, and/or Hasson)
Reducers
Fiber-optic laparoscope with camera and power (light) cord
Endoscopic instruments:
Electrosurgical suction irrigator/dissector with J hook tip or right angle tip, scissors (hook, straight, and micro), grasping clamps, e.g., 2 Babcock 5 mm and 2 10 mm, and 2 Allis)
Multifire ligating clip appliers
Loop sutures, e.g., Endoloop®

Supplies

Antiembolitic hose, if requested
Blades, (1) #10, (1) #15, or (1) #11
Basin set

Suction tubing
Silastic tubing for CO_2 insufflation
Culture tubes (aerobic and anaerobic)
Cystoscopy or similar straight tubing, e.g., K50, a 1000-ml bag normal saline, and three-way stopcock for irrigation
Endoscopic specimen retrieval bag, Endo Pouch, ENDOBAG™, optional

Special Notes

- Apply **Special Notes** from ***Abdominal Laparoscopy***, p. 140, as indicated.
- Take appropriate measures to maintain patient's body temperature. Consider that the patient may be febrile; infrequently, measures to decrease body temperature are employed, e.g., with cold packs that may be placed under the axilla and the groin. Consult with surgeon regarding the need for the cold packs.
- Instruments used for amputation of the appendix are to be isolated in a basin.
- If a laser is employed, instrumentation must be ebonized and all laser precautions must be employed; see p. 94 for mandatory laser precautions.

Colostomy

Definition

Formation of a permanent or temporary opening into the colon brought out onto the abdominal wall as a stoma.

Discussion

A **colostomy** is intended to be either permanent or temporary. A **temporary colostomy** is performed to divert the fecal stream from the distal colon, which may be obstructed by tumor or inflammation or which may require being "put at rest" because of an anastomosis or a pouch procedure performed distally. A temporary colostomy may be created in the transverse colon or the sigmoid colon. The proximal and distal limbs of the colon at the site of the colostomy remain connected (loop colostomy) or separated (double barrel colostomy). In a ***Hartmann procedure***, a **sigmoid colostomy** is formed, and the distal end of the colon is either brought out as a mucous fistula or closed and returned intraperitoneally.

A **permanent colostomy** is performed to treat malignancies of the colon, the rectum, and is obligatory when the distal rectum including the anus is excised; other indications include irrevocable rectal stricture, irrevocable anal incontinence, and inflammatory bowel disease. A permanent colostomy can be fashioned similar to a temporary colostomy, but most often, is an end colostomy.

A colostomy may be performed as an independent procedure or in conjunction with additional procedures, as colon resection, treatment of colonic trauma, presence of gynecologic malignancy, etc.

Laparoscopic approach or laparoscopic-assisted technique may be employed.

Procedure

An "open" procedure for creation of a colostomy is described. The incision depends on the segment of the colon to be used, unless performed in conjunction with another procedure. The segment of colon (to be formed into the colostomy) is mobilized. The colon can be brought out through the main incision or through a preselected adjacent site, from which a disc of skin and subcutaneous tissue has been excised. The underlying rectus fascia and muscle and peritoneal layers are incised to accommodate the colon. The appropriate segment of the colon is divided between clamps, atraumatic GI (e.g., Glassman) or vascular clamps, used on the retained portions of bowel), or an automatic stapling device may be employed. An "end" segment or loop of colon is brought through the stoma site and (usually) sutured to the peristomal skin.

In a loop colostomy, a rod or bridge may be placed under the colon to avoid retraction or the loop incised so that the proximal portion of the stoma is larger ("dominant") than the distal. Both proximal and distal portions are sutured ("matured") to the abdominal wall.

The wounds are closed, and a colostomy pouch is applied over the stoma (the skin around which has been protected with tincture of benzoin, karaya paste, etc.).

Preparation of the Patient

Antiembolitic hose may be put on the legs. The patient is supine; arms may be extended on padded armboards. A pad may be placed under the sacrum, or a pillow may be placed under the knees to avoid back strain. Apply electrosurgical dispersive pad. Pad all bony prominences and areas vulnerable to skin and neurovascular trauma or pressure. The anesthesia provider passes a lubricated nasogastric tube. A Foley catheter may be inserted.

Skin Preparation

Begin at the intended site of incision (check with surgeon), extending from nipples to upper thighs and down to the table at the sides.

Draping

Folded towels and a laparotomy or transverse sheet (depending on incision)

Equipment

Sequential compression device with disposable leg wraps, if requested
ESU
Suction

Instrumentation

Major procedures tray
Long instruments tray
Gastrointestinal procedures tray
Self-retaining retractor (e.g., Balfour), optional
Basic/Minor procedures tray (for "clean" closure), if requested

Supplies

Antiembolitic hose
Foley catheter with continuous drainage unit, if requested
Basin set
Blades, (2) #10
Suction tubing
Electrosurgical pencil and cord with holder and scraper
Penrose drain, 1″ (for retraction on colon)
Glass rod and tubing or a plastic bridge
Colostomy pouch (e.g., Karaya Seal)

Special Notes

- **Reminder:** The circulator must always use the JC Universal Protocol to identify that the patient is the correct patient, anticipating the correct surgery on the correctly marked side (laterality) and site. See the JC's Universal Protocol, p. 18, as necessary.
- **Reminder:** Before every surgery begins, an official "*time out*" must be taken; it is a safety measure. A '*time out*' is required and must be documented on the Perioperative Record for medicolegal reasons.
- See the suggested **Patient Care Plan** (p. 9) for care of the patient in surgery. The circulator adapts care to meet the individual patient's needs by implementing the nursing interventions that will result in the most optimal desired outcomes. Use the **Special Notes** to augment the plan of care to ensure that all considerations are explored.
- **Reminder:** The circulator will assist the anesthesia provider during the induction of anesthesia, e.g., during endotracheal intubation (by applying pressure to the cricoid cartilage), during the administration of a block (e.g., by holding the patient in position for an

epidural anesthetic), or by injecting medications the anesthesia provider has prepared (at his/her direction). For a description of the circulator's role during the administration of anesthesia, see p. 81.

- All care must be documented in the **Perioperative Record** (p. 12) for continuity of patient care and medicolegal reasons.
- The patient may have fear and anxiety regarding the surgical procedure and the unfamiliar environment; answer questions in a knowledgeable manner whenever possible and refer questions to surgeon, as necessary.
- The circulator can provide a measure of emotional support to the patient regarding feelings of altered body image by permitting the patient an opportunity to express his/her feelings.
- Provide emotional support to the patient by keeping the patient adequately covered and exposing only those areas involved in the procedure.
- Check chart for patient sensitivities and allergies, including to latex products, e.g., gloves, drains, or elasticized dressings. Note that simple drains (e.g., Penrose) and pressure bandages contain latex, among many other items in general use. Check the chart for allergies related to iodine; iodine is found in many prep solutions.
- Take appropriate measures to maintain patient's body temperature, e.g., a warmed blanket (from the blanket warmer), or adjust the room temperature accordingly. When ordered, a forced-air warming blanket may be placed over legs and/or chest.
- Antiembolitic hose should be applied when the patient arrives in the room, if requested. A sequential compression device with leg wraps may be applied over the antiembolitic hose, when ordered, to prevent deep-vein thrombosis.
- The electrosurgical pad should be applied to skin that is relatively hair-free (to obtain good contact) and as close to the surgical site as possible. It may be necessary to shave the area.
- The electrosurgical pencil tip should be kept free of debris and eschar (use the scratch pad) and kept in its holder when not in use.
- Large amounts of noxious smoke and fumes resulting from thermal destruction are a health hazard; smoke should be suctioned away by the room suction with an in-line filter or with a smoke evacuation system (e.g., Clear View® 350).
- Masks with a filtering capacity of between 2 and 5 microns should be worn by all persons in the OR during an operative procedure to prevent inhalation of toxic matter.

- Laparotomy pads (lap pads) are used once the abdominal cavity has been entered. All lap pads must have a radio-opaque strip incorporated in the fabric (making them x-ray detectable).
- Once the abdominal cavity has been entered, raytec sponges (4″ × 4″ sponges with a visible blue radio-opaque thread) are not placed on the sterile field, except when mounted on a sponge forceps (or other clamp) for use in the abdominal (or other) cavity; there should be no "free" raytec sponges on the sterile field.
- A raytec sponge, when mounted on a sponge forceps, is frequently referred to as a *spongestick*.
- Most surgeons prefer to have the lap pads lightly moistened with warm saline once the peritoneal cavity has been entered.
- Just prior to closure, the peritoneal cavity may be irrigated with copious amounts of normal saline that may be suctioned with a Poole suction.
- Instruments used on the bowel are considered contaminated and are isolated in a basin.
- "Clean" closure of the abdomen may be requested (discuss with surgeon as the procedure progresses). Regowning, regloving, redraping, and a "new" basic/minor procedures tray will be required, if clean closure is requested.

Closure of Colostomy

Definition

Reestablishment of colonic continuity and the repair of the abdominal wall.

Discussion

This procedure can be simple or involved depending on adhesion formation and the area of anastomosis, e.g., between a sigmoid end colostomy and the proximal rectal remnant.

Laparoscopic approach or laparoscopic-assisted approach may be employed.

Procedure

For an **end colostomy,** an incision circumscribes the stoma, which is dissected free of abdominal wall structures. An appropriate incision is made to enable intraabdominal dissection, permitting anastomosis at the site of the distal colon. The distal segment is mobilized and anastomosed to the proximal end; an end-to-end automatic stapling device transanally can facilitate the procedure when the end colostomy can be mobilized into the pelvis. The wound is closed; subcutaneous tissue and the skin of the stoma site can be left open to avoid infection.

For a **loop** or **double-barrel colostomy**, an elliptical incision is made about the stoma(s). The colonic loop is dissected free of scar tissue and skin, and the anastomosis is performed. The proximal and distal segments may need to be resected in order to perform anastomosis on a well-vascularized segment of satisfactory diameter. The abdominal wall is closed, often leaving the subcutaneous tissue and skin packed open to prevent wound infection.

Preparation of the Patient

Apply antiembolitic hose to the legs, as requested. The patient is supine with arms extended on padded armboards. A pad may be placed under the sacrum, or a pillow may be placed under the knees to avoid back strain. Apply electrosurgical dispersive pad. Pad all bony prominences and areas vulnerable to skin and neurovascular trauma or pressure. The anesthesia provider may pass a lubricated nasogastric tube. A Foley catheter is inserted.

Skin Preparation

Gently remove the existing stoma appliance and discard; carefully remove any gross fecal debris. Cover colostomy stoma with a sponge soaked in prep solution, or the stoma may be covered with a sterile plastic adhesive drape to isolate it from the sterile field, according to the surgeon's preference. Begin abdominal prep just beyond the perimeter of the stoma, extending from nipples to mid-thighs and down to the table at the sides. Cleanse the area immediately around the stoma and the stoma itself last. Discard each sponge after cleansing the stoma.

Draping

Folded towels and a laparotomy or transverse sheet

Equipment

Sequential compression device with disposable leg wraps, if requested
ESU
Suction

Instrumentation

Major procedures tray
Long instruments tray, available
Gastrointestinal procedures tray
Automatic disposable stapling device (optional)
Self-retaining retractor, e.g., Balfour (optional)
Basic/minor procedures tray (for "clean" closure)

Supplies

Antiembolitic hose, if requested
Foley catheter with continuous drainage unit, if requested

Basin set
Blades, (3) #10 and (1) #15
Needle magnet or counter
Suction tubing
Electrosurgical pencil and cord with holder and scraper
Sterile plastic adhesive drape, e.g., Steridrape 2037, optional
Packing (e.g., Adaptic dressing, 4″ × 4″ sponges), optional

Special Notes

- Apply **Special Notes** from ***Colostomy***, p. 240, as indicated.
- The method for doing the skin prep and use of the Steridrape™ will vary according to the surgeon's preference.
- Instruments used on the bowel are contaminated and should be isolated in a basin.
- "Clean" closure of the abdomen requires regowning, regloving, redraping, and a "new" Basic/Minor procedures tray.

Right Hemicolectomy

Definition

Resection of the right half of the colon (the cecum, ascending colon, and a portion of the transverse colon) and a segment of the terminal ileum and their mesenteries. An anastomosis is performed between the ileum and the transverse colon (ileocolostomy).

This procedure may be performed as an "open" procedure, laparoscopically, or as a laparoscopically-assisted procedure, see laparoscopic colostomy, p. 254.

Discussion

Indications for **right hemicolectomy** are tumors, bleeding, inflammation, or trauma. Obstruction is less often encountered in the right half than in the left half of the colon.

Procedure

A right paramedian, midline, or oblique right midabdominal incision is made. The distal small bowel and the midtransverse colon are identified, and their vascular attachments are ligated and divided. The appropriate segment of colon is excised between clamps (atraumatic GI clamps may be used on the portions of the retained bowel), or an automatic stapling device may be employed. An anastomosis is made between the terminal ileum and midtransverse colon employing various suture techniques or staples. Care is taken to avoid injury to structures including the right ureter, duodenum, inferior vena cava, and common bile duct. Clean closure technique is usually employed. The incision is then closed in layers in the usual manner.

Preparation of the Patient

Antiembolitic hose are applied to the legs. The patient is supine; arms may be extended on padded armboards. A pad may be placed under the sacrum and/or under the knees to avoid straining back muscles. Pad all bony prominences and areas vulnerable to skin and neurovascular trauma or pressure. The anesthesia provider may pass a lubricated nasogastric tube. A Foley catheter is inserted before the abdomen is prepped. Apply electrosurgical dispersive pad.

Skin Preparation

A Foley catheter is inserted and attached to continuous drainage before the skin prep.

Begin at the site of the intended incision for the skin prep (right paramedian, midline, or oblique right midabdominal), extending from nipples to upper thighs and down to the table at the sides.

Draping

Folded towels and a laparotomy sheet

Equipment

ESU
Suction

Instrumentation

Major procedures tray
Long instruments tray
Gastrointestinal procedures tray
Hemoclip or similar clip appliers (various sizes and lengths)
Disposable automatic stapling device (optional)
Harrington retractor
Self-retaining retractor, e.g., Balfour (optional)
Basic/Minor procedures tray (for "clean" closure)
Disposable automatic stapler, e.g., GIA or TA

Supplies

Antiembolitic hose
Foley catheter with continuous drainage unit
N/G tube to anesthesia provider, if requested
Basin set
Blades, (3) #10 and (1) #15
Electrosurgical pencil and cord with holder and scraper
Suction tubing

Needle magnet or counter
Hemoclips or similar ligating clips (various sizes)

Special Notes

- Apply **Special Notes** from ***Colostomy***, p. 240, as indicated.
- The scrub person may receive the specimen in a large basin.
- Instruments used on the colon and intraluminally are isolated in a basin.
- "Clean" closure of the abdomen requires regowning, regloving, redraping, and a "new" Basic/Minor procedures tray.

Transverse Colectomy

Definition

Resection of a segment of the transverse colon with an end-to-end anastomosis to reestablish continuity of the colon.

Discussion

Transverse colectomy is usually performed as treatment for a malignancy or a stricture caused by inflammatory bowel disease.

Transverse colectomy may be performed laparoscopically or as a laparoscopically assisted procedure, see p. 254.

Procedure

A vertical or transverse incision may be used. The transverse colon and hepatic and splenic flexures are mobilized by dividing the vascular mesenteric attachments and supporting connective tissues. The appropriate segment of colon is excised between clamps (atraumatic GI clamps may be used on the portions of the retained bowel), or an automatic stapling device may be employed. An anastomosis is fashioned between the proximal and distal colon, and the mesenteric defect is closed; sufficient mobility must be achieved to enable the anastomosis to be tension free (as need to "mobilize" the hepatic and/or splenic flexures). Injury to the stomach, pancreas, spleen, and superior mesenteric vessels is avoided. The wound is closed (clean closure technique employed) in the usual manner in layers.

Preparation of the Patient

Antiembolitic hose are applied to the legs. The patient is supine; arms may be extended on padded armboards. A pad may be placed under the sacrum, and/or a pillow may be placed under the knees to avoid back strain. A Foley catheter is inserted into the bladder and connected to continuous drainage before beginning the skin prep. Apply electrosurgical dispersive pad. Pad all bony prominences and areas vulnerable to skin and neurovascular trauma or pressure. The anesthesia provider may pass a lubricated nasogastric tube.

Skin Preparation

Begin at the site of the intended incision (midline or transverse), extending from nipples to upper thighs and down to the table at the sides.

Draping

Folded towels and a transverse or laparotomy sheet (depending on incision)

Equipment

Sequential pressure device with disposable leg wraps, as requested
ESU
Suction

Instrumentation

Major procedures tray
Gastrointestinal procedures tray
Disposable automatic stapling devices, EEA & TA or GIA & TA (optional)
Hemoclip or similar clip appliers (various sizes and lengths)
Harrington retractor
Self-retaining retractor (e.g., Balfour)
Basic/Minor procedures tray (for "clean" closure)

Supplies

Antiembolitic hose
Foley catheter with continuous drainage unit, if requested
N/G tube to anesthesia provider
Basin set
Blades, (3) #10
Suction tubing
Electrosurgical pencil and cord
Hemoclips or similar ligating clips (various sizes)
Needle magnet or counter

Special Notes

- Apply **Special Notes** from *Colostomy*, p. 240, as indicated.
- Instruments used on the colon intralumenally are contaminated and must be isolated in a basin.
- Specimen can be received in a large basin.

- Ends of the bowel may be covered with lap pads or surgical gloves and tied with umbilical tape to avoid contamination of the abdomen, or the surgeon's preferred method to avoid contamination is followed.
- "Clean" closure of the abdomen requires regowning, regloving, and redraping and a "new" Basic/Minor procedures tray.

Anterior Resection of the Sigmoid Colon and Rectum

Definition

Excision of the sigmoid colon (and when applicable, the rectosigmoid and the proximal two-thirds of the rectum) with the anastomosis of the distal descending or proximal sigmoid colon to the remaining segment of the rectosigmoid or rectum.

Discussion

Anterior resection of the sigmoid colon and rectum is performed for benign (e.g., diverticulitis) or malignant conditions. When the proximal or middle third of the rectum is to be resected, the procedure is referred to as **"low anterior resection."** In this situation, the patient is placed in a modified lithotomy position; in this way access is provided to both the abdomen and the perineum to permit transanal stapling anastomotic technique. When the resection includes the middle third of the rectum, a **colonic J-pouch** may be constructed (stapled) and anastomosed to the distal rectum to provide reservoir function not provided by an end-to-end anastomosis.

This procedure may be performed laparoscopically or as a laparoscopically-assisted procedure, see p. 255 (laparoscopic low anterior resection).

Procedure

Anterior resection of the sigmoid colon and rectum is described. A vertical or transverse incision can be used. The lower descending, sigmoid, and rectosigmoid colon (and proximal rectum) are mobilized by dividing mesenteric vascular attachments. In procedures for malignancy, greater portions of the mesentery are excised to include additional lymph node-bearing tissue (complete mesorectal excision). The ureters are identified and protected. The appropriate segment of colon is excised, and the proximal colon (or ileum) is anastomosed end to end with sutures or staples to the rectum. Tension is avoided on the anastomosis by mobilizing more proximal colon (e.g., splenic flexure) as necessary. When the proximal and middle thirds of the rectum are excised, a stapled J-pouch (of more proximal colon) may be anastomosed to the remaining distal rectum. When the anastomosis is made more distally than the rectosigmoid junction, a circular end-to-end stapling device (EEA, ILA) of appropriate diameter is passed transanally by the assistant surgeon. The tissue discs excised by the stapler are inspected for completeness. Suture repair may be needed if the tissue discs are incomplete. The anastomosis may be inspected with a sigmoidoscope and/or air tested for integrity by instilling air into the rectum via a sigmoidoscope with the pelvis filled with fluid. The abdomen is closed (employing clean closure technique) in the usual manner in layers.

Preparation of the Patient

Antiembolitic hose are applied to the legs. The patient is in modified lithotomy position with the feet placed in stirrups (padded); arms may be extended on padded armboards. A pad may be placed under the sacrum, to avoid back strain. A Foley catheter is inserted and attached to continuous drainage before the skin prep. Apply electrosurgical dispersive pad. Bony prominences and all areas vulnerable to skin and neurovascular trauma or pressure are padded. Anesthesia provider may pass a lubricated nasogastric tube.

Skin Preparation

Begin at the intended site of incision, extending from nipples to midthighs and to the table at the sides. Follow with a prep of the thighs, perineum, and the anus last, discarding each sponge after wiping the anus. **For women,** add prep of the vagina.

Draping

A drape sheet is tucked under the buttocks; leggings, folded towels, and a laparotomy sheet (lower part) goes over the perineum. An opening is cut during the perineal phase of the procedure to provide access to the anus.

Equipment

ESU
Suction
Padded stirrups, e.g., Allen or Lloyd-Davies
Extra Mayo stand (for perineal phase)

Instrumentation

Major procedures tray
Long instruments tray
Gastrointestinal procedures tray
Hemoclip or similar ligating clip appliers (various sizes and lengths)
Disposable automatic stapling device (optional)
Harrington retractor
Self-retaining retractor, e.g., Balfour (optional)

Sigmoidoscopy tray
Basic/Minor procedures tray (for "clean" closure)
Disposable automatic stapler, e.g., GIA™, TIA™, and EEA™ or ILA™ (with sizers), as requested

Supplies

Antiembolitic hose
Foley catheter with continuous drainage unit
N/G tube to anesthesia provider, if requested
Basin set
Blades, (3) #10 and (1) #15
Electrosurgical pencil and cord
Suction tubing
Needle magnet or counter
Hemoclips or similar ligating clips (various sizes)

Special Notes

- Apply **Special Notes** from ***Colostomy***, p. 240, as indicated.
- A sigmoidoscope may be requested to check the integrity of the anastomosis directly and/or the anastomosis may be "air tested" by instilling air into the rectum while there is irrigation fluid in the peritoneal cavity.

Abdominoperineal Resection of the Rectum

Definition

Excision of the rectum, usually including a portion of the sigmoid colon, through an abdominal (anterior) and a perineal approach.

Discussion

Abdominoperineal resection of the rectum is performed most often for the treatment of rectal malignancy, but also for inflammatory bowel disease, severe destructive rectal infection (e.g., lymphogranula venereum), irreversible sphincter injuries, etc. **Abdominoperineal resection of the rectum** may be combined with resection of the proximal colon as well.

The abdominal portion of this procedure can be performed laparoscopically.

Procedure

Abdominoperineal resection of the rectum is described. A vertical or transverse abdominal incision is made. The extent and level of the pathology is determined. The portion of the proximal colon to be removed is mobilized by dividing the mesenteric vascular attachments to the bowel, carrying the dissection to the rectum. The ureters and other adjacent organs are identified and otherwise avoided, unless they are to be removed. The colon is transected proximally.

The distal portion (the transected end of which is protected from spillage by use of lap pads, clamps, and/or a rubber glove secured by umbilical tapes) is dissected into the depths of the pelvis transecting the lateral rectal stalks (middle hemorrhoidal vessels) to the level of the coccyx. Perirectal connective and adipose tissue and lymph node-bearing tissues are removed with malignancies (complete mesenteric excision). In benign disease, the dissection stays close to the bowel wall.

A premarked stoma site is fashioned by excising a disc of skin and a segment of anterior rectus sheath, and tunneling into the peritoneum through the rectus muscle. The end of the proximal portion of the colon is passed through the tunnel (without tension and assuring good vascularity) and sutured ("matured") to the peristomal skin. The abdomen may then be closed, or if simultaneous perineal dissection is performed, the "abdominal" surgeon remains to assist from above.

As the perineal portion is completed, the surgeon above closes the abdomen in layers in the usual fashion (employing clean closure technique). The "perineal" surgeon begins by closing the anus with a heavy-gauge pursestring suture. An elliptical saggital incision is made into the perianal and perineal tissues and deepened, incising the levator muscles, freeing attachments of the anus and distal rectum; hemostasis is secured with ligatures, clips, and the ESU. The pelvis is entered, and the previously divided distal colon and proximal rectum is passed into the perineal wound. The rectal excision is completed, avoiding the urethra and prostate or vagina. When hemostasis is achieved, the perineal wound is closed in layers over one or more drains (as paired 30-ml Foley balloon catheters). A colostomy pouch is placed over the stoma, the skin about which is protected with tincture of benzoin (or other agent).

Preparation of the Patient

The patient is usually in a modified lithotomy position with the sacrum elevated on folded towels or a sandbag to provide better exposure to the perineum, or the procedure is begun with the patient supine and later moved to a lithotomy or modified lateral/Sims' position; see p. 24 for positions' considerations. A Foley catheter is inserted before beginning the skin preparation. Pad all bony prominences and areas vulnerable to skin and neurovascular trauma or pressure. Antiembolitic hose are applied to the legs. Anesthesia provider may pass a lubricated nasogastric tube. Apply electrosurgical dispersive pad.

Skin Preparation

Modified Lithotomy. Begin at the intended site of abdominal incision (midline, left paramedian, or transverse), extending from the nipples to lower thighs and down to the table at the sides.

Modified Lithotomy. Prepare genitalia (add a vaginal preparation for females), extending to the table at the perineal area; prepare anus last and discard each sponge.

Supine. Continue at the pubic symphysis, extending downward over the labia. Cleanse each inner thigh, working toward the perineum. Prep vagina, then perineum, and anus last (discarding each sponge).

Modified Lateral/Sims'. Continue at suprapubic area, extending from the iliac crest to mid-thighs and down to the table anteriorly and posteriorly. Prep genitalia and anus last.

Draping

Modified Lithotomy. Drape sheet (under buttocks), leggings, folded towels (abdomen), and a laparotomy or transverse sheet (an opening will be cut for perineal exposure).

Supine. Folded towels and a laparotomy or transverse sheet

Modified Lateral/Sims'. Folded towels and a laparotomy or transverse sheet

Lithotomy. Same as modified lithotomy.

Equipment

Sequential pressure device with disposable leg wraps, as requested
ESU
Suction
Padded stirrups, e.g., Allen; Lloyd-Davies (modified lithotomy position)

Instrumentation

Major procedures tray
Long instruments tray
Gastrointestinal procedures tray
Hemoclip or similar ligating clip appliers (various sizes and lengths)
Large retractors (e.g., Harrington, Israel, Balfour)
Basic/Minor procedures tray (for perineal approach when both abdominal and perineal approach are performed)
Basic/Minor procedures tray (additional for "clean" closure)

Supplies

Antiembolitic hose
Foley catheter with urimeter and continuous drainage unit
N/G tube to anesthesia provider, if requested
Basin set

Blades, (4) #10 and (1) #15
Needle magnet or counter (2) for simultaneous approach, (3) including "clean closure" setup
Electrosurgical pencils and cords with holders and scrapers (2) for simultaneous approach, (3) for "clean closure" setup
Suction tubing (2)
Hemoclips or similar ligating clips (assorted sizes)
Extra glove and umbilical tape (for proximal end of a specimen before it is passed through the perineal wound)
Vessel loop or umbilical tape (for retraction)
Heavy-gauge nonabsorbable sutures for anal closure, e.g., #2 silk
Marking pen (stoma site), optional
Colostomy pouch (with Karaya Seal)
Drainage supplies (e.g., Penrose, Hemovac, Foley catheter)

Special Notes

- Apply **Special Notes** from ***Colostomy,*** p. 240, as indicated.
- Consult the surgeon regarding choice of position for the patient. See the surgical position indicated, p. 239.
- For modified lithotomy position, prevent risk of positioning injury with stirrups that are padded and positioned correctly to avoid skin and neurovascular pressure or trauma.
- Prevent trauma to patient's fingers when lithotomy position is employed, i.e., when the lower section of the table is returned to level position.
- The modified lithotomy position is preferred as it enables abdominal and perineal approaches; the procedure is performed using a two-team approach working simultaneously (a second scrub nurse is necessary). Alternatively, after the abdominal phase is completed, the patient is prepared and draped for the perineal phase after the abdomen is closed.
- Isolate all instruments used on the colon in a basin; any instrument that touches the interior lumen of the colon is contaminated.
- The scrub person may receive the large specimen in a basin.
- **N.B.** *Because there are two separate surgical fields, additional care must be exercised to avoid confusion when counting sponges, needles and sharps, and instruments.*
- "Clean" closure of the abdomen requires regowning, regloving, redraping, and a "new" Basic/Minor procedures tray.
- Using a pouch for each electrosurgical pencil prevents accidental (inadvertent) activation of the second electrosurgical pencil when not in use, thereby avoiding burn injury.

Laparoscopic-Assisted Colon Resection

Definition

Excision of a segment of the large intestine incorporating endoscopic technique and a minilaparotomy incision or large-bore laparoscopic handport.

Discussion

Laparoscopic approach with an enlarged handport or laparoscopic-assisted approach may be employed for **colon resection**. Laparoscopic approach may not be appropriate in cases of severe obesity, extensive adhesions, severe inflammation, or colonic perforation with peritonitis or in malignancy when the primary tumor is large or associated with adjacent organ involvement or when wide dissection is necessary. When there is excessive bleeding, the laparoscopic procedure must be promptly converted to an "open" procedure.

Colon resection may be completed entirely by laparoscopic approach (with use of a handport or a large port for specimen retrieval) or may be performed laparoscopically, combined with a minilaparotomy incision. Similarly, creation or elimination of a stoma and procedures in which instruments may be inserted transanally may be combined with the laparoscopic approach. The selection of trocar sites will vary with the patient's habitus, pathology, previous surgery, and the preference of the surgeon; the trocar sites may need to be repositioned during the course of the procedure.

Should the involved colonic segment be mobile (or in a redundant loop) and a limited procedure is indicated, the segment may be delivered extracorporeally via a minilaparotomy incision and the procedure (resection, anastomosis, etc.) accomplished without further laparoscopic maneuvers.

When a small lesion requiring segmental excision has been identified colonoscopically, the endoscopist or surgeon can inject methylene blue dye into the adjacent bowel wall to facilitate identification on laparoscopic exploration. Similarly, if laparoscopic visualization cannot identify a smaller lesion or its regional location is not established with respect to deciding procedure of choice, intraoperative ***colonoscopy***, p. 185 can be performed to verify the level of pathology.

The more commonly performed laparoscopic (or laparoscopic-assisted) colonic procedures will be described.

Procedure

Laparoscopic-assisted Right Hemicolectomy is described. Pneumoperitoneum is established through the umbilicus. Three additional 10- to 11-mm ports are placed: suprapubic, right subcostal at the midclavicular line, and right subziphoid. The table is adjusted with the right side elevated to allow gravity to assist in the exposure of the immediate operative area and later placed in reverse Trendelenburg.

After assessment of the pathology, the cecum and proximal ascending colon are placed on traction as the lateral attachments are dissected. Care is taken to avoid injury to the ureter and duodenum as the dissection is continued about the terminal ileum, hepatic flexure, and proximal transverse colon. Division of the mesenteric vessel is then accomplished. Employing appropriate stapling devices, the segment of colon is resected and the specimen removed via a large port or minilaparotomy incision in the right upper quadrant. The anastomosis can be performed intracorporeally following resection or extracorporeally by delivering the bowel through the minilaparatomy incision onto the abdomen. The mesenteric defect is repaired, and after hemostasis is assured, the pneumoperitoneum is released. The incisions are closed.

Left Hemicolectomy or Sigmoid Resection is described. This procedure is similar to ***right hemicolectomy***. Pneumoperitoneum is established; the ports are placed on the left side (umbilical, left upper quadrant midclavicular line, left paraumbilical, left midclavicular line, and left suprapubic). The table is adjusted with the left side up and later placed in reverse Trendelenburg. The left colon is mobilized (avoiding injury to the spermatic or ovarian vessels, ureter, stomach, and spleen). After dissection has been completed, resection and anastomosis are performed as in right hemicolectomy. If the distal sigmoid colon is included in the resection, see Low Anterior Resection (to follow).

Low Anterior Resection. The patient is positioned in modified lithotomy, providing access to the anterior abdomen and perineum. Pneumoperitoneum is established. Patient is placed in Trendelenburg. Ports are similar to that of left hemicolectomy. The sigmoid colon and rectum are mobilized, taking care to avoid injury to gonadal vessels, ureters, and internal female genitalia. The mesenteric structures are divided, and the specimen is resected and delivered through a large-bore port, minilaparatomy incision or transanally via the distal rectal remnant.

Anastomosis is performed employing an intraluminal end-to-end stapler inserted transanally. The anastomosis is begun following extraction of the segment of resected bowel via a large-bore port or minilaparatomy incision. The staple line placed at the time of division of the colon (i.e., at the distal end of the proximal segment) is excised and the separated anvil of the stapler secured by hand-sewn pursestring suture or automatic pursestring suture device. The stapler is inserted transanally, and its trocar is extended perforating the stapled end of the rectal segment. Employing a modified anvil grasper to stabilize the proximal segment, end-to-end anastomosis is completed in the standard fashion. The tissue rings are inspected and the anastomosis tested employing a sigmoidoscope or bulb syringe. After hemostasis is assured, the pneumoperitoneum is released and the access ports closed.

Hartmann Procedure and Reversal of Hartmann Procedure are described. The conduction of the Hartmann procedure is identical to low anterior resection as described above with the exception that the distal rectal segment is closed or on occasion is brought out onto the abdominal wall as a mucous fistula. The proximal segment is brought out as an end colostomy. To reverse this procedure, that is, to restore continuity, the colostomy bearing proximal segment is anastomosed to the rectal remnant.

The pelvis is inspected and the closed rectal remnant identified. If visualization is inadequate, adherent viscera and adhesions must be dissected to expose the proximal portion of the rectal segment. To facilitate identification of the rectal segment, a blunt instrument, large-bore catheter, or sigmoidoscope is inserted transanally to "tent" the apex of the segment. When this dissection is complete, the previously established colostomy stoma is dissected free from the abdominal wall with laparoscopic assistance if necessary. Any questionably viable colon is excised. The anvil of the intraluminal stapler is placed within this proximal segment secured by a pursestring suture. This segment with the anvil is replaced intraperitoneally. The assistant surgeon then passes the trocar of the intraluminal stapler through the apex of the closed rectal segment. Care is taken to assure that no extraneous tissues or structures overlie the site of the anastomosis. The anastomosis is completed as in a low anterior resection above. Access ports are closed.

Laparoscopically Assisted Abdominoperineal Resection of the Rectum is described. The surgery is initially identical to low anterior resection except that the distal dissection is performed as low as feasible; the specimen is left in situ as the proximal end is transected. The proximal segment is then brought out as an end colostomy at a previously selected stoma site in the left lower quadrant. The perineal portion of the procedure is performed per usual (see Abdominonoperineal Resection, p. 250). Access ports are closed.

Preparation of the Patient

Consult the surgeon and anesthesia provider regarding the position. Antiembolitic hose are applied to the legs. A Foley catheter is inserted. All bony prominences and areas vulnerable to skin and neurovascular trauma or pressure are padded. Anesthesia provider may pass a lubricated nasogastric tube. An electrosurgical dispersive pad is applied.

For **right and left hemicolectomy,** the patient is supine with the table in Trendelenburg to establish pneumoperitoneum; patient may be repositioned in reverse Trendelenburg (if requested).

With **laparoscopic low anterior resection,** the patient is in modified lithotomy with the table in Trendelenburg.

The patient is supine for the **Hartmann procedure**. To reverse the Hartmann procedure (i.e., closure of colostomy), the patient is placed in modified lithotomy using Allen or Lloyd-Davies stirrups.

Skin Preparation

For the **right and left hemicolectomy and Hartmann procedure,** begin at the umbilicus, extending from nipples to upper thighs and down to the table at the sides. For peristomal prep, ***Closure of Colostomy***, p. 243.

For the **low anterior resection and reversal of Hartmann's procedure,** begin at the umbilicus extending from nipples to the pubic symphysis and down to the table at the sides.

Follow with prep of the thighs, perineum, and anus last, discarding each sponge after wiping the anus. **For women,** add a vaginal prep.

Draping

For right and left hemicolectomy and Hartmann procedures, folded towels and a laparotomy sheet.

For low anterior resection and reversal of Hartmann procedure, drape sheet under buttocks and a laparoscopy sheet with attached leggings.

Equipment

MUL-T-thermia pad or mattress or
Forced air warming blanket
Padded stirrups Allen or Lloyd-Davies stirrups (modified lithotomy position)
Sequential compression device with disposable leg wraps, as requested when applicable
Suction
ESU
Endoscopy cart:
Fiber-optic light source, e.g., Xenon 300 W
Video monitors (2)
VCR
Printer
CD burner
CO_2 insufflator-irrigator (CO_2 and water, respectively)
Pressure bag to facilitate irrigation
Camera console

Instrumentation

Limited procedures tray
Major procedures tray, available
Long instruments tray, available

Gastrointestinal procedures tray, available
Verres needle
Fiber-optic laparoscope with camera and cord
Blunt tip trocar
Trocars (4 each, 10 to 11 mm or 10 to 12 mm)
Endoscopic instruments:
(2) Babcock forceps, (3) scissors (curved, hook, straight), right angle dissector, Kelly clamp, fan retractor and Nathanson retractor, grasping forceps (2) , dissecting forceps, right angle and hook irrigation-suction-electrosurgical dissectors
Suturing device and sleeve, e.g., Endoloop
Multifire ligating clip applier
Disposable automatic stapler-cutter of choice

For Low Anterior Resection and Reversal of Hartmann's Procedure, Add

Sigmoidoscopy tray
Disposable stapler, e.g., EEA or ILA with sizers

Supplies

Antiembolitic hose
Foley catheter with urimeter and continuous drainage unit
Nasogastric tube (e.g., #16) to anesthesia provider
Basin set
Suction tubing
Silastic tubing for (1) CO_2 insufflation and (1) irrigation
Fog reduction agent, e.g., FRED, ELVIS
Blades, (2) #10, (1) #15, (1) #11
Methylene blue dye
Medicine cup, syringe, needle
Sterile marking pen and labels
Hand port, e.g., LAP DISC, HANDPORT, Intromit, Omniport Dexterity Device for laparoscopic-assisted procedures, if requested
Extra-large endoscopic impermeable specimen retrievable bag, Endo Pouch II, ENDOBAG, LAP-BAG, LAPSAC, GRABAG (optional)

Special Notes

- Apply **Special Notes** from ***Abdominal Laparoscopy***, p. 140, as indicated.
- **Reminder:** Padded shoulder braces are secured to the table when table is in Trendelenburg. The table is positioned this way to encourage organs to slide cephalad; to reduce the danger of inadvertently puncturing an organ or vital structure.

- Prevent musculoskeletal injuries to personnel and the patient by employing ergodynamic measures (see p. 51) when positioning the patient, as necessary.
- **N.B.** Ascertain that accessory equipment has been properly secured onto the table to ensure patient safety.
- After the patient is in the room, position and connect the monitors; circulator needs to recheck position of monitors to ensure that they can be easily viewed.
- Circulator connects remaining items (irrigation tubing, suction tubing, and electrosurgical cord) after the team is in position (to avoid tripping over the cords).
- For perineal phase for **low anterior resection or reversal of Hartmann's procedure,** add an additional Mayo stand.
- Endoscopic instruments and some laparoscopes may be flash-sterilized; see manufacturer's specifications regarding sterilization requirements.

Proctocolectomy with Ileal Pouch Anal Anastomosis

Definition

Excision of the colon and the rectum with creation of a distal ileal pouch (reservoir) attached to the anal canal.

Discussion

This restorative procedure is designed for patients with ulcerative colitis who require colectomy but in whom the anal canal is not severely diseased and fecal continence is not significantly impaired. The patients must be prepared to sustain potential complications of the procedure and to accept the possibility of multiple daily bowel movements.

Patients with familial adenomatous polyposis are also candidates for the procedure to avoid a permanent ileostomy. Patients with Crohn's disease or colonic malignancy are usually excluded from this surgery.

Several anatomical variations of pouch configuration (a fecal reservoir which permits intervals in defecation) are used, including "side to side," "W," "S," and "J". "J" is most commonly used. A temporary ileostomy to divert the fecal stream is frequently established during the procedure, allowing the pouch and ileo-anal anastomosis to heal satisfactorily prior to restoring intestinal continuity. The precise level of rectal transection, whether or not to excise all of the mucosa to the level of the dentate line or to leave a short transitional zone, and whether or not to staple or hand sew the ileo-anal anastomosis differs in practice. An important technical aspect of the procedure is to ensure sufficient mobility of the ileal mesentery while preserving adequate blood supply.

Procedure

The patient is placed in a modified lithotomy position to permit access to the anterior abdomen and perineum. (Some surgeons will perform the perineal dissection in prone jackknife poison and turn the patient for the abdominal phase.)

Through a generous incision, the distal ileum, entire colon, and proximal rectum are mobilized. If the distal ileum is relatively free of disease, transection is done at the ileocecal junction and the rectum transected 4 cm proximal to the dentate line. The colon is excised and the rectal dissection is maintained close to the bowel wall to spare pelvic nerve plexuses. The distal rectal mucosa is removed employing a pelvic and perineal approach. The ileal mesentery is mobilized, preserving adequate blood supply while enabling the intended pouch to reach to the depths of the pelvis.

A **"J" pouch** is fashioned using a linear intestinal stapler. The apex of the pouch is anastomosed to the anal canal, having been passed through the rectal remnant stripped of mucosa. Either a circular stapler or hand-sewn technique may be used. Drains may be placed in the pelvis and trans-anally into the pouch. A loop ileostomy is placed in the right lower quadrant at a preselected site. The abdomen is closed in layers in the usual manner.

Alternatively, much of the intra-abdominal dissection can be accomplished laparoscopically, allowing the pouch to be fashioned through a smaller incision (laparoscopically-assisted). Preoperative factors, such as the patient's general status, use of steroids, multiple medications, immune compromise, inflammation of the colon, intraoperative factors, etc., influence the ultimate choice of the variations in technique.

Preparation of the Patient

Antiembolitic hose are applied to the legs. Consult the surgeon for the desired patient position; most often the patient is in a modified lithotomy position with the buttocks slightly elevated on a pad to provide better access to the perineum; arms may be extended on padded armboards. The legs are placed in padded stirrups and the buttocks are slightly elevated (on a pad). Insert a Foley catheter before beginning the skin prep. Apply electrosurgical dispersive pad. Pad all bony prominences and areas vulnerable to neurovascular trauma or pressure. Anesthesia provider may pass a lubricated nasogastric tube.

Skin Preparation

Begin at the intended site of the abdominal incision (midline, left paramedian, or transverse), extending from the nipples to the thighs and down to the table at the sides.

Next, using a second prep set, prep the genitalia area (add a vaginal preparation for females), extending down to the table at the perineal area; prepare anus last, discarding each sponge afterward.

Equipment

Sequential pressure device with disposable leg wraps, as requested
ESU
Suction
Stirrups, padded (depending on position)
For laparoscopic approach, add:
Endoscopy cart:
Monitor(s)
VCR
Printer
CD Burner
Fiber-optic light source, e.g., Xenon 300W
Insufflator-Irrigator
Camera console

Instrumentation

Major procedures tray (open)
GI tray
Long instruments tray/Basic/Minor procedures tray (for "clean closure")
Disposable endoscopic stapler, e.g., GIA (additional reload staples available)
Sigmoidoscopy tray
For Laparoscopic Approach, add:
Verres needle
Hasson trocar
Trocars, 10 or 11 mm (2 or 3)
Trocars, 5 mm (2 or 3)
Reducer caps
Fiber-optic laparoscope and power cord
Endoscopic instruments:
electrosurgical suction irrigator/dissector with J hook tip or right angle tip, scissors (hook, straight, and micro), ligating clip appliers, Babcock 5 mm (2) and 10 mm (2), Allis (2)
Suturing device with sleeve, Endoloop

Supplies

Antiembolitic hose
Foley catheter with urimeter and continuous drainage unit
Nasogastric tube (e.g., #16) to anesthesia provider
Blades, (2) #10, (1) #15, (1) #11
Basin set
Suction tubing
Electrosurgical pencil and cord

Ileostomy appliance (with Karaya Seal™); peristomal skin-protecting agent

Special Notes

- Apply **Special Notes** from ***Colostomy***, p. 240, as indicated.
- For modified lithotomy position, prevent risk of positioning injury with stirrups that are padded and positioned correctly to avoid skin and neurovascular pressure or trauma.
- Prevent trauma to patient's fingers when lithotomy position is employed, i.e., when the lower section of the table is returned to level position.
- A sigmoidoscope may be requested for inspection of the anastomosis.

Transanal Endoscopic Microsurgery

Definition

Application of endoscopic surgical techniques via transanally placed rectoscope.

Discussion

For rectal and rectosigmoid lesions to the level of 20 cm proximal to the anus, which otherwise would be excised by an open (transperitoneal or transsacral) approach, or for a lesion not technically feasible to be adequately treated by the usual transanal exposure, special instrumentation has been devised permitting the use of endoscopic surgical instruments in a well-visualized gas-distended operative field.

Up to four instruments may be manipulated in parallel fashion simultaneously by the operator and assistant. A unit is utilized that continuously monitors intrarectal pressure and insufflates with carbon dioxide to maintain an appropriate pressure to keep the rectum distended, thus permitting visualization and responding to the introduction of instruments and need for suctioning blood or fumes as well. Visualization is by means of binocular stereoscopic optics, to which a side arm or teaching attachment or video monitor can be adapted.

An irrigating device to cleanse the lens is also a part of the system. A Martin arm retractor stabilizes the scope after it is positioned transanally. Most often this technique is employed for sessile lesions too large to be safely and/or adequately excised or electrofulgurated via a standard sigmoidoscope. Benign and limited malignancies may be so treated.

Preoperative evaluation may, in addition to biopsy, include transrectal ultrasonography to determine the depth of mural invasion and lymph nodal involvement, which would influence the operative approach. The position of the lesion will also influence the positioning of the patient for ease of access (i.e., prone, lithotomy, or lateral). Transanal endoscopic rectopexy in which the posterior rectal wall is incised and the rectum fixed to the presacral ligaments has been described. In most instances when violation of a full-thickness segment of rectal wall is anticipated, preoperative preparation and postoperative care is similar to that for a formal colon surgery. If during the course of the procedure the peritoneum is entered, immediate repair is performed.

Procedure

This procedure would be performed on a patient with a sessile tumor of the midrectum. After induction of anesthesia, the patient is positioned to best visualize the lesion with respect to the operative field (e.g., prone for an anterior lesion). The special rectoscope (Richard Wolf Medical Instrument Corporation) is inserted and secured. Carbon dioxide pressure of 150 mbar is maintained. Employing various grasping and electrosurgical cutting instruments, the lesion is circumscribed and excised. Depending on the size and depth of the defect thus created, after hemostasis is obtained, suture repair is then undertaken. Clips are used to secure the suture ends rather than standard knots. If the procedure cannot easily be accomplished, a standard surgical procedure may have to be performed.

Preparation of the Patient

Antiembolitic hose are applied to the legs prior to positioning. The patient is in prone, lithotomy, or lateral positioning, depending on the orientation of the lesion. See the descriptions of patient positions on p. 20. All bony prominences and areas vulnerable to skin and neurovascular trauma or pressure are padded. A Foley catheter is inserted prior to positioning when necessary. Apply electrosurgical dispersive pad.

Skin Preparation

Cleanse the area from the level of the umbilicus to the level of midthighs. Work from just outside the anus to the outer borders. Then prep the area around the anus, ending with the anus. Discard each sponge after wiping the anus.

Draping

Drapes used for ***transurethral resection of the prostate*** (p. 404) with integrated pouches and openings

Equipment

Stirrups with padding (for lithotomy position)
Pillow for between the legs (for lateral position)
ESU
Suction
Martin arm self-securing adjustable retractor mount

Endoscopic combination unit (monitors intrarectal pressure, provides gas insufflation to maintain desired pressure with connections for optic rinsing and suction)
Monitor (one)
VCR (optional)
CD burner
Printer
Camera console
Special roller pump suction device (e.g., Wolf, functions without causing total decompression)

Instrumentation

Special operating endoscopic rectoscope with binocular optics with rigid (for video adaptation) and flexible sideport viewing with camera and cord

Endoscopic instruments:
Grasping forceps, electrosurgical suction-irrigator, scissors (straight, hook, and micro), needle drivers, ligating clip appliers, camera (if not inside the rectoscope), and teaching arm attachment (flexible or rigid)

Supplies

Antiembolitic hose
Foley catheter with continuous drainage unit
Needle magnet or counter
Small basins (2)
Hemostatic agent (e.g., Surgical, Gelfoam)
Suction tubing
Electrosurgical cord
Lubricant (water soluble)

Special Notes

- Apply **Special Notes** from ***Hemorrhoidectomy***, p. 267, as indicated.
- The endoscopic combination unit is positioned on the surgeon's left side. The unit is controlled by the surgeon using the double footswitch.
- The optic irrigator, controlled by a single footswitch, is used by the assistant.
- The light source, monitor, and camera are positioned on the surgeon's right side.
- The U-shaped double ball joint (Martin arm) is attached to the table with the V-groove clamp approximately 20 cm below the anus.

- The surgeon sits on an adjustable chair.
- The scrub person sits on the right behind the surgeon and passes instruments from the right; the surgeon wears a back vest.

Hemorrhoidectomy, Anal Fissurectomy, Anal Fistulotomy

Definition

Hemorrhoidectomy. Excision of the veins of the anus and associated overlying skin and anoderm (externally) and mucous membrane (internally).

Anal Fissurectomy. Excision of an anal fissure or anal ulcer (chronic fissure).

Anal Fistulotomy. Incision into an anal fistula; may be followed by excision of the fistula (fistuleotomy).

Discussion

Hemorrhoidectomy refers to the removal of the hemorrhoidal tissues, including the enlarged veins within. Hemorrhoids may be treated with concomitant anal conditions, such as fissure (anal ulcer) and fistula. Numerous modalities are employed for internal hemorrhoids and associated rectal mucosal prolapse (latex band ligation, sclerosing injections, laser, cryotherapy, and others), most often performed as an office procedure without anesthetic (*not* to include external hemorrhoidal tissue). A circular intraluminal stapler, as used for intestinal anastomosis, can be employed for rectal mucosal prolapse performed as a formal transanal surgical procedure.

Anal Fissurectomy

An **anal fissure,** a disruption of the anodermal skin, acute or chronic, linear or ovoid, which does not resolve with nonoperative therapy, requires surgical excision, including surrounding inflamed scarified tissue if present (anal ulcer), an incision of the distal margin of the often scarified internal anal sphincter (to relieve spasm or stenosis), or a combination of these modalities. Subcutaneous left posterolateral internal sphincterotomy, usually performed as an office procedure, if failed, may require more formal treatment as above.

Anal Fistulotomy

An **anal fistula** presents as an abnormal opening of the anal skin, usually resulting from local infection. There are numerous causative entities that lead to this condition, in the most common of which, the intersphincteric fistula, an anal abscess which when drained, either spontaneously or surgically, leaves a residual tract (fistula) from the initial site of the infection to the skin. More complex presentations, such as in *Crohn's disease*, radiation, trauma, intraperitoneal sepsis, e.g., diverticulitis, etc., may demonstrate more than a single skin opening, may not necessarily be related to the sphincter muscles, and require comprehensive therapy. Preoperative evaluation, as gastrointestinal x-rays, ultrasound scan, endoscopy, fistulography, etc., are performed accordingly. Once a fistula is established, surgery is (almost always) required.

Consideration is given to the extent of the sphincter mechanism through which the fistula traverses. Significant division of the sphincter may need to be done with later reconstruction after the septic process resolves; see **Anal Sphincteroplasty**, p. 268, to follow. A temporary diverting colostomy may be required in severe cases.

Anesthesia may be regional, local, or general (or a combination). Following the induction of anesthesia, proctosigmoidoscopy is performed.

Procedure

Hemorrhoidectomy. The proximal portions of the hemorrhoidal complex are suture-ligated, and the hemorrhoid is excised by scalpel, electrosurgery, or laser. Less often, cryosurgery is employed (usually reserved for limited outpatient procedures). If the anus is stenotic, the distal internal sphincter may be incised. A mucous membrane flap and/or skin flaps may be employed to cover denuded areas. Care is taken not to excise too much skin, anoderm, or mucous membrane and to avoid injury to the sphincter mechanism.

Anal Fissurectomy. The distal margin of the internal sphincter is incised (percutaneously or subcutaneously via limited skin incision) in the left posterolateral position (or posteriorly if the fissure so presents). The fissure (or ulcer) itself may be excised. A mucosal flap may be advanced to cover denuded surfaces.

Anal Fistulotomy. For the presentation of an intersphincteric fistula, a malleable probe is passed from the skin opening into the anal canal at the cryptline. When this is not possible, deliberate dissection of the tract must be done. An incision is made over the probe (or grooved director), a fistulotomy. The exposed tract may be excised (fistulectomy) or curetted and tissue sent for histological evaluation. When a significant portion of the sphincter mechanism is involved, instead of complete division, a seton may be placed and/or the operation staged.

Preparation of the Patient

See ***Sigmoidoscopy***, p. 186. Antiembolitic hose may be applied to the legs. A Foley catheter may be inserted. Bony prominences and areas vulnerable to skin and neurovascular trauma or pressure are padded. Apply electrosurgical dispersive pad. Tincture of benzoin is applied to the buttocks over which wide adhesive is applied prior to sigmoidoscopy.

Skin Preparation

Begin inside tape margins, discarding each sponge after wiping the anus.

Draping

Jackknife. Folded towels and a laparotomy sheet. Tapes are attached to table sides.

Lithotomy. Drape sheet under buttocks, leggings, folded towels, drape sheet over abdomen. Tapes are attached to stirrups.

Modified Lateral/Sims. Folded towels and a laparotomy sheet. Tapes are attached to table sides.

Equipment

Stirrups or pillow and roll for positioning
ESU
Suction

Instrumentation

Rectal procedures tray
Rectal retractors, including Sims, Hill-Ferguson, and Sawyer (small, medium, large)
Curettes

Supplies

Antiembolitic hose
Foley catheter with continuous drainage unit, as requested
Blades, (1) #10 and (1) #15
Needle magnet or counter
Small basin
Hemostatic agent (e.g., Surgical, Gelfoam)
Suction tubing
Electrosurgical pencil and cord
Lubricant
Pressure dressing (e.g., petrolatum-impregnated gauze, 4″ × 4″ sponges)
Seton material (large-gauge suture or rubber band) as per surgeon's preference for fistula procedure
Dye and injection equipment (surgeon's preference) in fistula surgery, if requested

Special Notes

- Apply **Special Notes** from ***Sigmoidoscopy***, p. 189, as indicated.
- **N.B.** Be prepared for sigmoidoscopy prior to procedure.

- Lubricate retractors with water-soluble agent.
- A carbon dioxide laser may be used. All laser safety precautions must be observed; see p. 94.
- If the primary pathology is anal fissure or fistula, the basic setup is essentially the same as when hemorrhoids are the primary pathology.

Anal Sphincteroplasty

Definition

Repair of or substitution for the anal sphincter mechanism.

Discussion

Anal incontinence is due to congenital abnormalities (e.g., meningomyelocele, absence of sphincter, etc.), accidental, surgical, or obstetrical trauma, radiation therapy, local infection, neoplasm, stretching of related neuromuscular structures due to chronic constipation with straining, prolapse, aging, etc. In the adult, incontinence is graded according to the control of flatus, liquids, and solid stool. In lesser presentations, what is intolerant to some patients may not be a problem to others.

Nonoperative measures include bowel control, biofeedback training, and the occasionally effective anal incontinence plug. Digital examination, defecography, anal manometry, ultrasound exam, etc. help to delineate which component of the continence mechanism is at fault. Most often, direct sphincter repair is performed. A sphincter surrounding gracilis muscle sling, either as a tonic restraint or dynamically with the implantation of electrodes, and a pacemaker-like device (deactivated by an external magnet to permit defecation), a gluteus maximus muscle sling, or the implantation of an artificial device similar to that used in urinary incontinence have been employed with varying degrees of success. Ultimately, if continence is not achieved, an end colostomy is indicated.

Procedure

Direct sphincter repair will be described. Local, regional, or general anesthesia may be administered with the patient in jackknife prone, lithotomy, or modified lateral position. A hemicircumferential perianal incision is made over the site of the sphincter disruption (e.g., anteriorly, following obstetrical injury). The scarified ends of the sphincter are dissected, preserving the scar. After suitable mobilization, the ends (including the scar, which holds sutures better than muscle alone) are approximated, utilizing overlapping technique when length permits to allow an appropriate degree of anal patency. When indicated, the perineal body is reconstructed by approximating the levator ani and transverse perineal muscles and the residual scar. The anoderm may be directly sutured to the underlying sphincter and the remainder of the skin incision closed loosely or left open to avoid tension and permit drainage.

Preparation of the Patient

Antiembolitic hose may be put on the patient's legs prior to positioning. A Foley catheter may be inserted. Local, regional, or general anesthesia may be employed with the patient in the jackknife prone, lithotomy, or modified lateral position. See a description of each position, p. 187 to 188. All bony prominences and areas vulnerable to skin and neurovascular trauma or pressure are padded. Apply electrosurgical dispersive pad.

For Skin Preparation, Draping, Equipment, Instrumentation, Supplies, and **Special Notes,** see ***Hemorrhoidectomy***, p. 267.

Add to Instrumentation:
Skin hooks (2)
Senn retractors (2) sharp

Thiersch Procedure

Definition

Placement of a circumanal device to restrict complete rectal prolapse (procidentia).

Discussion

Prosthetic materials include various sutures, fascia, Mersilene tape, folded Marlex mesh, vascular prostheses, etc. The Thiersch procedure often ultimately fails when the prosthetic material extrudes, with ensuing local infection. The procedure may be repeated after the infection subsides.

This procedure is reserved primarily for poor-risk elderly patients.

Procedure

Two incisions, 1 cm each, are made diametrically opposite around the anus. A large curved hemostat is passed deep in the perianal tissues external to the sphincter (avoiding the vagina), encircling the sphincter, and exiting the opposite incision. The prosthetic material is passed through the tunnel created by the clamp. This maneuver is repeated for the other hemicircumference (prosthesis completely encircles the anal canal). The prosthetic ends are sutured (or stapled) after an appropriate degree of constriction is determined. The sutured segment is replaced deep in the wound. Wounds may be irrigated with an antibiotic solution. The incisions are closed.

Preparation of the Patient

Antiembolitic hose may be put on the patient's legs prior to positioning. A Foley catheter may be inserted. The procedure may be performed under regional, local, or general anesthesia. The patient may be in the jackknife, lithotomy, or modified lateral position; see a description of each position, pp. 187 to 188. Bony prominences and all areas vulnerable to skin and neurovascular trauma or pressure are padded. Apply electrosurgical dispersive pad. Apply distracting tapes to buttocks, see Hemorrhoidectomy, p. 266.

A sigmoidoscopy may be performed prior to the procedure; see Sigmoidoscopy, p. 186.

Skin Preparation

Preparation is minimal. Begin inside tape margins, working from the outside inward, discarding each sponge after wiping the anus.

Draping

Jackknife. Folded towels and a laparotomy sheet

Lithotomy. Drape sheet under buttocks, leggings, towels, drape sheet over abdomen

Modified Lateral. Folded towels and a laparotomy sheet

Equipment

- ESU
- Suction
- Pillow and roll or padded stirrups (for positioning)

Instrumentation

- Rectal procedures tray
- Rectal retractors, including Sims, Hill-Ferguson, and Sawyer (small, medium, large)
- Ligature carrier (optional)

Supplies

- Antiembolitic hose
- Foley catheter with continuous drainage unit, if requested
- Blades, (1) #10 and (2) #15
- Needle magnet or counter
- Small basin
- Suction tubing
- Electrosurgical pencil and cord
- Water-soluble lubricant
- Prosthesis, as requested

Antibiotic irrigation, (optional)
Bulb syringe

Special Notes

- Apply **Special Notes** from ***Hemorrhoidectomy***, p. 267.
- Check with the surgeon regarding prosthesis material and need to immerse in antimicrobial solution (such as dilute Betadine®).
- These patients are often frail; extra precautions on positioning.

Ripstein Procedure (Presacral Rectopexy)

Definition

An anterior (abdominal) approach to correct complete rectal prolapse (procidentia) by mobilizing the rectum within the abdomen (and pelvis) and fixing it to the presacral fascia and periosteum by an encircling (or partially encircling) band of material, such as a Teflon, Marlex, or Mersilene mesh.

Discussion

If the sigmoid colon is extremely redundant, a portion of it may be resected. A low anterior resection (see p. 248) with extensive mobilization of the distal rectum may be performed without requiring placement of a prosthetic mesh altogether and is currently considered by some to be the procedure of choice for complete rectal prolapse. A suture rectopexy may be performed with the low anterior resection. Accordingly, the Ripstein procedure is very seldom employed.

Procedure

A vertical or transverse incision is used. The rectum is dissected from its supporting tissue attachments. A mesh of Marlex (or Mersilene, Teflon, etc.) is sutured (or stapled) to the presacral periosteum, taking care to avoid the local venous plexus. If presacral venous bleeding cannot easily be controlled, a hemostatic surgical tack (Hemorrhage Occluder pin) with its applicator provides direct compression of the bleeding site. The mesh is placed around the bowel to anchor it to the sacrum without restricting the rectum too tightly. A resection proximally may be performed. The abdomen is closed in layers.

Preparation of the Patient

The patient is supine; arms may be extended on padded armboards. Bony prominences and all areas vulnerable to skin and neurovascular trauma or pressure are padded. Antiembolitic hose may be put on the legs. Check with the surgeon regarding insertion of a Foley catheter. Apply electrosurgical dispersive pad.

Skin Preparation

Begin at the intended site of incision (vertical or transverse), extending from nipples to upper thighs and down to the table at the sides.

Draping

Folded towels and a laparotomy or transverse sheet

Equipment

ESU
Suction
Sequential compression device, if requested

Instrumentation

Major procedures tray
Long instruments tray
Gastrointestinal procedures tray (available)
Harrington retractor
Self-retaining retractor (e.g., Balfour)
Hemoclip or other ligating clip appliers (assorted sizes and lengths)
Stapler (fascia)

Supplies

Antiembolitic hose
Basin set
Electrosurgical pencil
Blades, (3) #10
Suction tubing
Needle magnet or counter
Hemoclips or similar ligating clips (variety of sizes)
Hemorrhage Occluder pins (available; do not open unless requested)
Mesh or banding materials per surgeon's preference
Staples (optional)

Special Notes

- Apply **Special Notes** from *Colostomy*, p. 240, as indicated.
- **N.B.** Be prepared for sigmoidoscopy prior to procedure.

Perineal Resection of the Rectum for Complete Rectal Prolapse (Procidentia)

Definition

Excision of the prolapsed segment of the rectum, perineal approach.

Discussion

Complete excision of the prolapsed rectal segment may be accomplished by a perineal approach. This is particularly applicable in medically compromised patients in whom an abdominal procedure entails an undue risk yet with a satisfactory long term result anticipated (rather than an encirclement procedure; see Thiersch Procedure, p. 269).

Procedure

The lithotomy position is preferred as the prolapse is accentuated. The prone position can be employed. The patient has been prepared as for formal colon resection; a Foley catheter is placed. A circumferential incision is made proximal to the dentate line through the full thickness of the rectum. The prolapse is distracted and amputated at an appropriate level, taking care to obtain hemostasis of themesenteric vessels. A peritoneal defect, if created, is repaired. As indicated, a levatorplasty is preferred. The rectal continuity is then restored by primary anastomosis.

For Preparation of the Patient, Skin Preparation, Draping, Equipment, Instrumentation, and **Supplies,** see ***Hemorrhoidectomy***, p. 266.

Special Notes

- Apply **Special Notes** from ***Hemorrhoidectomy***, p. 267, as indicated.
- **In addition to the hemorrhoidectomy instrumentation, a pediatric Deaver and malleable retractors may be required.**
- **Antimicrobial irrigation (e.g., Betadine) of the operative field may be requested.**

Pilonidal Cystectomy and Sinusectomy

Definition

The removal of a cystic mass containing hair, skin, and tissue debris most often located in the sacrococcygeal area.

Discussion

Pilonidal cyst disease is not related to the gastrointestinal tract, but it is included here for convenience; however, this entity must be distinguished in certain presentations from anal fistula disease.

Pilonidal cysts are most frequently found in the sacrococcygeal region, but they can occur about the perineum, hands, etc. When acutely or chronically infected, surgical treatment is indicated. These cysts may be very extensive with multiple and deep side tracts (sinuses). Numerous procedures and approaches have been devised for this entity; recurrence (or nonhealing) to a greater or lesser degree is not uncommon, sometimes requiring further surgery.

Procedure

Anorectal examination may be done prior to preparation and draping to verify that an anal fistula, Crohn's disease, etc. is not present (this exam is usually performed prior to hospitalization but may be rechecked with the patient anesthetized).

An incision is made about the cyst or into the cyst directly. Necrotic tissue, hair, tissue debris, etc. are curetted and/or excised. The cyst wall, if discrete, is usually excised. Sinus extension(s) may be delineated by injection of methylene blue (or similar) dye. The wound can be packed open, partially closed, or completely closed directly or by means of mobilized tissue flaps.

Preparation of the Patient

Antiembolitic hose are put on the patient before positioning, if requested. The patient is in a jackknife position (the table is flexed) with arms extended on padded armboards angled toward the head of the table with the forearms pronated. A pillow may be placed under the head for comfort. A pillow is placed in front of the legs, and a roll in front of the ankles. Bony prominences and all areas vulnerable to skin and neurovascular pressure or trauma are padded. Following application of tincture of benzoin, buttocks are distracted by 3- or 4-inch adhesive tapes (after checking chart for patient's allergies) anchored to the underside of the table.

N.B. *The tapes are pulled toward patient's head (cephalad) before anchoring for maximal exposure.*

N.B. *Apply tapes to buttocks before the patient undergoes rectal examination, as tapes will not adhere to the skin where lubricant has been applied.*

Skin Preparation

Begin at the sacrum, extending from the iliac crests to the upper thighs. Cleanse anus last, discarding each sponge afterward.

Draping

Folded towels and a laparotomy sheet

Equipment

Pillow and roll for positioning
ESU
Suction

Instrumentation

Rectal procedures tray
Extra probes (available)
Curettes

Supplies

Antiembolitic hose, optional
Basin set
Blades, (3) #10
Suction tubing
Electrosurgical pencil and cord
Needle magnet or counter
Methylene blue with needle and syringe (optional, if sinus tract injection is performed)
Pressure dressing

Special Notes

- Apply **Special Notes** from ***Hemorrhoidectomy,*** p. 267, as indicated.
- **Reminder:** Check chart for patient sensitivities and allergies, particularly to latex products, e.g., gloves, drains, or elasticized dressings. Note that simple drains (e.g., Penrose) and pressure bandages (e.g., Elastoplast) contain latex, among many other items in general use.
- The circulator should obtain positioning aids prior to bringing patient into room.
- **Reminder:** The electrosurgical pad should be applied to skin that is relatively hair-free (to obtain good contact) and as close to the surgical site as possible. It may be necessary to shave the area.
- Multiple sinuses or tracts may be treated; have "extra" blades and ESU pencil tips available.
- The electrosurgical pencil tip should be kept free of debris and eschar (use the scratch pad) and kept in its holder when not in use.
- Large amounts of noxious smoke and fumes resulting from thermal destruction are a health hazard; smoke should be suctioned away by the room suction with an in-line filter or with a smoke evacuation system. Masks with a filtering capacity of between 2 and 5 microns should be worn by all in the room during an operative procedure to prevent inhalation of toxic matter.

- **N.B.** Be prepared with extra probes and curettes; have ready methylene blue dye in a syringe with a blunt tip to locate sinus tracts.
- If the wound is to be closed, the surgeon may request that the buttock distracting tapes be released prior to closure.
- A pressure dressing may be applied; check chart for patient's allergies before applying the elasticized tape, e.g., Elastoplast.

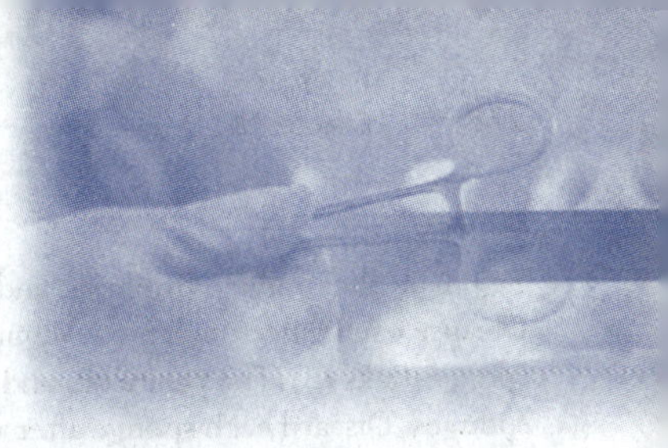

CHAPTER 18 Gynecologic and Obstetric Surgery

Dilatation of the Cervix and Curettage of the Uterus (D&C)

Definition

The gradual enlargement of the cervical canal and the removal (by scraping) of endocervical or endometrial tissue.

Discussion

The procedure is usually performed to diagnose cervical or uterine malignancy, control dysfunctional uterine bleeding, effect an abortion, complete an incomplete abortion, aid in evaluating infertility, and relieve dysmenorrhea. Fractional curettage differentiates between *endocervical* and *endometrial lesions.*

Procedure

A weighted speculum is placed in the vaginal vault. The cervix is grasped with a tenaculum. A sound is passed through the cervical canal into the uterine cavity to determine its depth and angulation. The cervix is dilated with graduated dilators. The uterine cavity may be explored with stone forceps. The uterine cavity is then curetted. Curettings are removed with stone forceps and collected on a nonadherent dressing sponge (e.g., Telfa™) placed in the posterior fornix. A small, serrated curette is used to scrape the uterine walls again, or when a D&C is performed to remove placental tissue, a large, blunt curette and ovum forceps are used.

Scrapings removed from the uterus are endometrial curettings. If *"fractional curettage"* is performed, endocervical curettings are obtained with a small curette ***before*** the uterus is sounded. By obtaining the endocervical curettings first, bringing endometrial tissue into cervical os is avoided, preventing misdiagnosis.

Preparation of the Patient

Antiembolitic hose may be placed on the legs, if requested, before anesthesia is administered. Following the administration of general, regional, or, less often, endocervical block anesthesia, the patient is positioned in lithotomy (using padded stirrups), with the buttocks positioned just over the edge of lower break in the table. Arms may be extended on padded armboards. Bony prominences and all areas prone to skin and neurovascular pressure or trauma are well padded.

Skin Preparation

Begin at the pubic symphysis and extend downward over the labia. Cleanse each inner thigh next. Vaginal vault and cervix are cleansed using spongesticks (3). The perineum and anus are cleansed with the remaining sponges. Discard each sponge after wiping the anus. The patient's bladder is drained with a straight catheter.

Draping

Drape sheet tucked in under the buttocks, followed by leggings, and a drape sheet over the abdomen

Equipment

Padded stirrups

Instrumentation

Dilatation and curettage (D&C) tray

Supplies

Antiembolitic hose, if requested
Straight catheter to drain the bladder (e.g., Robinson)
Small basin
Water-soluble lubricant
Telfa (for specimen)
T-binder or sanitary napkin belt
Perineal pad

Special Notes

- Apply **Special Notes** from ***Abdominal Laparotomy***, p. 134, as indicated. Because ***D&C*** is the first procedure in this chapter, **Gynecologic and Obstetrical Surgery,** many points from the **Special Notes** are reiterated here.
- The circulator must always use the **Joint Commission's (JC) (formerly the Joint Commission on Accreditation of Healthcare Organizations)** *Universal Protocol* to identify that the patient is the correct patient anticipating the scheduled surgical procedure. See the **JC**'s *Universal Protocol,* p. 18, as necessary.
- Before every surgery begins, an official "***time out***" must be taken; it is a safety measure. Taking a ***time out*** before every surgery is required and must be documented on the Perioperative Record for medicolegal reasons.
- See the suggested **Patient Care Plan,** p. 9, for care of the patient in surgery. The circulator adapts care to meet the individ-

ual patient's needs by implementing nursing interventions that will result in optimal desired outcomes for the patient. Use the **Special Notes** to augment the plan of care to ensure that the many considerations have been taken into account.

- All care that is given and observations made regarding the patient (e.g., condition of the skin preoperatively and postoperatively) must be documented in the operative record for continuity of care and for medicolegal reasons.
- The circulator, conveys to the patient that he/she will act as the patient's advocate by speaking for him/her while the patient is in surgery.
- The patient may have fear and anxiety regarding the surgical procedure and the unfamiliar environment. Explain nursing procedures before performing them and the sequence of perioperative events.
- Assess and document patient's anxiety level and level of knowledge regarding the intended procedure. Clarify misconceptions by answering the patient's questions in a knowledgeable manner and refer questions to the surgeon, as necessary.
- The circulator demonstrates emotional support to the patient by his or her presence, maintaining eye contact, and using caring gestures, such as holding the patient's hand during the administration of anesthesia.
- Provide emotional support to the patient regarding feelings of altered body image by providing the patient an opportunity to express her feelings.
- Check the chart for patient's sensitivities and allergies, e.g., allergy to iodine (frequently contained in prep solutions). Document sensitivities or allergies noted preprocedure and document the alternative used.
- Assess hemodynamic factors. Keep patient's legs uncrossed. Apply antiembolitic hose before anesthesia is administered.
- Prevent musculoskeletal injuries to team members by employing ergodynamic measures when positioning the patient.
- Prevent risk of positioning injury to the patient with stirrups that are adequately padded and positioned correctly to avoid skin and neurovascular pressure or trauma. Document appearance and condition of the skin preoperatively and postoperatively.
- Lift both legs at the same time when putting the patient's legs in stirrups to prevent postoperative lumbosacral strain.

- Raise and lower legs slowly to prevent cardiovascular disturbances, e.g., rapid alterations in venous return.
- **N.B.** *Avoid injury to the patient's fingers by preventing them from being caught in the table mechanism when the foot of the table is raised following the procedure.*
- Take appropriate measures to maintain patient's body temperature, e.g., offer a warmed blanket (from blanket warmer), raise room temperature, as necessary. Place a warmed blanket over the patient following surgical intervention.
- Keep the patient adequately covered to maintain patient's privacy; expose only the immediate area involved for the procedure.
- A straight catheter (e.g., Robinson) to drain the urinary bladder is added to the skin prep set. Catheterize the patient at the completion of the skin and vaginal prep; document that the patient was catheterized and the size catheter that was used. Draining the patient's bladder prevents the bladder from compromising the operative field and helps to avoid urinary distention postoperatively.
- The scrub person sets up the instruments on the back table for the surgeon. Usually, the surgeon takes the instruments directly off the table himself/herself; a scrub person is not required. Sterile, water-soluble lubricant should be placed on the back table near the cervical dilators for the surgeon to use as a lubricant before the dilators are inserted; this avoids injury to the cervix.
- **N.B.** *If "fractional curettage" is performed, there are two separate biopsy specimens; the specimens should be placed in separate containers, labeled "endocervical" and "endometrial," respectively.*
- Place the perineal pad dressing on the patient before removing the drapes to avoid bringing contaminants into the area of the surgical site.
- Prior to leaving the OR, the circulator assures that the patient is properly positioned on the gurney and that measures necessary to maintain the patient's body temperature have been taken (e.g., with a blanket from the warmer).
- The circulator accompanies the anesthesia provider and the patient to the Post Anesthesia Care Unit (PACU); he/she gives the PACU perioperative practitioner a detailed intraoperative patient report regarding the course of events as they apply to the individual.
- In the PACU, the perioperative practitioner observes the patient's breathing, monitors blood pressure and vital signs, and

documents all pertinent information (e.g., the amount of blood on the peri pad) in the **Perioperative Record** in the **Postoperative Record**. Documentation is vital for patient safety regarding continuity of care and for medicolegal reasons.

- In the PACU, the perioperative practitioner assumes the role as the patient's advocate.
- In the **PACU,** the perioperative practitioner observes the patient for vaginal bleeding (alert for excessive bleeding, e.g., hemorrhage). The amount of vaginal bleeding is recorded when the patient arrives in the PACU and at intervals (according to the amount of bleeding); the surgeon is notified if excessive bleeding occurs. Documentation (in the **Perioperative Record** in the **Postoperative Record** section) is necessary for patient safety and for medicolegal reasons.

Conization of the Uterine Cervix

Definition

The excision of tissue about the cervical os (opening).

Discussion

This procedure is performed to diagnose and/or treat conditions such as cervicitis, epithelial dysplasia, carcinoma in situ, and invasive carcinoma. Cervical dysplasia occurs most frequently in women between the ages of 25 and 35. The dysplasia is excised using scalpel, cervatome, electrosurgery, laser (e.g., CO_2), etc. Observe all mandatory laser safety precautions; see p. 94. Regarding hemostasis, the laser is the most reliable modality.

Cold conization refers to the scalpel and scissors dissection of the cervical cone. *Hot conization* refers to tissue removal by electrosurgery or laser. In the *loop electrosurgical excision procedure (LEEP)*, a loop electrode (using the electrosurgical unit [ESU]) is employed to excise a core of tissue from the *endocervical canal*. *Large loop excision of the transformational zone (LLETZ)* of the cervix is done with an extra-large loop electrode. In addition, a laser endofiber may be employed to perform an **excisional cone** procedure. While these "hot" procedures are essentially bloodless, the specimen is inferior, as it is altered somewhat by desiccation.

Procedure

A weighted speculum is placed in the vaginal vault. The outer portion of the cervix is grasped with a tenaculum. Dilatation and Curettage, p. 277, is performed after the uterine canal is carefully sounded and dilated. The cervix may be stained with Schiller's solution or Lugol's solution. Dysplasia can be noted in the areas that absorb the stain in high concentration. Sutures may be placed at 3 o'clock and 9 o'clock positions. The sutures are placed for purposes of orientation. The cervix may be initially injected circumferentially, with a phenylephrine/Neosynephrine solution 1:20,000 to reduce bleeding. An incision is made circumferentially around the cervical os using a scalpel, scissors, electrosurgery, or an endo-laser fiber. If a laser is employed, all laser safety precautions must be observed; see p. 94. For cold conization, bleeding may be controlled with sutures, cryosurgery (freezing), electrosurgery, or a hemostatic agent (e.g., Surgicel™) may be employed. When "hot" conization is performed, there is minimal bleeding. For wide excisions of cervical tissue, suturing the cervix may be necessary. Following the procedure, the vagina is packed with gauze and a Foley catheter is inserted, connected to straight drainage. The unit is placed below the level of the patient's bladder to prevent reflux. A perineal pad is applied before removing the drapes.

In addition, *excision of a cervical cyst* may be performed by utilizing cryosurgery or electrosurgery. When electrosurgery is employed, electrodesiccation of the cyst is done by means of an electrosurgical needle, a ball electrode, or an endo-laser fiber.

An endoscope may be inserted into the pelvic cul de sac to identify abnormal epithelial cells requiring biopsy. Acetic acid (3–5%), wiped over the cervix, causes the abnormal tissues to turn white (repeat application of the acetic acid may be necessary during the procedure as its effect is transient). A microscope (*microcolposcope*) is focused on the vulva, introitus, vaginal wall, and cervix at magnification 2X–30X (most commonly, 15X). Additional lesions as vaginal condylomata and other epithelial changes can be identified by this modality. Biopsies, local excision, or electrosurgical or laser (or other modality) destruction of tissues can be performed.

Preparation of the Patient

Antiembolitic hose may be placed on the legs, if requested, before anesthesia is administered. Following the administration of general (usually) or regional anesthesia, the patient is positioned in lithotomy (using padded stirrups), with the buttocks positioned just over the edge of lower break in the table. Arms may be extended on padded armboards. Bony prominences and all areas prone to skin and neurovascular pressure or trauma are well padded. Apply electrosurgical dispersive pad.

Skin and Vaginal Preparation

Consult the surgeon; skin prep is done, but the internal vaginal preparation may be omitted. If a skin and vaginal prep is to be done, follow directions for the prep for D&C; see p. 278.

Draping

Drape sheet under the buttocks, followed by leggings, and a drape sheet over the abdomen
Back vest, as necessary
Drape sheet for microcolposcope, when used

Equipment

Padded stirrups
ESU
Cryosurgery unit, optional
Laser, e.g., Nd:YAG, optional
Microcolposcope, optional

Instrumentation

D&C tray
Cervical conization tray

Supplies

Antiembolitic hose, if requested
Straight catheter to drain the bladder (e.g., Robinson)
Small basin
Water-soluble lubricant
Telfa (for specimen)
Electrosurgical pencil and cord with blade, needle, loops (regular and large loop), and/or ball electrode
Blade, (1) #11 Medicine cups
Labels and marking pen
Schiller's solution or Lugol's solution, optional
Neosynephrine, 1:20,000, to reduce bleeding
#22-gauge needle and Luer lok syringe
Hemostatic agent, e.g., Surgicel, Thrombostat™, optional
Gauze packing, 1″, plain or iodophor (check chart for patient's allergies)
Vaginal cream, antibiotic or hormonal (check chart for patient's allergies) applied to plain gauze packing, optional
Foley catheter with continuous drainage unit, optional
Perineal pad
T-binder or sanitary napkin belt
Acetic acid (3%) in a labeled medicine cup (when endoscopy into the cul de sac is performed)

Special Notes

- **N.B.** *Consult with surgeon regarding the internal vaginal preparation*. Usually the vaginal mucosa is **not** prepped (as not to alter the appearance of the cells to be stained in the biopsy specimen). The skin may be prepped.

- Apply **Special Notes** from ***D&C,*** p. 278, as indicated.
- Scrub person usually works directly off the back table; a Mayo stand is not used.
- The surgeon may be seated for the procedure; if so, he/she may need to wear a back vest to prevent contamination of the back table; this depends on positioning of the back table.
- Use safety precautions to identify, label, and dispense medications or solutions to avoid medication errors; see p. 30. It is mandatory that all medications and solutions on the sterile field be labeled by name and strength.
- Circulator shows the bottle of Neosynephrine 1:20,000 (used to help control bleeding) to the scrub person and surgeon. He/she reads the name and strength of the drug aloud, showing the label. The bottle is placed in plain view and retained in the room until the procedure has concluded.
- If a laser is employed, observe all mandatory laser safety precautions; see p. 94.
- Noxious smoke and fumes resulting from thermal cell destruction caused by electrosurgical (electrodessication) or laser are a health hazard; smoke should be suctioned away by the room suction with an in-line filter or with a smoke evacuation system (e.g., Clear View®).
- Masks (that filter smoke particles between 2 and 5 microns) should be worn by all staff in the room during procedure to prevent inhalation of toxic matter.
- **Reminder:** Ask the patient, in addition to checking the patient's chart, about sensitivities and allergies (especially to iodine), as prep solutions, vaginal packing, and vaginal cream ingredients may contain iodophor.
- Document any sensitivity or allergy noted and the product that replaced the one usually used. Also, document the appearance of the tissues before the application of a solution and following application.
- Pathology requisitions must indicate the source from which the tissue specimen was taken. The curettings are *endocervical or endometrial*; a cervical smear (Pap) may also be taken and sent to cytology. Sutures may be placed on the specimen to indicate orientation; appropriate indication regarding suture placement should be noted on the pathology requisition.

- **Reminder:** Place the perineal pad dressing on the patient before removing the drapes to avoid bringing contaminants into the area of the surgical site.
- **Reminder:** In **PACU** the perioperative practitioner observes the patient for vaginal bleeding (alert for excessive bleeding, e.g., hemorrhage). The amount of vaginal bleeding is recorded when the patient arrives in the PACU and at intervals (according to the amount of bleeding); the surgeon is notified if excessive bleeding occurs. Documentation (in the **Perioperative Record** in the **Postoperative Record** section) is necessary for patient safety and for medicolegal reasons.

Therapeutic Abortion by Suction Curettage

Definition

The vacuum aspiration of uterine contents performed to terminate an early (usually) pregnancy.

Discussion

This procedure is also performed for missed and incomplete abortions. Suction curettage is the safest and most frequently chosen method for the evacuation of uterine contents, as the uterus is more easily perforated (by other methods utilizing a sharp curette) during pregnancy. This method for abortion is performed preferably within the first 3 months of pregnancy. To effect an abortion for a fetus of longer gestation, abortion is done using a hypertonic saline solution.

Abortion by any method may be against the religious beliefs of individuals working in the operating room (OR); this should be taken into consideration when room and patient assignments are made. Personnel need to advise their supervisor of their religious beliefs. In addition, the feelings of the patient must also be considered; statements made regarding value judgments of a patient's "right to choose" are inappropriate in the OR at the time of surgery.

Procedure

This procedure is similar to ***dilatation and curettage (D&C)***. A weighted speculum is placed in the vaginal vault. The cervix is grasped with a toothed tenaculum. The cervix is carefully measured by uterine sound and dilated. The surgeon passes one end of the tubing to the scrub person or the circulator. An appropriately sized suction curette (attached to the other end of the tubing) is inserted through the dilated cervix into the uterine cavity. The controlled suction apparatus (vacuum unit) is activated by either the scrub person or the circulator at the direction of the surgeon. The vacuum curette is rotated 360°, with a back-and-forth motion, while traction is maintained on the cervix until most of the uterine contents are emptied. The endometrial cavity is *carefully* curetted with a sharp curette, and a brief suction curettage is repeated. Uterine contents are collected in a gauze bag within the unit.

For Preparation of the Patient, Skin and Vaginal Preparation, and Draping, see *Dilatation and Curettage (D&C),* pp. 277–278.

Equipment

Padded stirrups
Controlled-suction apparatus (vacuum unit), e.g., Berkeley Vacurette, Synevac™

Instrumentation

Dilatation and curettage (D&C) tray
Disposable vacuum curettes (assorted sizes, curved and straight) and tubing

Supplies

Antiembolitic hose, if requested
Straight catheter (e.g., Robinson) to drain the bladder, added to the prep tray
Water-soluble lubricant
Disposable aspiration tubing
Gauze tissue bag (for specimen)
Perineal pad
T-binder or sanitary napkin belt

Special Notes

- Apply **Special Notes** from ***D&C***, p. 278, as indicated.
- Evacuation is done using all available vacuum pressure when turning on the unit. In the Berkeley unit, recommended pressure should be used at a pressure higher than 73 cm of mercury to effect suction.
- The surgeon connects a vacuum curette to the aspiration tubing. The circulator or scrub person attaches the tubing to the controlled suction unit and activates the unit *on the surgeon's request.*
- A gauze tissue bag is attached to the inside of the collection bottle (to collect the specimen). The gauze tissue bag with its contents is sent to the pathology laboratory.
- **N.B. Reminder:** Place the perineal pad dressing on the patient before removing the drapes to avoid bringing contaminants into the area of the surgical site.

- **Reminder:** In the **PACU,** the perioperative practitioner observes the patient for vaginal bleeding (alert for excessive bleeding, e.g., hemorrhage). The amount of vaginal bleeding is recorded when the patient arrives in the PACU and at intervals (according to the amount of bleeding); the surgeon is notified if excessive bleeding occurs. Documentation (in the **Perioperative Record** in the **Postoperative Record** section) is necessary for patient safety and for medicolegal reasons.
- The suction unit is cleaned immediately following the procedure (before any blood residue becomes dry and hardened), and the gauze tissue bag is replaced. The vacuum curettes and aspiration tubing are disposable.

Marsupialization of Bartholin's Gland Duct Cyst

Definition

Incision and drainage of a Bartholin's gland duct cyst (vulvovaginal cyst) and the suturing the wall of the cyst to the edges of the incision (the vestibular mucosa), as applicable.

Discussion

Bartholin's glands, vaginal vestibular glands, located at the introitus of the vagina, provide vaginal lubrication. A cyst(s), characterized by a painful swelling of the vulva, occurs most frequently in young women (<30 years) as the result of a distal obstruction of the duct. Bacterial infection of the cyst may occur, resulting in an abscess. The cyst(s) wall is composed primarily of the duct of the gland. By incising the wall of the cyst and by not excising the gland, the secretory function of the gland may be preserved. As necessary, the entire gland may be excised. Marsupialization is performed with incision and drainage of the cyst in absence of abscess formation. Alternatively, a Word™ catheter (by Milex) may be employed to keep the shrinking cyst patent until a new orifice is formed. Adjunctive treatment includes sitz baths and antibiotic therapy.

Procedure

A vertical incision is made in the vaginal mucosa over the center of the cyst. The cyst is incised and drained. Marsupialization refers to the eversion of the lining of the cyst and the suturing of the lining to the vaginal mucosa with interrupted absorbable stitches. If *cystectomy* is necessary, the cyst is mobilized using blunt dissection and plastic scissors for sharp dissection. The intact cyst is excised. A drain may be inserted when the mucosa is approximated. When a Word catheter (10 Fr to 12 Fr) is to be inserted, a small incision is made into the cyst with a #11 blade. The retention balloon is inflated with 2 to 3 ml of saline. The catheter may be left in place 4 to 6 weeks. A perineal pad is placed.

Preparation of the Patient

Antiembolitic hose may be placed on the legs, before anesthesia is administered, if requested. Following the administration of local, regional, or general anesthesia, the patient is positioned in lithotomy (using padded stirrups), with the buttocks positioned just over the edge of lower break in the table. Arms may be extended on padded armboards. Bony prominences and all areas prone to skin and neurovascular pressure or trauma are well padded. Apply electrosurgical dispersive pad.

Skin and Vaginal Preparation

Begin 3 to 4 inches above the pubic symphysis and extend downward over the labia. Cleanse each inner thigh. Vaginal vault and cervix are cleansed using spongesticks (3). The perineum and anus are cleansed with the remaining sponges. Discard each sponge after wiping the anus. The patient's bladder is drained with a straight catheter.

Draping

Drape sheet under the buttocks, followed by leggings, and a drape sheet over the abdomen

Equipment

Padded stirrups
ESU

Instrumentation

Cervical conization tray

Supplies

Antiembolitic hose, if requested
Straight catheter to drain the bladder (e.g., Robinson)
Small basin
Blades, (1) #15 and (1) #11
Luer lok syringe and large gauge needle, e.g., #15
Culture tubes with swabs (2) for aerobic and anaerobic cultures
Smear slides (2)
Electrosurgical pencil and cord with holder and scraper
Drain, e.g., Penrose 1/4″ or Word catheter (10 or 12 Fr) with a 2 to 3 ml balloon (available in a kit with syringe)
Perineal pad
T-binder or sanitary napkin belt

Special Notes

- Apply **Special Notes** from ***D&C***, p. 278, as indicated
- Scrub person should be prepared with a slide and culture tubes for a smear and cultures to be taken.
- Circulator needs to prepare requisitions for a Pap smear and aerobic and anaerobic cultures.
- Cultures should be dispensed to the lab as soon as possible to prevent their drying out.
- Consult surgeon regarding the type of drain to be used, if any.

Culdoscopy

Definition

Culdoscopy is the introduction of an endoscope through the posterior vaginal wall to provide visualization of the pelvic structures.

Discussion

Once frequently employed as a diagnostic tool, Culdoscopy is rarely performed today. **Culdoscopy** has, for the most part, been replaced by ***pelvic laparoscopy/pelviscopy***. In pelvic laparoscopy, the positioning of the patient is safer and easier for the patient to maintain, and the surgeon has better visualization of the pelvic structures.

Vaginal Hysterectomy

Definition

Removal of the uterus through a vaginal approach.

Discussion

Vaginal hysterectomy is performed for benign and early or limited malignant conditions of the uterus. The approach depends on the size of the uterus, in conjunction with the various aspects of the pathology. Performing the procedure is usually limited to endocervical, endometrial, and early cancers. Malignancies that have not been detected early are an indication for ***abdominal hysterectomy***, as the abdominal approach affords the operator visualization of the entire pelvic cavity.

Indications for **vaginal hysterectomy** include diseases of the uterus once restricted to benign conditions, e.g., irregular bleeding or menorrhagia, uterine prolapse in which the uterus is not greatly enlarged, and conditions in which severely poor pelvic muscular support is present. Early, endocervical, and endometrial malignancies may be removed via this approach when the spread to other organs is not suspect (according to preoperative evaluation).

In addition to the **vaginal hysterectomy**, *anterior and posterior colporrhaphy* may be necessary to correct additional conditions involving pelvic support (e.g., *cystocele, rectocele*, and *enterocele*); see ***Anterior and Posterior Colporrhaphy***, p. 293.

Procedure

A weighted vaginal speculum is placed in the vaginal vault. The cervix is grasped with a tenaculum. Dilatation and curettage may be performed. A phenylephrine/Neosynephrine solution may be injected into the area for the intended vaginal incision site to reduce bleeding. An incision is made anterior to the cervix in the vaginal wall. The bladder is reflected from the cervix using sharp, then blunt dissection, exposing the peritoneum of the anterior cul-de-sac, which is then incised posteriorly. The uterosacral and round ligaments are ligated and divided. The uterus is placed on traction. The cardinal ligaments and uterine arteries are ligated and divided, and the uterus is delivered. If the fallopian tubes and ovaries are to be preserved, the ovarian vessels are preserved, and the remaining structures in the broad ligament are ligated and divided. After the specimen is removed, the incisions into the cul-de-sac and vaginal apex are approximated. The uterosacral and round ligament stumps may be sutured to the angles of the vaginal vault closure.

In addition to the vaginal vault repair, an ***anterior and/or posterior colporrhaphy,*** p. 293, may be performed. A Foley catheter is inserted at the conclusion of the procedure and connected to continuous straight drainage (unit). The vagina is packed with gauze packing, iodophor, or plain, to which a hormonal cream is often added. A perineal pad dressing is applied before the drapes are removed.

Vaginal hysterectomy may also be performed as a laparoscopic-assisted procedure (LAVH); see p. 295.

Preparation of the Patient

Antiembolitic hose may be placed on the legs, if requested, before anesthesia is administered. Following the administration of regional or general anesthesia, the patient is positioned in lithotomy (using padded stirrups) with the buttocks positioned just over the edge of lower break in the table. Arms may be extended on padded armboards. Padded shoulder braces are secured to the table. The table may be placed in Trendelenburg position. Bony prominences and all areas prone to skin and neurovascular pressure or trauma are well padded. Apply electrosurgical dispersive pad.

Skin Preparation

Begin 3 to 4 inches above the pubic symphysis and extend downward over the labia. Cleanse each inner thigh. The vaginal vault and cervix are then cleansed using spongesticks (3). The immediate perineum and anus are cleansed with the remaining sponges. Discard each sponge after wiping the anus. The bladder is drained with a straight catheter.

Draping

Drape sheet under the buttocks, followed by leggings, and a laparotomy sheet
Additional drape sheet
Back vests (2)
Extra Mayo stand cover (for "lap tray")
***Note:** Usually, the surgeon and his/her assistant don back vests; they are seated. The additional drape sheet is fastened across the bottom of the patient's buttocks, and the opposite end of the drape is placed on the surgeon's lap, followed by the instrument "lap tray." Some surgeons prefer to stand, eliminating the need for the extra drape sheet and lap tray.*

Equipment

Sequential compression device with disposable leg wraps,* if requested
Forced-air warming blanket, if ordered
ESU
Suction
Padded stirrups (e.g., Allen)
Padded shoulder braces
Sitting stools

Instrumentation

Vaginal hysterectomy tray
Additional hysterectomy forceps (clamps), as requested

Supplies

Antiembolitic hose, as requested
Straight catheter to drain the bladder (e.g., Robinson)
Blades, (2), #10
Needle magnet or counter
Basin set
"Lap tray," sterile (placed inside the extra Mayo stand cover), optional
Neosynephrine 1:20,000 to reduce bleeding

Luer lok syringe and #22-gauge needle
Medicine cup
Labels and marking pen
Suction tubing
Electrosurgical pencil and cord with holder and scraper
Foley catheter with continuous drainage unit (at the surgery's conclusion)
Gauze packing, e.g., 1″ iodoform or plain
Vaginal cream, antibiotic or hormonal (for plain gauze packing), optional
Perineal pad
T-binder or sanitary napkin belt

Special Notes

- Apply **Special Notes** from ***D&C***, p. 278, as indicated.
- **N.B.** *In addition to the signed surgical permit (e.g.,* **Authorization for and Consent to Surgery,** *p. 6) for* **vaginal hysterectom,** *a signed permit for sterilization e.g.,* **Authorization for and Special Consent to Surgical Sterilization Procedure,** *p. 7 must also be on the chart; the document is required before the patient may be brought into the room. The patient needs to indicate in her own words that she understands that she will no longer be able to have children. The patient's statement is documented (in her own words) in the* **Perioperative Record,** *see p. 12; this is done for patient safety and medicolegal reasons.*
- Use safety precautions to identify, label, and dispense medications and medicated solutions and to *avoid medication errors*; see p. 30. It is mandatory that all medications and solutions on the sterile field be labeled by name and strength. The medication bottle is retained in the room until the procedure has concluded.
- Circulator must show the bottle of Neosynephrine 1:20,000 (used to help control bleeding) to the scrub person and surgeon. He or she reads the name and strength of the drug aloud and then shows the label. Apply safety precautions to avoid medication errors; see p. 30.
- A needle, syringe, and the Neosynephrine in a *labeled* medicine cup are placed on the "lap tray" (surgeon injects incision sites to reduce bleeding).
- Instruments for the lap tray often include a weighted speculum, a tenaculum, retractors, curved Mayo scissors, and hysterectomy clamps of the surgeon's choice (e.g., Heaney, curved Kocher, etc.).

- A Mayo stand is not often used; the scrub person works from the back table.
- The surgeon and his/her assistant don back vests to prevent contamination of the back table.
- Initially, the scrub person should be prepared with suture (e.g., "stick tie") for use to retract the labia before the weighted speculum is placed, if necessary.
- A Foley catheter connected to a continuous drainage unit is inserted at the conclusion of the surgery to prevent urinary retention resulting from swollen tissues around the operative site.
- The straight drainage tubing of the Foley catheter should be patent (without kinks); the level of the bag should be kept below the level of the patient's bladder to prevent a reflux of urine that could lead to a urinary tract infection (URI).
- At the conclusion, the vagina is packed with gauze packing, plain or iodophor. **Remember:** Ask the patient and check the chart for patient sensitivities or allergies regarding iodophor (iodine) and latex preprocedure; many products used in the OR may contain these substances, e.g., gloves, drains, bandages, prep solution, packing, and/or vaginal cream. Document that the patient's sensitivity or allergy was noted in the chart or referred to by the patient and the substitute products used; also document the appearance of the area involved (where product was used) preoperatively and postoperatively in the **Perioperative Record,** p. 12.

Anterior and/or Posterior Colporrhaphy

Definition

Repair and reinforcement of the musculofascial support of the urinary bladder and the urethra (anteriorly) and the distal rectum (posteriorly) to prevent protrusion of these structures through the vaginal wall.

Discussion

Cystocele (or cystourethrocele) presents anteriorly, with symptoms of urinary retention and/or stress incontinence due to herniation of the urinary bladder into the vagina through a defect in the anterior vaginal wall. *Rectocele* presents posteriorly due to the herniation of the rectum into the vagina through a posterior wall defect and may be associated with difficulties in defecation. These conditions may present simultaneously or independently and to varying degrees. An associated *enterocele*, a (usually small) herniation of the small bowel through the rectouterine pouch, may also occur. This latter entity can also present with uterine prolapse or in patients in whom hysterectomy has been performed. Multiparity is the most common cause for these entities; they may also be the result of an inherent defect, aging, or trauma. Repair may be performed to correct any of these conditions alone or in combination or to complement vaginal hysterectomy.

Procedure

The patient is in lithotomy position; the cervix (if present) is grasped with a tenaculum. For **anterior colporrhaphy**, the anterior vaginal mucosa is incised in the midline. The incision is deepened into the musculofascial wall, reflecting the bladder anteriorly, mobilizing the urethra, and exposing the urethrovesical junction. Plication sutures are placed in the musculofascial tissues to restore the urethrovesical angle and support of the bladder. Care is taken not to overtighten the repair. Excess tissue from the previously stretched vaginal mucosa is excised, and the mucosal incision is approximated.

For **posterior colporrhaphy,** an incision is made at the mucocutaneous junction, reflecting the attenuated vaginal mucosa proximally to expose the rectocele. Perirectal fascia is separated from the mucosa and plicated. The levator muscles are approximated at the midline to an appropriate degree of tension. The excess vaginal mucosa is excised, and the mucosal incision is closed. A vaginal pack is often placed. When necessary, repair of an **enterocele** involves opening the hernia sac, reducing the hernia, excising the sac (excess tissue), and closure of the opening; the closure is reinforced to prevent recurrence. Approximation of the uterouterosacral ligaments and the levator ani is accomplished. A Foley catheter is inserted (with continuous drainage unit attached) and gauze packing is inserted. A perineal pad dressing is applied before the drapes are removed.

Preparation of the Patient

Antiembolitic hose may be placed on the legs, if requested, before anesthesia is administered. Following the administration of regional or general anesthesia, the patient is positioned in lithotomy using padded stirrups, with the buttocks just over the edge of lower break in the table. Arms may be extended on padded armboards. Padded shoulder braces are secured to the table. The table may be placed in Trendelenburg position. Bony prominences and all areas prone to skin and neurovascular pressure or trauma are well padded. Apply electrosurgical dispersive pad.

Skin and Vaginal Preparation

Begin 3 to 4 inches above the pubic symphysis and extend downward over the labia. Cleanse each inner thigh. The vaginal vault and cervix are then cleansed using spongesticks (3). The perineum and anus are cleansed with the remaining sponges. Discard each sponge after wiping the anus. Catheterize patient's bladder with a straight catheter.

Draping

Drape sheet under the buttocks, leggings, and laparotomy sheet or
Drape sheet under the buttocks and laparoscopy sheet

Equipment

Sequential compression device with disposable leg wraps, if requested
Padded stirrups
Padded shoulder braces
Suction
ESU

For **Instrumentation, Supplies,** and **Special Notes,** see *Vaginal Hysterectomy,* pp. 291–292.

Gynecologic Laparoscopy/Pelviscopy

Definition

The introduction of an endoscope (illuminated metal tube) through the anterior abdominal wall following the establishment of a pneumoperitoneum to visualize intraabdominal and pelvic structures for purposes of diagnosis and treatment. The term **"pelviscopy"** may be employed when referring to **gynecologic laparoscopy**.

Discussion

Laparoscopy, when employed for gynecologic purposes, is useful to diagnose causes of infertility, ectopic pregnancy, pelvic masses (benign and malignant), endometrial implants, etiology of the acute abdomen, pelvic pain, etc. It is also employed to perform an expanding number of therapeutic modalities, including various fertility procedures such as *ovarian drilling, laser-assisted neosalpingostomy* and *fimbrioplasty, salpingo-ovariolysis,* and *in-vitro fertilization.* Endo-ovarian procedures for sterilization, treatment of ectopic pregnancy and endometrial cysts, and *drainage of tubo-ovarian abscess* can be performed laparoscopically. *Uterine nerve ablation* for intractable dysmenorrhea, myomectomy, colposuspension, and pelvic lymphadenectomy can also be performed laparoscopically.

Hysterectomy, vaginal hysterectomy, and other treatments for endometriosis may be performed as laparoscopic and laparoscopic-assisted procedures. **"Incidental" appendectomy** and other general surgery procedures may be combined with the gynecologic surgery, as applicable.

Procedure

For most gynecological laparoscopic procedures, the patient is in a modified lithotomy position that affords access to the anterior abdomen and to the introitus of the vagina. ***D&C*** may be performed; see p. 277.

The table may be placed in Trendelenburg position. Pneumoperitoneum is established via the inferior margin of the umbilicus; see Abdominal Laparoscopy, p. 136. Usually a10-mm or 11-mm trocar is placed, and a laparoscope with a 30° angle (most commonly used) is inserted. Additional ports (5 and 12 mm) are placed in either lower quadrant at the lateral aspect of the rectus muscle, as necessary.

D&C may be performed. The anterior cervical os is grasped by a toothed tenaculum. A lubricated intrauterine manipulator/cannula is inserted into the uterus to permit transvaginal manipulation during the procedure, as necessary. For ***chromotubation,*** methylene blue or indigo carmine is injected into the uterus via a flexible catheter placed in the cervical canal (for fertility detection). Laparoscopically, if the dye is seen to escape the fimbriated fallopian tube (into the peritoneal cavity), the tube is patent. When the tube is not patent, multiple conditions may be responsible, requiring surgical treatment.

In **gynecologic laparoscopy/pelviscopy,** multiple definitive procedures may be performed. ***Tubal insufflation*** may be performed to test tubal patency; it may also be effective in disrupting minor adhesions. ***Salpingolysis***, the release of adhesions, usually due to an inflammatory process, can be done with a laser. ***Salpingostomy***, the creation of an opening into the distal end of a fallopian tube, is performed, employing plastic or eye scissors and fine suture (e.g., 6-0). A laser fiber is utilized for tuboplasty, tubal reconstruction, and/or tubal anastomosis to reestablish continuity of a fallopian tube, thereby restoring tubal patency when previous sterilization has been done. ***Tubal reimplantation*** into the uterus may also be performed. ***Salpingectomy,*** the removal of a fallopian tube (or part of a tube), and ***salpingo-oopherectomy***, the removal of the fallopian tubes and ovaries, may be done when fertility is not a concern. ***Oophorectomy,*** the removal of the ovaries for benign and malignant conditions may also be performed laparoscopically. Tissue may be excised and the biopsy specimen sent for frozen section. In ***ovarian cystectomy***, a benign ovarian cyst, the cyst may be aspirated and/or excised, preserving the ovary.

For the above procedures, an operating microscope may be attached (coupled) to the laparoscope. A laser fiber (e.g., Nd:YAG, Ho: YAG, or KTP) may be used in conjunction with the operating microscope to divide adhesions and to open blocked tubes, etc. Observe all laser safety precautions. When endometrial implants are treated, an *argon beam coagulator* (see p. 111) may be utilized. ***Hydrodissection*** may be employed to remove cysts, ectopic pregnancies, and/or clots from fallopian tubes using fluid under pressure; the openings made into the fallopian tubes are left open.

Upon completion of the procedure, any intraabdominal blood or fluid is aspirated, pneumoperitoneum is released, and incisional sites are closed and dressed. The transvaginal manipulator/cannula is removed and a perineal pad dressing is applied.

Preparation of the Patient

Antiembolitic hose may be placed on the legs, as requested. Following the administration of regional or general anesthesia, the patient is placed in modified lithotomy position using padded stirrups (e.g., Allen), with the buttocks just over the edge of the lower break in the table. The arms are extended on padded armboards. Shoulder braces are secured to the table. The table may be placed in Trendelenburg position. Pad all bony prominences and areas vulnerable to skin and neurovascular trauma or pressure. Apply electrosurgical dispersive pad.

Skin and Vaginal Preparation

Add extra sponges, prep solution, and a straight catheter before starting to prep. Stand at the foot of the table between the patient's legs and begin cleansing at the umbilicus, extending from the nipples to the mid-thighs and down to the table at the sides. Continue with a vaginal prep, as for ***D&C***, p. 278. Catheterize patient's bladder with a straight catheter (e.g., Robinson).

Draping

Drape sheet under the buttocks, folded towels on the abdomen (optional), and a laparoscopy sheet, or drape sheet under the buttocks, leggings, folded towels (optional) and a laparotomy sheet

Microscope drape, optional

Equipment

Padded shoulder braces

ESU

Suction

Endoscopy Cart:

CO_2 insufflation device, EndoFlo™ pump

Pressure regulating device for irrigation, e.g., HydroFlex™

Fiber-optic light source, e.g., Xenon™ 300 W

Camera console

VCR

Printer

CD burner

Monitor(s) (1 or 2)

Argon beam coagulator console, optional

Hydrodissector console, optional
Microscope (e.g., Zeiss), optional
Stirrups (if D&C performed)

Instrumentation
D&C tray (if performed)
Tenaculum
Uterine retractors
Uterine manipulator

Laparoscopy
Limited procedures tray
Mosquito hemostats (6) curved, (2) straight
Frazier suction tips (assorted)
Beaver knife handle
Verres needle (disposable available)
Trocars (5 mm, 10 or 11 mm, 12 mm, or Hasson)
Reducers and connectors
Coupler for microscope, if used
Fiberoptic laparoscope, 30°, and cord, usually used; 0° scope, optional
For **chromotubation** (infertility detection)
Intrauterine cannula (e.g., Cohen)
Endoscopic instruments:
Babcock forceps (2); (3) scissors curved, hook, and straight; right angle dissector; Kelly clamps; dissecting forceps; (straight, right angle, and hook), irrigation-suction-electrosurgical dissector, sponge holder
Multifire ligating clip applier

Supplies

Antiembolitic hose, as requested
Suction tubing (2) for uterine manipulator and abdominal suction
Electrosurgical cord
Basin set
Water-soluble lubricant
Blades, (1) #10, (1) #15, (1) #11, and Beaver
Needle magnet or counter
Silastic™ tubing for CO_2 insufflation
Cystoscopy or similar straight tubing, e.g., K50 (add 1000-ml bag normal saline and three-way stopcock, for irrigation)
Loop ligation sutures, e.g., Endoloop™ (with introducer sleeve available for ties), if requested
Fog reduction agent, e.g., FRED®, ELVIS™
For ***infertility detection chromotubation,*** 1000 ml bag normal saline and 3-way stapcock, plastic, Silastic, or polyethylene

tubing (e.g., K50), labeled syringe containing dye (e.g., methylene blue or indigo carmine)
Perineal pad
T-binder or sanitary napkin belt
Band Aids or skin closure strips (optional)

Special Notes

- Apply **Special Notes** from ***Abdominal Laparoscopy***, p. 140, as indicated.
- Consult the surgeon regarding whether **D&C** will first be performed. The scrub person should prepare a separate back table with D&C instrumentation, as necessary.
- Stents may be inserted into the fallopian tubes to help maintain patency. The circulator should record information regarding the stent(s) insertion in the **Perioperative Record**.

Uterine Myomectomy

Definition

Excision of uterine leiomyomata (fibroid tumors).

Discussion

Leiomyomata (also known as *fibroids,* myofibromata, *fibroleiomata,* etc.) are common benign smooth muscle uterine tumors that rarely degenerate into sarcomata. The leiomyomatas can be located intramurally, subserosally, or submucosally; they may be interligamentous or pedunculated; they may attach to adjacent organs (parasitic). These tumors can be single or multiple; most are small, asymptomatic, and require no treatment. Dependent on the patient's estrogen level, tumor growth can occur, leading to interference with fertility and concurrent pain, pressure, bleeding, and urethral and rectal compression.

Approaches to **Myomectomy** include: transabdominal as an "open" procedure, laparoscopic and/or hysteroscopic. Prior to surgery, abdominal and vaginal ultrasound scans are made to delineate the lesion(s); intravenous pyelogram (IVP), computed tomography (CT), and magnetic resonance imaging (MRI) scans, and hysterosalpingography can be performed as well. Some authorities recommend the use of gonadotropin-releasing hormone (GnRH) for 3 months to reduce the size of the tumors and to lessen intraoperative bleeding.

Uterine fibroid embolization (UFE) is an alternative method used to treat uterine fibroids that is less invasive. Appropriate branches of the uterine artery are embolized (blocked) with polyvinyl alcohol particles or acrylic spheres, "embospheres." Embospheres result in the degeneration and shrinkage of the fibroids due to loss of blood supply. Only the blood supply to the affected myometrium (i.e., the fibroids) is blocked; blood supply to the unaffected myometrium is maintained by collateral circulation. UFE is most often performed in the radiology department, but it may be done in the operating room (OR), employing fluoroscopic control.

Procedure

The table may be placed in Trendelenburg position for any of these approaches. Padded shoulder braces are secured to the table.

Transabdominal Approach Myomectomy. Via Pfannensteil or midline incision, the peritoneal cavity is entered and a large self-retaining retractor (e.g., Balfour) is placed. The bowel is packed away with warm moist (saline) lap pads, and the ureters are noted and protected as well. The lesions are identified. The uterine arteries may be isolated and encircled with vessel loops for temporary occlusion as necessary. Pitressin®/vasopressin or Pitocin®/oxytocin in very dilute in normal saline solution (labeled, including strength) may be injected about the lesions to minimize bleeding. The lesions are then excised from the myometrium. The laser may be used for dissection and hemostasis; observe all mandatory laser safety precautions, p. 94. If the lesions are adjacent to the fallopian tubes, stents may be passed via the tubes during uterine repair. The abdominal cavity is irrigated with warm saline and the fluid is aspirated. The abdomen is closed in layers. An abdominal dressing and a perineal pad are placed.

Transcervical Hysteroscopic Approach Myomectomy. This approach is used for submucosal and pedunculated lesions that present intravaginally. The uterus is distended with an appropriate medium, and the lesions are excised with a resectoscopic cutting loop. Extra care is taken near the tubal ostia. The KTP or argon laser may be employed, as well as the operating microscope.

Concurrent ***laparoscopy*** may be performed as a protective measure to identify and avoid blood vessels, ureters, and injury to the bladder or bowel. Intravaginal packing or a pressure balloon may be used for hemostasis. A perineal pad is placed.

Laparoscopic Approach Myomectomy. This approach may be employed in selected cases (not for large or deep lesions or those next to the cornua). Pneumoperitoneum is established; see ***Abdominal Laparoscopy***, p. 136. Lower abdominal ports are established. Oxytocin may be injected around the lesions to reduce bleeding. The specimens are sometimes morcellated (Semm morcellator) after they are retrieved and placed in a specimen bag, e.g., Endo Pouch™, etc.

Wounds in the myometrium are closed by suture repair. The abdominal wounds are closed, and Band Aids or Steri Strips are applied. A perineal pad is placed.

Preparation of the Patient

Antiembolitic hose may be placed on the legs, as requested. Regional or general anesthesia is administered. Padded shoulder braces are secured to the table. The table may be placed in Trendelenburg position during the procedure for better visualization of the pelvic contents (as the organs fall cephalad). Pad all bony prominences and areas vulnerable to skin and neurovascular trauma or pressure. Apply electrosurgical dispersive pad.

Abdominal Momectomy. The patient is supine; arms may be extended on padded armboards. A pillow may be placed under the lumbar spine and/or knees (to avoid straining back muscles).

Laparoscopic Myomectomy. The patient is positioned in modified lithotomy, see surgical positions, p. 20.

Transcervical Hysteroscopic and Simultaneous Laparoscopic Myomectomy. The patient is placed in modified lithotomy position using padded stirrups, with the buttocks positioned just over the edge of the lower break in the table, and the arms extended on padded armboards. Pad all bony prominences and areas vulnerable to skin and neurovascular trauma or pressure.

Skin Preparation

Abdominal Approach. A vaginal and an abdominal prep (separate trays) are required. The patient's legs are placed in a froglike position; prep as for ***D&C***, p. 278. Insert a Foley catheter and connect to continuous drainage. Return the patient's legs to their original position, place the drainage unit below the level of the table, and replace the safety belt. For the abdominal preparation, begin at the intended site of incision (usually Pfannenstiel), extending from nipples to mid-thighs and down to the table at the sides.

Laparoscopic Approach and Transcervical Hysteroscopic and Simultaneous Laparoscopic Approach. A combined abdominal and vaginal preparation is done. Add extra sponges, prep solution, and a straight catheter (e.g., Robinson) to the prep set. Stand between the patient's legs, after the lower section of the table is removed. Begin cleansing at the umbilicus, extending the prep from nipples to the mid-thighs. Continue the prep over the labia, discarding each sponge after wiping the labia. Cleanse each inner thigh and discard the sponge. Prep the vaginal vault and cervix using three spongesticks. Prep perineum and anus last; discard each sponge after wiping the anus. Catheterize patient's bladder with the straight catheter.

Draping

Abdominal Approach. Folded towels and laparotomy sheet

Transcervical Hysteroscopic and Laparoscopic Approach. Drape sheet under buttocks, leggings, and laparotomy sheet, or drape sheet under the buttocks and laparoscopy sheet.

Equipment

Abdominal, Laparoscopic, and Hysteroscopic Approaches

Sequential compression device with leg wraps, if requested
ESU
Suctions (2)
Padded shoulder braces
Cell-saver console, optional
Scales (2), for weighing sponges, available
Laser, e.g., Argon, KTP, or Nd:YAG, optional

Transcervical Hysteroscopic and Laparoscopic Approach

Padded stirrups (e.g., Allen)
ESU
Monitors (1 or 2)
Endoscopy Cart:
Laparoscopic CO_2 insufflator, e.g., Surgiflator™ 25
Laparoscopic irrigator system with pressure sensor for fluid distention, e.g., HydroFlex
Fiber-optic light source (2), e.g., Xenon 300 W tw (1) for laparoscope (1) for hysterscope
Camera console
VCR
Printer
CD burner
Laser, optional

Transcervical Hysteroscopic

Monitor
VCR
CD burner
Camera console
Hysteroscopic CO_2 insufflator, e.g., EndoFlo (**not** the laparoscopic CO_2 insufflator) Pressure infusion pump/roller pump console (e.g., Hamou Hysteromat II measures

intrauterine pressure) or Syringe (50 ml) may be used to infuse pressure within the uterus
Hysteroscopic irrigator system with pressure sensor for fluid distention, e.g., HydroFlex HD
SEMM macromorsellator console

Instrumentation

Abdominal Approach

Major procedures tray
Abdominal hysterectomy tray
Self-retaining retractor (e.g., Balfour)
Myomectomy 5-mm corkscrew (WISAP)

Transhysteroscopic and Laparoscopic Approaches

Limited procedures tray
D&C tray
Verres needle (disposable available)
Trocars (5 mm, 10 or 11 mm, 12 mm, or Hasson)
Fiber-optic laparoscope, e.g., 30° and 0°, and cord
Camera and coupler (if not integrated into scope)
Reducers and connectors
Smoke evacuator, e.g., Smoke Evac™ with trumpet valve Dorsey™ or in-line filter for smoke evacuator
CD burner
Printer

Laparoscopic (endoscopic) instruments:

Dissectors, graspers, scissors (blunt and sharp), electrosurgical suction-irrigator and electrosurgical cord
Multifire ligating clip applier
Semm morcellator handpiece and cord with myoma drill and rotary drill, optional

Note: Laparoscopy may be done concurrently, as noted above, as a protective measure during **hysteroscopy**. Laparoscopic instruments are seldom used in this combined procedure, but they should be available on back table ready for use (in case needed).

***Transcervical Hysteroscopic instruments*:**

D&C tray
Cervical cone tray
Self-retaining vacuum cannula with obturator (e.g., Cohen)

***Hysteroscopic instruments*:**

Probes, alligator cup forceps (assorted), biopsy forceps (rigid and flexible), light cord, cannulas (e.g., aspirating), micro scissors, rigid resectoscope with loop electrosurgical electrodes (tips

and loops) and "rollerball" electrodes, insulated electrosurgical coagulating electrode (e.g., GynePro™), Babcock forceps, micro-scissors, and rotary knife
Rigid fiber-optic hysteroscope (operating) and cord
Camera and coupling device
Electrosurgical cord
Loop resector electrodes, e.g., Gyne-Pro®
Laser handpiece and fiber tip, optional

Supplies

Antiembolitic hose
Basin set
Luer lok syringe with #22-gauge needle
Medicine cups, labels, and marking pen
Pitressin/vasopressin or Pitocin®/oxytocin labeled, in very dilute solution in N/S; the vasopressin may come in a preloaded syringe that is prelabeled
Needle magnet or counter

Abdominal Approach, Add

Blades, (2) #10, (1) #15, (1) #11
Suction tubing
Electrosurgical pencil with loop tip, cord, holder, and scrapers
Vessel loops, optional
Stents for fallopian tubes, optional
Foley catheter or special intrauterine balloon catheter for applying pressure, (tamponade) available
Sanitary napkin belt or T-binder
Perineal pad

Laparoscopic Approach, Add

Electrosurgical cord
Suction tubing
Straight tubing, e.g., K50, add: 1000-ml bag normal saline and three-way stopcock, for irrigation or
HydroFlex irrigation tubing, casette
Silastic tubing for laparoscopy insufflator
Loop ligation sutures, e.g., Endoloop (with introducer sleeve), if requested
Fog reduction agent, e.g., FRED, ELVIS
Specimen retrieval bag, e.g., Endo Pouch, ENDOBAG™, etc., optional
Band Aids or similar dressing for incisions

Hysteroscopic Approach

Water-soluble lubricant

Silastic tubing for hysteroscopy insufflator only (insufflators are not interchangeable)
Electrosurgical cord
Suction tubing
Polyethelene tubing, e.g., K50, add: 1000-ml bag normal saline and three-way stopcock, for hysteroscopy medium with syringe or
Single use tubing and cassette, e.g., GyneFlo™
Hysteroscopy viscid medium (to distend uterus, pre-warmed): Hyskon, Ringer's lactate, 1.5% glycine, 3% sorbitol, 5% mannitol. Additional media that may be used include: normal saline (0.9%), water, D5W, or CO_2 (40 to 60 ml/min at 100 mm/Hg)
Sanitary napkin belt or T-binder
Perineal pad

Special Notes

- Apply **Special Notes** from ***Gynecologic Laparoscopy/Pelviscopy***, p. 299, and ***Hysteroscopy***, p. 325, as indicated.
- **Reminder:** Use safety precautions to identify, label, and dispense medications or solutions and to avoid medication errors; see p. 30. It is mandatory that all medications and solutions on the sterile field be labeled by name and strength.
- Monitor the amount of medium being used during the procedure to distend the uterus. The circulator should carefully monitor output and consult the anesthesia provider regarding fluid output to avoid systemic overload.
- In the abdominal approach, vessel loops are used; they are included in *the count* and documented in **Perioperative Record**.
- The laser fiber of the KTP Nd:YAG, or argon, may be employed for dissection, hemostasis, adhesiolysis, and to open blocked fallopian tubes; see p. 94 for mandatory laser safety precautions.
- Suction smoke away using room suction with an in-line filter or with a smoke-evacuation system (e.g., Smoke Evac with trumpet valve).
- In the abdominal approach, when stents are placed to maintain fallopian tubal patency, the stent information is documented on the **Perioperative Record**.
- **N.B. Note:** *The hysteroscopic CO_2 insufflator (e.g., HydroFlex with pressure relief valve, e.g., GyneFlo) is* **not** *the same as the laparoscopic insufflator.* **Use the insufflator made**

specifically for hysteroscopy; the hysteroscopic insufflator provides higher CO_2 pressure at a lower rate.

- Instruments, especially optics, must be cleaned immediately following use, to prevent debris and agents in the solution from hardening, particularly if Hyskon has been used as the distending medium. A proteolytic enzyme wash is available for cleansing.
- Excision of leiomyomata (fibroids) may result in significant blood loss (hemorrhage). The patient usually makes an autologous blood donation preoperatively. The circulator should ascertain that the blood is ready and available, i.e., verify availability with the blood bank.
- Ascertain if cell saver will be needed; set up the console in advance as much as possible. Notify personnel as necessary to run the cell-saver.
- There must be two working suctions in the room (in addition to the suction on the anesthesia cart) in case significant blood loss (hemorrhage) should occur.
- The circulator must be prepared to assist anesthesia provider in checking the units of blood (or blood products) and comparing identification numbers on units to the patient identification number. A blood pump and blood warmer should be brought into the room prior to bringing the patient into the room.
- The circulator keeps an accurate record of irrigation fluid used to assist in determining replacement of total fluid loss.
- Weigh sponges as necessary to assist in determining blood and fluid loss replacement, as necessary. To see procedure for weighing sponges, see **Special Notes** from ***Pancreaticoduodenectomy (Whipple procedure),*** p. 161.
- Inspect instruments after use for breakage with possibility of retention of a foreign body in the uterine cavity. If a part of an instrument is missing, the surgeon is alerted (before closure begins) and supervisor of the department is notified. When the piece is not found, an x-ray must be taken of the cavity, and the information regarding the loss is documented in an **Incident Report** that becomes part of the patient's chart.

Total Abdominal Hysterectomy

Definition

Removal of the whole (total) uterus through an abdominal incision.

Discussion

Some indications for **total abdominal hysterectomy (TAH)** are endometriosis, adnexal disease, postmenopausal bleeding, dysfunctional uterine bleeding, and benign and malignant tumors. TAH was, until recently, considered an absolute necessity to avoid cancer of the cervix. Currently, some gynecologists perform supracervical hysterectomy (instead of TAH) in order to preserve the secretory function of the cervix and to aid in supporting the structures in the pelvis, thereby avoiding prolapse. In conjunction with TAH, gynecologists performing TAH can perform colporrhaphy procedures to correct anterior and posterior prolapse.

Hysterectomy may be performed laparoscopically (p. 318) and as a laparoscopic-assisted procedure (p. 318).

Procedure

A transverse, Pfannenstiel, midline, or paramedian incision is employed, depending on the diagnosis, anatomical considerations, and preference of the surgeon. The peritoneal cavity is entered, and a self-retaining retractor is placed. The table is placed in Trendelenburg position (the organs fall cephaled, e.g., towards the head) to facilitate viewing the pelvic contents. The intestines are protected with warm moist (saline) lap pads. The fundus of the uterus is grasped with a multi-toothed tenaculum for manipulation (by retracting cephalad); this, too, facilitates pelvic exposure. The round ligaments of the uterus are ligated and divided (by scalpel or Mayo or Jorgensen scissors), and ligatures are tagged with a hemostat, **not cut**. After identifying the ureters, the broad ligaments are ligated and divided. The bladder is reflected from the anterior aspect of the cervix using blunt and sharp dissection. The infundibulopelvic ligaments are ligated and divided. If the ovaries are to be preserved, the ovarian vessels are ligated and divided adjacent to the uterus (avoiding the ureters). The uterosacral ligaments are ligated and divided. The cardinal ligaments are likewise ligated and divided. Suture ligatures are employed on the patient side of the division. The cervix is grasped anteriorly (with a Kocher or similar clamp), and the vagina is incised circumferentially. The specimen (uterus) is removed. A free raytec sponge (soaked in prep solution) may be placed in the vagina with long smooth forceps prior to closure. Hemostasis is secured. The vaginal cuff is closed with a continuous absorbable suture; a drain may be placed (infrequently). The stumps of the uterosacral and round ligaments are sutured to the angles of the vaginal closure. The peritoneum is approximated, and the wound is closed in layers. Dressings are placed. The free raytec sponge is removed transvaginally; in order for the sponge count to be correct, the free raytec sponge must be retrieved before the patient is taken from the OR to PACU.

Preparation of the Patient

Antiembolitic hose are put on the legs, as requested. The patient is supine; arms may be extended on padded armboards. A pillow may be placed under the lumbar spine and/or under the knees to avoid straining back muscles. Padded shoulder braces are secured to the table. The table may be placed in Trendelenburg position. Pad all bony prominences and areas vulnerable to skin and neurovascular trauma or pressure. Apply electrosurgical dispersive pad.

Skin Preparation

A vaginal and an abdominal prep (separate trays) are required. The patient's legs are placed in a froglike position; prep as for ***D&C***, see p. 278. Insert a Foley catheter and connect to continuous drainage unit. Return the patient's legs to their original position, place the drainage unit below the level of the table, and replace the safety belt. For the abdominal preparation, begin at the intended site of incision (usually Pfannenstiel), extending from nipples to mid-thighs and down to the table at the sides.

Draping

Folded towels and a transverse or laparotomy sheet

Equipment

- Sequential compression device with disposable leg wraps, if requested
- Forced-air warming blanket, if ordered
- Padded shoulder braces
- Suction
- ESU

Instrumentation

- Major procedures tray
- Abdominal hysterectomy tray
- Self-retaining retractor (e.g., Balfour or O'Connor-O'Sullivan)

Supplies

- Antiembolitic hose
- Blades, (3) #10
- Basin set
- Needle magnet or counter
- Suction tubing

Electrosurgical pencil with blade, cord, holder, and scraper
Foley catheter with tubing and drainage unit
Sanitary napkin belt or T-binder
Perineal pad

Special Notes

- **N.B.** *A signed special permit for any* **sterilization procedure, p. 7,** *must be on the chart in addition to the signed surgical permit required for the procedure,* **Total Abdominal Hysterectomy,** *before the patient may be admitted to the room.* The patient needs to indicate in her own words that she understands that she will no longer be able to have children. The patient's words are documented in the **Perioperative Record.**
- Apply **Special Notes** from **Abdominal Laparotomy**, p. 134, as indicated.
- **N.B. Remember:** *Check with the patient before surgery and check the chart for patient sensitivities and allergies, particularly to iodine or latex products; many brands of prep solution and packing may contain iodophor; gloves, drains (e.g., Penrose), and elasticized dressings and pressure bandages contain latex.*
- The patient may have made an autologous blood donation preoperatively. The circulator should verify that the blood is ready and available, i.e., check with the blood bank.
- **N.B.** *Before bringing the patient into the room, the circulator should ascertain that there are two working suctions in the room (in addition to the suction on the anesthesia cart) in case hemorrhage should occur.* Keep an accurate record of irrigation used to assist in determining total fluid loss replacement.
- Weigh sponges, as necessary, to assist in determining blood and fluid loss replacement, as indicated.
- ***"Spongesticks"*** (raytec sponge on ringed forceps) may be requested throughout the surgery for blunt dissection.
- A ***"stick tie"*** refers to a suture ligature with a swaged-on needle; the needle may be loaded onto a curved Heaney needle holder. The needle tip protrudes from the convex aspect of the needle holder.

- Instruments that come in contact with the cervix or vagina are isolated in a basin.
- The specimen is most conveniently received in a basin due to its large size.
- **N.B. Three closure counts** *are taken for* **TAH:** *1) at closure of vaginal cuff, 2) at closure of peritoneum, and 3) at closure of skin.*
- **N.B.** *A "free sponge" is placed in the vagina prior to closure; the sponge is included in the sponge count, and its placement is noted in the* **Perioperative Record.** The sponge *must* be removed transvaginally at the termination of the procedure, before the patient leaves the room.
- A Foley catheter (connected to a continuous straight drainage unit) is inserted at the conclusion of the surgery to prevent urinary retention resulting from swollen tissues around the operative site.
- The drainage tubing of the Foley catheter should be patent (without kinks); the level of the bag should be kept below the level of the patient's bladder to prevent a reflux of urine that could lead to a urinary tract infection (UTI).

Salpingo-Oophorectomy

Definition

Removal of the fallopian tube(s) and the corresponding ovary or ovaries.

Discussion

Salpingo-oopherectomy is performed for a variety of nonmalignant diseases that include acute and chronic infections, cysts, tumors, and hemorrhage (tubal pregnancy, see p. 326). When a fallopian tube or an ovary is found to contain a malignancy, hysterectomy with excision of the both adnexae is indicated.

Procedure

A low midline, paramedian, or Pfannenstiel incision is employed. The peritoneal cavity is entered, and a self-retaining retractor is placed. The table is placed in Trendelenburg position. The intestines are protected with warm, moist (saline) lap pads. The abdomen is explored. If adhesions are present, a hydrodissector (see p. 298) may be employed. When the affected fallopian tube is blocked, a laser fiber may be used to open it and a stent may be placed to maintain patency. For excision, the infundibulopelvic ligament is ligated and divided, as are the broad ligament attachment and the blood vessels of the affected tube and ovary. The tube and ovary are excised. The site of adnexal excision may be reperitonealized. The wound is closed in layers. A dressing is applied to the wound and a perineal pad is placed.

For the laparoscopic approach, see ***Gynecologic Laparoscopy/ Pelviscopy***, p. 295.

Preparation of the Patient

Apply antiembolitic hose, as requested. The patient is supine; arms may be extended on padded armboards. A pillow may be placed under the lumbar spine and/or under the knees (to avoid straining back muscles). Padded shoulder braces are secured to the table. The table is placed in Trendelenburg position. Pad all bony prominences and areas vulnerable to skin and neurovascular trauma or pressure. Apply electrosurgical dispersive pad.

For **Skin Preparation and Draping,** see ***Total Abdominal Hysterectomy***, p. 308.

Equipment

- Sequential compression device with disposable leg wraps, if requested
- Forced-air warming blanket, if ordered
- Padded shoulder braces
- Suction
- ESU
- Hydrodissector console, optional
- Laser (e.g., Nd:YAG, KTP, or Argon) optional

Instrumentation

- Major procedures tray
- Self-retaining retractor (e.g., Balfour or O'Connor-O'Sullivan)
- Somer's clamp
- Hydrodissector hand piece and cord

Supplies

- Antiembolitic, as requested
- Blades, (2) #10, (1) #15
- Basin set
- Needle magnet or counter
- Suction tubing
- Electrosurgical pencil and cord with holder and scraper
- Sanitary napkin belt or T-binder
- Perineal pad

Special Notes

- N.B. *A* **sterilization procedure** *permit, in addition to the signed surgical permit for the procedure,* **bilateral salpingo-oophorectomy,** *is required before the patient may be brought into the room.* The patient needs to indicate in her own words that she understands that she will no longer be able to have children. Her statement to this effect should be included in the **Perioperative Record**.
- Apply **Special Notes** from ***Abdominal Laparotomy***, p. 134, as indicated.
- **"Spongesticks"** (raytec sponge on ringed forceps) are often used for blunt dissection and may be requested throughout the surgery.
- A Foley catheter connected to a continuous straight drainage unit is inserted at the conclusion of the surgery.
- Tubing attached to the Foley catheter should be patent (without kinks); the level of the bag should be kept below the level of patient's bladder to prevent a reflux of urine that could lead to a UTI.

Tubal Sterilization

Definition

Interruption in the continuity of the lumen of the fallopian tubes, resulting in sterilization.

Discussion

Tubal sterilization, also referred to as **tubal ligation,** can be accomplished by resection, desiccation or cauterization, lumenal obstructing device (e.g., Essure), clip application (e.g., using Filschie™ or Hulka™ clips, etc.), silicone banding, or ligation of the fallopian tubes. Puerperal sterilization is best performed 24 to 36 hours after vaginal delivery, although it may be performed at other times; i.e., immediately following ***Cesarean section*** or as an elective surgery. This elective procedure is a safe and especially effective means of performing sterilization. Patients need to be aware that the procedure may sometimes be reversed by tuboplasty, but the possibility of reversal cannot be guaranteed.

Approaches include minilaparotomy, posterior colpotomy via hysteroscopy, and laparoscopy (when the procedure does not follow childbirth).

Procedure

The table may be placed in Trendelenburg position for these approaches.

Minilaparotomy Approach. The patient's legs are placed in frog-leg position and a bivalved vaginal speculum (e.g., Graves) is employed to place a uterine manipulator. A small incision is made suprapubically and is extended into the peritoneal cavity. Each fallopian tube is individually grasped with a Babcock forceps, and the tubal procedure is performed (excision of, desiccation or cauterization of, silicone banding of, or the application of a suture or clip, e.g., ***Filschie clip*** or ***Hulka clip,*** on a section of each fallopian tube). The peritoneum is approximated. The wound is closed in layers. The wound is dressed and a perineal pad is placed.

Posterior Colpotomy Approach. A weighted speculum is placed in the vagina. The cervix is retracted anteriorly with a tenaculum. A transverse incision is made into the vaginal mucosa posterior to the cervix and extended through the peritoneum to enter the cul-de-sac. Each tube is grasped individually with a long Babcock forceps, and the tubal procedure is performed. The colpotomy site is closed with through-and-through sutures, including vaginal mucosa and peritoneum. A perineal pad is placed.

Hysteroscopy Approach (Essure Procedure). The Essure procedure may be performed in a doctor's office without anesthesia. It may also be performed as a hospital outpatient procedure. ***Hysteroscopy*** (p. 322) is done using a flexible hysteroscope; see p. 323. A thin tube-like instrument is threaded into each fallopian tube and the tiny inert Essure™ device is inserted. This device causes scarring that creates a barrier preventing sperm from traveling through the fallopian tube. Upon completion of the procedure, the distending medium is evacuated from the uterus and the hysteroscope is removed. A perineal pad dressing is placed.

For **Laparoscopic Approach,** see ***Gynecologic Laparotomy/Pelviscopy***, p. 295.

Preparation of the Patient

Antiembolitic hose are not often used (unless patient's history indicates a special need), as the procedure is short. Padded shoulder braces are secured to the table. Pad all bony prominences and areas vulnerable to skin and neurovascular trauma or pressure. Apply electrosurgical dispersive pad.

Minilaparotomy Approach. Patient is supine; arms may be extended on padded armboards. A pillow may be placed under the lumbar spine and/or under the knees (to avoid straining back muscles).

Laparoscopic approach and **Posterior Colpotomy and Hysteroscopic approaches.** Patient is in modified lithotomy position with the buttocks positioned just over the lower break in the table, legs bent at the knees, with the feet placed in padded stirrups. Arms may be extended on padded armboards.

Skin and Vaginal Preparation

Minilaparotomy. Begin at site of intended incision (usually Pfannenstiel) and extend area prepped from nipples to mid-thighs.

Laparoscopy. A combined abdominal and vaginal preparation is done. Add extra sponges, prep solution, and a straight catheter (e.g., Robinson) to the prep set. Stand at the foot of the table, between the patient's legs, after the lower section of the table is removed. Begin cleansing at the umbilicus, extending the prep from nipples to the mid-thighs. Continue the prep over the labia, discarding each sponge after wiping the labia.

Cleanse each inner thigh and discard the sponge. Prepare the vaginal vault and cervix using three spongesticks. Prep perineum and anus last; discard each sponge after wiping the anus. Catheterize patient's bladder with the straight catheter.

Posterior Colpotomy and Hysteroscopy. Begin at pubic symphysis and extend downward over the labia. Cleanse each inner thigh. Use three spongesticks to cleanse vaginal vault and cervix. The perineum and anus are cleansed with remaining sponges; discard each sponge after cleansing the anus.

Draping

Minilaparotomy. Folded towels and a laparotomy sheet

Laparoscopy and Posterior Colpotomy and Hysteroscopy. Drape sheet under buttocks, folded towels (optional), and laparoscopy sheet, or drape sheet under buttocks, leggings, and a laparotomy sheet

Equipment

Minilaparotomy
ESU
Suction
Padded shoulder braces
Laparoscopy: see *Gynecologic Laparoscopy/Pelviscopy,* p. 295.
Padded stirrups (e.g., Allen)
Fiber-optic light source, e.g., Xenon 300W
Monitor
Printer
CD burner
VCR
CO_2 insufflator for laparoscope, e.g., Laparoflator™, Thermoflator™, Endolap™ or
Pump powered by nitrogen or air, e.g., Endo Flo
Laparoscopic irrigation system, e.g., HydroFlex with fluid distention sensor, e.g., AquaSens™

Electrosurgical coagulator, e.g., GynePro™, Endo Coagulator™
Hysteroscopic CO_2 insufflator, e.g., Hysteroflator™, Endo Flo (for hysteroscope, **<u>not laparoscopic insufflator</u>),** if CO_2 is the medium
Fiber-optic light source, e.g., Xenon 300 W for laparoscope or hysteroscope
Roller pump system, e.g., Hamou Hysteromat II™ to measure intrauterine pressure **(hysteroscopy)**
Hysteroscopic fluid monitoring system, e.g., GyneFlo
Laser fiber, e.g., Nd:YAG, KTP, optional

Instrumentation

Minilaparotomy

Basic/Minor procedures tray
Abdominal self-retaining retractor
Bivalved speculum
Uterine manipulator, e.g., Cohen cannula
Tenaculum

Laparoscopy

Limited procedures tray
D&C tray
Uterine manipulator
Verres needle (disposable available)
Trocars (5 mm, 10 or 11 mm, 12 mm, or Hasson)
Fiber-optic laparoscopes, 30° and 0°, and cord
Camera and coupler or laparoscope with built-in camera
Reducers and connectors, as necessary
Laparoscopic irrigating handpiece, e.g., HydroFlex
***Laparoscopic instruments*:**
Electrosurgical dissector, Babcock forceps (2) scissors (blunt and sharp), electrosurgical suction-irrigator
Electrosurgical cord
Multifire ligating clip applier with clips
Loop suture, e.g., Endoloop (infrequent), optional
Spring clip or Silastic band

Posterior Colpotomy and Hysteroscopy

Cervical Cone Tray
D&C tray
Coagulating electrosurgical forceps, Babcock forceps (2) long, scissors (fine, sharp)
Hemoclip or similar clip appliers, optional
Rigid fiber-optic hysteroscope and cord

Irrigator, e.g., EndoFlo with special tips and probes and suction cannula

Hysteroscopic instruments:

Electrosurgical suction-irrigator dissector, cannulas, electrosurgical scissors, Babcock forceps (2), scissors (fine, sharp)

Essure device kit, optional

Supplies

Suction tubing

Perineal pad

Sanitary napkin belt or T-binder

Basin set

Needle magnet or counter

Silicone banding, Hemoclip®, Filschie™, or Hulka™, clip appliers, e.g., Hemoclips (small, medium), optional

For Minilaparotomy and Colpotomy Approaches, Add

Electrosurgical pencil and cord with holder and scraper

Water-soluble lubricant

Blades, (2) #15 **(minilaparotomy)**, (1) #10 **(posterior colpotomy)**

For Hysteroscopy and Laparoscopy Approaches, Add

Electrosurgical cord

Antifog agent, e.g., ELVIS, FRED

Silastic tubing for CO_2 insufflation (when CO_2 is the medium) or

Straight tubing, e.g., K50, add 1000-ml bag normal saline and three-way stopcock for irrigation or tubing cassette, single use for laparoscopic irrigation, e.g., HydroFlex LI

Pre-warmed high-viscosity fluid (e.g., Hyskon 32% Dextran 70% in dextrose, Dextran 10, and 1.5% glycine, 3% sorbitol, or 5% mannitol)

Loop ligation sutures, e.g., Endoloop **(laparoscopy)**

Special Notes

- **N.B. A sterilization procedure** *permit, in addition to the signed surgical permit for the procedure,* **tubal sterilization** *is required before the patient may be brought into the room.* The patient needs to indicate in her own words that she understands that she will no longer be able to have children. Her statement to this effect should be included in the **Perioperative Record**.
- For Minilaparotomy approach to tubal ligation, apply **Special Notes** from *Salpingo-Oophorectomy*, p. 312, as indicated.

- For Posterior Colpotomy approach to tubal ligation, apply **Special Notes** from ***Vaginal Hysterectomy***, p. 292.
- **N.B.** The circulator carefully monitors the amount of medium being used during the hysteroscopic approach to distending the uterus. When an excessive amount of fluid is used, fluid overload may result.
- **N.B.** The hysteroscopic specific CO_2 insufflator is **not** the same as the laparoscopic insufflator. The hysteroscopic insufflator provides higher pressure with lower flow.
- The tissue specimens (e.g., the fallopian tube sections) are placed in separate containers labeled "right" and "left" fallopian tube segment.

Laparoscopic Hysterectomy and Laparoscopic-Assisted Vaginal Hysterectomy With Or Without Salpingo-Oophorectomy

Definition

Excision of the uterus (with or without the excision of the fallopian tubes and ovaries) by laparoscopic approach with varying components of transvaginal manipulation and/or intraoperative maneuvers.

Discussion

Vaginal hysterectomy minimizes postoperative morbidity with the avoidance of a large laparotomy incision while directly identifying pelvic structures. When malignancy is suspect, the surgeon must have a view of the entire peritoneal cavity; either an "open" or a laparoscopic approach is employed. Whereas **vaginal hysterectomy** avoids an abdominal incision, in situations where the uterus is unduly enlarged (e.g., fibromyomata), uterine descensus is minimal, prior cesarean section has been performed, and pelvic adhesions (secondary to surgery or inflammatory disease), endometriosis, intestinal pathology, etc., are present, the vaginal approach may be either unsafe (because exploration for further disease is not possible) or technically infeasible. In these circumstances, mobilization of pelvic structures is done under direct visualization laparoscopically, with delivery of the specimen vaginally or laparoscopically-assisted through a large-bore port (e.g., Endoport™). In addition, certain phases of the procedure are less traumatic to the body by making the colporrhaphy incision, securing uterine vessels, and closure of the vaginal cuff via the vaginal approach, i.e., *laparoscopic or* **laparoscopic-assisted vaginal hysterectomy (LAVH)**. Finally, measures to repair pelvic support by *anterior and posterior colporrhaphy* (p. 293) may be performed in conjunction with hysterectomy with this approach.

Supracervical hysterectomy, in which the epithelium of the endocervical canal is ablated, but the cervix and its supporting ligaments are retained, has been reintroduced. The employment of laparoscopic hysterectomy and laparoscopic-assisted hysterectomy in cases of malignancy is currently controversial.

Procedure

Laparoscopic Approach. Patient is in modified lithotomy position. The table is placed in Trendelenburg position. Following the establishment of pneumoperitoneum (see ***Gynecologic Laparoscopy/Pelviscopy***, p. 295) with a 10- or 11-mm trocar, additional 12-mm trocars are inserted at the lateral borders of the rectus muscles, inferior to the level of the umbilicus and suprapubically (optional). The abdomen is explored. Optional intrauterine cannulas for uterine manipulation (*Kronner Manipujector or Valtchev uterine mobilizer*) may be placed transvaginally. If intra-abdominal adhesions are present, enterolysis is performed so that the uterus and adenexal structures can be freely moved (directly or by means of the uterine manipulator). The various supporting ligaments are transected. The ligaments are divided employing a linear endoscopic multiple clip applier. The fallopian tubes and ovaries may be preserved or excised accordingly. The uterovesical fold is placed under tension directly or by employing the intrauterine manipulator, and a peritoneal bladder flap may be developed using electrosurgical endoscopic scissors. A hydrodissector may be used for this maneuver as well. Once the ureters are identified, the uterosacral and cardinal ligaments are transected. The uterine vessels are tied and cut close to the uterine wall, leaving adequate amounts of tissue for repair. The uterus is excised and may be morcellated (Semm morcellator) within a specimen bag (e.g., ENDOBAG, Endo Pouch) and withdrawn through a large-bore port (HandPort)™.

Laparoscopic-Assisted Approach. Pneumoperitoneum is established. Pressure is placed on the vagina superiorly, and a posterior colotomy incision is made electrosurgically. Moist packing is inserted vaginally to minimize the loss of pneumoperitoneum. ***Colpotomy*** is completed anteriorly and laterally, and following excision, the uterine specimen is delivered vaginally or transabdominally through a large-bore port (e.g., 30 mm). When the nonmalignant uterine specimen is too large to be passed intact through the colpotomy incision, it can be morcellated (Semm morcellator) within a specimen bag (e.g., ENDOBAG, Endo Pouch) and withdrawn vaginally or through a large-bore port. The colpotomy incision is closed transvaginally or by endoscopic suture technique, suspending the corners to the uterosacral ligament remnants, when applicable. Pneumoperitoneum is restored and the bladder flap may be reapproximated laparoscopically with an endoscopic hernia stapler. In addition, the vaginal cuff may be closed via intraabdominal approach employing a disposable automatic stapler, e.g., transverse anastomosis (TA™). Alternatively, as in **vaginal hysterectomy**, the colpotomy incision, division of uterosacral and cardinal ligaments, and ligation of the uterine vessels, extraction of the specimen (as noted), and closure of the vaginal cuff may be performed transvaginally.

If ***supracervical hysterectomy*** is performed, after the uterine corpus is amputated, the epithelium of the endocervical canal is ablated as a cancer preventative measure; improved support and preservation of sexual sensation is achieved by retaining the cervix (controversial).

The various procedures involving the tubes and ovaries are performed according to the general format described above with additional instrumentation as necessary. As the definitive portions of these procedures are performed as in the corresponding open procedures, they will not be further addressed here. After the pelvis is irrigated and suctioned, the pneumoperitoneum is released and the incisions are repaired. ***Anterior and posterior colporrhaphy*** (see p. 293) may be performed. A Foley catheter is inserted at the conclusion of the procedure and connected to continuous drainage unit.

Preparation of the Patient

Antiembolitic hose are put on the legs, if requested. Following the administration of general anesthesia, the patient is placed in a modified lithotomy position using padded stirrups with the buttocks positioned just over the lower break in the table. The arms may be extended on padded armboards or one arm may be padded and tucked in at the patient's side and the other arm is extended on a padded armboard. Padded shoulder braces are secured to the table. Pad all bony prominences and areas vulnerable to skin and neurovascular trauma or pressure. The table may be placed in Trendelenburg position; this position encourages organs in the peritoneal cavity to fall cephalad, permitting a better view of the operative area. Apply electrosurgical dispersive pad.

Skin and Vaginal Preparation

A combined abdominal and vaginal prep is done. Add extra sponges, prep solution, and a straight catheter (e.g., Robinson) to the prep set. Stand between the patient's legs, after the lower section of the table is removed. Begin cleansing at the umbilicus, extending the prep from nipples to the mid-thighs. Continue the prep over the labia, discarding each sponge after wiping the labia. Cleanse each inner thigh and discard the sponge. Prepare the vaginal vault and cervix using three spongesticks. Prep perineum and anus last; discard each sponge after wiping the anus. Catheterize patient's bladder with the straight catheter.

Draping

Drape sheet under the buttocks, followed by a laparoscopy sheet, or drape sheet under the buttocks, leggings, and a laparotomy sheet

Equipment

Padded stirrups (e.g., Allen)
Padded shoulder braces
Camera console
CD burner
VCR
Printer
ESU or Electrocoagulator generator, e.g., GynePro™, Endo Coagulator™
Suction
Video monitors (1 or 2)
Fiber-optic light source, e.g., Xenon 300 W
CO_2 insufflator (laparoscopic), e.g., Laproflator™, Thermoflator™, Endolap or
Insuffflator pump powered by nitrogen or air, e.g., Endo Flo
Laparoscopic irrigation system, e.g., HydroFlex with pressure rate control
Laser, e.g., argon (observe all mandatory laser safety precautions)
Morcellator console
SEMM macromorcellator console, optional
Plume evacuator console or in-line filter, e.g., Plume Away™

Instrumentation

Limited procedures tray
D&C tray (tenaculum)
Intrauterine manipulator, e.g., Kronner Manipujector or Valtchev uterine mobilizer
Filschie or Hulkaclip
Cannula, e.g., Cohen
Verres needle (disposable available)
Trocars (5 mm, 10 or 11 mm, 12 mm, or Hasson)
Connectors, as needed

Electrosurgical cord
Fiber-optic laparoscope, 0°, and cord
Camera and coupler camera (or built in to laparoscope)
Plume evacuator, e.g., Plume Away, Smoke Evac (Dorsey) with trumpet valve
Endoscopic instruments:
Electrosurgical suction-irrigator-dissector, electrosurgical scissors, electrocoagulating probe, Babcock forceps, scissors (blunt and sharp)
Multifire clip appliers with medium and large clips
Endoscopic suture, e.g., Endo Stitch
Macromorcelator (e.g., Semm), with drill tip and cord, optional
Specimen retrieval bag, e.g., Endo Sac, Endo Pouch
Disposable automatic stapler for intraabdominal cuff closure with TA, optional **(laparoscopic-assisted)**

Supplies

Antiembolitic hose, as requested
Suction tubing
Basin set
Medicine cup, vasopressin, labels, and sterile marking pen
Syringe, e.g., Luer lok (1) #22 needle or
Vasopressin (in kit, predrawn in a syringe, labeled, with the needle)
Electrosurgical pencil and cord with holder and scraper ***(laparoscopic-assisted)***
Blades, (1) #10 and/or (1) #15
Needle magnet or counter
Silastic tubing for CO_2 insufflation or
Single use tubing cassette for laparoscopic CO_2 insufflation, e.g., Endolap 25
Straight tubing, e.g., K50, add 1000-ml bag normal saline and three-way stopcock for irrigation or
Laparoscopic irrigator with automatically protected fluid levels, e.g., Hydro Flex
Loop ligation sutures, e.g., Endoloop (with introducer sleeve, intracorporeal available for ties), if requested
Specimen retrieval bag, e.g., Endo Pouch, Endo Sac
Hand port, e.g., Endoport™, Lap Port™
Antifog agent, e.g., ELVIS, FRED
Foley catheter with tubing and drainage unit
Perineal pad
Sanitary napkin belt or T-binder

Special Notes

- *A signed permit for a sterilization procedure must be on the chart, in addition to the signed surgical permit* **for Laparoscopic Vaginal Hysterectomy,** *p. 7* **or Laparoscopic-Assisted Vaginal Hysterectomy** *is required before the patient may be brought into the room.* The patient needs to indicate in her own words that she understands that she will no longer be able to have children. The Patient's statement is documented in the **Perioperative Record.**
- Apply **Special Notes** from ***Gynecologic Laparoscopy/Pelviscopy,*** p. 299, for laparoscopic procedure, as indicated. Be prepared for surgeon to perform a ***D&C,*** p. 277 before the laparoscopic or laparoscopic-assisted procedure. The scrub person sets up the instruments for ***D&C*** on a separate back table.

Hysteroscopy

Definition

The visual examination of the uterine cavity by means of a hysteroscope.

Discussion

Hysteroscopy is performed for diagnostic and therapeutic purposes, as well as in conjunction with hysterosalpingography, laparoscopy, and laparotomy. Indications include evaluation of bleeding (after nondiagnostic ***D&C),*** directed biopsy, evaluation of the endocervical versus the endometrial mucosa, and infertility evaluation. ***Tubal sterilization*** can be accomplished hysteroscopically; see Essure, p. 313.

Excision or ablation of polyps and other lesions (including submucosal fibromyomata), division of a congenital uterine septum, lysis of adhesions, retrieval of a retracted intrauterine device, etc., can be performed. Visualization of the endometrial surfaces depends on the ability to distend the uterus with a variety of media. The rigid scopes, similar to the urologic resectoscope (used to excise benign prostatic hypertrophy), are employed for surgical purposes. When diagnosis only and/or limited biopsy are indicated, a flexible fiber-optic scope similar to the choledochoscope is employed.

Complications include perforation of the uterus, excessive bleeding, embolization or dissection of the distensive media, and laser injury to adjacent structures. Concomitant laparoscopy can be useful to observe and correct these problems. Contraindications include hemorrhage, acute infection, cervical stenosis, and malignancy.

Procedure

Antiembolitic hose is applied. **Hysteroscopy** is usually performed under general anesthesia; paracervical blocks with sedation and other modalities are less often employed. The cervix is carefully dilated using graduated cervical dilators to the diameter of the hysteroscope. A pre-warmed high-viscosity fluid (e.g., Hyskon 32% Dextran 70 in dextrose, Dextran 10, and 1.5% glycine, 3% sorbitol, or 5% mannitol) may be employed to distend the uterus. Other media include normal saline (N/S), water, D5W, and CO_2; the type of medium depends on the procedure to be performed and the surgeon's preference.

A self-retaining vacuum cannula (with obturator) is inserted into the cervical canal, held in place at the cervix by negative pressure. The obturator is removed and the rigid (operating) hysteroscope with a 10°- to 45°-angle is used. The scopes with multiple channels permit the circulation of the media and up to three endoscopic instruments. The pressure and flow rate of the media distending the uterus must be monitored to prevent injury by extravasation. Osmotic-related fluid changes and embolization through intrauterine absorption or extravasation into the peritoneum are complications.

When CO_2 is the distending medium, pressures must not exceed 100 mm Hg or a flow rate greater than 40 to 60 ml/min during ***hysteroscopy***. *Equipment specific for* ***hysteroscopy*** *only,* is used, as hysteroscopic insufflator requires higher CO_2 pressure but lower flow rate than laparoscopic insufflator. As smoke, foam, and bleeding are produced during various operative procedures, a fluid medium is preferable, as it provides better visibility. Intrauterine pressure (IUP) can be carefully controlled using a roller pump system, e.g., Hamou Hysteromat™ II or Hydro Flex with Aqua Sens fluid protector. The uterus is distended with the medium of the surgeon's choice under direct visualization. Excessive dilatation is avoided, as it leads to a loss of the distending medium and possible embolization. The uterus is explored and diagnostic, therapeutic, and surgical measures may be performed under direct vision. When using a laser, observe all laser safety precautions; see p. 94. At the conclusion of the procedure, the medium is evacuated and the hysteroscope and the self-retaining retractor are removed. A perineal pad is placed.

A microscope may be requested.

Preparation of the Patient

Antiembolitic hose is put on the legs, as requested. General or regional anesthesia is administered. The patient is placed in lithotomy position using padded stirrups; the buttocks are positioned just over the lower break in the table. The arms may be padded and tucked in at the patient's sides or extended on padded armboards. Padded shoulder braces are secured to the table. The table may be placed in Trendelenburg position. Pad all bony prominences and areas vulnerable to skin and neurovascular trauma or pressure. Apply electrosurgical dispersive pad.

Skin and Vaginal Preparation

Antiembolitic hose are applied to the legs, as requested. Begin cleansing at the pubic symphysis, extending downward over the labia. Cleanse each inner thigh. The vaginal vault and cervix are then cleansed using sponge-sticks (3). The perineum and anus are cleansed with the remaining sponges. Discard each sponge after wiping the anus. Catheterize patient with a straight catheter.

Draping

Drape sheet under the buttocks, leggings, and drape sheet over the abdomen
Microscope cover, optional

Equipment

Padded stirrups
Padded shoulder braces
Suction
ESU
Monitor
CD burner
Printer
Fiber-optic light source, e.g., Xenon 300 W
Hysteroscopic CO_2 insufflation unit, GyneFlo **(not** laparoscopic type)
Roller pump system, e.g., Hamou Hysteromat II, to measure IUP
Camera console
VCR
Laser (e.g., Argon, KTP 532 nm, Nd:YAG 1064 nm), available
Microscope (e.g., Zeiss), optional

Instrumentation

D&C tray
Self-retaining vacuum cervical cannula (with obturator)
Limited procedures tray
Hysteroscopic insufflator, e.g., GyneFlo with pressure relief valve
Flexible hysteroscope and cord (for diagnosis and biopsies <3 mm)
Fiber-optic rigid hysteroscopes 10° and 45° and cord (for operating and biopsies)

Resectoscope

Hysteroscopy endoscopic:

Probes, electrosurgical suction-aspirator, electrosurgical biopsy forceps, graspers, micro-scissors, electrosurgical tips, loops, alligator cup forceps (assorted)

Camera and coupler

Supplies

Antiembolitic hose, as requested

Suction tubing

Electrosurgical cord

Basin set

Water-soluble lubricant

Knife blade, (1) #10

Needle magnet or counter

Silastic tubing for laparoscopic CO_2 insufflation or Luer lok syringe and straight tubing, e.g., K50 for dye, and flexible needle, optional or tubing may be available in a cassette

Cystoscopy or Silastic straight tubing, e.g., K50, add 1000-ml bag normal saline and three-way stopcock for distending medium

Essure device kit, optional

Labels and marking pen, optional

Distending media: viscid fluid (e.g., Hyskon 32% Dextran 70% in dextrose, Dextran 10, and 1.5% glycine, 3% sorbitol, 5% mannitol) or N/S, Ringer's lactate, water, or CO_2

Luer lok™ syringe and #22-gauge needle

Foley catheter or special intrauterine balloon catheter, available

Perineal pad

Sanitary napkin belt or T-binder

Special Notes

- Apply **Special Notes** from ***Gynecologic Laparoscopy/Pelviscopy***, p. 299, as indicated.
- Monitor the amount of medium being used during the procedure to avoid distention of the uterus.
- Have catheter (Foley or intrauterine) available for intrauterine tamponade, should excessive bleeding occur. The catheter may be left in the uterus, to be deflated gradually postoperatively.
- **N.B.** Be aware that a sudden loss of intrauterine pressure may indicate perforation, resulting in shock.
- Prophylactic antibiotics may be requested. The circulator should be certain that the drug is the correct one, at the correct strength. Observe safety precautions to avoid medication errors; see p. 30.

- Lasers, such as KTP or argon may be employed for dissection, hemostasis, adhesiolysis, and to open blocked fallopian tubes. Observe all mandatory laser safety precautions; see p. 94.
- When the microscope is employed, the scrub person should pass all instruments carefully, placing them in the surgeon's hands, ready for use, to avoid taking the surgeon's attention away from the field.
- If stents are placed to maintain fallopian tubal patency, the stent information is documented in the **Perioperative Record;** stent placement may also be recorded in the hospital log book (according to hospital policy).
- Inspect instruments after use for breakage with possible retention of a foreign body in the uterine cavity. The scrub person should report the breakage and loss if the object is not found; the loss must be reported to the surgeon and the circulator. An x-ray should be taken of the operative site and the supervisor notified. The incident should be filed in an **Incident Report** signed by both the scrub person and the circulator; it is placed in the patient's chart as part of the permanent record, e.g., **Perioperative Record** (see p. 12).
- Instruments, especially the optics, must be cleaned immediately following use, particularly if Hyskon is used, as any debris hardens and becomes difficult to remove. A proteolytic enzyme wash is available for cleansing endoscopic instruments.

Surgery for Ectopic Pregnancy

Definition

Surgical treatment of a pregnancy established at a site other than within the uterine cavity, e.g., fallopian tube.

Discussion

The fertilized ovum may implant (rarely) within the uterine tube, ovary, peritoneal surface, broad ligament, and cervix. The fallopian tube is the most frequently involved other site, usually within the ampullary portion. Many small ectopic pregnancies abort and go undetected, with minimal abdominal pain the only symptom. If pregnancy is suspect, hCG titers are elevated, and an adnexal mass is palpated, transvaginal ultrasound scan, culdecentesis, and laparoscopy are used to confirm the diagnosis. Laparoscopy is the preferred surgical treatment.

In small presentations, in the medically stable patient, methotrexate (with leucovorin) can be given systemically, or methotrexate, potassium chloride, prostaglandin fraction, or hypertonic glucose can be injected directly into the fallopian tube *(salpingocentesis)* under laparoscopic or transvaginal ultrasound guidance. Other agents, as dactinomycin and etoposide, may also be employed. When these agents are unsuccessful, surgical intervention is indicated. Laparoscopic treatment is preferred when there are no contraindications, although simultaneous fine-suture tuboplasty to preserve fertility is not often successful. When feasible, the gestational tissues can be expressed from the fimbriated end of the tube, but this is not usually recommended unless spontaneous abortion has begun. Otherwise, the tube can be unduly traumatized or trophoblastic tissues will not be completely removed. ***Fallopian tubal rupture*** with hemorrhage requires laparotomy, with fine suture repair of the tube or primary tubal anastomosis after partial tubal resection. Preservation of fertility may be dependent upon status of the contralateral tube, size of the pregnancy, previous history of ectopic pregnancy, and the availability of in vitro fertilization to the patient. Indications for salpingectomy include hemorrhage, tubal rupture, lack of desire for further pregnancy, and history of prior ectopic pregnancies.

Procedure

Laparoscopic Approach. Pneumoperitoneum is achieved and two or three laparoscopic ports are established; see ***Gynecologic Laparoscopy/Pelviscopy***, p. 295. If the pregnancy occurs in the ampullary portion and the tube is to be preserved, a linear incision is made and the gestational tissues are removed. Hemostasis is achieved; the tube may be left open (to heal by second intention) or fibrin glue may be applied, or fine sutures may be placed. For *salpingectomy,* a dilute solution of vasopressin (4 u/20 ml saline) may be injected into the intended line of incision (to reduce bleeding). The mesosalpinx is divided, ligating larger vessels, and the tube is excised at the isthmus by Endoloop ligation. Alternatively, a segment of traumatized tube can be resected with plastic repair secondarily. Suturing a portion of broad ligament or round ligament to the tubal stump is thought to minimize adhesions. The peritoneal cavity is irrigated and blood and tissue debris are aspirated. Pneumoperitoneum is released and the incisions are closed. Band Aid or Steristrip dressing may be applied. A perineal pad is placed.

Laparotomy Approach. Laparotomy affords the ability to rapidly aspirate blood, detect and control bleeding, and perform salpingectomy. A lower abdominal incision is made; the operative field is cleared of tissue debris, and the bleeding is controlled. Tubal preservation can be attempted with fine-suture (6-0, 7-0) repair of the tube, or if a traumatized section is excised, direct reanastomosis can be performed if the tissues are deemed salvageable. Otherwise, resection and secondary repair of the tube can be done. For *salpingectomy*, the procedure is similar to that described above, using ordinary surgical techniques. The abdomen is irrigated and the irrigation (and tissue debris) is aspirated. The wound is closed in layers. In the rare presentation of interstitial ectopic pregnancy, especially if rupture has occurred, wedge resection of the involved area or even hysterectomy (see p. 289) is performed. When the uterus has been operated upon, Cesarian section for subsequent pregnancy may be advised.

Preparation of the Patient

Antiembolitic hose may be put on the legs when requested.

Laparoscopic Approach. Following the administration of general anesthesia, the patient is placed in a modified lithotomy position using padded stirrups (e.g., Allen) with the buttocks positioned just over the lower break in the table. The arms may be extended on padded armboards. Padded shoulder braces are secured to the table. Pad all bony prominences and areas vulnerable to skin and neurovascular trauma or pressure. The table is placed in Trendelenburg position; this position encourages organs in the peritoneal cavity to fall cephalad, permitting a better view of the operative area. Apply electrosurgical dispersive pad.

Laparotomy Approach. The patient is supine; arms may be extended on padded armboards. A pillow may be placed under the lumbar spine and/or under the knees (to avoid straining back muscles). Padded shoulder braces are secured to the table. The table may be placed in Trendelenburg position. Pad all bony prominences and areas vulnerable to skin and neurovascular trauma or pressure. Apply electrosurgical dispersive pad.

Skin and Vaginal Preparation

Laparoscopic Approach. A combined abdominal and vaginal prep is done. Add extra sponges, prep solution, and a straight catheter (e.g., Robinson) to the prep set. Stand between the patient's legs, after the lower section of the table is removed. Begin cleansing at the umbilicus, extending the prep from nipples to the mid-thighs. Continue the prep over the labia, discarding each sponge after wiping the labia. Cleanse each inner thigh and discard the sponge. Prep the vaginal vault and cervix (as for **D&C**) using three spongesticks. The perineum and anus are prepared last; discard each sponge after wiping the anus. Catheterize patient's bladder with a straight catheter.

Laparotomy Approach. A vaginal and an abdominal prep are required; use two separate trays. The patient's legs are placed in a froglike position; prep as for ***D&C,*** p. 278. Insert a Foley catheter and connect to continuous drainage. Return the patient's legs to their original position, place the drainage unit below the level of the table, and replace the safety belt. For the abdominal prep, begin at the intended site of incision (usually Pfannenstiel), extending from nipples to mid-thighs and down to the table at the sides.

Draping

Laparoscopic Approach. Drape sheet under the buttocks, followed by a laparoscopy sheet, or drape sheet, leggings, and a laparotomy sheet

Laparotomy Approach. Folded towels and a transverse or laparotomy sheet
Microscope cover, optional

Equipment

Laparoscopic and Laparotomy

Forced-air warming blanket, if ordered
Sequential compression device with disposable leg wraps, if requested
Padded shoulder braces
Suction
ESU

Laparoscopic Approach Only

Padded stirrups (e.g., Allen)
Monitor(s)
Fiber-optic light source (e.g., Xenon 300 W)
CO_2 insufflator, e.g., Endo Lap™ F 25, Laparoflator™
Camera console
VCR
Irrigation system, e.g., HydroFlex with pressure control of the rate
Microscope, optional
CD burner
Printer

Instrumentation

Laparoscopic Approach

Limited procedures tray
D&C tray
Verres needle (disposable available)
Trocars (5 mm, 10 or 11 mm, 12 mm, or Hasson)
Fiber-optic laparoscopes, 30° and 0°, and cord
Camera and coupler
Endocoagulator generator with footswitch

Reducers and connectors
Microscope coupler
Endoscopic instruments:
Babcock forceps, (3) scissors (curved, hook, straight), right angle dissector, Kelly clamp, grasping forceps (2), dissecting forceps, right angle and hook irrigation-suction-electrosurgical dissectors or electrocoagulator
Connectors, as necessary

Laparotomy Approach

Major procedures tray
Somer's clamp
Mosquito hemostats (6) curved, (2) straight
Frazier suction tips (assorted)
Beaver knife handle, available

Microtuboplasty

Lacrimal duct probes, jeweler's forceps (straight, with and without teeth), tying forceps, Castroviejo needle holder, iris scissors

Supplies

Antiembolitic hose, as requested
Suction tubing
Basin set
Blades, (2) #10 and (1) #15
Needle magnet or counter
Medicine cups, paper labels, and marking pen
Suction tubing
Perineal pad
T-binder or sanitary napkin belt

For Laparoscopic Approach, Add

Electrosurgical cord
Silastic tubing for CO_2 insufflation or
Tubing (in a cassette) pressure line with relief valve, e.g., Gyne Flo™
Straight tubing, e.g., K50 (add 1000-ml bag normal saline and three-way stopcock for irrigation) or
Tubing (in a cassette) for irrigation
Loop ligation sutures, e.g., Endoloop (with introducer sleeve available for ties), if requested
Fog reduction agent, e.g., FRED, ELVIS
Band Aids or skin closure strips (optional)

For Laparotomy Approach, Add

Electrosurgical pencil and cord with holder and scraper

Special Notes

- Apply **Special Notes** from ***Gynecologic Laparoscopy/Pelviscopy***, p. 299, for *laparoscopy approach*.
- Apply **Special Notes** from ***Abdominal Laparotomy***, p. 134, for *laparotomy approach*.
- The laparoscopic approach is considered *only* when the ectopic is **not** ruptured, i.e., the tubal pregnancy has not ruptured the fallopian tube.
- "Spongesticks" (raytec sponge on ringed forceps) may be requested throughout the surgery.
- **N.B.** *Emergency situation exists for ruptured ectopic pregnancy.* Check with blood bank regarding the status of blood for transfusion.
- Patient may have made an autologous blood donation when the surgery is elective (patient's own blood will be available). The circulator should ascertain that blood is ready, i.e., check with the blood bank.
- The circulator assists the anesthesia provider in administering a transfusion by setting up perfusion set as needed, checking identification number on unit of blood and comparing the number to the number on the patient's identification armband, and by obtaining a blood pump and blood warmer.
- **N.B.** ***There must be two working suctions (in addition to the one on the anesthesia cart) in the room in case hemorrhage should occur. Keep an accurate record of irrigation fluid used to assist in determining blood loss and fluid replacement.***
- Determine if the cell saver will be used. If so, prepare console for use stat and notify personnel required to operate unit
- The surgeon may wear magnifying loupes or use the microscope for tubal reconstruction (laparotomy).
- The scrub person passes all instruments carefully, placing them in the surgeon's hands, ready for use, to avoid taking the surgeon's attention away from the field.
- The Somer's clamp is used to grasp the ovary (without crushing or damaging tissue).
- A Foley catheter connected to a continuous straight drainage unit is inserted at the conclusion of the surgery.

- The drainage tubing of the Foley catheter should be patent (without kinks); the level of the bag should be kept below the level of the patient's bladder to prevent a reflux of urine that could lead to a UTI.

Tuboplasty of the Fallopian Tubes

Definition

The reestablishment of patency to the fallopian tubes.

Discussion

Tuboplasty is usually performed when the patient seeks a reversal of a sterilization procedure. Success depends on the amount of fallopian tubal destruction. Tuboplasty is also performed to surgically treat (excise and reanastomose the fallopian tube) where there is an unruptured tubal pregnancy.

Procedure

General or conductive anesthesia (e.g., spinal block) is employed. A Pfannenstiel incision is made. The peritoneal cavity is entered, and a self-retaining retractor is placed. Warm, moist (saline) lap sponges are used to protect the bowel and ureters. The table may be placed in Trendelenburg position. Tubal patency may be demonstrated by the injection of dye (e.g., methylene blue, indigo carmine) through a cervical cannula (e.g., Cohen) that is placed in the cervix by the surgeon following the vaginal prep. When a fallopian tube is not patent, the operating microscope is often employed to perform a tuboplasty procedure. The circulator may be requested to inject the dye. Care is taken not to contaminate the drapes or to dislodge the cannula. According to the type of site obstruction, cornual resection with reimplantation, tubal resection with anastomosis, or fimbrioplasty is performed. A laser beam may be directed through the microscope to open adhesions of the fimbria and to lyse lesions within the fallopian tubes. When the laser is employed, observe all laser safety precautions; see p. 94. When the microscope is not employed, loupes are used and mini instruments as a probe, iris scissors, and a #11 blade are used. A sterile tongue depressor may be requested to be the flat surface placed under the tube when it is cut. The tongue blade is moistened with normal saline to prevent the tubal tissue from sticking to it. Fine sutures may be employed, as necessary. Upon completion of the procedure, the abdomen is closed in layers. The cervical cannula is removed transvaginally. A perineal pad is placed.

Preparation of the Patient

Apply antiembolitic hose, as requested. The patient is in supine position; arms may be extended on padded armboards. A pillow may be placed under the lumbar spine and/or under the knees (to avoid straining back muscles). Padded shoulder braces are secured to the table. The table may be placed in Trendelenburg position. Pad all bony prominences and areas vulnerable to skin and neurovascular trauma or pressure.

Note: A vaginal prep is necessary.

D&C may be performed. A catheter or cannula is inserted into the cervical canal by the surgeon for the subsequent instillation of dye to determine fallopian tubal patency. When this step is to be included, the patient must initially be placed in lithotomy position using padded stirrups. The buttocks are positioned just over the lower break in the table. After the surgeon inserts the catheter (connected to extension tubing and a syringe filled with dye) and it is secured, the patient is returned to the supine position. The safety belt is replaced. Care is taken to avoid injury to the patient's fingers when the bottom of the table is raised and also not to dislodge the catheter. Apply electrosurgical dispersive pad.

Skin and Vaginal Preparation

A vaginal and an abdominal preparation (separate trays) are required. The patient's legs are placed in a froglike position; prep as for ***D&C***, p. 278. Insert a Foley catheter and connect to continuous drainage. Return the patient's legs to their original position, place the drainage unit below the level of the table, and replace the safety belt. For the abdominal preparation, begin at midline, extending from nipples to mid-thighs and down to the table at the sides.

Draping

Folded towels, transverse or laparotomy sheet
Microscope cover, optional

Equipment

Sequential compression device with disposable leg wraps, if requested
Forced-air warming blanket, if ordered
Padded stirrups for cannula insertion
Padded shoulder braces
Suction
ESU and bipolar ESU
Microscope, e.g., Zeiss, optional
Laser (e.g., Argon, KTP 532 nm, Nd:YAG 600 nm), available

Instruments

D&C tray
Major procedures tray [includes (1) probe]
Micro-instrumentation
Lacrimal duct probes, eye forceps (straight, with and without teeth), tying forceps, Castroviejo needle holder, iris scissors
Beaver knife handle
Mosquito hemostats (6) curved, (2) straight
Frazier suction tips (assorted)

Supplies

Antiembolitic hose
Water-soluble lubricant
Basin set
Blades, (2) #10 and (1) #11
Beaver knife blade, optional per surgeon's request
Needle magnet or counter
Electrosurgical pencil with blade, needle tips, and cord or (bipolar) electrosurgical forceps
Suction tubing
Pediatric Foley or special flexible cannula, extension tubing, syringe
Dye (e.g., methylene blue, indigo carmine)
Sanitary napkin belt or T-binder
Perineal pad

Special Notes

- Apply **Special Notes** from ***Surgery for Ectopic Pregnancy***, p. 331, as indicated.
- The patient is positioned in lithotomy following induction of anesthesia (before the abdominal skin prep); the surgeon inserts a cannula with attached extension tubing.
- **Reminder:** ***Avoid injury to the patient's fingers by preventing them from being caught in the table mechanism when the foot of the table is raised following the insertion of the cannula.***
- When returning patient to supine position, reassess positioning aids, as necessary to avoid pressure injury, etc.
- A syringe filled with dye solution is attached to the catheter. During the procedure, the circulator may be requested to inject the dye (slowly). Care must be taken not to contaminate the field or to dislodge the cannula. Document information regarding the cannula and positioning considerations in the **Perioperative Record**. Document the appearance of the skin

pre- and immediate postoperatively, because comparison rash may indicate allergic reaction to the dye.

- The scrub person should drape the microscope in advance, whenever possible (so that it is immediately ready when needed).
- When the microscope is employed, pass all instruments carefully, placing them in the surgeon's hands, ready for use, to avoid taking the surgeon's attention away from the field.
- When the laser is employed, observe all laser safety precautions; they are mandatory, see p. 94.

Cytoreductive Surgery for Ovarian Cancer ("Debulking Procedure")

Definition

Surgical excision or destruction of macroscopic ovarian cancer metastases.

Discussion

Ovarian cancers (of the several cell types) comprise 4% of new cancers and 6% of cancer deaths in the female, according to the American Cancer Society in 2004. The effects of chemotherapy (with agents such as cisplatin-cyclophosphamide, peclitaxel-cisplatin, etc.) are variable, as these tumor cells develop resistance or become relatively dormant and nonsusceptible to the drugs. On that basis, it has been found that minimizing the residual tumor tissue surgically, i.e., employing a ***cytoreductive or a "debulking" procedure***, can prolong the patient's survival and sometimes permit chemotherapy to be more effective subsequently. Cytoreductive surgery is done primarily after the diagnosis and staging are determined or in response to a second-look procedure after a course of chemotherapy. Unfortunately, ovarian cancer can spread directly in the pelvis, including genitalia, bladder, and rectosigmoid colon, and to pelvic and paraaortic lymph nodes (requiring **lymphadenectomy**), greater omentum, small intestine (especially terminal ileum), spleen, liver, diaphragm, and peritoneal surfaces, etc. The goal of the surgery is to excise or ablate as much of the gross metastatic tumor and involved organs as possible. The procedure can be formidable, and clinical judgment must guide the extent of the procedure.

After additional chemotherapy (and radiotherapy), a CT scan may show tumor residual, or, if negative, a laparoscopic or open exploration is performed to assess the situation. When additional malignant tumor is found, further surgery is indicated. Open exploration is generally preferred, as laparoscopy may be compromised by adhesion formation, affording a lesser ability to view the retroperitoneal structures safely. If no gross tumor is encountered, multiple biopsies are taken and washings are done.

To destroy metastatic deposits (>1.5 to 2.0 cm) and to facilitate the dissection, in addition to surgical and electrosurgical technique, the Cavitron ultrasonic surgical aspirator (CUSA), the argon beam coagulator, and, less often, the Nd-YAG laser can be used.

Procedure

Laparoscopy can be performed before laparotomy to determine the extent of the metastastatic disease and the feasibility of performing a cytoreductive procedure. The peritoneal cavity is entered by a lower midline incision (that can be extended cephalad, as necessary). The entire peritoneal cavity is explored, and any ascitic fluid is sent for cytologic exam. In the absence of ascites, washings taken in the pelvis, paracolic gutters, and subdiaphragmatic spaces are sent for cytological examination. Tissue samples may also be sent. If ovarian cancer is confirmed, ***hysterectomy*** and ***bilateral salpingo-oophorectomy*** is performed. In special circumstances, oocytes may be harvested for fertility considerations (in vitro fertilization with surrogate implantation). If no gross metastases are found, multiple biopsies are taken in the peritoneal cavity and retroperitoneally. If metastatic disease is present, the surgery may be terminated and chemotherapy instituted with subsequent ***cytoreductive surgery***, or the procedure to be performed initially is undertaken.

The greater omentum is resected, separating it from the transverse colon and stomach. If splenic deposits are noted, the superficial lesions can be coagulated or ***splenectomy*** (p. 171) can be performed. After incising the hepatic ligaments, the peritoneum can be stripped from the diaphragm. If the diaphragm is perforated, these wounds are repaired and a thoracostomy tube is placed. Iliac and paraaortic nodes can be excised. If the distal ureter is involved, the proximal segment can be transplanted into the bladder, or if the bladder if involved, ***partial cystectomy*** is done. When necessary, ***total cystectomy*** is done with formation of an ***ileal conduit*** (see p. 425). The rectosigmoid colon can be resected (see p. 238) with primary anastomosis or ***Hartmann procedure*** (see p. 238), etc. If segments of the small bowel are involved, especially if a pending obstructive situation can be determined, local limited resection (or bypass) can be done.

Isolated small metastatic implants (which may be numerous) can be destroyed by electrosurgical technique, CUSA, argon beam coagulator, etc. The abdomen is closed in layers.

Preparation of the Patient

Apply antiembolitic hose. Patient is in modified lithotomy position with the buttocks positioned just over the lower break in the table and the arms extended on padded armboards. Padded shoulder braces are secured to the table. The table may be placed in Trendelenburg position. Pad all bony prominences and areas vulnerable to skin and neurovascular trauma or pressure. CVP and arterial lines may be required; consult surgeon and anesthesia provider. Apply electrosurgical dispersive pad.

Skin Preparation

Both a vaginal and an abdominal prep are required; two separate prep trays are require used. The patient's legs are placed in a froglike position; prep as for ***D&C***, p. 278. Insert Foley catheter and connect it to drainage unit. Return the patient's legs to their original position, place the drainage tubing and unit below the level of the table, and replace the safety belt. For the abdominal preparation, begin at the midline, extending from nipples to mid-thighs and down to the table at the sides.

Draping

Folded towels and a transverse or laparotomy sheet

Equipment

- Sequential compression device with disposable leg wraps, if requested
- Forced-air warming blanket, if ordered
- Central venous pressure (CVP) equipment, optional
- Padded shoulder braces
- Suctions (2)
- ESU
- Scales (2) for weighing sponges
- Cavitational Ultra Sound Aspirator (CUSA) console, optional
- Argon beam coagulator console, optional

Instrumentation

- Major procedures tray
- Long instruments tray, available
- Vascular procedures tray, available
- Gastrointestinal tray, available
- Gastrointestinal staplers (with staples in unit), e.g., EEA, TA, GIA, available
- Multifire Hemoclip applicators with clips
- CUSA handpiece with tip (aspiration, irrigation, ultrasound vibration) and cord, optional
- Argon beam coagulator handpiece and cord, optional

Supplies

- Antiembolitic hose
- Blades, (3) #10

Basin set
Needle magnet or counter
Suction tubing with in-line filter, e.g., Clear View
Electrosurgical pencil and cord with holder and scraper
Foley catheter with tubing and drainage unit
Aspiration tubes for washings, several, as needed
Labels for aspiration tubes
Pleurevac™, if diaphragm is perforated, optional
Chest tube, e.g., Argyle, optional
Connector 5-in-1 (for chest tube)
Colostomy pouch (Karaya Seal™), optional
Sanitary napkin belt or T-binder
Perineal pad

Special Notes

- **N.B.** *A signed permit for a* **sterilization procedure** *must be on the chart in addition to the signed surgical permit for the procedure,* **Cytoreductive Surgery,** *p. 335; it is required before the patient may be brought into the room.* The patient needs to indicate in her own words that she understands that she will no longer be able to have children. Her statement is written in the **Perioperative Record**.
- Apply **Special Notes** from ***Abdominal Laparotomy***, p. 134, as indicated.
- **Cytoreductive Surgery** may be lengthy; personnel assignments must be considered, particularly to keep patient care consistent.
- **N.B.** Many samples of cell washings and tissue biopsies may be taken. Scrub person needs to take care not to allow aspiration (by suction) of washings intended for cytologic exam by pinching off the suction. Scrub person and circulator need to know the site(s) from which specimen(s) was (were) obtained.
- Circulator needs to correctly identify the washings and the areas from which tissue samples were taken on the requisition slip; be certain that specimen bottles correspond, are labeled correctly, accordingly.
- **N.B.** *Ascertain that there are two working suctions in the room before starting the surgery in case hemorrhage should occur.* Keep an accurate record of irrigation fluid used to assist in determining blood and fluid loss replacement.
- Circulator must verify with the blood bank that the correct number of units of blood ordered is ready and available.

- The circulator assists anesthesia provider in administering transfusion by setting up perfusion set as needed, checking identification number on unit of blood or blood product and comparing it to the patient identification number, and by obtaining a blood pump and blood warmer.
- The circulator weighs sponges as necessary to assist in determining blood and fluid loss replacement.
- If there is a perforation of the diaphragm, a chest tube, connector, and closed-suction drainage unit, e.g., Pleurevac, is needed.
- Keep all soiled instruments isolated in a basin.
- When necessary, "clean" closure of the abdomen requires regowning, regloving, redraping, and a basic/minor procedures tray.
- A Foley catheter connected to a continuous straight drainage unit is inserted at the conclusion of the surgery to prevent urinary retention resulting from swollen tissues around the operative site.
- The drainage tubing of the Foley catheter should be patent (without kinks); the level of the bag should be kept below the level of the patient's bladder to prevent a reflux of urine that could lead to a UTI.
- Do not open surgical staplers until specific items are requested, as they are expensive.

Pelvic Exenteration

Definition

The en bloc removal of the rectum, distal sigmoid colon, urinary bladder and distal ureters, internal genitalia, pelvic lymph nodes, pelvic peritoneum, and a portion of the levator muscles, and the creation of an ileal or colonic loop urinary diversion and colostomy; the hypogastric vessels are no longer removed.

Discussion

The primary indication for **Pelvic Exenteration** is radio-resistant or recurrent cervical carcinoma. **Total pelvic exenteration** implies the excision of the internal genitalia, rectum, and bladder, necessitating a permanent colostomy and a urinary diversion. If malignancy has spread beyond the pelvis or there are significant medical risks, this procedure is abandoned. The rectum may be spared, and *anterior exenteration* is performed. *Posterior exenteration* is usually not performed for gynecologic malignancy, but it may be done for rectal malignancy. The morbidity and mortality for this procedure is significant.

Procedure

A generous midline incision is employed. A large self-retaining retractor is placed. The abdomen is explored. Multiple frozen sections may be done. The order of the procedure varies with the surgeon. The urinary diversion (see ***Ileal Conduit***, p. 425) may be done first or later in the procedure. ***Pelvic lymphadenectomy*** is done, removing the fatty tissues about the iliac vessels extending into the obturator fossa. The ligamentous attachments of the uterus and adnexae are separated from the pelvic wall, and the rectum is mobilized from its posterior and lateral attachments (see ***Abdominoperineal Resection***, p. 250). The bladder and urethra are mobilized and excised (see ***Cystectomy***, p. 399). From the perineal approach (often by a second team), the anus and distal rectum are excised (see Abdominoperineal Resection, p. 250). The distal vagina may be preserved or reconstructed later on. The specimen is removed en bloc. A ***colostomy*** (p. 238) is created and the pelvic floor closed. Perineal (and other) drains may be placed. The abdomen is closed in layers. Appropriate stomal pouches are applied.

Preparation of the Patient

Antiembolitic hose are put on the legs. A nasogastric tube, Foley urinary catheter (with drainage unit), and rectal tube may be inserted before the surgical procedure begins. The circulator assists the anesthesia provider with establishing IV and CVP lines, and other lines (e.g., arterial) as necessary. Following the administration of general anesthesia, the patient is placed in a modified lithotomy position with the legs tilted forward (using padded stirrups) and the buttocks positioned just over the lower break in the table. Folded towels may be used to elevate the buttocks. Arms may be extended on armboards. The legs and feet are padded with towels or foam pads to avoid injury at pressure points, as are all bony prominences and areas vulnerable to skin and neurovascular trauma or pressure. Padded shoulder braces are secured to the table. The table may be placed in Trendelenburg position. Apply electrosurgical dispersive pad.

Skin Preparation

Use two prep sets. Standing at the foot of the table between the patient's legs (the lower section has been removed), begin cleansing at the midline, extending from nipples to knees and down to the table at the sides. Cleanse the anus last, discarding each sponge after use. Drain the patient's bladder with a straight catheter (e.g., Robinson).

Draping

Drape sheet under the buttocks, followed by a laparoscopy sheet, or drape sheet, leggings, and a laparotomy sheet

Note: The laparotomy sheet will be cut (as necessary) to expose the patient's perineum.

Equipment

Sequential compression device with disposable leg wraps, as requested
Forced-air warming blanket, if ordered
CVP unit
Padded stirrups (e.g., Allen)
Padded shoulder braces
ESU
Suctions (2)
Scales to weigh sponges (2)

Instrumentation

Major procedures tray
Long instruments tray
Abdominal hysterectomy tray
Self-retaining retractors (e.g., Balfour, O'Connor-O'Sullivan, Bookwalter)
Multifire Hemoclip appliers (all sizes and lengths)
Vascular procedures tray, available
GI procedures tray, available
Gastrointestinal staplers, as requested

Supplies

Antiembolitic hose
Straight catheter, to drain bladder (prep), e.g., Robinson
Blades, (4) #10 and (1) #15
Basin set
Needle magnet or counter
Suction tubing
Electrosurgical pencils and cords with holder and scraper (2)
Dissectors (e.g., peanuts, Kittners)
Penrose drains, umbilical tapes, and vascular loops (for retraction)
Hemoclips, all sizes
Graduate and asepto syringes (2)
Pouches for colostomy and urostomy (e.g., Karaya Seal), optional
Perineal drains, as requested
T-binder

Special Notes

- **N.B.** *In addition to the signed surgical permit for the procedure,* **Pelvic Exenteration,** *a signed permit for a* **steril-**

ization procedure *must be on the patient's chart p. 7; it is required before the patient may be brought into the room.* The patient indicates in her own words that she understands that she will no longer be able to have children; her words should be quoted on the **Perioperative Record**.

- Apply **Special Notes** from **Abdominal Laparotomy**, p. 134, as indicated.
- *Avoid injury to the patient's fingers by preventing them from being caught in the table mechanism when the table is returned to its original position.*
- Prevent risk of positioning injury to the patient with stirrups that are adequately padded and positioned correctly to avoid skin and neurovascular pressure or trauma. Document appearance and condition of the skin preoperatively and immediately postoperatively.
- **N.B.** *Ascertain that there are two working suctions in the room before starting the surgery in case hemorrhage should occur.* Keep an accurate record of irrigation fluid used to assist in determining blood loss and fluid loss replacement.
- Patient may have made an autologous blood donation preoperatively. Confirm with laboratory that blood and blood products are ready and available, as ordered.
- Assist anesthesia provider in administering transfusion by setting up perfusion set as needed, checking identification number on units, and obtaining a blood pump and blood warmer.
- Anesthesia provider may request additional items, e.g., setup for arterial line.
- Basic/Minor procedures tray and second Mayo stand may be requested for the simultaneously performed perineal phase of the procedure.
- **N.B.** Extra caution must be taken for counting of sponges and instruments, etc. in light of two surgical fields. A second scrub person may be necessary.
- **N.B.** The scrub person should advise the surgeon when a blade has been changed, e.g., indicate a "new" blade.
- The circulator weighs sponges and keeps an accurate record of the amount of irrigation used to help to correct fluid imbalance.
- The scrub person should be prepared for many frozen sections to be taken. Specimens may be labeled by marking pen on a label attached to a towel or similar.

- The circulator must correctly identify the area from which the specimen was taken when writing the requisitions. Identifying the "right specimen" from the designated area, "right area," from the correctly identified patient, "right patient."
- Keep all soiled instruments isolated in a basin.
- Clean closure of the abdomen requires regowning, regloving, redraping, and the use of a basic/minor procedures tray.
- Do not open staplers until requested; this is done to effect cost effectiveness. These items are costly and should only be opened when specifically requested.
- Instruments must be completely accounted for during the counts in their entirety, as they have multiple parts.

Radical Vulvectomy With Regional Lymphadenectomy

Definition

Extensive excision of the vulva and its lymphatic drainage in the inguinal, femoral, and pelvic areas.

Discussion

Radical Vulvectomy with Regional Lymphadenectomy is most often performed for invasive squamous cell carcinoma of the vulva, labia majora more than labia minora, or clitoris and perineum (other less-common lesions may include melanoma, *Paget's disease,* Bartholin gland carcinoma, sarcoma, etc.). These often-neglected lesions, seen mostly in the postmenopausal patient, present at the time of detection with 30% metastatic disease to regional lymph nodes, necessitating a radical procedure. However, each case is individualized. In instances when lymph nodes exhibit metastatic disease, en bloc removal of the vulva, clitoris, distal urethra, distal vagina, bulbocavernosus, ischiocavernosus, superficial transverse perineal muscles (as are the anus and distal rectum with necessity for permanent colostomy if involved) is done with inguinal, femoral, and pelvic lymphadenectomy. If the ipsilateral nodes are clear, the contralateral dissection may be omitted.

Preoperative biopsy, colposcopy, and CT scan of the pelvis are performed to establish the diagnosis and identify local involvement and lymph nodal enlargement. Lymphatic mapping using intralesional injection of isosulphan blue and lymphoscintigraphy (Tc^{99} sulfur colloid) may identify sentinel node involvement guiding the extent of the procedure. Lesser presentations (lesions less than 1 mm of stromal invasion in depth) may require only wide local excision or, if very superficial, local excision alone. In advanced cases, preoperative radiotherapy may be employed as well postoperatively (with chemotherapy). The patient must be prepared to accept common postoperative difficulties, as lower-extremity lymphedema and psychological problems related to compromised sexuality and loss of body image. When the procedure is extensive and wound closure is a problem, myocutaneous grafts (gracilis, gluteus maximus, tensor fascia lata), thigh rotation flaps, etc., may be employed, sometimes using the assistance of a plastic surgeon.

Procedure

The patient is placed in a modified lithotomy position to give access to the lower abdomen and perineum. A urinary catheter is inserted; pneumatic hose are applied. If bilateral dissection is anticipated, two surgical teams may be used. A butterfly-shaped incision is made, incorporating a wide suprapubic incision extending the lateral aspects of same inferiorly across the groin over the femoral triangles and then posteriorly across the perineum. Alternatively, three separate incisions can be used, two inferior to the inguinal folds and one about the vulva. Ipsilateral inguinal and femoral flaps are raised, preserving the subcutaneous fat. In the inguinal dissection, the round ligament (uterine) is divided; in the femoral triangle, the proximal saphenous vein is divided and the femoral nerve protected. If positive nodes are detected, pelvic **lymphadenectomy** (retroperitoneal approach) is done as well as the contralateral groin and pelvis. During the pelvic node dissection, the ureters and major vessels are protected. Hemoclips are used, which also may serve as markers for subsequent radiotherapy. The vulvar tissues and distal urethra (catheter replaced after the dissection and reconstruction) and vagina are excised. Wound reconstruction is then performed; suction drains are placed in the groin incisions and beneath wound flaps. Rotational flaps or myocutaneous grafts are employed as needed as noted above. Pneumatic hose are continued.

Preparation of the Patient

Antiembolitic hose are put on the legs, as requested. Following the administration of general anesthesia, the patient is placed in a modified lithotomy position using padded stirrups (e.g., Allen) with the buttocks just over the lower break in the table. The arms are padded and may be tucked in at the patient's sides or extended on padded armboards. Padded shoulder braces are secured to the table. Pad all bony prominences and areas vulnerable to skin and neurovascular trauma or pressure. The table is placed in Trendelenburg position. Apply electrosurgical dispersive pad.

Skin and Preparation

Begin prep by standing at the foot of the table between the patient's legs, (as the lower section of the table has been removed), and start at the umbilicus, extending the prep from the nipples to the mid-thighs, down over the labia, discarding each sponge after wiping the labia. Cleanse each inner thigh. A vaginal prep is performed. The perineum and anus are prepared last; discard each sponge after wiping the anus. Insert Foley catheter with drainage unit.

Equipment

Sequential compression device with disposable leg wraps, as requested
Forced-air warming blanket, if ordered
Padded stirrups (e.g., Allen)
Padded shoulder braces
ESU
Suctions (2)
CVP unit
Scales to weigh sponges (2)

Instrumentation

Major procedures tray
Long instruments tray
Abdominal hysterectomy tray
Self-retaining retractors
Multifire Hemoclip appliers (assorted sizes and lengths)
Vascular procedures tray, available

Supplies

Antiembolitic hose
Foley catheter with drainage unit
Blades, (2) #10 and (1) #15
Basin set
Needle magnet or counter
Suction tubing
Electrosurgical pencils and cords with holders and scrapers (2)
Dissectors (e.g., peanut, Kittner)
Penrose drains, umbilical tapes, and vascular loops (for retraction)
Graduate and asepto syringe
Perineal drains, e.g., Hemovac™, optional
T-binder

Special Notes

- Apply **Special Notes** from ***Abdominal Laparotomy***, p. 134, as indicated.
- **N.B.** *Avoid injury to the patient's fingers by preventing them from being caught in the table mechanism when the table is returned to its original position.*

- Obtain patient's x-ray studies, verify identification (e.g., "right x-rays," for "right patient" of the pertinent area, the "right area"); have the x-rays in the room before bringing the patient into the room
- A sequential compression device with leg wraps may be applied over the antiembolitic hose, when ordered, to prevent deep vein thrombosis.
- Prevent risk of positioning injury to the patient with stirrups that are adequately padded and positioned correctly to avoid skin and neurovascular pressure or trauma. Document appearance and condition of the skin preoperatively and postoperatively.
- **N.B.** *Ascertain that there are two working suctions (in addition to the suction on the anesthesia provider's cart) in the room before starting the surgery in case hemorrhage should occur.*
- The circulator should keep an accurate record of irrigation fluid; the record is used to assist in determining fluid loss replacement.
- Patient may have made an autologous blood donation preoperatively. Confirm with the blood bank that blood and blood products are ready and available, as ordered.
- The circulator assists the anesthesia provider in administering transfusions by setting up perfusion set as needed, checking identification number on the blood or blood product unit and comparing it to the patient's identification number, and by obtaining a blood pump and blood warmer.
- The circulator weighs sponges and keeps an accurate record of the amount of irrigation used to help correct fluid imbalance. For the procedure for weighing sponges, see p. 162.
- The scrub person and circulator should be prepared for many frozen sections to be taken. He/she must know the origin of the specimen; when in doubt, the scrub person or the circulator should ask the surgeon.
- The circulator must correctly identify the area from which the specimen was taken when preparing the requisitions.

Cerclage Procedures

Definition

The placement of an encircling tape ligature at the level of the internal os to maintain the integrity of the cervical canal during pregnancy.

Discussion

Cerclage is performed to correct an incompetent cervix during mid or latter pregnancy to prevent spontaneous abortion. Incompetency is related to previous laceration or congenital weakness. The procedure is best performed before the cervix actually dilates. The two most commonly performed cerclage procedures are the **Shirodkar** and the **McDonald.**

Procedure

In the *Shirodkar* procedure, a transverse incision is made in the vaginal mucosa at its junction with the anterior aspect of the cervix. The bladder is reflected away. A similar incision is made posteriorly. A tape ligature of heavy material is passed on a ligature carrier to encircle the cervix, with both ends exiting in the anterior incision. Thus, a tape ligature encircles the cervix ("cerclage"). The tape is tightened and sutured. The posterior portion of the tape loop may be sutured to the vaginal mucosa. The mucosal wounds are closed.

In an alternate procedure, the *McDonald,* a suture of Mersilene (4 mm tape) is placed in pursestring fashion around the four quadrants of the cervix and tied to effect competency.

Preparation of the Patient

Following the administration of regional or general anesthesia, the patient is placed in a lithotomy position. Arms may be extended on padded armboards. Apply electrosurgical dispersive pad.

Skin Preparation

N.B. Extreme care must be taken to do the vaginal preparation ***very gently***. Begin at the pubic symphysis and extend down over the labia. Cleanse each inner thigh. Gently cleanse vaginal vault and cervix with spongesticks (3). The perineum and anus are cleansed with the remaining sponges. Discard each sponge after wiping the anus.

Draping

Drape sheet under the buttocks, leggings, and a drape sheet over the abdomen

Equipment

Padded stirrups
ESU

Instrumentation

Weighted vaginal speculum
Limited procedures tray

Short Heaney retractors (2)
Ligature carrier

Supplies

Antiembolitic hose, as requested
Small basin
Blade, (1) #15
Needle magnet or counter, optional
Tape ligature (e.g., 4-mm Mersilene tape)
Nonabsorbable suture material, 2-0, to secure Mersilene tape
Perineal pad
T-binder

Special Notes

- Apply **Special Notes** from ***Dilatation and Curettage (D&C)***, p. 278, as indicated.
- Circulator may take this opportunity to explain that he/she will act as the patient's advocate. The circulator explains the course of the perioperative events and nursing actions before doing them to decrease patient's anxiety about the surgery and the unfamiliar environment.
- Assess and document patient's anxiety level and level of knowledge regarding the intended procedure. Clarify misconceptions by answering the patient's questions in a knowledgeable manner and refer questions as necessary to the surgeon.
- **N.B.** The circulator must perform the vaginal prep *very carefully*, so as not to provoke uterine contraction (reflex stimulation).

Cesarean Section

Definition

Delivery of the fetus through incisions in the abdominal wall and the uterus.

Discussion

There are numerous indications for Cesarean section (also spelled: caesarian) of surgical delivery, including mechanical (cephalopelvic disproportion), fetal distress, malrotation, malpresentation, toxemia, multiple pregnancies, placenta previa, and prolapsed cord. When performed as an emergency (necessitated because delay could seriously compromise the infant), the goal is to deliver the infant promptly, while avoiding injury to both mother and infant. Additional reasons for this type of surgical delivery might be cervical dystocia, active herpes simplex in the birth canall, or metabolic disease, as diabetes. Previous cesarean section or other uterine surgery (e.g., ***myomectomy***) is no longer regarded as an absolute indication for this procedure.

Procedure

Regional anesthesia is most frequently administered to the patient, who is awake. A low transverse *(Kerr)* or vertical (*Krohnig*) incision consistent with the estimated size of the fetus is made. The rectus muscles are separated and the peritoneum incised. Hemostasis is assured. The bladder is reflected from the lower uterine segment, and the uterus is incised. The amniotic sac is spontaneously entered, and fluid must be aspirated immediately. Some surgeons prefer to use the suction tubing without a tip to avoid injury. The fetal head is delivered using manual pressure or by obstetric forceps and counter-pressure on the fundus. Retractors are removed.

As soon as the head is delivered, the newborn's nares are aspirated by bulb syringe *immediately* **but *very gently***; the delivery is completed. Oxytocin is administered intravenously to encourage the uterus to contract and to decrease blood loss. The umbilical cord is clamped and cut. The infant is received in a sheet and transferred to a gowned and gloved member of the neonatal team, e.g., the pediatrician. ***Standard Precautions*** (see p. 33) are observed. Resuscitative measures are provided to the neonate under warming lamps. The pediatrician determines the infant's Apgar score. Vernix, etc., are wiped from the infant's skin. Ointment (erythromycin 0.5%) is applied to the conjunctival sacs of the newborn by a member of the neonatal team. The placenta is delivered. The uterus is massaged to encourage it to contract. ***Tubal ligation*** (see p. 312) may be performed. Blood, amniotic fluid, etc., are aspirated. Hemostasis is assured. The edges of the uterine incision are clamped to aid in its closure; the uterus and bladder are closed in a single or a double layer. The peritoneum at the lower uterine segment is sutured to its anatomic position. The wound is closed in layers. An abdominal dressing and perineal pad are applied. Warmed blankets (from blanket warmer) are placed over the mother.

The mother and infant, in good condition, are given a moment to bond on the gurney. The infant is rushed to the neonatal unit to be further cleaned, weighed, etc.

Preparation of the Patient

Antiembolitic hose are put on the legs. The patient is supine with the right side slightly elevated to displace pressure from the inferior vena cava. Arms may be extended on padded armboards. A pillow may be placed under the lumbar spine and/or under the knees (to avoid straining back muscles). Pad all bony prominences and areas vulnerable to skin and neurovascular trauma or pressure. Very carefully insert Foley catheter and connect it to continuous drainage.

Skin Preparation

Do not prep the vagina.

Draping

Folded towels and a laparotomy (or transverse) sheet
Additional drape sheet to cover a second back table for care of the infant

Equipment

Suction (two), available
ESU
Heat lamps and bassinet with a warmer
Identification bands (3)
Ink pad (for infant's footprint, single use) (optional)

Instrumentation

Cesarean section tray
Delivery forceps
Head extractor, available

Supplies

Basin set
Electrosurgical pencil and cord with holder and scraper
Suction tubing
Blades, (2) #10
Needle magnet or counter
Bulb syringe (to aspirate infant's nose and mouth)
Resuscitation equipment for infant
Erythromycin ointment (0.5%) for infant's eyes (conjunctival sacs)
Oxytocin, usually 20 mg in a syringe (to the anesthesia provider)
Medicine cup, paper labels, marking pen
Test tubes (2) for cord blood
Drain (e.g., Penrose), optional

Special Notes

- Apply **Special Notes** from ***Abdominal Laparotomy***, p. 134, as indicated.
- The circulator ascertains that the pediatrician is present in the labor and delivery (L&D) department.
- ***Standard Precautions*** (see p. 33) must be observed, at all times during the delivery, as exposure to body fluids may be encountered

at any time. ***Standard Precautions*** are the minimally accepted precautions regarding protection of personnel from contamination from body fluids (e.g., wearing a head covering, mask, face shield, gown with an impermeable front, gloves, and shoe covers).

- **Reminder:** Use safety precautions to identify, label, and dispense medications or solutions; to avoid medication errors; see p. 30. It is mandatory that all medications and solutions within the sterile field be labeled.
- Circulator usually prepares the oxytocin, 20 units for the anesthesia provider to administer intravenously. Oxytocin will help the uterus to contract, minimize blood loss, and aid in expulsion of the placenta. The bottle is retained in the room until the procedure has concluded.
- **N.B.** Once the uterus is surgically opened, immediate suctioning of amniotic fluid is necessary; particular care is taken to avoid injury to the fetus. Some gynecologists refer not to have a metal tip on the suction tubing.
- **N.B.** As soon as the infant's head is delivered, the scrub person hands the bulb syringe to the surgeon to aspirate amniotic fluid from the infant's nose and mouth. The bulb syringe is passed to the pediatrician with the infant.
- **N.B.** Following delivery of the infant, the nose and mouth are immediately suctioned with a bulb syringe, the cord is clamped and cut, and the infant is carefully handed to the pediatrician.
- Apgar scores are obtained from the pediatrician and recorded by the circulator in the **Perioperative Record**. Records pertaining to the birth are completed according to hospital policy, as soon as possible.
- Newborn identification bands are placed on the infant (usually around the ankle) and another newborn identification band is placed on the wrist of the mother (in addition to her own armband) before either mother or infant leaves the delivery room. Care is taken to be certain that circulation to the infant's foot is not compromised.
- Cord blood is sent to the laboratory in two test tubes; the tubes must be labeled with the identification of the mother and the indication that the blood is infant cord blood.
- Prophylactic treatment of gonococcal or Chlamydial ophthalmia neonatorum is achieved with erythromycin 0.5% ointment placed in the conjunctival sacs of the newborn.
- Closure counts are taken at three intervals; 1) prior to the closure of the uterus, 2) prior to the closure of the peritoneum, and 3) prior to the closure of the skin.

- The infant is taken in a pre-warmed isolettte to the nursery and the mother is taken to the postpartum recovery room. All measures necessary to maintain the infant's temperature and to assure breathing is unobstructed in mother and infant are taken.
- The circulator accompanies the anesthesia provider and the patient to the Post Anesthesia Care Unit (PACU); he/she gives the PACU perioperative practitioner a detailed intraoperative patient report regarding the course of events as they apply to that patient.
- In the postoperative postpartum unit and the newborn nursery, respectively, the patient's breathing is observed, blood pressure and vital signs are monitored, and documentation of all pertinent information (e.g., the amount of blood on the mother's peri pad) are documented. Observations of the patient and documentation of nursing interventions are vital for patient safety regarding continuity of care and for medicolegal reasons.
- The infant and mother are observed closely following the delivery. Documentation is made of all pertinent patient information (e.g., vital signs, breathing, etc.). The gynecologist is notified of irregularities as is necessary for patient safety and for medicolegal reasons.

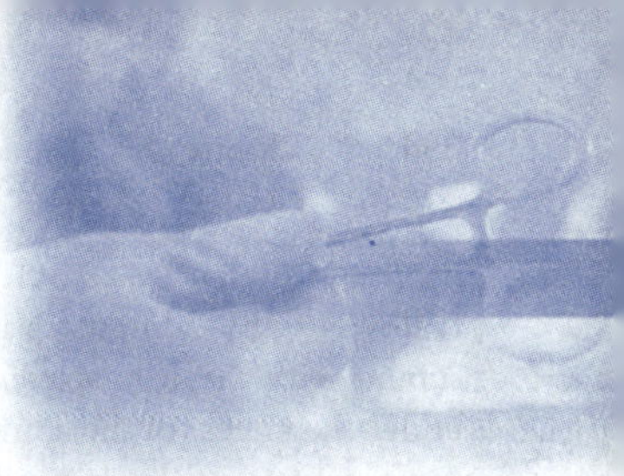

CHAPTER 19 Genitourinary Surgery

Hypospadias Repair

Definition

Reconstruction of the distal urethra and meatus from the ventral surface of the penis to the normal position.

Discussion

This condition is a relatively common congenital anomaly. In *hypospadias*, the urethral meatus may open on the distal end, midshaft, at the penoscrotal junction, or on the perineum. The ventral aspect of the penis is often shortened with a downward curvature (chordee) that may be caused by fibrous bands; in some presentations of chordee, the fibrous bands may not be present. Depending on the degree of hypospadias, ***meatoplasty, glanuloplasty, urethroplasty, orthoplasty*** (straightening of the urethra), and/or ***scrotoplasty*** may be indicated. Very distal deformities may not require correction; proximal locations necessitate surgery to avoid difficulty in urination and coitus. The surgeon determines if the procedure can be performed in a single-staged repair or if a two-staged repair is necessary; tissue graft or a rotational skin flap may be required. Continence is usually not affected because the urinary sphincters are not involved.

Hypospadias repair is most often performed on infants and children. ***Circumcision*** should **not** be performed on infants and children with hypospadias in order to preserve skin useful in correcting the deformity. This anomaly infrequently occurs in the female, with the urethra opening into the vagina.

Procedure

To correct the chordee, repair is accomplished by cutting the fibrous tissue bands on the ventral aspect of the penis. The absent portion of the urethra may be reconstructed out of the foreskin. In circumcised patients, a tissue graft, e.g., a segment of vein or skin from a nonhair-bearing area, such as the inner aspect of the arm, may be used. An incision is made on the ventral aspect of the penis. The reconstructed urethra, splinted from within by a catheter (e.g., Foley), is placed in the tunnel that is constructed, over which the remaining foreskin is grafted. According to the severity of the defect, the meatus, glans, urethra, and/or scrotum may require repair; some presentations require a *second stage* to restore urethral continuity.

Preparation of the Patient

Following the administration of general anesthesia, the patient is supine with the legs apart (well-separated). A pillow may be placed under the knees (of the adult patient) to help maintain the position and to prevent lower back strain. For the adult (or large child), the arms may be extended on padded armboards and the safety strap is replaced above the knees following positioning. Pad all bony prominences and areas vulnerable to skin and neurovascular pressure or trauma. Apply electrosurgical dispersive pad.

For infants and small children, the lower segment of the table and pad are removed; this will permit closer access to the child in supine position. Adhesive tape-to-tape or hypoallergenic tape may be used to help maintain the froglike position of the legs; a pillow support may be used as well. The arms are secured with softly padded nonconstricting restraints. Particular care must be taken to adequately secure the child, while preventing trauma to areas vulnerable to skin and neurovascular trauma or pressure. Apply pediatric-sized electrosurgical pad.

Skin Preparation

A small sterile plastic adhesive drape may be placed over the anus to isolate it. Cleanse entire pubic area (penis, scrotum, and perineum), extending from the umbilicus to the mid-thighs.

Draping

Cuffed towel under the scrotum, folded towels around pubic area, and a sheet with a small fenestration

Equipment

Electrosurgical unit (ESU)

Instrumentation

Adults

Vasectomy tray
Urethral sounds

Infants and Children

Pediatric plastic procedures tray
Lacrimal duct probes

Supplies

Small plastic adhesive drapes
Blades, (2) #15
Small basin
Water-soluble lubricant

Needle magnet or counter
Catheter, e.g., Foley
Sterile marking pen
Electrosurgical pencil with needle tip and cord with holder and scraper
Dressing pad (e.g., Adaptic, DuodermR™, Owen's gauze), gauze "fluffs," and dressing sponge(s). Dressing is applied with light pressure, when applicable to graft site
T-binder or scrotal support (adult or large child)

Special Notes

- The circulator must always use the **Joint Commission's (JC) (formerly the Joint Commission on Accreditation of Healthcare Organizations)** *Universal Protocol* to identify the patient, site, and side and the correct procedure; see the **JC's** *Universal Protocol*, p. 18, as necessary. Obtain the aid of parents to identify the pediatric patient.
- *"The child is not a small adult"; therefore, it is imperative that persons administering care to the child patient, see Pediatric General Information, p. 978, for the many special concerns regarding the pediatric patient.* ***Give assurances and information as necessary. Refer questions to the surgeon when appropriate.***
- Before every surgery begins, an official "***time out***" must be taken; it is a *safety measure*. A *time out* is required and must be documented on the **Perioperative Record** for patient safety and medicolegal reasons.
- See the suggested **Patient Care Plan,** p. 9; adapt care to meet the patient's needs; this is especially true regarding infants and children. Implement and document nursing interventions that will result in optimal desired outcomes for the child. Use the **Special Notes** to augment the plan of care.
- Apply **Special Notes** from ***Abdominal Laparotomy,*** p. 134, as it applies to the pediatric patient, in general.
- The circulator assists the anesthesia provider during the induction of anesthesia. For the circulator's role, see p. 60. Induction of anesthesia for children is usually by mask, followed by intravenous (IV) sedation.
- For measures to take regarding anesthesia administered to infants and children, see p. 984. Assorted pediatric-sized intravenous catheters, endotracheal tubes, breathing circuit and bag,

as well as suction catheters, humidifier, temperature probe (axillary or rectal), and appropriately sized electrodes for electrocardiogram (EKG) are necessary.

- The circulator conveys to the patient (and/or parents, as appropriate) that he/she will act as the patient's advocate and demonstrates emotional support by his or her presence during the administration of anesthesia. This is demonstrated to the child by comfort measures such as holding or speaking softly.
- **N.B.** *When using tape-to-tape adhesive tape restraints for children, the central portion (of adhesive tape) is prepared "tape-to-tape" to avoid direct contact of the adhesive with the skin, or hypoallergenic tape may be used.* Apply tincture of benzoin to the areas on the legs where the hypoallergenic tape will be applied. Document the appearance of the skin on the legs in the areas where the tape will be placed preoperatively and immediately postoperatively.
- All care must be documented in the **Perioperative Record** for continuity of care and for medicolegal reasons. Documentation contains the record of nursing care that explains what has been done for the (child) patient. The care given by each caregiver is recorded. It acts as a safety measure in that the next person to assume care for the (child) patient knows what treatments have been administered so that particular "ordered care measures" are not duplicated.
- Take appropriate measures to maintain patient's body temperature, e.g., **for adults**: a warmed blanket (from the blanket warmer, if the patient is cold) and; when ordered, a forced-air warming blanket may be placed over legs and/or chest or a warming blanket may be placed on the table. **For infants and children:** the room temperature may be adjusted, accordingly; see next measure.
- **Neonates and infants are transported in isolettes,** *warming lamps placed overhead are used to maintain the pediatric patient's temperature while on the operating table, and the room temperature is adjusted according; see Pediatric General Information, p. 978, for room temperature recommendations.*
- Prevent hyperextension and hyperflexion positioning injuries by correctly positioning the patient. The patient should be positioned in good body alignment. Supply adequate support (e.g., pads, pillows, etc.) for the patient's limbs and joints to provide stability and comfort. Bring into the room before the patient is

brought into the room, the necessary pads, pillows, etc. used to support the patient's position on the OR (bed) table.

- When applicable, avoid injuries to the staff when positioning the patient by having adequate assistance and by employing ergonomic measures; see p. 51. The patient, when awake, is instructed how to move to the table. When the patient is unable to move on his/her own, secure an adequate number of persons to help to move the patient as necessary. Special devices as lifts (Hoyer) or rollers (Davis) may be employed for moving patients. If the patient has an IV, and other types of lines, prevent the lines from becoming kinked, tangled, or pulled out when one of these devices are used.
- Avoid pooling of prep solutions, as this results in excoriation of the skin (particularly in the pediatric patient) and to prevent burns when electrosurgery is employed. Document in the Perioperative Record, the appearance of the skin and all measures taken when positioning and prepping, repositioning, etc. the patient preoperatively and postoperatively. The appearance of the skin is documented; should the patient suffer a pressure injury, the documentation of the appearance of the skin provides proof of injury or not. When a patient is moved to a different position on the OR table, documentation is done to provide a record and the patient's pressure points are rechecked, and this, too, is documented.
- The electrosurgical pad should be applied to skin that is relatively hair-free in order to obtain good contact. Apply the pad as close to the surgical site as possible. It may be necessary to shave the contact area in the adult patient. In the pediatric patient, use an appropriately-sized pad, as well.
- The adult, as well as the child patient, may have fear and anxiety regarding the surgery and the unfamiliar environment. The circulator should explain nursing procedures before performing them and describe the sequence of perioperative events, as appropriate for the patient's age. Explanations prevent fear of the unknown by advising the patient as care is administered. The explanation serves as emotional support of the patient in surgery.
- It is important to provide emotional support to the adult patient regarding feelings of altered body image. Give the patient an opportunity to express his feelings. Respect the patient's right to his/her feelings. Consider parent's position and concerns regarding their infant. When a question is asked, perioperative person-

nel answer to the best of his/her ability with factual information. Keep the patient adequately covered to avoid loss of body heat and to avoid embarrassment by overexposure of the body. The circulator should be certain to adequately expose the area necessary to perform the surgery, but only that area.

- Assess and document patient's anxiety level and level of knowledge regarding the intended procedure. Clarify misconceptions by answering the patient's (or patient's parents') questions knowledgably when possible. Redirect questions to the surgeon, as necessary. Speak to the infant and small child patient in a soft soothing voice.
- **Reminder:** Check the chart for patient sensitivities and allergies, including to iodine and latex products (e.g., gloves, drains, or elasticized pressure dressings). For infants and children, obtain this information from parent(s). Document the appearance of the skin and any aberrations noted before using tape or prep solution and follow with the use of the alternate product if substitution is necessary.

Epispadias Repair

Definition

Correction of a congenital absence of the dorsal wall of the urethra proximal to the glans.

Discussion

The urethral meatus opens on the dorsal aspect of the penis. This deformity most often occurs at the abdominopenile junction and can be associated with deformities of the bladder and urinary sphincter. Repair is necessary to effect continence and the ability to copulate. Circumcision should ***not*** be performed on infants with epispadias in order to preserve skin useful in correcting the deformity. The procedure may be staged; the first stage involves the rotation of the foreskin to cover the defect created by mobilizing the distal urethra. A second stage addresses the creation of the distal urethra and meatus. If defective, the bladder and prostatic urethra are repaired.

Procedure

When epispadias occurs in the distal penis, the tissues are mobilized and sutured over the defect. The urethral meatus is opened at the tip of the glans. A suprapubic incision is made to expose the prostatic urethra. Redundant tissue of the prostatic urethra is excised. Absorbable sutures, e.g., catgut approximate the prostatic urethra and vesical neck over a probe or catheter, recreating the continence mechanism. A suprapubic cystostomy tube is placed to provide temporary urinary diversion. The skin is closed.

When the defect in the urethra is proximal, correction is similar to that employed for hypospadias; see p. 353.

For **Preparation of the Patient, Skin Preparation, Draping, Equipment,** and **Instrumentation, Supplies,** and **Special Notes,** see ***Hypospadias Repair***, p. 354.

Supplies

Add suprapubic cystostomy catheter, e.g., Pezzer, Malecot.

Urethroplasty

Definition

Excision of urethral stricture(s) with reconstruction of the urethra to reestablish genitourinary continuity.

Discussion

Urethral strictures occur in males as the result of infectious or inflammatory processes, trauma (including iatrogenic), and congenital abnormalities. Correction or repair may be done following the treatment of the infection (if present) using serial dilatations, laser (CO_2, argon, KTP, Nd:YAG, Ho:YAG, or excimer) vaporization of scar tissue, internal *throtomy*, or placement of urethral stent. When none of these treatments is successful, plastic reconstruction of the urethra provides long-term relief. Numerous procedures, done in one or two stages, correct various presentations of stricture. ***Free grafts (full or split-thickness***, nonhair-bearing skin), bladder epithelium, buccal mucosa, or island pedicle grafts from the penile shaft, perineum, and scrotum can be employed to construct a ***neourethra.*** Preoperative evaluation includes urodynamic studies, *intravenous pyelogram (IVP)*, cysto-*urethroscopy*, and *urethrography* with visualization proximal and distal to the stricture. Urosepsis is corrected prior to surgery. The most direct form of reconstruction is performed when the stricture is short. After mobilizing the corpus spongiosum and membranous urethra, the stricture can be excised. A direct tension-free anastomosis may be performed. More often, a procedure involving tissue transfer will be necessary.

Procedure

Antiembolitic hose may be applied. The adult is positioned in modified lithotomy on the "cysto" table, or the standard operating room (OR) table (e.g., Ritter™) is used with padded stirrups. Placement of the incision varies according to the presentation of the stricture: at the base of the scrotum, laterally on the penile shaft, or on the anterior aspect of the penis, extending to the glans. The stricture is incised and the scar tissue excised, if possible. The proximal urethra is sounded to ascertain that additional strictures are not present.

In a single-stage procedure, a free graft of tissue (from a source as described above) or an island pedicle graft (from penile or scrotal skin) is sutured proximally and distally to the existing urethra and to the "bed" of the excised stricture. A tube graft (epithelial side to the lumen) is sewn about a catheter. The graft ("free" or pedicle) is reinforced by approximation of the corpus spongiosum and the surrounding tissues. The graft donor site is closed; a pressure dressing (when applicable) is applied. A ***urinary diversion*** may be performed (e.g., ***suprapubic cystostomy***). Prior to wound closure, the neourethral construction is tested for leakage.

When ***urethroplasty*** is staged, only the graft is placed initially. The neourethral tube is not fashioned, but urinary diversion is established (i.e., by suprapubic catheter). During the healing phase, epilation on the skin transfer site is performed as necessary. The patient is returned to surgery 2 to 6 months later, and construction of the neourethral tube, by mobilizing the healed epithelial and surrounding tissues, is performed accordingly.

Preparation of the Patient

Adults. A warming blanket/mattress pad may be placed on the table, or a forced-air warming unit may be employed when requested. Antiembolitic hose may be applied. Following the administration of regional or general anesthesia, the patient is positioned in modified lithotomy using padded stirrups, with the buttocks positioned just over the lower break in the table. A folded towel may be placed under the buttocks to elevate the scrotum to provide full access to the scrotum and perineum. Arms may be extended on padded armboards, or they may be padded and tucked in at the patient's side. The lower portion of the table and pad are removed when the patient is placed in lithotomy. Pad all bony prominences and areas vulnerable to skin and neurovascular pressure or trauma. An electrosurgical dispersive pad is applied.

Infants and Small Children. General anesthesia is administered to the supine child by mask initially, followed by IV sedation. Heating lamps are placed over the table to help maintain the body temperature of neonates and infants. The lower segment of the table and pad are removed for closer access to the patient. Adhesive tape-to-tape or hypoallergenic tape may be used to help maintain the froglike position of the legs; a small pillow support may be used as well. The arms are secured with softly padded nonconstricting restraints. Particular care must be taken to adequately secure the child while preventing trauma to areas vulnerable to skin and neurovascular trauma or pressure. Apply *pediatric* electrosurgical dispersive pad.

Skin Preparation

A small sterile plastic adhesive drape may be placed over the anus to isolate it from the surgical field. Cleanse entire pubic area (penis, scrotum, and perineum), extending from the umbilicus to the mid-thighs.

Draping

Cuffed towel under the scrotum, folded towels around pubic area, and a sheet with a small aperture; when necessary,

Equipment

Sequential compression device with disposable leg wraps, when requested (adults)
Forced-air warming unit or warming blanket, when requested (adults and older children)
Warming lamps (neonates and infants)
Small sterile, plastic adhesive drape to isolate the anus
Padded stirrups, e.g., Allen (adult)
ESU
Fiber-optic light source, e.g., Xenon™ 300 W (for cystoscope)
Extra IV standard for hanging cystoscopy irrigation fluid
Laser, e.g., CO_2, Argon, KTP, Nd:YAG, Ho:YAG, or the excimer, optional

Instrumentation

Adults

Cystoscope (telescope, obturator, sheath) and cord
Basic plastic procedures tray
Urethral sound, dilators, stopcock
Laser hand piece, fiber, and cord, (use of laser is optional)

Infants and Children

Pediatric cystoscope (telescope, obturator, sheath) and cord
Pediatric minor procedures tray
Lacrimal duct probes
Laser hand piece, tip, and cord (use of laser is optional)

Supplies

Antiembolitic hose (optional, adult)
Small plastic adhesive drape (to isolate the anus)
Water-soluble lubricant
Cystoscopy tubing

Irrigation fluid, e.g., 2000 to 3000 ml sterile water (adult); 1000 ml sterile water (pediatric)
Blades, (2) #15
Needle magnet or counter
Basin set
Electrosurgical pencil with needle tip and cord and holder and scraper
Sterile marking pen
Urethral catheter, e.g., Foley and drainage unit or catheter plug
Suprapubic cystostomy catheter, e.g., Pezzer, Malecot, and drainage unit
Dressing pad, e.g., Adaptic, Duoderm®, or Owen's gauze and pressure dressing (when applicable) to graft site
Bulky dressing, e.g., gauze fluffs, Kerlix™, and scrotal support or T-binder

Special Notes

- Apply **Special Notes** from ***Hypospadias Repair***, p. 355, as indicated.
- **Reminder:** *For all pediatric surgeries, refer to* **Pediatric General information,** *p. 978.*
- Provide emotional support as is demonstrated by one's presence at the patient's side. Assess and document patient's (adult's, older child's, and/or parents') anxiety level and level of knowledge regarding the intended procedure. Document measures taken to ease anxiety.
- Document the presence of pedal pulses (or absence of same) that are taken preoperatively, intraoperatively, and postoperatively when the patient has been positioned in lithotomy. Report lack of pulse to surgeon.
- Lift both legs at the same time when putting the patient's legs in stirrups to prevent postoperative lumbosacral strain. Ideally, two persons are best suited to put the patient's legs in stirrups; however, one person can put the legs in stirrups by lifting both legs simultaneously and placing one leg on his/her shoulder while placing the other leg in stirrups.
- Raise and lower legs slowly to prevent cardiovascular disturbances, e.g., rapid alterations in venous return.
- **Reminder:** *Avoid injury to the patient's fingers by preventing them from being caught in the table mechanism when the foot of the table is returned to the raised position following the procedure.*

- *Cystoscopy may be performed as the first procedure.* The lubricant, a clamp or hemostat, cystoscopy tubing, and a stop-cock, cystoscope, and cord should be available on a separate back table. The surgeon will work directly off this back table without a scrub person for the cystoscopy. Keep the cystoscopy set up on the table in the room until the conclusion of the procedure.
- The circulator connects the cystoscopy tubing to the irrigation and the fiber-optic cystoscopy cord (cable) to the fiber-optic light source.
- When the laser is employed, observe all laser safety precautions; see p. 94. Laser safety precautions are mandatory.

Circumcision

Definition

Excision of the foreskin of the penis.

Discussion

This procedure is performed in the adult, as well as the pediatric patient; however, it is a far more traumatic procedure for the adult patient, both physically and emotionally. Circumcision may be performed as a prophylactic health measure, to correct phimosis (constriction of the foreskin), to treat recurrent balanitis (inflammation of the glans penis), and/or to fulfill a religious rite.

Procedure

Adults and Older Children. The preputial opening is stretched. If phimosis is present, a slit is made on the dorsal side of the penis. Adhesions underlying the foreskin are lysed, as necessary. A circumferential incision is made at the reflection of the foreskin, taking care before excising the tissue to ensure adequate tissue remains for the repair. Hemostasis is achieved, usually by needle-tip electrosurgery. The wound is approximated using individual fine absorbable sutures on a cutting needle. Care must be taken not to penetrate the urethra. Antiseptic ointment (e.g., Betadine) and a dressing pad (e.g., Telfa or Adaptic) or a petrolatum-impregnated gauze dressing are applied.

Infants and Small Children. An anesthetic cream, e.g., EMLA, may be applied 1 hour before the procedure. Other measures such as a honey-dipped pacifier and soft music may be employed to reduce the perception of pain. The procedure is often performed using a circumcision clamp, e.g., Gomco or Plastibell. Each of these devices requires the use of lubricant to prevent the glans from sticking to the clamp. The bell-shaped plunger is applied over the glans and the prepuce tissue is compressed by tightening the clamp. Care must be taken to avoid a tangential cut through the urethra and also to avoid excising so much tissue that the repair is not relaxed and supple. Compression of the blood vessels makes the tissue blood-free. A circumferential incision is made by cold knife, *not* electrosurgery. Time is allotted for clotting and coagulation to occur; removing the clamp prematurely will cause bleeding to occur. Should bleeding occur, the tissue is repaired with fine absorbable suture on a small curved cutting needle. Again, care must be taken not to penetrate the urethra with the sutures. Antiseptic ointment (e.g., Betadine) and a dressing (e.g., telfa, Adaptic, or petrolatum impregnated gauze) are applied.

For **Preparation of the Patient, Skin Preparation, Draping,** and **Equipment,** see *Hypospadias Repair,* p. 354.

Instrumentation

Adults

Limited procedure tray
Probe, optional

Infants and Children

Circumcision clamp (e.g., Gomco, Plastibell)
Pediatric limited procedures tray
Lacrimal duct probe, optional

Supplies

Antiembolitic hose (adult)
Forced-air warming blanket or warming mattress, when requested (adult)
Warming lamps (infants and children)
Blades, (1) #15
Electrosurgical pencil with needle tip and cord with holder and scraper
Water-soluble lubricant
Needle magnet or counter
Small basin
Urethral catheter, e.g., Foley and drainage unit (adult)
Antiseptic ointment, e.g., Betadine, optional
Dressing pad, e.g., telfa, Adaptic, or petrolatum-impregnated gauze
Bulky dressing, e.g., gauze fluffs, Kerlix, and scrotal support or T-binder

Special Notes

- Apply **Special Notes** from *Hypospadias*, p. 355, as directed.
- **Reminder: See Pediatric General Information** *for infants and children, p. 978.*

- **Reminder**: Provide emotional support by keeping the patient adequately covered to avoid loss of body heat and embarrassment of the adult patient caused by overexposure of the body. Expose only the area necessary to perform the surgery.
- **Reminder**: Assess and document patient's (and/or parents') anxiety level, depending on the age of the patient and level of knowledge regarding the intended procedure. Clarify misconceptions by answering questions knowledgeably when possible; redirect questions to the surgeon when necessary.
- Consider the special needs of a patient and parents of the pediatric patient for whom circumcision is a religious ritual (e.g., Jewish, Moslem).

Penile Implant

Definition

Insertion of a prosthetic device into the penis for the treatment of impotence.

Discussion

Although the procedure permits the patient to engage in sexual intercourse, it does not treat the underlying cause of impotence. The most important concern regarding the implant is the prevention of infection. Prostheses are highly susceptible to infection. Extreme urethral constriction is avoided, as it may result in urinary retention that could lead to infection.

There are two major categories of penile implants (prostheses):

- **Rigid, semi-rigid, or malleable rods**: Produce varying degrees of rigidity and are placed in the penile shaft only.
- **Inflatable or dynamic prosthesis**: There are two types of inflatable: *multi-component* and *self-contained*. In both types the cylinders are placed in the shaft of the penis and the pump is placed in the scrotal sac. At the top of the pump is the inflation site; it is squeezed to push fluid into the cylinders. At the bottom of the pump is the deflation site; it is squeezed to allow the fluid to return to the reservoir.

The approach can be *penoscrotal*, utilizing an incision at the base of the penis, *perineal* with the incision under the scrotum, *dorsopenile* on the dorsal aspect of the penis, or *infrapubic* above the penis on the abdominal wall. The type of prosthesis employed depends on the recommendation of the surgeon, the patient's choice, and the surgeon's surgical experience.

The most important factor in prosthesis selection is obtaining the proper length and diameter. Meticulous attention to detail is required to avoid contamination during preoperative preparation and intraoperative insertion of the prosthesis. Copious amounts of irrigation are used. Prophylactic antibiotics may be employed systemically and/or as an antibiotic irrigation.

Complications include infection, reservoir, or prosthesis migration due to perforation, kinked tubing, fluid leaks, dilatation of the cylinders, loss of rigidity, wire breakage, and spontaneous deflation or inflation. Perforation and migration of the prosthesis can be minimized when a Dacron graft is used.

Procedure

Foley catheter is usually inserted at the beginning of the procedure for the insertion of any of the prostheses.

Rigid, Semi-Rigid, or Malleable Prosthesis. When a single-rod prosthesis is used, a dorsal incision is made on the penis proximal to the glans and a tunnel is constructed between the corpora cavernosa. Hemostasis is achieved. A double-rod prosthesis requires incisions to be made into the corpora cavernosa. The tunnel is dilated using a clamp or hemostat and dilators, e.g., Hegar. The prosthesis is inserted. The incision is closed.

Inflatable or Dynamic Prosthesis. For insertion, a penoscrotal incision is made. The corpora cavernosa are dilated, and the prosthesis cylinders are placed. A second incision is made in the tunica albuginea toward the base of the penis or in the low suprapubic region. The reservoir is placed in the prevesical space, and the pump is placed in the scrotum via subcutaneous tunnels made through the initial incision. The wounds are closed.

Preparation of the Patient

A warming mattress or forced-air warming blanket may be requested. Antiembolitic hose may be applied. A sequential compression device with leg wraps may be applied over the antiembolitic hose when ordered to prevent deep vein thrombosis. The patient is in supine position with the legs separated; a small pad is placed under the buttocks to maximize visualization. Modified lithotomy position is employed using padded stirrups with the buttocks positioned just over the lower break in the table. A pad is placed under the scrotum to maximize visualization. Arms may be padded and tucked in at the patient's sides or extended on padded armboards. The safety strap is replaced above the knees for supine position. All bony prominences and areas vulnerable to skin and neurovascular pressure or trauma are padded. Apply electrosurgical dispersive pad.

Skin Preparation

A sterile, plastic adhesive drape is placed to isolate the anus. Cleanse the entire pubic area (penis, scrotum, and perineum), extending from the umbilicus to the lower thighs and down to the table at the sides.

Draping

Cuffed towel under the scrotum, folded towels around pubic region, and a laparotomy sheet

Equipment

Sequential compression device with disposable leg wraps, when requested
Forced-air warming blanket or warming mattress, as requested
Padded stirrups, e.g., Allen
Padded shoulder braces
ESU
Suction

Instrumentation

Limited procedures tray
Ruler and/or caliper, Andrews suction tip 9½″, dilators (e.g., Heagar), Senn retractors (2), blunt, and Metzenbaum scissors, long, 9″

Supplies

Antiembolitic hose, as requested
Small sterile, plastic adhesive drape
Blades, (1) #10 and (2) #15
Basin set
Needle magnet or counter
Suction tubing
Electrosurgical pencil with needle tip and cord with holder and scraper
Water-soluble lubricant
Sterile marking pen and labels
Foley catheter and drainage unit
Dissectors (e.g., peanut)
Antibiotic solution, graduate, and bulb syringes (2), optional
Prosthesis and necessary sterile equipment for insertion (e.g., syringes, needles, connectors)
Dacron graft material, optional
Antibiotic ointment, optional
Bulky dressing, e.g., dressing pad (telfa), gauze fluffs, Kerlix and scrotal support, or T-binder

Special Notes

- Apply **Special Notes** from ***Hypospadias Repair*** (adults), p. 355, as indicated.
- Necessary sterile equipment for insertion of the implant (e.g., syringes, needles, connectors, or a custom kit) is usually supplied with the prosthesis.
- ***Excessive handling and exposure of prepackaged sterile implants are to be avoided. Do not allow glove powder, lint from sponges, or any other foreign material to come in contact with the prosthesis.***
- Should the prosthesis require sterilization, pay strict attention to manufacturer's recommendations. Again, handle prosthesis as little as possible. Extreme precautions must be observed to avoid contamination of the prosthesis and to minimize reaction to and rejection of a foreign body in regard to the implantation of the prosthesis.
- Meticulous attention to detail is required to avoid infection during the preoperative preparation and the intraoperative insertion.
- Anticipate the need for antibiotic irrigation; copious amounts of irrigation may be used. Consult the surgeon regarding the type of antibiotic he/she would like to use. Be certain the scrub person has two bulb syringes to avoid delay.
- The scrub person needs a small basin for the antibiotic, labels, and a marking pen, as all medications on the sterile field must be labeled.
- Avoid medication errors (see p. 30) in the administration of prophylactic antibiotics added to the irrigation.
- Prepackaged sterile prostheses should not be opened until the surgeon confirms the size. This will avoid excessive exposure of the prosthesis to the environment and the unnecessary expense regarding resterilization and repackaging (when possible) of a prosthesis that will not be used.

Marshall-Marchetti-Krantz Procedure

Definition

Suspension of the bladder neck and proximal urethra in females to the symphysis pubis to correct urinary stress incontinence.

Discussion

This procedure is performed when incontinence is caused by weakness in the structures that support the bladder neck and proximal urethra (including loss of the urethrovesical angle). Elevation of the bladder neck is performed to restore continence. If there are other causes of incontinence, e.g., neurological problems, this surgery is not appropriate. An alternative procedure preferred by many surgeons is the ***Burch procedure,*** p. 371.

A laparotomy approach is described.

Procedure

A Pfannenstiel incision is made. After displacing the muscles, the peritoneal cavity is entered and a self-retaining retractor is employed. Warm, moist lap pads are placed. The prevesical space of Retzius is entered. The bladder is identified and reflected from the vagina. The urethra is exposed. Sutures are placed in the paraurethral tissues, suspending them to the periosteum at the symphysis pubis. Care is taken to avoid injury to the urethra when the sutures are placed. At intervals, counterpressure is applied by the assistant's gloved hand vaginally. The space of Retzius may be drained, e.g., with a Penrose, Hemovac™ or Jackson-Pratt™ drain. The wound is closed in layers.

Preparation of the Patient

Apply antiembolitic hose, as requested. Following administration of general or regional anesthesia, the patient is supine or in modified lithotomy position (using padded stirrups) with the buttocks just over the lower break in the table, according to surgeon's preference. Arms may be extended on padded armboards. Padded shoulder braces are secured to the table. The table may be placed in Trendelenburg position. All bony prominences and areas vulnerable to skin and neurovascular pressure or trauma are padded. Apply an electrosurgical dispersive pad.

Skin and Vaginal Preparation

Supine. Vaginal and abdominal preparations are required (separate trays). Add a Foley catheter and drainage unit to the vaginal preparation. The patient's legs are placed in a froglike position; prepare as for ***dilatation and curettage (D&C),*** p. 277. Insert the Foley catheter and connect to drainage unit. Return the patient's legs to their original position; place the drainage unit below the level of the table, and replace the safety belt. For the abdominal preparation, begin at the intended site of incision (usually Pfannenstiel), extending from nipples to mid thighs and down to the table at the sides.

Modified Lithotomy. Use one tray; add extra sponges, prep solution, Foley catheter, and drainage set before starting to prep. Stand at the foot of the table between the patient's legs and begin cleansing at the umbilicus, extending from the nipples to the mid thighs and down to the table at the sides. Continue with a vaginal prep, as for ***D&C***, p. 278. Catheterize patient's bladder with the Foley catheter and connect to drainage unit; place the drainage unit below the level of the bladder.

Draping

Drape sheet under the buttocks, leggings, folded towels, and a transverse sheet

Equipment

Sequential compression device with disposable leg wraps, when requested
Warming blanket or forced-air warming unit, when ordered
Padded shoulder braces
Padded stirrups for modified lithotomy, e.g., Allen
ESU
Suction

Instrumentation

Major procedures tray
Self-retaining retractor (e.g., Balfour)
Ligating clip appliers, e.g., Hemoclip® appliers (assorted sizes and lengths)
Heaney needle holders, optional
Uterine manipulator, optional

Supplies

Antiembolitic hose, as requested
Foley catheter and drainage unit
Basin set
Blades, (2) #10, (1) #15
Needle magnet or counter
Electrosurgical pencil and cord with holder and scraper
Suction tubing
Ligating clips, e.g., Hemoclips (assorted)
Drain, e.g., Penrose, Hemovac, or Jackson-Pratt
Perineal pad and sanitary napkin belt, in addition to the abdominal dressing

Special Notes

- Apply **Special Notes** from ***Abdominal Laparotomy***, p. 134, as indicated.
- When the uterine manipulator is requested, the patient's position on the table must be modified lithotomy (to manipulate the

uterus). If the patient has had a hysterectomy, it follows that the uterine manipulator is unnecessary.

- **Reminder:** Prevent risk of positioning injury to the patient in the modified lithotomy position by using stirrups that are padded and positioned correctly to avoid skin and neurovascular pressure or trauma. Document appearance and condition of the skin preoperatively and immediately postoperatively for patient safety and for medicolegal purposes.
- Document the presence of pedal pulses (with modified lithotomy position) preprocedure, intraprocedure, and postprocedure for patient safety and for medicolegal purposes.
- Lift both legs at the same time when putting the patient's legs in stirrups to prevent postoperative lumbosacral strain; see urethroplasty for technique for placing legs in stirrups.
- Raise and lower legs slowly to prevent cardiovascular disturbances, e.g., rapid alterations in venous return.
- The urinary drainage unit is placed below the level of the bladder to prevent a reflux of urine; this may avoid potential urinary tract infection (UTI).
- Extra gloves are required for the change of gloves for the assistant who applies vaginal counterpressure.

Burch Procedure (Retropubic Colposuspension)

Definition

A paravaginal suspension to correct stress incontinence.

Discussion

Numerous procedures have been devised to correct urinary stress incontinence in the patient who has an intact sphincter but with poor urethral support and a displaced urethrovesical junction. In this procedure, the paravaginal fascia is sutured to Cooper's ligament (iliopectineal tract) on either side. The Burch procedure may be performed as "open" laparotomy or laparoscopically. The procedure may be performed in conjunction with *hysterectomy.* Obliteration of the cul-de-sac may be performed (*Moschcowitz purse-string suture* or *Halban sagittal suture technique*) with nonabsorbable sutures to prevent subsequent rectocele or enterocele.

Several means of suspension are employed: direct suture, use of a *Stamey needle (percutaneous and vaginal suture technique),* and use of a hernia repair mesh strip, which is stapled to the paravaginal fascia and Cooper's ligament in lieu of sutures. A transperitoneal or preperitoneal approach may be used. For many practitioners, the **Burch procedure** has supplanted the traditional ***Marshall-Marchetti-Krantz Procedure*** (p. 368). The laparoscopic approach is described.

Procedure

The patient is in a modified lithotomy position to provide access to the lower abdomen and perineum at the same time. *Cystoscopy* is performed. A Foley catheter (30 ml) is placed, and methylene blue or indigo carmine dye is injected into the bladder to demonstrate intraoperative perforation.

When the transperitoneal approach is used, the pelvis is examined and the various viscera are protected with warm moist (saline) lap sponges.

Pneumoperitoneum and laparoscopic ports are established. If ***hysterectomy*** was performed earlier in the procedure, the vaginal cuff is closed. Otherwise, an additional port is placed in the suprapubic area through which the retropubic space is entered. The bladder is mobilized, the paravaginal tissues are identified, and fatty tissues are dissected away to expose the fascia. A carbon dioxide (CO_2) or Nd:YAG laser, the CUSA™ (cavitational ultrasonic surgical aspirator), or the harmonic scalpel (p. 109) may be utilized. The dissection is kept to 2 to 2.5 cm from the urethra. One or two nonabsorbable sutures are placed in the paravaginal fascia midway between the midurethra and urethrovesical juncture and into Cooper's ligament.

Palpation of the catheter balloon, with transvaginal pressure applied by the assistant surgeon (or surgeon), helps to ascertain the anatomical landmarks. The anterolateral vaginal wall is tented towards Cooper's ligament and the suture(s) tied by extracorporeal technique (*Clark-Reich knot pusher* may be used) without applying undue tension (and not necessarily with direct apposition). Again, transvaginal manipulation facilitates the tying of the sutures by relieving some degree of pressure. Care is taken not to compress or kink the urethra or injure the ureters. Hemostasis is confirmed; the site is irrigated. A suprapubic catheter is inserted and any remaining dye is evacuated. *Cystoscopy* is performed to assure that no suture has penetrated the bladder wall. Indigo carmine dye (5 ml) and furosemide 20 mg may be given intravenously by the anesthesia provider to confirm the integrity of the ureters. Wound closure is performed in the usual manner.

Preparation of the Patient

A warming blanket/mattress may be placed on the table when ordered. Apply antiembolitic hose, as requested. Following the administration of general or regional anesthesia, the patient is in modified lithotomy position using padded stirrups (e.g., Allen) with the buttocks positioned just over the lower break in the table. The arms are padded and may be tucked in at the patient's side. All bony prominences and areas vulnerable to skin and neurovascular pressure or trauma are padded. The anesthesia provider often inserts a nasogastric tube. A Foley catheter (#16) with a 30-ml balloon (filled with 20 ml) is placed in the bladder to allow continuous drainage and to facilitate the delineation of urethra and bladder neck.

Skin and Vaginal Preparation

An abdominal and a vaginal prep are required; use one prep set. Add additional sponges, prep solution, and a Foley catheter with 30-ml balloon to the prep tray. Stand between the patient's legs (last section of the table and pad have been removed), and prep the abdomen. Begin at the umbilicus, extending from nipples to mid-thighs and down to the table at the sides. Continue with the vaginal prep as for ***D&C*** (p. 278). Drain the patient's bladder with a Foley catheter using 20 ml to fill the 30-ml balloon and attach to continuous drainage.

Draping

Drape sheet under the buttocks, folded towels (optional), and a laparoscopy sheet, or drape sheet under the buttocks, folded towels (optional), leggings, and a laparotomy sheet

Equipment

- Sequential compression device with disposable leg wraps, when requested
- Warming blanket or mattress (under patient, on table), optional
- N/g tube to the anesthesia provider, as requested
- Padded shoulder braces
- Padded stirrups (e.g., Allen)
- Suction
- ESU, (1) bipolar forceps and (1) unipolar pencil, each with cords
- Extra IV standard/pole for hanging irrigation fluid
- Monitors (2)
- CO_2 insufflator for laparoscope, e.g., Laparoflator™, Thermoflator™, Endolap™ or
- Pump powered by nitrogen or air, e.g., Endo Flo™
- Laparoscopic irrigation system, e.g., HydroFlex™ with fluid distention sensor, e.g., AquaSens™
- Fiber-optic light source (2), e.g., Xenon 300 W
- Camera console
- VCR
- Printer

CD burner
Laser unit, e.g., CO_2, Nd:YAG, optional
Harmonic scalpel console, optional
Ultrasound cutting device console, e.g., Ultracision™, CUSA, optional

Instrumentation

Cystoscope with obturator, sheath, and cord
D&C tray
Limited procedures tray
Verres needle
Trocars (5 mm, 10 or 11 mm, 12 mm, or Hasson)
Fiber-optic laparoscopes, 30° and 0° with cords (cable)
Cameras and couplers, if not incorporated into scopes
Reducers and connectors
Electrosurgical cords (2)

Laparoscopic Instruments

Dissectors, graspers, scissors (blunt and sharp), electrosurgical suction-irrigator, multifire ligating clip applier, unipolar electrosurgical hook, bipolar electrosurgical scissors, bipolar electrosurgical forceps, loop ligation sutures (e.g., Endoloop™ 2-0 with introducer sleeve), and endoscopic sutures with needle holder, e.g., EndoStitch™, Clark-Reich (extracorporeal) knot pusher
Nd:YAG laser hand piece with cord, optional
Harmonic scalpel hand piece with cord, optional
CUSA (cavitational ultrasonic surgical aspirator) hand piece with flue and cord, optional

Supplies

Antiembolitic hose
N/G tube to anesthesia provider
Foley catheter (#16Fr with 30-ml balloon) and drainage unit
Water-soluble lubricant
Suction tubing
Electrosurgical cords (2)
Straight tubing, e.g., K50, add 1000-ml bag normal saline and three-way stopcock for laparoscopic irrigation
Silastic™ tubing for laparoscopy insufflator
Suprapubic catheter, e.g., Pezzer, Malecot, and drainage unit
Fog reduction agent, e.g., FRED®, ELVIS™
Mesh, e.g., Prolene™ and staples, optional
Medicine cup, syringe, needle, methylene blue dye
Labels and marking pen
Stamey needle

Medications to anesthesia provider, as requested:

Indigo carmine (5 ml) dye is used to validate the integrity of the ureters

Furosemide 20 mg is a diuretic

Nonabsorbable suture, e.g., 2-0

Perineal pad and sanitary napkin belt in addition to abdominal dressing

Special Notes

- Apply **Special Notes** from ***Pelvic Laparoscopy/Pelviscopy***, p. 299, as indicated.
- Antiembolitic hose should be applied when the patient arrives in the room when requested. A sequential compression device with leg wraps may be applied over the antiembolitic hose, if ordered, to prevent deep vein thrombosis.
- **Reminder:** Document pedal pulses preoperatively, intraoperatively, and postoperatively when the patient is positioned in lithotomy for patient safety and medicolegal reasons. Should a pedal pulse be absent, notify the surgeon.
- *When cystoscopy is not going to be performed initially, the circulator inserts a Foley catheter (with a 30-ml balloon inflated to 20 ml) and connects it to a drainage unit following the prep.* The drainage unit is placed below the level of the patient's bladder to avoid reflux of urine and potential urinary tract infection.
- **N.B.** *Cystoscopy (p. 391) may be performed prior to the procedure if it was not performed at an earlier date.* A separate back table should be prepared for the cystoscopy (p. 391); a scrub person is not required.
- **Reminder:** *Avoid injury to the patient's fingers by preventing them from being caught in the table mechanism when the foot of the table is raised following the procedure.*
- **N.B.** *Cystoscopy may be performed first.* The lubricant, a clamp or hemostat, cystoscopy tubing and a stopcock, cystoscope, and cord should be available on a separate back table. The surgeon will work directly off this back table without a scrub person for the cystoscopy. Keep the cystoscopy set up on the table in the room until the conclusion of the procedure.
- All fluids should be warmed prior to use to help maintain patient's body temperature.

- The most convenient room set up has surgeon on patient's left, assistant on the right side, and scrub person to the surgeon's left. The video monitor and ancillary equipment are placed between the patient's legs.
- **N.B.** When choosing the laparoscopic insufflator, a high-flow insufflation system delivering 15 l/min CO_2 is preferred. (A different insufflator is used for hysteroscopic propcedures.)
- Cystoscopy may be performed at the end of the procedure to assure that no suture has penetrated the bladder wall; 5 ml of indigo carmine dye and furosemide 20 mg may be administered intravenously by the anesthesia provider to confirm the integrity of the urethra.
- The suprapubic catheter is inserted using the skin knife through a separate stab wound to divert the stream of urine temporarily.

Tension-Free Vaginal Tape (TVT) Procedure for Bladder Suspension

Definition

Suspension of the bladder and the proximal urethra in the female by placing a tension-free "sling" under the mid-urethra.

Discussion

TVT procedure is performed to treat urinary stress incontinence. The soft Prolene (polypropylene) mesh tape sling (pubourethral) is held in place primarily by scarring. TVT is performed on older women, i.e., women who are not pregnant and do not intend to become pregnant. Advantages of the TVT procedure over the **Marshall-Marchetti-Krantz** procedure or the **Burch** procedure include:

- TVT is less invasive
- There is less postoperative pain following TVT
- Results of TVT are more durable
- TVT is performed with smaller incisions
- Only local anesthetic is necessary for TVT
- TVT requires shorter hospitalization (same day or overnight stay)

Possible complications of TVT include vascular injury, mesh erosion, urethral erosion, and bladder perforation (cystotomy). A similar procedure, *TOT (transobturator tape)* procedure, in which the mesh sling is introduced through the obturator foramen, may provide an even lower complication rate.

Procedure

TVT may be performed using local anesthetic and conscious sedation. Local anesthetic (e.g., Marcaine 0.25%) and pitressin (to control bleeding) are injected into tissues surrounding the symphysis pubis and suburethrally into the anterior vaginal mucosa. ***Cystoscopy*** is performed. A weighted vaginal speculum is placed. The anterior vaginal tissue is incised. Sharp and blunt dissection are used to form tracts on both sides of the urethra. A catheter is inserted via catheter guide to identify the urethra. Special trocars of the TVT device permit the Prolene tape to be transferred from the vagina to the retropubic area with minimal manipulation. The long needle of the TVT tape is guided up to the symphysis pubis on one side (the TVT device is attached to a nondisposable handle for ease of insertion) and pulled up through the skin over the sysphysis pubis. The procedure is repeated on the other side. With both tapes now in position, the surgeon pulls the tapes through the tissue. Cystoscopic examination of the bladder confirms that neither the bladder nor the urethra has been punctured. The trocars on the TVT device are removed and the tapes are tied tightly. The vaginal incisions are closed with a running absorbable suture. The abdominal incisions (puncture wounds) may be repaired with nonabsorbable suture or tape strips (e.g., Steri-Strips™).

Preparation of the Patient

A warming blanket may be placed on the table when ordered. Apply antiembolitic hose as requested. Following the administration of *conscious sedation*, the patient is positioned in modified lithotomy using padded stirrups (e.g., Allen) with the buttocks positioned just over the lower break in the OR table, or the "cysto" table is used with the patient in lithotomy using padded (table-incorporated) crutch leg holders. The arms may be extended on padded armboards, or they are padded and tucked in at the patient's side. All bony prominences and areas vulnerable to skin and neurovascular pressure or trauma are padded. An electrosurgical pad is placed.

Skin Preparation

Begin at the pubic symphysis and extend from above the umbilicus downward over the labia. Follow by cleansing each inner thigh. Vaginal vault and cervix are cleansed using three spongesticks. The perineum and anus are cleansed with the remaining sponges. Discard each sponge after wiping the anus. Consult the surgeon regarding draining the patient's bladder with a straight catheter.

Draping

Drape sheet under the buttocks, folded towels (optional), leggings, and a cystoscopy drape (with built-in trough).

When the "cysto" room is not available, the draining fluid is directed into a kickbucket.

Equipment

Forced-air warming blanket or warming mattress, when ordered
Sequential compression device with disposable leg wraps, as requested
ESU
Suction
Padded stirrups (e.g., Allen) or padded crutch leg holders on "cysto" table
Monitor
Extra IV standard/pole for hanging irrigation fluid
Fiber-optic light source, e.g., Xenon 300 W
Camera console
VCR

Instrumentation

Cervical cone tray
Fiber-optic cystoscope with obturator, sheath, and cord
TVT device with nondisposable handles

Supplies

Antiembolitic hose
N/g tube to anesthesia provider
Foley catheter (#16Fr with 30-ml balloon) and drainage unit
Water-soluble lubricant
Local anesthetic (e.g., Marcaine 0.25%) and pitressin (to control bleeding)
Cystoscopy tubing and irrigation solution (e.g., 2000 to 3000 ml sorbitol)
Suction tubing
Electrosurgical cord
Sterile labels and marking pen
Medicine cup and syringe
Methylene blue or indigo carmen dye
Perineal pad and sanitary napkin belt in addition to abdominal dressing

Special Notes

- Apply **Special Notes** from ***Anterior and Posterior Repair,*** p. 293, as indicated.
- Antiembolitic hose should be applied when the patient arrives in the room when requested. A sequential compression device

with leg wraps may be applied over the antiembolitic hose, if ordered, to prevent deep vein thrombosis.

- Use safety precautions to identify, label, and dispense medications or solutions and to avoid medication errors; see p. 30. It is mandatory that all medications and solutions on the sterile field be labeled by name and strength. The medication bottle is retained in the room until the procedure has concluded.
- **Cystoscopy** *(p. 391) is usually performed prior to the procedure, if it was not performed at an earlier date.* A separate back table should be prepared for the cystoscopy (p. 392); a scrub person is not required.
- **Reminder:** *Avoid injury to the patient's fingers by preventing them from being caught in the table mechanism when the foot of the table is raised following the procedure.*
- **N.B.** *Cystoscopy may be performed first.* The lubricant, a clamp or hemostat, cystoscopy tubing and a stopcock, cystoscope, and cord should be available on a separate back table. The surgeon will work directly off this back table without a scrub person for the cystoscopy. Keep the cystoscopy set up on the table in the room until the conclusion of the procedure.
- *When cystoscopy is not going to be performed initially, the circulator will insert a Foley catheter (with a 30-ml balloon inflated to 20 ml) and connect it to a drainage unit following the prep.* The drainage unit is placed below the level of the patient's bladder to avoid reflux of urine and potential urinary tract infection.
- To maintain patient's body temperature, all fluids should be warmed prior to use.
- *Cystoscopy* is performed at the end of the procedure to assure that no suture has penetrated the bladder wall; 5 ml of indigo carmine dye and furosemide 20 mg may be administered intravenously by the anesthesia provider to confirm the integrity of the urethra.
- A Foley catheter is not routinely inserted at the end of the procedure.

Varicocelectomy

Definition

Excision of dilated pampiniform venous plexus.

Discussion

In an estimated 15% of males, the pampiniform plexus (branches of the internal spermatic or testicular vein) that drain the testis and epididymis are dilated and often asymptomatic. When this condition progresses, pain, impeded testicular growth, and subfertility result. The left side is more often involved than the right (due to the difference in the anatomical course of the veins proximally); accordingly, if a varicocele develops on the right side acutely or increases in size rapidly on the left, studies such as ultrasound and CT scan should be performed to assure that no retroperitoneal tumor is compressing the internal spermatic vein proximally. Strictly speaking, varicocele can occur in the female involving dilatation of the plexus of the ovarian vein in the broad ligament, but this is rarely treated.

Most often, elective treatment is instituted to increase fertility; bilateral procedures are done when indicated. Ligation of the internal spermatic vein and percutaneous injection of sclerosants or embolization of the vein with Gelfoam, coils, balloons, clips, etc. can be done. Surgery is indicated when, aside from any desire to increase fertility, the size of the varicocele causes local symptoms.

The laparoscopic approach, once frequently performed, is being replaced by the microsurgical approach that employs techniques through limited incisions. Local anesthesia with *conscious sedation* may be appropriate for the microsurgical approach for select patients.

Procedure

Inguinal (or Scrotal) Approach. Following regional or general anesthesia, an inguinal or scrotal incision is made with high ligation of the internal spermatic vein by retroperitoneal approach. Following appropriate local dissection, the internal spermatic artery is protected and the dilated venous plexus is ligated and excised. The wounds are closed.

Laparoscopic Approach. Following the establishment of pneumoperitoneum, three ports are employed, supraumbilical, infraumbilical, and inguinal on either affected side. The branches of the internal spermatic vein are separated from the artery; an endoscopic Doppler probe may be utilized to aid in distinguishing between artery and vein. The veins are clipped and divided.

Microsurgical Approach. A small (2- to 3-cm) inguinal or subinguinal incision is made, through which the spermatic cord is delivered. Under magnification, the appropriate venous structures are ligated while avoiding injury to adjacent structures, such as small arteries and lymphatics.

Preparation of the Patient

All Approaches. Antiembolitic hose may be requested. Following the administration of general or regional anesthesia, the patient is in supine position with legs separated; a small pad may placed under the buttocks to maximize visualization, and a pillow may be placed under the knees (for comfort). Arms may be extended on padded armboards, or they may be padded and tucked in at the patient's sides. All bony prominences and areas vulnerable to skin and neurovascular pressure or trauma are padded. Apply electrosurgical dispersive pad.

Skin Preparation

Begin at the intended site of incision (either inguinal or scrotal) and include the penis and scrotum, extending from the umbilicus to lower thighs and down to the table at the sides.

Draping

Cuffed towel under the scrotum, folded towels around the pubic area, and a sheet with a small aperture and laparotomy sheet or individual drape sheets

Microscope cover (if microscope used)

Equipment

Antiembolitic hose, if requested

ESU

Suction (optional) with in-line filter, e.g., Clear View

Microscopic Approach

Microscope

Doppler

For Laparoscopic Approach, add:

Monitor

Insufflator for CO_2 for laparoscope, e.g., Laparoflator, Thermoflator, Endolap or

Laparoscopic irrigation system, e.g., HydroFlex with fluid distention sensor, e.g., AquaSens

Fiber-optic light source, e.g., Xenon 300 W

Camera console

VCR

CD burner

Printer

Instrumentation

Limited Procedures Tray

Doppler

Handpiece and cord

For Microscopic Approach

Microscopic instruments:

Tissue forceps (2), curved smooth forceps (2), curved tying forceps (1), Castroviejo needle holder (1), jeweler's forceps, iris scissors

Laparoscopic Approach

Verres needle (disposable available)
Trocars (5 mm, 10 or 11 mm, 12 mm, or Hasson)
Fiber-optic laparoscopes, 30° and 0°, and cord
Camera, coupler, and cord
Reducers and connectors, as necessary
Laparoscopic instrumentation:
Fiber-optic laparoscope 30° and 60° with camera and power cord, electrosurgical dissector, grasper, scissors, (blunt and sharp), Babcock forceps (2), electrosurgical suction/irrigator, multifire clip applicator, electrocoagulating forceps, unipolar electrosurgical hook, loop ligation sutures (e.g., Endoloop, needle holder)

Supplies

Antiembolitic hose, if requested
Small basin
Medicine cup, local anesthetic, Luer lok syringe, and # 25 needle
Blades, (1) #10 (inguinal approach), (2) #15 (adult), (2) #15 (child)
Needle magnet or counter
Penrose drain, small (retraction)
Electrosurgical pencil with needle tip and cord with scraper
Suture for venous ligation, e.g., 2-0 silk, optional
Syringe (30 ml) and needle (20 gauge)
Dressing pad, e.g., telfa and "gauze fluffs" and scrotal support or T-binder

For Laparoscopic Approach, add:

Silastic tubing for CO_2 insufflation
Electrosurgical cord
Silastic tubing, e.g., k50, add 1000 ml bag normal saline (N/S) and 3-way stopcock

Special Notes

- Apply **Special Notes** from ***Abdominal Laparoscopy***, p. 140, for laparoscopic approach, p. 236, as indicated.
- Apply **Special Notes** from ***Abdominal Laparotomy*** for microsurgical approach, p. 134, as indicated.
- The circulator advises the patient that he/she will be the patient's advocate while in surgery.
- Emotional support is demonstrated to the patient during the administration of anesthesia by the presence of the circulator.

- Recognize patient's feelings regarding altered body image, and give the patient an opportunity to express his/her feelings. Use a nonjudgmental attitude regarding patient's feelings.
- **Reminder:** Assess and document patient's anxiety level and level of knowledge regarding the intended procedure. Clarify misconceptions by answering the patient's questions in a knowledgeable manner when possible, or redirect the question to the physician. Document nursing interventions and patient outcome.
- Be prepared by draping the microscope as early as convenient (when its use is anticipated).
- The surgeon may wear magnifying loupes or use the microscope. Pass all instruments carefully, placing them in the surgeon's hands, ready for use, to avoid taking the surgeon's attention away from the field.

Hydrocelectomy

Definition

Excision of a portion of the tunica vaginalis testis with evacuation of fluid contained therein.

Discussion

A *hydrocele* is an accumulation of serous fluid around the testis within the tunica vaginalis that may occur spontaneously or may result from trauma or infection. Hydrocele may be treated by needle aspiration that usually offers temporary relief; recurrence is frequent and requires surgical intervention. In children, ***indirect inguinal hernia*** may accompany the hydrocele.

Procedure

Following the administration of anesthesia, an inguinal or scrotal incision is made. In the inguinal approach, the testis and spermatic cord are delivered into the inguinal wound. The hydrocele fluid is aspirated through a small incision or with a needle and syringe. Excessive sac wall is excised or may be wrapped around and sutured behind the epididymis. Hemostasis is achieved before closure. A small drain (e.g., ¼″ Penrose) may be placed. The incision is closed. A bulky dressing is applied. When a hernia is present, repair is performed; see ***Adult Herniorrhaphy,*** p. 142, and ***Pediatric Herniorrhaphy,*** p. 1013.

Preparation of the Patient

Antiembolitic hose may be applied to the legs of the adult patient. The patient is supine with legs apart; a small pad may be placed under the buttocks to maximize visualization. A pillow may be placed under the knees (for comfort and support). Arms may be extended on padded armboards, or they may be padded and tucked in at the patient's sides. All bony prominences and areas vulnerable to skin and neurovascular pressure or trauma are padded. Apply electrosurgical dispersive pad.

Skin Preparation

Scrotal Approach. Begin at the scrotum and include the penis, extending from umbilicus to lower thighs and down to the table at the sides.

Inguinal Approach. Begin at the inguinal region on the affected side, extending from the umbilicus to lower thighs (including genitalia) and down to the table at the sides.

Draping

Cuffed towel under the scrotum, folded towels around the pubic region, and a laparotomy sheet

Equipment

ESU
Suction

Instrumentation

Basic/Minor procedures tray (adult)
Pediatric minor procedures tray (child)

Supplies

Antiembolitic hose (adult), optional
Basin set
Blades, (1) #10, (2) #15 (adult), (2) #15 (child)
Needle magnet or counter
Suction tubing
Electrosurgical pencil with needle tip and cord with holder and scraper
Penrose drains (2), small, e.g., ¼″ (for retraction and for drainage)
Syringe, 30 ml, and #20 needle (for aspiration) and test tube(s) for aspiration specimen
Dressing, e.g., telfa, "gauze fluffs," and scrotal suspensory support (adults)

Special Notes

- Apply **Special Notes** from ***Hypospadias***, p. 355, as directed.

Vasectomy

Definition

Excision and ligation of the vas deferens.

Discussion

The distal and proximal ends of the vas are ligated, and a segment of the vas deferens is excised. The procedure is done bilaterally for the purpose of male contraception or to prevent orchitis prior to prostatectomy. Occasionally, the vasal ducts may be multiple or may be absent on either side.

Procedure

The vas is palpated through the scrotum. A scrotal incision is made, the vas is seized, and it is freed of surrounding tissue. A segment of vas is excised and the ends are ligated, cauterized, or crushed with a clamp or clip prior to ligation. The severed ends may be allowed to retract, or they may be buried within the scrotal connective tissue and sutured in place. The wound is closed. The procedure is repeated on the other side. A bulky dressing is applied.

"No needle and/or no scalpel vasectomy" is an optional method described as being less painful. However, for this approach, local anesthesia is administered via "jet" spray (injection system without needles); see p. 53. A specialized clamp is used to grasp and fix the vas transcutaneously. A puncturing forceps exposes the vas; the vas is divided, ligated, clipped and/or cauterized. The vas is returned to the scrotum. The small puncture wounds "*self-close*" and do not require sutures.

Preparation of the Patient

Antiembolitic hose may be applied. The patient is supine with legs apart; a small pad may be placed under the buttocks to maximize visualization. A pillow may be placed under the knees for comfort and to avoid lower back pain. Arms may be extended on padded armboards, or they may be padded and tucked in at the patient's sides. All bony prominences and areas vulnerable to skin and neurovascular pressure or trauma are padded. Apply electrosurgical dispersive pad.

Skin Preparation

Begin at the scrotum, extending from above the pubic symphysis to the lower thighs. Prepare perianal area last, discarding each sponge after wiping over the anus or use a small sterile, plastic adhesive drape to isolate the anus.

Draping

Folded towels and a sheet with a small aperture and drape sheets or laparotomy sheet

Equipment

ESU

Instrumentation

Vasectomy tray

Supplies

Small basin
Medicine cup, local anesthetic, Luer lok syringe, and #25 needle
Label and sterile marking pen
Electrosurgical pencil with needle tip
Blade, (1) #15
Dressing, e.g., telfa, "gauze fluffs," and scrotal support
Ice pack (at conclusion)

Special Notes

- Apply **Special Notes** from ***Hypospadias***, p. 355, as indicated.
- **N.B.** In addition to the signed surgical permit (e.g., **Authorization for and Consent to Surgery**, p. 6), a signed surgical permit for **Vasectomy**, and a signed sterilization permit is required to be on the chart before the patient is brought into the room, e.g., **Authorization for and Special Consent to Surgical Sterilization Procedure,** p. 7 must also be on the chart. The patient's statement is documented in the **Perioperative Record**, see p. 12; this is done for patient safety and medicolegal reasons.
- All medications used in the sterile field must be labeled. Scrub person should use a sterile marking pen to identify all solutions. To avoid medication errors, see p. 30.
- All medication containers should be kept in the room until the completion of the procedure. Follow all safety precautions to avoid medication errors; see p. 30.
- Be prepared with an ice pack that will be applied to the scrotum immediately postoperatively before leaving the OR.

Vasovasostomy

Definition

Restoration of continuity of the previously interrupted vas deferens.

Discussion

The procedure is performed to reestablish continuity of the vas deferens after vasectomy or to correct a stricture, as from iatrogenic trauma (e.g., *pediatric herniorraphy*) to restore fertility. Prior to the procedure, gynecologic fertility status of the spouse should be established when applicable. At the beginning of the procedure, testicular biopsy with immediate examination of fluid from the proximal end of the transected vas may be performed to assess the presence of spermatogenesis. This procedure produces successful results 70% of the time.

When only one segment of the remaining vas is viable, *epididymovasostomy* may be performed to restore continuity by using a segment of the epididymis as a substitute for one segment of the vas.

Procedure

A scrotal incision exposes the vas deferens above and below the site of the previous ligation. A needle biopsy, or preferably incisional testicular biopsy, may be performed. Under magnification, scar tissue is excised from both ends of the vas and the vas is mobilized to avoid tension on theананstomosis. Care is taken to avoid undue trauma to the local blood supply. A two-layer anastomosis (9-0 nylon for the seromuscular layer and 10-0 nylon for the mucosal layer) or a single layer of suture (e.g., 9-0 nylon for both layers) may be used. The wound is closed. A bulky dressing is applied.

For Preparation of Patient, Skin Preparation, and **Draping,** see *Vasectomy*, pp. 385–386.

Draping

Add microscope cover, as necessary.

Equipment

ESU

Magnifying loupes or microscope, as requested

Instrumentation

Limited procedures tray

Microscopic instruments:

Tissue forceps (1), curved smooth forceps (2), curved tying forceps (1), Castroviejo needle holder (1), vas holding forceps (1)

Supplies

Antiembolitic hose
Small basin
Blades, (1) #15 and (1) #11
Needle magnet or counter
Electrosurgical pencil with needle tip
Suture (fine), e.g., 9-0 and 10-0 nylon
Dressing, e.g., telfa, "gauze fluffs," and scrotal support
Ice pack (as requested)

Special Notes

- Apply **Special Notes** from ***Abdominal Laparotomy***, p. 134, as indicated.
- Check with the surgeon regarding use of loupes or microscope. A special drape sheet is required for the microscope (when used).
- ***When the surgeon wears magnifying loupes or uses the microscope, all instruments should be carefully placed in the surgeon's hands ready for use to avoid taking the surgeon's attention away from the operative field.***
- Be prepared with an ice pack following the application of the bulky dressing (optional).

Cutaneous Vasostomy

Definition

Establishment of an opening of the vas onto the scrotal skin.

Discussion

Cutaneous vasostomy is performed to drain an infected epididymis or testis by incising a loop of the vas and suturing it to the scrotal skin. The wound or wounds usually close spontaneously after the precipitating episode subsides.

Vasography may be done by injection of contrast media into the severed end(s) of the vas.

Procedure

An incision is made over the vas; the vas is grasped and freed of surrounding tissue. The vas is divided, and the severed ends are sutured to the scrotal skin. A bulky dressing is applied.

For Preparation of the Patient, Skin Preparation, Draping, Equipment, Instrumentation, Supplies, and **Special Notes,** see **Vasectomy,** pp. 385–386.

Spermatocelectomy

Definition

Excision of a benign cystic swelling or mass located in the tubular testicular ductal system that conveys sperm.

Discussion

A spermatocele usually occurs when the epididymis is obstructed. The etiology may be congenital in origin or it may be infectious (post epididymitis), as a complication resulting from vasectomy. When fertility is a consideration, excision of the cystic mass and/or the area of stenosis with *vasoepididymostomy* is performed.

Procedure

A scrotal incision is made and the pathology assessed. The cystic mass is excised. If an obvious interruption of the ductal system is created, an end-to-side anastomosis is performed with the aid of magnifying loupes or a microscope. Repair is made with fine suture (e.g., 9-0 nylon). The incision is closed. A bulky dressing is applied.

For Preparation of the Patient, Skin Preparation, Draping, Equipment, Instrumentation, Supplies, and **Special Notes,** see **Vasovasostomy,** pp. 387–388.

Orchiectomy

Definition

Removal of one or both testicles.

Discussion

Orchiectomy may be performed for benign disease as the result of irreversible vascular compromise due to severe testicular tortion, trauma, or infection. It may also be performed for endocrine control of prostatic carcinoma and primary tumors of the testes. Intra-abdominal undescended testicles (particularly if atrophic) are assumed to be precancerous and are removed as a preventative measure as are undescended testes if not surgically corrected or if there is a failure to descend after a few years of age (not responsive to hormonal therapy as chorionic gonadatropin). Even testes that are surgically relocated to the scrotum present a greater subsequent cancer risk than the naturally descended testis (requiring indefinite monitoring). The decision to remove these testes is made easier when the problem is unilateral (i.e., with a normal contralateral testis). Following bilateral orchiectomy, the patient is no longer able to produce testosterone (responsible for secondary sex characteristics); hormone replacement therapy will be necessary when the procedure is performed on a child. The patient (or the patient's parents) must sign an informed consent for sterilization in addition to the permit for bilateral orchiectomy. The patient (or the patient's parents) must indicate verbally the understanding that he will be rendered sterile by the procedure.

Some patients may elect to have ***testicular prostheses*** implanted for cosmetic reasons, although this is not generally recommended by surgeons, as the implant may mask future pathology. Complications that may result from testicular implants are infection, shifting or migration of the implant, thick scarring, and the formation of a hard capsule surrounding the implant. In the United States, the implantation of saline-filled prostheses has been approved by the Food and Drug Administration, and in other countries, silicone gel implants are available. Some physicians advocate ***subcapsular orchiectomy*** as an alternative to implantation so that the testicular sac is not left completely empty.

Procedure

The incision can be made transcrotally or inguinally. The testis is identified, the spermatic cord is ligated, and the testis is removed. This procedure is repeated on the other side, as indicated. For primary testicular malignancy, high ligation of the spermatic cord is done. *Radical lymphadenectomy* may be performed through an abdominal incision or laparoscopically, or as a stated procedure after administration of chemotherapy. Lymph node-bearing fatty tissues from the level of the renal vessels and around the aorta to the level of the transection of the spermatic cord are removed. A testicular prosthesis may be placed at the time of orchiectomy, at a later date, or not at all. The incision is closed. A bulky dressing is applied.

For Preparation of the Patient, Skin Preparation, Draping, Equipment, Instrumentation, and **Supplies,** see *Hydrocelectomy,* p. 383.

Skin Preparation

When *lymphadenectomy* is anticipated, an abdominal skin preparation (from nipples to mid-thighs and down to the table at the sides) should be included.

Supplies

Add testicular prostheses when ordered.

Special Notes

- Apply **Special Notes** from ***Hydrocelectomy***, p. 385, as indicated.
- In addition to the surgical permit for **Orchiectomy**, e.g., a signed sterilization permit for **Bilateral Orchiectomy** is required to be on the patient's chart before the patient is brought into the room. The two documents are a medicolegal necessity. The circulator should be certain that the patient understands that he will no longer be able to father progeny; the patient's statement should be quoted on the **Perioperative Record**.
- **Reminder:** The circulator demonstrates particular emotional support to the patient considering the nature of the surgery. Emotional support during the administration of anesthesia is demonstrated by the presence of the circulator. The circulator needs to recognize the patient's right to feelings regarding altered body image. He/she should give the patient an opportunity to express these feelings.
- **Reminder:** Assess and document patient's anxiety level and level of knowledge regarding the intended procedure. Clarify misconceptions by answering the patient's questions in a knowledgeable manner when possible or redirect the question to the physician. Nursing interventions and outcomes should be documented.
- When a testicular prosthesis is placed, precautions must be observed to avoid infection by handling the prosthesis as little as possible and by preventing lint, powder, etc., from coming in contact with the prosthesis. Document special measures taken in the **Perioperative Record** for medicolegal reasons.
- Do not open the prosthesis until the surgeon has determined the size to avoid unnecessary expense to the patient (when he is charged for a unit not used).
- Record the type, size, serial number, etc., of the prosthesis in the **Perioperative Record.** Record the prosthesis data in the hospital log book, according to hospital policy.

Cystoscopy

Definition

Endoscopic examination of the urethra, bladder, and the ureteral orifices.

Discussion

Cystoscopy can be a valuable diagnostic tool. Indications for performing cystoscopy are hematuria, frequent bouts of cystitis and other urinary tract infections, incontinence, urinary retention, and calculi discovered on incidental x-ray. Cystoscopy may also be performed to catheterize the ureters, to obtain a biopsy specimen, to treat lesions, and/or to follow-up the examination of an operative or endoscopic procedure. Most surgical facilities have a "cysto room" complete with a "cysto" table with built-in knee holders useful for placing the patient in lithotomy position; the table has x-ray capabilities to deliver fluoroscopy, as needed.

When resection is to be performed, a resectoscope with a working element (electrical wire loop) is used to cauterize and coagulate tissue.

Procedure

Insertion of a well-lubricated cystoscope into the urethra is attempted. In the presence of a stricture, the urethra may be dilated with filiform sounds. Once the stricture has been cleared, the urethra is inspected and the cystoscope is advanced into the bladder. The obturator is removed, and a urine specimen is obtained. The bladder is filled with irrigation fluid, and under direct visualization, the bladder, ureteral orifices, bladder neck, and urethra are examined. A panendoscope, a resectoscope, and/or a ureteral catheterizing endoscope may be required depending on the procedure to be performed.

Preparation of the Patient

Antiembolitic hose are applied when requested. When general or spinal anesthesia is employed, it is administered before the skin prep. Local anesthetic may be inserted into the urethra of the male patient and applied to the urethral meatus of the female patient following the skin prep. The patient is usually on the cystoscopy table (in the "cysto" room) in lithotomy position. The customized "cysto" table has special built-in padded crutch supports for the knees that should be padded. If a "cysto" table is unavailable, padded stirrups (e.g., Allen) are used. All bony prominences and areas vulnerable to skin and neurovascular pressure or trauma are padded. When a procedure in addition to cystoscopy is performed requiring electrosurgery, application of an electrosurgical dispersive pad is necessary.

Skin Preparation

A sterile screen is placed over the drain or a drain is incorporated into disposable drapes following the skin prep. The table may be tilted downward to permit easy drainage of prep solution. Care is taken to prevent prep solutions from pooling under the patient to avoid excoriation of the skin and to avoid burns when using the ESU. Extend the prep from umbilicus to mid-thighs.

Males. Cleanse entire pubic area, including the penis, scrotum, and perineum. Discard each sponge after wiping the anus.

Females. See skin and vaginal preparation for ***D&C***, p. 278.

Draping

Drape sheet under the buttocks and a "cysto" drape (drain and screen incorporated), or drape sheet under the buttocks, leggings, a laparotomy sheet, and a sterile screen and drain

Equipment

- Padded "cysto" table crutch leg holders or padded stirrups (e.g., Allen) on OR table
- Extra IV standard/pole for hanging irrigation fluid
- Fiber-optic light source, e.g., Xenon 300 W
- ESU

Instrumentation

- Sterile screen unless cystoscopy drape used (sterile screen incorporated)
- Rigid fiber-optic cystoscope (Brown-Berger) and panendoscope (McCarthy) or cystourethroscope (Wappler) for bladder visualization
- Lateral and foroblique fiber-optic telescopes (interchangeable with all sheaths) and (power) cord
- Resectoscopes, e.g., Iglesias, Nesbit, Baumrucher, and Stern-McCarthy (sheath, Timberlake obturator, telescope [composed of Bakelite], and working element (cutting electrode) to cut and coagulate
- Bridge (e.g., short, Alberran) required for telescope to fit into the sheath
- Stopcock, hemostat, and catheter nipples
- Penile clamp (used following local anesthetic instillation in males)
- Urethral sound

Add

- Resectoscope (for *bladder fulguration*)
- Ureteral lithotrite and corresponding scope (for *lithopaxy*)
- Catheterizing telescope (for catheterization of the ureters), add ureteral catheters

Note: A flexible fiber-optic cystoscope is employed for patients unable to tolerate the lithotomy position.

Supplies

Antiembolitic hose
Sterile screen ("cysto" drape has sterile screen incorporated)
Medicine cup, syringe (20 ml)
Topical anesthetic (e.g., lidocaine hydrochloride/Anestacon 1% or 2%) for males
Medicine cup, syringe, and dye (optional)
ESU cord (for procedures in addition to cystoscopy)
Water-soluble lubricant
Irrigation solution, usually sterile water (available in 2000- or 3000-ml bags)
Disposable cystoscopy tubing
Filiform urethral sounds, available
Graduated pitcher
Test tubes with screw tops (for urine specimen collections)

Special Notes

- Apply **Special Notes** from ***Abdominal Laparotomy***, p. 134.
- Ensure and verify that all x-ray, IVP, etc. reports are in the room and that they belong to the *correct* patient.
- For the female patient, local anesthetic is placed into the urethral meatus with a cotton-tipped applicator (or cone-shaped syringe) following the skin and vaginal prep. The applicator stick is to remain in the meatus until the surgeon inserts an instrument.
- For the male patient, a disposable syringe with acorn tip is used to instill the anesthetic agent into the urethra. A penile clamp is placed for a few minutes to retain the anesthetic.
- A perioperative RN, in addition to the circulator, may be requested to monitor the patient when an anesthesia provider is not required to be present. See the perioperative RN's responsibilities for monitoring the patient during *conscious sedation*, p. 74.
- **Reminder:** Assess and document patient's anxiety level and level of knowledge regarding the intended procedure. Circulator can provide a measure of comfort by clarifying misconceptions by answering the patient's questions in a knowledgeable manner when possible or redirect the question to the physician.
- **Reminder:** All medications used in the sterile field must be labeled. Scrub person should use a sterile marking pen to identify all solutions. To avoid medication errors, see p. 30.

- **Reminder:** All medication containers should be kept in the room until the completion of the procedure. Follow all safety precautions to avoid medication errors; see p. 30.
- A flexible fiber-optic cystoscope is used for patients who cannot tolerate the lithotomy position (e.g., patients with arthritis, etc.); the patient may not require an anesthetic. Position patient carefully to avoid injury.
- An imaging system is an integral part of the "cysto" table; often fluoroscopy is incorporated into the table. Employ x-ray safety protection, as necessary, e.g., the room should be lead-lined, personnel should wear lead aprons (donned before scrubbing) and stand behind lead walls during x-ray exposure; see p. 52.
- Care must be taken to position patients on the "cysto" table correctly; particular care should be taken for patients with hip problems or arthritis (if they can tolerate the lithotomy position at all). The built-in knee crutch supports on the "cysto" table help to avoid pressure damage on neurovascular structures in the popliteal space when legs are padded adequately and positioned correctly. Customized gel pads with Velcro® are available. When using a standard OR table, employ the same considerations; use padding for the Allen stirrups.
- Note and document pedal pulses when the patient is positioned in stirrups preoperatively and postoperatively for patient safety and medicolegal reasons.
- When positioning patient, prevent employees straining muscles by showing them how to employ ergo dynamic techniques (see p. 51).
- Lift both legs at the same time when putting the patient's legs in stirrups to prevent postoperative lumbosacral strain. This is best done by two persons; however, one person can do this by placing one leg on his/her shoulder while placing the other foot in the stirrup.
- Raise and lower legs slowly to prevent cardiovascular disturbances, e.g., rapid alterations in venous return.
- The "cysto" table has a drainage pan that can be pulled out of the lower break in the table after the patient is positioned. When the standard OR table must be used instead, a kickbucket is used to catch the irrigation fluid.
- The scrub person or the circulator prepares the instrument table from which the surgeon works. A Mayo stand is not used; a scrub person is not required during the procedure.

- The surgeon usually dons a sterile disposable plastic apron that is worn under the sterile gown or a gown with an *impermeable* inset is worn when working in the "cysto" room to prevent (strike-through) contamination.
- Sterile water is the solution of choice when *only* cystoscopy will be performed. When a procedure in addition to cystoscopy is performed, the irrigation solution should be *nonelectrolytic and isotonic* (e.g., glycine, sorbitol) to prevent burning the patient.
- Observe the level of irrigation as it is used and replace irrigation bags, as necessary. Always be prepared with a new bag of irrigation, as necessary.
- Special care is taken not to damage the fragile lensed telescopes and fiber-optic light cords by placing a pad in the sink before cleaning them.
- High end disinfection (p. 43) is the minimal requirement (of the Centers for Disease Control) for processing endoscopic instrumentation. Cystoscopes are usually disinfected using a 2% aqueous glutaraldehyde solution (e.g., Cidex™). As Cidex is very irritating, rinse instruments well.
- Many facilities prefer to sterilize the instrumentation; aqueous glutaraldehyde (e.g., Cidex), peracetic acid, and/or hydrogen peroxide gas plasma, in addition to ethylene oxide, may be used. Each disinfection or sterilization process has particular time restraints; see methods of disinfection and sterilization, p. 41.
- Instruments that have blood on them need to be scrubbed with a brush. The inside channel of tubular instruments must be cleaned. Instruments cannot be left soaking longer than necessary, as the seals will be affected. Moving parts of the instruments should be lubricated with an instrument "milk."
- When a "cysto" drape is available, a screen is incorporated into it. Otherwise, a sterile screen is required to capture resected tissue.
- Depending on the procedure performed, a urinary drainage unit may be attached to the Foley catheter. The unit should be placed below the level of the bladder to prevent a reflux of urine; this may prevent a potential urinary tract infection.
- When the ESU is used *(for procedures in addition to cystoscopy),* an electrosurgical dispersive pad is required. It should be placed on skin that is relatively hair-free (the area may require shaving) and as close to the area of the surgery as possible, without being in the sterile field.

- The power control settings of the ESU should be set as low as possible while still being effective.
- Check and replace the wire loops (disposable) used with resectoscopes as necessary for breakage, as they are malleable and fragile.

Cystostomy

Definition

An opening made into the bladder.

Discussion

Cystostomy is performed for purposes of urinary diversion to relieve an obstruction and to "protect" the site of a more distal surgical procedure (e.g., *vesicourethral anastomosis*). This procedure may be done as an independent procedure or as an adjunct to another procedure.

Percutaneous cystostomy is usually performed at the patient's bedside.

Procedure

A low vertical or transverse incision is used. The bladder is distended using a urethral catheter (e.g., Foley) when there is no obstruction. The dome of the bladder is incised, and a Pezzer or Malecot catheter is inserted into the incision. The catheter is secured with absorbable sutures to obtain a watertight closure around the catheter. The catheter may exit the main incision or (preferably) a stab wound; it is secured to the skin with a nonabsorbable suture. The wound is closed in layers; additional drainage is optional.

"Tube cystostomy" (i.e., catheter cystostomy) often complements other open bladder procedures (e.g., *ureterolithotomy*). A urethral catheter, e.g., Foley is usually placed until the cystostomy tract matures to minimize leakage.

Preparation of the Patient

Antiembolitic hose may be applied when requested. Following the administration of regional or general anesthesia, the patient is supine; a pad may be placed under the lumbar spine and a pillow may be placed under the knees (to avoid straining back muscles and for comfort). The arms may be extended on padded armboards. Padded shoulder braces are secured to the table; the table may be placed in Trendelenburg position to facilitate exposure. All bony prominences and areas vulnerable to skin and neurovascular pressure or trauma are padded. Check with the surgeon regarding the insertion of a Foley catheter. Electrosurgical dispersive pad is placed.

Skin Preparation

Males. Ascertain if a Foley catheter should be inserted prior to the skin prep. Begin at the intended site of the incision, extending from the nipples to the lower thighs and down to the table at the sides; the genitalia are included.

Females. Ascertain if a Foley catheter should be inserted. A Foley catheter may be inserted following the vaginal prep, prior to the abdominal prep (when requested). Both vaginal and the abdominal skin preps are required; use two prep sets (see preparation for Total Abdominal Hysterectomy, p. 308).

Draping

Folded towels and a laparotomy sheet

Equipment

Padded shoulder braces
ESU
Suction

Instrumentation

Major procedures tray
Long instruments tray
Trocar, catheter stylet, and urethral sounds (e.g., filaform), available
Ligating clip appliers, e.g., Hemoclip appliers (assorted sizes and lengths)

Supplies

Antiembolitic hose
Foley catheter and sealed drainage unit
Basin set
Blades, (2) #10, (1) #15, and (1) #11
Needle magnet or counter
Electrosurgical pencil and cord with scraper
Suction tubing
Irrigation solution (e.g., 1.5% glycine or sorbitol) and asepto syringe
Ligating clips, e.g., Hemoclips (small, medium, large)
Cystostomy catheter (e.g., Pezzer, Malecot) and sealed drainage unit

Special Notes

- Apply **Special Notes** from *Cystoscopy*, p. 394, as indicated.
- The circulator may be requested to unclamp urethral catheter when the bladder is incised.

Cystectomy

Definition

Total or partial removal of the urinary bladder.

Discussion

A *partial cystectomy* may be performed when the lesion is localized. *Total radical cystectomy* is performed depending on infiltration of the lesion, evidence of metastases, and the ability of the patient to tolerate the procedure. A urinary diversion procedure, e.g., *ureteroileostomy (ileal-loop)* or *cutaneous ureterostomy,* may be performed concomitantly or as a prior separate procedure.

This procedure is performed most often for malignancy primary to the bladder or in adjacent organs. Other indications include neurologic disorders, radiation injury, congenital defects, intractable infection, and severe trauma. When malignant disease is present, the depth of infiltration, presence of metastases, and general condition of the patient will dictate the extent of the procedure. Superficial bladder lesions are treated transcystoscopically by various modalities, e.g., with radiation therapy or partial cystectomy.

Total radical cystectomy is performed when an infiltrating lesion is restricted to the bladder and there are no distant metastases. In conjunction with cystectomy, a urinary diversion procedure is performed (either a *cutaneous ureterostomy* or, preferably, an *ileal conduit, e.g., ureteroileostomy (Kock pouch, see p. 232), or colonic conduit, e.g., ureterocolostomy*). Alternatively, the *ureteroileostomy* or *ureterocolostomy,* instead of draining to an abdominal wall stoma, may be fashioned into a pouch and anastomosed to a urethral remnant in the pelvis. Drains and proximal urinary diversion ureteral stents are employed to keep the remnant patent. Postoperatively, the patient will need to perform self-catheterization to empty an intestinal pouch reservoir. *Pelvic lymphadenectomy* (p. 340) may be performed as well.

Procedure

A midline or low transverse incision is made, the abdomen is explored, and the extent of the pathology is assessed. The bladder is dissected from its vascular supply. In males, the prostate and seminal vesicles are included in the specimen. The distal ureters, urethra, and vasa are divided and ligated. In the female, hysterectomy (see *Total Abdominal Hysterectomy,* p. 307), including the proximal vagina, urethra, and distal ureters, are resected and included in the specimen. *Urinary diversion* (see *Ileal Conduit,* p. 425) is then performed, or it may have been performed prior to cystectomy. A closed-system wound drain may be employed. When the *ileal or colonic conduit (intestinal urinary reservoir)* is anastomosed to the urethral remnant, the pouch can be fashioned into an ***"M" configuration*** with an additional proximal ***"T" limb*** attached, into which the ureters are implanted. Drains and proximal urinary diversion ureteral stents are needed, as well as a urethral catheter. The wound is closed in layers.

Preparation of the Patient

Antiembolitic hose are applied when requested. Following the administration of general anesthesia, the patient is *supine*; a pad may be placed under the lumbar spine and a pillow may be placed under the knees to avoid straining back muscles and for comfort. Arms may be extended on padded armboards. Pad all bony prominences and areas vulnerable to skin and neurovascular pressure or trauma. A Foley catheter is not routinely placed. Electrosurgical dispersive pad is applied.

Skin Preparation

Begin at the intended site of incision, extending from nipples to lower thighs and down to the table at the sides.

Male. Include external genitalia in the preparation.

Female. Both vaginal and abdominal preparations are required; use two prep sets. (See Skin and Vaginal Preparation for Abdominal Hysterectomy, p. 308).

Draping

Folded towels and a transverse sheet

Equipment

Forced-air warming blanket or a warming mattress, when requested
Sequential compression device with disposable leg wraps, as ordered
ESU
Suction
Blood warmer, optional

Instrumentation

Major procedures tray
Long instruments tray
Kidney tray
Gastrointestinal procedures tray
Abdominal hysterectomy tray (available)
Self-retaining retractor (e.g., Balfour, O'Connor-O'Sullivan)
Ligating clip appliers, e.g., Hemoclip appliers (assorted sizes and lengths)
Automatic stapling devices, e.g., TA, GIA, and EEA

Supplies

Antiembolitic hose
Basin set
Blades, (2) #10, (1) #15, (1) #11, (1) #12
Needle magnet or counter
Suction tubing
Electrosurgical pencil and cord with holder and scraper
Dissectors (e.g., peanuts, Kittners)
Ligating clips, e.g., Hemoclips (assorted sizes)
Additional staple cartridges, as necessary
Stents, optional (for urinary conduit)
Urostomy or ileostomy pouch, e.g., Hollister Karaya seal pouch (depending on procedure performed)
Drain (e.g., Hemovac, Jackson-Pratt, Penrose)
Foley catheter and drainage unit
Perineal pad and T-binder or sanitary napkin belt (female), in addition to abdominal dressing

Special Notes

- Apply **Special Notes** from **Abdominal Laparotomy**, p. 134, as indicated.
- The circulator should verify with blood bank that blood ordered is ready and available.
- The circulator should bring the blood administration set, blood pump, and blood warmer into the room and assist the anesthesia provider as necessary to administer blood. Compare identifying numbers on the blood (or blood product) with the numbers on the patient's wrist band identification.
- Antiembolitic hose should be applied when the patient arrives in the room, if requested. A sequential compression device with leg wraps may be applied over the antiembolitic hose, when ordered, to prevent deep vein thrombosis.
- An automatic stapling device may be used to perform the intestinal anastomosis and/or to construct the ileal or colonic conduit. Be prepared with automatic stapling devices available, as requested.
- The circulator should not open automatic stapling devices until the surgeon is assured of the size and type wanted, as they are expensive.
- Determine if an external collection device (e.g., Hollister urostomy pouch with a karaya seal) will be needed; obtain type requested from central supply before it is needed.

- Ureteral stents are needed when a urinary diversion is created to keep the conduit patent.

Transurethral Resection of the Prostate (TURP) and/or Lesions of the Bladder or Bladder Neck (TURB)

Definition

The transcystoscopic piecemeal electrodissection of benign hypertrophied prostatic tissue (leaving the prostatic capsule intact) and/or lesions of the bladder or bladder neck.

Discussion

This procedure is particularly desirable when the patient is a poor surgical risk, as it eliminates the need for *open prostatectomy.* If carcinoma is present following the histological studies of the resected specimen, open prostatectomy may be indicated in the good-risk patient. The goal of prostate surgery for benign prostatic hypertrophy (BPH) is to remove the obstruction, minimize the damage to surrounding structures, and cause the patient as little discomfort as possible. The accessibility of the obstruction via resectoscope affords the removal of the obstruction transcystoscopically. This approach also protects the surrounding organs from injury (by not spreading cancerous cells inadvertently during laparotomy), as tissue is removed intralumenally (through the urethra), not intra-abdominally (through an abdominal incision).

Symptoms of BPH include slow, intermittent, or weak urinary stream; the sensation of incomplete bladder emptying, postvoid dribbling; urinary frequency, and nocturia. Patients may also present with acute or chronic urinary retention, urinary tract infections, gross hematuria, renal insufficiency, bladder pain, a palpable abdominal mass, or overflow incontinence. The absolute indications for primary surgical management of BPH are:

- Refractory urinary retention
- Recurrent urinary tract infections due to prostatic hypertrophy
- Recurrent gross hematuria
- Renal insufficiency secondary to bladder outlet obstruction
- Bladder calculi
- Permanently damaged or weakened bladders
- Large bladder diverticula that do not empty well secondary to an enlarged prostate

TURP is performed less frequently today because alternative medical and surgical treatment options are available. TURP is reserved for patients with symptomatic prostatic hyperplasia who have acute, recurrent, or chronic urinary retention. TURP is also appropriate for the sexually active man in whom the obstruction is not overly large. A major disadvantage of TURP is that occult tumors in the prostate may be overlooked. Alternative surgical procedures, as ***transurethral microwave therapy (TUMT),*** in which the tumor is destroyed by the thermal destruction of microwaves, ***transurethral needle ablation (TUNA),*** in which radio waves transmitted through needles placed under telescopic guidance (fluoroscopy) are used to destroy the tumor, and ***prostatic laser surgery,*** which employs a laser fiber for interstitial coagulation of selected tissue, are performed more frequently than TURP, although the treatments may not be as durable or effective as TURP.

An effective treatment for carcinoma of the prostate, ***brachytherapy*** is performed by radiation oncologists in specially licensed facilities. In brachytherapy, a template is made and seeds of radioactive iodine^{125} or palladium^{103} (encased in titanium rods) are implanted percutaneously under ultrasonic guidance; only tumor cells are destroyed by the radiation, see p. 963. ***Cryoablation,*** a nonsurgical therapy is performed for treating an enlarged prostate, utilizes liquid nitrogen passed through percutaneously inserted probes. Should further treatment become necessary, all of the aforementioned surgical approaches may be performed.

Procedure

The urethra may be dilated, as necessary. The irrigation tubing, fiberoptic light cord, and eletrosurgical cord are connected and the bladder is continuously irrigated during the procedure. Cystoscopy is performed to assess the hypertrophy and to inspect the bladder. A resectoscope is passed into the bladder using a water-soluble lubricant. The urethra and bladder trigone are reexamined. Electrodissection (monopolar or bipolar) is employed to excise pieces of hypertrophied prostatic tissue. At intervals, the fragments of tissue and blood clots are washed out of the bladder using an Elik evacuator or Toomey syringe. Total removal of all tissue fragments is desired. When resection is complete, the bladder and prostatic fossa are examined for residual unattached fragments of tissue. When adequate hemostasis is assured, the resectoscope and sheath are removed. A Foley catheter (30-ml balloon) is inserted into the bladder, filled with 5 to 10 ml of fluid, and then drawn into the prostatic fossa, where an additional 12 to 25 ml of fluid is introduced to provide pressure for hemostasis.

Preparation of the Patient

The room of choice is the "cysto" room with the "cysto" table. A forced-air warming blanket may be placed. Antiembolitic hose are applied, when ordered. Following the administration of regional (preferred) or general anesthesia, the patient is positioned in lithotomy using padded knee crutches on the "cysto" table. Arms may be extended on padded armboards. All bony prominences and areas vulnerable to skin and neurovascular pressure or trauma are padded. Electrosurgical dispersive pad is placed.

Skin Preparation

Cleanse entire pubic area (including scrotum and perineum), extending from the umbilicus to the mid-thighs. The anus is prepped last; discard each sponge after wiping the anus.

Draping

Impervious drape sheet under the buttocks, leggings, and transverse sheet or "cysto" drape

Equipment

Sequential compression device with disposable leg wraps, when requested
Forced-air warming blanket, as ordered
"Cysto" table knee crutches (padded) or padded stirrups (e.g., Allen) on standard OR table (Ritter)
Extra IV standard pole for hanging irrigation fluid
ESU (bipolar)
High-flow fluid warmer for irrigation
Fiber-optic light source, e.g., Xenon 300 W

Instrumentation

Sterile screen unless cystoscopy drape used (sterile screen incorporated)
Rigid fiber-optic cystoscope (Brown-Berger) and panendoscope (McCarthy) or cystourethroscope (Wappler) for bladder visualization
Lateral and foroblique fiber-optic telescopes (interchangeable with all sheaths) and (power) cord
Resectoscopes (continuous flow), e.g., Iglesias, Nesbit, Baumrucher, and Stern-McCarthy (sheath, Timberlake obturator, telescope [composed of Bakelite], working element, and cutting electrode) to cut and coagulate tissue
Bridge (e.g., short, Alberran) required for telescope to fit into the sheath
Stopcock, hemostat, and catheter nipples
Penile clamp (used following local anesthetic instillation in males)
Urethral sound

Add

Resectoscope (for *bladder fulguration*)
Catheterizing telescope (for catheterization of the ureters), add ureteral catheters
Sounds (e.g., Van Buren), urethral dilators, hemostat, Toomey syringe, stopcock
Bipolar resectoscope (e.g., McCarthy, Nesbit, Iglesias) with sheath, obturator, and cutting loops
Adaptors, short bridge, evacuator (e.g., Ellik), rubber tips, electrosurgical cord, 30-ml glass syringe
Foroblique and lateral telescopes and (fiber-optic light) cords with rotating contact

Note: A flexible fiber-optic cystoscope is employed for patients unable to tolerate the lithotomy position.

Supplies

Antiembolitic hose
Sterile screen ("cysto" drape has sterile screen incorporated)
Medicine cup, syringe (20 ml)
Topical anesthetic (e.g., lidocaine hydrochloride/Anestacon 1% or 2%) for males
Medicine cup, syringe, and dye (optional)
Water-soluble lubricant
Isotonic nonhemolytic irrigation (e.g., sorbitol, mannitol, or 1.5% glycine)
Disposable irrigation tubing
Cord for bipolar electrosurgery (resectoscope)
Graduated pitcher with N/S (Toomey syringe or Ellik evacuator)
Various collection devices with screw tops
Filiform urethral sounds, available
Foley catheter with 30-ml balloon and drainage unit

Special Notes

- Apply **Special Notes** from ***Cystoscopy,*** p. 394, as indicated.
- A belladonna and opium (B&O) suppository may be requested for insertion just before taking the patient's legs down at the end of the procedure. The suppository reduces immediate postoperative bladder spasms and provides some analgesic relief as the (spinal) anesthetic wears off.
- **Reminder:** Before the suppository is inserted, verify the name and amount of the drug contained in the suppository. Avoid medication errors by administering the "right drug" to the "right patient," see p. 30.

- **Reminder:** All medication containers should be kept in the room until the completion of the procedure. Follow all safety precautions to avoid medication errors; see p. 30.
- When assisting the surgeon performing cystoscopy, prepared instrumentation for additional procedures should be readily available.
- The patient is grounded with an electrosurgical dispersive pad when any urological procedure in addition to cystoscopy is performed, e.g., when a resectoscope is employed.
- Solutions that are safe for use when employing electrosurgery are 1.5% glycine, mannitol, and sorbitol.
- A generator (specially redesigned) operates safely using isotonic saline irrigation during TURP. Use only glycine, mannitol, or sorbitol unless certain that the ESU is specifically designed for use with saline during cystoscopic electrosurgery so that the patient will not be burned inadvertently.
- When a catheter guide has perforated the prostatic urethra, the Foley catheter may enter the retroperitoneal space. Considerable morbidity may result if the perforation is not recognized and quickly corrected. Be alerted to this; a cystogram is taken "stat" to verify the location of the catheter when perforation is suspected.
- TURP irrigation fluids must be warmed prior to use to avoid hypothermia. Use the high-flow fluid warmer specifically designed for TURP irrigating fluid.

Prostatectomy

Definition

Excision of the prostate gland.

Discussion

Prostatectomy is usually performed to relieve urinary obstruction caused by benign or malignant disease. The approaches to prostatectomy include the following.

1. *Transurethral prostatectomy/TURP* (p. 402) is performed most often when disease is benign.
2. *Suprapubic (open) prostatectomy* is performed through a bladder incision, which also permits correction of associated conditions such as calculi and diverticula. This procedure is not used for malignancy.

3. *Retropubic prostatectomy* avoids entry into the bladder and allows good visualization of the field. Limited malignancies may be treated by this approach.
4. *Perineal prostatectomy* affords excellent visualization and access to the prostate and seminal vesicles. This approach permits a more *radical prostatectomy* in which the capsule, seminal vesicles, and portions of the vasa are excised; however, the approach is inadequate to perform *iliac node dissection.* Perineal prostatectomy may result in impotency, and the possibility of injury to the rectum is increased when using this approach. "*Nerve sparing prostatectomy*" can be performed only when the suprapubic or laparoscopic approach is performed.
5. *Laparoscopic prostectomy* can be performed intraperitoneally or extraperitoneally. Radical prostactectomy can be performed laparoscopically; chances of retaining sexual potency may be excellent.

Prior to **radical prostatectomy**, *suprapubic lymphadenectomy* or *laparoscopic lymphadenectomy* is performed. If lymph node metastasis is present, a lesser resection is performed and/or adjunctive chemotherapy and radiotherapy are instituted. *Bilateral vasectomy* (p. 385) is usually performed in conjunction with prostatectomy to avoid retrograde infection. The laparoscopic approach (intraperitoneal or extraperitoneal) may be used to perform prostatectomy. *Laparoscopic robotic radical prostatectomy* using the **da Vinci robotic system** has been modified to include four functional operating arms that are remotely controlled from a console. The laparoscopic robotic approach, in an increasing number of facilities, supplants the traditional retropubic and perineal approach.

Procedure

Vasectomy (p. 385) may be performed prior to prostatectomy to decrease the potential for epididymoorchitis when potency is not a factor.

Suprapubic Approach. A transverse or vertical suprapubic incision is made and the dome of the bladder is incised. An additional incision is made through the bladder over the prostatic capsule. The external urinary sphincter, just distal to the verumontanum, is specifically used as the distal resection border (and landmark) to prevent injury to the sphincter. The prostate is enucleated by finger dissection. The bladder is explored for additional pathology. Hemostasis is achieved. A transurethral Foley catheter is placed. A suprapubic catheter exits a stab wound incision through the abdominal wall. A drain may be placed in the prevesical space. The anterior bladder and the abdomen are closed.

Retropubic Approach. A suprapubic incision is made; the prostate and bladder neck are exposed in the prevesical space. When possible, dissection is performed close to the prostatic capsule to preserve the neurovascular bundles (that maintain potency). More often, the prostatic capsule is incised and the gland is enucleated by digital dissection. Hemostasis is achieved. Urethrovesical anastomosis is performed after a transurethral Foley catheter is positioned. The prostatic capsule is repaired. A drain may be employed. The wound is closed.

Perineal Approach. A tractor is placed in the bladder transurethrally to displace the prostate toward the perineum. A curvilinear incision is made in the perineum. In benign disease the prostate is enucleated from its capsule. For malignancy the entire gland, its capsule, the seminal vesicle, and a distal portion of the vasa are excised. Care is taken to avoid injury to the rectum. Urethrovesical anastomosis is performed after a transurethral Foley catheter is placed. The wound is drained and the incision is closed.

Laparoscopic Approach. Following established pneumoperitoneum, six ports are placed. The table may be placed in Trendelenburg position. When the da Vinci robot is employed, four of the laparoscopic ports are used for robotic instrumentation (or camera). ***Lymphadenectomy*** may be performed, as indicated. The extraperitoneal space is entered, exposing the prostate, seminal vesicles, vasa, and bladder neck. Care is taken to preserve the neurovascular bundles. The bladder neck is transected. The prostatectomy is completed and urethrovesicle anastomosis is performed. The anastomosis is tested for leaks. A Foley catheter is inserted transurethrally. Hemostasis is assured. The specimen is retrieved and the ports closed.

An alternative to the da Vinci robot, the **Aesop robotic arm** (voice/pedal/hand activated) can be employed to control the camera, providing greater viewing stability than that afforded by a human assistant.

Preparation of the Patient

A forced-air warming blanket or a warming mattress may be placed when ordered. Antiembolitic hose are applied, as requested. Regional or general anesthesia is administered. Arms may be extended on padded armboards. All bony prominences and areas vulnerable to skin and neurovascular pressure or trauma are padded. A Foley catheter is not routinely placed. Shoulder braces are secured to the table. The table may be positioned in Trendelenburg position. Apply electrosurgical dispersive pad.

Suprapubic, Retropubic, and Laparoscopic. The patient is **supine** with the legs separated (abducted); a pad may be placed under the buttocks to maximize visualization.

Perineal. The patient is in **exaggerated lithotomy** (using padded stirrups), positioned with the knees touching the chest. The buttocks are tilted and elevated (e.g., with folded bath towels).

Skin Preparation

Suprapubic, Retropubic, and Laparoscopic. Begin in the suprapubic region, extending from below the nipples (well above the umbilicus) to the lower thighs (including genitalia) and down to the table at the sides.

Perineal. Cleanse entire pubic area (including scrotum and perineum), extending from the umbilicus to the mid-thighs. The anus is prepped last; discard each sponge after wiping the anus.

Draping

Suprapubic and Retropubic. Cuffed towel and an impervious sheet under the scrotum (extending to the foot of the table), folded towels, sheet with a small aperture and then a laparotomy or transverse sheet (depending on incision) or individual drape sheets to complete the draping

Perineal. A sheet under the buttocks, leggings, towels (optional), and a laparotomy sheet

Laparoscopic. Folded towels and a laparotomy sheet

Equipment

Forced-air warming unit or warming mattress when requested
Sequential compression device with disposable leg wraps, as ordered
ESU
Suction
Padded shoulder braces

Perineal Approach
Padded stirrups, e.g., Allen

Laparoscopic Approach
Monitors (1 or 2)
CO_2 insufflation device
Fiber-optic light source, e.g., Xenon 300 W
CD burner
Printer
Camera console
VCR
Irrigation system with pressure control, e.g., HydroFlex™

Instrumentation

Major procedures tray
Long instruments tray
Abdominal prostatectomy instruments, long,
Camera
Boomerang suture passer, Heaney needle holders (2)
Lahey clamps (4)
Otis prostatic urethral sounds
Prostatic lobe forceps, prostatic enucleator
Ligating clip appliers, e.g., Hemoclip appliers (assorted)

For Suprapubic, add:

Self-retaining abdominal retractor (e.g., Judd-Mason in abdominal prostatectomy tray) or straight and curved Lowsley tractors

For Retropubic, add:

Millin retropubic bladder retractor

For Perineal, add:

Retractors: lateral, anterior, bifurcated, and perineal self-retaining (e.g., Denis-Browne) and/or Doyen vaginal retractors, Roux retractors, and Young retractors

For Laparoscopic Approach, add:

Limited procedures tray
Verres needle (disposable)
Trocars (5 mm, 10 or 11 mm, 12 mm, or Hasson)
Fiber-optic laparoscopes, 30° and cord, usually used; 0° scope and cord
Camera
Reducers and connectors

Endoscopic for laparoscopy:

(2) Babcock forceps, (3) scissors (curved, hook, straight); right angle dissector; Kelly clamps; multifire ligating clip applier; dissecting forceps; straight, right angle, and hook irrigation-suction-electrosurgical dissectors

da Vinci robot, optional
Aesop robotic arm, optional

Supplies

Antiembolitic hose
Sterile screen ("cysto" drape has sterile screen incorporated)
Water-soluble lubricant
Disposable cystoscopy tubing
Medicine cup, syringe (20 ml)
Topical anesthetic (e.g., lidocaine hydrochloride/Anestacon 1% or 2%) for males
Medicine cup, syringe, and indigo carmine dye (optional)

Basin set
Blades, (2) #10, (1) #15, (1) #11, (1) #12
Needle magnet or counter
Electrosurgical cord for resectoscope
Suction tubing
Graduated pitcher
Test tubes with screw tops (for urine specimen collections)
Dissectors (e.g., peanut)
Ligating clips, e.g., Hemoclips (assorted sizes and lengths)
Irrigation syringe, 30 ml with cone tip, for catheters
Catheter to apply hemostasis within prostatic capsule (e.g., 22Fr or 24Fr Foley with 30-ml balloon)
Filiform urethral sounds, e.g., suprapubic catheter (Malecot or Pezzer) and drainage unit
Foley catheter and drainage unit
Drain, e.g., Penrose 1″, Hemovac, or Jackson-Pratt

Laparoscopic
Electrosurgical cord
Silastic tubing for CO_2 insufflation
Cystoscopy or similar straight tubing, e.g., K50 (add 1000-ml bag normal saline and three-way stopcock for irrigation)
Loop ligation sutures, e.g., EndoLoop (with introducer sleeve available for ties), if requested
Fog reduction agent, e.g., FRED, ELVIS
Specimen collection bag, e.g., Endopouch
Band Aids or skin closure strips (optional)

Special Notes

- **Apply Special Notes** from ***Cystoscopy***, p. 394, as indicated.
- **N.B.** *In addition to the signed surgical permit (e.g., Authorization for and Consent to Surgery) for Prostatectomy, permission for Vasectomy (p. 385) may also be indicated on the permit. When vasectomy is performed, a signed permit for sterilization (e.g., Authorization for and Special Consent to Surgical Sterilization Procedure) must be on the chart before the patient is admitted to the room.*
- Scrub person should be prepared for vasectomy to be performed first (to decrease the potential for orchitis resulting from prostatectomy).
- The drape sheet placed under the scrotum during draping must be *impervious*.

- The patient is grounded with an electrosurgical dispersive pad for all cystoscopic procedures employing electrosurgical dissection.
- Bladder irrigation fluid should be warmed to body temperature to maintain patient's body temperature using the specially designed warmer (for use during prostatectomy).
- Scrub person should be prepared with the suction as soon as the bladder is incised.
- During the suprapubic approach, the surgeon may place a finger in the rectum to facilitate enucleation of the prostate. In order to maintain aseptic technique, he/she is either double-gloved and one glove is removed following this maneuver or the circulator removes the surgeon's glove and the surgeon is regloved by the scrub person.
- When perineal prostectomy is performed, the surgeon may request a "frozen section." A biopsy of the prostate is made to determine if malignancy is present; malignancy indicates the need for performing a more radical procedure. Be prepared for frozen section.
- A Foley catheter with a large balloon is used to effect hemostasis within the capsule of the enucleated prostate.
- When a laparoscopic robotic procedure is performed, a representative from the company is often present in the OR to direct the surgeon regarding use of the robot.
- A permit signed by the patient must be on the chart acknowledging the representative's presence during the surgery.
- The circulator is responsible for verifying the salesperson's credentials. The Association of periOperative Registered Nurses (AORN) offers a class and written guidelines for salespersons regarding what the salesperson must know before being admitted to an OR; give information regarding this class to salespeople, as necessary.

Nephrectomy

Definition

Removal of a kidney.

Discussion

This procedure is performed for numerous conditions including hydronephrosis, pyelonephritis, renal atrophy, renal artery stenosis, trauma, and tumors of the kidney and ureter. *Radical Nephrectomy* is performed for malignant lesions; when the major portion of the ureter is also excised, the procedure is termed *nephroureterectomy. Bilateral nephrectomy* is performed in preparation for renal transplantation. The patient will require dialysis until a functioning transplanted kidney is established.

The approach employed depends on the location of the pathology, extent of the pathology, the procedure to be performed, and the condition of the patient. Approaches employed include flank, transperitoneal, and thoracoabdominal.

Nephrectomy can also be performed laparoscopically; the specimen can be morcellated and removed in an endoscopic specimen collection bag, or nephrectomy can be a laparoscopic-assisted procedure and the specimen is removed via a mini-laparotomy incision.

Procedure

Nephrectomy for benign disease most often employs a *flank approach* that avoids entering the peritoneal cavity. An incision is made along the border of the 11th or 12th rib with or without rib resection according to the amount of exposure needed. Gerota's fascia is incised and the kidney and ureter are mobilized. The vascular pedicle is ligated. The distal ureter (may be exposed by an additional lower flank or extraperitoneal incision) is divided; the distal end is ligated.

For malignant disease, *radical nephrectomy* is performed via *transperitoneal* or *anterior retroperitoneal approach. Thoracoabdominal approach* may be employed for large upper-pole lesions. The duodenum is protected with moistened laparotomy pads. The vascular pedicle is transected, and lymph node-bearing tissue is excised (*lymphadenectomy*). Gerota's fascia is dissected from surrounding tissues. The ureter is divided, and the kidney and surrounding fat, adrenal gland, and fascia are removed en bloc. If tumor is present in the renal vein, the vena cava is mobilized and the tumor embolus is removed as well. When the lower ureter is involved in the malignant process, *ureterectomy* is included in the excision. The distal ureter is dissected free of surrounding tissues, and a small cuff of bladder is excised with the intramural portion of the ureter. The bladder incision is repaired, a suprapubic cystostomy catheter is placed, and the distal ureter and bladder cuff are delivered into the flank wound and removed with the kidney. The flank incision may be closed with or without drainage. For traumatic conditions and some presentations of calculus disease involving only a portion of the kidney, *partial nephrectomy* may be performed.

Preparation of the Patient

Antiembolitic hose are applied when requested. Following the induction of general anesthesia with endotracheal intubation, a Foley catheter is inserted. The patient is positioned; all bony prominences and areas vulnerable to skin and neurovascular pressure or trauma are padded. Electrosurgical dispersive pad is applied.

The patient is in the *lateral position* for a *flank approach* with the affected side up. The patient's waist is positioned over the middle break in the table; the table is flexed. The torso is stabilized with padded kidney rests; the larger blade is placed in front, and/or pillows or sandbags may be necessary. The arm on the unaffected (down) side is extended on a padded armboard; the arm on the affected side may be supported by a Mayo stand padded with a pillow, or a padded double armboard may be used. The leg on the unaffected side (down) is flexed, and the upper-most leg is extended with a pillow between the legs; adequate padding is needed around the feet and ankles. Following the application of tincture of benzoin to protect the skin, the position is secured by wide adhesive tape applied at the shoulder, thigh, and leg of the affected side fastened to the underside of the table.

When *nephroureterectomy* is performed, a *secondary lower flank (or inguinal) incision* is employed. The patient is turned from the *lateral to the supine* position at the direction of the anesthesia provider. Before the second incision is made, a sponge count is taken preoperatively (and postoperatively). Care is taken to protect the first incision with sponges, towels, and/or drapes. Some surgeons prefer a single incision extending from beneath the twelfth rib to the suprapubic region.

For the **abdominal, transperitoneal, or anterior retroperitoneal approach,** the patient is **supine;** arms may be extended on padded armboards. The thorax on the affected side may be elevated for optimal exposure. Padded shoulder braces are secured to the table. The table may be placed in modified Trendelenburg position.

Skin Preparation

Lateral. Begin at the level of the 12th rib, extending from the axilla to several inches below the iliac crest and down to the table anteriorly and posteriorly.

Supine. Begin at the intended site of incision, extending from the axilla to the mid-thighs and down to the table at the sides. This preparation includes the area to be prepared when the second incision is necessary (nephroureterectomy).

Draping

Nephrectomy. Folded towels and a transverse sheet (lateral)

Nephroureterectomy. Folded towels, two transverse sheets, and additional drapes to cover the first flank incision (when two incisions are used), or folded towels and a transverse sheet may be cut for a single long incision

Equipment

Hypothermia mattress, when requested
Sequential compression device with disposable leg wraps, as ordered
Padded kidney rests (with the larger blade in front), pillows, etc. **(lateral)**
Padded shoulder braces **(supine)**
Suction
ESU

Instrumentation

Major procedures tray
Long instruments tray
Kidney tray
Vascular procedures tray
Gastrointestinal procedures tray
Thoracotomy tray, optional (**lateral position**)
Ligating clip appliers, e.g., Hemoclip appliers, assorted sizes and lengths

Supplies

Antiembolitic hose
Basin set
Blades, (2) #10, (1) #15, (1) #11, (1) #12
Suction tubing
Needle magnet or counter
Graduated pitcher
Ligating clips, e.g., Hemoclips (assorted sizes)
Dissectors (e.g., peanuts, Kittners)
Vessel loops, umbilical tapes
Penrose drains, long, (2) 1″ (for retraction and drainage)
Closed-suction drainage unit, e.g., Hemovac or Jackson-Pratt (available)
Chest tube, e.g., Argyle
Closed-chest drainage unit, e.g., Pleurevac and connector (**trans-thoracic approach**)
Suprapubic catheter, e.g., Pezzar or Malecot and drainage unit (for *nephroureterectomy*)

Special Notes

- Apply **Special Notes** from ***Abdominal Laparotomy,*** p. 134, as indicated.
- The circulator should be certain the urologic x-ray studies are available in the room, e.g., IVP, for the *correct* patient.

- Hypothermia measures are employed (e.g., hypothermia blanket/mattress) to minimize the effects of ischemia when nephrectomy is performed to provide a (viable) kidney for transplantation.
- When positioning the patient in the lateral position, protect patient's skin under adhesive tape with tincture of benzoin. Document the appearance of the skin preoperatively and immediately postoperatively in the **Perioperative Record** for continuity of care and for medicolegal purposes.
- **Reminder:** The patient is moved into the position required for the surgical procedure when the anesthesia provider indicates readiness. The patient's position is *never* moved without the expressed permission of the anesthesia provider.
- Hemorrhage must be anticipated during nephrectomy. Verify with blood bank that blood is available as ordered before starting the procedure.
- The circulator should be prepared to assist the anesthesia provider as necessary to obtain, check identification, and prepare for the administration of blood.
- **N.B.** All resected perirenal fat is collected by the scrub person and placed in a small basin of normal saline. The fat may be used as a bolster to stop bleeding.
- When two incisions are employed, the patient is repositioned, reprepared, and redraped. An additional instrument tray is unnecessary.
- Vessel loops, umbilical tapes, instruments and their removable parts must be included in the sponge count. The scrub person must take care to notice if any part of an instrument is broken or missing. These counts are considered for all surgeries. Missing pieces of instruments must be reported to the surgeon. An x-ray is taken; this is reported to the OR supervisor and an Incident Report must be completed (pp. 48–49).
- Extra care must be taken when the counts are done when there are two separate incisions. Additional counts are taken for the opening and closing of the second incision (when made).

Upper Tract Urolithotomy (Ureterolithotomy, Pyelolithotomy, Nephrolithotomy)

Definition

Removal of calculi from the ureter, renal pelvis, and/or kidney.

Discussion

Numerous techniques are available for removing calculi from the urinary tract. If lithotriptic procedures, e.g., ***extracorporeal shock wave lithotripsy (ESWL),*** ultrasonic, electrohydraulic, and other nephroscopic and transcystoscopic modalities are unsuccessful or unavailable, or there are contraindications to these techniques, "open" surgery is required.

Laparoscopic or laparoscopic assisted technique can be employed for appropriate presentations. See also ***Percutaneous Nephrostomy***, p. 420.

Procedure

Proximal Calculi. A *flank incision* is made (with the patient in the ***lateral position***); rib resection (twelfth) is optional. For stones within the renal parenchyma (requiring *nephrolithotomy*), temporary interruption of the renal circulation is achieved by occluding the main vessels atraumatically. After the position of the stone is ascertained, the parenchyma is incised and the calculus is removed; the kidney is repaired. Fatty tissue may be used to bolster the suture line.

Stones in the renal pelvis require *pyelolithotomy,* while stones in the proximal ureter require *ureterolithotomy* and are extracted through incisions overlying the stones. Atraumatic clamps, tapes, or vessel loops occlude the distal ureter to prevent migration of stone fragments. The collecting system is irrigated and sutured closed. Drainage may be employed. The wound is closed in layers.

Distal Calculi: The patient is *supine* when the calculi are located in the distal ureters. The approach may be retroperitoneal, employing an inguinal, lower midline abdominal, or transverse oblique incision. The stone is palpated, noting that the ureter proximal to it may be dilated. Control of the ureter proximal and distal to the stone is achieved with vessel loops or atraumatic clamps. The ureter is opened and the stone retrieved. The ureter is irrigated and closed. Wound drainage may be employed. The wound is closed in layers.

N.B. The surgeon may inject a mixture of calcium chloride, thrombin, and cryoprecipitate to form a "clot" around the calculus to prevent its migration.

A double J ureteral stent may be placed prior to closure of the ureterotomy. Dye (e.g., indigo carmine) instilled into the bladder via Foley catheter is employed to determine the integrity of the ureteral closure.

Preparation of the Patient

Antiembolitic hose is applied, when requested. A Foley catheter is inserted. The patient is positioned in the *lateral* position when the stone is located in the kidney or proximal ureter. The *supine* position is indicated for stones located in the distal ureter. See *Nephrectomy,* p. 413, for patient positioning. Apply electrosurgical dispersive pad.

Skin Preparation

Lateral Position for Flank Approach. Begin at the level of the 12th rib, extending from the axilla to several inches below the iliac crest and down to the table anteriorly and posteriorly.

Supine Approach. Begin at the site of the intended incision, extending from axilla to mid-thighs and down to the table at the sides. This preparation includes the area to be prepared when the second incision is necessary (nephroureterectomy).

Draping

Folded towels and a transverse sheet (*lateral* or *abdominal approach*)

Equipment

Sequential compression device with disposable leg wraps, as ordered
Forced-air warming blanket or warming mattress, when requested
Padded kidney rests with larger blade in the front, pillows, etc. (*lateral approach*)
Suction
ESU
Fiber-optic light source, e.g., Xenon 300 W (for percutaneous lithotomy), optional

Instrumentation

Major procedures tray
Long instruments tray
Kidney tray
Thoracotomy instruments tray (*lateral approach*)
Nephroscope or nephroureteroscope and cord, bridge, and grasping forceps (available for percutaneous lithotomy) or substitute choledochoscope (refer to ***Cholecystectomy***, p. 151)
Vascular procedures tray
Gastrointestinal procedures tray (available)
Ligating clip appliers, e.g., Hemoclip appliers (assorted sizes and lengths)

Supplies

Antiembolitic hose
Blades, (2) #10, (1) #15, (1) #11, (1) #12

Basin set
Suction tubing
Electrosurgical pencil and cord with holder and scraper
Needle magnet or counter
Graduated pitcher
Ligating clips, e.g., Hemoclips (assorted sizes)
Vessel loops and umbilical tapes
Dissectors (e.g., peanut)
Calcium chloride, thrombin, and cryoprecipitate for "clot" preparation, optional
Syringe and needle for injecting "clot" material, optional
Disposable tubing for irrigation when scopes are used (optional)
Penrose drain, 1″ (retraction)
Stent (e.g., double J ureteral), optional
Dye (e.g., indigo carmine), syringe, and medicine cup (optional)
Sterile labels and marking pen (optional)
Closed-suction wound drainage unit, e.g., Hemovac or Jackson-Pratt (optional)

Special Notes

- Apply **Special Notes** from ***Abdominal Laparotomy***, p. 134, as indicated.
- Be certain urologic x-ray studies are available in the room, e.g., IVP, for the *correct* patient. Employ principles of **JC's** *Universal Protocol*.
- To facilitate calculus extraction, the surgeon may inject a mixture of calcium chloride, thrombin, and cryoprecipitate to form a "clot" around the calculus and thereby prevent its migration. Supplies to form the "clot" should be readily available in the room.
- **Reminder:** All medication containers should be labeled and kept in the room until the completion of the procedure. Follow all safety precautions to avoid medication errors; see p. 30.
- Record the insertion of a stent, including type, size, etc., on the **Perioperative Record** and the hospital log book, according to hospital/flexible policy.
- Stone specimens are placed in a dry container and sent to the lab; do not place stones in fixative solution.
- Fiber-optic nephroscope or nephroureteroscope, bridge, cord, with appropriate grasping instruments and disposable irrigation

tubing, irrigation solution, and fiber-optic light source should be available.

- An open lithotomy procedure is performed when an ultrasonic, laser, or ***electrohydraulic lithotripsy*** via ***cystoscopy*** is unsuccessful.
- When a percutaneous incision is made, additional counts are taken for the opening and closing of the second incision.

Percutaneous Nephrostomy and Nephrolithotomy

Definition

Removal of renal calculi by percutaneous insertion of a progression of instrumentation into the renal pelvis.

Discussion

This procedure is performed in an attempt to avoid "open" surgery. Minimally invasive surgery for the upper urinary tract is made possible by placing a catheter percutaneously into the renal pelvis. The initial insertion is performed in the radiology suite employing appropriate imaging modalities (contrast urogram, CT and ultrasound scans, etc.).

Indications include urinary diversion for obstruction due to stone, infection, tumor, etc., not amenable to transcystoscopic and ureteroscopic techniques or as an adjunct to prior lithotripsy procedures (such as ESWL, p. 430) and for access otherwise to the renal pelvis. Once a tract is established, larger-bore catheters, nephroscopes, stone removal instrumentation, and various types of lithotriptors may be introduced. When the immediate problem is resolved, a stent may be placed to maintain the patency of the collecting system. The definitive procedures may be performed in stages as influenced by the presence of sepsis or the general status of the patient. In addition, ureteral stricture may be excised and a ureteral stent is placed.

Procedure

A guide wire is introduced via needle insertion into the kidney. The guide wire is used for the initial placement of a catheter by the interventional radiologist in the radiology department. The patient is *prone* with the affected side slightly elevated; local anesthesia is employed. Imaging modalities help to avoid false entry into major vessels, the pleural cavity, an intestinal segment, etc. Contrast dye (indigo carmine) is injected retrograde transcystoscopically or transureteroscopically; in azotemic or dye-allergic patients, CT and ultrasound scans are used. If the initial insertion of the catheter achieves satisfactory drainage of the kidney with an obstruction, an appropriate self-retaining catheter is left in the renal pelvis affixed to the skin, with further intervention done subsequently.

When a larger-bore catheter or if a (rigid or flexible) nephroscope is to be inserted, additional anesthesia and the OR team are employed. The established tract is enlarged with serially graduated dilators, and a nephroscope is inserted. Direct inspection and biopsy may be performed. Stone crushing (lithopaxy) and stone retrieval instruments (stone forceps, baskets, irrigators, etc.) are employed under visual guidance.

Similarly, a laser fiber, ultrasound, and *electrohydraulic lithotripsy probes* can be placed adjacent to the stone in the renal pelvis or ureter. The calculi are fragmented and retrieved or the ureter is irrigated until returns are clear. At the completion of these maneuvers, a ureteral stent may be positioned and a nephrostomy tube left in place, affixed to the skin. If these procedures cannot be accomplished, an open procedure is performed (see *Ureterolithotomy,* p. 416) at that time or the procedure may be delayed.

Preparation of the Patient

Antiembolitic hose are applied when requested. The ***lateral position*** is chosen when the approach is flank or transthoracic; the affected side is up. The patient's waist is over the middle break in the table; the table is flexed. The arm on the unaffected side is extended on a padded armboard. The arm on the affected side may be supported by a Mayo stand padded with a pillow, or a padded double armboard may be used. The torso is stabilized using padded kidney rests (larger blade in front) and/or pillows or sandbags. The leg on the unaffected (down) side is flexed, and the upper-most leg is extended with a pillow between the legs. Adequate padding is placed around the feet and ankles. All bony prominences and areas vulnerable to skin and neurovascular pressure or trauma are padded. Following the application of tincture of benzoin to protect the skin, the position is secured by wide adhesive tape at the shoulder, thighs, and legs, fastened to the underside of the table.

Skin Preparation

Care is taken during the skin prep not to dislodge any catheter that was placed in the radiology suite. Begin at the level of the 12th rib, extending from the axilla to 2 to 3 inches below the iliac crest and down to the table anteriorly and posteriorly.

Draping

Folded towels and a transverse sheet

Equipment

Forced-air warming blanket, when requested
Sequential compression device with disposable leg wraps, as ordered
Padded kidney rests with larger blade in front, pillows, etc. (*lateral*)
Suction
ESU
Fiber-optic light source, e.g., Xenon 300 W, available
Laser, electrohydraulic, or ultrasonic lithotripter, optional
ESWL (transportable) or electrohydraulic lithotripter (available)

Instruments

Limited procedures tray
Serially graduated dilators for tract enlargement
Rigid fiber-optic nephroscope or flexible fiber-optic nephroscope, with cord and variety of stone-grasping forceps and baskets, etc., and suction
Laser fiber, ultrasonic probe and flue, or electrohydraulic lithotripter (available)

Supplies

Antiembolitic hose
Small basin
Blades, (1) #15
Local anesthesia, medicine cup, syringe, #25 and #22 needle (optional)
Sterile labels and marking pen
Graduated pitcher
Irrigating catheter
Ureteral stent, e.g., double J, as requested
Dye (e.g., indigo carmine), syringe, and medicine cup, optional
Sterile labels and marking pen
Foley catheter and drainage unit

Special Notes

- The circulator must always use the **JC's** *Universal Protocol* to identify that the patient is the correct patient, anticipating the correct surgery on the correctly marked side (laterality) and site. See the **JC's** *Universal Protocol,* p. 18, as necessary. Before every surgery begins, an official "*time out*" must be taken; it is a safety measure. A "*time out*" is required and must be documented on the **Perioperative Record** for medicolegal reasons.

- All care that is given must be documented in the **Perioperative Record** for patient safety for continuity of care (e.g., to avoid following orders twice) and for medicolegal reasons.
- To provide emotional support to the patient, the circulator, conveys to the patient that he/she will act as the patient's advocate while the patient is in surgery.
- If a laser fiber is employed, all laser safety precautions (p. 94) must be observed. Document this.
- A drainage collection device (e.g., Hollister with karaya seal) is required for the nephrostomy tube.
- **N.B.** Stone specimens are placed in dry containers and sent to the lab; **do not** place in a preservative.
- When a ureteral J stent is inserted, dye (e.g., indigo carmine) may be instilled into the bladder via Foley catheter to test the integrity of the ureteral closure. The insertion of the stent and use of the dye are indicated in the **Perioperative Record** by the circulator. Any reaction to this or absence of a reaction is recorded for medicolegal reasons

Cutaneous Ureterostomy

Definition

Establishment of a ureteral stoma on the anterior abdominal wall.

Discussion

Cutaneous ureterostomy is a urinary diversion performed for distal ureteral obstruction caused by tumor (e.g., carcinoma of the cervix, bladder, rectum, prostate, testes, and ovaries), radiation injury, fibrosis, and intractable infection. The procedure is usually temporary; the stoma is later incorporated into an *ileal-loop conduit* or the affected ureter is anastomosed to the opposite ureter, creating a *ureteroureterostomy.*

Procedure

A *flank extraperitoneal* incision is made according to the level of the obstruction. Gerota's capsule is freed of surrounding tissue, but not the vascular pedicle. The ureter is exposed and dissected free. ***Nephropexy*** to the anterior or lateral abdominal wall is performed. The obstruction may or may not be dealt with at this time (depending on the condition of the patient). The ureter is transected as far distally as possible to prevent retraction of the ureter and stomal stenosis. The stoma site is chosen to exit at a site that is comfortable for the patient to reach when sitting. The stoma is matured (sutured) to the abdominal skin. A urostomy pouch is placed. The incision is closed.

A ***continent ileal conduit*** or ***Kock pouch*** (see p. 425) with ***cutaneous ureterostomy*** has a one-way catheterizable nipple valve at the insertion site of the stoma. The continent conduit acts as a storage receptacle and is catheterized at intervals by the patient.

Pediatric cutaneous ureterostomy is often a temporary measure prior to a more definitive procedure.

Preparation of the Patient

Antiembolitic hose are applied when requested. Following the administration of general anesthesia, the patient is supine. A pad may be placed under the sacrum, and a pillow may be placed under the knees to avoid straining back muscles and for comfort. Arms may be extended on padded armboards. All bony prominences and areas vulnerable to skin and neurovascular pressure or trauma are padded. A Foley catheter is not routinely placed. Electrosurgical dispersive pad is applied.

Skin Preparation

Begin at the intended site of incision, extending from nipples to mid-thighs and down to the table at the sides.

Draping

Folded towels and a laparotomy sheet

Equipment

Forced-air warming blanket or warming mattress, when ordered
Sequential pressure device with disposable leg wraps, if requested
ESU
Suction

Instrumentation

Major procedures tray
Long instruments tray
Self-retaining abdominal retractor (e.g., Balfour)
Ligating clip appliers, e.g., Hemoclip appliers (various sizes and lengths)

Supplies

Antiembolitic hose
Basin set
Blades, (2) #10, (1) #15, (1) #11, and (1) #12
Needle magnet or counter
Suction tubing
Electrosurgical pencil and cord with holder and scraper
Dissectors (e.g., peanuts, Kittners)

Ligating clips, e.g., Hemoclips (assorted)
Splinting urostomy catheter (usually Silastic)
Ureteral stent, optional
Urostomy pouch, e.g., Hollister with karaya seal

Special Notes

- Apply **Special Notes** from ***Abdominal Laparotomy***, p. 134, as indicated.
- **N.B.** *Ask the patient, in addition to checking the patient's chart, regarding sensitivities and allergies, particularly to iodine or latex products.* Prep solutions may contain iodine, and many gloves, drains, and collection devices contain latex. Document any sensitivity or allergy noted and the product that replaced the one usually used.
- Document the condition of the skin preprocedure and postprocedure, particularly at the intended site of the stoma placement for patient safety and for medicolegal purposes.

Ileal Conduit

Definition

An isolated segment of ileum into which the ureters are implanted, exiting as a urostomy stoma on the abdominal wall.

Discussion

This procedure is performed in conjunction with *cystectomy*, p. 399. Creation of an ileal conduit has superseded ureterosigmoidostomy and cutaneous ureterostomy in order to avoid potential ascending urinary tract infection, diarrhea, skin problems, etc. Most often the ileal segment is brought out as a urostomy stoma, but a continent pouch with a nipple valve may be constructed (*Kock pouch*). In selected cases when urinary sphincter function remains intact, the ileal segment may be anastomosed as a bladder substitute to the proximal urethra, preserving "anatomical" urinary function. An isolated loop of the sigmoid colon may be used instead of ileum.

Procedure

See *Cystectomy*, p. 399. The ileal conduit may be constructed prior to or after the excision of the bladder. The distal ileum is exposed; a segment (approximately 15 cm) is divided from the ileum, maintaining its mesentery. The continuity of proximal and distal ileum is reestablished. The mesentery is closed over the intervening mesentery of the isolated loop to avoid internal herniation. The proximal end of the isolated loop is closed. The ureters are dissected and anastomosed to the ileal loop. The distal end of the ileal loop is brought out to the stoma site (right lower quadrant of the abdomen). The stoma is sutured *(matured)* to the skin, and a urostomy pouch is applied. The abdominal wound is closed. Drainage is optional. Stapling devices may be employed to perform the intestinal anastomoses and closure of the proximal end of the isolated loop.

When a Kock pouch (there are variants, such as Indiana pouch and those which include the cecum and part of the ascending colon) is created, a 50 cm ileal segment is folded on itself as a "U." The U limbs are anastomosed side to side on the antimesenteric border and the common wall divided establishing the pouch. The GIA stapler is most useful for this maneuer. The proximal end is closed; the distal is intussuscepted into itself to form a nipple valve to admit an 8Fr catheter. The ureters are anastomosed to the pouch and the stoma matured to the skin. A combination of stapling and hand sewn techniques are employed.

Preparation of the Patient

Antiembolitic hose are applied when requested. Following the administration of general anesthesia, the patient is supine; a pad may be placed under the sacrum and a pillow may be placed under the knees to avoid straining back muscles and for comfort. Arms may be extended on padded armboards. Pad all bony prominences and areas vulnerable to skin and neurovascular pressure or trauma. A Foley catheter is not routinely placed. An electrosurgical dispersive pad is applied.

Skin Preparation

Begin cleansing at the intended site of the incision (check with the surgeon). Extend preparation from the nipples to mid-thighs and down to the table at the sides.

Draping

Folded towels and a laparotomy sheet

Equipment

Forced-air warming blanket or warming mattress, when ordered
Sequential pressure device with disposable leg wraps
ESU
Suction

Instrumentation

Major gastrointestinal procedures tray
Gastrointestinal procedures tray

Long instruments tray
Self-retaining abdominal retractor (e.g., Balfour)
Ligating clips, e.g., Hemoclip appliers (assorted sizes and lengths)
Ruler
Automatic (disposable) stapling device with contained staples, e.g., TA, GIA, and EEA, optional

Supplies

Antiembolitic hose
Basin set
Blades, (2) #10, (1) #15, (1) #11, (1) #12
Needle magnet
Suction tubing
Electrosurgical pencil and cord with holder and scraper
Dissectors (e.g., peanut)
Ligating clips, e.g., Hemoclips
Ureteral stent (e.g., Silastic ureteral catheter), optional
Urostomy pouch, e.g., Hollister with karaya seal
Drain, e.g., Penrose, Hemovac, or Jackson-Pratt, optional

Special Notes

- Apply **Special Notes** from *Cystectomy*, p. 401, as indicated.
- When a disposable stapler is requested, do not open the package until the surgeon is certain about the size and type, as they are expensive and the cost would have to be passed on to the patient.
- Document the insertion of a ureteral stent and the type, size, etc., on the **Perioperative Record**.

Adrenalectomy

Definition

Excision of either or both of the adrenal glands.

Discussion

This procedure is done to excise primary tumors of the adrenal glands, benign or malignant (usually unilaterally), or to modify an endocrine-dependent tumor, as in breast or prostatic malignancy. During the entire perioperative period, corticosteroid replacement must be administered. When the adrenal lesion is a pheochromocytoma, antihypertensive agents as nitroprusside, phentolamine, or β-blocking agents are employed to keep the blood pressure controlled. Small fragments of the adrenal cortex may be implanted in the patient's thigh musculature so that some glandular function is preserved.

Adrenalectomy is most often performed employing an anterior or posterior approach. The posterior approach is less traumatic to the patient, but it does not permit exploration of the abdomen, concomitant oophorectomy when indicated, or other coincidental intra-abdominal procedures. The anterior approach also affords the opportunity to search for ectopic adrenal tissues.

N.B. Laparoscopic adrenalectomy can be performed with the patient turned to a **semi-lateral** position following the establishment of pneumoperitonem, with the patient repositioned to the opposite **semi-lateral** position if a bilateral procedure is done.

Alternatively, a **posterior** approach can be employed using a balloon trocar to develop the space about the adrenal. When the adrenal lesion is large or other local contraindications to a laparoscopic approach exist (prior local surgery, metastatic spread with need for en bloc and lymph node excision, etc.), an open procedure is done.

Procedure

Posterior Approach. The patient may be in the **lateral** position for unilateral adrenalectomy. For bilateral adrenalectomy, the patient is prone in the **jackknife position**. An incision is made from the lower ribs (the 12th rib is resected after the muscles are separated) to the posterior iliac crest. The fascia is incised and Gerota's capsule exposed. The adrenal gland is identified and excised, taking care not to injure the kidney. The left adrenal vein is divided from the renal vein, and the right adrenal vein is divided from the inferior vena cava. Careful hemostasis of the fragile vasculature is required; clips may be employed. The incision is closed in layers. If the pleural cavity was entered, drainage may be necessary.

Anterior Approach. An upper-abdominal longitudinal incision is made. The peritoneal cavity is explored, and additional procedures are performed as indicated. The retroperitoneal space is entered on the right after reflecting the duodenum and on the left through the lesser sac. Precautions are taken to assure that hemostasis is maintained, as noted above. The adrenal gland(s) is/are excised, and the wound is closed in layers.

Preparation of the Patient

A forced-air warming blanket or a warming mattress may be placed. Antiembolitic hose are applied. General anesthesia with endotracheal intubation is employed. The anesthesia provider places a nasogastric tube. All bony prominences and areas vulnerable to skin and neurovascular pressure or trauma are padded. Ask about a Foley catheter (not routinely placed, but may be requested). Electrosurgical dispersive pad is applied.

The patient is in the **lateral** position with the affected side up for unilateral adrenalectomy. For a bilateral adrenalectomy, the **anterior approach** (supine position) or **posterior approach** (jackknife position) may be employed.

Anterior Approach. Following the administration of general anesthesia, the patient is supine. Arms may be extended on padded armboards.

Posterior Approach. The patient is **prone** in the jackknife position. An IV is inserted, and general anesthesia (with endotracheal intubation) is inducted while the patient is on the gurney. The patient is carefully rolled over to prone position onto the OR table. The patient is placed in jackknife position with arms extended on padded armboards, angled toward the head of the table with the hands pronated. Chest rolls are placed under the patient from the acromioclavicular joint to the level of the iliac crests to facilitate breathing. Female breasts and male genitalia are protected. A pillow(s) is placed in front of the ankles. Pads may be placed under the elbows and knees. The safety strap is secured across the patient's thighs.

Skin Preparation

Lateral Position. Begin cleansing at approximately the level of the 12th rib, extending from the axilla from 5 to 7.5 cm (2 to 3 inches) to below the iliac crest and down to the table at the sides.

Anterior Approach. Begin cleansing for an upper midline incision, extending from the axilla to mid-thighs and down to the table at the sides.

Prone Position. Begin cleansing under the ribcage for bilateral curvilinear incisions that begin at the level of the 10th rib and extend to the superior border of the iliac crests. Prepare the skin from the axilla to the upper thighs and down to the table at the sides.

Draping

Folded towels and a transverse sheet (**all positions**); sheet may be cut to accommodate the incisions for a bilateral procedure

Equipment

Forced-air warming blanket or warming mattress, when ordered
Sequential compression device with disposable leg wraps
Pillow and padded kidney rests with larger blade in front, pillow, etc. **(lateral)**
Pillow and chest rolls **(prone)** .
ESU
Suction
Blood warmer for transfusion (available)

Instrumentation

Major procedures, long instruments, and kidney trays
Thoracotomy, vascular, and gastrointestinal procedures trays (available)
Ligating clip appliers, e.g., Hemoclip appliers (assorted sizes and lengths)

Supplies

Antiembolitic hose
Basin set
Blades, (2) #10, (1) #15, (1) #11, and (1) #12
Suction tubing
Electrosurgical pencil and cord with holder and scraper
Needle magnet or counter
Dissectors (e.g., peanuts, Kittners)
Penrose drain, 1″ (for retraction)
Ligating clips, e.g., Hemoclips (assorted, optional)

Special Notes

- Apply **Special Notes** from ***Abdominal Laparotomy***, p. 134, as indicated.
- Ascertain which approach will be used and obtain necessary positioning equipment before bringing the patient into the room.
- **Reminder:** All medication containers should be kept in the room until the completion of the procedure. Follow all safety precautions to avoid medication errors; see p. 30.
- N.B. Hormonal drugs as hydrocortisone (e.g., Solu-Cortef™) or other corticosteroids and antihypertensives may be requested.

Extracorporal Shockwave Lithotripsy

Definition

Disintegration of upper urinary tract calculi by precisely directed shock waves generated by an electromagnet through water-filled cushions that couple with the patient; additional energy modalities include electrohydraulic and piezoelectric.

Discussion

Dornier Delta II or the Compact S ESWL portable lithotripter provides shock waves that are discharged in coordination with ECG monitoring to avoid cardiac distress. The surgeon initiates the shockwaves (70 to 120/min). The total number of shock waves depends on the size, composition, and location of the calculus, as well as the physique of the patient. The isocentric design permits the imaging system to revolve around the stone. X-ray and/or *isocentric ultrasound* guidance minimizes energy dosage to a specific pinpoint area.

ESWL is preferred for stone disintegration within the renal pelvis and over ureteroscopic lithotripsy whenever possible because ESWL is noninvasive and requires a lesser level of anesthesia. However, ESWL is less efficient in treating ureteral stones, and the clearance of stone fragments may take as long as 4 months. Contraindications (or relative contraindications) to ESWL include larger stones (>2 cm), obesity, patients with bony deformities or immobility, urinary tract infection, cystine stones, and stones in the mid-ureter or lower pole renal calyces, for which ureteroscopic or nephroscopic procedures are preferred. Alternative minimally invasive procedures include **ultrasonic, laser**, or **electrohydraulic lithotripsy**.

Procedure

The physician, sitting at the ESWL console, positions the stone on the crosshairs and releases the shock waves that coincide with the ECG to avoid arrhythmias. The voltage is read continuously and altered to change the intensity of the shocks. For calculi in the proximal portion of the ureter (superior to the pelvic brim), the surgeon may attempt to reposition the calculus back into the kidney (renal pelvis) to achieve the maximum effect of ESWL.

Transcystoscopically under fluoroscopic control, a ureteral catheter may be positioned in the ureter immediately distal to the calculus. The ureter is filled with a lidocaine mixture (e.g., 2% Xylocaine jelly and sterile water 3:1). If the calculus cannot be repositioned into the renal pelvis, the physician may elect to perform ESWL with the stone in the ureter. In that case, two or three additional ureteral catheters may be positioned just distal to the stone to prevent its premature passage while still intact (to prevent possible injury to the ureter). ESWL is performed.

Preparation of the Patient

Antiembolitic hose are applied, when ordered, as long as the procedure is not performed in a water bath. Regional anesthesia is usually administered. The patient is awake (with *conscious sedation*) and supine; a pad may be placed under the lumbar spine and a pillow may be placed under the knees to avoid straining back muscles and for comfort. Arms may be comfortably positioned on the patient's lap; softly padded restraints may be applied. Pad all bony prominences and areas vulnerable to skin and neurovascular pressure or trauma. Ultrasound gel is put on the shockhead and on the patient's skin. The shockhead is positioned. The patient is then alerted that the shocks are going to commence. Cystoscopy or ureteroscopy may precede ESWL and/or be employed during the lithotripsy.

Skin Preparation

For ESWL, the only preparation required is ultrasound gel applied to the patient's skin where the shockhead will be directed.

For additional procedures, see Skin Preparation for Cystoscopy, p. 392.

Draping

The patient is covered with a sheet and/or blanket for ESWL. For additional procedures, see draping for **Cystoscopy**, p. 393.

Equipment

Sequential compression device with disposable leg wraps, when ordered
ESWL portable unit with high-frequency generator, e.g., Dornier Delta II or Compact S
ESWL table with fluoroscopy capabilities
Computer with a main control panel
Monitor(s)
Digital camera
VCR
Ultrasound generator
Extra standard for hanging cystoscopy irrigation, optional
Fiber-optic light source, e.g., Xenon 300 W, for scopes as necessary, optional

Instrumentation

Ultrasound wand and hand device with flue

When Cystoscopy and Additional Procedures are Performed, add:

Sterile screen unless cystoscopy drape is used (sterile screen incorporated)
Rigid fiber-optic cystoscope (Brown-Berger) and panendoscope (McCarthy) or cystourethroscope (Wappler) for bladder visualization
Lateral and foroblique fiber-optic telescopes (interchangeable with all sheaths) and (power) cord
Bridge (e.g., short, Alberran) required for telescope to fit into the sheath
Assorted grasping forceps and baskets
Stopcock, hemostat, and catheter nipples
Penile clamp (used following local anesthetic instillation in males)
Urethral sound

Add

Ureteral lithotrite and corresponding scope (for *lithopaxy*)
Catheterizing telescope (for catheterization of the ureters), add ureteral catheters

Note: A flexible fiber-optic cystoscope is employed for patients unable to tolerate the lithotomy position.

Supplies

Antiembolitic hose
Ultrasound gel
Foley catheter and drainage bag

For Cystoscopy, Retrograde Pyelography, or Ureteroscopy, add:

Sterile screen ("cysto" drape has sterile screen incorporated)
Medicine cup and topical anesthetic (e.g., lidocaine hydrochloride/Anestacon 1% or 2%)
Syringe (20 ml) for males
Water-soluble lubricant
Disposable irrigation tubing
Suction tubing
Coated malleable core guidewire (e.g., 0.035″ × 150 cm) and hollow needle
Urethral catheter, Xylocaine jelly, 2%, and adaptor (to connect to drainage)
Filiform urethral sounds, available
Ureteral stent (e.g., double-J stent to avoid obstruction from large calculi)
Medicine cup, syringe, and dye (optional)
ESU cord (for procedures in addition to cystoscopy)
Graduated pitcher
Test tubes with screw tops (for urine specimen collections)
Foley catheter and drainage unit

Special Notes

- Apply **Special Notes** from ***Abdominal Laparotomy***, p. 134, as indicated.
- A lithotripter supervisor is responsible for checking and preparing the ESWL equipment, assisting the surgeon and anesthesia provider, and documenting nursing care of the patient.

- Care is taken to position the patient correctly. Pad all bony prominences and areas vulnerable to skin and neurovascular trauma or pressure.
- Document the appearance of the skin preoperatively and immediately postoperatively for patient safety and for medicolegal reasons.
- **N.B.** *It is extremely important for the patient to be told/warned when shockwaves are to begin.* Alerting the patient is paramount so that the patient is not startled; it is important for the patient not to move.
- X-ray precautions (p. 52) are observed during fluoroscopy. Lead aprons are worn in the room during fluoroscopy, donned prior to scrubbing, or personnel may stand behind a leaded wall.
- When an anesthesia provider is not present, an additional perioperative RN is required to monitor the patient's blood pressure, heart rate, respirations, EKG, and oxygen saturation and to administer medications, see *conscious sedation (by RN)* p. 74.
- All personnel working with the ESWL must be thoroughly familiar with its operation.
- Anticipate that cystoscopy, retrograde pyelography, or ureteroscopy may precede the ESWL.

Ultrasonic Lithotripsy

Definition

Disintegration of urinary tract calculi located in the ureter by means of ultrasonic waves delivered by a probe inserted transureteroscopically.

Discussion

The **ultrasonic lithotripter** generates ultrasonic waves that shatter a calculus within the ureter. The pulverized particles are eliminated in the urine. This procedure may be extended to include stones in the renal pelvis that are approached by percutaneous nephrostomy. ESWL is the preferred method for the disintegration of stones in the renal pelvis when applicable.

Alternatively, when ultrasonic lithotripsy does not shatter the stone, lithotripsy may be performed with laser or electrohydraulic lithotripsy.

Procedure

Cystoscopy, p. 391 is performed. Under fluoroscopic control, a guide wire is passed into the affected ureter. An ureteroscope is passed into the ureter over the guide wire when possible. The ureter may require dilation using serially graduated catheters or a dilating pressure balloon catheter. Once the ureter is sufficiently dilated, the ureteroscope is passed over the guide wire. The ultrasonic wand is passed through the ureteroscope, and the stone is either shattered or dislodged by ultrasonic waves and removed with irrigation and suction.

Preparation of the Patient

Antiembolitic hose are applied when requested. When general or spinal anesthesia is employed, it is administered before the skin prep. Local anesthetic may be inserted into the urethra of the male patient and applied to the urethral meatus of the female patient following the skin prep. The patient is usually on the cystoscopy table (in the "cysto" room) in lithotomy position. The customized "cysto" table has special built-in crutch supports for the knees that should be padded. If a "cysto" table is unavailable, padded stirrups (e.g., Allen) are used. All bony prominences and areas vulnerable to skin and neurovascular pressure or trauma are padded. Apply electrosurgical dispersive pad.

Skin Preparation

A sterile screen is placed over the drain or a drain is incorporated into disposable drapes following the skin prep. The table may be tilted downward to permit easy drainage of prep solution. Care is taken to prevent prep solutions from pooling under the patient to avoid excoriation of the skin and to avoid burns when using the ESU. Extend the prep from umbilicus to mid-thighs.

Males. Cleanse entire pubic area, including the penis, scrotum, and perineum. Discard each sponge after wiping the anus.

Females. See Skin and Vaginal prep for D&C, p. 278.

Draping

Drape sheet under the buttocks, leggings, and a "cysto" drape (drain and screen incorporated), or drape sheet under the buttocks, leggings, a laparotomy sheet, and a sterile screen and drain

Equipment

Forced-air warming blanket or warming mattress, as ordered
Sequential compression device with disposable leg wraps
"Cysto" table with padded crutch leg holders or padded stirrups (e.g., Allen) on OR table
Ultrasonic lithotripter generator with foot switch
Fiber-optic light source for cystoscope or ureteroscope, e.g., Xenon 300 W
Extra IV standard for irrigation fluid
ESU

Instrumentation

Ultrasonic wand and cord

Sterile screen unless cystoscopy drape used (sterile screen incorporated)

Rigid fiber-optic cystoscope (Brown-Berger) and panendoscope (McCarthy) or cystourethroscope (Wappler) for bladder visualization

Lateral and foroblique fiber-optic telescopes (interchangeable with all sheaths) and (power) cords

Bridge (e.g., short, Alberran) required for telescope to fit into the sheath

Assorted grasping forceps

Stopcock, hemostat, and catheter nipples

Penile clamp (used following local anesthetic instillation in males)

Urethral sound

Ureteral lithotrite (stone crusher) and corresponding scope (for *lithopaxy*), as necessary

Catheterizing telescope (for catheterization of the ureters), add ureteral catheters), as necessary

N.B. A flexible fiber-optic cystoscope is employed for patients unable to tolerate the lithotomy position.

Supplies

Antiembolitic hose

For Cystoscopy, add:

Sterile screen ("cysto" drape has sterile screen incorporated)

Medicine cup, syringe (20 ml) and topical anesthetic (e.g., lidocaine hydrochloride/Anestacon 1% or 2%) for males and penile clamp

Water-soluble lubricant

Irrigating solution and disposable irrigation system

Suction tubing

Coated malleable core guidewire (e.g., 0.035″ × 150 cm)

Urethral catheter, Xylocaine jelly, 2%, and adaptor (to connect to drainage)

Filiform urethral sounds, available

Ureteral stent (e.g., double-J stent to avoid obstruction from large calculi)

Medicine cup, syringe, and dye (optional)

ESU cord (for procedures in addition to cystoscopy)

Graduated pitcher

Test tubes with screw tops (for urine specimen collections)

Foley catheter and drainage unit

Special Notes

- Apply **Special Notes** from ***Cystoscopy***, p. 394, as indicated.
- The ultrasonic lithotripter wand is connected to suction.
- The irrigating solution for performing cystoscopy, *only*, may be water, normal saline, or lactated Ringer's solution.
- Any stone (calculus) matter retrieved is labeled and sent to the laboratory in a dry container.

Electrohydraulic Lithotripsy

Definition

Fragmentation of urinary tract calculi in the bladder by means of electrohydraulic shockwaves delivered by a probe inserted transcystoscopically.

Discussion

An electrohydraulic lithotripter releases a series of high-voltage sparks that, when placed in a 0.15% or (1/6 normal) saline solution, produce a series of sharp, high-amplitude shock waves that crack and fragment bladder calculi. The fragments may then be eliminated in the urine. These shock waves have minimal adverse effect on tissue due to tissue flexibility. This procedure may be employed for the fragmentation of ureteral calculi, employing appropriate instrumentation accordingly.

Alternatively, when **electrohydraulic lithotripsy** does not shatter the stone, lithotripsy may be performed with ***laser*** or ***ultrasonic lithotripsy***.

Procedure

Cystoscopy is performed. The electrohydraulic lithotripter probe is passed through the cystoscope so that the electrode tip lies 1 to 2 mm from the calculus and 1 to 2 mm from the tip of the cystoscope. The stone is cracked and fragmented by the hydraulic shock waves. Fragments are removed via irrigation of the bladder.

Preparation of the Patient

Antiembolitic hose are applied when requested. When general or spinal anesthesia is employed, it is administered before the skin prep. Care is taken to prevent prep solutions from pooling under the patient to avoid excoriation of the skin and to avoid burns when using the ESU. Extend the prep from umbilicus to mid-thighs. The patient is usually on the cystoscopy table (in the "cysto" room) in lithotomy position. The customized "cysto" table has special built-in crutch supports for the knees that should be padded. If a "cysto" table is unavailable, padded stirrups (e.g., Allen) are used. When positioning the patient, all bony prominences and areas vulnerable to skin and neurovascular pressure or trauma are padded. An electrosurgical dispersive pad is applied.

Males. Local anesthetic may be inserted into the urethra of patient (and the penile clamp is applied) following the skin prep.

Females. Local anesthetic is applied to the urethral meatus of the patient following the skin prep.

Skin Preparation

Extend the prep from umbilicus to mid-thighs. A sterile screen is placed over the drain or a drain is incorporated into disposable drapes following the skin prep. The table may be tilted downward to permit easy drainage of prep solution. Care is taken to prevent prep solutions from pooling under the patient to avoid excoriation of the skin and to avoid burns when using the ESU.

Males. Cleanse entire pubic area, including the penis, scrotum, and perineum. Discard each sponge after wiping the anus.

Females. Extend prep from the umbilicus to the mid-thighs and down to the table at the sides. Continue with a vaginal prep and extend the prep downward over the labia. Cleanse each inner thigh next. The vaginal vault and cervix are prepared using three spongesticks. The perineum and anus are cleansed with the remaining sponges. Discard each sponge after wiping the anus.

Draping

An impervious sheet under the buttocks, leggings, and a "cysto" sheet

Equipment

Electrohydraulic lithotripter generator, foot switch, and extender cable
Fiber-optic light source for cystoscope, e.g., Xenon 300 W
Extra IV standard for irrigation fluid

Instrumentation

Electrohydraulic lithotripter hand piece and probe (electrode)
Sterile screen unless cystoscopy drape used (sterile screen incorporated)
Cystoscopy instrumentation (e.g., assorted grasping forceps and baskets) and cord

Alligator forceps, Wappler forceps, Ellik evacuator, Toomey syringe (for fragments)
Disposable probes
Rigid fiber-optic cystoscope (Brown-Berger) and panendoscope (McCarthy) or cystourethroscope (Wappler) for bladder visualization
Lateral and foroblique fiber-optic telescopes (interchangeable with all sheaths) and (power) cord
Bridge (e.g., short, Alberran) required for telescope to fit into the sheath
Stopcock, hemostat, and catheter nipples
Penile clamp (used following local anesthetic instillation in males)
Urethral sound
Ureteral lithotrite and corresponding scope (for *lithopaxy*), as requested
Catheterizing telescope (for catheterization of the ureters), add ureteral catheters, as necessary
Extender cable

Note: A flexible fiber-optic cystoscope is employed for patients unable to tolerate the lithotomy position.

Supplies

Antiembolitic hose

For Cystoscopy, add:
Sterile screen ("cysto" drape has sterile screen incorporated)
Medicine cup, syringe (20 ml), and topical anesthetic (e.g., lidocaine hydrochloride/Anestacon 1% or 2%) for males
Water-soluble lubricant
Irrigating solution, usually saline solution 0.15% (1/6 normal saline)
Suction tubing
Disposable irrigation system
Urethral catheter, Xylocaine jelly, 2%, and adaptor (to connect to drainage)
Filiform urethral sounds, available
Ureteral stent (e.g., double-J stent to avoid obstruction from large calculi)
Medicine cup, syringe, and dye (optional)
ESU cord (for procedures in addition to cystoscopy)
Graduated pitcher
Test tubes with screw tops (for urine specimen collections)
Foley catheter and drainage unit

Special Notes

- Apply **Special Notes** from *Cystoscopy*, p. 394, as indicated.
- **Do not** reuse the electrohydraulic probe (electrode).
- Sterilize lithotripter extender cable using ethylene oxide gas *only*.
- N.B. **Do not** use the electrohydraulic lithotripter for patients with a pacemaker, as using the lithotripter will cause these patients to suffer cardiac arrhythmias.
- The irrigating solution is to be kept at room temperature; keep solutions in a warming cupboard.
- The irrigating solution of 0.15% (1/6 normal) saline may be prepared in the OR by adding 500 ml of normal saline to a 3-l bag of sterile distilled water from which 500 ml has been discarded. Alternatively, 6 ml of concentrated sodium chloride solution (23.4%) can be added to each liter of sterile water.
- Any stone (calculus) matter retrieved is labeled and sent to the laboratory in a dry container.

Implantation of an Artificial Urinary Sphincter

Definition

The insertion of a prosthetic device to maintain urinary continence.

Discussion

This procedure is performed when other measures for urinary incontinence (including suburethral sling procedure) have failed. Patients include those who have had radical prostatectomy, spinal cord injury, radiation therapy, congenital conditions (as myelomeningocele), pelvic fractures, etc. The implanted device includes a cuff that surrounds the bulbous urethra (male) and/or the bladder neck (male and female); a reservoir (containing isotonic radio-opaque dye) is placed beneath the rectus adbdominis muscle, and a pump activator is placed in the scrotum or labium majorum with connecting tubes placed between the components. Compression of the pump releases the constricting effect of the cuff, and reversal occurs when the pump is released. The newer devices can accommodate to changes in intra-abdominal pressure. This procedure may be combined with bladder augmentation and is usually performed in stages.

Contraindications include adult (and pediatric) patients who are unable to control the device or those patients in whom bladder compliance is poor or hyper-reflexic. Self-catheterization may be necessary. The patient must be prepared to agree to removal should it become necessary, e.g., in cases of infection, local tissue pressure changes, or mechanical failure. Surgical approach is via a suprapubic incision combined with a perineal incision for males, and for females a transvaginal approach is employed.

Procedure

Males are placed in **modified lithotomy** position. A midline incision is made in the perineal body to expose the bulbous portion of the urethra, taking care to avoid nerve injury when dissecting it from the bulbocavernosus muscle. A suprapubic incision is made on the dominant hand side over the inferior portion of the rectus muscle. The reservoir is placed beneath the rectus and a tunnel made subcutaneously into the scrotum (e.g., employing dilators or tunneling instruments). The pump is placed, the cuff wrapped, and interconnecting tubes are attached. Antibiotic solutions are used to irrigate all sites. The system is tested, and the incisions are closed.

Females, males with bladder augmentation, or children are placed in supine position. The procedure is performed via suprapubic approach. The bladder neck is exposed, taking care to avoid nerve injury to the vagina (or rectum). Enough room (usually 2 cm) is allowed for wrapping the cuff. The reservoir is placed in the prevesical space, the pump is inserted into the labium or scrotum via subcutaneous tunnel, and the connecting tubes are attached.

Preparation of the Patient

Antiembolitic hose are applied when requested. When general or spinal anesthesia is employed, it is administered before the skin prep. All bony prominences and areas vulnerable to skin and neurovascular pressure or trauma are padded. An electrosurgical dispersive pad is applied.

Males are placed in modified lithotomy position using padded stirrups, e.g., Allen.

Females, males with bladder augmentation, or children are placed in supine position.

Skin Preparation

Extend the prep from umbilicus to mid-thighs. Care is taken to prevent prep solutions from pooling under the patient to avoid excoriation of the skin and to avoid burns when using the ESU.

Males. Cleanse entire pubic area, including the penis, scrotum, and perineum. Extend the prep from above the umbilicus to the lower thighs. Discard each sponge after wiping the anus.

Females, Males with Bladder Augmentation, or Children. Begin cleansing the suprapubic region, extending from 7.5 to 10 cm (3 to 4 inches) above the umbilicus to the lower thighs and down to the table at the sides. Cleanse perineum and anus last, discarding each sponge after wiping the anus.

Draping

Males. An impervious sheet under the buttocks, leggings, and a "cysto" sheet

Females, Males with Bladder Augmentation, or Children. Folded towels and a transverse sheet

Equipment

Forced-air warming blanket, when ordered
Sequential compression device with disposable leg wraps, if requested
ESU
Suction
Padded stirrups, e.g., Allen **(males)**
Padded shoulder braces **(females, males with bladder augmentation, or children)**

Instrumentation

Major procedures tray or Pediatric major procedures tray
Long instruments tray
Ligating clip appliers, e.g., Hemoclip appliers (assorted sizes and lengths)
Prosthesis and components, as ordered

Supplies

Antiembolitic hose, as requested
Water-soluble lubricant (males)
Basin set
Blades, (2) #10 and (1) # 15
Needle magnet or counter
Electrosurgical pencil and cord with holder and scraper
Suction tubing
Dissectors (e.g., peanuts, Kittners)
Ligating clips, e.g., Hemoclips (assorted)
Irrigation syringe, 30 ml with cone tip, and normal saline

Special Notes

- Apply **Special Notes** from *Abdominal Laparotomy*, p. 134, as indicated.
- **Reminder:** The circulator is able to demonstrate emotional support to the patient during the administration of anesthesia by his or her presence. He or she recognizes the patient's feelings regarding

altered body image and gives the patient an opportunity to express his/her feelings. The circulator's attitude is nonjudgmental. Especially with children, circulator uses a gentle, reassuring attitude.

- **Reminder:** Assess and document patient's level of anxiety and knowledge regarding the intended procedure. The circulator may help the patient feel more secure if he/she is understanding regarding the patient's anxiety and offers an explanation, as necessary. Clarify misconceptions by answering the patient's questions in a knowledgeable manner when possible or redirect the question to the physician.
- For male patients in lithotomy position, pedal pulses must be documented preprocedure and postprocedure for patient safety and for medicolegal reasons. Avoid musculoskeletal injuries to personnel by employing ergodynamic measures when positioning the patient in lithotomy position for the perineal approach.
- Prevent risk of positioning injury to the patient with stirrups that are adequately padded and positioned correctly to avoid skin and neurovascular pressure or trauma. Document appearance and condition of the skin preoperatively and immediately postoperatively for patient safety (e.g., checking pressure points and pedal pulses) and medicolegal reasons.
- Lift both legs at the same time when putting the patient's legs in stirrups to prevent (patient's) postoperative lumbosacral strain. Ideally, two persons are best suited to put the patient's legs in stirrups; however, one person can put the legs in stirrups by lifting both legs simultaneously and placing one leg on his/her shoulder while placing the other leg in stirrups.
- Raise and lower legs slowly to prevent cardiovascular disturbances, e.g., rapid alterations in venous return.
- *Avoid injury to the patient's fingers by preventing them from being caught in the table mechanism when the foot of the table is raised following the procedure.*
- *Ask the patient, in addition to checking the patient's chart, regarding sensitivities and allergies, particularly to iodine or latex products.* Prep solutions may contain iodine, and many gloves, drains, and collection devices may contain latex. This procedure may be performed in children with Spina Bifida who are predisposed to latex allergy. Document any sensitivity or allergy noted and the product that replaced the one usually used. Also, document the condition of the skin preprocedure and postprocedure; check and record adequately padding of pressure points and

appearance rashes, etc. indicating sensitivity or more symptoms that may indicate allergic reaction to iodine-based prep solution.

- Document the condition of the skin preprocedure and postprocedure, particularly at the intended site for the insertion of the prosthesis for patient safety to verify the condition of the skin and to have a level for comparison and for medicolegal purposes.
- Check prior to surgery with the surgeon for the type and size prosthesis to be used. Several sizes and varieties of the prosthesis are available; keep one size larger and one size smaller prosthesis in the room.
- Handle prosthesis as little as possible to prevent tissue reaction to foreign body. Glove powder, lint from sponges, etc. act as foreign bodies to which the body will react (e.g., rejection).
- Do not open sterile packaging of prosthesis until the surgeon is certain of the size, as the prostheses are expensive.
- If rectal injury occurs during the dissection (male), the procedure is abandoned. The injury must be reported to the OR supervisor and documented in the **Perioperative Record,** p. 12. An **Incident Report** (see p. 48–49) must be completed and signed that describes the incident. The Incident Report becomes a part of the patient's permanent record.
- If bladder injury is suspect during the dissection, indigo carmine dye may be instilled into the bladder to identify the perforation, and repair the defect; likewise report and document in **Perioperative Record** and complete an **Incident Report.**
- Document type, manufacturer, size, and serial number of prosthesis in the **Perioperative Record** and in the hospital log according to policy.

CHAPTER 20
Thoracic Surgery

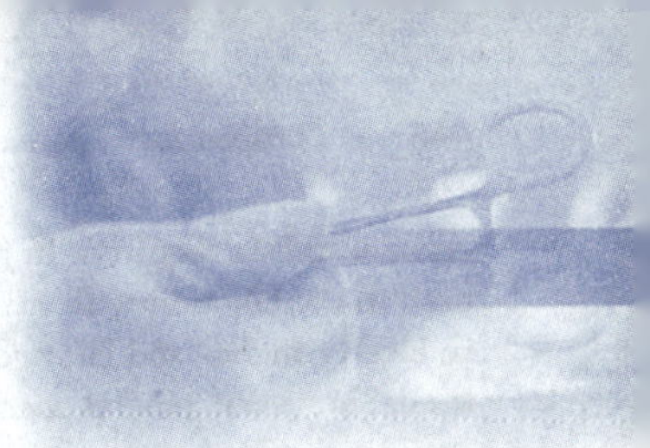

Bronchoscopy

Definition

Endoscopic visualization of the trachea, mainstem bronchi, most of the segmental bronchi, and lungs.

Discussion

Bronchoscopy is performed for diagnosis and treatment. Indications for bronchoscopy include infections, presence of foreign objects, trauma, and tumors. Rigid or flexible fiber-optic bronchoscopy may be performed. When the patient's neck has limited range of motion or as an urgent bedside procedure, the flexible scope is employed. In the pediatric patient, the rigid scope is preferred (general anesthesia).

Rigid fiber-optic bronchoscopes are best used for treatment, permitting aspiration of secretions and/or bronchial washings, identification of a source of bleeding, biopsy of lesions, removal of foreign objects, and placement of stents. Ventilation is maintained throughout the procedure. With the rigid scope, there is a better chance of success retrieving a foreign object in an emergency. A negative consequence of using the rigid scope is that the tissues may be more easily traumatized, resulting in bleeding and pneumothorax.

Flexible fiber-optic bronchoscopes are best used for diagnostic purposes, as flexible scopes are more easily passed, permitting the surgeon/endoscopist a more comprehensive inspection of the area with access to small, otherwise inaccessible areas. Mediastinal lymph nodes can be aspirated using a flexible scope transbronchial needle aspiration (TBNA) under computed tomography (CT) or transesophageal ultrasound guidance. A disadvantage of flexible scopes is that larger foreign objects and copious, viscid mucous cannot be removed through the small lumen. There are various collection tubes, cytology brushes, forceps, and aspirators available for both types of bronchoscopes. Bronchoalveolar lavage can be accomplished with either type of scope. Lasers (e.g., Nd:YAG or argon) may be used in conjunction with either type of scope.

Procedure

General anesthesia is most often employed for rigid endoscopy. Topical anesthesia may be used in conjunction with the general anesthesia to reduce broncho- and laryngospasm and may reduce the depth of general anesthesia required. In flexible bronchoscopy, topical anesthesia is used in conjunction with *conscious sedation* to control the gag reflex and reduce broncho- and laryngospasm without the need for general anesthesia; however, general anesthesia may be necessary in some instances. Atropine is used most often to reduce secretions, and lidocaine 1% or 2% is used in the nebulizer/atomizer. Glycerine may be applied to the patient's lips with a cotton-tipped applicator sponge to prevent drying and cracking following the procedure.

Rigid. Topical anesthetic is administered by spray and instillation (see topical anesthetic tray following), concomitantly with *conscious sedation,* or general anesthesia is employed. The head section of the table is removed while the patient's head is cradled in the assistant's hands as the patient's head is lowered, as directed by the surgeon/endoscopist. A guard is placed to protect the teeth. A well-lubricated bronchoscope is inserted into the mouth. The epiglottis is elevated using the end of the bronchoscope as the scope is passed through the vocal cords into the trachea. The scope is advanced into the bronchi. Secretions, washings, and biopsies are obtained, as necessary. Other treatments may be performed, e.g., extraction of foreign objects. When the laser is employed, all laser safety precautions (p. 94) are observed. Following treatment, the patient is well suctioned and the scope is removed slowly.

Topical Anesthetic Tray

A topical anesthetic "clean" tray is set up on an extra Mayo stand to include:

- Luer lok syringe
- Medicine cups (drugs of choice), include:
  - atropine is employed to reduce secretions
  - lidocaine 1 or 2%
- Paper labels and marking pen
- Atomizer
- Laryngeal syringe with straight and curved cannulas (instillation)
- Forceps and bronchoscopy sponges (application of topical anesthetic)
- Laryngeal mirrors
- Basin, small with saline
- Tongue depressor (or lingual spatula)
- Raytec sponges (moistened with saline to wipe lips and hold tongue)
- Paper tissues
- Emesis basin
- Glycerine and cotton-tipped applicator sponge

Flexible. Following administration of spray and instillation of topical anesthetic, the well-lubricated flexible bronchoscope is inserted transnasally or orally with a guard placed to protect the scope. The bronchoscope is advanced visualizing the larynx and trachea and into the bronchi. Bronchoscopy washings may be aspirated and collected in a Luken's tube; *care is taken to immediately pinch off suction to prevent the specimen from being aspirated.* Biopsies (not to exceed 3 mm) are excised using forceps or cytology brush, and foreign objects are removed using foreign body forceps and graspers. The patient is suctioned well, and the scope is removed slowly. Foreign objects may be seized and controlled by a grasping forceps through the flexible scope, and then the entire scope is withdrawn as the foreign object cannot be withdrawn through the scope channel. The scope may be reinserted, as necessary, for further inspection, etc. Advantages to the flexible scope include: less traumatic for the patient and it may also avoid the need for general anesthetic. A disadvantage to using the flexible scope is the narrow lumen of the instrumentation channel.

Preparation of the Patient

Topical Anesthesia. The patient sits at the edge of the operating room (OR) table facing the surgeon/endoscopist (a footstool is needed). Offer a warmed blanket, as the patient wearing only a hospital gown may be cold. The circulator or the scrub person stands by to support the patient from behind to prevent falls and to assist the surgeon as necessary. An electrosurgical dispersive pad is applied.

General Anesthesia. The patient is supine. The anesthesia provider moves with the anesthesia equipment to the patient's side, permitting the surgeon/endoscopist to work at the head of the table. The patient's shoulders are positioned just above the top break in the table so that the head may be lowered. An electrosurgical dispersive pad is applied.

Skin Preparation

None required.

Draping

The patient is covered with a drape sheet. A drape sheet covers the back table and another drape sheet covers the patient. Sterile gloves (only) are required to be worn; however, wearing a gown prevents soiling of OR garb. Wearing a mask and a face shield prevents accidental contamination of eyes and mucous membranes of scrubbed members of the OR team.

Equipment

Suction
Electrosurgical unit (ESU)
Fiber-optic light source, e.g., Xenon™ 300 W high intensity with
 multipurpose adaptor
Monitor
VCR
Printer
CD burner

Camera console
Footstool (for patient during topical anesthesia)
Fiber-optic headlight and cord, e.g., topical
Sitting stool for surgeon (during the procedure)
Laser (e.g., Nd:YAG), optional

Instrumentation

Rigid Bronchoscopy

Rigid fiber-optic bronchoscope (check regarding size wanted) and adaptor (to anesthesia provider)

Endoscopic instruments:

Fiber-optic telescope, fiber-optic light cords, suction-electrosurgical cannulas, cytology brush, two sponge carriers (loaded with bronchoscopy sponges), biopsy forceps, grasping forceps [e.g., Jackson serrated, side grasping, fenestrated forceps (foreign body extractor); Clerf-Arrowsmith safety pin closer; and Gordon bead grasper]

Flexible Bronchoscopy

Endoscopic instruments:

Flexible fiber-optic bronchoscope with camera and fiber-optic light cord, endotracheal adaptor (for anesthesia provider), cytology brush, suction-electrosurgical cannula, biopsy forceps and foreign body grasper
Laser fiber, e.g., Nd:YAG, optional

Supplies

Guard for teeth (**rigid**)
Guard for scope (**flexible**)
Water-soluble lubricant
Bronchoscopy sponges
Small basins with sterile saline syringe for bronchial washings and to defog mirror
Sterile labels and marking pen to label drugs
Suction tubing
Specimen collection device (e.g., Luken's tube)
Telfa and 25-gauge needle for removing specimen from forceps without damaging it
Glycerine, cotton-tipped applicator sponges (for lips at the conclusion of the procedure)

Special Notes

- Apply **Special Notes** from ***Abdominal Laparoscopy***, p. 140, as they apply (in general to the surgical patient).

- Always follow ***Universal Protocol*** mandated by the Joint Commission (JC) (formerly the Joint Commission on Accreditation of Healthcare Organizations) for identifying the correct patient for the correct procedure at the correct site (location) and side (laterality).
- Ascertain that a signed **Authorization and Consent for Surgery** is in chart before bringing the patient into the room.
- Before every surgery begins, an official "***time out***" is required to ensure that the correct patient is on the table for the correct surgery (site and laterality); all members of the team must participate. A "time out" is required and must be documented on the **Perioperative Record** for patient safety and medicolegal reasons.
- See suggested **Patient Care Plan**, p. 9 and adapt care given to meet patient's needs. Adjust plan of care using these **Special Notes** to ensure that all reasonable considerations have been taken into account.
- The circulator assists the anesthesia provider during the induction of anesthesia. He/she makes certain the anesthesia provider is supplied with an adapter for the bronchoscope prior to the start of general anesthesia when rigid bronchoscopy is to be performed.
- A **topical anesthetic tray** ("clean," not sterile) is prepared on an extra Mayo stand when topical anesthesia is used; the topical agent may also be used during general anesthesia. **Bronchoscopy** is a "clean" procedure, as the respiratory tract is not sterile.
- Use safety precautions to identify and label all medications on the topical anesthetic tray and the back table. Retain medication containers in the room until procedure has concluded. Apply all safety precautions to avoid medication errors; see p. 30.
- **N.B.** Provide a headlight for the surgeon/endoscopist when topical anesthetic will be administered. The headlight is plugged into the xenon light source and the cord to the headlight is safety pinned to the back of the surgeon/endoscopist's gown to keep it out of the way.
- As circulator, advise the patient that you will act as his/her advocate. Provide emotional support by maintaining eye contact and by standing near the patient during administration of either topical or general anesthesia.
- Sterile gloves (only) are required to be worn; however, wearing a gown prevents soiling of OR attire. Also, wearing a mask and a face shield prevents accidental contamination of eyes and mucous membranes of scrubbed members of the OR team.

- The circulator must question the patient regarding any loose teeth or permanent dental work (e.g., permanent bridges); document this information and advise the anesthesia provider. Documentation is made for the patient's protection and for medicolegal reasons.
- The circulator helps the patient cope with anxiety regarding the procedure and the unfamiliar environment by relating the course of perioperative events and by explaining procedures before performing them.
- The circulator assesses and documents the patient's anxiety level and level of knowledge regarding the intended procedure. Misconceptions are clarified by answering the questions knowledgeably whenever possible or redirecting questions to the surgeon/endoscopist as necessary.
- When a laser fiber (Nd:YAG, optional, flexible scope) is used to excise a lesion, employ all laser safety precautions; see p. 94.
- During application of the anesthetic spray, the mirror may be dipped in the bowl of saline or a defogging agent may be used; antifogging or defogging agents are applied to and wiped off the lens before the bronchoscope is used to prevent fogging of the lens.
- Protect the patient's upper lip with a damp sponge and his or her teeth with a plastic mouth guard when rigid bronchoscopy is performed. During flexible bronchoscopy, protect the bronchoscope with a mouth guard that is placed just prior to insertion of the scope.
- During bronchoscopy (rigid or flexible), a syringe filled with approximately 5 ml of saline must be available for washings; once injected, the washings are collected in a Luken's tube.
- **N.B.** ***The specimen-collecting device (e.g., Luken's tube) is held upright as the specimen is obtained.*** The suction tubing must be pinched closed ***immediately*** after specimen is obtained to prevent its aspiration into the suction unit.
- The scrub person guides instruments into the bronchoscope to prevent the surgeon's attention from being distracted from the field of vision. Biopsy forceps should be passed with tips closed.
- Care is taken not to crush specimens. A #25 needle should be used to remove a specimen from the forceps. Specimen(s) is/are placed on a nonsticking surface (e.g., telfa). Specimens should be placed in formalin unless directed otherwise by the surgeon.
- A bronchoscopy cart complete with bronchoscopes, instrumentation, and necessary supplies and equipment in the OR department facilitates faster preparation for bronchoscopy pro-

cedures. An endoscopy cart may be used to provide a source of suction or xenon light source.

- **N.B. Reminder:** *A protective face shield should be worn by scrubbed persons to prevent becoming contaminated by the patient's secretions and so irrigation fluids are not splashed or sprayed into the eyes and mucous membranes.*
- Careful adherence to ***Standard Precautions*** (p. 33) mandated by the **JC** should be observed during all surgical procedures. In addition, ***Standard Precautions*** are observed to prevent contamination by airborne contaminants or droplet infection (e.g., when patient is suspected to have a highly transmissible disease).
- Following the procedure, the patient is taken to the Post Anesthesia Care Unit (PACU). When the patient has received general anesthesia, the patient's head is turned to the side to promote drainage of secretions and prevent their aspiration. Fluids should be restricted until the patient's gag reflex returns.
- In PACU, the patient, who has undergone bronchial biopsy is closely observed for signs of hemorrhage. Vital signs and blood pressure are recorded every few minutes at first, then every 5 minutes, and if stable, at increasing intervals for about two hours. Observations and graphed vital signs are documented in the **Postoperative Record** portion of the **Perioperative Record.**
- Carefully handle fiber-optic scopes, instruments, and cords to avoid damage (i.e., do not over-bend or fold cords or drop instruments, etc. as the fiber-optic fibers are fragile and break easily). Pad the sink before cleaning scopes.
- Instruments are washed thoroughly and sterilized following use; see p. 41 for methods of high-level disinfection and sterilization. To sterilize endoscopes, carefully follow manufacturer's recommendations.

Mediastinoscopy

Definition

Endoscopic (direct) visualization of the mediastinum.

Discussion

The mediastinum includes the tracheobronchial junction, bronchi, aortic arch, bases of the great vessels, pericardium (and heart), thymus, nerves, and regional lymph nodes. Thorough diagnostic evaluation, including a variety of scans and other imaging studies, are completed prior to undertaking this procedure. **Mediastinoscopy** is performed when there is a mediastinal mass or adenopathy or when bronchogenic carcinoma, sarcoidosis, etc., are suspected. Mediastinal tissue biopsies are taken to confirm the diagnosis. The flexible mediastinoscope is preferred (its smaller diameter instrument channel may present a limitation in selected cases). Mediastinoscopy may be performed as a video-assisted procedure.

An alternative to the standard cervical suprasternal notch approach to mediastinoscopy is the ***Chamberlain procedure*** in which the incision is (usually) made at the left sternal border in order to more readily access lymph nodes and masses in the central mediastinum. There is a somewhat higher incidence of pneumothorax with this modification.

Procedure

A transverse incision is made over the suprasternal notch and extended down to the pretracheal fascia. Hemostasis is achieved. Using blunt dissection, the superior mediastinum is entered. The mediastinoscope is passed. When a video-mediastinoscope (flexible) is used, the camera is incorporated into the scope. The assistant controls the video-mediastinoscope, permitting the surgeon to operate using both hands. Care is taken to avoid injury to vascular structures. Biopsy may be taken from lymph node tissue or a mass. Needle (e.g., Stamey) aspiration may be employed to identify a nonvascular structure. Specimens are obtained with biopsy forceps. Hemostasis is achieved. The mediastinoscope is removed. The wound is closed.

During the course of the procedure, if significant bleeding occurs or injury to named structures occurs, conversion to an open procedure is necessary on an emergent basis.

Preparation of the Patient

Antiembolitic hose are applied. General anesthesia is administered via endotracheal intubation. The patient is supine; a pillow may be placed under the knees to avoid strain on the back muscles and for comfort. The arm on the side of the anesthesia provider is padded and tucked in at the patient's side; the other arm may be extended on a padded armboard. After the patient is anesthetized, at the direction of the anesthesia provider, a rolled towel is placed between the shoulder blades to extend the patient's neck. Bony prominences and all areas prone to skin and neurovascular pressure or trauma are padded. An electrosurgical dispersive pad is applied. The anesthesia provider and the anesthesia equipment move to patient's side, permitting the surgeon to operate at the head of the table.

Skin Preparation

Begin at the suprasternal notch; prep the entire neck and shoulders down to the table at the sides, extending from chin to 3″ to 4″ below the umbilicus. Sterile towels may be tucked in at the sides of the neck during the prep to prevent prep solution from pooling under the patient; they are carefully removed prior to draping.

Draping

Folded towels, a sheet with a small fenestration (e.g., thyroid sheet), and additional drape sheets, as necessary

Equipment

Rolled towel (place under shoulders)
ESU
Suction
Fiber-optic light source, e.g., Xenon 300 W

Video-assisted Mediastinoscopy, Add
Endoscopy cart:
Monitor(s), 1 or 2
CD burner
VCR
Printer
Camera console
Laser console (e.g., Nd YAG)
Emergency sternotomy
Power saw, oscillating (e.g., Sarns or Stryker) and power source

Instrumentation

Rigid
Mediastinoscopy tray contains ***rigid endoscopic instruments:***
Rigid fiber-optic mediastinoscope and camera with coupler; fiber-optic light cable and fiber-optic light cord; biopsy forceps; graspers; electrosurgical suction; electrosurgical cord; etc., see p. 181)
Multifire clip applier

Flexible
Limited procedures tray
Flexible endoscopic instruments:
Flexible fiber-optic video-mediastinoscope with camera and cord, electrosurgical cord and a variety of flexible instruments such as biopsy forceps and graspers and electrosurgical suction
Laser handpiece (e.g., Nd YAG)
The following trays must be available for emergency conversion to fully "open" surgical procedure:

Emergency sternotomy
Major procedures tray (available in room)
Open heart basic instruments tray

Supplies

Antiembolitic hose, as requested
Basin set
Blade, (1) #10
Suction tubing
Electrosurgical pencil and cord with holder and scraper
Ligating clips, e.g., Hemoclips® (small, medium, large), available
Drain, e.g., mediastinal tube (Redon™), optional
Telfa and #25 gauge needle (for specimen removal from biopsy forceps)

Emergency sternotomy
Umbilical tapes and vessel loops
Hemostatic agents (e.g., Avitene, Surgicel, etc.)

Special Notes

- Apply **Special Notes** from ***Bronchoscopy***, p. 448, as indicated.
- The circulator should verify that ordered blood is available. Ascertain that the correct number of units is ready.
- The circulator should have readily available a blood administration set, a blood pump, and blood warmer. Assist the anesthesia provider as necessary to administer blood; compare identifying numbers on the blood (or blood product) with the numbers on the patient's wrist band identification.
- Note that the approach is both endoscopic and surgical.
- A sponge count is taken before the scope is removed and at closure of the wound.
- When emergency sternotomy is performed, particular care is taken to assure that counts are correct.
- **Reminder:** Remove specimens from biopsy forceps with a #25 needle only to avoid damage to cells.
- **N.B.** *The circulator must ascertain that there are two working suctions in the room (in addition to the suction on the anesthesia cart in case of hemorrhage).*
- **N.B.** *Since hemorrhage is a realistic possible complication the patient should be prepped and draped for a "stat" thoracotomy via sternotomy, as soon as the surgeon acknowledges need to convert to "open" surgery.* Instrumentation and supplies must be in the room immediately available. In some facilities, all the instrument trays (see above) are opened before the mediastinoscopy begins in case of emergency bleeding.

- If the surgery is converted to an open procedure, the circulator should summon help, to avoid delay in the preparing for the emergency sternotomy.

Segmental Resection of the Lung

Definition

Excision of an anatomical subdivision (bronchopulmonary segment) of the pulmonary lobes.

Discussion

Only segments that contain benign lesions or diseased tissues contained within the lung parenchyma that present in a segmental distribution are removed. Indications for this procedure include conditions such as bronchiectasis (common), tuberculosis, benign lesions/tumors, cysts, or blebs, or conditions characterized by chronically inflamed tissue.

In addition to **segmental resection**, ***mediastinal lymph node dissection*** may be performed.

Segmental resection can be performed as a video-assisted thoracoscopic surgery (VATS).

See *(VATS) Thoracoscopic Wedge Resection*, p. 479.

Procedure

The affected lung is exposed through a posterolateral incision. The diseased segment is identified. The visceral pleura is dissected free from blood vessels and bronchi of the appropriate bronchiopulmonary segment. The segmental pulmonary vein and segmental branches of the pulmonary artery are ligated and clipped. The segmental bronchus is isolated, doubly clamped, and transected. The area is suctioned prior to clamping to prevent blood and fluid from entering the unaffected lung. The bronchial stump is sutured or stapled; if stapled, Peri-Strips Dry® may be used to enhance sealing of the staple line. The suture line is tested for air leaks. The pleural space is irrigated. Hemostasis is achieved. A chest tube (one or more) is inserted. The wound is closed in layers. The chest tube is connected to a sealed drainage unit.

Preparation of the Patient

A forced-air warming blanket may be requested. Antiembolitic hose are applied. The anesthesia provider may place Swan-Ganz and central venous pressure (CVP) lines. Following the administration of general anesthesia with endotracheal intubation, the patient is in the lateral position with the affected side uppermost. The torso is stabilized with padded kidney rests (the larger blade in front), and/or pillows or sandbags. The arm on the unaffected side is extended on a padded armboard, and the arm on the affected side is supported by a Mayo stand, padded with a pillow (or a padded double armboard may be used). The leg on the unaffected side (down) is flexed, and the leg on the affected side (uppermost) is straight or slightly flexed (to stabilize the position) with a pillow placed between the legs; padding is placed around the feet and ankles. All bony prominences and areas prone to skin and neurovascular pressure or trauma are padded. Tincture of benzoin is applied to protect the skin, as the position is secured by wide adhesive tape at the shoulder, hip, and legs (check chart for sensitivity or allergy) anchored to the underside of the table. Check with the surgeon regarding insertion of a Foley catheter. Apply electrosurgical dispersive pad.

Skin Preparation

Begin cleansing for a posterolateral incision (mid-thorax), extend the prep from the shoulder (include the axilla) to the iliac crest and down to the table anteriorly and posteriorly.

Draping

Folded towels, a sterile, adhesive plastic drape (optional), a transverse sheet, and magnetic instrument pad (optional, recommended)

Equipment

Forced-air warming blanket or warming mattress, when ordered
Sequential compression device with disposable leg wraps, as requested
ESU
Suction
Fiber-optic light source, e.g., Xenon 300 W (headlight)
Fiber-optic headlight and cord
Scales (2) to weight sponges

Positioning Aids

Padded kidney rests (larger blade in front), pillows, padding, sandbags or beanbags (suction required for hardening)
Tincture of benzoin
Adhesive tape 4 or 5″ (check the patient's chart for sensitivity or allergy to tape; skin is painted with tincture of benzoin on the areas that will be taped to protect it before applying tape)

Instrumentation

Major procedures tray
Thoracotomy tray
Vascular procedures tray
Cushing vein retractors
Ligating clip appliers, e.g., Hemoclip appliers, assorted sizes, long-handled
Long Pean clamps
Automatic (disposable) stapling devices with staples, e.g., TA (optional)

Supplies

Antiembolitic hose
Swan-Ganz intravenous (IV) line set up to anesthesia provider, as requested
CVP set up to anesthesia provider, as requested
Sterile, plastic adhesive drape (optional)
Magnetic instrument pad (optional)
Basin set
Suction tubing
Electrosurgical pencils and cords with holders and scrapers (2)
Needle magnet or counter
Blades, (3) #10 and (1) #15
Dissectors (e.g., peanuts or Kittners)
Asepto syringes (2) and graduated pitcher
Automatic (disposable) stapler with staples (optional)
Peri-Strips Dry (staple line reinforcement), optional
Ligating clips, e.g., Hemoclips (assorted sizes)
Vessel loops, umbilical tapes
Chest drainage tube(s), e.g., Argyle; with connector, (e.g., straight [5 in 1] or large Y, if two tubes are used)
Sealed drainage unit (e.g., Pleurevac™)

Special Notes

- The circulator must always use the JC's *Universal Protocol* to identify that the patient is the correct patient, anticipating the correct surgery on the correctly marked side (laterality) and site. See the JC's *Universal Protocol,* p. 18, as necessary.
- Before every surgery begins, an official "***time out***" must be taken; it is a safety measure. A *time out* is required and must be documented on the Perioperative Record for patient safety and medicolegal reasons.
- Apply **Special Notes** from ***Bronchoscopy,*** p. 448, and **Abdominal Laparotomy,** p. 134, as they apply (in general to the surgical patient).
- Antiembolitic hose should be applied when the patient arrives in the room, when requested. A sequential compression device with leg wraps may be applied over the antiembolitic hose to prevent deep vein thrombosis, when ordered.
- The circulator questions the patient and checks the chart for patient sensitivities and allergies, particularly to latex products (found in gloves or drains) and to iodine preparations (contained in many prep solutions). Note and document sensitivity and product that was substituted. Document the condition of

the skin preoperatively and immediately postoperatively for patient safety and medicalegal reasons.

- The circulator must verify with the blood bank that ordered blood is available, ascertaining that the correct number of units is ready.
- Verify that the patient's x-ray studies are in the room for the *correct* patient.
- **N.B.** *The circulator should ascertain that there are two working suctions in the room, in addition to the one on the anesthesia cart, in case of hemorrhage.*
- The circulator can help to prevent musculoskeletal injuries to personnel and the patient by obtaining adequate assistance to move the patient and by employing ergodynamic measures (see p. 51) when positioning the patient, as necessary.
- Ascertain and document in the **Perioperative Record** that accessory equipment (e.g., padded kidney rests) have been properly secured onto the table to ensure patient safety.
- See the suggested **Patient Care Plan** (p. 9) for care measures to consider regarding care of the individual patient, The circulator adapts nursing care interventions (according to this patient's needs) that will result in optimal desired outcomes. Use the **Special Notes** for considerations noted in this procedure to augment the plan of care.
- All care that is given must be documented in the **Perioperative Record**, p. 12 for patient safety regarding continuity of care and for medicolegal reasons.
- The circulator should assess hemodynamic factors as they pertain to this individual patient particularly in regard to the patient's surgical procedure, e.g., weigh sponges to help to determine blood loss and keep accurate record of the amount of irrigation used to help determine fluid loss replacement. To weigh sponges, see p. 162.
- The electrosurgical pad is applied (to skin that is relatively hair free to obtain good contact) as close to the surgical site as possible. It may be necessary to shave the area.
- The electrosurgical pencil tip should be kept free of debris and eschar (use the scratch pad) and kept in its holder when not in use.
- Smoke and fumes from thermal destruction are a health hazard; smoke should be suctioned away using the room suction with an in-line filter or with a smoke-evacuation system.

- Everyone present in the room should wear a mask (with a filtering capacity of between 2 and 5 microns) to prevent inhalation of toxic matter.
- **N.B.** *The scrub person should have spongesticks ready and mounted (raytec sponge mounted on a sponge forceps) available at all times for applying pressure in case of sudden bleeding.*
- **Reminder:** *A protective face shield should be worn by scrubbed persons to prevent the splashing or spraying of the patient's secretions and irrigation fluids into their eyes and /or mucous membranes.*

Wedge Resection of the Lung

Definition

Excision of a small wedge-shaped section with adequate margins of the parenchyma of the lung.

Discussion

Excision of the small wedge-shaped section of tissue containing a peripheral pulmonary lesion (of limited size) is performed for either diagnostic or therapeutic purposes. A frozen section is performed on the specimen. If the lesion is benign, the wound is closed in the usual manner. When the lesion is malignant, a more extensive procedure is performed (e.g., ***pulmonary lobectomy***, p. 460).

In addition to segmental resection, ***mediastinal lymph node dissection*** may be performed.

Wedge resection of the lung can be performed as a VATS; see ***Thoracoscopic Wedge Resection***, p. 479.

Procedure

The anesthesia provider may place Swan-Ganz and CVP lines. Following the administration of general anesthesia with endotracheal intubation, the patient is placed in the lateral position with the affected side uppermost. The affected lung is exposed through a posterolateral thoracotomy. The lesion is identified. A wedge of peripheral lung tissue containing the lesion is grasped with a lung clamp (e.g., Duval or Pennington) and excised over clamps (e.g., Sarot), or an automatic linear stapler may be used. The lung tissue held in the clamps is sutured. The suture line is tested for air leaks. Additional sutures or ligating clips may be required to achieve hemostasis. When a stapler is employed, the staple line may be reinforced with Peri-Strips Dry. A chest tube is inserted. The wound is closed in layers. The chest tube is connected to a sealed suction drainage unit.

For **Preparation of the Patient, Skin Preparation, Draping, Equipment, Instrumentation, Supplies,** and **Special Notes,** see ***Segmental Resection of the Lung,*** p. 455.

Pulmonary Lobectomy

Definition

Excision of one or more lobes of the lung.

Discussion

Pulmonary lobectomy is performed to excise benign or (primary) malignant or metastatic malignant lesions. When the lesion is malignant, it must be limited to the periphery of the lobe(s) of the lung with the margins of the tumor specimen tumor-free. If the malignancy is not contained, ***pneumonectomy,*** p. 461, is indicated. The procedure performed varies according to the type of lesion, the location of the lesion, and the condition of the patient. Other conditions for which lobectomy is appropriate are bronchiectasis, blebs or bullae (emphysematous), benign tumors (any location), and fungal infections.

In addition to lobectomy, ***mediastinal lymph node dissection*** is performed.

Pulmonary lobectomy can be performed as a VATS.

Procedure

A forced-air warming blanket may be requested. Antiembolitic hose are applied. The anesthesia provider may place Swan-Ganz and CVP lines. Following the administration of general anesthesia with endotracheal intubation, the patient is in the lateral position. The affected lung is exposed through a posterolateral incision. A rib retractor is placed, with or without the resection of a rib, and the surrounding tissues are protected by warm, moist laps. The diseased lobe is identified. The visceral pleura is dissected free from the hilus. The pulmonary artery and vein of the diseased lobe are ligated and divided, e.g., with clips. The bronchus is isolated, doubly clamped, and transected; an automatic (disposable) stapler may be used. The area is suctioned prior to clamping to prevent blood and fluid from entering the unaffected bronchus. The bronchial stump is sutured, or, more frequently, a stapling device may be employed. The suture line is tested for air leaks. When a stapler is employed, the staple line may be reinforced with Peri-Strips Dry. The pleural cavity is irrigated. Hemostasis is achieved. Chest tubes are inserted. The chest is closed in layers. Chest tubes are connected to a sealed drainage unit.

For **Preparation of the Patient, Skin Preparation, Draping, Equipment, Instrumentation, Supplies,** and **Special Notes**, see *Segmental Resection of the Lung*, p. 455.

Pneumonectomy

Definition

Excision of the lung.

Discussion

Chief indications for **pneumonectomy** are bronchogenic carcinoma and extensive benign conditions, e.g., bronchiectasis, tuberculosis (unilateral), some benign tumors, and multiple lung abscesses. When the malignancy is not contained, the procedure is abandoned and other types of treatment (e.g., radiotherapy) are instituted.

At the completion of this procedure, the affected pleural cavity is empty and the mediastinal structures are liable to "shift," causing central circulatory compromise. Measures are employed to stabilize the mediastinum at the end of the procedure by adjusting the pressure in the affected pleural space (e.g., not to exceed greater than negative 10 cm of water).

Procedure

Antiembolitic hose are applied. The anesthesia provider may place Swan-Ganz and CVP lines. Following the administration of general anesthesia with endotracheal intubation, the patient is in the lateral position with the affected side uppermost. The affected lung is exposed through a posterolateral thoracotomy incision. A rib retractor is placed, with or without the resection of a rib, and the surrounding tissues are protected by warm, moist laps. The chest is explored, and the feasibility of the procedure is determined. Advanced metastases contraindicate resection; chest tubes are inserted, the wound is closed, and chest tubes are connected to a sealed suction drainage unit.

The mediastinal pleura is dissected free. The bronchus, pulmonary artery, and superior and inferior pulmonary veins are isolated. Care is taken to avoid injury to the vagus nerve. The pulmonary artery and veins are ligated. The bronchial stump is clamped, transected, and sutured or stapled. The area is suctioned to prevent blood and fluid from entering the unaffected lung. Lymph node-bearing tissues are excised, as necessary. Hemostasis is achieved. The chest is closed in interrupted layers. A chest tube is not employed unless there is anticipated contamination from the underlying pulmonary condition that would lead to infection of the postoperative effusion. In this instance, a small-bore catheter is placed higher in the chest that is used to introduce or withdraw air to stabilize the mediastinum and to introduce antibiotics until the danger of infection has passed.

For **Preparation of the Patient, Skin Preparation, Draping, Equipment, Instrumentation, Supplies,** and **Special Notes,** see **Segmental Resection of the Lung,** p. 455.

Special Notes, add:

- Ascertain whether a chest tube or large syringe with a large-bore needle will be necessary at the conclusion of the procedure to create the slightly negative pressure in the affected pleural space necessary for stabilization of the mediastinum.

Decortication of the Lung

Definition

The stripping away of a restrictive membrane that forms on the visceral pleura and interferes with respiration.

Discussion

Decortication is performed to remove the restrictive membrane that may form as a result of empyema due to pneumonia or a lung abscess, clotted hemothorax, and tuberculosis. When empyema is detected and drainage instituted immediately, a restrictive membrane may not have time to form, obviating the need for subsequent decortication. When thoracotomy is indicated, rib resection is avoided whenever possible so that chest movement during respiration is easier following the procedure.

Procedure

A forced-air warming blanket may be requested. Antiembolitic hose are applied. The anesthesia provider may place Swan-Ganz and CVP lines. Following the administration of general anesthesia with endotracheal intubation, the patient is in the lateral position with the affected side uppermost. The affected lung is exposed through a posterolateral incision. A rib retractor is placed, with or without the resection of a rib, and the surrounding tissues are protected by warm, moist laps. When necessary, rib resection may be indicated for adequate exposure. The fibrous membrane is carefully peeled away from the visceral pleura. Cultures (aerobic and anaerobic) taken from the specimen may be requested. Hemostasis may be difficult but must be achieved. Topical hemostatic agents may be employed. Chest tubes are inserted. The wound is closed in layers. Chest tubes are connected to a sealed drainage unit.

For **Preparation of the Patient, Skin Preparation, Draping, Equipment, Instrumentation,** and **Supplies,** see **Segmental Resection of the Lung,** p. 455.

Supplies, Add:

Culture tubes (aerobic and anaerobic)
Topical hemostatic agents, e.g., Avitene™, Surgicel™, topical thrombin, Tisseel™

Special Notes, Add:

- Apply **Special Notes** from ***Segmental Resection*** of the lung, p. 457.
- Instruments that are in contact with the empyema process are isolated in a basin.

Insertion of Implantable Transvenous Endocardial Pacemaker

Definition

The insertion of an electrode into the endocardium via the cephalic, subclavian, or jugular vein (under fluoroscopic guidance) that is attached to a pulse generator.

Discussion

A *temporary external pacemaker* may be employed in acute situations. An *epicardial pacemaker* is employed when the chest is open during cardiac surgery, or the epicardial electrodes may be inserted via a subxiphoid incision for mediastinoscopy. When a permanent pacemaker is to be placed, a **transvenous endocardial pacemaker** (with leads inserted transvenously) is indicated. The purpose of a permanent transvenous endocardial pacemaker is to maintain circulatory integrity by providing standby pacing when there is a disturbance in the conduction of impulses. A permanent pacemaker can initiate atrial or ventricular (or both types of) contractions. Insertion of a **transvenous endocardial pacemaker** does not require general anesthesia, nor does it require an "open" surgical procedure. Both reasons make the choice ideal for "at-risk" patients.

Indications for a permanent pacemaker include myocardial infarction with complete heart block, bradycardia, metabolic abnormalities, drug side effects, surgical trauma, and tachyarrhythmias. The permanent pacemakers are programmed to respond physiologically to dysrhythmias and neuroconductive disturbances. They may be unipolar or bipolar.

Asynchronous. Stimulates ventricular contraction when a specified rate (fixed rate) of pacing is required.

Demand. Initiates ventricular contraction only when the heart rate falls below a preset rate.

Physiologic. Synchronizes atrial and ventricular activity to improve cardiodynamics.

In ***cardiac resynchronization therapy,*** both ventricles are paced at the same time with the ***biventricular pacemaker,*** increasing the amount of blood pumped by the heart.

Complications include infection in the generator pocket and/or wire tract, phlebitis, nonsustained arrhythmias, and increased pacing threshold. Infrequently, migration of a lead occurs postoperatively. When there is a malfunction in the system, it is usually due to improper connections, faulty lead placement, or improper set up.

Procedure

Local anesthetic is injected into the areas of lead and generator placement. Trendelenburg position may be requested (to accentuate venous filling, providing an easier target for access). A cut down is performed to expose the subclavian, cephalic, or external jugular vein; the right side is preferred. A *pacing electrode* is inserted through a venotomy and advanced (under fluoroscopy) into the right atrium or ventricle. The distal tip of the electrode may be screwed into the endocardium (coiled tip) or simply placed. The proximal end of the electrode is attached to an external pacemaker generator and tested. The pacemaker's pulse generator is programmed for the patient. An incision is made in the chest wall and deepened down to the fascia, creating a "pocket" for the pulse generator. A tunneling instrument is used to make a path for the electrode, which is attached to the pulse generator. The pulse generator is placed in the pocket. Both incisions may be irrigated with antibiotic solution and closed.

Pacemakers are powered by lithium battery and require battery change in the OR about every 5 years; this information is given to the patient along with the instructions for programming the pacemaker.

Preparation of the Patient

Antiembolitic hose are applied. The patient is supine with the head turned to the left (side opposite the dominant hand). A pillow may be placed under the knees to avoid straining back muscles and for comfort. Usually the left arm is padded and tucked in at the patient's side (check pressure point at the elbow); the right arm is extended on a padded arm table. All bony prominences and areas prone to skin and neurovascular pressure or trauma are padded. The procedure is often performed under local anesthesia. The patient is closely monitored continuously (usually by an anesthesia provider). An electrosurgical dispersive pad is applied.

Skin Preparation

Begin cleansing the right chest and right axilla including the shoulder and arm, down to the elbow. Extend the prep from the chin to lower ribs; prep well beyond the midline on the left border and down to the table on right side.

Draping

Impervious tube, stockinette, drape sheet, folded towels, and a laparotomy sheet The hand is grasped in an impervious tube stockinette. A large sheet is draped over the hand table (under the arm) and tucked under the shoulder. Folded towels and a fenestrated sheet (laparotomy) or individual drape sheets complete the draping.

Equipment

ESU
Suction
Padded hand table
Image intensifier and C-arm or fluoroscopy
External pacemaker

Instrumentation

Pacemaker tray
Permanent transvenous endocardial pacemaker ***(internal)*** with leads, electrodes, and accessory items for insertion (includes screwdriver, etc.) in sterile packaging
Ligating clip appliers, e.g., Hemoclip appliers (small and medium)

Supplies

Antiembolitic hose
Impervious tube stockinette
Medicine cup for local anesthetic (e.g., Marcaine), 10-ml c
Control syringe, 10 ml and needles (e.g., #25- and #22-gauge needle)
Sterile labels and marking pen
Basin set
Blades, (2) #10, (1) #15, (1) #11
Needle magnet or counter
Electrosurgical pencil and cord with holder and scraper
Suction
Ligating clips, e.g., Hemoclips
Vessel loops
Antibiotic irrigation and bulb syringe (optional)

Special Notes

- Apply **Special Notes** from **Bronchoscopy**, p. 448 and ***Abdominal Laparotomy***, p. 134, as applicable (in general to the surgical patient).
- The procedure, performed using local anesthetic, may be lengthy; position the patient as comfortably as possible; use pillows and padding as necessary. Particular care is taken to pad all pressure points.
- The circulator ascertains that the x-ray department has been advised and is prepared to be present for the surgery.
- **Reminder:** Use safety precautions to identify, label, and dispense medications or solutions and to avoid medication errors; see p. 30. It is mandatory that all medications and solutions on the sterile field be labeled by name and strength. The medication bottle is retained in the room until the procedure has concluded.
- Check with the surgeon (or procedure credentialed cardiologist) regarding availability of the sterile generator and leads. Most often, a pacemaker company representative brings the pacemaker, the tunneling lead wire, and the accessory equipment in sterile packaging. The representative is usually present in the OR to direct the surgeon in the use of the particular company's pacemaker.
- The circulator verifies that a permit signed by the patient acknowledging the representative's presence in the OR during the surgery is in the patient's chart.
- The circulator is responsible for verifying credentials of the representative. The Association of periOperative Registered Nurses (AORN) offers a class and written guidelines for company representatives regarding basic information they must know before being admitted to an OR.
- When x-ray or fluoroscopy is in use, all x-ray safety precautions must be followed; see p. 52. The scrub person dons a lead-lined vest before scrubbing.
- For the most convenient room arrangement, x-ray equipment is set up on the patient's left side. The scrub person positions the back table on the patient's right side and assists the surgeon side to side.
- **N.B.** *Document the type and serial numbers of the pacemaker on the* **Perioperative Record** *and in the hospital log book, according to hospital policy.* Also, complete the forms from the manufacturer, including the serial numbers, as this serves as a form of warranty.

- **N.B.** *Details of how the pacemaker has been programmed must be included in the patient's chart.* A copy of the instructions for programming the pacemaker and battery information should be given to the patient when leaving PACU or the floor unit.

Insertion of Implantable Cardioverter Defibrillator (ICD)

Definition

The transvenous insertion of endocardial leads attached to a generator that senses (detects) and defibrillates the heart to reestablish normal rhythm.

Discussion

The **implantable cardioverter defibrillator (ICD)** is effective for heart monitoring and treatment of ventricular tachycardia; some models are also effective for treating atrial fibrillation. Surgically implanted, the ICD senses dangerous arrhythmias (or arrest) and delivers electrical shocks to repace the heart to prevent "sudden cardiac death" due to sustained ventricular tachyarrhythmia. When the heart is in tachycardia, a shock is delivered by cardioversion or defibrillation, depending on the severity of the tachycardia.

The surgical procedure is similar to insertion of **transvenous endocardial pacemaker.** The distal end of the electrode lead is transvenously inserted into the right ventricle. The proximal end of the electrode is tunneled subcutaneously to a pocket and attached to the generator. The generator delivers the defibrillating shock. If during testing the shock is not strong enough via the transvenous electrode alone, a second "patch" electrode is placed subcutaneously on the chest wall. Should the defibrillation still be inadequate, the cathode (tip of the electrode) is inserted via sternotomy, limited thoracotomy, or subxiphoid incision with incision of the pericardium. It is fastened to the myocardium by screwing in the coiled tip or and the electrode attached proximally to the generator in a subcutaneous pocket adjacent to the umbilicus.

For **Procedure, Preparation of the Patient, Skin Preparation, Draping, Equipment, Instrumentation, Supplies,** and **Special Notes,** see *Insertion of Implantable Transvenous Endocardial Pacemaker*, p. 464.

Correction of Pectus Excavatum

Definition

The correction of a "funnel" chest deformity refers to the straightening of a deformity of the anterior chest wall in which there is a depression of the sternum and costal cartilages.

Discussion

Pectus excavatum occurs most frequently in males (3:1); association of the deformity in other family members is approximately 35%. A worsening of the appearance of the chest and the symptoms that occur happens during periods of rapid growth, e.g., puberty. The need for corrective surgery for pectus excavatum may be considered "cosmetic" until the asymptomatic child reaches late teens or adulthood. In reality, this procedure is performed to alleviate circulatory and/or respiratory symptoms. Variations of the procedure are performed according to the extent of the deformity. The ideal age to have this correction procedure is 12 to 18 years old. Many procedures have been devised to correct pectus excavatum, including reversal of a wedge osteotomy. The most frequently employed surgical corrections include the following.

1. In the ***Ravitch Approach,*** a sternal bar (Adkin's strut) is positioned behind the sternum after mobilization of the deformed cartilage. The bar is removed in about 12 months.
2. The ***Nuss Procedure*** involves the insertion of a large curved bar that is removed after 2 to 3 years.
3. In the ***Leonard Procedure,*** a wedge resection is taken from the lower sternum (wedge sternotomy) and the chest is repositioned. Wires through the sternum are fitted to a plastic external Jewitt brace to provide traction. The brace is worn for 6 weeks to secure the correct position during healing and removed after that time.
4. The ***Lorenz procedure*** is a minimal access thoracoscopically-assisted procedure in which a curved bar is inserted through a transverse substernal tunnel extending from the anterior axillary line to the opposite anterior axillary line.

A modification of the ***Ravitch procedure*** obtains good long-term results, with less patient discomfort and a shorter hospital stay than previously performed procedures. The Lorenz procedure, employing a thoracoscopic-assisted technique, is less invasive and though patient discomfort is similar, avoids a large incision with less concomitant morbidity. The procedure is performed ideally with a combination of general anesthesia and thoracic epidural block. The patient receives prophylactic antibiotics.

Procedure

Modified Ravitch Procedure is described. Approach is through a vertical presternal incision or through transverse submammary incisions. The origins of the pectoral muscles are reflected. Small segments of rib cartilages (three to six) are separated from the sternum, medially and laterally. An incision is made into the anterior mediastinum, and the pericardium is dissected from the sternum. The sternum is elevated to a desired position. A metal bar is positioned from behind (to correct the pectus excavatum) and is attached to a rib on each side. The costal cartilages are sutured back to the sternum medially, and small chips of the patient's own cartilage are placed into the prechondral sheaths bilaterally to encourage cartilage regeneration. The wound is closed. The reconstructed sternum will become solid within 4 to 6 weeks.

The Lorenz Procedure is described. The surgeon marks the chest to designate where the bar will be inserted. The surgeon measures and then bends the Lorenz pectus bar to fit the patient's chest. An incision (approximately 2 cm) is made on the mid-axillary line at the level of the deepest point of the depression on the right and left sides. A skin tunnel is raised on each side to facilitate passage of the bar. On the right, 1 to 2 interspaces below the level of the incisions a thoracoscope is inserted thru a 5 mm port. A long instrument (e.g., Crawford vascular clamp or a Lorenz pectus introducer) is inserted under direct endoscopic vision at the correct intercostal level (previously determined), traversing the thorax substernally, to exit the opposite side. Care is taken not to injure mediastinal structures. Umbilical tapes are seized and withdrawn retrograde as the clamp is removed. The umbilical tapes are then used to guide the placement of the curved Lorenz bar through the previously created tunnel (under thoracoscopic visualization). Initially, the convex curve of the bar faces posteriorly and when in appropriate position, the bar is turned with a Lorenz bar rotational instrument so that the convexity faces anteriorly elevating the sternal depression. More than one attempt at positioning may be required with the bar rebent as needed; sometimes a second bar is required. The bar position is then maintained with suture loops about the adjacent ribs and chest wall musculature. In the female patient, breast symmetry is considered in the various maneuvers. Pulmonary function is assessed by the anesthesia provider including a chest x-ray which also notes the position of the bar. Postoperatively, general movement is restricted for several days. The bar usually remains in place for two years and is removed by a simple procedure.

Preparation of the Patient

A forced-air warming blanket may be requested. The patient is supine and the chest is slightly elevated with a rolled sheet. Arms are extended on padded armboards to allow maximum access to the patient's chest. A pillow may be placed under the knees to avoid straining back muscles and for comfort. All bony prominences and areas prone to skin and neurovascular pressure or trauma are padded. An electrosurgical dispersive pad is applied.

Skin Preparation

Begin at the middle of the chest for a **vertical incision,** extending from the chin to below the umbilicus and down to the table at the sides.

For **submammary incisions,** begin by preparing the area across the chest (at the nipple line), extending from the chin to below the umbilicus and down to the table at the sides.

Draping

Folded towels, a sterile, plastic adhesive drape (optional), and a laparotomy sheet or separate drape sheets may complete the draping

Equipment

Forced-air warming blanket, when ordered
ESU
Suction
Power source for saw, e.g., nitrogen tank for Stryker® saw **(modified Ravitch procedure)**

Lorenz Procedure, Add
Monitor
Endoscopy cart:
VCR
Printer
CD burner
Camera console
Fiber-optic light source
Suction
CO_2 insufflator (generally not used)

Instrumentation

Basic orthopedic procedures
Bone-holding instruments trays
Thoracotomy tray
Vascular procedures tray (available)
Bar bender (Zimmer™)

Modified Ravitch Procedure, Add
Gigli saw set, bone single-hook tenacula (2), awl with fenestration, and pliers
Lebsche sternal knife and mallet
Power saw, e.g., Stryker (with circular blade) and cord, optional
Sternal bar(s) and tunneling instrument for leads, as requested

Lorenz procedure, Add
Crawford vascular clamp 15″ or Lorenz pectus introducer (tunnelling)
Lorenz Pectus bar rotational instrument

Lorenz pectus bar (2 sizes)
Thoracoscope with camera and cord

Supplies

Antiembolitic hose (adults, optional)
Foley catheter with continuous drainage unit
Sterile, plastic adhesive drape, optional
Basin set
Blades, (2) #10 and (1) #15
Electrosurgical pencil and cord with holder and scraper
Suction tubing
Needle magnet or counter
Bone wax
Umbilical tapes (2), Lorenz procedure
Closed chest drain (e.g., Pleurevac)
Chest tube (e.g., Argyle), and straight connector (5 in 1)

Special Notes

- Apply **Special Notes** from **Abdominal Laparotomy** (adults), p. 134 as they apply (in general to the surgical patient). If the patient is a child, apply **Pediatric General Information**, p. 978. Employ special pediatric considerations, e.g., warming devices, small endotracheal tubes, etc., for anesthesia administration; padded extremity restraints, smaller drapes and instruments, etc., are mandatory. Circulator should check with the blood bank to determine that the correct number of units of blood is available and ready. He/she should bring a blood administration set, blood warmer, and blood pump into the room for use in case of inadvertent hemorrhage.
- **Reminder:** Consult the suggested Patient Care Plan, p. 9, and **Special Notes** for this procedure to deliver the best care resulting in optimal patient outcomes.
- **N.B.** *Thoracotomy tray and Vascular procedures tray should be available in the room (unopened) in case the pleural space is entered inadvertently or vascular injury results in hemorrhage.*
- **Reminder:** The electrosurgical pencil tip should be kept free of debris and eschar (use the scratch pad) and kept in its holder when not in use.
- **Reminder:** Large amounts of noxious smoke and fumes resulting from thermal destruction are a health hazard; smoke should be suctioned away by the room suction with an in-line filter or with a smoke-evacuation system.

- **Reminder:** All persons in the room should wear masks (with a filtering capacity of between 2 and 5 microns) during the operative procedure to prevent inhalation of toxic matter.
- In the **Ravitch modified procedure,** the scrub person should be prepared with a mallet for use with the sternal knife (e.g., Lebsche) to split the sternum, if a power saw is not requested.
- In the **Ravitch modified procedure,** the small bone chips should be collected in a small medicine cup (moistened with normal saline).
- When two incisions are used, a sponge count is taken before the closure of each incision.

Thymectomy

Definition

Excision of the thymus gland.

Discussion

This surgery is performed in an attempt to alleviate myasthenia gravis or to remove benign or malignant tumors. The thymus gland is largest in infancy and atrophies in adulthood. When a thymectomy is performed to treat myasthenia gravis, the possibility of respiratory compromise must be anticipated. Prolonged endotracheal intubation or a tracheostomy may become necessary with the concomitant administration of neostigmine methyl sulfate (Prostigmin) and other agents.

Thymectomy can also be accomplished by ***video-assisted thoracoscopic surgery (VATS).***

Procedure

The patient is in supine position as general anesthesia is administered via endotracheal intubation. The approach is usually through a sternal splitting incision made with a power saw or a sternal splitting knife. The mediastinal fat pad is incised and the thymus gland dissected from it and the underlying pericardium. Vascular attachments are ligated. Care is taken to avoid the great vessels and the parathyroid glands. Hemostasis is achieved. A drain may be inserted. If either pleural space has been entered, a chest tube(s) and a sealed drainage unit may be necessary.

Preparation of the Patient

A forced-air warming blanket or a warming mattress pad (placed on the table before the patient enters the room) may be used. Antiembolitic hose are applied. The patient is supine; a pillow may be placed under the knees to avoid straining back muscles and for comfort. Arms may be extended on padded armboards. All bony prominences and areas vulnerable to skin and neurovascular pressure or trauma are padded. Apply electrosurgical dispersive pad. Determine whether insertion of a Foley catheter is necessary (not routinely placed). Electrosurgical dispersive pad is applied.

Skin Preparation

Begin at the midline of the upper chest, extending from the chin to below the umbilicus and down to the table at the sides. Lap pads may be placed at the sides of the neck to prevent prep solution from pooling under the patient. The pads are carefully removed when the prep is completed.

Draping

Folded towels, plastic adhesive drape (optional), and sheet with a small fenestration, e.g., "thyroidectomy" sheet

Equipment

Forced-air warming blanket or warming mattress pad, when ordered
ESU
Suction
Power source for saw (e.g., Stryker, Sarns)

Instrumentation

Basic/Minor procedures tray
Vascular procedures tray
Thoracotomy tray
Tracheostomy tray (available)
Lebsche sternal knife and mallet
Sternal saw (power), e.g., Stryker, Sarns
Rake retractors (4- and 6-prong)
Ligating clip appliers, e.g., Hemoclip appliers

Supplies

Antiembolitic hose
Adhesive plastic drape, optional
Basin set
Blades, (2) #10 and (1) #15 (adult); (2) #15 (children)
Electrosurgical pencil and cord with holder and scraper
Suction tubing
Umbilical tape (for retraction)
Dissectors (e.g., peanuts or Kittners)
Needle magnet or counter
Bone wax
Ligating clips, e.g., Hemoclips

Chest tube(s), argyle and connector, with sealed drainage unit, e.g., PleurevacDrain, e.g., Penrose (optional)

Special Notes

- Apply **Special Notes** from ***Abdominal Laparotomy***, p. 134, as the notes apply to surgical patient care in general.
- **N.B.** Clarify with the anesthesia provider as to immediate availability of drugs related to treatment of myasthenia gravis as discussed preoperatively with the internist, surgeon, and anesthesia provider.
- If lap pads are used during the skin prep, they are discarded into the kickbucket; the lap sponges are included in the count.
- Prep solution is not permitted to pool under the patient as it may be flammable. Also, prep solution that pools under the patient excoriates the skin.
- Umbilical tape and peanut or Kittner dissectors are included in the sponge counts.
- Heavy-gauge wire sutures can be used to effect a (sturdy) repair of the sternum.

Thoracoscopy

Definition

Endoscopic visualization of the pleural spaces.

Discussion

Thoracoscopy is performed to diagnose and treat pleural and intrapleural conditions including diseases of the pleura, mediastinum, pericardium, esophagus, and lungs. Assessment of thoracic trauma, tissue sampling, drainage of fluid collections, and diverse surgical procedures can be performed via this route. Procedures such as wedge resection, lobectomy, pneumonectomy, treatment for pneumothorax (secondary to pulmonary blebs and empyema), dissection of the esophagus for benign and malignant conditions, hiatal herniorrhaphy, vagotomy, or transhiatal esophagectomy via **video-assisted thoracoscopic surgery (VATS)** approach have also been performed. Esophagomyotomy, pericardial window creation, thymectomy, sympathectomy (for hyperhydrosis and for various vasospastic syndromes), and mediastinal cystectomy have been performed as well.

VATS is indicated when noninvasive or minimally invasive procedures (such as x-rays, scans, bronchoscopy, etc.) have not yielded sufficient information for diagnosis. VATS approach is ideal for patients with reduced pulmonary function for whom the risk of open thoracotomy is great. With VATS, postoperative morbidity is greatly diminished when compared to open "limited" thoracotomy. Another significant advantage to the VATS approach is that the entire hemithorax can be viewed without performing an "open" procedure.

The risks of VATS include hemorrhage, air embolism, diaphragmatic injury, or injury to adjacent organs, etc., in which case prompt conversion to open thoracotomy is required. There is questionable evidence regarding tumor seeding via the port used for specimen retrieval during VATS. Contraindications include lesions in close proximity to major central vessels and patients in whom the anesthesia provider cannot safely maintain unilateral pneumothorax. In postoperative anticoagulated cardiac patients, VATS drainage of pericardial effusion may be preferable to a repeat of the open sternotomy approach.

Robotic techniques have been introduced to thoracoscopic procedures with increasing applications.

Procedure

VATS is usually performed under general anesthesia; limited VATS may be performed employing local anesthesia at the port site, with the patient receiving *conscious sedation*. General anesthesia is administered via double-lumen endotracheal tube; the tube permits ventilation of the nonoperative lung, while permitting pneumothorax on the operative side. When the double lumen tube cannot be inserted (e.g., due to a small trachea), pneumothorax on the operative side can be increased by the judicious insufflation of CO_2 and the use of pneumatic seals (such as for laparoscopy). A nasogastric tube may be placed. Patients are monitored with an arterial line, continuous oximetry, central venous line, and urinary catheter. A thoracic epidural catheter is placed preoperatively and used for postoperative pain control.

An initial port is established at the fourth to seventh intercostal space, midaxillary to the posterior axillary line (according to the pathology and the surgeon's preference). Prior to insertion of the port, digital exploration confirms clear entrance into the pleural cavity. The telescope is inserted, the situation assessed, and the feasibility of VATS is determined. Two or three additional ports are established according to the location of the lesion. Large specimens may be retrieved through an ancillary incision (limited thoracotomy or "thoracoscopically-assisted procedure"), usually without a need to spread the ribs, although an endoscopic morcellator may be used. The specimen is retrieved in a specimen pouch (e.g., Endo Pouch™) and morcellated in the pouch before it is removed. In limited thoracotomy, VATS endoscopic instruments are employed to retract, dissect, ligate, excise, and suture tissues, but standard thoracotomy instruments may be used as well. The Nd:YAG laser may be used to excise small lesions not amenable to stapling. Specimens can be retrieved in a specimen bag (e.g., Endo Pouch or LapSac®) to avoid seeding of malignant cells or spreading infectious matter. Upon conclusion of the procedure, a chest tube is inserted through a port; it is connected to a closed drainage unit. The incisions are closed in the usual manner. The chest tube may be removed prior to the patient's leaving the OR, or it may be removed in the PACU after a lesser procedure has been performed.

Preparation of the Patient

Antiembolitic hose are applied. A sequential compression device with disposable leg wraps may be applied over the antiembolitic hose. A forced-air warming blanket may be used in conjunction with the fluoroscopy. General anesthesia is administered through a double-lumen endotracheal tube. The patient is usually in the lateral position with the affected side uppermost. The arm on the unaffected side is placed on a padded armboard (pressure points are padded). A small axillary roll may be placed under the patient's dependent arm. The arm on the affected side is angled toward the head and supported by a Mayo stand padded with a pillow (or a padded double armboard may be used). The torso is stabilized with padded kidney rests (larger blade in front) and/or pillows, sandbags, or a beanbag. The leg on the unaffected side (down) is flexed; the leg on the affected side (uppermost) may be extended, or it may be slightly flexed. A pillow is placed between the legs, and pressure points at the knee, ankle, and foot are padded. After the skin is sprayed with tincture of benzoin, the position is secured by wide adhesive tape at the shoulder, hip, and legs and anchored to the underside of the table. All bony prominences and areas vulnerable to skin and neurovascular pressure or trauma are padded. Check with the surgeon regarding the insertion of a Foley catheter. Apply electrosurgical dispersive pad.

Skin Preparation

Begin cleansing at the level of the nipple on the affected side, extending from the shoulder and axilla to the iliac crest and down to the table anteriorly and posteriorly.

Draping

Folded towels, a sterile, adhesive plastic drape, and a laparotomy or transverse sheet

Additional drape sheets may be requested.

Equipment

Sequential compression device with leg wraps

Forced-air warming blanket

CVP line (to anesthesia provider)

Arterial line (to anesthesia provider)
Padded kidney rests, pillow(s), padding for positioning and tincture of benzoin
ESU (bipolar) and (unipolar)
Suction
Endoscopy cart:
ESU
Suction
Irrigator system with pressure sensor
CD burner
Fiber-optic light source, e.g., Xenon 300 W
Video monitors (2)
CO_2 insufflation device to increase pneumothorax pressure (infrequent)
Camera console
Printer
VCR
CD burner
Argon beam coagulator unit (optional)
Nd:YAG laser fiber (noncontact), optional

Instrumentation

Endoscopic:
Trocars, 2 10- to 11-mm blunt, 2 10- to 12-mm sharp (available as disposable); 0° and 30° telescopes, flexible with cameras and cords, reducers, lung retractor (e.g., Naticoke), electrosurgical suction-irrigator and cord, dissectors, graspers (Allis, Babcock, tonsil, right angle, Pennington), vascular forceps, scissors (hook, micro, and straight blunt and sharp), disposable
Multifire ligating clip applier, as requested
Semm morcellator

Limited incision, Add
Modified ring forceps, lung retractor, and ligating clip applier preloaded with clips
Argon beam coagulator hand piece and flue
Laser, fiber, e.g., Nd:YAG, optional

For Limited Thoracotomy or Should the Procedure Need to Be Converted to an "Open" Procedure, Add
Major procedures tray, available
Thoracotomy tray, available
Vascular procedures tray, available
Ligating clip appliers, e.g., Hemoclips, available

Supplies

Antiembolitic hose
Foley catheter and drainage unit (optional)
N/G tube to anesthesia provider, optional
Sterile, adhesive plastic drape, optional
Magnetic instrument pad
Basin set
Blades, (1) #10 and (1) #15
Suction tubing
Electrosurgical pencil and cord with holder and scraper
Ligating clips, e.g., Hemoclips, available
Trocars (available as disposable, optional)
Electrosurgical cord for bipolar endoscopic electrosurgical forceps
Defogging agent, e.g., ELVIS™ or FRED®
Sealed drainage unit (e.g., Pleurevac)
Chest drainage tube (e.g., Argyle #28, adult) with straight or "Y" connector
Loop sutures (e.g., Endoloop®), suturing device with introducer sleeve (intracorporeal)
Impervious specimen retrieval bag (e.g., Endo Pouch)
Skin suture, staples, or adhesive skin closure strips (e.g., Steristrips™), optional

Special Notes

- Apply **Special Notes** from **Bronchoscopy**, p. 448 and ***Segmental Resection***, p. 455, as indicated.
- **Reminder:** The circulator must ascertain that there are two working suctions in the room, in addition to the one on the anesthesia cart, before bringing the patient into the room in case of hemorrhage.
- The circulator and scrub person must be prepared to convert to an "open" procedure at any time. A crucial principle: the procedure is "convert to an open procedure if proper treatment of the pathologic condition or patient safety is compromised by reduced exposure."
- Conversion to an open procedure requires additional sponge, needle, and instrument counts for the second procedure with documentation in the Perioperative Record.
- ***Observe all laser safety precautions, p. 94, when the laser is employed.***
- **N.B.** If the opposite side is also to be operated on, the patient is repositioned, reprepped, and redraped; the anesthesia provider repositions endobronchial tubes accordingly.

- Care is also taken not to over-flex or damage flexible fiber-optic instrumentation. Rigid fiber-optic scopes, instruments, and light cables must also be handled with great care to avoid breaking the light fibers.
- Strict observance of manufacturer's recommendations for disinfection and sterilization must be followed (e.g., using ethylene oxide, peracetic acid, or hydrogen peroxide gas plasma).
- NOTE: All nondisposable thoracoscopy instruments may be flash-sterilized.
- Steris 20™ (peracetic acid) solution system (most frequently employed) may be used to sterilize instruments; the instrument must be completely submerged for 12 minutes at 122°F to 131°F (50°C to 55°C) for sterilization conditions to be met; see p. 43. Rinse instrumentation well, as Steris is caustic.

Video-Assisted Thoracoscopic (VATS) Wedge Resection of the Lung

Definition

Excision of a wedge-shaped section from the periphery of the lung via thoracoscopy (VATS).

Discussion

VATS wedge resection of the lung can provide a large biopsy specimen when diffuse pulmonary disease is present. An isolated lesion may be excised in its entirety during (VATS), sparing the patient an open thoracotomy procedure. The excision of lesions thoroscopically, such as primary benign and malignant lesions, metastatic malignant lesions, or localized infectious lesions or bullae, may be treated by this modality. Specimens can be retrieved in a specimen bag (e.g., Endo Pouch or LapSac) to avoid seeding of malignant cells or spreading of infectious matter.

Procedure

A forced-air warming blanket may be used in conjunction with the fluoroscopy. The patient is in supine position. General anesthesia is established with a double-lumen endotracheal tube. A nasogastric tube may be placed. Patients are monitored with an arterial line, continuous oximetry, central venous line, and urinary catheter. A thoracic epidural catheter may be placed preoperatively and used for postoperative pain control.

The ports are established. The pathology is assessed. When surgical excision is the determination, the tissue surrounding the lesion is grasped. A staple line is placed to provide an appropriate margin of clearance surrounding the lesion. Alternating approaches with a grasping forceps and stapler are made (through different ports, if necessary). A third staple line completes the wedge for resection, and the specimen is retrieved using an endoscopic specimen bag (e.g., Endo Pouch or LapSac) to avoid seeding of malignant cells or spreading infectious matter. Hemostasis is ascertained by checking for air leakage using saline while partially inflating the collapsed lung. An Nd:YAG laser fiber may be employed to achieve local hemostasis and seal air leaks. Whereas the laser can be used to excise the specimen altogether, the stapler is faster and gives more satisfactory hemostasis and control. Peri-Strips Dry can be applied to the stapler jaws to enhance sealing of the staple line. A chest tube is placed through one of the port sites. The incisions closed. The chest tube is connected to a closed-suction drainage unit.

For **Preparation of the Patient, Skin Preparation, Draping, Equipment, Instrumentation, Supplies,** and **Special Notes,** see **Thoracoscopy (VATS),** p. 476.

Instrumentation, add: (disposable) automatic endostapler, e.g., EZ 45 or Endo GIA

Special Notes, add:

- Apply **Special Notes** from ***Segmental Resection,*** p. 457.
- A thoracic epidural catheter may be placed preoperatively and used for postoperative pain control when the patient is in the **PACU** and later on the floor unit.

Video-Assisted Thoracoscopic (VATS) Pneumonectomy

Definition

Transthoracoscopic (VATS) pneumonectomy (excision of the entire lung).

Discussion

The indications for VATS pneumonectomy are malignant neoplasms and extensive unilateral pulmonary disease resulting from trauma, congenital deformity, extensive bronchiectasis, or chronic abscess. Lymph node-bearing tissues are excised, as necessary. Potential complications arise due to a mediastinal "shift" when the affected pleural cavity is empty, causing central circulatory compromise. Special measures may be employed to stabilize the mediastinum at the end of the procedure by adjusting the pressure in the affected pleural space (e.g., not to exceed greater than negative 10 cm of water). The mediastinum is stabilized by measuring the intrathoracic pressure and aspirating the residual air in the chest until the desired pressure is reached in the pleural cavity.

Procedure

General anesthesia is established with a double-lumen endotracheal tube. A nasogastric tube may be placed to facilitate identification of the esophagus during the posterior extrapleural dissection. Patients are monitored with an arterial line, continuous oximetry, central venous line, and urinary catheter. A thoracic epidural catheter may be placed preoperatively and used for postoperative pain control. The patient is placed in the lateral position. Three ports are established. Ports are made at the posterior and anterior axillary lines; in addition, a submammary incision (6 cm) may be made (limited thoracotomy). Following an assessment of the pathology, lung tissue is seized with grasping and forceps, and the lung is retracted anteriorly and inferiorly. Major vessels are dissected, stapled, and divided. (Prior to division of major vessels, a vascular clamp is loosely placed proximal to the site of division in case of mechanical failure of the staple line.) Division of the inferior pulmonary ligament permits exposure of the inferior pulmonary vein. The main stem bronchus is exposed, peribronchial nodes removed, and the bronchus stapled and divided. The superior pulmonary vein is divided, periaortic nodes are excised, and the specimen is removed through the inframammary incision. During the procedure, standard instruments may be introduced through this incision. The incisions are closed after placement of a chest tube through the lower posterior port site. Measures are taken to stabilize the mediastinum; see above.

For **Preparation of the Patient, Skin Preparation, Draping, Equipment, Instrumentation, Supplies,** and **Special Notes,** see **Video-Assisted Thoracoscopy (VATS),** p. 476.

Video-Assisted Thoracoscopic (VATS) Esophagogastromyotomy

Definition

Division of the longitudinal and circular muscles of the distal esophagus employing VATS.

Discussion

This procedure is performed to treat achalasia of the esophagus, a neuromuscular disorder characterized by failure of the lower esophageal sphincter to relax. Initial symptoms include dysphasia and, later, as the esophagus dilates above this functional obstruction, regurgitation and weight loss. After a thorough investigation and failure of pharmacologic agents and balloon dilation, surgical division of the distal esophageal muscle fibers gives lasting relief. This procedure (**modified Heller procedure**) is performed transabdominally (see p. 191) or transthoracically and by thoracoscopic approach (VATS). Proponents of this latter approach believe that it provides a more complete visualization of the operative field with less trauma to surrounding structures than the open procedure. The laparoscopic approach may be used, but thoracoscopy is more direct and probably less destructive to the structures about the esophageal obstruction. Prophylactic antibiotics are administered immediately prior to surgery.

Procedure

General anesthesia via a double-lumen endotracheal tube is administered. Patients are monitored with an arterial line, continuous oximetry, central venous line, and urinary catheter. A thoracic epidural catheter may be placed preoperatively for postoperative pain control. The patient is in the right lateral position. Five ports are employed. A flexible fiber-optic gastroscope is passed to aid in the identification of the esophagus. Traction and manipulation are employed to minimize the extent of dissection. The lung is retracted and the inferior pulmonary ligament divided. The esophagus is identified, and the outer longitudinal and inner circular muscle fibers are divided (using an electrosurgical hook or scissors) from the level of the inferior pulmonary vein to the diaphragm. Care is taken to avoid injury to the mucosa. Pressure on the diaphragm reveals the esophagocardiac junction, and the final division of fibers is continued onto the cardia of the stomach. The divided muscle is bluntly separated to 40% of the circumference of the esophagus to prevent adherence during the healing process. The esophageal hiatus is repaired as necessary. The adequacy of the myotomy is assessed. Careful hemostasis is achieved. A chest tube is placed through a lower port. The incisions are closed. At the completion of the procedure, the effect of the repair can be directly visualized. The chest tube is connected to a closed-suction unit.

For **Preparation of the Patient, Skin Preparation, Draping, Equipment, Instrumentation, Supplies,** and **Special Notes,** see **Thoracoscopy,** p. 476.

Equipment, Add

Fiber-optic light source for the gastroscope (e.g., Xenon 300W)

Instrumentation, Add

Fiber-optic gastroscope and cord

***Endoscopic instruments*:**

Electrosurgical suction irrigator/dissector with J hook or right angle tip, scissors (hook, straight, and micro), multifire ligating clip appliers, grasping clamps, and suturing device with sleeve

CHAPTER 21
Vascular Surgery

Carotid Endarterectomy

Definition
Excision of plaque from the intima (inner lining) of the carotid artery.

Discussion
Plaque that forms on the intima of arteries is caused by arteriosclerosis. Fragments of (inflamed) plaque or adherent blood clots migrating distally can cause transient ischemic attacks (TIA) or complete blockage of the larger carotid artery branches, resulting in stroke/cerebrovascular accident (CVA). **Carotid endarterectomy (CEA)** restores carotid arterial blood flow, enhances cerebral circulation, and often prevents CVA. In postendarterectomy patients, "restenosis" may result from radiation therapy. Carotid endarterectomy with angioplasty was thought for many years to be best treatment for stenotic cerebral arteries. When the patient's condition requires a bilateral procedure, the second surgery is performed a week after the first. Restenosis can be treated by endarterectomy and the application of a patch graft made of synthetic material (e.g., woven Dacron or other fabric), or an autologous (e.g., saphenous vein) patch graft was applied and fixed with fine vascular nonabsorbable suture. Plaque embolization may occur during or following carotid endarterectomy.

Except when the diagnosis is acute carotid obstruction, the surgeon must spend adequate time making a careful assessment of the patient's condition. To optimally time the surgery for the patient, the surgeon evaluates circulatory, neurological, and general medical considerations as they pertain to the individual patient. If there is concomitant coronary artery disease (CAD), this must be corrected by angioplastic (endovascular) or surgical means, e.g., ***coronary artery bypass graft (CABG)*** (p. 521) before the carotid procedure. Also, before and during carotid endarterectomy, the need for an intraoperative shunt must be evaluated. Arteriographic studies of the contralateral carotid, backflow as observed surgically, and neurological response of the patient (if under local block) help the surgeon to assess the patient's status.

Today, many surgeons believe the best treatment for carotid artery stenosis is the insertion of a drug-coated *endovascular stent* inserted percutaneously via femoral artery puncture (or less often via direct carotid artery cut down) under fluoroscopic guidance, avoiding open surgery. The choice to proceed with the endovascular stent is an especially important option for patients at "high risk." The endovascular stent does not require suture because it is either self-expanding or it exerts intravascular pressure. The stent inherently creates hemostasis. This procedure is performed in a special procedure room in the radiology department.

For some patients in whom the artery is either completely obstructed by plaque or the plaque is too hard to permit the insertion of a stent (with a large enough lumen for it to be effective), **carotid endarterectomy** with the insertion of a polytetrafluroethylene (PTFE) or Dacron patch graft remains the best treatment. In situations where the state of the carotid arterial wall is deemed too fragile to hold sutures to perform endarterectomy, a prosthetic graft or vein may be placed from the common carotid to the internal carotid as an extraluminal bypass around the site of the obstruction.

Vein harvesting for an autologous graft may be performed as an endoscopic procedure.

Procedure

An incision is made along the anterior border of the sternomastoid muscle. The carotid sheath is exposed and incised. Care is taken to identify and prevent injury to cranial nerve branches (X, XI, XII) and ansa cervicalis. Proximal and distal control of the carotid artery and its bifurcation is achieved with vascular clamps and/or umbilical tapes and vessel loops. Arteriotomy is made with a #11 blade and continued with Pott's scissors. At this time, if a shunt is to be placed, it is passed proximal and distal to the arteriotomy and secured by tapes (or Rummel tourniquet). Plaque is freed from the arterial wall by blunt dissection. Care is taken to extract all plaque and debris to prevent subsequent embolization. A *bypass graft patch* is applied from the common carotid artery to the internal carotid artery. If an intimal flap has developed, it is tacked to the vessel wall with fine sutures to prevent dissection when blood flow is restored. The arterial lumen is flushed with a heparinized saline solution. The arteriotomy is closed, or if the lumen appears stenotic, a patch graft (autogenous, e.g., saphenous vein graft or synthetic graft) may be employed. Prior to placement of the final sutures when a shunt has been used, the shunt is removed and the arterial lumen is flushed once again with heparinized saline solution to remove any residual debris or air bubbles. Hemostasis is assured. The wound is closed in layers. A drain may be employed.

Preparation of the Patient

A forced-air warming blanket may be used when requested. Central venous pressure (CVP), arterial, and venous pressure lines are placed. Continuous electroencephalography (EEG) to monitor brain activity and transesophageal echocardiography is employed to monitor cardiac function. When an autograft will not be taken, antiembolitic hose and a sequential compression device with disposable leg wraps may be employed. The disposable leg wraps are applied over the antiembolitic hose. The patient may receive a local block or general anesthesia via endotracheal intubation. Prior to the arteriotomy, systemic heparinization may be requested. The patient is in supine position with the neck slightly extended; a rolled towel may be placed transversely between the scapulae. The head is supported by a padded headrest (doughnut) and turned toward the unaffected side. Excessive rotation of the head and extension of the neck is avoided because this significantly decreases blood flow to the carotid and vertebral arteries. Arms may be extended on padded armboards (that permit vascular access). A pillow may be placed under the knees to avoid strain on back muscles and for comfort. All bony prominences and areas prone to skin and neurovascular pressure or trauma are padded. Foley catheter is not routinely placed. An electrosurgical dispersive pad is applied.

Skin Preparation

When a synthetic graft "patch" is used, before starting the prep, place a cotton ball in the patient's ear on the affected side. Towels or lap sponges may be placed at the sides of the neck to prevent prep solution from pooling under the neck. Begin at the neck on the affected side, extending from just above the infra-auricular border to just below the level of the axilla (include the axilla), and prep down to the table at the sides.

Circulator should remove the towels or lap sponges very carefully; the lap sponges are part of the count.

For an autologous "patch" graft, in addition to prep above, both legs are usually prepared; a second prep tray is needed. Two people are required to prepare the legs (front and back), including the feet, or one person can prep using a leg holder and sterile towels, as necessary.

Draping

When a synthetic "patch" graft is used, folded towels and a sheet with a small fenestration (e.g., thyroid sheet) are placed.

For an autologous "patch" graft, both saphenous veins usually need to be available for "autografting"; a folded towel (thirds lengthwise) is placed over the genital area after placing towels around the operative site, followed by the thyroid drape. The bottom end of the thyroid drape is brought down over the genital area while the legs are held up. The feet are covered with impervious tube stockinettes or rubber gloves (placed over the feet). Two large drape sheets are tucked under the legs covering the distal end of the table, and the sheets are clipped around the thighs.

Drape for microscope, when used.

Equipment

Forced-air warming blanket, optional
Sequential compression device with disposable leg wraps, as requested
Leg holder (for ***autograft***), optional
Padded headrest (e.g., doughnut)
Electrosurgical unit (ESU)
Suction
Headlight and fiber-optic light source (optional)
Doppler box (with coupling gel), optional
Scales (2) to weigh sponges (available)
Magnifying loupes or microscope (e.g., Olympus, optional)
Power source for Hall drill

Instrumentation

Basic/minor procedures and shunt trays
Self-retaining retractor, e.g., Weitlaner (without teeth)
Ligating clip appliers, e.g., Hemoclip® appliers, short (small and medium)
Rummel tourniquet, optional
Doppler probe and cord, optional
High-speed drill, e.g., Hall oscillating endarterectomy valvutome
Microscopic instruments:
Micro tissue forceps, curved smooth forceps (2), curved tying forceps, micro-dissector, and Castroviejo needle holder (optional)

Supplies

Antiembolitic hose (if synthetic graft is used)
CVP and vascular pressure line accessories to anesthesia provider
Impervious stockinettes or gloves to cover the feet (for **autograft**)
Basin set
Blades, (2) #10, (1) #15, (1) #11
Electrosurgical pencil and cord with holder and scraper
Suction tubing
Umbilical tapes, vessel loops (for retraction)
Dissectors (e.g., peanut)
Heparin (interferes with blood clotting mechanism) administered intravenously (IV) (to anesthesia provider) or diluted with normal saline for irrigation

Antibiotics IV or diluted for irrigation
Protamine sulfate (heparin antagonist, reverses action of heparin)
Sterile labels, marking pen, and medicine cups
Graduate and disposable syringes, including bulb for heparinized saline
Hemostatic agents (e.g., Gelfoam, Hemopad, Helistat, Avitene, Surgicel™, Oxycel, Thrombin, or fibrin glue)
Ligating clips, e.g., Hemoclips (small, medium)
Shunt (e.g., Javid or polyvinyl tubing may be customized to fit), available
Drain, e.g., closed-suction, Hemovac™

Special Notes

- Apply **Special Notes** from ***Abdominal Laparotomy***, p. 134, as indicated.
- Determine that the patient's x-ray studies are in the room for the *correct* patient.
- **N.B.** *Verify that there are two working suctions in the room before starting surgery.*
- The circulator assists the anesthesia provider during induction of anesthesia, e.g., during endotracheal intubation (by applying pressure to cricoid cartilage) or by injecting medications the anesthesia provider has prepared (at his/her direction), etc. For the circulator's role during anesthesia administration, see p. 81.
- Care is taken during the skin prep not to allow prep solution to pool under the patient, as it may cause excessive excoriation to the skin; it also may be flammable. A cotton ball is placed in the ear on the affected side to prevent prep solution from dripping into the ear. Document the condition of the skin preoperatively and postoperatively.
- Both legs are usually prepped when an autograft will be taken. Two people are required to prepare the legs (front and back), including the feet, or one person may prep using a leg holder and sterile towels, as necessary.
- The circulator assists the anesthesia provider to obtain vascular access for intravenous lines for measuring arterial and venous pressures and CVP and documents the treatments.
- Circulator ascertains that blood is available and ready for immediate use as ordered by calling the blood bank. When the surgery is elective, the patient may have given blood in advance for an auto infusion.

- The circulator should ascertain if the cell-saver is required before starting the surgery. If additional (specialized) assistance is necessary, notify the supervisor (or the person in charge or the qualified person), according to hospital policy. It should be set up in advance of the surgery.
- When the cell-saver is used, all intraoperative blood is suctioned, filtered, and reinfused into the patient. The scrub person should squeeze blood out of sponges following use, before discarding them into the kick bucket. The cell-saver is used only when the blood is free of contamination; it cannot be employed once antibiotic irrigation or any other drug is used.
- Circulator anticipates the possibility of blood transfusion(s) and obtains items necessary for administration (e.g., tubing set, blood warmer, pressure bag) and assists the anesthesia provider to monitor hemodynamics and to administer blood (identify patient and blood type, etc.).
- Circulator documents blood administration and any reaction or lack of reaction to the transfusion in the **Perioperative Record**.
- The circulator and the anesthesia provider continuously monitor the patient's neurological status. When local block anesthetic is used, the neurological status of the patient can be determined by conversing with the patient. When the patient receives general anesthesia, neurological status must be viewed by continuous monitoring of EEG. Assessment and documentation of the patient's neurological status is done for patient safety (and continuity of care) and for medicolegal reasons.
- **Reminder:** Use safety precautions to identify, label, and dispense medications or solutions and to avoid medication errors; see p. 30. It is mandatory that all medications and solutions on the sterile field be labeled by name and strength. The medication bottle is retained in the room until the procedure has concluded.
- When the surgeon uses a headlight, the circulator safety pins the cord to the back of the gown. The circulator attaches the cord to the fiber-optic light source when the surgeon indicates that the light is needed.
- The circulator notes the time and documents both carotid pulses (manually or by Doppler) before starting the skin prep.
- Using the Doppler requires coupling gel to effectively transmit sound. The Doppler probe and cord of some devices may be sterilized and used in the operative field.

- The circulator should obtain sterile grafts (various types and sizes); grafts should be *available* in the room before the surgery is started. Consult the surgeon regarding the type of graft preferred.
- The scrub person may be asked to "prepare the shunt for insertion." The graft is usually prepared by "clotting," i.e., immersing the graft in a small amount of blood (in an emesis basin) before its insertion.
- Fibrin glue may be requested to obtain hemostasis. Fibrin glue is composed of cryoprecipitate (bovine), thrombin, and calcium; it is applied directly onto a bleeding area to form a fibrin patch.
- **N.B.** *The circulator (in addition to the anesthesia provider) notes and documents the time at which the aortic artery is cross-clamped.*
- **N.B.** *Every effort is made by the surgical team to minimize the amount of time the carotid artery is clamped; organization of equipment, efficiency of movement, and attention to the wound site by the scrub person are extremely important.*
- Scrub person chooses self-retaining retractors (e.g., Weitlaner) with dull teeth to avoid injury to blood vessels.
- Umbilical tapes and vessel loops used for retraction are pre-moistened with normal saline before they are passed on a clamp (e.g., tonsil forceps/clamp).
- **N.B.** *Scrub person* **should not** *cut double-armed sutures used in vascular surgery.*
- When a femoral incision is made for saphenous vein "harvesting," counts are taken before the second incision is made and at the closure of each incision.
- Maintain an accurate record of irrigation used and weigh sponges (when indicated) to determine blood loss and fluid replacement.
- **Reminder:** *Persons scrubbed should wear a protective face shield to prevent injury from splashing or spraying of the patient's blood and irrigation fluids that are used.*
- Document the type, size, and serial numbers of a synthetic graft in the **Perioperative Record** and in the hospital's log for insertion of an implant, according to policy.
- The circulator accompanies the patient to the postanesthesia care unit (PACU) and reports intraoperative information and any other significant information regarding the patient, e.g., allergies to medications (for patient safety and for continuity of care) to the PACU perioperative practitioner.
- The patient's neurological status, in addition to the patient's vital signs, is continuously monitored in the PACU.

Abdominal Aortic Procedures (Abdominal Aortic Aneurysmectomy, Abdominal Aortic Endarterectomy) with Aortoiliac Graft

Definitions

Aortic Aneurysmectomy is the excision of an attenuated (dilated and weakened) widening of the aorta (aneurysm).

Aortic Endarterectomy is the removal of plaque from the intima (lining) of the aorta.

Aortic Bypass is the anastomosis of an aortic graft directly to iliac or femoral vessels *bypassing* any blockage or stenosis in the aorta.

Discussion

In patients with abdominal aortic aneurysm (AAA), the aortic wall has weakened and dilation has occurred. A thrombus may fill most of the increased lumen, creating a potential source of embolus; the aneurysm may rupture *freely* with massive bleeding into the retroperitoneal space, or may rupture *intramurally* and produce a dissection with significant bleeding and obstruction of aortic branches. These latter presentations constitute an extreme surgical emergency. In *abdominal aortic aneurysmectomy,* the diseased portion of the aorta is excised and a tubular graft (synthetic) is inserted to reestablish vascular continuity. When the iliac arteries are involved, aortoiliac bifurcated Y-graft is employed. Aortic and iliac "extender cuffs" are available for use, as necessary. Suitable veins are not always available for use as grafts. Dacron or PTFE grafts are employed for bypass. Dacron grafts are available coated with protein (collagen/albumin) that reduces blood loss and antibiotics that prevent graft infection. Impregnated grafts are considerably more expensive than the noncoated grafts. PTFE grafts are often preferred by the surgeon, as they are composed of Teflon velour with a smooth inner surface and are less thrombogenic than the Dacron grafts. Neointimal hyperplasia that may occur at the distal anastomosis is reduced when a segment of vein is incorporated as either a Millar Cuff or Taylor Patch. Complications that arise from using synthetic grafts include occlusion or infection and the formation of true or false aneurysms at the graft site, embolization of plaque fragments, and erosion of the graft into adjacent structures, e.g., aorto-enteric fistulae.

Patients with AAA frequently have concomitant coronary artery disease that can lead to myocardial infarction following surgery. AAA occurs more frequently in men and is often detected by routine chest x-ray. AAA does not usually rupture spontaneously but may dissect acutely (as noted above) with severe symptoms (such as back pain, hypotension, etc.). When surgery is appropriate, it is most often done as an elective procedure under controlled circumstances. Should the aneurysm rupture during surgery, the most important factor is controlling the hemorrhage. Postoperatively, patients are at risk for renal damage.

Endovascular stent/endoluminal stent (e.g., SMART®, Acculink™, Guidant, or AneuRx®) is utilized in appropriate patients, especially "high-risk" patients who are unable to tolerate an open procedure. The endovascular stent graft may be inserted in patients in whom there is a proximal renal "neck" of at least 1 to 2 cm. The stent graft is inserted via bilateral femoral artery cut downs and is fixed by self-expanding stent, or a "balloon" type stent exerts intravascular pressure on "mini-hooks" at the terminal ends of each segment (creating a hemostatic seal). For patients with aortic rupture caused by blunt force, endovascular stent graft insertion may be appropriate treatment. The advantages of placing an endovascular stent graft are shorter operating time, avoidance of ***cardiopulmonary bypass*** (if thoracoabdominal), decreased need for general anesthesia, lack of aortic cross clamp time, and the avoidance of an open procedure when feasible.

Endovascular stent placement is not an appropriate treatment for all patients, as the site (location) of the aneurysm may make insertion difficult. Tortuous arteries may be impossible to cannulate. For these patients, incorporation of a graft must be considered.

Procedure

The open procedures are described. AAA is approached by a long midline incision. The intestines are mobilized, protected, and packed out of the field. The posterior parietal peritoneum is incised, and the aorta is exposed. Care is taken to identify and protect the inferior vena cava, renal artery, and ureters. When AAA involves the inferior mesenteric artery, the artery may be sacrificed (or preserved if backflow is brisk). Proximal and distal control is obtained with vascular forceps (e.g., DeBakey). The aneurysm is opened, endarterectomy is performed, the vessel is flushed with heparinized saline, and clot(s) are evacuated. The lumbar vessels are sutured, leaving the posterior portion of the aneurysm in situ. The common iliac arteries (when involved) are transected and anastomosed to the aorta utilizing a bifurcated graft/prosthesis (autologous or synthetic) for the *bypass*. If the aneurysm is located higher in the abdomen, a tubular graft/prosthesis is employed. When appropriate, the inferior mesenteric artery (distally) or renal artery (proximally) may require reimplantation. When the graft has been sewn into place, the vascular control clamps are removed and the anastomoses are tested for leakage. The shell of the aneurysm may be sutured about the graft for "reinforcement." Hemostasis is assured. The abdomen is closed in the usual manner.

When a section of the aorta is bypassed, a graft is anastomosed from a location on the aorta (according to the level of patency) directly to iliac or femoral vessels, *bypassing* any blockage or stenosis, and the need for extensive endarterectomy is eliminated. In endarterectomy of the aorta and iliac vessels, the vessels are incised, plaque and clots are removed, and the vessels are repaired (with or without patch graft). Various combinations of these techniques can be employed. Local anticoagulation with heparinized saline is used prior to closure of the anastomoses; blood clots are flushed out by the transient release of the control clamps. The posterior peritoneum is closed, and the wound is closed.

Preparation of the Patient

A forced-air warming blanket may be requested. Antiembolitic hose are applied when the graft used is synthetic; antiembolitic hose cannot be used when an autograft (using the saphenous vein) is performed. The anesthesia provider, assisted by the circulator, inserts lines to monitor arterial, central venous, and pulmonary artery pressures. Continuous transesophageal echocardiography is employed. The patient is placed in supine position; a pillow may be placed under the knees to avoid strain on the back muscles and for comfort. Arms may be extended on padded armboards (that permit venous access). All bony prominences and areas prone to skin and neurovascular pressure or trauma are padded. Consult with the surgeon regarding insertion of a Foley catheter. Apply electrosurgical dispersive pad.

Skin Preparation

Begin at the midline, extending from axilla to mid-thighs and to the table at the sides.

Draping

A folded towel (thirds lengthwise) placed over pubic area, folded towels around the operative site, followed by two sterile, plastic adhesive drapes (optional) and a laparotomy sheet (which may be cut with straight Mayo scissors).

A drape is needed for the microscope, when used.

Equipment

Forced-air warming blanket, when requested
Sequential compression device with disposable leg wraps, optional
CVP or Swan-Ganz, and vascular pressure line accessories to anesthesia provider
Cell-saver, optional
ESU
Suctions (2)
Scales (2) for weighing sponges
Headlight and fiber-optic light source, optional
Doppler box with coupling gel, optional

Instrumentation

Major procedures tray
Abdominal and thoracic vascular procedures tray
Sterile Doppler probe, optional
Self-retaining retractors, e.g., Bookwalter (large) and Weitlaner (2 small)
Harrington retractors (2)
Extra towel clips for draping
Ligating clip appliers, e.g., Hemoclip appliers (various sizes and lengths)
Sterile Doppler probe and cord, optional

Supplies

Antiembolitic hose
Foley catheter and continuous drainage unit
Sterile, plastic adhesive drapes (2), optional
Basin set
Blades, (2) #10, (1) #15, (1) #11
Needle magnet or counter
Suction tubings (2)
Electrosurgical pencil and cord with holder and scraper
Penrose drains, umbilical tapes, vessel loops (for retraction)
Dissectors (e.g., peanut)
Hemostatic agent (e.g., Avitene, Surgicel, Thrombostat)
Needle, 18-gauge (to vent the vena cava, to prevent air embolus)
Ligating clips, e.g., Hemoclips (all sizes)
Sterile marking pen with indelible ink, labels, and medicine cups and syringes
Heparin (anticoagulant) diluted to surgeon's preference is added to normal saline for heparinized saline
Graduated pitcher and assorted syringes, including bulb (for heparinized saline)
Protamine sulfate (heparin antagonist, reverses action of heparin)
Antibiotic (intravenous or for irrigation), optional
Shunt graft may be autologous or synthetic, sterilized, e.g., Dacron "patch" or collagen-impregnated graft
Endovascular stent graft, e.g., AneuRX, Acculink, Guidant, or SMART (shape memory alloy recoverable technology), etc.

Special Notes

- Apply **Special Notes** from **Abdominal Laparotomy**, p. 134.
- **Reminder:** Ascertain that the patient's x-ray studies are in the room for the *correct* patient.

- **Reminder:** *Verify that there are two working suctions in the room before starting the surgery.*
- **Reminder:** Circulator assists the anesthesia provider in establishing vascular access for CVP, arterial, and venous lines and assists in hemodynamic monitoring.
- The anesthesia provider and the circulator continuously monitor and assess the patient's neurological status. Documentation of the patient's neurological status is done for patient safety (continuity of care) and for medicolegal reasons.
- **N.B.** *The circulator (in addition to the anesthesia provider) notes and documents the time at which the aortic artery is cross-clamped.*
- **N.B.** Every effort is made by the surgical team to minimize the amount of time the carotid artery is clamped; organization of equipment, efficiency of movement, and attention to the wound site by the scrub person are extremely important.
- **Reminder:** Circulator ascertains that blood is available as ordered and ready for immediate use. Blood for transfusion may have been given to the blood bank in advance in anticipation of the need.
- Circulator anticipates possible blood transfusion(s) and obtains items for blood administration (e.g., tubing set, blood warmer, pressure bag). Circulator assists the anesthesia provider to administer blood and to monitor hemodynamics.
- The circulator and anesthesia provider (together) verify that the blood (and type) is *correct* for the *correctly* identified patient. Compare the blood type and identification number on each unit with the patient's identification. Document that this has been done.
- Document any reaction to blood administered (or the absence of a reaction) for medicolegal purposes.
- **N.B.** *Circulator marks (with indelible pen) both pedal pulses before preparing the skin. Documentation is made of pulses and times taken (either manually or by Doppler).*
- **Reminder:** When an incision is made for saphenous vein "harvesting," counts are taken before the second incision is made and at the closure of each incision.
- **Reminder:** Use safety precautions to identify, label, and dispense medications or solutions and to avoid medication errors; see p. 30. It is mandatory that all medications and solutions on the sterile field be labeled by name and strength. The medication bottle is retained in the room until the procedure has concluded. Document medications used and precautions taken.

- **Reminder:** The electrosurgical pad is applied to skin that is relatively hair-free to obtain good contact (as close to the surgical site as possible). It may be necessary to (wet) shave the area.
- The electrosurgical pencil tip should be kept free of debris and eschar (use the scratch pad) and kept in its holder when not in use.
- Smoke and fumes from thermal destruction are a health hazard; smoke should be suctioned away using the room suction with an in-line filter or with a smoke-evacuation system. Everyone present should wear a mask (with a filtering capacity of between 2 and 5 microns) to prevent inhalation of toxic matter.
- **N.B.** *The scrub person should keep a spongestick (raytec sponge mounted on a sponge forceps) available at all times for applying pressure in case of hemorrhage.*
- Assorted grafts should be in the room before surgery is started. Consult with surgeon to determine the type and size of graft to be used. Sterilize and prepare the synthetic graft for use according to surgeon's directions.
- Document the type, size, and serial numbers of the graft in the **Perioperative Record** and in the facility's log for insertion of an implant, according to hospital policy.
- **N.B.** Scrub person notes that double-armed sutures used in vascular surgery are **not** cut.
- The circulator should have a variety of irrigation and balloon embolectomy catheters in the room prior to starting the procedure, e.g., Fogarty.
- Warm saline is used for irrigation and to moisten sponges to be used intra-abdominally. Umbilical tapes and vessel loops are moistened with normal saline before passing them on a clamp (e.g., tonsil forceps/clamp).
- Note the amount of urinary drainage (output) and document the amount at the start of the procedure, as requested during the procedure, and at the conclusion of the procedure for patient safety (continuity of care) and medicolegal purposes.
- Weigh sponges to assist in determining blood loss and fluid replacement.
- Keep an accurate record of the amount of irrigation used to assist in determining blood loss and fluid replacement.
- **N.B. Reminder:** *All persons scrubbed should wear a protective plastic face shield to prevent injury from the splashing or spraying of the patient's blood and irrigation fluids used.*

- Document the type, size, and serial numbers of a commercial graft in the **Perioperative Record** and in the hospital log, according to hospital policy.
- When an endovascular stent is to be inserted, be certain of the surgeon's selection of these very expensive items before opening the package. Document the data pertinent to the stent.
- The circulator should be prepared to give a report to the PACU practitioner regarding medications used, transfusions, patient's allergies, intraoperative observations and nursing care implemented (actions taken), outcomes, and any information necessary to provide continuity of care of the patient.
- In the PACU, the perioperative nurse continuously monitors and assesses the patient's neurological status. The nurse in the PACU should know how to use somatosensory evoked monitoring for early detection of abnormal signals indicating spinal cord ischemia. Documentation of the monitoring is done for patient safety (continuity of care) and for medicolegal purposes.
- The perioperative practitioner in PACU documents evidence of the patient's mental status.

Femoropopliteal Bypass

Definition

The restoration of arterial circulation to the leg by interposition of a graft to bypass an occluded segment of the femoral artery.

Discussion

Patency of the popliteal artery is determined prior to surgery by ultrasound and later confirmed by angiography. When the popliteal artery is occluded, shunting the blood flow to a more distal artery becomes necessary; the exploration of tributary vessels (e.g., posterior tibial artery) may require use of a microscope. The graft may be autologous (e.g., saphenous vein) or a synthetic prosthesis, e.g., Dacron. Woven Dacron grafts are available coated with protein (collagen/albumin) that reduces the blood loss and antibiotics that prevent graft infection. Impregnated grafts are considerably more expensive than the noncoated grafts.

Risks associated with the surgery are bleeding, stroke, myocardial infarction, pulmonary embolus, and infection. If bypass fails, amputation may become necessary.

An *ultrasonic angioscope system* is currently being developed that uses intra-balloon fluorescence in conjunction with photodynamic therapy for the prevention of restenosis. The scope may also be employed to visualize the lumen and send ultrasonic waves ahead of a stricture within a vessel to cause plaque breakdown that can further be treated by laser.

Vein harvesting for an autologous graft may be performed as an endoscopic procedure.

Procedure

A vertical incision is made in interrupted segments over the course of the femoral artery, from the inguinal area along the medial aspect of the thigh to below the knee; there may be several interruptions in the incision. The common femoral artery and its bifurcation are exposed. The distal popliteal artery is exposed, retracting the gastrocnemius and soleus muscles (posteriorly) and adductor muscles (anteriorly). The posterior tibial nerve is protected. A tunneling instrument is used to make a passage from the femoral triangle to the popliteal space under the sartorius muscle. For an autograft, the saphenous vein is harvested and its multiple branches are divided and ligated. The segment is flushed with heparinized saline, tested for leakage, and set aside in an emesis basin. The femoral artery, controlled by vascular clamp, is flushed with heparinized saline. The autograft (saphenous vein segment) is sutured to the common femoral artery in reversed anatomical position to avoid the action of the valves, or the valves are removed. Endarterectomy and "patch" angioplasty may be performed at the origin of the deep femoral artery. The autograft is passed through the tunnel (avoiding kinking or tension) and anastomosed to the popliteal artery. Prior to placing the final sutures, the graft is flushed with blood and controlled by pressure or further sutures. Intraoperative angiography may be performed. The incisions are closed. If vessels distal to the popliteal artery are used, similar maneuvers are performed.

Vein harvesting may be performed as an endoscopic procedure.

Preparation of the Patient

An antiembolitic stocking may be applied to the unaffected leg. Epidural or spinal block anesthetic or general anesthesia may be employed. The patient is supine with the affected hip and thigh slightly externally rotated and abducted, and the knee is flexed. A pillow or roll may be requested to maintain the patient's position. Arms may be extended on padded armboards. All bony prominences and areas prone to skin and neurovascular pressure or trauma are padded. Check with the surgeon regarding insertion of Foley catheter (usually requested). Apply electrosurgical dispersive pad.

Skin Preparation

The entire abdomen is routinely prepared for the harvesting of saphenous vein(s); when in doubt, consult with surgeon. The genital area is excluded from the prep by covering it with a towel folded in thirds.

Unilateral. Begin at the groin on the affected side, extending from the umbilicus to the toes (including front and back of thigh, leg, and foot). Prepare down to the table on both sides, including to midthigh on the unaffected side.

Bilateral. Prepare both groin regions, extending from the umbilicus to the toes (including front and back of thighs, legs, and feet). Two persons are required to complete the preparation, or one person may prep using a leg holder and sterile towels, as necessary.

Draping

Unilateral. The affected extremity is held up and abducted. A large sheet is draped over the end of the table. A towel (folded in thirds, lengthwise) is placed over the pubic area. A split sheet is draped under the thigh. Two towels are placed on the table, the foot is lowered onto the towels, and the towels are fashioned into a boot and clipped, or sterile impervious stockinette or a large glove is placed on the foot. The foot is held up and the affected leg may be passed through a laparotomy sheet and lowered to the table, or a large sheet is draped under the legs and over the top of the patient with individual drape sheets, as necessary, to complete the draping.

Bilateral. The legs are held up and abducted. A large drape sheet is placed over the end of the table. A towel (folded in thirds, lengthwise) is placed over the pubic area. A large sheet is draped under the thighs. Sheets are draped along the sides of the patient and fastened. Two towels for each foot are placed on the table, the feet are lowered onto the towels, and the towels are fashioned into boots and clipped, or sterile impervious stockinettes or large gloves are placed on the feet. The feet are held up, and a large drape sheet is placed under the legs; the legs are lowered. A large sheet is draped over the top of the patient, and individual drape sheets, as necessary, complete the draping.

Equipment

- Pillows or rolls
- Leg holder, optional
- ESU
- Suction
- Doppler and cord with coupling gel (not sterile) used prior to prep, if requested
- C arm for x-ray angiography
- Magnifying loupes, optional

Instrumentation

- Basic/minor tray
- Peripheral vascular procedures tray

Tunneling instrument
Ligating clip appliers, e.g., Hemoclip appliers, short, medium
Self-retaining retractors, e.g., Weitlaner or Gelpi
Sterile Doppler probe and cord, optional
Valvutome, e.g., Mills, to excise valves from saphenous vein (optional)
Doppler and cord with coupling gel (sterile)

Supplies

Antiembolitic hose (for unaffected leg)
Foley catheter, optional
Basin set
Blades, (2) #10, (1) #15, (1) #11
Suction tubing
Electrosurgical pencil and cord with holder and scraper
Umbilical tapes, Penrose drains, vessel loops for retraction
Needle magnet or counter
Dissectors (e.g., peanut)
Ligating clips, e.g., Hemoclips (small, medium, and large)
Hemostatic agents, e.g., Gelfoam, Surgicel, Thrombostat, Collastat, Oxycel, and/or Avitene, etc. (available)
Synthetic graft (according to surgeon's choice of type and size)
Heparin and heparinized saline (diluted to surgeon's preference)
Graduate pitcher and bulb syringe
Protamine sulfate (heparin antagonist, reverses action of heparin)
Medicine cups and syringes
Sterile labels and marking pen
Contrast media for angiography, optional
Antibiotic (intravenous or for irrigation), optional

Special Notes

- Apply **Special Notes** from ***Carotid Endarterectomy***, p. 487.
- **Reminder:** *The circulator should verify that there are two working suctions in the room in addition to the one on the anesthesia cart before starting the surgery.*
- Assorted grafts should be in the room before surgery is started. Consult with the surgeon to determine the type and size of graft to be used. Sterilize and prepare the synthetic graft for use according to surgeon's directions.
- **N.B. Reminder:** Circulator ascertains that blood is available as ordered and ready for immediate use. Blood for transfusion may have been given to the blood bank in advance in anticipation of the need.

- **N.B.** Circulator anticipates possible blood transfusion(s) and obtains items for blood administration (e.g., tubing set, blood warmer, pressure bag). Circulator assists the anesthesia provider to administer blood (identify patient and blood type, etc.) and to monitor hemodynamics. All information is documented.
- The surgeon may choose to perform intraoperative angiography. The circulator should notify the x-ray department as soon as this is known. Check with the surgeon for type of catheters needed; have available syringes and contrast medium. Observe all x-ray safety precautions; see p. 52.
- During draping, the foot may be grasped with a tube stockinette or a glove may be placed over the distal portion of the foot.
- **Reminder:** Use safety precautions to identify, label, and dispense medications or solutions and to avoid medication errors; see p. 30. It is mandatory that all medications and solutions on the sterile field be labeled by name and strength. The medication bottle is retained in the room until the procedure has concluded. Document medications used, precautions taken, and their effect.
- **N.B.** *The scrub person should keep a spongestick (raytec sponge mounted on a sponge forceps) available at all times for applying pressure in case of hemorrhage.*
- Document the type, size, and serial numbers of the graft in the Perioperative Record and in the facility's log for insertion of an implant, according to hospital policy.
- When a laser is employed, observe all laser safety precautions, p. 94.
- **N.B. Reminder:** Scrub person notes that double-armed sutures used in vascular surgery are **not** cut.

Femoral Arterial Thromboembolectomy

Definition

Extraction of a propagated thrombotic mass obstructing the femoral artery.

Discussion

Contrary to the insidious onset of an atherosclerotic or gradual thrombotic disease process or developing stenosis of an arterial graft, an embolic blockage is an *acute* cause of arterial ischemia. The embolus may be derived from a thrombus in the left atrial appendage associated with atrial fibrillation or from the thrombus in a left ventricular aneurysm following myocardial infarction. Cardiac valvular prostheses may likewise be a source of embolism, especially if the induced anticoagulant status is disturbed. The common sources previously, as rheumatic mitral valve disease or endocarditis, have become much less frequent (except in younger patients with endocarditis from intravenous drug use). Atrial tumor (e.g., myoma) fragments, metastatic cancer which has invaded into the great vessels, atheromata from proximal large vessels or an aortic aneurysm (sometimes provoked by angiography), or venous thrombi that can pass through a right-to-left cardiac shunt defect are causative. Less often, fat particles following an injury or the migration of a bullet or other foreign body can be responsible. Prompt recognition of the symptoms of local pain, paresthesiae, pallor, paralysis, and loss of pulse require initiation of anticoagulation to prevent propagation of thrombus fragments distal to the embolus and development of venous thrombosis, especially in older patients with established peripheral vascular disease.

Alternatives to surgery include thrombolytic drug therapy delivered by catheter to the thromboembolus, percutaneous suction catheters that include rotation devices, and ultrasound accelerated thrombolysis.

However, surgical treatment remains the standard approach. The use of local anesthesia and limited incision (when feasible) is most helpful with often critically ill patients with concomitant disorders. If endovascular maneuvers with Fogarty catheters do not adequately restore flow, a bypass procedure or other technique is required (see ***Femoropopliteal Bypass,*** p. 496).

Procedure

Thromboembolectomy of the femoral artery is described. The common femoral artery is exposed through a vertical incision. A self-retaining retractor is employed, enabling the placement of vascular clamps and vessel loops around the artery and the superficial and deep femoral artery branches. An arteriotomy is made; any gross thrombotic material is directly extracted. A succession of appropriately sized Fogarty balloon and irrigating catheters (usually #3Fr or #4Fr) are passed proximal and distal to site of obstruction, being manipulated to extract the embolic particles, taking care to avoid undue fragmentation or distal dislodgement of the embolic matter. If necessary, a radiologically controlled guide wire can be passed, over which the catheters are placed, when the course of the arteries is tortuous or otherwise uncertain. Several passes may be made to ensure removal of all of the thrombotic material until backflow is reestablished. Intravascular ultrasound can be used to identify residual thrombus. When a vascular prosthesis is present, special latex covered or bare wire coil-covered catheters can be used to facilitate the thrombectomy. Heparinized saline is injected. Distal pulses are palpated, and angiography (or angioscopy) can be performed. The arteriotomy and wound are closed. Thrombolytic agents may be administered.

Preparation of the Patient

Following the administration of the anesthetic, the patient is supine, with the thigh on the affected side externally rotated and abducted and the knee flexed. A pillow or roll may be requested to maintain the patient's position. Arms may be extended on padded armboards. The patient is secured to the table with the safety belt fastened over the unaffected thigh. All bony prominences and areas prone to skin and neurovascular pressure or trauma are padded. Check with the surgeon regarding insertion of Foley catheter. Apply electrosurgical dispersive pad.

Skin Preparation

Begin at the groin on the affected side, extending from the umbilicus to the toes (including front and back of thigh, leg, and foot). Prep down to the table on affected side and well beyond midline on opposite side.

Draping

The affected extremity is held up and abducted. A large sheet is draped over the end of the table. A towel (folded in thirds, lengthwise) is placed over the pubic area. A split sheet is draped under the thigh. Two towels are placed on the table, the foot is lowered onto the towels, and the towels are fashioned into a boot and clipped, or sterile impervious stockinette or a large glove is placed on the foot. The foot is held up, and the affected leg may be passed through a laparotomy sheet and lowered to the table, or a large sheet is draped under the legs and over the top of the patient with individual drape sheets, as necessary, to complete the draping.

Equipment

ESU
Suction
Doppler and cord with coupling gel
C arm for x-ray angiography, as requested
Magnifying loupes, optional

Instrumentation

Basic/Minor procedures tray
Peripheral vascular procedures tray
Ligating clip appliers, e.g., Hemoclip appliers short, medium

Self-retaining retractors, e.g., Weitlaner (sharp) or Gelpi
Sterile Doppler probe and cord, optional
Guide wire, optional

Supplies

Antiembolitic hose (for unaffected leg)
Foley catheter, optional
Basin set
Blades, (1) #10, (1) #15, (1) #11
Suction tubing
Electrosurgical pencil and cord with holder and scraper
Umbilical tapes or vessel loops for retraction
Needle magnet or counter
Dissectors (e.g., peanut)
Fogarty balloon catheters, e.g., #3Fr or #4Fr
Ligating clips, e.g., Hemoclips (small, medium, and large)
Hemostatic agents, e.g., Gelfoam, Surgicel, Thrombostat, Collastat, Oxycel, or Avitene (available)
Heparinized saline diluted to surgeon's preference, e.g., 1000 U/50 ml
Graduate pitcher and bulb syringe
Protamine sulfate (heparin antagonist, reverses action of heparin)
Local anesthetic, medicine cups, and syringes
Sterile labels and marking pen
Contrast media for angiography, optional

Special Notes

- Apply **Special Notes** from ***Femoropopliteal Bypass***, p. 499.

Greater Saphenous Vein Ligation and Stripping

Definition

Excision of the greater saphenous vein and its tributaries.

Discussion

This procedure is indicated to treat severe varicose vein disease secondary to venous valvular incompetence. Another indication is superficial thrombophlebitis of the lower extremities. The lesser saphenous vein system may also be excised, as indicated.

When the condition is less severe, varicose veins may be treated by endovenous laser (EVLT), endoluminal radio-frequency ablation (ERFA), or high-frequency electrocoagulation. Sclerotherapy, usually performed as an outpatient procedure, may be employed for small cutaneous varices (e.g., "spider" veins). Subfascial endoscopic perforator vein surgery (SFPS) is an additional surgical modality.

Procedure

An oblique incision is made in the groin overlying the saphenofemoral junction. The superficial fascia is incised and the proximal portion of the saphenous vein is mobilized, divided, and ligated close to the saphenofemoral junction. Tributaries are divided and ligated as indicated. A transverse incision is made over the saphenous vein distally anterior to the medial malleolus; tributaries are exposed, divided, and ligated. The probe end of the internal stripper is inserted into the distal end of the saphenous vein and threaded proximally. A ligature is tied about the distal end, securing the vein about the acorn end of the stripper. The surgeon withdraws the stripper proximally (with vein attached) through the femoral incision, as the assistant applies pressure over the course of the vein with a folded towel. The vein may be removed segmentally, or sections of it may be removed with external strippers. Saphenous vein branches and perforating veins (usually marked by the surgeon preoperatively) are stripped, excised, or ligated using external strippers. This might entail numerous small incisions. The lesser saphenous vein (posterior aspect of the leg) may require similar treatment. All incisions are closed and dressed. The leg(s) are wrapped with cotton batting (optional) and an elastic bandage.

Preparation of the Patient

Epidural or general anesthesia is administered. The patient is supine with the thigh on the affected side externally rotated and abducted, and the knee is flexed. For a bilateral procedure, the legs are slightly apart, i.e., abducted. Arms may be extended on padded armboards. The patient is secured to the table with the safety belt fastened over the unaffected thigh. All bony prominences and areas prone to skin and neurovascular pressure or trauma are padded. When the procedure is bilateral, the safety belt is fastened about the waist; care is taken not to interfere with respiration. Foley catheter is not routinely inserted. Electrosurgical dispersive pad is applied.

Skin Preparation

Unilateral. Begin at the groin on the affected side, extending from the umbilicus to the toes (including front and back of thigh, leg, and foot). Prep down to the table on the affected side and well beyond the midline on the opposite side proximally.

Bilateral. Prepare both groin regions, extending from the umbilicus to the toes (including front and back of thighs, legs, and feet). Two persons are required to prep, or one person can prep using a leg holder and sterile towels, as necessary.

Draping

Unilateral. Following the prep, the affected extremity is elevated and abducted. A large sheet is draped over the end of the table. A towel (folded in thirds lengthwise) is placed over the pubic area. A split sheet is draped under the leg. Two towels are placed on the table, the foot is lowered onto the towels, and the towels are fashioned into a boot and clipped. A large sheet is draped over the top of the patient's body. The affected leg is passed through a laparotomy sheet and lowered to the table, or individual drape sheets may complete the draping.

Bilateral. Following the prep, the legs are elevated and abducted. A large drape sheet is placed over the end of the table. A towel (folded in thirds lengthwise) is placed over the pubic area. Sheets are draped along the sides of the patient and fastened. A large sheet is draped under the legs. Two towels for each foot are placed on the table, the feet are lowered onto the towels, and the towels are fashioned into boots and clipped. Another large sheet (or more) is draped over the top of the patient.

Equipment

Leg holder
ESU
Suction

Instrumentation

Basic/minor tray; peripheral vascular procedures tray, optional
Internal and external vein strippers
Weitlaner (sharp) or Gelpi retractor
Skin hooks (2), small sharp rakes (2)
Ligating clip appliers, e.g., Hemoclip appliers, short (small, medium, large)

Supplies

Basin set
Marking pen (indelible)
Blades, (2) #10, (1) #15
Needle magnet or counter
Suction tubing
Electrosurgical pencil and cord with holder and scraper
Ligating clips, e.g., Hemoclips
Cotton batting, optional, and elastic bandages, e.g., Ace

Special Notes

- Apply **Special Notes** from ***Abdominal Laparotomy***, p. 134, as applicable.

- A tube stockinette or a glove may be placed over the distal portion of the foot instead of a boot.
- Immediately preoperatively, with the patient erect, indelible ink is used to mark the varicose veins, as the vein sites may become less easy to detect when the patient is lying down.
- The scrub person should remove the vein from the internal stripper by cutting the suture as soon as possible. This is done so that the stripper is available for continued use.
- With multiple incisions, additional scalpel blades may be required. Additional counts must be taken, according to the number of incisions.
- Cotton batting may be applied to the leg after dressings have been placed, before the elastic bandages.

Portosystemic Shunt

Definition

Diversion of portal venous blood to the systemic venous system.

Discussion

This procedure is performed to relieve elevated portal venous pressure (portal hypertension), which can result in bleeding from esophageal or gastric varices, ascites, and hepatic failure. Preoperative angiography (splenoportagram) is useful for diagnosis. The primary cause is cirrhosis. The portal blood may be shunted into the inferior vena cava from the portal vein (end to side or side to side), from the splenic vein (with splenectomy), from the distal splenic vein (retaining the spleen), or mesocaval shunt from the superior mesenteric vein (with or without an interposing prosthetic graft). An additional procedure is a distal *splenorenal shunt,* in which the splenic vein is anastomosed to the left renal vein. The particular type of shunt is determined by the patient's condition and the surgeon's preference.

Procedure

Portacaval Shunt is described. A right subcostal incision is made, extending across the midline as necessary. Less often, a thoracoabdominal incision may be employed. Careful dissection is performed because even minor vessels may bleed significantly. The duodenum is reflected, exposing the inferior vena cava. The hepatoduodenal ligament is incised; the common bile duct and hepatic artery are protected. The portal vein is exposed from the porta hepatis to the superior border of the pancreas. Portal pressure is measured (for a reference) by manometry through a needle inserted in a small mesenteric vein. Partial occlusion of the vena cava and the portal vein are obtained with vascular clamps. Anastomosis is made side to side after excising a generous window in either vein. For end-to-side anastomoses, the portal vein is transected at the porta hepatis, ligating the (hepatic) stump securely. The distal end is anastomosed to the side of the vena cava. Repeat manometry is performed. The wound is closed in layers.

Preparation of the Patient

Antiembolitic hose are applied. Following the administration of general anesthesia with endotracheal intubation, the patient is in supine position with the right side elevated. Anesthesia provider inserts a nasogastric tube and CVP line. A folded sheet or roll is placed under the right shoulder to facilitate visualization. The table may be positioned in Trendelenburg position. Arms may be extended on padded armboards. All bony prominences and areas prone to skin and neurovascular pressure or trauma are padded. Foley catheter is inserted and connected to drainage unit. Apply electrosurgical dispersive pad.

Skin Preparation

Begin at the right subcostal region, extending from the axillae to the upper thighs and down to the table at the sides.

Draping

Folded towels and a laparotomy sheet

Equipment

Forced-air warming blanket, optional
Sequential compression device with disposable leg wraps, as requested
ESU
Suction
Spinal manometer (for measuring portal pressure)
Blood pump and blood warmer
Scales for weighing sponges (2)
Cell-saver (optional, check with surgeon)

Instrumentation

Major procedures tray
Abdominal and thoracic vascular procedures tray
Long instruments tray
Ligating clip appliers, e.g., Hemoclip appliers (assorted sizes and lengths)

Supplies

Antiembolitic hose
N/G tube to the anesthesia provider

Basin set
Foley catheter and drainage unit
Extra lap sponges
Blades, (2) #10, (1) #15, (1) #11
Electrosurgical pencil and cord with holder and scraper
Suction tubing (2)
Needle magnet or counter
Three-way stopcock, polyethylene tubing (e.g., angiocath), and syringe
Ligating clips, e.g., Hemoclips (assorted sizes)

Special Notes

- Apply **Special Notes** from ***Hepatic Resection***, p. 169, as applicable.
- **Reminder:** Ascertain that the *correct* x-ray studies and scan reports are in the room for the *correct* patient.
- Be prepared for possible significant blood loss. Verify that at least two suction units in the room are operational.
- Circulator consults the surgeon regarding the use of the cell-saver. If needed, bring unit into the room before the patient. Notify supervisor or necessary personnel regarding its use.
- Circulator confirms with blood bank that the correct number of units of blood (or blood products) have been ordered and are ready and available.
- Circulator assists in verifying identification of the patient number and compares it to the identification number on the blood or blood products.
- The circulator should obtain blood administration set, warmer, and blood pump in advance to be used as needed.
- The circulator should obtain extra lap sponges for back table; they should be counted in advance to prevent delay in case of emergency.
- Keep strict accounting of lap sponges, as a saturated sponge could be overlooked.
- Use warm moist lap sponges after entering abdominal cavity and warm irrigation fluids to maintain patient's temperature and to avoid hypothermia.
- A fibrin glue/sealant may be employed at suture lines, e.g., Tissucol™ or Tisseel VH™ (optional).
- Keep an accurate record of the amount of irrigation used to determine replacement of fluid loss.

- Circulator weighs sponges accurately to help in determining fluid loss replacement. Weigh sponges to determine fluid loss replacement. To weigh sponges, two scales are used, one for raytec sponges and one for lap pads. To weigh sponges, calculate the weight of the dry sponge and set the scale to 0 after weight adjustment.
- **N.B.** To measure portal pressure, polyethylene tubing inserted into a jejunal mesenteric vein is attached to a three-way stopcock and a spinal manometer. The scrub person should have these items on the back table to avoid delay.
- Portal pressure is remeasured following the portacaval anastomosis to determine if the shunt is functioning.

Arteriovenous Shunt or Arteriovenous (Bridge) Fistula

Definition

Establishment of a direct connection between an artery and a vein.

A communicating prosthetic loop between an artery and a vein (shunt) or a direct communication between an artery and vein (fistula).

Discussion

The procedure is performed to provide easy access for venipuncture with a large-bore needle for purposes of renal dialysis or infusion chemotherapy. **Arteriovenous (AV) shunts or arteriovenous (bridge) fistulas** involve the creation of a connection between an artery and a vein. When patients are in the late stages of renal disease, an arteriovenous shunt (Cimino shunt) is created for them in anticipation of their receiving dialysis. An anastomosis of the artery and vein form an internal connection (side to side, side to end, or end to end). The anastomosis on the venous side bulges under the greater pressure from the artery. The site of the venous dilatation formed at the anastomosis site thickens over the period of a few weeks. When the walls of the vein become thick (like arteries), the vein is strong enough to endure the repeated venipuncture required by dialysis.

Bridge fistulas are the creation of a connection between an artery and a vein by means of a bridge. A bridge may be created from a saphenous vein graft, an umbilical vein graft, or a bovine artery prosthesis (usually enzymatically treated) or PTFE (Teflon) graft. A modification of the PTFE graft has tapered ends. The size of the bridge, whether straight or curved, depends upon the proximity of the vessels to each other.

Procedure

Arteriovenous shunt or arteriovenous bridge fistula is performed following injection of local anesthetic. An incision is made over a selected artery and adjacent vein (often the radial artery and cephalic vein of the proximal forearm). Use of the nondominant forearm is preferable; lower extremities can be used if forearm sites cannot be used (e.g., previous surgery). Vascular clamps or bulldogs are used to control the vessels. An incision is made into the lumen of the artery (arteriotomy). The artery is usually dilated with coronary artery dilators. The venous side is ligated distally. A shunt (e.g., saphenous vein graft, umbilical vein graft, or bovine artery prosthesis) is anastomosed to the artery and to the vein. When these vessels are inadequate, a synthetic PTFE graft may be positioned between the artery and the vein. Usually a loop fistula is created in the antecubital fossa by interposing a bridge between the brachial artery and the cephalic or basilic vein. Heparin solution is instilled into the shunt. Alternatively, a fistula may be created in the arm between the brachial artery and the axillary vein. The wound is closed, and a protective dressing is placed.

Preparation of the Patient

Antiembolitic hose may be applied. The patient is supine; a small pad may be placed under the lumbar spine and/or a pillow may be placed under the knees to avoid straining back muscles and for comfort. The affected forearm is extended on a padded hand table; the other arm may be extended on an armboard or padded and tucked in at the patient's side. All bony prominences and areas prone to skin and neurovascular pressure or trauma are padded. Apply electrosurgical dispersive pad.

Skin Preparation

Begin at the proposed site (e.g., nondominant forearm), extending from 3″ to 4″ above the elbow to include the entire hand (fingers, nails, and interdigital spaces).

Draping

The hand is elevated in a doubled tube stockinette. A large cuffed sheet is draped over the table and under the arm. A folded towel is wrapped around the arm and clipped. A drape (or split) sheet is draped under the arm and clipped. A drape sheet covers the shoulder and is clipped under the arm. A fenestrated sheet (e.g., laparotomy or transverse) or additional drape sheets complete the draping.

Equipment

ESU
Hand table

Sitting stools (2) for surgeon and scrub person
Loupes, optional

Instrumentation

Shunt tray
Coronary artery dilators

Supplies

Antiembolitic hose, optional
Small basin
Electrosurgical pencil with needle tip and cord
Needle magnet or counter
Blades, (1) #15, (1) #11
Shunt, e.g., PTFE cannulas (2) or surgeon's preference
Shunt connector
Heparin
Heparinized saline (diluted to surgeon's preference)
Graduated pitcher and syringe
Shunt clamps (2)

Special Notes

- Apply Special Notes from **Carotid Endarterectomy**, p. 487, as applicable.

CHAPTER 22
Cardiac Surgery

Cardiac Surgery

Introduction

Cardiac surgery involves the correction of congenital anomalies, acquired diseases of the heart, pericardium, and great vessels (including repair and replacement of diseased valves, **resection of ventricular aneurysm, pericardiectomy, pulmonary embolectomy, and replacement of segments of the great vessels), and the revascularization of ischemic myocardium**. To fully comprehend cardiac abnormalities and the function of ***cardiopulmonary bypass (CPB)***, knowledge of anatomy and the circulation is invaluable.

Cardiac surgery is in a constant state of evolution. When performed as a minimally invasive procedure, aortic valve replacement is achieved through a mini-sternotomy. Saphenous vein for the coronary artery bypass surgery or grafts (CABS or CABG) can be obtained endoscopically, and coronary artery segments can be endoscopically replaced. **"Hybrid procedures"** are being performed with the minimal-access approach. A hybrid procedure involves **CABS and stented angioplasty**. The procedures are not new, but combining them is possible when an operating room (OR) has a catheterization lab in the same OR.

Some cardiac procedures are performed utilizing CPB; however, ever-evolving interventions are making it possible to perform these surgeries without bypass. Utilizing *minimally invasive techniques* in the OR and cardiac catheterization lab, including lasers, ultrasound, cryosurgery, radio-frequency ablation, robots, and other state of the art modalities, heart surgery has become an option for many patients whose conditions could not tolerate an open bypass procedure. **Endoscopic CABS** may eliminate the use of CPB. Prolonged time on the pump can potentially result in renal failure, pulmonary insufficiency, and neurological sequelae.

Approaches to cardiac surgery include standard sternotomy, mini-sternotomy, and minimally invasive endoscopy. Using a mini-sternotomy approach depends on the structures to be exposed and the existing pathology. Advantages of the mini-incision access include cosmesis, less bleeding, less pain, fewer infections, and a more rapid rate of recovery. The disadvantage of mini-sternotomy is that the approach is technically more demanding, with lesser overall exposure of the operative field, and some surgeons may lack experience for these modifications. In patients whose myocardium cannot recover from corrective surgery, an **intra-aortic balloon counterpulsation catheter or**

implanted left ventricular assist pumping device (see p. 516) may be employed. If independent myocardial recovery still does not occur, a **mechanical heart or cardiac transplantation** (not to be presented in this text) is required to sustain the life of the patient.

The advantages of performing cardiac procedures "off pump" likewise include quicker recovery, decreased need for blood transfusion, and fewer side effects and complications. Today, bypass machines are making the mechanics of circulatory support less harmful for those patients whose condition requires bypass. With these machines, venous drainage is achieved with vacuum-assisted cannulas that are smaller. The machines require less priming (normal saline or lactated Ringer's) solution. That results in less hemodilution and hemolysis. The smaller cannulas are small enough to be used during minimal-access procedures.

All cardiac surgeries performed off pump are especially valuable for high-risk patients. **Off-pump CABG** is sometimes performed with **transmyocardial laser revascularization procedure** through a keyhole incision via left thorocotomy, making comprehensive revascularization of the myocardium possible for these patients. For patients who have had previous cardiac surgery, this approach encounters fewer adhesions and better myocardial exposure. When safe, anticoagulation is reinstituted postoperatively.

During cardiac surgery, the patient's hemodynamics and other physiologic functions are monitored continuously. In addition to those monitors employed for most major surgeries, such as the electrocardiogram (ECG), pulse oximeter, urimeter, etc., invasive hemodynamic catheters are placed. These include an arterial line to measure blood pressure directly and to serve as a ready access for blood gas determination sampling and a central venous pressure (CVP) or Swan-Ganz line to measure intracardiac pressures. Transesophageal echocardiography (TEE) and electroencephalogram (EEG) are also monitored.

Hypothermia and/or pharmacologic agents may be employed to slow or arrest the heart to reduce the body's oxygen demands and to preserve neurological function. ***Hypothermia*** (low-core body temperature) reduces the body's metabolic and oxygen requirements, permitting the body to tolerate periods of decreased perfusion. Hypothermia may be induced using a temperature-controlled blanket (e.g., Blanketrol® II Hypothermia System) placed within a specialized mattress of alternating cold air cushions (e.g., TheraKair®), a water-circulating mattress (e.g., PlastiPad®), the direct application of iced saline, and/or by cooling the blood being returned to the patient from the pump's oxygenator. Both head and body cooling can be achieved with a Bair Hugger® blanket (lightweight mattress with tiny holes) that delivers constant cold air-flow *(Polar Bair). MUL-T-Blanket®*, a hyperthermia/hypothermia blanket, is an alternate method of temperature control.

While the heart is on pump, icy sterile saline slush is packed around the heart. Some cardiac surgeons are proponents of "*warm-arrest techniques*" to reduce trauma to the circulatory system.

Cardioplegic drugs, alone or in combination with other modalities (e.g., buffering agents to counteract acidosis), may be injected directly into the coronary arteries to arrest the heartbeat. The cardioplegic agent contains potassium (induces hyperkalemia), resulting in electrochemical cardiac arrest. The ECG monitor shows a flat line when procedures are performed on-pump. When electrical activity reappears on the monitor screen, additional cardioplegia is administered (about every 15 to 20 minutes) until arrest is no longer required.

In certain procedures involving the aortic arch and in which CPB must be interrupted, cerebroplegia can be prevented by cooling and by the retrograde pumping of blood through the superior vena cava cannula until the repair is completed. When body temperature is restored at the conclusion of the cardiac procedure, the potassium preparation is flushed out. The heartbeat may resume spontaneously, or electrical ***cardioversion by defibrillator*** (see p. 467) may be employed to restore effective activity to the heart (in its state of arrest or ventricular fibrillation). Pacemaker wires may be sewn onto the epicardium at the completion of CPB. The heart and the patient as a whole are gradually warmed (returned to normothermia) as water-filled thermic coils in the CPB machine pumps the blood back into the arterial circulation.

The approach to cardiac surgery, as in other types of surgery, is becoming less invasive as techniques and technology evolve. In the minimally invasive cardiac approach, selected procedures permit the surgeon to operate through a "keyhole" incision under direct vision using a thoracoscope/videoscope, and in some centers, under robotic control. Discussions regarding procedures to correct congenital anomalies in pediatric patients, cardiac transplantation, and insertion of an artificial heart are beyond the scope of this text. Procedures involving repair and replacement of valves, **Ross procedure, pulmonary embolectomy, coronary artery bypass grafts, MAZE procedure, transmyocardial revascularization (TMR)**, and minimal access procedures are discussed, and the procedures are described. **Preparation of the Patient, Skin Preparation, Equipment, Supplies**, and **Special Notes** are combined for cardiac procedures, as applicable.

Cardiopulmonary Bypass (CPB)

Definition

The technique by which the patient's blood is diverted from the body, oxygenated, and reperfused, bypassing the heart and lungs.

Discussion

This artificial means of diverting and oxygenating the blood and recirculating it through the body may be employed for intracardiac procedures, coronary artery bypass, and procedures on intrathoracic major vessels. Prior to instituting CPB, the patient is anticoagulated with heparin to prevent blood clot formation. For patients with heparin intolerance, ancrod/Arvin may be used. This (anticoagulated) status is reversed following the procedure with protamine sulfate. Protamine sulfate can cause catastrophic pulmonary vasoconstriction in some patients undergoing CPB; therefore, it is advisable to have prostaglandin E on hand to reverse the reaction.

CPB may be either total or partial. For *total bypass* (when used for some approaches to intracardiac procedures, such as valve replacements, septal defects, major anomalies, and ventricular aneurysm resection), all the blood is diverted from the heart and pulmonary circulation, except intrinsic cardiac circulation, by means of bypass cannula. *Partial bypass* (may be used for coronary artery bypass surgery, thoracic aortic aneurysms, etc.) can be achieved with several configurations, including cannulation of the right atrium via the femoral vein and the aorta via the femoral artery. *Vacuum-assisted venous drainage* (VAVD) is used to enhance venous return. The left ventricle via the right superior pulmonary vein, ascending aorta, and pulmonary artery are vented with catheters connected to suction lines of the pump to prevent potential air bubble emboli.

There are several anatomical sites at which CPB can be established. The femoral vein, inferior vena cava, and right atrium are examples of sites from which blood is diverted from the patient to the pump. Blood is returned to the patient through the femoral artery, subclavian artery, or ascending aorta. The preference of the surgeon, the nature of the surgery, and the condition of the vessels will determine the arterial sites chosen for each patient. A commonly used configuration is the cannulation of the right atrium by a single multi-holed cannula, the tip of which inserts into the inferior vena cava, transporting the venous return from the patient to the pump. A cannula inserted in the ascending aorta returns blood to the patient from the pump. Prior to cannulation, heparin is administered intravenously. Purse-string sutures are placed prior to cannulation to secure the cannulas.

CPB initiates a cascade of inflammatory processes that may result in end-organ damage. These include noncardiac complications such as fluid imbalance, electrolyte imbalance, damaged red blood cells, damaged platelets, problems with blood clotting mechanism, hemolysis, need for transfusion, kidney and lung complications, and microemboli to the brain. *Hypovolemia* may result from nonblood products that are added to the circulation (to increase the intravascular volume) while on CPB. Hypovolemia triggers release of stress hormone secretion that may induce edema in the brain; however, brain damage may not ensue if the condition is promptly corrected and the edema is transient. "*Post Pump Psychosis*" may promote temporary visual and auditory hallucinations and delusions. Prolonged time on CPB results in renal failure, pulmonary dysfunction, and neurological dysfunction. *Acute Respiratory Distress Syndrome* is a type of respiratory failure characterized by the inability of the lungs to provide adequate oxygenation and CO_2 excretion. The condition has been likened to adult hyaline-membrane disease. CPB may be used for conditions other than adult cardiac disease, e.g., infant conditions including pulmonary hypertension, meconium aspiration in newborns, sepsis, pneumonia, and respiratory distress syndrome.

Considering the negative effects of performing surgery "on pump," it follows that cardiac surgeons have introduced "off-pump" technology into their practices. The approach to cardiac surgery is becoming, as previously mentioned, less invasive. In a minimally invasive cardiac approach, selected procedures permit the surgeon to operate through limited incisions under direct vision via thoracoscope/videoscope. In addition, robots are being used to hold lights, cameras, and retractors in addition to their being used to perform surgical maneuvers in areas that are too small for the human hand (guided by the surgeon per console).

Intra-Aortic Balloon Catheterization (IABC)

Definition

The insertion of a balloon-tipped catheter into the aorta that forcibly, by means of a *counterpulsation pump,* increases blood flow to the coronary arteries and peripheral blood vessels.

Discussion

A balloon catheter is inserted into the femoral artery and passed to a level distal to the left subclavian artery. During diastole, as the aortic valve closes, the balloon activates (counterpulsation), forcing arterialized blood within the aorta to distribute with adequate pressure for coronary artery and organ and tissue perfusion. IABC is often performed in the OR following open-heart procedures to support the circulation during a gradual weaning from CPB and as an adjunct when left ventricular function is inadequate. IABC can also be performed in the special procedure room in the radiology department (independent of CPB) following myocardial infarction. The size of the balloon (volume displacement) varies from 20 to 40 ml of helium or CO_2. Additional indications for IABC include cardiac instability and ventricular arrhythmias not responsive to medical treatment, mitral valve disease (prior to corrective surgery), pre-bypass, and as a bridge to cardiac transplantation. Complications associated with the procedure are thrombus formation resulting in emboli, gas emboli, perforation, and decreased circulation in the ipsilateral lower extremity. In the postanesthesia care unit (PACU) following the procedure, the lower extremities are observed frequently and assessed for signs of impaired circulation. The appearance of the lower extremity in regard to moisture, color, and temperature is documented in the **Postoperative Record** section in the **Perioperative Record.**

When left ventricular assist is required for a prolonged period (weeks) prior to cardiac transplantation or insertion of a mechanical heart, a *ventricular assist device (VAD)* may be employed. Its principle is similar to that of the IABC. There are several utilized, including Abiomed BVS 5000, HeartMate LVAS (air pump or battery driven), and Thoratec system (employs an external blood pump within a large console for left and right ventricular assist). In a common configuration, a battery pump is implanted below the diaphragm, receiving oxygenated blood from a cannula inserted via the apex of the left ventricle. The blood from the ventricle is then pumped into the proximal aorta via an implanted cannula. A cable exits the abdominal wall and is connected to a monitoring and drive console (which is portable, enabling some patients to ambulate and perform some daily functions).

Procedure

The skin at the selected side (groin site) is prepped. **IABC** (with the cylindrical balloon) is inserted percutaneously by needle (with guide-wire) into the femoral artery. The needle is removed. Arterial dilators are inserted over the guide-wire to increase the lumen of the artery. The catheter (with the balloon deflated) is advanced into the descending aorta distal to the level of the left subclavian artery. The IABC is connected to the pump console and the balloon. The femoral arteriotomy site may be reinforced with prosthetic graft material. The pump works automatically or may be triggered by ECG, or it can be adjusted manually. The pump is usually coordinated with the patient's ECG so that the balloon inflates during diastole, forcing blood retrograde to better perfuse the coronary arteries. IABC also forces the blood antegrade into the distal aorta and its branches. This improves oxygenation of the myocardium and increases peripheral blood flow, thus diminishing the workload of the ventricle. The position of the catheter is observed by x-ray in the OR; in the radiology department, the patient is on a radiolucent table and the catheter is observed fluoroscopically. When counterpulsation assist is no longer necessary, the catheter is removed by opening the arteriotomy site.

Aortic Valve Replacement

Definition

Excision and replacement of a nonfunctioning aortic valve.

Discussion

When *aortic stenosis* due to arteriosclerotic hardening, infection, or any other disease process that damages the aortic valve occurs, a restriction in the ability of the valve to open occurs and repair or replacement is indicated. In the early stages of aortic valve disease, patients may be asymptomatic. Symptomatology that develops as the disease becomes more severe includes fatigue, angina, and syncope following exertion that eventually leads to *congestive heart failure* (CHF) and death. **Balloon valvuloplasty** (for treatment of aortic stenosis) is usually performed in the cardiac catheterization lab.

Aortic valve replacement surgery can be an open procedure employing CPB, or it can be performed as a minimally invasive procedure (i.e., via mini-sternotomy), depending on the patient's condition and the surgeon's experience.

A variation of aortic valve replacement is the *Ross Procedure,* in which the patient's own pulmonary valve (along with a segment of the pulmonary artery) is excised and replaced with a homograft (valve). The aortic valve is excised and replaced with an autologous pulmonary valve. In children, this procedure permits the autograft to grow as the child grows. With a minimal access incision (videoscopically assisted), aortic valves can be isolated and exposed (p. 516) after placing a shunt that bypasses the ascending aorta. Valve replacements are classified as biological (autografts, allografts, or xenografts) or mechanical grafts. An autograft is the individual's own pulmonary valve that is excised and grafted into position to replace the aortic valve. Aortic valve allografts are tissue grafts taken from human cadavers. Xenografts are tissue valves taken from pigs (and less often bovine), because a pig's heart structure is similar to the human heart. The tissue valves are chemically impregnated with a protein (collagen/albumin) coating that reduces blood loss and antibiotics that prevent graft infection. Mechanical aortic valve prostheses require patients to take coumadin for the rest of their lives. Patients who are allergic to coumadin are placed on Ximelgatran, a blood-thinning substitute. The general consensus of cardiac surgeons is that tissue valves should be placed in patients over age 65 only, as the "bio" valves usually require replacement after 10 years. Some patients object to having a mechanical valve because they are noisy (related to the heartbeat). Bioprosthetic™ valves are often used for patients in whom coumadin use is contraindicated; they are also recommended for patients who want to bear children. ADIAM is a polymeric valve that does not require anticoagulation therapy.

There is considerable technical difficulty for the surgeon in learning how to operate through the keyhole incision (minimal-access) procedure; reoperation is even more difficult with that approach. Cardiac surgeons use the EuroSCORE to predict mortality for the patient when all the variables regarding the patient's condition are factored into an equation. The EuroSCORE is used to provide the patient with a surprisingly accurate percentage of risk that is assumed by having the surgery. Risk factors include CVA resulting from emboli from the calcified valve and the cannulation sites. As with all cardiac procedures, other risks include hypoperfusion (from CPB hemodilution), hemorrhage, chest infection, and pleural effusion. Postoperative hemorrhage requires resternotomy that can be contributory to infection and acute renal failure, etc.

Procedure

The standard approach for **Aortic Valve Replacement** is through a median sternotomy incision, extending from the sternal notch to the xiphoid process. The sternum is divided by oscillating saw, and a sternal self-retaining retractor is placed. Cannulation for total CPB is achieved. A venting catheter is inserted through an incision in the right pulmonary vein and advanced to the left ventricle. The aorta is occluded distal to the valve. A cardioplegic solution is infused through the aortic root into the coronary arteries. **Aortotomy** is performed. The valve is excised (avoiding injury to the annulus). The annulus is measured, and the "appropriate size" prosthesis is inserted. If necessary, annuloplasty may be performed to accommodate an appropriate-sized prosthesis. If the annulus is too small to accept a mechanical prosthesis (and mechanical prosthesis is to be used), the aorta is enlarged with a patch graft. The valve may be sutured into place; some surgeons advocate the use of fibrin glue to supplement sutures. Air is vented from the left ventricle and the aorta. The aortotomy is closed. The cross-clamped aorta is released. The anesthesia provider inflates the lungs. When the surgeon is satisfied with the hemostasis, CPB is discontinued. If the heart does not resume beating spontaneously, *defibrillation* is performed. The wound may be irrigated with warm saline or an antibiotic solution. The patient is gradually warmed to normothermia. ***Temporary pacemaker*** electrodes (epicardial) are sutured to the heart. Mediastinal drains may be inserted. The sternum is closed with heavy wire suture. The wound is closed.

Mitral Valve Replacement

Definition

Excision and replacement of the mitral valve.

Discussion

Repair rather than replacement of the **mitral valve** is performed whenever possible, as repair avoids anticoagulation therapy "for the rest of one's life" and the complications associated with a prosthetic replacement valve. Repair of the mitral valve may be performed as **commissurotomy, annuloplasty, chordoplasty, or leaflet repair (plication)**. When the damage from leaking and regurgitation is too extensive for repair of the mitral valve, replacement of the valve with prosthesis is performed. As mitral stenosis progresses, it causes a rise in pressure and dilatation of the left atrium, resulting in pulmonary hypertension, right ventricular hypertrophy, and possibly tricuspid regurgitation. Initial symptoms exhibited are dyspnea, fatigue, and orthopnea. Later symptoms include more severe pulmonary congestion and right ventricular failure.

Mitral valve replacements are classified as biografts (allografts) or mechanical grafts. Like aortic valve replacement, allografts are tissue grafts taken from human cadavers. Xenografts are tissue valves taken from mammals (e.g., pig). Also, like aortic valves, mitral valves are chemically impregnated to reduce damage to red blood cells and to prevent graft infection (with antibiotics). Lifelong anticoagulation therapy is required for the patient with a mechanical mitral valve prostheses. Ximelgatran, one of several blood thinning agents, may be prescribed for patients who cannot take Coumadin. Since the tissue valves get worn out and require replacement approximately every ten years, they are placed only in patients over age 65. The standard approach for **mitral valve replacement** is through a median sternotomy with the patient supine. When mitral valve replacement is performed as a minimally invasive procedure, the approach is via right thoracotomy. The minimally invasive approach avoids splitting the sternum with a thoracotomy (lateral) approach. Mitral valve may also be performed using a mini-sternotomy incision with the patient in the supine position. Robotics may be employed. Mitral valve replacement surgery with CPB is performed utilizing either approach, depending on the patient's condition and the surgeon's experience.

Mitral valve replacement by standard approach is described. Cannulation for total CPB is achieved. The ascending aorta is occluded. Cardioplegic solution is infused through the aortic root into the coronary arteries. (Cardioplegia may be delivered by direct antegrade infusion into the coronary arteries or retrograde through the right atrium into the coronary sinus, depending on the pressure within the coronary arteries.) The left atrium is incised to expose the mitral valve. Any part of the mitral valve that is not diseased (as much as possible) is left in place. A portion of the annulus is usually retained for the insertion of fixation sutures. When possible, chordae tendineae and papillary muscles are left intact. The immediate area is debrided of calcifications, employing rongeurs when necessary. The valve is excised, the annulus is measured, and the "appropriate size" prosthesis is selected. Interrupted sutures (nonabsorbable) are placed first into the annulus and next into the outer edge of the prosthesis (circumferentially) before the prosthesis is lowered into place. The sutures and the prosthesis are kept moist until placed in the annulus. To prevent stitches around the new valve (prosthesis) from tearing through tissue, *Teflon pledgets* may be placed to bolster the stitches. The sutures may be placed in alternating colors. Air is aspirated from the left ventricle as the cardiotomy incision is closed and the aortic cross clamp is removed. CPB is discontinued. The wound may be irrigated with an antibiotic solution (at room temperature) or warmed saline as the heart and the whole patient are gradually rewarmed. ***Temporary pacemaker*** electrodes (epicardial) are sutured to the heart's surface. Mediastinal drains may be inserted. The wound is closed. There are many types of cardiac valve prostheses available, including preserved biological valves (porcine) or totally fabricated prostheses of various sizes, shapes, and mechanics. A patient may have more than one valve requiring replacement.

Coronary Artery Bypass Graft (CABG)

Definition

Occluded coronary arteries are bypassed with autologous or synthetic grafts.

Discussion

CABG is performed to relieve chest pain from coronary artery disease and to prevent ischemic myocardial injury. The ischemic myocardium is revascularized bypassing the obstructed coronary artery(ies) with a graft(s). The graft(s) may be fashioned from segments of the saphenous vein, the internal mammary artery (internal thoracic artery), the radial artery, or a combination of these. Usually, segments of the saphenous vein (taken from one or both lower extremities) are employed when multiple grafts are needed. Infrequently, synthetic grafts may be employed.

Coronary artery bypass grafts may be performed in conjunction with another procedure, e.g., valve replacement.

Procedure

CABG may be performed using the standard approach through a median sternotomy; additional approaches (e.g., MIDCAB, OPCAB, and TECAB) are described below. CABG is described here using the standard approach.

A single or multiple grafts may be placed with this fully open approach. In the standard approach, the graft (most often, the saphenous vein) is harvested (dissected to obtain maximal length) endoscopically and its tributaries are clipped. The distal end of the (vein) graft is marked by clips, etc., as it must be positioned in reverse before grafting. Saphenous veins may be harvested bilaterally. The (vein) grafts are evaluated regarding adequate blood flow and tested for leaks. The prepared grafts are kept moist with heparinized saline or blood until needed for grafting. The lower extremity wounds are closed. The legs may be wrapped with elastic bandages (e.g., Ace) to prevent swelling. When feasible, the left internal mammary (thoracic) artery is directly anastomosed to the left anterior descending (LAD) (or can be harvested as an interposition graft). Cannulation for partial CPB is achieved, and mild hypothermia is instituted. The aorta is occluded; cardioplegic solution is infused. The occluded coronary artery is isolated; it may be dilated (e.g., with Garrett dilators) to increase the size of the artery's lumen. The grafts are anastomosed to the coronary artery and tested for leaks. Multiple grafts may be necessary. The grafts are placed sequentially; that is, one graft segment can be anastomosed to more than one coronary artery. The aortic cross-clamp is released, and a portion of the aorta is then occluded. At a site on the proximal portion of the aorta (where occluded), the aortotomy is made using an aortic punch. The grafts are measured, cut, and anastomosed to the aorta. The positions of the graft sites are marked with clips for future location identification. The clamp on the aorta is removed. (Some surgeons prefer to perform the aortic anastomoses for CABG prior to the coronary artery anastomoses. The sequence of anastomoses varies with each surgeon, particularly when multiple grafts are performed.) Temporary pacemaker electrodes are sutured to the heart. Grafts are again inspected for leaks. All sources of air bubble accumulation are vented. CPB is discontinued; sometimes the patient will require weaning from CPB. The wound may be irrigated with an antibiotic solution or warmed saline. Mediastinal drains may be inserted. The wound is closed.

Minimally invasive direct coronary artery bypass (MIDCAB) is performed for revascularization of the LAD using a partial anterior mini-sternotomy with a lower-end sternal splitting (LESS) approach as opposed to completely splitting the sternum, employing minimally invasive CPB. Surgery is performed through a "keyhole"-sized opening.

Off-pump coronary artery bypass (OPCAB) can be performed using a partial or complete sternotomy approach; off-pump can be performed for multi-vessel revascularization on the beating heart. Procedures on the beating heart are facilitated by the use of retractor systems that isolate and stabilize the immediate operative site. Vessel conduits (e.g., radial a. or saphenous v.) are harvested with patient in supine position prior to lateral positioning of the patient for OPCAB.

Totally endoscopic coronary artery bypass (TECAB), including robotics, can be performed using total endoscopic access off-pump for harvesting the internal mammary artery (IMA) and gastroepiploic artery (GEA) to bypass the LAD, coronary artery, and right coronary artery (RCA). The endoscopic approach permits the harvesting and grafting of these vessels via only the mini-incisions needed for introducing the scope and a few accessory instruments. The IMA can be harvested using *robotic telemanipulation* using three ports. Robotic ports can be employed to introduce retractors, etc. The radial artery can be harvested endoscopically, when necessary.

The *Hybrid procedure* combines MIDCAB to bypass blockages in the LAD plus the minimally invasive endovascular angioplasty technique with stenting to restore patency to additional coronary arteries. Patients receive a more complete revascularization without having additional procedures.

Pulmonary Embolectomy

Definition

Extraction of thrombi (blood clots) from the pulmonary arteries.

Discussion

Pulmonary emboli most often result from migration of thrombi from the deep veins of the pelvis and lower extremities to the main or larger pulmonary arteries. Thrombophlebitis, trauma, or surgery of the abdomen or the lower extremities, estrogen therapy, pregnancy, and unduly prolonged bed rest, etc., predispose the formation of blood clots. Pulmonary emboli may be asymptomatic and only incidentally detected; however, more extensive presentations include chest pain, dyspnea, blood-tinged sputum, and hypotension in the more severe presentations. Death may occur soon after a "massive" embolization.

Intervention includes general medical support, anticoagulation, antithrombolytic therapy (when not medically contraindicated, such as in presence of recent surgical wounds, blood dyscrasias, etc.), transvenous thrombectomy (employing suction and irrigation, with mechanical disruption of the thrombi), and institution of extracorporeal life support in more severe cases. When nonoperative measures cannot maintain hemodynamic stability, surgery is indicated. Studies including ventilation/perfusion, computed tomography, or magnetic resonance imaging must be instituted promptly when the patient does not respond medically. Arteriography is most definitive but is infrequently done due to time factors and the instability of the patient's condition. If surgery is indicated, prompt intervention is mandatory. When time and the status of the patient permit, transesophageal echocardiography is performed as a final diagnostic measure prior to making the incision. CPB is instituted with cardioplegia. After the blood clots are extracted and the arterial incisions closed, a *venous filter* is placed in the inferior vena cava. Postoperative anticoagulation is maintained.

In circumstances when the patient sustains pulmonary embolism and subsequently develops pulmonary hypertension due to retained organized thrombi or thickened intima, pulmonary endarterectomy is indicated. **Pulmonary endarterectomy** is performed electively with CPB and hypothermic cardioplegia. Both left and right arteries are explored, and the obstructing matter in these fragile vessels is carefully removed. The pleural cavities are avoided. The procedure is similar otherwise to acute ***arterial embolectomy***.

Procedure

A sternal splitting incision is made; CPB is instituted. The pulmonary artery is incised and thrombi are removed with forceps or suction catheter. The left and right pulmonary arteries are explored for additional clots. A sterile pediatric bronchoscope may be employed to explore the lesser arterial tributaries. Any clot in the right atrium or ventricle is removed. The pleura may be entered to massage the lungs to express peripheral clots more centrally to facilitate their extraction. The arteriotomies are closed. CPB is discontinued. Chest tubes may be placed, and the wound is closed in the usual manner. An *inferior vena caval filter* (e.g., Greenfield) is placed transvenously.

MAZE Procedure

Definition

A maze of surgical incisions is made in the atria to interrupt aberrant nerve conduction pathways.

Discussion

This procedure corrects atrial arrhythmias, particularly atrial fibrillation, which is unresponsive to medical treatment and various cardiac catheterization lab ablative procedures. A number of incisions are made in the atria at various angles so as to describe a "maze" pattern. These incisions interrupt aberrant electrical impulses that interfere with the normal physiologic stimulation through the atrioventricular node necessary for regular ventricular contraction. The "standard" **MAZE III** (evolving from the original procedure, James Cox, MD) procedure is performed on bypass with cardioplegia, with incisions made in both atria, excising the left atrial appendage, incisions about the pulmonary veins, and, in some circumstances, incisions within the atria about the coronary sinus and tricuspid valve and the mitral valve annulus. The surgery is often done in conjunction with *mitral valve surgery*.

Modifications of the procedure are also performed, including the *CryoMAZE* technique, a minimally invasive procedure via a "keyhole" incision employing thoracoscopic approach (utilizing the freezing capacity of an argon probe, e.g., SurgiFrost®); similarly, high-intensity focused ultrasound wave ablation can be done under minimally invasive access, off-pump technique. *Microwave therapy* employs energy to create incisions performed concurrently with CABG. A percutaneous technique employing *radio-frequency wave* energy has been used in the cardiac catheterization lab for the right and left atria; however, this modification may take 8 to 12 hours to complete with a lesser success rate than the open procedure or minimally invasive approach.

Procedure

Following the establishment of CPB with cardioplegia, incisions are made in the atrial wall and within the atria in a mazelike pattern (as noted above). The atrial wall incisions are suture repaired. Epicardial pacemaker leads are sewn onto the surface of the heart. The electrical conduction patterns are monitored. As noted, *mitral valve surgery* may be done simultaneously. CPB is reversed, drains placed, and the parietal incisions closed.

Transmyocardial Laser Revascularization Procedure (TMLR)

Definition

A laser is employed to form channels in the myocardium to effect local neovascularization in the healing process with improved oxygenation of the ventricular muscle.

Discussion

By creating (1-mm) channels in the myocardium of an ischemic, but not scarified, left ventricle, vascularity and local perfusion are improved as a capillary network seeks to communicate with the channels, and/or neoangiogenesis during the healing process creates a new capillary network. The procedure is undertaken when medical treatment (e.g., drugs) or CABG has been unsuccessful in relieving angina or when the obstructed coronary arteries are too small to be bypassed (directly). Channels of 1-mm diameter (20 to 40) are created with the CO_2 laser (or holmium:YAG laser), extending from the epicardium into the ventricle (approximately one channel per square centimeter of ischemic ventricular surface). The procedure can be performed via left anterolateral thoracotomy using a limited incision without bypass (i.e., off-pump). It can also be performed using a thoracoscopic "keyhole" approach off-pump when circumstances permit, in the absence of adhesions, noting that many of these patients have undergone prior cardiac surgery. A double-lumen endotracheal tube permits deflation of the lung on the operative side to enhance exposure.

Procedure

Under general anesthesia after placement of Swan-Gans catheter and transesophageal echocardiogram probe (TEE) and insertion of a double-lumen endotracheal tube, a left anterolateral thoracotomy is performed (fifth to sixth interspace). A "heart cradling" retractor is employed. Adhesions are carefully lysed and the pericardium opened. After mapping out the sites of channeling, the CO_2 laser probe is placed on the epicardium and fired during end-systole (to minimize creation of a ventricular arrhythmia). The laser is set from 15 to 60 J for 20 to 50 milliseconds. On TEE, evidence of successful channeling is noted by bubbles or steam within the tracts created. Bleeding from the channels is usually controlled by pressure (or suture). Mediastinal (and pleural) drains are placed, and the incision is closed.

Considerations for Perioperative Nursing Care of the Cardiac Patient

Probably no other surgery is as intimately associated with the fear of death and dying as cardiac surgery. Similarly, perioperative nursing care of the cardiac patient demands more than that of most other surgeries. The perioperative RN allays the patient's fears by offering emotional support without deemphasizing the serious nature of the proposed surgery. As the RN assesses the patient's physical condition, he/she converses with the patient to determine the patient's comprehension level (knowledge deficit) regarding the surgery. The perioperative RN clarifies misconceptions and answers questions in a knowledgeable manner whenever possible, refers questions to the surgeon, as necessary, and explains perioperative events and treatments ahead of time to ease anxiety associated with the unfamiliar environment. He/she indicates a willingness to act as the patient's advocate.

The surgical team members must recognize that even minor lapses in concentration or inattention to details can lead to irreversible consequences for the patient. In addition to the usual exercise of diligence, the perioperative team must be familiar with a wide spectrum of life support and monitoring devices not usually utilized for other types of surgeries. The perioperative RN, the scrub technologist, and the anesthesia provider (usually an anesthesiologist/intensivist specializing in cardiac surgery) must be experienced in assisting during cardiac surgery and thoroughly familiar with the routine of the surgeon and the "open-heart" procedure. Specialized care of the cardiac patient involves continuous perioperative assessment of the patient's physical condition and the institution of nursing measures or interventions that will contribute to the best outcomes for the patient. Review laboratory and test results, the **Surgical Assessment and Preoperative Checklist**, p. 9, the suggested **Perioperative Care Plan**, p. 12, and the **Special Notes** to develop a plan of care, and document, document, document!

The perioperative practitioner in the surgical holding (preop) area may perform the initial skin prep with a depilatory or clippers when ordered. Razors and "wet" shave are to be avoided, as the risk from infection in the surgical wound is greater when the skin is broken. The OR is prepared before the cardiac patient is brought into the room, as extensive preparations are necessary and observing this activity may cause undue anxiety to the patient. The open-heart room is usually the largest OR, to accommodate the necessary equipment. When the procedure will be performed on-pump, perfusionists set up the apparatus in advance. When the procedure is performed off-pump, the cell-saver is employed; the pump perfusionists should be available (present).

Preparation of the Patient

A hyperthermia/hypothermia mattress, e.g., MUL-T-Blanket may be placed on the table for temperature control. The patient is positioned in the supine or the lateral position for cardiac surgery, depending on the procedure to be performed and the surgeon's preference. See Segmental Resection of the Lung, p. 455, for particulars regarding lateral positioning of the patient.

The supine approach will be described. The patient receives general anesthesia (such as high-dose narcotics and short- and intermediate-acting anesthetic agents) via a double-lumen endotracheal tube. A pillow may be placed under the knees to avoid strain on the back muscles and for comfort. ECG leads (9 to 12) and a pulse oximeter (to measure oxygen saturation) are placed. When harvesting the saphenous vein for grafting, a pillow is placed under the knees to maintain slight flexion and to facilitate access. The circulator assists the anesthesia provider in placing vascular lines in the upper extremities: arterial lines (e.g., radial artery) to directly monitor arterial blood pressure and to obtain samples for blood gas analysis, venous lines (peripheral and central) to infuse drugs and fluids, and a Swan-Ganz catheter to measure intracardiac pressures. The arms may be extended on padded armboards or are padded and tucked in at the patient's sides. The anesthesia provider establishes continuous TEE; ultrasound technology displays the interior of the heart. A temperature probe is inserted into the esophagus. Antiembolitic hose are applied when harvesting the saphenous vein is *not* required. A sequential compression device with disposable leg wraps may be employed to prevent thrombus formation. The disposable wraps are applied over the antiembolitic hose. All bony prominences and areas prone to skin and neurovascular pressure or trauma are padded. The electrosurgical dispersive pad is applied to a relatively hair-free site; the skin may require hair removal. A Foley catheter is inserted and connected to a urimeter or urometer.

Skin Preparation

For standard sternotomy approach for valve replacement and other cardiac procedures that do not require access to the saphenous veins, begin at the midline of the chest, extending from the chin to just above the knees and down to the table at the sides. The genitalia are prepped last.

For standard sternotomy approach for cardiac procedures that require access to the saphenous veins, usually both lower extremities are prepped to facilitate access for harvesting an adequate length of saphenous vein (in case several grafts are needed). Two prep trays are used; one tray has adequate supplies for the circulator to prep the abdomen. Begin at the midline of the chest, extending from the chin to the symphysis pubis and down to the table at the sides. The genitalia are prepped last. The tray is discarded. A second tray (with additional prep solutions and sponges) is used to prep the lower extremities. The prep is best performed by two persons; however, one person may perform the prep when a leg holder is used (attachment to the table) with sterile towels. Begin the prep on the inside of the thighs (where the vein grafts will be harvested). Extend the prep from the thighs to the toes. Prep the front and back of the lower extremities. The feet are prepared last, include toes and interdigital spaces, and each sponge is discarded after cleansing the toes. When the prep is completed, the legs are elevated and abducted as the end of the table is draped by sterile team members.

Draping

Large drape sheets, folded towels, and sterile, adhesive plastic drapes (2)

For standard sternotomy approach for valve replacement and other cardiac procedures that *do not* require access to the saphenous veins, a large drape sheet (impervious, some surgeons prefer a sheet with plastic liner be placed over the legs and the end of the table). A towel (folded in thirds lengthwise) is placed over the genitalia. Towels folded longitudinally are placed along the patient's sides and across the sternal notch. Sterile, adhesive plastic drapes may be applied across the chest and abdomen. Large drape sheets are placed at the sides and across the top of the patient.

For standard sternotomy approach for cardiac procedures that require access to the saphenous veins, the legs are held up and abducted by the persons who performed the prep as sterile team members place a large drapc sheet on the end of the table. The feet are lowered onto the towels (two each), and the towels are fashioned into boots and clipped. A towel (folded in thirds lengthwise) is placed over the genitalia. A split sheet is placed under and around both legs. Towels are folded longitudinally and placed along the patient's sides and across the sternal notch. Sterile, adhesive plastic drapes may be applied across the chest and abdomen. Large drape sheets are placed at the sides and across the top of the patient.

Equipment (depending on the procedure and the surgeon's preference)

MUL-T-Blanket (hyperthermia/hypothermia blanket or mattress pad)
Arkive™ touch screen oscilloscope displays
Temperature probe (esophageal)
Transesophageal echocardiograph monitor and probe
ECG (12 leads) and EEG monitors
CVP or Swan-Ganz manometry
Headrest or support, e.g., donut
Small roll placed between the scapulae, pillow, pad, and additional padding, as necessary
Extra intravenous line standards
Suctions (4 working), available
Cell-saver (autotransfusion) for "off-pump"
CPB machine, pump oxygenator, blood filter, temperature sensor (with thermal adjuster), slush machine
External pacemaker and external defibrillator
ESU
Laser (CO_2, holmium:YAG)
Fiber-optic headlight with camera and fiber-optic power source (combined unit where available)
Video monitor
Fiber-optic light source for endoscope

Instrumentation

Oscillating saw, sternal, e.g., Sarns®, Stryker®
Cardiac procedures instrument trays
Phrenic nerve pad
Tube clamps
Hemoclip® appliers (assorted sizes and lengths)
DeBakey "bulldog" clips and appliers (1.25 and 1.5 mm)

Cell-saver suction
Epicardial pacemaker leads
Defibrillator paddles and cord (internal use)

Minimally Invasive

The following are examples of the myriad of instrumentation developed to facilitate procedures performed "off-pump"

Retractors and stabilizers, e.g., mini-thoracotomy retractor, mammary self-retaining retractor with Teflon tip, Octopus® and Starfish™ retractors (Medtronics), CTS Access Ultima Retractor (CardioThoracic Systems), ESTECH retractor system (Estech, Inc.), ACROBAT Systems (suction exposure device)

Device to lift heart, e.g., Myoloft Flexsite retractor and stabilizer or AXIUS and Xpose, Symmetry Bypass System

Miscellaneous: Heartstring II aortic cutter, CO_2 mister-blower (controlled saline and CO_2), Clearglide Endovascular Vessel Harvester System, anastomosis assist device (CABG), extracorporeal membrane oxygenator (EMCO)

Long-handled dissectors, vascular clamps, scissors, knife handles, suturing device (e.g., Semb), alligator forceps (valves)

Endoscope, e.g., thoracoscope and cord

Endoscopic Redo Sternotomy Retractor

Robotic systems, e.g., Aesop 3000, Hermes, da Vinci

Endoscopic:

Babcock forceps (2), scissors (3) (curved, hook, straight), right angle dissector, Kelly clamps, multifire ligating clip applier, dissecting forceps (straight, right angle, and hook), irrigation-suction-electrosurgical dissectors

Supplies

Antiembolitic hose (saphenous vein graft **will not** be harvested)

Cardiac valve either biologic or mechanical (range of sizes of the type requested should be in the room)

Intraaortic balloon catheter (IABC), ventricular assist device (VAD), optional

Cannulas and associated supplies for vascular pressure lines arterial, venous, CVP, and Swan-Ganz lines

Foley catheter with drainage tubing and urimeter

Impervious stockinette tubes or towels with towel clips (to fashion into boots, i.e., foot drapes)

Sterile, adhesive plastic drapes (2)

Basin set

Knife blades, (2) #10, #15, #11, and Beaver blade

Electrosurgical pencils, (2) (1 spatula and 1 needle point), cords with holders and scrapers

Bone wax
Suction tubing
Needle magnets or counters
Assorted syringes and needles, sterile labels and marking pen, medicine cups

Medications

Heparin IV and heparin added to 0.9% saline for irrigation to prevent blood clot formation
Topical papaverine solution (60 mg in 40 ml) to prevent vasospasm (mammary artery)
Cardioplegic agents contain potassium and buffering agents to arrest the heart
Nitroglycerine prophylaxis for ischemia
Antibiotic for irrigation solution or for IV use

Large graduate pitchers (2) with Asepto or bulb syringes (2)
Ligating clips, e.g., Hemoclips (assorted sizes)
Cell-saver suction tubing for auto transfusion (off-pump) and auto transfusion system
Bypass circuit tubing
Fibrin sealant or "glue" (thrombin, calcium, and cryoprecipitate) may be injected over bleeding site
Hemostatic agents (e.g., Gelfoam, Oxycel, Surgicel™)
Teflon felt strips and pledgets or suture boots, Silastic® suture (inflow occlusion), or Silastic tape
Cardioplegia administration set, as requested
Pacemaker wires (epicardial)
Elastic bandages for lower extremities (saphenous vein grafts)
Mediastinal drains (2) with Y-connector
Defibrillator paddles and power cord
Heavy-gauge wire suture and wire cutter for sternal closure
Argyle chest tube(s) with tubing connector (straight or "Y") and intrapleural sealed drainage unit, e.g., Pleurevac™

CryoMAZE, Add

Argon cryo probes
Laser, e.g., CO_2 or holmium:YAG hand piece, consoles, safety equipment
Mediastinal drains, e.g., Jackson-Pratt™

Special Notes

- Apply **Special Notes** from ***Abdominal Aortic Aneurymectomy***, p. 493.
- Specialized care of the cardiac patient involves continuous perioperative assessment and documentation of the patient's

physical condition. All nursing care administered (intervention) is documented for patient safety through continuity of care and for medicolegal reasons.

- Emotional support is also vital, particularly considering the serious nature of cardiac surgery. Answer patient's questions in a calm manner or refer questions to the surgeon. Explain actions before performing them.
- The circulator(s) and scrub person(s) must be thoroughly familiar with the routine of the surgeon and the "open-heart" team. Persons not familiar with cardiac surgery or the surgeon's routine should work with someone who is experienced until the person "new" to the open-heart team feels confident about working alone.
- A bag fashioned out of a Mayo stand cover is fastened to the head of the table for the defibrillator paddles. This bag should be placed as soon as possible.
- Circulator ascertains that blood is available as ordered and ready for immediate use. Circulator obtains items necessary for administration (e.g., tubing set, blood warmer, pressure bag) and assists the anesthesia provider to monitor hemodynamics and to administer blood (identify patient and blood type, etc.). When the surgery is elective, the patient may have given blood in advance for an autotransfusion.
- The circulator assists the anesthesia provider in obtaining vascular access for intravenous lines for measuring arterial and venous pressures and CVP and documents these treatments.
- Circulator documents the administration of blood and any reaction or lack of reaction to the transfusion in the **Perioperative Record.**
- When the cell-saver is used, all intraoperative blood is suctioned, filtered, and reinfused. The scrub person should squeeze blood out of sponges before discarding them into the kick bucket. The cell-saver is used only when the blood is free of contamination; it cannot be employed once antibiotic irrigation is used.
- The scrub person should keep instruments free of blood clots, plaque, and tissue debris.
- Several liters of iced saline slush may be needed when going on the pump.
- **Reminder:** Care must be taken to maintain patient's body temperature. Off-pump temperature is maintained with a

warming mattress, warm IV fluids, and by adjusting the room temperature; *hypothermia is required on pump*.

- Avoid risk for infection by maintaining sterile technique; use a separate (isolate) instrument set for saphenous vein harvesting, change gown and gloves when moving from the extremity incisions to the chest incision, etc.
- **N.B.** The prosthesis is delivered to the surgeon on a prosthesis holder; it is handled as little as possible to avoid contamination. Do ***not*** open prosthesis until the surgeon is sure of the size.
- **N.B.** Scrub person should have the appropriate sizers (according to type) on the Mayo stand as the diseased valve is being removed. The valve holder on which the valve is placed (before handing same to the surgeon) should also be visible on the Mayo stand in anticipation of use.
- **N.B.** *Scrub person* **should not** *cut double-armed sutures used in vascular surgery.*
- **N.B.** Scrub person should have a pair of French-eyed needles available should another stitch be required of a suture placed earlier (when the needles have been cut off); additional sutures should be readily available.
- Great care must be taken to ensure that the needle count is correct, as many small double-armed swaged on needles will be used.
- "Cryo"-preserved heart valves (e.g., allografts or xenografts) must be carefully thawed and thoroughly rinsed of any remaining glutaraldehyde according to the manufacturer's directions.
- Mechanical valves are placed in antibiotic solution prior to insertion.
- Circulator documents blood administration and any reaction or lack of reaction to the transfusion in the **Perioperative Record**.
- Circulator maintains an accurate record of irrigation used and weighs sponges to determine blood loss and fluid loss to estimate requirements for fluid replacement.
- Measure urine every 15 minutes while on the pump.
- **N.B.** *Saline is used instead of water on the back table to ensure that only saline,* **not** *water, is used to fill the cannula, as water causes hemolysis.*
- **Reminder:** Use safety precautions to identify, label, and dispense medications or solutions and to avoid medication errors;

see p. 30. It is mandatory that all medications and solutions on the sterile field be labeled by name and strength. The medication bottle is retained in the room until the procedure has concluded.

- **Reminder:** Persons scrubbed should wear a protective face shield to prevent injury from splashing or spraying of the patient's blood and irrigation fluids that are used.
- Circulator documents the type, size, and serial numbers of a synthetic graft (valve) in the **Perioperative Record** and in the hospital's log for insertion of an implant, according to policy.
- When a femoral incision is made for saphenous vein "harvesting," counts are taken before the second incision is made and at the closure of each incision.
- Femoral artery (and vein) access is usually chosen for the patient having a repeat cardiac procedure with partial CPB and minimal access procedure.
- **N.B.** The scrub person should ***always*** maintain the sterility of the back table until the patient leaves the room. At the conclusion of the procedure, the scrub person should have a sterile wire cutter and a sternal retractor "on hand" (e.g., on the Mayo stand); all instrumentation should remain sterile in case the chest has to be reopened.
- **N.B.** Scrub person should be prepared to go back "on pump" at any time. Cannula, sutures, etc., are kept sterile until the patient leaves the room, should CPB be renewed.
- The circulator accompanies the patient to the cardiovascular recovery unit (CVRU) and reports intraoperative information that has been documented in the **Perioperative Record** to the CVRU RN for safety and for medicolegal reasons. This may include details about transfusions, medications administered, and any information necessary to provide continuity of care of the patient, e.g., stability of condition, neurological status, allergic reaction to medications, intraoperative observations, and nursing care implemented (interventions) with outcomes (results).
- **N.B.** The patient's vital signs and blood pressure are charted on the vital signs graph; they are continuously monitored and documented in CVRU. Any deviations from the "norm" that might indicate hemorrhage are reported to the surgeon "stat."

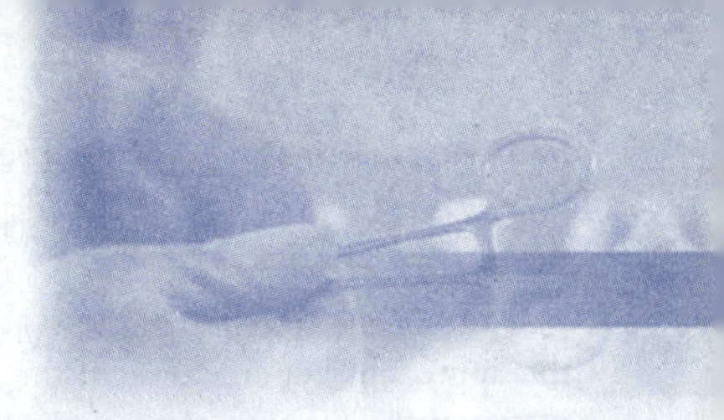

CHAPTER 23
Orthopedic Surgery

Open Reduction and Internal Fixation of a Carpal Bone Fracture

Definition

Surgical realignment and fixation of carpal bone fractures (or a fracture dislocation).

Discussion

Most fractures of the wrist are treated by closed reduction and immobilization (cast). Surgery is required when the fracture is displaced or dislocated or when there is a nonunion. Fixation may be achieved with a number of devices, including pins, wires, and a compression plates and screws. Persistent nonunion may necessitate an autologous bone graft (from the forearm or the iliac crest). More severe injuries may require excision of carpal bones and/or the radial or ulnar styloid process to prevent restricted mobility. ***Arthrodesis*** of the wrist may be preferable in patients who engage in manual labor. Numerous permutations of fractures and dislocations can present. The most common fracture is of the scaphoid (navicular) bone. When indicated, if the scaphoid is severely traumatized or osteonecrosis develops, an implanted prosthesis (made of silicone, plastic, materials, or metal) can be employed. Closed reduction with transcutaneous pin insertion can be facilitated by ***arthroscopy of the wrist***; see p. 544.

Pneumatic tourniquets are often employed for fractures of the extremities. Care is taken to avoid pressure injury over bony structures. Following the skin prep, the arm is abducted and elevated, as an Esmarch rubber bandage is wrapped around it (distally to proximally) to achieve exsanguination.

For additional tourniquet safety measure guidelines, see p. 45. Tourniquet ends must overlap by about 3 inches, but not more than 6 inches. Do not apply the tourniquet near or at the elbow. *The tourniquet should always be inflated for the least amount of time possible.* Recommended tourniquet time suggests less than 1 hour on the upper extremity for an adult and 1.5 hours on the lower extremity. Setting for an adult is approximately 250 to 300 mm Hg for the upper extremity (lower extremity at the thigh, 350 mm Hg). Alternative pressure guidelines are: 50–75 mm Hg above patient's systolic blood pressure for the upper extremity in adults; 100–150 mm Hg for the lower extremity. Thin adults and children will require less pressure.

Procedure

The site of the fracture and the preference of the surgeon determine the approach. For fractures of the scaphoid bone, an incision may be made on the dorsum of the wrist distal to the radiocarpal joint. Tendons and nerve roots are protected. Small bone fragments (chips) are excised; the bone chips may be saved (kept moist in blood or saline), and later the bone chips (in the barrel of a syringe may be compacted by pressure exerted on the plunger) may be used as a bone graft to replace a bone defect. Larger fragments are aligned and fixed with Kirschner wires to maintain the correct anatomical position. When bone graft pegs are employed, they may be obtained with a tubular gouge. Herbert or Acutrak™ screws or a small compression plate with screws are employed for fixation. An "auto" bone graft requires an additional incision made (usually to expose the radial styloid), from which the bone graft may be taken. In some cases of nonunion, such as necrosis, larger fragments or the entire bone segment (or fragment) may be excised. The wound may be cleansed of debris with pulsed lavage of lactated Ringer's solution or irrigated with normal saline prior to closure; antibiotics may be added to either solution. The wound is closed. A short arm splint or cast is applied.

Preparation of the Patient

Antiembolitic hose are applied (adult), as requested. Regional (e.g., Bier block) anesthetic or general anesthesia may be employed. The patient is in supine position, close to the ipsilateral edge of the table, with the affected arm extended on a padded hand table (radiolucent, when available). The unaffected arm may be extended on a padded armboard, or the arm is padded and tucked in at the patient's side. A pillow may be placed under the knees to prevent lower back strain and for comfort. Webril and a tourniquet are applied to the affected arm. Pad all bony prominences and areas vulnerable to skin and neurovascular pressure or trauma. Apply electrosurgical dispersive pad.

Skin Preparation

Begin at the wrist; extend the prep from the fingertips to the level of the tourniquet (include the arm, forearm, hand, fingers, and interdigital spaces).

Draping

The extremity (covered with tube stockinette) is abducted and elevated. A sheet is draped over the hand table. A split sheet is draped under the arm. A folded towel (thirds, longitudinally) is wrapped around the top of the arm (over the stockinette) and secured. A drape (or split) sheet covers the shoulder and is fastened under the arm. The extremity is passed through a fenestrated sheet (transverse or laparotomy), or additional drape sheets complete the draping.

Equipment

Padded hand table, radiolucent preferred (e.g., Multilok™ or Tenet)
Positioning device for hand, optional
Suction
Generator for pulsed lavage suction irrigator, e.g., Simpulse, MicroAire optional
Electrosurgical unit (ESU)
Tourniquet and pneumatic insufflator with microprocessor regulator
Sitting stools (3) (surgeon, assistant, scrub person)
Power source for power drill (optional, depends on type of drill)
Cast cart

Instrumentation

Minor orthopedic procedures tray (wire cutter, included)
Multilok tabletop with accessories (optional)
Hand holder/stabilizer (single use, sterile)
Micro power drill (e.g., Stryker®, Hall, or 3M self-contained) or with cord, drill sheath, chuck, drill sleeve, and drill bits
Fixation device, e.g., Kirschner wires, compression plate and screws, Herbert screws, Acutrak screws, or Steinmann pins
Bone grafting instruments, e.g., Dowel tubular gouge for bone peg, Cloward bone graft double-ended impactor
Lexer gouges, Cobb gouges, periosteal bone elevator (small), bone tamp, awl, pin cutter
Pulsed lavage suction irrigator and tip, e.g., Simpulse®, MicroAire® (optional)

Supplies

Antiembolitic hose, as requested
Webril (unsterile, under the tourniquet)
Tube stockinette
Esmarch bandage
Blades, (1) #10 and (2) #15
Electrosurgical pencil and cord with holder and scraper
Needle magnet or counter
Suction tubing (2) or cojoined suction and irrigation tubing for pulsed lavage (available)
Irrigation solution (lactated Ringer's solution) in 3000-ml bags for pulsed lavage or normal saline in 3000 ml irrigation bags with K50 polyethylene cystoscopy tubing and 3- way stopcock
Antibiotic may be added to the irrigation bags or a graduated pitcher, bulb syringe, antibiotic irrigation
Casting supplies

Special Notes

- Apply **Special Notes** from ***Abdominal Laparotomy***, as they apply to all patients in surgery (e.g., regarding correct identification of the patient, observing "time out," etc.); see p. 134. All nursing care interventions and outcomes are documented in the **Perioperative Record** for patient safety regarding continuity of care and for medicolegal reasons.
- **Reminder:** Ascertain that the *correct* x-ray films for the *correctly identified* patient are in the room prior to starting the surgery.
- Circulator must notify x-ray department that fluoroscopy is anticipated for this surgical procedure. The hand table is made of radiolucent materials to facilitate fluoroscopy.
- Observe x-ray safety precautions; see Chapter 3, p. 52.
- A padded hand table is an accessory to the standard Ritter operating room (OR) table. A Multilok hand table (radiolucent) may be requested. Multilok system components include a base locking onto the table, a hand rest (for surgeon), presterilized tabletop (single use), and accessories (thumb post, finger posts, wrist wrap, Silicone™ ties, and retractors). A combination of the components can provide stabilization of the hand in an infinite number of positions. Document the use, serial number on the pieces used, and placement (position) of the components when Multilok is used.
- **Reminder:** Do not permit preparation solutions to pool under tourniquet, to avoid excoriation the skin. Document the appearance of the skin before and after skin prep and preoperatively and immediately postoperatively.
- The circulator places the tourniquet as high on extremity as possible. Webril (sheet wadding) is wrapped smoothly around the extremity (under tourniquet). The limb is elevated and an Esmarch bandage is wrapped proximally, i.e., from the fingertips proximally, to exsanguinate the limb. Document the location of tourniquet placement, the name of the person who placed it, and the appearance of the skin before and after the tourniquet use on the **Perioperative Record**.
- Monitor the amount of time the tourniquet is on. Document the unit number, setting, and times starting and ending for tourniquet use. Observe safety precautions regarding pneumatic tourniquet use; see Chapter 2, p. 45.
- Take appropriate measures to maintain patient's body temperature (e.g., offer a warmed blanket, adjust room temperature).

When ordered, a hyperthermia/hypothermia MUL-T-Blanket® may be placed over the patient; a heated mattress pad is not used, as it interferes with taking x-rays.

- **Reminder:** Use safety precautions to identify, label, and dispense medications or solutions and to avoid medication errors; see p. 30. It is mandatory that all medications and solutions on the sterile field be labeled by name and strength. The medication bottle is retained in the room until the procedure has concluded.
- When available, a fluid-control drape (with pouch) should be used to collect the irrigation solution (as necessary) to prevent contamination of the sterile field.
- Wearing a protective face shield or goggles is recommended to protect those scrubbed from the splashing of irrigation fluid, blood, bone chips, etc.
- Document the application of the fixation device, according to type, size, and serial numbers, in the Perioperative Record.
- Be prepared to assist the surgeon with the application of a splint or cast. A "cast cart" complete with supplies needed for making a plaster cast is available in most hospitals; casts can be made of other materials, e.g., fiberglass.
- The circulator obtains the "cast cart" at the conclusion of the surgery. All supplies for making a cast should be assembled before application of the cast is begun, as the plaster dries hard very quickly. As plaster casts are heavy, they may later be exchanged for one composed of lighter material (fiberglass) to facilitate patient mobility.
- **N.B.** For cast application: Webril is wrapped around the hand, wrist, and forearm (including dressing) to a level 3″ above the anticipated proximal extent of the cast or splint. Various lengths of plaster material are dipped in a disposable bucket of lukewarm water. When the material no longer bubbles under water, it is ready for use. Heavy-duty scissors should be readily available.
- The circulator accompanies the patient to the PACU with the anesthesia provider and provides a report to the perioperative RN in the PACU with information necessary for continuity of care for the safe care of the patient.
- Upon the patient's arrival, and at intervals in the PACU, the RN monitors the patient's vital signs. He/she continuously assesses the patient's pain level, level of consciousness, and neurological status (i.e., strength and movement of extremities). The dressing (or cast) is observed for bleeding.

- In the PACU, the perioperative practitioner notes the circulation in the fingers and the patient's ability to move the fingers and perceive light touch. He/she checks that the cast is not constricting blood flow or causing neurological symptoms (e.g., paresthesias) and documents observations, nursing interventions, and patient outcomes.

Excision of Ganglion

Definition

Removal of a cystic dilation in a joint capsule or tendon sheath.

Discussion

The dorsal wrist is most frequent site of origin; it may also be noted about the finger joints, volar aspect of the wrist, dorsum of the foot, and about the knee and ankle. A ganglion usually occurs as the result of trauma or tissue degeneration due to disease, e.g., Raynaud's disease, but may appear de novo. Occasionally the cyst may spontaneously resolve. Aspiration (only) of the cyst usually results in recurrence. Careful, complete excision makes recurrence rare. A ganglion about the wrist can also be excised endoscopically.

Procedure

Regional anesthetic (i.e., block) or general anesthesia may be employed. The tourniquet is inflated. A transverse incision is made over the location of the ganglion. Soft tissue dissection exposes the ganglion. Care is taken to avoid injury to local nerves, tendons, and vascular structures. The ganglion is mobilized and excised (including a generous border at its base). The wound may be irrigated. The tendon sheath is repaired as necessary. The wound is closed. A dressing and an elastic pressure bandage are applied (after checking the chart for patient allergies). A splint may be utilized.

For **Preparation of the Patient, Skin Preparation,** and **Draping,** see ***Open Reduction of a Carpal Bone Fracture***, p. 536.

Equipment

Padded hand table (Matlock table), radiolucent preferred Multilok Modular System padded hand table
ESU
Suction (available)
Tourniquet and insufflator (tank of compressed air) with microprocessor regulator
Magnifying loupes, as requested
Sitting stools (2) for surgeon and scrub person
Cast cart

Instrumentation

Minor orthopedic procedures tray
Hay's metacarpal retractors, pediatric Deaver retractor (available)
Multilok tabletop hand holder (single use, sterile) and accessories, optional

Supplies

Webril (unsterile, under tourniquet)
Tube stockinette
Esmarch bandage
Blades, (2) #15
Electrosurgical pencil with needle tip and cord
Needle magnet or counter
Small basin, bulb syringe, and irrigation solution (antibiotic, optional)
Suction tubing (optional)
Elastic bandage, e.g., Ace

Special Notes

- Apply **Special Notes** from ***Open Reduction of a Carpal Bone Fracture***, p. 538, as applicable.

Carpal Tunnel Release

Definition

Decompression of the median nerve at the wrist.

Discussion

Carpal tunnel syndrome (CTS) is one of the most frequently incurred work-related injuries. Computer operators, assembly line workers, meat packers, construction workers, and cashiers are the most likely casualties of this repetitive strain injury. Symptoms of CTS (compression of the median nerve) include pain, numbness and tingling of the fingers, and weakness of intrinsic thumb muscles. By dividing the deep transverse carpal ligament, decompression of the median nerve results, relieving the symptoms.

Carpal tunnel release may be performed as an "open" or an endoscopic procedure.

Procedure

The open procedure is described. A curved incision is made parallel to the thenar crease in the palm and angled toward the volar aspect of the wrist. Care is taken to avoid injury to sensory branches of the median nerve. After the skin and subcutaneous tissues are excised and reflected, the deep transverse carpal ligament (flexor retinaculum) is divided, decompressing the nerve. The wound is closed. A compression dressing and a short arm splint are usually applied.

Preparation of the Patient

Regional (e.g., Bier block) or general anesthesia is employed. The patient is in supine position near the ipsilateral edge of the table for ease of access to the extremity. The affected arm is extended on a padded hand table. The unaffected arm is extended on a padded armboard, or it may be padded and tucked in at the patient's side. A pillow may be placed under the knees to prevent strain on the lower back and for comfort. Sheet wadding and a tourniquet are applied high on the affected arm. Bony prominences and areas vulnerable to skin and neurovascular pressure or trauma are padded. An electrosurgical dispersive pad is applied.

Skin Preparation

Begin the prep with the palm; include fingers and interdigital spaces. Prep the wrist and forearm, extending the prep to the elbow.

For **Draping, Equipment, Instrumentation, Supplies, and Special Notes,** see ***Open Reduction and Internal Fixation of a Carpal Bone Fracture***, p. 536.

Endoscopic Carpal Tunnel Release

Definition

Employing endoscopic visualization to decompress the median nerve at the wrist.

Discussion

The endoscopic procedure has certain advantages over the open procedure; it results in less scar pain, enhanced functioning of the hand, and increased pinch strength. There is no palmar incision; pain in the palm is not an issue. The disadvantages, however, include greater cost, a learning curve that must be overcome by the surgeon, and the increased chance for nerve injury. See "open" procedure, Carpal Tunnel Release, p. 541.

Procedure

The skin over the wrist lesion may be marked with indelible ink prior to the skin prep. Local anesthetic with or without epinephrine and conscious sedation are often administered, but general anesthesia may be employed as well. The tourniquet is inflated. A horizontal skin incision (1.5 cm) is made at the wrist anteriorly and deepened to the fascia. Dilators may be employed at the site, or approximately 6 ml of normal saline can be injected for ease of entry of the trocar. The scope (arthroscope) is introduced under the transverse carpal ligament. Local nerves and blood vessels are identified and avoided. An endoscopic hook knife is guided via the scope to release the transverse carpal ligament (decompressing the median nerve). The tourniquet is deflated. The incision is closed. A soft dressing and a short arm splint may be applied.

For **Preparation of the Patient, Skin Preparation,** and **Draping** see ***Open Reduction and Internal Fixation of a Carpal Bone Fracture,*** p. 536.

Equipment

Antiembolitic hose, optional
Padded hand table or Multilok Modular System padded hand table
ESU
Tourniquet and insufflator (tank of compressed air) with microprocessor regulator
Suction (available)
Sitting stools (2) for surgeon and scrub person
Arthroscopy tower with pump
Fiber-optic light source, e.g., Xenon™ 300 W
Monitor
VCR
Printer
CD burner
Camera console
Cast cart

Instrumentation

Minor orthopedic procedures tray
Arthroscope, 30° (2.4 mm) with camera and cord, sheath, bridge adaptor, camera
Endoscopic:
Cannulas, trocars, electrosurgical suction-irrigator and cord, meniscal hook blade, obturator, rasp, synovial elevator, sharp and dull probes, dilators (4, 6 mm), nerve hooks, knife (beaver) blade, knife handle
Multilok tabletop hand holder (single use, sterile) and accessories

Supplies

Indelible marking pen
Webril (unsterile under tourniquet)

Esmarch bandage
Tube stockinette
Marking pen (indelible ink), optional
Small basin, bulb syringe, suction tubing (available)
Needle, #18 spinal, 3½″, and 10-ml syringe
Silastic® intravenous (IV) tubing (2) for inflow and outflow
Irrigation bag (3000 ml) with lactated Ringer's solution (antibiotic may be added to the solution), optional
Splint materials

Special Notes

- Apply **Special Notes** from ***Open Reduction and Internal Fixation of a of Carpal Bone Fracture***, p. 538, as applicable.
- **N.B.** For all minimal access procedures, the patient must sign the surgical consent to include the possibility of conversion to an open procedure.
- When available, a fluid-control drape (with pouch) should be used to collect the irrigation solution as necessary to prevent contamination of the sterile field.
- The scrub person must monitor the temperature of the irrigation solution as it leaves the outflow tubing before the solution reaches the patient.
- Strict observance of manufacturer's recommendations for disinfection and sterilization of endoscopy scopes and instrumentation must be followed [e.g., using ethylene oxide, peracetic acid (Steris™) or hydrogen peroxide gas plasma].
- Using the Steris system, completely submerge scope in Steris™ 20 solution for 12 minutes, as recommended for sterilization; see p. 43.
- Most nondisposable endoscopic instruments may be carefully washed and flash sterilized.

Arthroscopy of the Wrist

Definition

Endoscopic visualization of the wrist joint.

Discussion

Wrist arthroscopy is performed to diagnose or clarify diagnoses regarding painful conditions of the wrist joint inadequately defined by arthrograms or magnetic resonance imaging (MRI) scans or to substantiate the need for an open procedure; scopes may permit up to a

115°-angle intra-articular view (e.g., TrueView™II). Loose bodies in the joint also can cause pain. In addition, the patient may have pain due to synovitis and/or disruption of ligamentous structures. Loose bodies detected during arthroscopy can be removed. Shortening or shaving the ulnar head, synovectomy, repair of the scapholunate ligament, excision of a ganglion, and repair of some fractures represent a few of the other procedures that can be performed arthroscopically. If articular surfaces are involved in the fracture, arthroscopic visualization can guide a satisfactory reduction with greater confidence than when fluoroscopy or MRI scan is employed. When assessment of wrist mobility and instability is needed, the procedure can be performed without distraction (the forearm lying freely on a padded table).

When treatment can be accomplished arthroscopically, it is usually performed as an outpatient procedure. Postoperative morbidity is reduced compared to an "open" procedure.

Procedure

Dorsal approach is discussed. The patient usually receives general anesthesia (regional anesthesia, e.g., brachial plexus block may be used). The surgeon may mark the dorsal wrist veins prior to the skin prep to provide a landmark (to avoid injury), as the veins are difficult to locate following elevation of the extremity and the inflation of pneumatic tourniquet. The forearm is wrapped with a carefully applied sterile Coban to prevent extravasation of irrigation solution into the forearm. Incision for primary port entry is made approximately 1-cm distal to the dorsal radial tubercle, between the radius and the lunate bone. The incision is enlarged, and approximately 6 ml of local anesthetic (with epinephrine to reduce bleeding) is injected to distend the capsule. An 18-gauge needle is inserted at the medial aspect of the wrist, adjacent to the extensor carpi ulnaris tendon, and used as an inflow site; gravity assists the inflow of the irrigation solution. The joint is entered (indicated by the flow of irrigation fluid); additional flow is necessary to maintain clear visualization without air bubbles.

A thorough examination is made of the various structures as the scope is advanced to assess the ulnar side of the wrist. Additional ports are established, as necessary. When systematic examination is completed, arthroscopic probes, joint shaver, etc., are employed to debride the joint and repair disruptions of ligamentous structures, and loose bodies are excised. Kirschner wires may be inserted to stabilize a fracture site. Repair is performed, as necessary (see Discussion above). A short arm splint is applied.

Preparation of the Patient

The patient usually receives general anesthesia. The supine position is employed, with the patient near the extreme ipsilateral edge of the table. A pillow may be placed under the knees to prevent lower back strain and for comfort. The affected arm is positioned "free" of the table; the forearm is flexed to 90° (at the elbow). An overhead traction device, a pulley system with two finger traps (index and middle fingers), exerts 10 pounds of traction to facilitate positioning of the limb and opening of joint spaces. This weight is counter-balanced by a forearm stabilizer (felt cuff with protective padding) that exerts 8 to 10 pounds of traction. A loop of traction rope connects a hook to the overhead device (above), and the finger traps (from below) suspend the hand. All parts of the equipment beneath the hook are sterile. Proper distention of the wrist should prevent excessive bleeding; therefore, a tourniquet is infrequently applied to the arm. The unaffected arm may be extended on a padded armboard, or the arm is padded and tucked in at the patient's side. A padded footboard supports the feet. Bony prominences and areas vulnerable to skin and neurovascular pressure or trauma are padded. Apply electrosurgical dispersive pad.

For **Skin Preparation** and **Draping,** see ***Open Reduction and Internal Fixation Carpal Bone Fracture,*** p. 536.

Equipment

Overhead traction device with hook, felt cuff (arm), 2 finger traps, and wrist stabilizer with protective padding, traction rope, traction weights (8 to 10 pounds)
Suction
ESU
Arthroscopy tower with power pump, optional
Shaver power system
Power source for drill or drill (with power pack batteries), e.g., Stryker
Monitor
VCR
Printer
Camera console
CD burner
Fiber-optic light source e.g., Xenon 300 W
Cast cart
Generator for pulsed lavage suction irrigator, e.g., Simpulse, MicroAire, optional

Instrumentation

Minor orthopedic procedures tray
Arthroscope (e.g., Olympus TrueView II) with camera (for the wrist, 2.4, 2.7, 2.9, or 3.0 mm) and cord, sheath and bridge adaptor, irrigation cannula (for inflow irrigation), sheath or

bridge adaptor, small irrigation cannula (2) with blunt obturator, conical ("Christmas tree") adaptor (for outflow cannula), high-speed power burr, circular rasp, suture passer, motorized shaver system with appropriate blades, blunt probe, pituitary rongeurs, grasping forceps, suture retriever, suture anchors, scissors, and microscissors
Fixation device, e.g., Kirschner wires, pins, screws
Power drill, drill bits, chuck, and key
Pulsed lavage suction irrigator, tubing, and tip, e.g., Simpulse, MicroAire, optional

Supplies

Antiembolitic hose, optional, adults
Sterile marking pen (indelible ink)
Tube stockinette
Coban, optional
Basin set
Blades, (1) #15 and (1) #11
Suction tubing
Electrosurgical cord
Needle, #18 spinal, $3\frac{1}{2}''$, and 10-ml syringe
Silastic IV tubing (2) for inflow and outflow
Suction tubing or cojoined suction and irrigation tubing for pulsed lavage
Bags of irrigation solution (lactated Ringer's) for pulsed lavage unit, or graduated pitcher, bulb syringe, and saline or antibiotic irrigation
Supplies for splint (cast cart)

Special Notes

- Apply **Special Notes** from ***Open Reduction of and Internal Fixation of a Carpal Bone Fracture,*** p. 538, as applicable.
- For all minimal access procedures, the patient must sign the surgical consent to include the possibility of conversion to an open procedure.
- All equipment should be checked regarding working order prior to surgery.
- Check with the surgeon regarding the type of the suspension device to be used for the skin prep.
- When available, a fluid-control drape (with pouch) should be used to collect the irrigation solution, as necessary, to prevent "strike through" contamination of the sterile field.

- The scrub person must monitor the temperature of the irrigation solution as it leaves the outflow tubing before the solution reaches the patient.
- **Reminder:** Strict observance of manufacturer's recommendations for disinfection and sterilization of endoscopy scopes and instrumentation must be followed [e.g. using ethylene oxide, peracetic acid (Steris) or hydrogen peroxide gas plasma].
- **Reminder:** Using the Steris system, completely submerge scope in Steris 20 solution for 12 minutes, as recommended for sterilization; see p. 43.
- **Reminder:** Most nondisposable endoscopic instruments may be carefully washed and flash sterilized.

Arthroplasty of the Wrist with Prosthetic Replacement of the Carpal Bones

Definition

Replacement of carpal bones or components by prosthesis.

Discussion

When wrist motion is restricted and painful, consideration is given to **wrist arthroplasty**. The most common diagnoses are osteoarthritis and rheumatoid arthritis. Cartilage is worn away due to bones rubbing together, or the bones have been damaged by injury, infection, or disease. To achieve pain relief and to maintain limited function of the hand and wrist, the affected bones in the wrist may be fused, or, infrequently, they may be replaced by wrist arthroplasty. This is performed in older patients who do not use their wrists for doing heavy labor or excessive exercise.

Procedure

The approach is often dorsal, but the volar approach may also be used. The damaged ends of the radius and ulna are excised; the proximal row of carpal bones may also be removed. The radial shaft is prepared (usually with a reamer). The shaft and surrounding tissues may be cleansed of debris with pulsed lavage of lactated Ringer's solution or irrigated with normal saline prior to closure; antibiotics may be added to either solution. The radial shaft is dried, and the radial prosthesis is seated with polymethylmethacrylate (PMMA) cement. Depending on the type of prosthesis, the distal component is inserted into the third metacarpal or the capitate, seated with PMMA cement or screwed into the remaining row of the carpal bones. An appropriate-sized spacer is placed between the metal components. The carpal bones may be fused together. When hemostasis is achieved, the wound is closed in the usual manner.

For **Preparation of the Patient, Skin Preparation, Equipment, Instrumentation, Supplies,** and **Special Notes,** see *Open Reduction and Internal Fixation Carpal Bone Fracture,* p. 536, as applicable.

Equipment

Generator for pulsed lavage suction irrigator, e.g., Simpulse, MicroAire, optional

Instruments add:

Reamers
Kirschner wires
Prostheses and associated instrumentation
Bone spacers
Pulsed lavage irrigator and tip

Supplies add:

Irrigation solution (lactated Ringer's) in 3000 mL bogs for pulsed lavage
Polymethylmethacrylate (PMMA) and supplies for mixing or use PMMA kit (to seat each prosthesis)

Special Notes add:

- Consult the surgeon regarding the type and size of prostheses, compression plates and screws, etc. Do not start procedure unless implant and necessary instrumentation for insertion and extraction are in the room.
- Record the insertion of the device(s) used in the Perioperative Record and the hospital log according to hospital policy.

Open Reduction and Internal Fixation of the Radius and/or Ulna Fractures

Definition

Realignment and open fixation of fractures of the forearm.

Discussion

When closed reduction produces unsatisfactory results or when there is a nonunion, open reduction and fixation may be achieved by employing a variety of devices, including intramedullary nail, pin, rod, or compression plate with screws. Fractures present as greenstick or a transverse, oblique, or comminuted configuration.

Two types of forearm fractures that occur most frequently, requiring an "open" procedure, include the **Monteggia,** a proximal fracture of the ulna and a dislocated head of the radius, and the **Colles',** a malaligned fracture of the radius with angular displacement of its dorsal end.

In addition to the trauma associated with fractures of the forearm, vascular injury that may occur leads to "compartment syndrome" as a result of local tissue swelling and the resulting pressure. Compartment syndrome requires prompt surgical treatment by decompression fasciotomy to prevent irreversible muscle and nerve injury.

Procedure

Open Reduction and Internal Fixation of the Radius and/or Ulna Fractures is described. An appropriate incision is made according to location of the fracture. Neurovascular structures are identified and protected. Dissection is continued down to the fracture site. Open fixation may be achieved with wires, pins, compression plate with screws, lag screw, rod, etc. A guide wire may be drilled through the fractured ends of the bone to stabilize the reduction. Fluoroscopy ensures proper alignment. When a rod, nail, or pin is inserted, the intramedullary canal is reamed prior to the insertion. A nail guide, when a nail is used, guides the pin as it is being driven into the canal. The length of the nail, rod, etc., is measured by comparing the lengths of the Kirschner wire accordingly. A transfixing screw may be placed at the end of the device to prevent migration of the pin or nail. Alternatively, a plate may be used to fix shaft fractures. Holes are drilled, gauged, and tapped as necessary for screw placement. The plate is secured with screws; a depth gauge is used to determine screw length. The wound may be cleansed of debris with pulsed lavage before closure and/or irrigated with saline or an antibiotic solution. Hemostasis is achieved. The wound is closed. A splint or bivalved cast is applied.

Displaced radial head fracture requiring excision of the radial head may be necessary to treat the adult patient. All fragments and debris are removed, including excess periosteum with pulsed lavage, or the wound may be irrigated with saline or an antibiotic solution. This type of fracture is infrequently seen in the pediatric patient. The radial head is ***not*** removed in the pediatric patient.

Radial shaft fractures are usually repaired by compression plate with screws or rod (Rush) may be inserted via the radial styloid.

For proximal ulna or the olecranon fractures, see ***Open Reduction of the Olecranon***, p. 553. Fractures of the forearm are often repaired by open reduction and fracture fixation with long lag screws. Kirschner wires may be used to stabilize the correct anatomical positioning of the bone fragments or to repair smaller fragments.

Fixation of distal forearm fractures is achieved with a specially shaped plate, e.g., T-plate and screws.

Preparation of the Patient

Antiembolitic hose are applied (adult), as requested. The patient usually receives general anesthesia; however, block (e.g., axillary) anesthetic may be employed instead or in addition. The patient is in supine position, close to the ipsilateral edge of the table. The affected arm is (draped "free") positioned across the chest and placed on a pillow on the patient's lap (secured temporarily with a soft restraint), or it is extended on a padded hand table. A pillow may be placed under the knees to prevent lower back strain and for comfort. The unaffected arm is usually extended on a padded armboard, or the arm may be padded and tucked in at the patient's side. Bony prominences and areas vulnerable to skin and neurovascular pressure or trauma are padded. Sheet wadding and a tourniquet are applied high (at the top) on the affected arm. Apply electrosurgical dispersive pad.

Skin Preparation

Begin with the forearm; include the hand, fingers, and interdigital spaces and beyond the elbow up to the level of the tourniquet.

Draping

The extremity is (in a tube stockinette) elevated and abducted. A large cuffed sheet is draped over the hand table (if one is used) tucked under the shoulder. The tube stockinette is brought up to the top of the arm. A towel, folded in thirds longitudinally, is wrapped around the top of the stockinette and secured. A cuffed drape (or split) sheet with collection pouch is draped under the arm and fastened. A drape sheet covers the shoulder and is secured under the arm. A fenestrated sheet or individual drape sheets complete the draping.

Equipment

- Padded hand table or Multilok radiolucent hand table (optional)
- Suction
- ESU
- Tourniquet and pneumatic insufflator with microprocessing regulator (compressed air tank)
- Power source for drill (as necessary, according to type)
- Pulsed lavage suction irrigator generator, e.g., Simpulse, MicroAire, optional
- Cast cart

Instrumentation

- Basic orthopedic procedures tray
- Bone-holding instruments tray

Bone hooks, wire, awl, depth gauge, bone tap, nail set, compression plate-holding forceps
Bone grafting instruments, e.g., Cloward (available)
Fixation device and accessory instrumentation, e.g., wire, straight compression or T plate with screws, stainless wire, lag screws, Rush rods, or Steinmann pins (with awl, reamers, and driver/extractor, etc.)
Power drill, chuck, drill sleeve, drill bits, and cord (or self-contained)
Pulsed lavage suction irrigator, and tip, e.g., Simpulse, MicroAire, optional

Supplies

Antiembolitic hose, optional
Webril
Tube stockinette
Esmarch bandage
Basin set
Blades, (2) #10
Electrosurgical pencil and cord with holder and scraper
Needle magnet or counter
Suction tubing or cojoined suction and irrigation tubing for pulsed lavage
Bags of irrigation solution (lactated Ringer's) for pulsed lavage unit, or graduated pitcher, bulb syringe, and antibiotic irrigation
Splint or cast materials

Special Notes

- Apply **Special Notes** from ***Open Reduction and Internal Fixation of a Carpal Bone Fracture***, p. 538, as indicated.

Open Reduction and Internal Fixation of an Olecranon Process Fracture

Definition

Realignment and open fixation of fractures of the elbow.

Discussion

The treatment indicated for almost all fractures about the elbow is open reduction and fixation. In patients with badly comminuted fractures, bone grafts ("autografts") may be obtained from the iliac crest. The surgeon may choose not to use a bone graft (as many patients complain of pain at the donor site) but instead to use bone chips (from the repair site). The patient's bone chips are compacted and pressed into place. Donated bone from the bone bank may provide an alternate bone graft. When the bone fragments (larger than bone chips) are adequate, they are held in place with tension bands and cancellous bone screws. The purpose of the surgery is to stabilize the elbow joint and to avoid the possibility of posttraumatic arthritis.

Procedure

Open Reduction and Internal Fixation of an Olecranon Process Fracture is described. An incision is made over the fractured olecranon. The ulnar nerve is protected. Small bone fragments are excised. Under fluoroscopic guidance, Kirschner wires may be drilled into bone fragments for correct anatomical positioning and for stabilization of the fracture site. Large fragments are usually fixed with a cerclage of wire; cancellous screws can be used to stabilize the fractured bone. For cerclage of wire repair, drill holes are made in the olecranon fragment and in the distal bone shaft. Bone-holding clamps maintain the fragment in anatomical position. Stainless steel wire is pulled through the holes and, using figure-of-eight technique, tightened. The triceps tendon, if attached to a smaller fragment (to be excised), is reattached to the ulnar shaft. The wound may be cleansed of debris with pulsed lavage prior to closure or irrigated with saline or an antibiotic solution. Hemostasis is achieved. The wound is closed. A long arm splint is applied.

Preparation of the Patient

Antiembolitic hose may be applied (adult), as requested. The patient usually receives general anesthesia and is placed in supine position, close to the ipsilateral edge of the table. The affected extremity is placed on a padded hand table, or it may be flexed and positioned across the chest on a pillow (temporarily secured by a soft restraint). A pillow may be placed under the knees to avoid straining the low back and for comfort. The unaffected arm may be extended on a padded armboard, or it may be padded and tucked in at the patient's side. Bony prominences and areas vulnerable to skin and neurovascular pressure or trauma are padded. Sheet wadding and a tourniquet are applied high on the affected arm. Apply electrosurgical dispersive pad.

Alternate positions that may be employed for this repair include prone and lateral.

Skin Preparation

Begin at the elbow; extend the prep from the bottom of the tourniquet to the fingertips; include fingers and interdigital spaces.

Draping

The extremity (covered with tube stockinette) is elevated and abducted. A large sheet is draped over the hand table. A split sheet is draped under the arm and secured above. The tube stockinette is brought up to the top of the arm. A towel folded in thirds longitudinally is wrapped around the top of the stockinette and secured. A split or drape sheet covers the shoulder and is fastened under the arm. A fenestrated sheet (e.g., lap or transverse) or additional individual drape sheets complete the draping. When available, a split sheet with a pouch is preferred to collect irrigation solution.

Equipment

Pad, sandbag, or rolled sheet
Padded hand table or Multilok radiolucent hand table (optional)
Pneumatic tourniquet and insufflator with microprocessor regulator (tank of compressed air)
Suction
ESU
Power source for drill (as necessary, according to type)
Shaver system, optional
Cast cart

Instrumentation

Basic orthopedic procedures tray (contains wire and pin cutter)
Bone-holding instruments tray
Multilok tabletop hand holder (single use, sterile) and accessories (optional)
Bone hooks, depth-gauge, wire tightener, Hibbs and Bennett retractors
Power drill and cord, chuck, drill bits, drill sleeve, awl
Fixation devices and required accessory instrumentation: automatic screwdriver, flat, Phillip's head, cancellous bone screws, stainless steel wire, e.g., 18 gauge (for cerclage of wire), Kirschner wires, or Steinmann pins (with awl, reamers, and driver/extractor)
Pulsed lavage suction irrigator and tip, e.g., Simpulse, MicroAire, optional

Supplies

Antiembolitic hose, as requested
Tube stockinette
Webril
Esmarch bandage
Basin set
Blades, (2) #10 and (1) #11
Electrosurgical pencil and cord with holder and scraper
Needle magnet or counter
Wire, e.g., 18- or 20-gauge stainless steel
Suction tubing or cojoined suction and irrigation tubing for pulsed lavage
Irrigation solution in bags (for pulsed lavage), optional

Graduated pitcher, bulb syringe, antibiotic solution (optional)
Penrose drain, 1/4″ (retraction of ulnar nerve)

Special Notes

- Apply **Special Notes** from ***Open Reduction and Internal Fixation of a Carpal Bone Fracture***, p. 538, as indicated.

Transposition of the Ulnar Nerve

Definition

Repositioning the ulnar nerve at the elbow from the posterior aspect of the medial epicondyle to the anterior aspect.

Discussion

Various forms of trauma, such as local fracture, dislocation, chronic soft tissue stress, and local congenital deformities, can lead to scarring, with resulting compression or traction injuries to the ulnar nerve. Ulnar nerve palsy and cubital tunnel syndrome not responsive to non-surgical measures (avoidance of excessive flexion, splinting, etc.) require surgical intervention. This procedure relieves numbness, pain, tingling, and atrophy in the hand, according to the distribution of the nerve. Clinical exam, electromyogram (EMG), and nerve conduction studies confirm the diagnosis. Neurolysis and transposition of the nerve to the subcutaneous, intramuscular, or submuscular anterior position is sometimes performed with medial epicondylectomy.

Procedure

Pneumatic tourniquet is applied with the arm abducted and externally rotated. A generous incision is made on the posteromedial aspect of the elbow, proximal to the medial epicondyle, passing distally anterior to the medial epicondyle. Cutaneous antebrachial nerves are protected, and the ulnar nerve is dissected from local scar and callus. The origin of the flexor carpi ulnaris m. is freed from the epicondyle. Muscular branches of the nerve are protected as further neurolysis is performed. The mobilized nerve is positioned anterior to the epicondyle to lie on the fascia of the flexor-pronator muscles (under fat). The medial intermuscular septum is incised proximally, and sutures are placed in the tissues surrounding the nerve to prevent posterior slippage. Alternatively, the nerve can be positioned beneath the flexor and pronator muscles. As indicated, the medial epicondyle can be lifted subperiosteally and replaced (or excised) to facilitate the nerve transfer. Any divided muscular origins are repaired. The tourniquet is deflated, hemostasis is achieved, and the wound is closed. A posterior splint is applied.

For **Preparation of the Patient, Skin Preparation, Draping, Equipment, Instrumentation, Supplies,** and **Special Notes,** see ***Open Reduction and Internal Fixation of a of Carpal Bone Fracture,*** p. 536.

Supplies

Add: Penrose drains, vessel loops, and umbilical tapes (for nerve traction/protection).

Arthroscopy of the Elbow

Definition

Direct visualization (arthroscopic) of the elbow joint.

Discussion

When various noninvasive diagnostic and treatment techniques are unable to achieve relief of elbow pain, arthroscopy of the elbow may be employed. Elbow arthroscopy is used to evaluate and treat conditions such as the presence of loose bodies, posttraumatic adhesions, osteophytes, osteochondral fractures, osteochondritis dissecans, synovitis, etc. The nature and extent of local fractures can be evaluated; pyarthrosis can be drained and irrigated. Severe posttraumatic injuries and alkylosis are contraindications to this modality. Caution must be exercised in this small operative field to avoid injuring the brachial artery, median and ulnar nerves, and main branches of the radial nerve.

Procedure

Arthroscopy of the Elbow is described. The OR with laminar air may be requested. The surgeon palpates and marks (with indelible ink) the skin over the bony landmarks (radial head, lateral and medial epicondyles, olecranon tip) prior to the prep. Commonly used ports include anterolateral, anteromedial, lateral, posterolateral, and posterior sites. Employing fluoroscopic guidance, the surgeon inserts an 18-gauge needle into the lateral aspect of the elbow to position the needle within the elbow joint. Following confirmation of the position, he/she distends the joint by injecting 25 to 30 ml of saline (or Ringer's lactate). The trocar is inserted to establish the anterolateral port; the obturator is removed from the trocar (sleeve), and the arthroscope is inserted. The surgeon's view through the arthroscope is projected on a monitor screen. Arthroscopic visualization is employed to avoid neurovascular injury, as additional ports are established, as necessary. The elbow joint is thoroughly inspected, and diagnoses may be confirmed. Treatments can be performed with endoscopic instrumentation, such as tissue debridement, removal of loose bodies, or osteophytes. Soft tissue is excised as needed. The areas of excision can be smoothed with a motorized burr. Bipolar radio-frequency ablation can be employed to smooth and shrink stretched, torn ligaments. The port incisions are closed, and a pressure dressing is applied.

Note: Until recently, bone joint replacement surgery was performed (whenever possible) in an OR equipped with laminar airflow. Surprisingly, studies have proven that ORs with laminar air-flow systems having *high-efficiency particulate-arresting* (HEPA) filters are no more effective at preventing intraoperative wound (or bone) infections than operating rooms routinely equipped with air-conditioning systems that provide 12 or more air exchanges per hour. Nevertheless, some orthopedic surgeons prefer to operate in the OR with laminar air.

Preparation of the Patient

Antiembolitic hose may be applied (adult), as requested. The patient is placed in supine position near the ipsilateral edge of the table. Following the administration of general anesthesia, an overhead shoulder holder or similar suspension device is used to suspend the arm from a wrist gauntlet, with the arm balanced by a 5- to 10-pound weight. The arm is positioned to hang free of the edge of the table, with the shoulder in neutral rotation and abducted to 90° and the elbow flexed to 90°. Maximum relaxation is achieved in this position. The balanced suspension permits elbow flexion and extension during the procedure. The contralateral arm may be extended on a padded armboard and tucked in at the patient's side. A pillow may be placed under the knees to avoid strain on back muscles and for comfort. Bony prominences and areas vulnerable to skin and neurovascular pressure or trauma are padded. Apply electrosurgical dispersive pad.

Skin Preparation

Begin at the elbow; prep from the tourniquet to the fingertips; include the arm, forearm, hand, fingers, and interdigital spaces.

Draping

See Draping, ***Open Reduction and Internal Fixation of Carpal Bone Fracture,*** p. 536, as indicated.

Equipment

Overhead shoulder holder with wrist gauntlet and 5- to 10-pound weight
Padded hand table (radiolucent), optional
Stools, optional

Tourniquet and insufflation tank (of compressed air) with microprocessor regulator
ESU
Fiber-optic light source, e.g., Xenon 300 W
Monitors (2)
VCR
Printer
CD burner
Camera console
Suction
Arthroscopy tower with power pump
Power source for drill or drill with power pack (batteries), e.g., Stryker
Shaver power system, optional
Cast cart

Instrumentation

Minor orthopedic procedures tray
Arthroscope with camera, 2.7 and 2.9 mm, and cord, sheath, bridge adaptor, blunt probe, pituitary rongeurs, small irrigation cannulas (2) with blunt obturators, conical ("Christmas tree") adaptor (for outflow cannula), blunt dissector, grasping forceps, suture retriever, suture anchors, scissors, micro scissors, circular rasp, suture passer
Motorized shaver with appropriate blades, high-speed power burr
Kirschner wires

Supplies

Antiembolitic hose, optional
Sterile marking pen (indelible ink), optional
Tube stockinette
Webril
Esmarch bandage
Basin set
Blades, (1) #10 and (1) #11
Electrosurgical pencil and cord with holder and scraper
Needle magnet or counter
Needles, #18 spinal 3½″ and 30-ml syringe
Silastic IV tubing (2) for inflow and outflow
Bags of irrigation (3000 ml) lactated Ringer's solution with antibiotic solution, optional
Pressure dressing
Cast cart
Splint, optional

Special Notes

- Apply **Special Notes** from ***Open Reduction and Internal Fixation of a Carpal Bone Fracture***, p. 538, as applicable.
- Ensure that all equipment is in working order prior to bringing patient into the room for surgery.
- Circulator checks with the surgeon regarding the type of suspension device before starting the skin prep.
- The scrub person must monitor the temperature of the irrigation solution as it leaves the outflow tubing before the solution reaches the patient.
- A system by Smith and Nephew Co. (and others) provides safe placement for working channels.
- Most arthroscopes may ***not*** be flash sterilized. When a scope requires soaking, completely submerge the scope in Steris 20 solution for 12 minutes, as recommended for sterilization; see p. 43.
- Nondisposable instruments may be carefully washed and flash sterilized.

Open Reduction and Internal Fixation of Fractures of the Humerus

Definition

Realignment and open fixation of an arm fracture.

Discussion

A variety of fractures of the humerus may present; the repair is determined by the type, level, and location of the fracture. Intra-articular involvement, bone displacement, bone quality, joint stability, and the necessity for adequate quality of soft tissue coverage must be considered to perform the repair. In pediatric patients, the fusion of the epiphyses must be taken into account. Whenever possible, pediatric patients (and older patients) with humerus fractures should be treated by closed reduction and percutaneous pin insertion employing fluoroscopic guidance. The treatment of supracondylar fractures may be closed reduction and the application of a cast, as there is no articular involvement with which to be concerned. Epicondylar and transepicondylar fractures, with or without articular involvement, often require internal fixation.

For patients of all ages, when closed reduction and immobilization by percutaneous pinning are unsatisfactory or when there is a nonunion, open reduction and internal fixation may be achieved with a variety of devices, such as lag screws, threaded Kirschner wires, intermedullary nail, rod, pin, a cerclage of wire, compression plate with screws, or T plate with screws. Most fixation devices require insertion instrumentation particular to that device, e.g., awl, reamers, and driver/extractor, etc. A cast is applied to keep the arm immobilized until the fracture heals. Patient compliance is an important factor influencing successful results.

Contraindications or factors predisposing to nonunion include poor nutritional status, age, steroid use, anticoagulation therapy, fractures located close to a burn injury, and prior radiation treatments.

Procedure

An incision is made over the fracture site, avoiding neurovascular structures. The anatomy is identified. Soft tissue structures are carefully preserved. In the anterolateral approach to treat mid-humerus fractures, the brachialis is dissected down to the bone anteriorly and laterally to the intermuscular septum. Care is taken to avoid injury to the antebrachial cutaneous nerve. The fracture is reduced; a guide wire may be drilled into the bone to stabilize the reduction. Fluoroscopy ensures proper alignment. The reamers, trial prosthesis, and implanted prosthesis are placed within the intermedullary canal. The length of the nail, rod, etc., is measured accordingly. The wound may be cleansed of debris with pulsed lavage. A nail guide, when a nail is used, guides the pin as it is being driven into the canal. A transfixing screw may be placed at the end of the device to prevent migration of the pin. Alternatively, a plate may be used to fix shaft fractures. The plate is secured with screws; screw length is measured by depth gauge.

If the humeral head is displaced, it is relocated into the glenoid, following stabilization of the head on the shaft. If the fractured humeral head cannot be stabilized, prosthetic replacement is required; see ***Open Reduction and Internal Fixation of Fractures of the Humeral Head (including Humeral Head Replacement by Prosthesis),*** p. 570, and *Arthroplasty of the Shoulder with Hemi (Partial) or Total Prosthetic Replacement of the Shoulder Joint,* p. 574. Fluoroscopy confirms bone alignment and correct positioning of the fixation device. The wound may be cleansed of debris with pulsed lavage prior to closure, or the wound may be irrigated with saline or antibiotic solution. The soft tissue is repaired. The wound is closed. A long arm cast is applied to keep the extremity immobilized.

When the posterior approach is employed to treat some distal fractures, the patient is placed in prone position. The tricipital heads are separated. Deep dissection involves splitting the medial head, with consideration given to protect the radial nerve and the brachial artery. If malunion has occurred, *osteotomy* is performed, alignment is restored, and repair is made with a cerclage of wire.

Preparation of the Patient

Antiembolitic hose are applied (adult) when requested. The patient usually receives general anesthesia and may be positioned in a modified sitting (30°) "beach chair" or semi-Fowler's position. An extension rest is used to support the patient's head and neck, after removing the top section of the table. An alternate position places the patient at the extreme ipsilateral edge of the table with the head and neck gently bent away from the shoulder; a pad, sandbag, or rolled towel is placed under the affected scapula medially to stabilize the shoulder and to project the shoulder forward. At the discretion of the anesthesia provider, adhesive tape may be placed across the forehead to support the head (after checking the chart for patient's allergies); the skin is protected with tincture of benzoin and a 4 × 4 pad. The affected arm is placed on the patient's lap on a pillow (temporarily held by soft restraint). The arm on the unaffected side may be padded and tucked in at the patient's side, or it may be extended on a padded armboard positioned alongside the patient. A padded footboard supports the feet. All bony prominences and areas vulnerable to skin and neurovascular pressure or trauma are padded. Care is taken to prevent injury to the fingers when the lower section of the table is returned to its original position. Apply electrosurgical dispersive pad.

Skin Preparation

Begin at the top of the arm; prep the area about the shoulder, extending the prep beyond the midline of the chest in front, to the inferior costal margin below, and down to the table at the back. Prep includes the axilla, arm, and forearm.

Draping

The extremity (covered with double tube stockinette) is elevated, abducted, and draped "free." A large drape sheet is cuffed and tucked under the patient's shoulder. The outer tube stockinette is brought up (unrolled) to the top of the arm. A towel, folded in thirds longitudinally, is wrapped around the top of the stockinette and secured; this permits access to the extremity for shoulder manipulation to assure proper fixation. A cuffed drape (or split) sheet (with a collection pouch) is placed under the arm. A split or drape sheet covers the area around the shoulder and is fastened under the arm. A fenestrated sheet (e.g., lap or transverse) or additional individual drape sheets complete the draping.

Equipment

Extension rest for head and neck or padded donut, pad, sandbag, and/or rolled sheet, optional
Padded hand table, e.g., Multilok radiolucent hand table, optional
Padded footboard

Suction
ESU
Power source for drill (according to type), optional
Cast cart, optional
Distal fractures: tourniquet and insufflator with microprocessor regulator (tank of compressed air)

Instrumentation

Basic orthopedic procedures tray
Bone-holding instruments tray
Bone grafting instruments (available)
Bone hooks, depth gauge, wire, Bennet retractors, plate holding forceps, automatic screwdriver
Fixation device(s) (as requested) with accessory instrumentation, e.g., stainless steel wire (18- or 20-gauge) straight compression or T plates with screws, Rush rods, Steinmann pins (with awl, reamers, and driver/extractor)
Power drill, chuck, drill sleeve, drill bits, and cord (optional)

Supplies

Antiembolitic hose, optional
Tube stockinettes (2)
Basin set
Blades, (2) #10
Electrosurgical pencil and cord with holder and scraper
Needle magnet or counter
Suction tubing
Stainless steel wire, 18 or 20 gauge (wire cutter is in bone tray)
Graduated pitcher, bulb syringe, and antibiotic irrigation, optional
Paper labels, sterile (label medications on the sterile field)
Distal fractures: Webril, unsterile (under tourniquet), and Esmarch bandage

Special Notes

- Apply **Special Notes** from ***Open Reduction and Internal Fixation of a Carpal Bone Fracture***, p. 538, as applicable.
- **Reminder:** Ascertain that x-ray films and studies are in the room for the *correct* patient prior to bringing the patient into the room.
- Circulator notifies x-ray department when fluoroscopy may be required before the patient enters the room (in order to save the patient the cost of some of the OR time).

- Ascertain adequate gas or air (under pressure) level in tank (or battery reserve) used to power the drill before bringing the patient into the room.
- **Reminder:** Do not permit prep solutions to pool under tourniquet, as they excoriate the skin. Document the appearance of the skin preoperatively and immediately postoperatively.
- When the fracture is distal and a tourniquet is used, observe tourniquet safety precautions, see p. 45.
- The scrub person must monitor the temperature of the irrigation solution as it leaves the outflow tubing before the solution reaches the patient.
- **Reminder:** Use safety precautions to identify, label, and dispense medications or solutions and to avoid medication errors; see p. 30. It is mandatory that all medications and solutions on the sterile field be labeled by name and strength. The medication bottle is retained in the room until the procedure has concluded.
- **Reminder:** Persons scrubbed should wear a protective face shield or goggles to prevent injury from splashing or spraying of the patient's blood and irrigation fluids.
- Document the application of the fixation device, regarding type, size, and serial numbers, in the Perioperative Record and hospital log according to hospital policy.
- **Reminder:** The circulator obtains the "cast cart" (with casting supplies) at the conclusion of the surgery. All supplies for making a cast should be assembled before application of the cast is begun, as the plaster dries hard quickly.
- **Reminder:** The orthopedic technician may assist in applying a cast; however, the scrub person or the circulator must be prepared to assist the surgeon in applying a cast or splint when necessary. To apply a cast or splint, a plaster roll or plaster sheets are dipped in lukewarm water; when the bubbling stops, the roll or sheets are ready for use.

Arthroscopy of the Shoulder

Definition

Endoscopic visualization of the shoulder joint.

Discussion

Diagnosis and treatment of shoulder joint pathology was difficult prior to arthroscope usage. Extensive arthroscopic visualization of the intra-articular aspect of the shoulder joint is possible. Indications for arthroscopy of the shoulder include removal of loose bodies, lysis of adhesions, synovectomy, bursectomy, biopsy of the synovium, stabilization of dislocation, correction of rotator cuff tears, and decompression of the subacromial area.

Procedure

Arthroscopy of the Shoulder is described. The bony anatomical landmarks are marked with indelible ink, as necessary. Usually three ports are employed; location of the ports is modified by the patient's size. The posterior port is inferior and medial to the posterolateral corner of the acromium. Under arthroscopic vision, the anterior port is placed inferior to the biceps tendon. A transarticular guide is inserted (with arthroscopic guidance) through the anterior capsule, tenting the skin (approximately 2 cm below the anterior edge of the acromium). A stab wound is made and a port is inserted over the rod into the joint. The lateral port is established 2 cm distal to the lateral border of the acromium. The trocar is passed through the deltoid muscle to the greater tuberosity. An additional port is directed into the bursal cavity beneath the anterior third of the acromium. Arthroscopic inspection of all aspects of the shoulder joint (employing the most direct and least traumatic modalities) is made to assess the pathology. Appropriate therapeutic measures are performed accordingly. The procedure can be performed as an *arthroscopically assisted* procedure, i.e., assisted by a "mini" incision to facilitate exposure, obtain the specimen, or insert a device. The patient must sign for both an arthroscopic and an open procedure; whenever difficulties are encountered during the endoscopic procedure, the surgeon has the prerogative to revert to an "open" procedure.

Note: Until recently, bone joint replacement surgery was performed (whenever possible) in an OR equipped with laminar airflow. Surprisingly, studies have proven that operating rooms with laminar air-flow systems having *high efficiency particulate arresting* (HEPA) filters are no more effective at preventing intraoperative wound (or bone) infections than operating rooms routinely equipped with standard air-conditioning systems that provide 12 or more air exchanges per hour. Nevertheless, some orthopedic surgeons prefer to operate in the OR with laminar air.

Preparation of the Patient

Antiembolitic hose are applied (adult), when requested. Following the administration of general anesthesia with endotracheal intubation, the patient is placed in modified sitting (30°) semi-Fowler's position ("beach chair") or lateral/kidney/lateral decubitus position. Pad all bony prominences and areas vulnerable to skin and neurovascular pressure or trauma. Apply electrosurgical dispersive pad.

Modified Semi-Fowler's Position. The patient is positioned close to the ipsilateral edge of the table with the body aligned over the breaks in the table. A padded headrest extension, secured to the table, can support the head and neck (when available), or a padded donut can be placed at the head of the table to stabilize the head (and protect the dependent ear). When the donut is employed, adhesive tape can be placed across the forehead to further stabilize the head (after checking the chart for patient allergies); the skin is protected with tincture of benzoin and 4×4 pad. The arm on the affected side is secured in a sterilized foam traction boot. The arm is supported in a position of approximately 70° of abduction and 10° of flexion. The arm on the unaffected side may be extended on a padded armboard placed alongside the patient, or it may be padded and tucked in at the patient's side. Care is taken to avoid injury to the fingers when the table is repositioned. A pillow may be placed under the knees and legs to avoid undue pressure on the heels. A blanket covers the patient's lap; the safety strap is secured.

Lateral (Decubitus) Position. The patient is turned to the lateral position (operative side up) with beanbag support on the table to maintain the position, or padded kidney rests can be used (larger blade in front). An axillary roll, placed beneath the dependent side of the (unaffected) thorax (near the axilla), protects the brachial plexus; the arm on the unaffected side is slightly flexed and extended on a padded armboard. A pillow is placed between the knees and legs; the ankles are padded to prevent pressure injuries.

Skin Preparation

Begin at the top of the shoulder; prep the area about the shoulder, extending from the submandibular region to the inferior costal margin. Prep beyond the midline on the front of the chest, down to the table at the back, and to the inferior costal margin below. Prep also includes the axilla, arm, and forearm.

Draping

When available, use the "shoulder drape pack" specifically made for this purpose; it includes a plastic "U" drape sheet and a drape sheet with a collection pouch. The (two) connectors are attached to the collection pouch on the drape; the pouch drains into a gravity reservoir.

If shoulder pack is unavailable, drape as for ***Repair of Recurrent Anterior Dislocation of the Shoulder***, p. 569.

Equipment

Modified Semi-Fowler's Position

Padded headrest extension or a padded donut, padded kidney rests, pillow, and extra padding, as necessary

Lateral Decubitus Position

Beanbag, e.g., Bair hugger™, axillary roll, pillow, extra padding, as necessary
Sterilized foam traction unit, optional
Weight for traction unit (approximately 10 pounds)
Finger traps (4 sizes available) to use with wrist traction
ESU
Suction
Video monitors (2)
VCR
Printer
CD burner
Camera console
Fiber-optic light source, e.g., Xenon 300 W
Arthroscopy tower with pump power system
Fluid standard (adjustable with sensors)

Instrumentation

Basic orthopedic procedures tray
Arthroscope with camera and cord, large irrigation cannula with blunt obturator, small outflow cannula with blunt obturator, conical ("Christmas tree") adaptor (for outflow cannula), switching stick or orthopedic guide rod, arthroscopic sheath or appropriate bridge adaptor, plastic operating cannula with diaphragm and side port, rotator cuff liberator-elevator, high-speed power burr, gauge punches (3), circular rasp, suture passer, suturing device (e.g., Smart Stitch™), suture passer and controller (Elite Pass Suture Shuttle™), automatic knot-tyers (Opus AutoCuff®), and suture anchor (BioRaptor™ 2.9)
Motorized shaver system with blades, acromionizer burr, full radius shaver blade
Fixation device with required insertion and extractior instrumentation

Supplies

Antiembolitic hose
Sterile marking pen (indelible ink)
Tube stockinettes (2)
Knife blades, (1) #10 and (1) #11
Electrosurgical cord
Basin set
Needle, #18 spinal, 3½″
Syringes (1) 10 ml and (1) 60 ml
Silastic IV tubing (2) for inflow and outflow

Irrigation bag (3000 ml) with lactated Ringer's solution, antibiotic (optional)
Suture for repairs, e.g., Ultrabraid™ polyethylene suture for mattress stitch
Skin closure strips
Soft dressing
Special shoulder brace

Special Notes

- Apply **Special Notes** from ***Open Reduction and Internal Fixation of a Carpal Bone Fracture***, p. 538, as indicated.
- For all minimal access procedures, the patient must sign the surgical consent to include the possibility of conversion to an open procedure. Check with the surgeon regarding the patient's position and positioning equipment in the room.
- All equipment and instrumentation should be checked as to working order prior to bringing the patient's into the room for surgery.
- A system provided by Smith & Nephew, Co. (and others) provides safe placement for working channels.
- Irrigation solution replacement bags must be immediately ready at all times; one bag should hang "in waiting."
- The scrub person must monitor the temperature of the irrigation solution as it leaves the outflow tubing before the solution reaches the patient.
- Sterilize arthroscopes according to manufacturer's specifications.
- To use Steris solution for sterilization, soak the completely submerged scope in Steris 20 solution as recommended for 12 minutes to achieve sterilization; see p. 43.
- The arthroscope (e.g., Olympus Goldtip™), shaver and power system (e.g., APS II Adapteur™), ESU (e.g., OPES Electrosurgical System™), and power pump (Continuous Wave Pump™) may be used to facilitate performing this procedure.
- Nondisposable endoscopic instruments must be carefully washed and may be flash sterilized.

Repair of Recurrent Anterior Dislocation of the Shoulder

Definition

Strengthening of the anterior joint capsule and musculotendinous support of the shoulder.

Discussion

There are many procedures and modifications of the procedures employed for the repair of recurrent anterior dislocation of the shoulder; posterior dislocations are rare.

Commonly performed procedures include:

Bankart Procedure. The glenoid labrum and the anterior part of the capsule (which should cushion and support the humeral head) are reattached to the rim of the glenoid cavity with heavy sutures or bone anchors.

Putti-Platt Procedure. This procedure provides a barrier that prevents the shoulder from repeat dislocation. The subscapularis tendon and capsule are detached from the humerus and sutured laterally on the humeral neck to strengthen the anterior supporting structures and to prevent excessive external rotation of the shoulder.

Bristow Procedure. This procedure is infrequently used. The coracoid process and attached muscles are detached, reinserted into the neck of the scapula, and transfixed. The transferred muscular origins serve as a buttress across the anterior and inferior aspect of the joint, anchoring the lower half of the subscapularis.

Rotator cuff repair may be performed as a minimally assisted arthroscopic procedure, utilizing a "mini" incision with the AutoCuff system.

Procedure

An anterior incision is made over the pectoral groove. The joint capsule is exposed; the extent of the injury is assessed. The coracoid process, with its muscular attachments, is osteotomized from the scapula. The subscapularis tendon is transferred to the anterior neck of the scapula with screw fixation. The lateral portion of the subscapularis tendon is sutured to the joint capsule, and the medial edge of the subscapularis is sutured to the rotator cuff or at the bicipital groove, overlapping the layers of the joint (Putti Platt). The osteotomized coracoid tip may be transfixed to the neck of the glenoid under the fibers of the subscapularis using a screw (Bristow). The soft tissues are repaired and the incision closed. A shoulder immobilizer, sling and swathe, or Velpeau dressing is applied.

Preparation of the Patient

Antiembolitic hose are applied (adult patient), when requested. The patient may be placed in a modified sitting (30° angle) "beach chair" or semi-Fowlers position, close to the extreme ipsilateral edge of the table, with the head and neck gently bent away from the shoulder; a padded donut supports the head (and protects the dependent ear). A pad, sandbag, or rolled towel is placed under the affected scapula medially to stabilize the shoulder and to project the shoulder forward. After checking the chart for patient allergies, adhesive tape can be placed across the forehead to stabilize the head (at the discretion of the anesthesia provider); the skin on the forehead is protected with tincture of benzoin and a 4 × 4 pad. The arm on the affected side will be draped "free"; however, prior to the skin prep, the arm may be placed in the patient's lap on a pillow. The arm on the unaffected side is padded and tucked in at the patient's side, or it may be extended on a padded armboard placed alongside the patient. Care is taken to avoid injury to the fingers when the table is repositioned. A pillow may be placed behind the knees and legs to avoid undue pressure on the heels. A padded footboard supports the feet. A blanket covers the patient's lap; the safety strap is secured. All bony prominences and areas vulnerable to skin and neurovascular pressure or trauma are padded. Apply electrosurgical dispersive pad.

Skin Preparation

Begin at the anterior aspect of the shoulder and prep the area around the shoulder. Extend the prep from the level of submandibular region to the inferior costal margin, beyond the midline of the chest in front, to the inferior costal margin below, and down to the table at the back. Prep includes the axilla, arm, and forearm.

Draping

The extremity (in a double tube stockinette) is elevated and abducted. A large, cuffed drape, split, or U drape (with collection pouch, when available) sheet is tucked under the patient's shoulder. The outer tube stockinette is brought up (unrolled) to the shoulder. A towel folded in thirds longitudinally and wrapped around the top of the stockinette and fastened. A split or U sheet is draped and fastened under the arm. A large drape (or split) sheet is draped around the shoulder and fastened below. The arm may be passed through a fenestrated sheet (laparotomy or transverse), or individual drape sheets may be used to complete the draping.

Equipment

- Padded donut, pillow, padded footboard, and pad (or sandbag or folded sheet)
- Suctions (2)
- ESU
- Power source for drill, as necessary
- Cast cart

Instrumentation

- Basic orthopedic procedures tray
- Retractors, e.g., Hibbs, Bennett, Bankart

Bone hooks, Cobb elevator, rasps, awl (Bankart), osteotome rack (curved)
Automatic screwdrivers for Phillips and flat-head screws
Power drill and cord (or self-contained), drill bits, chuck, bone screws, washer
Fixation devices, e.g., Kirschman or Steinmann pins, plates, screws, staples (and instrumentation)

Supplies

Antiembolitic hose, optional
Tube stockinettes (2)
Basin set
Blades, (2) #10 and (1) #11
Needle magnet or counter
Suction tubing
Electrosurgical pencil and cord with holder and scraper
Graduated pitcher, bulb syringe, antibiotic irrigation (optional)
Sling and swathe, shoulder immobilizer, or Velpeau dressing

Special Notes

- Apply **Special Notes** from ***Open Reduction and Internal Fixation of Fractures of the Humerus***, p. 562, as applicable.

Open Reduction and Internal Fixation of Fracture(s) of the Humeral Head (Including Humeral Head Replacement by Prosthesis)

Definition

Realignment and fixation of fractured and/or displaced humeral head.

Discussion

Most of these fractures do not require surgical treatment; repair is accomplished by closed reduction (fractured bones are manipulated into alignment manually without incising the skin) and percutaneous fixation by wire, pin, or nail insertion. Closed reduction is preferred over open reduction, as infection and wound problems would not be of concern. These injuries are often associated with dislocations, particularly in children. When the humeral head must be replaced, there is concern regarding the child's growth. When PMMA cement is necessary to secure the prosthesis, epiphyses may be closed prematurely in the pediatric patient. Following reduction of the fracture, fixation may be achieved with wire and/or special plates. If the fracture is severely comminuted, replacement of the humeral head by prosthesis may be necessary. Numerous humeral prostheses are available in single component or dual component; some have porous application to the stem portion to promote better fixation with or without cement. Each system has its set of jigs, templates, tools, etc. The desired outcome for patients with any type of fracture of the humeral head is to reestablish normal joint articulation and movement, as well as replace the soft tissues to correct anatomical position.

Procedure

Avulsion fractures of the tuberosities require a deltopectoral approach. Repair by fixation of the fractured humeral head may be accomplished with stainless steel wire to contain and support the fragments in alignment. Soft-tissue injury (e.g., rotator cuff) must also be repaired. When the humeral head is fractured, repair, containment, and support may be accomplished with a cerclage of stainless steel wire and/or T-compression plate to achieve the necessary union. Severely comminuted fractures may require humeral head prosthesis. The deltoid muscle is detached. Attachments of major tendons are preserved with adequate bone fragments. Loose fragments and debris may be pulse lavaged or irrigated with saline or an antibiotic solution. The prosthesis (e.g., Magnum Implant™) is driven into the humeral shaft, and the bone fragments are attached to the prosthesis with wire sutures. The Magnum Implant is one example that comes with sutures preloaded; it has built-in cinching and suture-fixation mechanisms that require less time to secure the prosthesis. PMMA cement may be used in seating the prosthesis. The rotator cuff and soft tissue are closed over the wire sutures. The long head of the biceps tendon, previously detached, may be sutured to the repaired rotator cuff or implanted into the bicipital groove. The deltoid muscle is reattached. The incision is closed. A sling and swathe are placed.

Preparation of the Patient

Antiembolitic hose are applied (adult) when requested. General anesthesia or a combination of general and interscalene block anesthesia may be used for more profound relaxation intraoperatively and to enhance pain relief postoperatively. The patient is placed in a semi-sitting, e.g., 30° angle (i.e., beach chair), or semi-Fowlers position with an extension rest that supports the patient's head and neck (after removing the top sections of the table). An alternate position places the patient at the extreme ipsilateral edge of the table with the head and neck gently bent away from the shoulder; a pad, sandbag, or rolled towel is placed under the affected scapula medially to stabilize the shoulder and to project the shoulder forward. At the discretion of the anesthesia provider, adhesive tape may be placed across the forehead to further support the head, after checking the chart for patient's allergies. The forehead skin is protected with tincture of benzoin and a 4 × 4 pad. The arm on the affected side will be draped "free"; however, prior to the skin prep, the arm may be placed in the patient's lap on a pillow (secured with soft restraint). The arm on the unaffected side is padded and tucked in at the patient's side, or it may be extended on a padded armboard, secured alongside the patient. Care is taken to prevent injury to the fingers when the sections of the table are returned to the original position. A padded footboard supports the feet. All bony prominences and areas vulnerable to skin and neurovascular pressure or trauma are padded. Apply electrosurgical dispersive pad.

Skin Preparation

Begin at the anterior aspect of the shoulder and prep the area around the shoulder. Extend the prep from the level of submandibular region to the inferior costal margin, beyond the midline of the chest in front, to the inferior costal margin below, and down to the table at the back. Prep includes the axilla, arm, and forearm.

Draping

The extremity grasped in double tube stockinette is elevated and abducted. A large, cuffed drape, split, or U sheet (with collection pouch, when available) is tucked under the patient's shoulder. The outer tube stockinette is brought up (unrolled) to the shoulder. A towel folded in thirds longitudinally is wrapped around the top of the stockinette and fastened. A split or U sheet is draped and fastened under the arm. A large drape (or split) sheet is draped about the shoulder and fastened below. The arm may be passed through a fenestrated sheet (laparotomy or transverse), or individual drape sheets may be used to complete the draping.

Equipment

- Extension rest for support of the head and neck or padded donut
- Pillow, padded footboard, padded arm restraint, and pad (or sandbag or folded sheet, optional)
- ESU
- Suction
- Power sources for drill and saw
- Pulsed lavage suction irrigation unit, e.g., Simpulse, MicroAire, optional
- Cast cart

Instrumentation

- Basic orthopedic procedures tray
- Osteotomes, Bennett and Hibbs retractors, Kirschner wires, wire tightener, threaded pins

Power drill, sheath, cord, drill bits, and burrs
Power saw, blades, chuck, and cord (optional)
Fixation devices, e.g., wire (stainless steel #20), T-compression plate, screws
Humeral head prosthesis with instrumentation, e.g., Magnum Implant (with pre-loaded sutures), and rasps, impactor, extractor, and reamers
Pulsed lavage suction irrigator and tip, e.g., Simpulse, MicroAire, optional

Supplies

Antiembolitic hose, optional
Tube stockinettes (2)
Basin set
Blades, (2) #10
Needle magnet or counter
Magnetic instrument pad, optional
Electrosurgical pencil and cord with holder and scraper
Suction tubing or cojoined suction and irrigation tubing for pulsed lavage
Irrigation solution in bags (for pulsed lavage), or graduated pitcher, bulb syringe, antibiotic solution
PMMA cement kit
Sling and swathe

Special Notes

- Apply **Special Notes** from ***Open Reduction and Internal Fixation of a Carpal Bone Fracture***, p. 538, as indicated.
- Circulator notifies the x-ray department when the patient is being positioned on the table. (Fluoroscopy will give views of fracture, guide pins, and position of nailing device.)
- All equipment should be checked as to working order prior to bringing the patient into surgery. Check amount of gas in tanks, as necessary.
- Some surgeons prefer to double-glove and remove the first pair following completion of draping.
- Irrigation solution replacement bags must be immediately ready at all times; the next bag should "hang in waiting."
- There is a system that provides safe placement of working channels by Smith and Nephew Co. (and others).
- Keep movement and conversation in the room to a minimum, especially during procedures involving placement of a prosthesis.

- When available, a fluid-control drape (with pouch) should be used to collect the irrigation solution as necessary to prevent "strike through" contamination of the sterile field.
- The scrub person must monitor the temperature of the irrigation solution as it leaves the outflow tubing before the solution reaches the patient.
- **N.B.** *The scrub person provides a moist lap sponge to protect the surface of an implant as the driver is used to seat it.*
- Document the date, patient's name, brand name, type, size, and serial numbers of the implanted prosthesis in the **Perioperative Record** and in the hospital's log (for insertion of an implant), according to hospital policy.

Arthroplasty of the Shoulder with Hemi (Partial) or Total Prosthetic Replacement of the Shoulder Joint

Definition

The release of soft tissues to restore the normal anatomy and range of motion to the shoulder joint with partial (humeral) or total (glenohumeral) prosthetic joint replacement.

Discussion

Arthroplasty of the Shoulder with Hemi (Partial) or Total Prosthetic Replacement of the Shoulder Joint is described. Total shoulder arthroplasty is performed in patients with restricted motion of the shoulder joint (due to pain) or painful conditions related to traumatic arthritis, osteoarthritis with osteophyte formation, osteonecrosis, etc., not responsive to nonoperative therapy. Prior to surgery, patients undergo medical evaluation, radiologic, EMG, and nerve conduction studies, as needed. The importance of restoring the anatomy and biomechanics of the patient's shoulder cannot be understated. Shoulder arthroplasty is successful when management of bone loss, rotator cuff dysfunction, and fracture alignment and stabilization are achieved. Proper exposure is obtained by removing osteophytes and performing soft-tissue releases as needed to restore normal range of motion. To perform shoulder arthroplasty with total shoulder joint replacement, a great deal of experience is required to meet the degree of difficulty encountered in performing the repair.

Contraindications (to shoulder arthroplasty) include patients with severe medical problems, current infection in the shoulder or other locations, neuropathy, bone deficiencies that prevent healing, paralysis of both the deltoid and rotator cuff, severe rotator cuff tears, uncontrolled seizure disorder, or lack of motivation to participate in postoperative rehabilitation, which may take as long as 18 to 24 months.

"Unconstrained" prostheses have replaced **"constrained."** Each type of "unconstrained" prosthesis has a variety of tools for insertion and extraction of that particular prosthesis. Depending on the integrity of the bone about the glenoid, the prosthetic component is seated with a peg or screw or, when the bone is compromised, a "keel" fixation. Bone grafts (often taken from the resected humeral head) may be used to support the glenoid component. Polymethylmethacrylate (PMMA) cement is used for humeral head and glenoid fixation (except in younger patients in whom the bone integrity otherwise is good). When PMMA cement is not used, a "press-in" prosthesis is employed. Numerous prosthetic systems are available; the humeral component may consist of a single piece or dual (stem and cap); some shafts are coated with porous application to promote more secure fixation with or without the use of cement. Each system comes with its own jigs, templates, tools, etc. (Some proprietary names include Biomodular™ by Biomet, Polaris™ by Acumed, Aequalis™ by Tournier, etc.)

Hemi-arthroplasty is the preferred procedure for younger patients, as the desired outcome may be achieved with this "lesser" approach. As a young patient will wear the prosthesis for years longer than the older patient, the concern regarding the young patient is that growing may "loosen" the glenoid prosthesis. Some surgeons prefer to start with the hemi-arthroplasty procedure because the total shoulder replacement procedure can always be considered a future alternative. **Total shoulder joint replacement** affords better pain relief than hemi-arthroplasty (replacement of humeral component only); however, the surgery takes longer, there is greater potential for blood loss, and the joint prosthesis is expensive. The results obtained with total shoulder joint replacement by prostheses are good.

Note regarding laminar airflow: Until recently, joint replacement surgery was performed (whenever possible) in an OR equipped with laminar airflow. Surprisingly, studies have proven that operating rooms with laminar air-flow systems having *high efficiency particulate arresting* (HEPA) filters are no more effective at preventing intraoperative wound (or bone) infections than operating rooms routinely equipped with air-conditioning systems that provide 12 or more air exchanges per hour. Nevertheless, some orthopedic surgeons prefer to operate in the OR with laminar air.

Procedure

Total shoulder joint replacement is described. The skin over the coracoid process is marked with indelible ink preoperatively (to serve as a landmark). The incision is extended from the acromioclavicular joint to the insertion of the deltoid muscle, along the deltopectoral groove. The cephalic vein and its branches are protected. The deltoid tendon is retracted (or detached with reattachment later). The subscapularis tendon is dissected to its humeral insertion, detached, and tagged for later reattachment and/or Z-plasty lengthening. The anterior humeral circumflex artery and the axillary nerve are protected as necessary when subcapsular dissection is performed. The anterior joint capsule is incised and the humeral head dislocated; manipulation of the extremity permits better visualization and access to the humeral head and rotator cuff. The long head of the biceps is retracted. Osteophytes are excised. The wound may be cleansed of debris with pulsed lavage. A portion of the humeral head is resected. Oscillating saw or an osteotome is used to resect the humeral head, according to the extent of underlying "good" bone and the type and size of the prosthesis to be used. Similarly, the type, size, and length of the neck of the prosthesis chosen is determined by drilling into the shaft with medullary reamers to the desired depth required to make the repair. The angulation of the neck (version) of the prosthesis is oriented with the elbow flexed. It is imperative for the surgeon to place a correct-sized prosthesis with version, according to the bony and tendinous anatomy of the individual patient.

When only repair of the rotator cuff is necessary, a shorter-necked prosthesis is used. Drill holes and sutures are placed for later reattachment of the subscapularis tendon and repair of rotator cuff. The glenoid is assessed and, if not eroded, preserved after local osteophytes are excised. Hemi-arthroplasty is completed. In most instances, PMMA cement is introduced into the reamed medullary canal after debris and blood are removed by pulsed lavage and the medullary canal dried. Hemostasis is assured with epinephrine or thrombin pledgets, as necessary. The PMMA cement is deposited and tamped into the cavity in increments; the excess cement is removed each time, until the properly positioned prosthesis is seated optimally. Use of the cement may be decided as per individual patient. Dual-component humeral prostheses are assembled after size and condition of the soft tissues have been assessed.

If the glenoid requires replacement, it is replaced prior to the humeral element. Cartilage and diseased bone about the neck are excised; if there is insufficient purchase for the prosthesis, a bone graft is fixed by cancellous screw. A hole may be drilled to accommodate the screw or peg of the prosthesis, or a drill burr trough is created with drill burr or reamer for a "keeled" prosthesis. Following pulsed lavage, the medullary canal of the bone is dried. Hemostasis is achieved (as above). The appropriate humeral component is seated with PMMA bone cement. The humeral head (prosthesis) is relocated. Repair is performed by reattachment of the rotator cuff, the subscapularis, and other tendon(s), using the previously placed sutures, as noted above. The subscapularis tendon, if contracted, may require lengthening [by ***Z-plasty (skin graft)***, p. 690] prior to reattachment. Again, care is taken to avoid injury to the axillary nerve. The joint capsule is not closed. The deltopectoral interval may be loosely approximated with absorbable suture. As necessary, additional procedures, including resection of the acromioclavicular joint or relocation of the long head of the biceps, may be performed. The wound is repaired, leaving a closed suction catheter/drain under the deltoid (protecting branches of the axillary vessels). Some surgeons prefer to inject the wound with local anesthetic to enhance pain control immediately postoperatively. The dressings are placed, and the extremity is immobilized with sling and swathe (e.g., Dujarrier strip) or shoulder immobilizer (e.g., abduction humeral splint).

Preparation of the Patient

Antiembolitic hose are applied (adult) when requested. General anesthesia or a combination of general and interscalene block anesthesia may be used for more profound relaxation intraoperatively and to enhance pain relief postoperatively. The patient is placed in a semi-sitting, e.g., 30° angle (i.e., beach chair), or semi-Fowlers position with an extension rest that supports the patient's head and neck (after removing the top sections of the table). An alternate position places the patient at the extreme ipsilateral edge of the table with the head and neck gently bent away from the shoulder; a pad, sandbag, or rolled towel is placed under the affected scapula medially to stabilize the shoulder and to project the shoulder forward. At the discretion of the anesthesia provider, adhesive tape may be placed across the forehead to further support the head, after checking the chart for patient's allergies. The forehead skin is protected with tincture of benzoin and a 4 × 4 pad. The arm on the affected side will be draped "free"; however, prior to the skin prep, the arm may be placed in the patient's lap on a pillow (secured with soft restraint). The arm on the unaffected side is padded and tucked in at the patient's side, or it may be extended on a padded armboard, secured alongside the patient. Care is taken to prevent injury to the fingers when the sections of the table are returned to the original position. A padded footboard supports the feet. All bony prominences and areas vulnerable to skin and neurovascular pressure or trauma are padded. Apply electrosurgical dispersive pad.

Skin Preparation

Begin at the top of the shoulder; extend the prep from the submandibular region to the inferior costal margin. Continue down to the table at the back, beyond the midline of the chest in front, and to the inferior costal margin below. Prep also includes the axilla, arm, and forearm.

Draping

The extremity (held in double tube stockinette) is elevated and abducted. A large cuffed drape sheet is tucked under the shoulder. The outer tube stockinette is brought up (unrolled) to the top of the arm. A towel, folded in thirds longitudinally, is wrapped around the top the stockinette and secured; this permits access to the extremity for shoulder manipulation to assure proper fixation. A cuffed split sheet is placed under the arm; when available, a split sheet with a collection pouch is used. A large sheet is draped around the shoulder. Folded towels are placed around the perimeter of the incision. A sterile, plastic adhesive drape (e.g., Steri-drape™) may be placed. A fenestrated sheet (e.g., lap or transverse sheet) or additional individual drape sheets complete the draping.

Equipment

Extension support for head and neck (optional) or padded donut
Pad, sandbag, or rolled sheet (under the affected scapula, optional)
Padded footboard
Suction
ESU
Power sources for saw, drill, and reamers (unless motor is self-contained, e.g., Stryker), optional
Cell-saver, or blood pump and blood warmer (as necessary)
Cast cart

Instrumentation

Basic orthopedic procedures tray
Bone hooks, Cobb elevator, burrs and burring template, rasps, broach
Retractors: Darrach, Richardson, Hobbs, Crego or Fukuda, Richardson, and/or glenoid neck retractor (pickle fork)
Self-retaining retractors, e.g., Hawkins-Bell retractor system (DuPuy)
Automatic screwdriver for Phillips and flat-head screws
High-speed burr drill and cord, drill bits, chuck, reamers, etc.
Reciprocating or oscillating saw (e.g., Stryker, Hall, or 3M) with cord or self-contained
Trial prostheses (include three, i.e., the prosthesis and one size larger and one size smaller), template, guide for humeral head and glenoid sizer
Prostheses of choice with insertion instrumentation, e.g., awl, reamers, driver-extractor, mallet

Supplies

Antiembolitic hose (adult), optional
Sterile marking pen (optional)

Tube stockinettes (2)
Sterile, plastic adhesive drape, e.g., Steri-drape (optional)
Basin set
Blades, (2) #10
Electrosurgical pencil and cord with holder and scraper
Suction tubing or cojoined suction and irrigation tubing for pulsed lavage, optional
Irrigation solution (lactated Ringer's) in 3000-ml bags for pulsed lavage unit, or graduated pitcher, bulb syringe, and antibiotic irrigation
Needle magnet or counter
Cotton pledgets
Epinephrine and thrombin to promote hemostasis
PMMA and cement supplies (kit available), optional
Sterile paper labels (to identify medications on the sterile field)
Local anesthetic with epinephrine, medicine cup, syringe, and needle (injected at end of surgery)
Closed suction drain, e.g., Hemovac™, optional
Sling and swathe or shoulder immobilizer (e.g., abduction humeral splint)

Special Notes

- Apply **Special Notes**, as applicable from ***Arthroplasty of the Wrist with Prosthetic Replacement of the Carpal Bones,*** p. 549, as indicated.
- **Reminder:** Prior to bringing the patient into the room, the circulator checks the chart and verifies the patient's identity, etc., (according to the **JC's *Universal Protocol***). He/she discusses allergies and sensitivities with the patient to avoid potential allergic reactions; e.g., for the patient with an allergy to rubber products, a substitute hypoallergenic tape for adhesive tape (used in positioning) is made. Document in the **Perioperative Record** that the allergy was noted, the alternative product used, and the appearance of the skin preoperatively and immediately postoperatively.
- **Reminder:** Maintain patient's body temperature with a warmed blanket or by adjusting the room temperature, as necessary. When ordered, a forced-air warming blanket may be used.
- **N.B.** *Prior to bringing the patient in the room, the surgeon is shown a variety of implants and chooses the type he/she prefers.* ***Do not*** start any procedure unless the implant and insertion instrumentation are in the room. The preoperatively

measured prosthesis (size), as well as implants a size above and a size below, must be sterilized, including insertion and extraction instrumentation required for that type of prosthesis.

- Keep movement and conversation in the room to a minimum, especially during procedures involving placement of a prosthesis to avoid distraction of the surgeon and/or inadvertent contamination.
- Ascertain that there are adequate levels of pressure (gas or compressed air) in the tank, when required, for power equipment.
- A pulsed lavage unit may be used to debride the wound prior to closure; follow safety precautions regarding its use, see Chapter 2, p. 46.
- A system provided by Smith and Nephew may be used to provide safe placement of working channels.
- The pulsed lavage unit (with dual channels) is used for controlled, powered irrigation with or without suction; bags of irrigation solution are necessary. The scrub person attaches the tubing with spike adaptor to the pistol grip handle and passes off the (single or dual spiked) tubing to the circulator. The tubing (either straight or a "Y") is connected to bag(s) of irrigation solution at one end and the suction at the other.
- The scrub person inserts the tip of choice (e.g., soft splash shield tip) into the handle of the pulsed lavage unit and primes the unit by squeezing the trigger until irrigation solution exits the tip. The circulator may squeeze the irrigation bag(s) to facilitate priming.
- Irrigation solution replacement bags must be immediately ready at all times; the next irrigation bag should "hang in waiting."
- When available, a fluid-control drape (with pouch) should be used to collect the irrigation solution, as necessary, to prevent contamination of the sterile field.
- The scrub person must monitor the temperature of the irrigation solution as it leaves the outflow tubing before the solution reaches the patient.
- **N.B.** *Reminder: The scrub person provides a moist lap sponge to protect the surface of the implant as the driver is used to seat it.*
- Document the date, patient's name, brand name, type, size, and serial numbers of the implanted prosthesis in the **Periopera-**

tive Record and in the hospital's log (for insertion of an implant), according to policy.

- A splint and a sling and swathe or a shoulder immobilizer will be applied. Cast supplies (cast cart) should be available at the conclusion of the surgery.
- **Reminder:** Wearing a protective face shield or goggles is recommended to protect those scrubbed from splashing of irrigation and other fluids.

Open Reduction and Internal Fixation of Fractures of the Hip

Definition

Alignment and open stabilization of fractures of the trochanteric region and femoral neck.

Discussion

Fractures of the hip include intertrochanteric and subtrochanteric; they are usually the result of a fall. If the fracture cannot be reduced or the patient cannot tolerate prolonged immobilization, surgical intervention is indicated. Open reduction and fixation is indicated for almost all patients, including the "poor-risk" patient, as this enables early postoperative ambulation. The procedure should be performed as soon as possible to avoid complications such as pulmonary congestion, thrombophlebitis, and avascular necrosis. The fracture table facilitates manipulation and reduction of the hip fracture, and the position is maintained to facilitate placement of the fixation device. Open reduction and internal fixation of hip fractures can be performed under local anesthesia, regional block including continuous epidural anesthesia, and general anesthesia. Fixation may be achieved with pins (Knowles), nail (e.g., Ender), or nail with plate (e.g., Omega Plus™), Gamma nail, and screws. Fractures of the femoral head will be addressed to follow; see p. 595.

Contraindications include active infection (local or systemic), osteoporotic bone too weak to sustain fixation, or poor tissue quality due to burns, surgical scars, etc.

Procedure

The fracture table is preferred. The patient is brought into the room in his/her hospital bed. Following endotracheal intubation with the administration of general anesthesia (or following the administration of regional block, e.g., continuous epidural anesthesia), at the discretion of the anesthesia provider, the patient is lifted from his/her hospital bed with the surgeon's supervision and transferred to the fracture table. Adequate assistance is necessary to assure the safe transfer of the patient and also to protect the employees involved in the transfer from personal injury. The circulator is responsible for obtaining adequate assistance for the transfer of the patient [or a lift may be used (e.g. Hoyer)] before anesthesia is induced. The surgeon and his/her assistant assume responsibility for supporting the affected extremity during the transfer. The patient is placed in supine position on the fracture table. The surgeon manipulates (or directs the manipulation of) the fracture table distraction components until the fracture is reduced; x-rays (in one plane) and fluoroscopy (in two planes) confirm the reduction; see **Preparation of the Patient** below. Prior to prepping and draping, the surgeon may indicate appropriate anatomical landmarks with indelible ink.

When local anesthesia is employed in conjunction with conscious sedation (usually for a poor-risk patient), the injections are administered prior to the transfer to the fracture table. A lateral (less often an anterior) incision is made to expose the fracture site. Threaded pins (e.g., Knowles), a cannulated nail, a compression screw, or a nail with a plate is placed after guide wires are inserted (for angle determination and length). Guide wires temporarily maintain alignment; x-ray confirms position and ascertains that the joint space has not been violated. A high-speed power drill is used to facilitate placement of the plate screws; specific instrumentation (drivers, guides, reamers, etc.) is employed according to the hardware selected. X-ray check again is performed. Following pulsed lavage (antibiotic, optional), hemostasis is obtained. The wound is closed. A closed suction drain may be employed.

Preparation of the Patient

The fracture table is preferred; the surgeon and his/her assistant assume responsibility for supporting the affected extremity and the table adjustments (as noted above). The patient is placed in supine position on the fracture table; the perineal post is padded and protected with an adhesive-backed plastic drape. The leg on the unaffected side is placed in a stirrup, somewhat flexed, to permit access of the C-arm to take the lateral x-ray view of the affected extremity. The foot on the affected side is padded and secured in a padded boot (with Velcro™ straps) attached to a traction bar. By manipulating the moveable components on the fracture table, closed reduction is achieved, often with abduction and internal rotation of the extremity. The position is confirmed by x-ray (anteroposterior [AP] and lateral views). Adequate padding is needed to protect bony prominences and any areas vulnerable to skin and neurovascular pressure and trauma. A sterile, plastic adhesive drape, e.g., Steridrape, may be placed to drape the perineum out of the field before the skin prep. Apply electrosurgical dispersive pad.

Skin Preparation

Fracture Table. A Foley catheter (with drainage unit) is usually inserted into the patient's bladder prior to the skin prep. Begin at the greater trochanter; extend the prep from the level of the nipples to below the knees. Prep beyond the midline of the abdomen or to the plastic adhesive drape (placed to isolate the perineal region), anteriorly, and down to the table on the affected side.

Standard Table (e.g., Ritter). When a fracture table is not used, the lower extremity is prepped (excluding the foot) in addition to the area noted above. The perineal area is isolated by a plastic drape prior to prepping.

Draping

Fracture Table. A large sheet is draped over the foot of the table. Folded towels (four) are placed; two are folded diagonally, one placed proximal and one placed distal to the incision site, and two are folded lengthwise, one across the top and one along the bottom border; the towels are secured, as necessary. A sterile plastic adhesive drape is placed over the intended incision site. A split sheet is placed proximal to the incision with the tails draped (adhesive-backed) along the superior and inferior borders of the incision site. A transverse sheet completes the draping.

Standard Table. The leg is abducted and the foot grasped in a double tube stockinette. A large drape sheet is placed over the end of the table. The tube stockinette is placed on the foot and the outer one is brought up (unrolled) to the top of the thigh. A split sheet is draped under the thigh, and the tube stockinette is brought up over the iliac crest and secured; the adhesive-backed tails of the split sheet are draped around the borders of the (intended) incision. Towels may be secured around the incision site. A large sheet is draped proximal to the incision. The leg is passed through a large fenestrated (e.g., laparotomy or transverse) sheet. An opening for the incision is cut out of the stockinette, towels may be placed around the incision borders, and a sterile, plastic adhesive drape is placed over the incision site.

A drape is required for the C-arm.

Equipment

Fracture table (e.g., Stryker, Chick, etc.) or standard Ritter table with radiolucent table extension
Fluoroscopy with C-arm (portable x-ray)
ESU
Suction (2)
Power sources for saw, drill, and reamers (e.g., Hall and 3M; unless motor is self-contained, e.g., Stryker), optional
Cast cart

Instrumentation

Basic orthopedic procedures tray, bone-holding instruments, and hip retractors trays
Beckman retractors
Power drill, cord (or self-contained), and drill bits
Fixation device and instrumentation necessary for insertion: pins (e.g., Knowles), nail with fixed angle screw plate (e.g., Gamma), or screw (lag, dynamic hip screw), compression screw with plate and instrumentation particular to each device, e.g., driver/extractor, reamers, etc.
Guide pins, osteotomes, broach, large mallet
Pulsed lavage suction irrigator and tip, e.g., Impulse™, Simpulse, MicroAire, optional

Supplies

Antiembolitic stocking, optional
Foley catheter tray (with drainage unit)
Sterile, plastic adhesive drapes (2); perineum and operative site, optional
Tube stockinettes (2) with standard table
Sterile marking pen
Basin set
Blades, (3 to 4) #10
Needle magnet or counter
Electrosurgical pencil and cord with holder and scraper
Sterile paper labels, medicine cup, needle, syringe, and antibiotic (for irrigation)
Antibiotic
Suction tubing (2) or cojoined suction and irrigation tubing for pulsed lavage, e.g., Simpulse with long lavage tip, with irrigation solution (lactated Ringer's) in 3000-ml bags for pulsed lavage unit (antibiotic added) or graduated pitcher, asepto syringes (2), and antibiotic irrigation
Closure of choice for skin, e.g., preloaded skin stapler
Pressure dressing, e.g., Elastoplast™ (check chart for allergy)

Special Notes

- Apply **Special Notes** from ***Abdominal Laparotomy***, p. 134, as they apply to all patients in surgery (e.g., regarding correct identification of the patient, observing "*time out*," employing comfort measures that make a difference, etc.). All nursing care interventions and outcomes are documented.

- **Reminder:** Be certain that x-rays are in the room prior to the start of the procedure. Verify that the correct x-ray films in the room are for the *correctly identified* patient.
- Notify the x-ray department when the patient is being positioned on the fracture table. If the fracture table is unavailable, a radiolucent extension is added to the standard table. Fluoroscopy is employed (or individual x-rays may be taken) to provide AP and lateral views of the reduced fracture site, provide guidance for the correct placement of guide wires, pins, etc., and to confirm proper placement of the fixation device.
- **Reminder:** Observe all x-ray safety precautions; see p. 52.
- Personnel positioning patients on the fracture table must have intimate knowledge of its mechanisms of operation for safe usage.
- Prevent risk of positioning injury to the patient with adequate padding and correct positioning to avoid skin and neurovascular pressure or trauma. Document appearance and condition of the skin at pressure points preoperatively and immediately postoperatively.
- **Reminder:** The circulator checks the chart to verify the patient's identity, etc., and discusses allergies with the patient to avoid potential allergic reactions; e.g., for allergy to rubber products, a substitute for adhesive tape (used in positioning) and tape for pressure dressing (e.g., Elastoplast) is made. Document in the **Perioperative Record** that the allergy was noted, that an alternative product used, and the appearance of the skin preoperatively and immediately postoperatively (where tape was placed).
- Some surgeons prefer to double-glove and remove the first pair following completion of draping.
- **Reminder:** Maintain patient's body temperature with a warmed blanket or by adjusting the room temperature, as necessary. When ordered, a forced-air warming blanket may be used; warming mattress pads are **not** placed, as they interfere with taking x-rays (radiopaque).
- Check gauge to ascertain that there are adequate levels of pressure (gas or compressed air) in the tank when required to operate power equipment or when power equipment uses batteries, check level of battery before starting surgery.
- A pulsed lavage unit may be used to debride the wound prior to closure; follow safety precautions regarding its use, see p. 46.

- When available, a fluid-control drape (with pouch) should be used to collect the irrigation solution as necessary to prevent strike-through contamination of the sterile field.
- Irrigation solution replacement bags must be immediately ready at all times; the next bag should "hang in waiting."
- The scrub person must monitor the temperature of the irrigation solution as it leaves the outflow tubing before the solution reaches the patient.
- **Reminder:** Wearing a protective face shield or goggles is recommended to protect those scrubbed from splashing of irrigation and other fluids.

Prosthetic Replacement of the Femoral Head

Definition

Prosthetic substitution for the head of the femur.

Discussion

Femoral head replacement is indicated when there is nonunion of femoral neck fractures or avascular necrosis of the femoral head and in degenerative changes of the hip postfracture or from arthritis (primarily fractures that cannot reasonably be expected to heal retaining the femoral head). One advantage of this procedure is that immediate weight bearing is permitted. Procedures that involve femoral head replacement are more extensive and entail more risks than procedures where the femoral head is retained, and older patients are at a higher risk for fixation device failure than young patients, but are also at a higher risk for osteonecrosis of the femoral head. It follows, then, that prosthetic head replacement surgery is often performed on older patients. Several prostheses are available, e.g., bipolar three component (by DuPuy, Richards, Zimmer, Stryker-Howmedica). The bipolar models have increased motion between the prosthetic component, and the femoral head leads to decreased motion at the acetabulum; this results in less acetabular wear and a lower rate of dislocation of the prosthesis.

Some orthopedic surgeons prefer to operate in the OR with laminar airflow.

Procedure

Prosthetic Replacement of the Femoral Head is described. A room with laminar airflow may be requested. The incision and the approach depend on the habitus of the patient, as well as the experience and discretion of the surgeon. When a posterior approach is used, the incision is made over the gluteus maximus superiorly and paralleling the proximal femur. The muscle fibers are split. The sciatic nerve is protected. The external rotators of the hip are freed from the femur, and the joint capsule is incised. Flexion, adduction, and internal rotation of the thigh are employed to dislocate the hip. A corkscrew may be employed to extract the femoral head. The excised femoral head is removed and measured; a similar-sized trial prosthetic head is chosen. The medullary canal is reamed with a rasp, particular to that prosthesis. The neck is shaped to receive the prosthesis without rotation, leaving enough of the calcar medially. Excess bone fragments are trimmed. After checking the size of the trial acetabular prosthesis in the acetabulum, the prosthesis is seated (using instrumentation special to that prosthesis). Care is taken not to fracture the thinned femoral shaft. If the proximal femoral shaft sustains a fracture, a circlage of wire is placed. PMMA cement may be employed to seat the prosthesis in the femoral shaft. When cement is used, it is introduced into the reamed medullary canal after debris and blood are removed by pulsed lavage. The medullary canal is dried. Hemostasis is assured. The PMMA cement is deposited and tamped into the cavity in increments. The excess cement is removed each time, until the properly positioned prosthesis is seated optimally. The components of the prosthesis are assembled and the hip relocated. Repair of divided soft tissues is performed when applicable. The incision is closed in the usual manner.

Use of PMMA cement may be decided as per individual patient.

Preparation of the Patient

Antiembolitic hose are applied, as requested. A Foley catheter is usually inserted into the patient's bladder prior to the skin prep. The approach may be anterior, lateral, or posterior. A posterior approach with the patient in the lateral position (most often used) is described. A sterile, plastic adhesive drape is placed to drape the perineum out of the field. The position can be supported with sandbags, Vac Pac, beanbags, or padded kidney rests. The arm on the affected side is flexed over the chest, with a pillow placed between the arms, and the arm on the affected side is secured by a padded restraint (or a double padded armboard may be used). The arm on the unaffected side is extended on a padded armboard; a pad may be positioned to relieve pressure on the brachial plexus. The affected leg is draped "free," and the unaffected leg may be extended under the drape. Adequate padding protects bony prominences and all areas vulnerable to skin and neurovascular pressure and trauma. After checking the chart for the patient's allergies, the patient's position is secured at the shoulder by wide adhesive tape (or when the patient is allergic, a substitute item is used) anchored to the underside of the table; the skin is protected with tincture of benzoin. A safety strap is secured over the blanket that covers the unaffected leg. An electrosurgical dispersive pad is applied.

Skin Preparation

Begin at the hip (area of the greater trochanter); extend the prep from the nipples to the tips of the toes. Prep the skin beyond the midline of the abdomen, in the front and down to the table at the back. Prep the lower extremity (excluding the foot).

Draping

The leg is abducted and the foot grasped in a double tube stockinette. A tube stockinette is placed on the foot; the outer tube stockinette is brought up (unrolled) to the top of the thigh. A large sheet is draped over the end of the table. A split sheet is draped under the thigh, as the tube stockinette is brought up and over the iliac crest and secured; the adhesive backed tails of the split sheet are draped around the borders of the (intended) incision. A large sheet is draped proximal to the incision. The leg is passed through a large fenestrated (e.g., laparotomy or transverse) sheet. An opening for the incision may be cut out of the stockinette, with a sterile, plastic adhesive drape placed over the incision site.

Alternatively, the leg is abducted and the foot is grasped in a double tube stockinette. The tube stockinettes are placed on the foot, and the outer stockinette is brought up (unrolled) to the top of the thigh. A large sheet is draped over the end of the table. A split sheet is draped under the extremity, and the tails are brought up on either side. A large sheet is draped proximal to the incision. Towels (4) are placed around the incision borders. A sterile, plastic adhesive drape is placed over the incision site. The extremity is passed through a fenestrated sheet, e.g., transverse or laparotomy.

The C-arm requires a drape.

Equipment

Sandbags, Vac Pac, or padded kidney rests (larger one in front); pillows and padded (arm) restraint
ESU
Suction (2)
Power sources for power drill and saw, as necessary
Generator for pulsed lavage suction irrigator, (e.g., Simpulse, MicroAire) optional

Instrumentation

Basic orthopedic procedures tray
Hip retractors tray
Osteotomes, bone hooks, broach, heavy mallet, automatic screwdriver for Phillips and flat-head screws

Extra guide pins
Femoral head extractor (corkscrew), acetabular knife, hip skid, femoral rasps, caliper, driver
High-speed power drill and cord (or self-contained), drill bits (including 1/4″ and 1/2″), burrs, reamers, chuck, and key
Reciprocating or oscillating power saw, cord (or self-contained), chuck, and key
Trial prostheses (include three, i.e., the prosthesis and one size larger and one size smaller), template, guide
Prosthesis, e.g., bipolar femoral head and specific instrumentation
Pulsed lavage suction irrigator and tip, e.g., Impulse, Simpulse, optional

Supplies

Antiembolitic hose; stocking (unaffected extremity), as requested
Foley catheter tray
Tube stockinettes (2)
Sterile, plastic adhesive drapes (2); perineum and operative site
Sterile marking pen (indelible ink), optional
Basin set
Blades, (3 to 4) #10
Electrosurgical pencil and cord with holder and scraper
Needle magnet or counter
Suction tubing (2) or cojoined suction and irrigation tubing for pulsed lavage, e.g., Simpulse with long lavage tip, optional
Irrigation solution (lactated Ringer's) in 3000-ml bags for pulsed lavage unit (antibiotic solution may be added), or graduated pitcher, asepto syringes (2), and antibiotic irrigation
PMMA cement, e.g., Simplex™ radio-opaque bone cement
Cement mixer with vacuum, e.g., Stryker with Kamvac
Cement restrictor

Special Notes

- Apply **Special Notes** from ***Arthroplasty of the Shoulder with Hemi (Partial) or Total Prosthetic Replacement of the Shoulder Joint,*** p. 579 as indicated.
- **Reminder:** All nursing care interventions and outcomes are documented in the **Perioperative Record**.

Total Hip Arthroplasty with Prosthetic Replacement of the Hip Joint

Definition

Reconstruction and replacement of the hip joint.

Discussion

Disorders of the hip joint for which total hip arthroplasty may be indicated include rheumatoid arthritis and degenerative diseases (e.g., osteoarthritis, posttraumatic conditions such as avascular necrosis, damage caused by infection, and failed reconstruction). Numerous modifications of prostheses are employed, including different metallic alloys, porous coatings (to encourage better bony adherence in noncemented stems), plastics (including cross-linked polyethylene with less wear and shedding of microdebris, which can lead to inflammatory changes), ceramics, and the bipolar cup. Various combinations of materials for either the acetabular or femoral element are available, each system with its "expert" advocates.

Some of the prostheses available include the bipolar endoprostheses (Gilberty & Bateman; Howmedica), which have a smaller femoral head that articulates by a snap-fit with a polyethylene liner within a metal acetabular shell. The bipolar prosthesis is thought to cause less erosion of the acetabulum, prolonging longevity of the arthroplasty. Johnson & Johnson (DuPuy) has a 360° femoral prostheses (porous, coated) in several stem lengths, and Biomet produces PLR (Proximal Load) that has a stem revision; these are some of the "cementless" prostheses available. PMMA cement is used in the "cemented" version; it is used primarily for seating the femoral head portion of the prosthetic joint. The cementless acetabular prosthesis uses a "press-fit" technique, e.g., DuPuy anatomic medullary locking (AML), Harris-Galante (porous coated metal), and others. In addition, there are instances when "resurfacing" rather than full replacement is applicable, wherein the femoral head is surface excised but otherwise left intact with application of a metallic shell (Buechel-Pappas, Smith & Nephew Birmingham Hip Resurfacing Device™). Biomet has a diamond-coated prosthetic surface that will be more resistant to wear.

Increasing application of minimal access approach with smaller incisions is in practice. Many well-known orthopedic proprietary companies (e.g., Zimmer, DuPuy, Howmedica, Smith & Nephew, etc.) manufacture a variety of these hardware modifications. Weight-bearing is within several postoperative days when the cemented version is employed; the "cementless" prosthesis is not weight-bearing for up to as long as 3 months. Of course, the "cementless" prosthesis can be removed more easily, should that become necessary. Long-term efficacy of the "cementless" hip prosthesis (versus cemented) is being reevaluated with consideration for the newer surfacing materials; the "Charnley type" cemented total hip prosthesis has been the standard.

Some orthopedic surgeons prefer to operate in the OR with laminar airflow.

Procedure

Total Hip Arthroplasty with Prosthetic Replacement of the Hip Joint is described. One of several techniques may be employed. The patient is brought to the OR in his/her hospital bed. General with endotracheal intubation, regional, or local anesthetic may be employed. Temporary traction devices are removed prior to the skin preparation. At the anesthesia provider's discretion and under the surgeon's supervision, the patient is transferred to the OR table (e.g., Ritter). (During the transfer, the surgeon and/or the assistant surgeon are responsible for the affected extremity.) In the lateral approach (most common), a longitudinal incision is made proximal to the greater trocanter, distally along the proximal femoral shaft. The fascia is incised, and the muscle fibers are separated. Scar tissue is freed. The insertions of the rotator muscles of the hip are divided (and tagged for later reapproximation).

The hip joint capsule is exposed. The hip is dislocated, employing adduction and internal rotation, as gently as possible. If this maneuver is difficult, scar tissue and/or additional tendons may be divided. The femoral neck is osteotomized and the femoral head extracted. The proximal femur is trimmed and the medullary canal reamed to accept the prosthesis. The acetabulum is then exposed, any remaining labrum excised, and the capsule detached from the anterior and inferior margins. Cartilage and soft tissues are curetted from the acetabulum. Acetabular reamers are employed to prepare the acetabulum to accept the cup prosthesis. Anchoring holes are drilled in the acetabulum. The proper position and angulation of the cup are determined. When PMMA cement is used, it is introduced into the reamed acetabulum after debris and blood are removed by pulsed lavage, the area dried, and hemostasis assured. PMMA cement is prepared and applied, and the cup is positioned. Excess PMMA cement is trimmed. Debris and blood are removed by pulsed lavage from the femoral canal. The canal is dried; hemostasis is assured. A trial prosthesis is inserted and test relocation is performed, making corrections, as necessary, to provide proper seating of the prosthesis. The trial prosthesis is then removed and the (actual) prosthesis is "seated again" after PMMA cement has been deposited and tamped into the medullary canal in increments. The excess cement is removed each time, until the properly positioned prosthesis is optimally seated.

When the PMMA cement is set, the hip is relocated. The previously incised soft tissue and osteotomized (or tendon) attachments are replaced and fixed, using nonabsorbable sutures. The wound is closed. A closed drainage system may be employed. Pillows are placed postoperatively to prevent adduction of the thighs.

Use of PMMA cement may be decided as per individual patient.

For **Preparation of the Patient, Skin Preparation,** and **Draping,** see *Open Reduction and Internal Fixation of Fracture(s) of the Humeral Head (Including) Prosthetic Replacement of the Femoral Head,* P. 571.

Equipment

Laminar airflow, optional
Sandbags, Vac Pac, padded kidney rests, pillows, and padded arm restraint
ESU
Scales (2) to weigh sponges
Suctions (2)
Pillows (for positioning postoperatively)

Instrumentation

Basic orthopedic procedures tray
Hip retractors tray
Hip gouges, hip skid, rasps, femoral head extractor, caliper (for measuring), bone hooks, guide pins
High-speed power drill (and cord, as necessary), drill bits (including 1/4″ and 1/2″), burrs, reamers, chuck, and key
Special drills: acromionizer, razor cutter, and stone cutter (Stryker, Dyonics, etc.) for cutting tubular channels
Reciprocating or oscillating saw (e.g., Stryker, Hall, or 3M) with cord (or self-contained), chuck, and key
Trial stem and cup prostheses (include 3, i.e., the prosthesis and one size larger and one size smaller), template, femoral head and acetabular guides, and specific insertion instrumentation, e.g., reamer, rasp for stem prosthesis, acetabular reamer, and acetabular knife
Total hip prosthetic implants and specific instrumentation
Pulsed lavage suction irrigator and tip, e.g., Impulse, Simpulse, MicroAire, optional

Supplies

Antiembolitic hose (stocking on unaffected extremity), as requested
Tube stockinettes (2)
Sterile, plastic adhesive drapes (2), perineum and operative site
Basin set
Suction tubing
Electrosurgical pencil and cord with holder and scraper
Blades, (3 to 4) #10
Needle magnet or counter

Suction tubing (2) or cojoined suction and irrigation tubing for pulsed lavage, e.g., Simpulse with long lavage tip, optional
Irrigation solution (lactated Ringer's) in 3000-ml bags for pulsed lavage unit (antibiotic, optional), or graduated pitcher, asepto syringes (2), and antibiotic irrigation
Gelfoam, thrombin, and cotton pledgets (available) to dry canal
PMMA cement, e.g., Simplex™ radio-opaque bone cement
Cement mixer with vacuum, e.g., Stryker with Kamvac
Cement restrictor
Closed drainage unit (e.g., Hemovac), optional
Abduction pillow

Special Notes

- Apply **Special Notes** from ***Arthroplasty of the Shoulder with Hemi (Partial) or Total Prosthetic Replacement of the Shoulder Joint,*** p. 579, as applicable.
- Surgeon may request that the procedure be performed in an OR equipped with laminar flow.
- **Reminder:** Be certain that x-rays are in the room prior to the start of the procedure. Verify that the correct x-ray films in the room are for the *correctly identified* patient.
- **Reminder:** Prior to bringing the patient into the room, the circulator checks the chart to verify the patient's identity, etc., and discusses allergies with the patient to avoid potential allergic reactions; e.g., for allergy to rubber products, a substitute for adhesive tape (used in positioning) is made. Document in the **Perioperative Record** that the allergy was noted and the alternative product used and the appearance of the skin preoperatively and immediately postoperatively.
- **N.B.** *Prior to bringing the patient into the room, the surgeon is shown a variety of implants and chooses the type he/she prefers.* ***Do not*** start any procedure unless the implant and insertion instrumentation are also in the room; they should be sterile. The preoperatively measured prosthesis (size) as well as implants a size above and a size below must be sterilized, including insertion instrumentation required for that type of prosthesis.
- Prevent risk of positioning injury to the patient positioned correctly to avoid skin and neurovascular pressure or trauma. Document appearance and condition of the skin preoperatively and immediately postoperatively.
- During positioning, protect patient's skin with tincture of benzoin under places to be covered with adhesive tape.

- **Reminder:** Keep movement and conversation in the room to a minimum, especially for total joint replacement.
- Some surgeons prefer to double-glove and remove the first pair following completion of draping.
- Fluoroscopy is employed (or individual x-rays may be taken) to provide AP and lateral views of the reduced fracture site, guidance for the correct placement of guide wires, pins, etc., and to confirm proper placement of the fixation device.
- **Reminder:** Observe all x-ray safety precautions; see p. 52.
- **Reminder:** Maintain patient's body temperature with a warmed blanket or by adjusting the room temperature, as necessary. When ordered, a forced-air warming blanket is used; warming mattress pads are **not** used as they are radio-opaque and interfere with taking x-rays.
- Ascertain that there are adequate levels of pressure (gas or compressed air) in the tank when required for power equipment; if self-contained power equipment is used, check the level of charge left in the battery.
- Check with the blood bank that blood ordered is available; for prescheduled cases, the patient may have donated blood for an "auto" transfusion.
- Maintain an accurate record of irrigation used and weigh sponges (when indicated) to determine blood loss and fluid replacement.
- Cotton pledgets and all small items that could be sequestered in the wound are included in the count.
- A pulsed lavage unit may be used to debride the wound prior to closure; follow safety precautions regarding its use; see Chapter 2, p. 46.
- There is a system that provides safe placement of working channels by Smith and Nephew.
- The pulsed lavage unit (with dual channels) is used for controlled, powered irrigation with or without suction; bags of irrigation solution are necessary. The scrub person attaches the tubing with spike adaptor to the pistol grip handle and passes off the (single- or double-) tubing to the circulator. A connector is added to the tubing that connects to bag(s) of irrigation solution at one end and the suction at the other (when used).

- The scrub person inserts the tip of choice (e.g., soft splash shield tip) into the handle of the pulsed lavage unit and primes the unit by squeezing the trigger until irrigation solution exits the tip. The circulator may squeeze the irrigation bag(s) to facilitate priming.
- An antibiotic may be added to the irrigation bags; add the correct amount of antibiotic to avoid medication errors, see p. 30.
- Irrigation solution replacement bags must be immediately ready at all times. Be prepared to change suction apparatus and tubing if it becomes clogged. The next bag of solution should "hang in waiting."
- The scrub person must monitor the temperature of the irrigation solution as it leaves the outflow tubing before the solution reaches the patient.
- **N.B.** *The scrub person provides a moist lap sponge to protect the surface of the implant as the driver is used to seat it.*
- Documentation regarding the date, patient's name, brand name, type, size, and serial numbers of the implanted prosthesis is made in the **Perioperative Record** and in the hospital's log (for insertion of an implant), according to policy.
- **Reminder:** Wearing a protective face shield or goggles is mandatory to protect those scrubbed from splashing of irrigation and other fluids.

Open Reduction and Internal Fixation of Fractures of the Femoral Shaft

Definition

Realignment and open fixation of fractures of the femoral shaft.

Discussion

Fractures of the femur result from trauma or may be pathologic, e.g., osteoporosis or lytic lesions, such as in metastatic cancer. In adults, a fractured femur is most often treated by internal fixation device. Fractures of the femoral shaft present as spiral, transverse, comminuted, or open. In children and young adults, a fractured femur is the result of trauma; fractures are often reduced by closed reduction and traction, followed by immobilization, e.g., spica cast. In fractures in children in which the epiphyses are displaced, pin fixation may be necessary. In adults, femoral shaft fractures are reduced, and fixation is performed with a nail, pin, or plate with screws. The fractured shaft may be stabilized with a Kirschner wire prior to placement of the fixation device. Intramedullary nails or rods are used, including Rush, Enders, Küntscher, and Gamma and Zickel nails. When a compression plate is used, it must have at least three holes above and below the fracture. Early mobilization is indicated following surgery.

Procedure

Open Reduction and Internal Fixation of Fractures of the Femoral Shaft is described. One of several techniques may be employed. The fracture table is preferred, although the OR table may be used with the patient in supine or lateral position. The patient is brought to the OR in his/her hospital bed. General with endotracheal intubation or regional anesthetic may be employed. Temporary traction devices are removed prior to the skin preparation. At the anesthesia provider's discretion and under the surgeon's supervision, the patient is transferred to the fracture table. (During the transfer, the surgeon and/or the surgeon's assistant are responsible for the affected extremity.) A posterolateral incision is made over the fracture site. A guide pin is driven proximally through the fracture site; it emerges subcutaneously, just proximal to the greater trochanter. A small counter incision is made over the prominence of the emerging guide pin. The cortical opening can be enlarged with a drill. An appropriate length and diameter rod is seated over the guide pin, such as when a Küntscher rod is used; the extractor eye is oriented posterolaterally. The rod is then introduced into the now-reduced distal segment and seated securely into the condylar region. The proximal end should protrude no more than 2.5 cm. If the fracture site is comminuted, wire loops are placed about the fragments, e.g., cerclage of wire. X-ray control (fluoroscopy) is employed as necessary to avoid creating false passages or malalignment. The wound is closed.

Preparation of the Patient

The patient is positioned on the fracture table in the supine position. The arm on the affected side is flexed across the chest; it may be positioned on a Mayo stand padded with a pillow (or a double armboard may be used). The arm on the unaffected side is extended on a padded armboard. Adequate padding around feet, ankles, and bony prominences must be taken into consideration to avoid neurovascular damage, particularly because the fracture table is very hard. When the lateral position is employed, the position can be maintained by padded kidney rests (larger one in front) or wide adhesive tape (check patient's chart for allergies first) placed at the shoulders, secured to the underside of the table. A safety strap is secured over the unaffected thigh. A sterile, plastic adhesive drape may be used to drape the perineum out of the field before the skin prep. Apply electrosurgical dispersive pad.

Skin Preparation

Begin over the fracture site; extend the prep from the umbilicus to below the knee, beyond the midline of the trunk, in front and down to the table at the back. When the extremity is draped "free" (i.e., the fracture table is not used), the leg and thigh are prepped. A leg holder may be used.

Draping

The site of the incision is draped with folded towels and a sterile, plastic adhesive drape (optional). Four sheets may be draped around the perimeter of the site; a fenestrated sheet (e.g., transverse or laparotomy) completes the draping. If the fracture table is not employed, the extremity is draped "free"; see **Draping for Femoral Head Prosthetic Replacement**, p. 588.

Equipment

Fracture table (e.g., Stryker, Chick), as requested
Leg holder (optional)
ESU
High-speed power source for drill
Suction or pulsed lavage suction unit

Instrumentation

Basic orthopedic procedures tray
Bone-holding instruments tray
Hip retractors tray
Power drill and cord (or self-contained unit), drill bits, including 1/4″ gauge
Extra guide pins, screw set
Fixation device: lag screws, nails or rods (e.g., Küntscher, Rush), including instrumentation particular to that device, or compression set
Pulsed lavage suction irrigator and tip, e.g., Impulse, Simpulse, MicroAire, optional

Supplies

Antiembolitic hose; stocking (unaffected extremity), as requested
Sterile, plastic adhesive drapes (two); perineum and operative site
Tube stockinette
Basin set
Blades, (2) #10

Suction tubing (2) or cojoined suction and irrigation tubing for pulsed lavage, e.g., Simpulse with long lavage tip, optional
Irrigation solution (lactated Ringer's) in 3000-ml bags for pulsed lavage unit (antibiotic may be added) or graduated pitcher, asepto syringes (2), and antibiotic irrigation
Electrosurgical pencil and cord with holder and scraper
Needle magnet or counter

Special Notes

- Apply **Special Notes** from ***Open Reduction and Internal Fixation of Fractures of the Hip***, p. 584, as applicable.
- **Reminder:** Irrigation solution replacement bags must be immediately ready at all times; the next bag should "hang in waiting."
- The scrub person must monitor the temperature of the irrigation solution as it leaves the outflow tubing before the solution reaches the patient.
- When available, a fluid-control drape (with pouch) should be used to collect the irrigation solution to prevent strike-through contamination of the sterile field.

Arthrotomy of the Knee

Definition

Incision into the knee joint.

Discussion

A variety of injuries can occur about the knee joint. These include fractures, meniscal tears, and ligamentous injuries related to torsion or tearing. Synovectomy may be performed for a variety of conditions, including: chronic synovitis, post-trauma, or after infectious conditions, in addition to rheumatoid arthritis, hemangioma, and villonodular changes.

- Procedures include: **Open reduction of femoral condyle and tibial plateau fractures.** Provide joint stabilization by aligning the articular surfaces of the distal femur and proximal tibia.
- **Menisectomy.** Excision of a torn meniscus and either/or both semilunar fibrocartilages.
- **Patellectomy.** Excision of all or a portion of the patella.
- **Synovectomy.** Excision of all or a portion of the synovial membrane of the knee.

- **Collateral or Cruciate Ligament Repair.** Repair of damaged ligaments of the knee, restoring them as closely as possible to the original anatomy.

The arthroscopic approach has supplanted the "open" surgical approach (arthrotomy) for many presentations of these conditions; see ***Arthroscopy of the Knee***, p. 602, for that approach.

Procedure

Open Reduction of Fractures of Femoral Condyles and Tibial Plateau is described. A longitudinal incision is made, exposing the fracture site. Debris and minor bone fragments are irrigated out. Temporary reduction may be achieved with Kirschner wires, which are removed following the insertion of Knowles pins, cancellous bone screws or bolts, etc., with penetration of the opposite cortex. "T-fractures" of the femoral condyles may be stabilized with a plate or screws. In tibial plateau fractures, the joint is explored after reflecting the iliotibial band and/or additional muscular attachments. Ligamentous and cartilaginous injuries are repaired. The fracture is reduced and fixed with hardware, as above. Cancellous bone from the proximal tibia may be packed into the fracture site. X-rays are taken to visualize and document the repair. The wound is closed. A posterior splint may be applied.

Lateral Menisectomy is described. An anterolateral incision is made from the level of the patella to the upper tibia. The quadriceps aponeurosis and joint capsule are incised. The meniscus is grasped and excised, taking care to avoid injury to the popliteus tendon, fibular collateral ligament, and vascular structures. A secondary posterolateral incision may be necessary to visualize and excise the posterior horn of the meniscus. The incisions are closed. A bulky compression dressing is applied.

Open Reduction of Fractures of the Patella and Patellectomy is described. A transverse prepatellar incision is made. The patellar tendon and joint are explored (and suture-repaired during closure). The fracture site is exposed. Debris and small fragments are irrigated from the joint. Major fracture fragments are approximated and repaired through a variety of techniques using wire and/or screws. Lesser fragments and the severely comminuted entire patella can be excised with shortening of the patellar tendon, or a patellar prosthesis can be inserted. The wound is closed, and a splint is applied.

Synovectomy is described. An anteromedial incision is made. The synovial membrane is excised from medial, lateral, and anterior aspect of the joint, including prepatellar fat pad and menisci (if they are degenerated). Using a sponge or curette, pannus is removed from the femoral condyles. By flexing the knee, posterior synovium is excised.

Optimal hemostasis is achieved. The wound is closed over a suction drain. The leg is immobilized.

Medial Collateral Ligament Repair is described. A medial longitudinal incision is made. The greater saphenous vein and sensory branches of the saphenous nerve are protected. The deep fascia is incised, and the sartorius muscle is retracted with the knee flexed. The tibial insertion of the medial collateral ligament is inspected. The joint capsule is incised, and the cruciate ligaments, menisci, and adjacent articular surfaces are inspected. Capsular tears and other ligamentous injuries are repaired; menisci, if injured, are excised. The medial collateral ligament and posterior cruciate ligament are repaired by sutures or staples at their midpoint or by staples or sutures to the bone at their origins or insertions. Tendons may be transferred if further strengthening is required. Hemostasis is achieved. The joint is closed. A long leg cast is applied.

Preparation of the Patient

The patient is supine with the knees over the lower break in the table; arms may be extended on padded armboards. The patient is secured with the safety belt over the thigh of the unaffected extremity. Webril (sheet wadding) and a tourniquet are applied to the top of the thigh of the operative leg. Apply electrosurgical dispersive pad.

Skin Preparation

Begin at the knee; extend the prep from immediately below the tourniquet (on the thigh) to the ankle.

Draping

The leg is abducted and elevated, grasped in a double tube stockinette. A sheet is draped over the end of the table. A split sheet is draped under the thigh. The outer stockinette is brought up (unrolled) to the top of the thigh. A folded towel (in thirds lengthwise) is wrapped around the top of the tube stockinette and fastened. The leg is passed through a fenestrated sheet with a rubberized extremity fenestration. The leg is passed through a fenestrated sheet (e.g., transverse or laparotomy).

An additional sheet will be necessary to cover the foot of the table, if the foot of the table is lowered (in order to flex the knee) during the procedure.

Equipment

Suction
ESU
Tourniquet and pneumatic insufflator with microprocessor regulator

Power sources for high-speed drill and saw or self-contained power device
Pulsed lavage unit
Cast cart

Instrumentation

Basic orthopedic procedures tray
Knee arthrotomy tray
High-speed power drill, cord, drill bits, chuck, and key
Power saw with blades, chuck, and key
Staples or other fixation device with insertion instrumentation for ligament repair
Kirschner wires

Supplies

Tube stockinettes (2)
Webril (sheet wadding)
Esmarch bandage
Basin set
Blades, (2) #10 and (1) #15
Electrosurgical pencil and cord with holder and scraper
Wire, e.g., stainless steel #18
Suction tubing (2) or cojoined suction and irrigation tubing for pulsed lavage
Needle magnet or counter
Asepto or bulb syringe and antibiotic irrigation, optional
Cast or splint

Special Notes

- Apply **Special Notes** from ***Open Reduction and Internal Fixation of Fractures of the Hip***, p. 584, as applicable.
- **Reminder:** Confirm correct identification of the patient, correct identification of extremity to be operated, observe "*time out*," employ comfort measures that make a difference, etc. All nursing care interventions and outcomes are documented in the **Perioperative Record**.
- Obtain the *correct* x-ray films in the room for the *correctly identified* patient.
- The circulator notifies x-ray department that films will be needed post-repair.
- Position the patient so that the knees are over the lower break in the table.

- **Reminder:** *Avoid injury to the patient's fingers by preventing them from being caught in the table mechanism when the foot of the table is raised following the procedure.*
- The circulator can help to prevent musculoskeletal injuries to team members by obtaining adequate assistance and by employing ergodynamic measures when positioning the patient.
- **Reminder:** Place tourniquet as high on the extremity as possible. Wrap Webril (sheet wadding) around the extremity smoothly. Tourniquet ends should overlap about 7.5 cm (3 inches).
- Obey all safety precautions regarding use of the tourniquet; see p. 45. The setting for the lower extremity on the average adult is approximately 350 mm Hg. Monitor tourniquet time and setting.
- **N.B.** Tourniquet **must** be released after 2 hours to avoid injury.

Arthroscopy of the Knee

Definition

Endoscopic visualization of the knee joint.

Discussion

Many procedures formerly requiring arthrotomy are performed arthroscopically. Indications for arthroscopy of the knee (as well as in other joints) include confirmation of radiographic studies and diagnostic and therapeutic procedures, which, when feasible, minimize postoperative morbidity compared to "open" arthrotomy. Visualization of intra-articular structures and anatomical diagnoses are ascertained. Therapeutic procedures include menisectomy, repair of meniscus, synovectomy, patellar shaving, prosthetic repair of ligaments (synthetics versus allografts/homografts), etc. Loose bodies may be removed directly or by irrigation. Biopsy specimens for conditions as rheumatoid arthritis and chondromalcia may be obtained.

Numerous synthetic materials are used for ligamentous grafting. Autografts, e.g., tissue obtained from the central portion of one's own patellar tendon is preferred, but, allografts, e.g., tissue from other human patellar tendons may be used., When the latter are employed, serologic testing of the donated tissue [for hepatitis, human immunodeficiency virus [(HIV), and syphilis] is done; antibiotics and cryopreservation are employed. The grafts are thawed immediately prior to use.

Procedure

Arthroscopy of the Knee is described. The knee joint is examined under anesthesia. Range of motion and stability are ascertained. (A tourniquet is applied to be immediately available, but not inflated as the tamponade effect of the distending medium, e.g., Ringer's lactate, will minimize local bleeding.) The knee joint is distended with Ringer's lactate through an inflow cannula inserted laterally into the suprapatellar pouch adjacent to the superior pole of the patella. An incision is made over the anterolateral aspect of the joint. A trocar and sheath are inserted; an obturator replaces the trocar in the sheath, and the obturator is advanced into the joint. The obturator is removed and replaced by the arthroscope with the attached camera. Inflow and outflow irrigation tubings are attached. A fluid management system, e.g., Intellijet, with the capability to automatically maintain the appropriate degree of distension, is used to provide a clear field and obviate the need for inflation of the tourniquet. The knee joint is thoroughly examined. Additional port(s) can be employed accordingly.

Procedures such as menisectomy, synovectomy, patellar shaving, or replacement of the anterior cruciate ligament may be performed. Numerous devices have been developed to facilitate these procedures. Examples include a power patellar shaver and other power smoothers. Also available are introducer and vector guides to create tunnels for ligamentous repairs. Fixation can be achieved with sutures, staples, interference screws (of metal or bioabsorbable composition) with their assorted screw holders, etc. Another instrument for intra-articular use is the Caspari suture punch that facilitates suture placement.

A carbon dioxide laser may be employed with some arthroscopes, in which case the knee joint is distended with carbon dioxide and the tourniquet is inflated to prevent dissection by the gas. For procedures utilizing the Nd:YAG and Ho:YAG laser, the liquid distention medium is needed. For laser safety precautions, see p. 94. Following completion of the procedure(s), the wound is simultaneously copiously irrigated with Ringer's lactate and the solution aspirated. The scope is withdrawn; the wounds are closed in the usual manner. A soft bandage is applied in addition to a pressure stocking, e.g., **T.E.D.**®

Preparation of the Patient

An antiembolitic stocking is applied to the unaffected extremity as requested. The patient is in supine position with the affected side close to the edge of the table. Arms are extended on padded armboards. Webril (sheet wadding) and a tourniquet are applied to the thigh of the operative leg. A leg holder or lateral post is secured to the table, placed on the side of the affected leg (which permits the leg to be angled off the lateral aspect of the table). Alternatively, the lower segment of the table is fully flexed and both knees are flexed over the table edge. All bony prominences and areas vulnerable to skin and neurovascular pressure or trauma are padded. Apply an electrosurgical dispersive pad.

For **Skin Preparation** and **Draping,** see ***Arthrotomy of the Knee***, p. 600.

Equipment

Leg holder for skin prep (optional)
Leg holding post (to help maintain positioning during surgery)
Tourniquet and pneumatic insufflator with microprocessor regulator
ESU
Video monitors (2)
Camera console, e.g., digital ConMed or Apex Camera system
VCR (optional)
Printer
CD burner
Arthroscopy tower: Main control unit front panel, fluid pump, cassette, Intellijet suction supply unit (suction level control unit), adjustable IV pole with level-alert sensors (2), waste containers (4), and power systems for shavers
Laser fiber, e.g., Nd:YAG or Ho:YAG

Instrumentation

Limited access procedures tray
Arthroscopes (0°, 30°, 45°, 70° angle) from 2.5, 2.7, 2.8, 3.5, 4.0 mm with cord, sheath, bridge, camera
QuickLatch 2.9- and 4.0-mm scopes with camera head and coupler

Endoscopic

Cannulas, trocars (short, blunt), electrosurgical suction-irrigator and cord, meniscal hook blade, obturator, rasp, synovial elevator, sharp and dull probes, grasping forceps, nerve hooks, acromionizer, Beaver (endo) blade handle, knife, and hook knife, pituitary forceps, osteotomes, guide, ligament passer
High-speed power drill, cord, drill bits and burrs, chuck, and key
Patellar shaver handle and motor (smoothing device)

For Patella Tendon Repair, Add

Osteotomes, saw with small blade (e.g., Dyonics), rongeurs, bone cutters, drill bits, bone button

For Anterior Cruciate Ligament, Add

Vector guide, guide pins, automatic drill, reamer, 6.5- and 10.0-mm drill bits, fastlok staple and buckle system (2 for allografts), staple inserter and remover, and tension device for allografts
Cottony dacron suture with needle for allografts and autografts

Supplies

Antiembolitic stocking (unaffected leg), optional
Tube stockinettes (2)

Esmarch bandage
Marking pen
Basin set
Blade, (1) #15
Needle, 18-gauge spinal
Disposable tubing and cassette (attached to main control unit)
Disposable operative cannula and tubing set
Ringer's lactate in 3000-ml bags (2 to 6 extra on hand)
Graft (allograft, frozen) and antibacterial solution (to soak the graft), type of solution is optional
Culture tube (anaerobic)
Fastlok staples for anterior cruciate ligament (ACL), optional
Skin closure strips, optional
Soft dressing (e.g., 4 × 4s, ABD pads, and TED stockings)
Leg brace for ACL repair
TEMPPAD, optional (cold application over the dressing)

Special Notes

- Apply **Special Notes**, as applicable, from ***Arthroscopy of the Shoulder***, p. 567.
- Position the monitors after everyone scrubbed is in position at the table (to avoid tripping over cords).

Suggested progression:

- The circulator turns (Intellijet) control unit on and gives tubing to scrub person.
  - The scrub person removes the cassette and waste and fluid bag tubing and passes it to the circulator.
  - The circulator attaches a cassette to the side of the unit, closes the pinch clamps on the tubing using fluid bag tubing spikes, connects the waste tubing to the waste containers, and turns the suction supply switch on.
  - The scrub person attaches arthroscope cannula and powered instruments to appropriate cords.
  - The circulator then selects pressure range using site-selection key and pushes pump to start. The key on the control unit displays "pump running."
  - Assorted abraders and shavers, endoblades, and acromionizers must be sterilized and readily available.
- **N.B.** Instruments may be washed and then flash sterilized; some brands of telescopes and cameras may be flash sterilized. DO NOT FLASH STERILIZE any telescopes unless there are direc-

tions from the manufacturer to do so. Check manufacturer's specifications. Steris™ 20 solution is recommended for those instruments requiring sterilization by soaking; see p. 43.

- Grafts (of ligaments) are thawed in sterile, warm normal saline; afterward they are soaked in an antibiotic solution before they are used.
- All medications, dyes, etc. on the operating field must be labeled. Scrub person should use a marking pen on labels to identify all solutions. All medication containers should be kept in the room until the completion of the procedure. Follow all safety precautions to avoid medication errors; see p. 30.
- The circulator is responsible for replacing empty irrigation bags. Irrigation solution replacement bags must be immediately ready at all times; the next bag should be "held in waiting."
- The scrub person must monitor the temperature of the irrigation solution as it leaves the outflow tubing before the solution reaches the patient.

Excision of Popliteal (Baker's) Cyst

Definition

Excision of a synovial or bursal cyst from the popliteal space.

Discussion

Baker's cysts are formed by the herniation of synovial membrane or the escape of synovial fluid from the knee joint with the accumulation of the fluid in one of several bursae in the popliteal space. The cysts also occur in rheumatoid arthritis. Other conditions affecting the knee may be associated (e.g., torn meniscus). Arthrography or arthroscopy may be used to delineate the cyst and to distinguish it from other lesions, such as tumors and popliteal artery aneurysm.

Procedure

Excision of Popliteal (Baker's) Cyst is described. An oblique incision is made over the mass at the posterior knee. Deep fascia is incised, exposing the sac that is then dissected free, tracing its attachment to the posterior aspect of the knee joint capsule. The pedicle is ligated and the cyst excised. Tendon bundles may be used to reinforce the closure. The wound is closed. A splint is applied.

Preparation of the Patient

Antiembolitic stocking is placed on the unaffected extremity. General anesthesia administered via endotracheal intubation or regional block is employed. At the discretion of the anesthesia provider and the supervision of the surgeon and the surgeon's assistant protecting the affected leg, the patient is turned to the prone position. Chest rolls are placed at the patient's sides to facilitate chest expansion, and a roll placed in front of the ankles to protect the toes. The arms are positioned on padded armboards angled toward the head of the table with the forearms pronated. A tourniquet is applied high on the thigh of the affected leg. A safety strap is secured over the blanket covering the unaffected thigh. An electrosurgical dispersive pad is placed.

Skin Preparation

A leg holder may be used. Begin at the back of the knee; extend the prep from the top of the thigh (to the tourniquet, if used) to the ankle.

Draping

The leg is abducted and elevated as the foot is grasped and covered by a double tube stockinette. A large sheet is draped over the end of the table. The outer stockinette is brought up (rolled) over the knee. A folded towel (thirds, lengthwise) is wrapped around the top of the stockinette and fastened. A split sheet is draped under the thigh and fastened. A split sheet is draped cephalad over the thigh and fastened, or a drape with a rubberized extremity aperture is employed. The extremity is passed through a fenestrated sheet (e.g., transverse or laparotomy), or individual drape sheets complete the draping.

Equipment

Chest rolls, ankle roll, pillows, padding (as necessary for positioning)
Leg holder for skin prep, optional
ESU
Tourniquet and pneumatic insufflator with microprocessor regulator (available)
Cast cart

Instrumentation

Vascular shunt tray
Knee arthrotomy tray (available)

Supplies

Antiembolitic stocking, as requested
Tube stockinettes (2)
Esmarch bandage
Basin set
Suction tubing (2), e.g., inflow-outflow
Blades, (2) #10 and (1) #15
Electrosurgical pencil and cord with holder and scraper

Needle magnet or counter
Bulb syringe and antibiotic irrigation, optional
Supplies for splint application (cast cart)

Special Notes

- Apply **Special Notes** from ***Abdominal Laparotomy***, p. 134, as indicated.
- In the adult patient, a popliteal cyst may be indicative of intra-articular disease; arthrotomy may be necessary.
- **N.B.** Circulator should obtain adequate assistance and supplies when the patient is turned to prone position.
- **Reminder:** *Have adequate padding readily available to pad the area around female breasts and male genitalia when positioning the patient.*

Arthroplasty of the Knee Joint with Unicompartmental or Total Knee Prosthetic Replacement

Definition

Prosthetic replacement of diseased articular surfaces of the femur, tibia, and/or patella.

Discussion

Bone deformity and joint instability are secondary to degenerative rheumatoid arthritis, osteoarthritis, and/or the consequence of post-traumatic events. The pain caused by these diseases can be so severe that it is disabling. When nonsurgical measures have proven unsatisfactory in relieving the pain, **total knee arthroplasty with joint replacement** surgery is recommended. The surgical procedure has given many disabled by severe pain a new lease on life. Articular surfaces of the femoral condyles, tibial plateau, anterior trochlear surface of the femur, and posterior surface of the patella can be replaced by prosthesis, as necessary. When the prosthesis, composed of cobalt/chromium or titanium alloy, polyethelene, and/or other polymeric materials, is fixed, it is ***"cemented"*** with PMMA. Alternatively, a ***"cementless"*** prosthesis may have a coated or textured surface, or it may require "press-fit" without cement, with the placement of screws or pegs for stability optional. Additionally, when a ***"hybrid"*** technique is employed, a ***"cementless"*** femoral component is used with a ***"cemented"*** tibial component. The longevity and performance of the implant depends on the patient's activity level and age, weight, and general health.

Use of PMMA cement is decided on a per-patient basis; generally, younger patients or patients who are very physically active do not receive ***"cemented"*** prostheses, as the "cemented" prostheses often loosen in these patients.

There are a large number prosthetic brands and designs available. Most systems provide a metallic surface (femoral) to articulate with a plastic surface (tibial and patellar). The surgeon chooses the appropriately engineered prosthesis according to the specific needs of the patient. He/she evaluates the amount of arthritic bone loss, the integrity of the remaining bone, and whether the quality of the ligaments will be sufficient to support the knee. Other factors include: the surgeon's experience, the total cost of the procedure, and the performance record of the specific prosthesis.

On occasion, a single component of the knee's articular surface (e.g., medial femoral and tibial condyles) requires replacement ***(unicompartmental)***. More commonly, the entire or total surface, i.e., medial and lateral condyles and patellofemoral tract, require replacement ***(tricompartmental)***.

Prostheses are categorized accordingly:

1. Constrained (hinged)
2. Nonhinged constrained (spherocentric)
3. Nonconstrained
4. Partially constrained

Partially constrained prostheses are used most often because they provide stability to the knee joint while allowing some degree of rotational motion. Whether the knee ligaments are retained is determined according to preoperative MRI findings and other studies. The results of the studies and the operative findings are important in determining prosthesis selection. At surgery, contracted ligaments can be released or excised; loose ligaments can be shortened to achieve "balancing." The femoral and tibial components must be aligned to articulate properly, maintain joint space and extremity length, and avoid rotational and varus or valgus deviations.

Intraoperative computer-based imaging has been introduced to simplify the various measurements taken to assure proper fitting of the prosthetic components. An example is the Stryker Knee Navigation System that employs three infrared emitters intraoperatively, screwed into the superior iliac spine, femur, and tibia in conjunction with a computed tomography scanner to eliminate the need for jigs to properly place the prostheses.

In increasing use is the minimally invasive technique that employs shorter incisions with the usual benefit to the patient postoperatively, with respect to less pain and faster rehabilitation. This technique is more demanding in that the entire joint cannot be visualized without revising the operative field; e.g., the excision of the femoral and tibial condyles are done in stepwise fashion rather than as single cuts.

Replacement of the prosthesis may not be necessary in patients (over age 40) who modify their activity levels; when necessary, replacement is 15 to 20 years after prosthesis insertion. Active patients unwilling to limit their activity and younger patients require replacement sooner. Difficulties encountered with the "cemented" fixation, such as loosening of the prosthesis from the bone (due to movement and weight bearing) and inflammation (local response to loose microscopic debris particles into surrounding tissues), result from wear and tear. When the weight load applied to the knees during walking is uneven, the prosthesis may "lift off" the bone. When carried loads are heavier than the bone can bear, the cemented prosthesis sinks or loosens, as cancellous bone into which the prosthesis is implanted is not as hard as the original cortical bone. Newer "cementless" versions have not obviated the problems of the cemented version. The time required for stabilization (dependent on new bone growth formation into the prosthesis) of the "cementless" version is much longer than the cemented version. Instability between bone and the "cementless" prosthesis causes microscopic particulate debris formation (similar to "cemented" version) that results in inflammation. Studies regarding these factors are ongoing.

Despite any difficulties, knee replacement surgery has proven very successful in relieving pain and restoring joint movement to countless numbers once disabled by advanced degenerative joint disease.

Note: Until recently, **bone joint replacement surgery** was always performed (whenever possible) in an OR equipped with laminar airflow; some orthopedic surgeons still prefer to operate in the OR with laminar airflow.

Procedure

Arthroplasty of the Knee Joint with Unicompartmental or Total Knee Prosthetic Replacement is described. The incisions may be medial parapatellar, quadriceps splitting, or subvastus (medialis). Less often, a lateral approach is employed. A longitudinal incision extends from over the patella to the tibial tuberosity. The quadriceps tendon is incised superiorly, the capsule is incised, the knee is flexed, and the knee joint exposed. The menisci, any osteophytes, and hyperplastic synovium are excised. Soft-tissue scarring (if any) is released, and the patellar fat pad may be excised. The ligaments are excised, preserved, lengthened, or shortened on an individual basis. Jigs, guides, templates, and spacers of varying sizes for each prosthetic type are employed. Lines may be marked with methylene blue dye, or a pen with indelible ink is used to indicate appropriate amounts of bone to be excised, usually employing system specific jigs and an oscillating saw. Slots or holes are cut or drilled to accept the prostheses. Loose fragments and debris may be pulse lavaged or irrigated with saline or an antibiotic solution. When the cemented technique is employed, PMMA cement is used to seat the prosthesis; excess cement is removed. The posterior surface of the patella, if irregular, is shaved; a polyethylene "button" or disc prosthesis is affixed with pegs or screws to restore the anatomical thickness. A check is made of stability, alignment, and range of motion. Realignment of the quadriceps mechanism and patella tendon is carefully performed. Hemostasis is achieved after the tourniquet is released. Quixil™, a fibrin sealant, may be sprayed on hemorrhagic surfaces prior to wound closure. X-rays may be requested to confirm and document the arthroplasty. Suction drains may be placed in the joint, and the wound layers are closed. A bulky dressing is applied. The extremity may be placed in a continuous passive motion (CPM) device when the patient reaches the post-anesthesia care unit (PACU) or several days postoperatively. (The CPM device may be used for other postoperative conditions of the knee, hip, shoulder, and elbow, as well.)

Preparation of the Patient

An antiembolitic stocking may be applied to the unaffected extremity when requested. The patient is supine, positioned with the knees over the lower break in the table. Arms may be extended on padded armboards placed alongside the patient or tucked in at the patient's sides. The patient's lap is covered with a blanket; a safety strap is secured over the thigh of the unaffected extremity. Care is taken to ensure that the correctly identified extremity on the correctly identified patient is prepped. Sheet wadding and a tourniquet are applied high on the thigh of the affected extremity. A tourniquet is *omitted* when the patient has a history of deep vein thrombosis or other vascular problems. Electrosurgical dispersive pad is applied.

Skin Preparation

A leg holder may be used. Begin at the knee; extend the prep from immediately below the tourniquet (on the thigh) to the ankles.

Draping

The extremity is elevated and abducted; the foot is grasped in a double tube stockinette. A large sheet is draped over the end of the table. A split sheet is draped under the thigh. The outer tube stockinette is brought up (unrolled) to the top of the thigh. A folded towel (thirds, lengthwise) is wrapped around the top of the tube stockinette and secured. A split sheet is draped cephalad, over the top of the thigh, and fastened underneath. An extremity sheet with a rubberized fenestration, a transverse or laparotomy sheet, or individual drape sheets complete the draping.

An additional drape sheet will be needed when the dropped end of the table is returned to standard position.

Equipment

Laminar airflow (optional)
Foot holder for skin prep, optional
Suction
ESU
Tourniquet and pneumatic insufflator with microprocessor regulator
Power sources for drill and saw

Instrumentation

Basic orthopedic procedures tray
Knee arthrotomy tray (available)
Fixation devices and insertion instrumentation, as necessary
High-speed power drill and cord (or self-contained), chuck, drill bits, and key
Osteotomes, gouges, automatic screwdriver, optional
Trial prostheses, total knee prosthesis, and necessary instrumentation, per surgeon's choice
Power oscillating saw and cord (or self-contained) with jigs and templates
Pulsed-lavage suction irrigator and tip, e.g., Impulse, Simpulse, MicroAire, optional

Supplies

Antiembolitic stocking
Tube stockinettes (2)
Esmarch bandage
Blades, (3) #10 and (1) #15
Basin set
Marking pen with indelible ink (optional)
Needle magnet or counter
Electrosurgical pencil and cord with holder and scraper
Quixil fibrin sealant, optional
Suction tubing or cojoined suction and irrigation tubing for pulsed lavage

Irrigation solution in bags (for pulsed lavage), or graduated pitcher, bulb syringes (2), and antibiotic solution
PMMA cement kit
Closed drainage system (e.g., Hemovac), optional
Bulky dressing

Special Notes

- Apply **Special Notes** from ***Total Hip Arthroplasty with Prosthetic Replacement of the Hip Joint***, p. 593, as indicated.
- **Reminder:** Record the date, type of prostheses, serial number, and size of implant on the **Perioperative Record** of the patient's surgery. Follow hospital policy for recording insertion of a prosthesis in the hospital log.
- **N.B.** *A knee immobilizer and a CPM device may be used following surgery.* This is usually applied in the PACU; however, the circulator should consult the surgeon regarding ordering the immobilizer once the surgery has begun.

Open Reduction and Internal Fixation of Fractures of the Tibial Shaft

Definition

Realignment and fixation of a tibial shaft fracture.

Discussion

The type of fixation device is determined by the anatomic considerations of the fracture (e.g., comminuted, spiral, or "open"). Severely comminuted fractures may have to be treated with prolonged traction rather than fixation.

Procedure

Open Reduction and Internal Fixation of Fractures of the Tibial Shaft is described. The fracture is exposed. Transverse bone screws or plates (including compression plates) may be applied to reduce fracture fragments. In addition, after the fragments have been reduced, an intramedullary nail or rod may be employed (e.g., Ender nail or Rush rod) to fix a fractured tibia and provide improved rotational stability. An Ender nail is slightly curved and semi-elastic. An incision about the tibial tuberosity is made. A drill reamer penetrates the medullary canal. The measured nail is inserted and aligned to avoid malrotation or shattering the shaft of the tibia. Loose fragments and debris may be pulse lavaged or irrigated with saline or an antibiotic solution. The Ender nail is then driven past the fracture site into the distal portion until the threaded end remains exposed (for later extraction). A counter incision over the fracture site may be needed to effect reduction. Again, care is taken during the driving of the nail to avoid injury to the shaft. Use of multiple Ender nails can improve rotational stability; fanning of the proximal end helps control rotation. Small bones or fractures at the insertion site may complicate use of Ender nails. X-rays are taken to visualize and document the repair. Hemostasis is assured before the wound is closed.

Preparation of the Patient

An antiembolitic stocking may be placed on the unaffected extremity, as requested. General anesthesia or regional block anesthetic may be employed. The patient is supine; arms may be extended on padded armboards. The safety strap is secured over the blanket-covered unaffected extremity. Sheet wadding and a tourniquet are placed high on the thigh of the operative leg. An electrosurgical dispersive pad is applied.

Skin Preparation

Care is taken to support the extremity to avoid further injury. Begin at the fracture site; prep the entire extremity. Include the leg, thigh (up to the tourniquet), and foot.

Draping

The supported leg is abducted and elevated; the foot is grasped and covered by a tube stockinette. A large sheet is draped over the end of the table. The stockinette is brought up (unrolled) to the level of the tourniquet. A folded towel (thirds, lengthwise) is wrapped around the top of the stockinette and secured. A split sheet is draped under the leg, or the leg may be passed through a sheet with a rubberized fenestration. A large drape (or split) sheet is draped cephalad, over the thigh, and secured underneath. The leg is passed through a fenestrated sheet (e.g., transverse or laparotomy), or additional drape sheets complete the draping.

Equipment

- Suction
- ESU
- Tourniquet and insufflator (tank of compressed air) with microprocessor regulator
- Power sources for drill and saw (unless power equipment is self-contained)

Instrumentation

- Basic orthopedic procedures tray
- Bone-holding instruments tray

Fixation device and insertion instrumentation
High-speed power drill, cord, chuck, key, and drill bits
Pulsed lavage suction irrigator and tip, e.g., Impulse, Simpulse, MicroAire (optional)

Supplies

Antiembolitic stocking, optional
Webril
Tube stockinette
Esmarch bandage
Blades, (2) #10
Electrosurgical pencil and cord with holder and scraper
Basin set
Needle magnet or counter
Suction tubing (2) or cojoined suction and irrigation tubing for pulsed lavage
Irrigation solution in bags (for pulsed lavage), or graduated pitcher, bulb syringes (2), antibiotic solution

Special Notes

- Apply **Special Notes** from ***Open Reduction and Internal Fixation of Fractures of the Hip,*** p. 584, as indicated.

Open Reduction and Internal Fixation of Fractures of the Ankle

Definition

Realignment and fixation of ankle fractures.

Discussion

Open reduction and internal fixation of ankle fractures may involve the medial malleolus (tibia), lateral malleolus (fibula), and/or posterior malleolus (posterior aspect of distal tibia). Many anatomic variations of ankle fractures and dislocations may occur. The procedure is performed to correct acute fractures or nonunion of fractures.

Procedure

Fracture of the lateral malleolus is discussed. An anterolateral incision is made over the fracture site. The sural nerve is avoided. The malleolus is exposed. The fracture is fixed with screws that engage bone from the opposite cortex. Care is taken not to compromise the tendon sheaths or other soft tissues. X-rays are taken to visualize and document the repair. After the incision is closed, a short leg cast is applied.

In addition to the standard screws, a radiolucent polycarbonate absorbable screw may be used; it obviates the need to remove the screw as is necessary, on occasion, with metallic screws.

Preparation of the Patient

Antiembolitic stocking is placed on the unaffected leg. General or regional block anesthesia is employed. The patient is supine; arms may be extended on padded armboards, and the safety belt is secured over the unaffected extremity. Webril and a tourniquet are applied to the thigh of the operative leg. An electrosurgical dispersive pad is placed.

Skin Preparation

The extremity is supported. Begin at the ankle; prep from the tips of the toes to include the knee.

Draping

The extremity is abducted and elevated as the foot is grasped and covered by a tube stockinette. A large sheet is draped over the end of the table. The tube stockinette is brought up to the top of the thigh. A folded towel (thirds, lengthwise) is wrapped around the top of the tube stockinette and fastened. A split sheet is draped under the thigh and fastened above. A split sheet is draped over the thigh proximally and fastened underneath. The extremity is passed through a fenestrated sheet (transverse or laparotomy), or additional drape sheets cover the field.

Equipment

Leg holder (optional)
Suction (available)
ESU
Tourniquet and insufflator (tank of compressed air) with microprocessor regulator
Power source for drill
Cast cart

Instrumentation

Basic orthopedic procedures tray
Power drill and cord (or self-contained), drill bits, chuck, and key
Kirschner wires and Steinmann pins
Selected screws

Supplies

Antiembolitic stocking (unaffected extremity, as requested)
Webril
Tube stockinette
Esmarch bandage
Basin set

Blades, (2) #10 and (1) #15
Needle magnet or counter
Suction tubing (optional)
Graduated pitcher, bulb syringe, and antibiotic irrigation, optional
Electrosurgical pencil and cord with holder and scraper
Casting supplies for short leg cast

Special Notes

- Apply **Special Notes** from ***Open Reduction and Internal Fixation of Fractures of the Hip***, p. 584.

Arthroscopy of the Ankle and Foot

Definition

Endoscopic visualization of the joints of the ankle and foot.

Discussion

Arthroscopy is indicated when other diagnostic modalities such as arthrography or MRI scan have not revealed the etiology of various painful ankle and foot problems, such as swelling, instability, or "locking." Ankle arthroscopy is employed for treatment of injuries to cartilage and soft tissue, excision of loose bodies, synovitis, and osteophytes, smoothing of osteochondral defects, and excision of arthrofibrosis. Triple arthrodesis (fusion of the bones) of the ankle can be performed; however, as this procedure limits flexibility, it is usually performed on older patient or a patient who has limited physical activity expectations. See Triple arthrodesis of the ankle, p. 619.

Contraindications to ankle arthroscopy include soft tissue (but not intra-articular) infection and severe degenerative joint disease.

Procedure

According to the pathology, three anterior ports (anterolateral, anterocentral, and anteromedial) and three posterior ports (posterolateral, transachilles tendon, and posterior medial) are placed. Care is taken to avoid neurotendenous structures. Transmalleolar ports may be employed for drilling osteochondrial lesions of the talus. An external (noninvasive) sterile support strap is applied. When the ankle joint is tight, invasive pins (e.g., Steinman) may be placed in the distal tibia and calcaneus or talus, penetrating only the lateral cortex of the bone. Care is taken to avoid injury to underlying structures by applying limited distraction, i.e., greater than 7 to 8 mm is avoided. Lactated Ringer's solution (10 ml) is infused through an 18-gauge spinal needle to establish the anteromedial port. A skin incision is made, and a clamp is inserted into the joint capsule to spread the soft tissue. A cannula is carefully inserted into the joint and more fluid is infused, as necessary. Under arthroscopic visualization, additional ports are established; enough fluid must be infused to maintain adequate distention. The joint is thoroughly examined in systematic fashion. Definitive procedures may be performed, e.g., loose body removal, debridement, synovectomy, shaving of osteochondral lesions, insertion of pins, or placement of fixation devices. A splint may be applied.

Preparation of the Patient

The patient is in the supine position with the arms extended on padded armboards, or either or both arms may be tucked in at the patient's side. The safety belt is secured over the unaffected extremity. A nonsterile thigh holder may be used to flex the affected hip 45° to 50°, supporting the extremity from the proximal thigh to the popliteal fossa. Foam padding is used with the thigh holder to avoid injury to the sciatic nerve. A sterile foot holder may be used to support the foot and ankle in the desired position during invasive distraction. A sterile strap used with noninvasive ankle distraction may be adequate. Pad all bony prominences and areas vulnerable to skin and neurovascular pressure or trauma. A tourniquet and Webril (sheet wadding) are applied to the proximal thigh. Apply an electrosurgical dispersive pad.

For **Skin Preparation and Draping,** see **Open Reduction of the Ankle,** p. 616.

Equipment

Tourniquet and pneumatic insufflator with microprocessor regulator
Sterile foot holder, optional
Sterile distraction device(s), optional
Thigh holder (nonsterile), optional
Foam padding
Suction (available)
ESU
Video monitor(s)
Arthroscopy tower with power pump
Camera console
Fiber-optic light source, e.g., Xenon 300 W
Power source for drill (unless self-contained, e.g., Stryker)
Cast cart

Instrumentation

Limited-access procedures tray
Hand and foot tray, available
Arthroscopes (e.g., 0°, 30°, 45°, and/or 70° angle) from 2.5, 2.7, and 2.8 mm with cord, sheath, bridge, camera
QuickLatch 2.9-mm scope, camera head, and coupler are **autoclavable**

Endoscopic

Cannulas, trocars (short, blunt) and obturators, electrosurgical suction-irrigator and cord, rasp, synovial elevator, sharp and dull probes, grasping forceps, nerve hooks, acromionizer, Beaver (endo) blade handle, knife, and hook knife, pituitary forceps, osteotomes, guide, ligament passer

High-speed power drill, cord, drill bits and burrs, chuck, and key

Steinman pins (optional)

Supplies

Antiembolitic stocking (unaffected extremity), optional

Webril

Basin set

Blades, (1) #11 and (1) #15

18-gauge spinal needle and syringe, 10 to 20 ml

Electrosurgical pencil and cord with holder and scraper

Suction tubing

Irrigation bags (3000 ml normal saline), K50 polyethylene (cystoscopy) tubing, and three-way stopcock

Antibiotic may be added to the irrigation, or graduated pitcher or small basin, bulb syringe, and antibiotic irrigation, optional

Special Notes

- Apply **Special Notes** from **Arthroscopy of the Knee**, p. 605, as applicable.
- Reminder: Some arthroscopes are autoclavable. Strict observance of manufacturer's recommendations for sterilization must be followed.

Triple Arthrodesis of the Ankle

Definition

Fusion of the bones of the ankle.

Discussion

Triple arthrodesis of the ankle is performed on the talocalcaneal (subtalar), talonavicular, and calcaneocuboid bone articulations. The bones of the ankle are fused together to relieve pain, provide stability, and arrest joint-destroying disease processes. Multiple combinations of ankle joint arthrodeses and techniques may be employed. They are classified accordingly as intraarticular, extra-articular, or a combination of the two. Repair is performed by placing two cannulated screws for each fusion.

The arthroscopic approach is employed in selected cases.

Procedure

An incision is made from the dorsal prominence of the lateral aspect of the foot to the midportion of the calcaneus. Tendons are retracted, exposing the floor of the sinus tarsi. The periosteum of the calcaneus is exposed, and the calcaneocuboid joint capsule is incised. The articular surfaces are excised; the bone fragments are saved. The talonavicular joint capsule is incised, and the head of the talus is excised. The proximal articular surface of the navicular is removed. The subtalar joint is incised, and the articular surface is removed with that of the sustenaculum tali and anterior facet of the talus. Bony surfaces are trimmed to correct deformity and to provide for maximum contact. An accessory medial incision may be required. Bone chips may be packed into the defect. Soft tissues are sutured to fill the sinus tarsi, obliterating dead space. Kirschner wires, pins, screws, and staples may be used to maintain alignment. X-rays are taken to visualize and document the arthrodesis. A long leg cast is carefully applied, molding the foot to correct shape and aligning the malleoli. Ten to 14 days postoperatively, remanipulation of the foot under anesthesia may be necessary.

For **Preparation of the Patient, Skin Preparation, Draping, Equipment,** and **Supplies,** see ***Open Reduction and Internal Fixation of Fractures of the Ankle,*** p. 616.

Instrumentation

Basic orthopedic procedures tray
Power drill, cord, drill bits
Osteotomes, curettes, gouges
Steinmann pins, Kirschner wires
Fixation device and instrumentation (e.g., screws, staples)
Vertebral spreader (small)
Pulsed lavage suction irrigator and tip, e.g., Simpulse, MicroAire (optional)

Special Notes

Apply **Special Notes** from ***Open Reduction and Internal Fixation of Fractures of the Hip***, p. 584.

Total Ankle Arthroplasty with Prosthetic Joint Replacement

Definition

Prosthetic substitution of the articular surfaces of the distal tibia and the talus.

Discussion

In general, younger, more active patients will have better ankle function with fusion; see ***Arthrodesis of the Ankle***, p. 619. Total ankle arthroplasty is performed when there is pain and instability due to post-traumatic (including postsurgical), degenerative, and rheumatoid arthritic changes. Elderly, less-active patients are usually better candidates for joint replacement. The prostheses are composed of high-density polyethylene and metal components, fixed with PMMA cement, and classified as constrained (restricted motion), semiconstrained (semirestricted motion), or nonconstrained (unrestricted motion). The long-term results of this procedure are not as durable as hip or knee total arthroplasty. Prostheses include Agility™ Total Ankle System (Dupuy), two components; STAR (Scandinavian Total Ankle Replacement); Buechel-Pappas, three components; TNK Ankle (Kyocera Corp.), two components.

Procedure

An anterolateral incision is made. Tendons and neurovascular structures are retracted. The tibiotalar joint and dome of the talus are exposed. Using special templates, osteotomy incisions for the tibia and talus are outlined and made with an oscillating saw. Care is taken to avoid injury to posteromedial neurovascular bundle and the anterior talofibular ligament. A template is used to cut a section of tibia to accept the stem of the prosthesis. Holes are made in the talus with a curette to provide fixation points for the cement. Trial insertion of the prosthesis is made, and range of motion is determined. The metallic tibial prosthesis is permanently seated after prepared PMMA cement is applied. Similarly, the polyethylene talar prosthesis is seated; excess PMMA cement is trimmed. The wound may be cleansed of debris with pulsed lavage of lactated Ringer's solution or irrigated with normal saline prior to closure; antibiotics may be added to either solution. The incision is closed over suction drains. A splint is applied over a bulky dressing.

For **Preparation of the Patient, Skin Preparation,** and **Draping,** see ***Open Reduction Internal Fixation of Fractures of the Ankle,*** p. 616.

Equipment

Laminar airflow, optional
Suction
ESU
Tourniquet and pneumatic insufflator with microprocessor regulator
Cast cart
Power source for power drill (optional, depends on type of drill)

Instrumentation

Basic orthopedic procedures tray
Osteotomes, curettes
High-speed drill with power burr set (available)
Power oscillating saw and cord (or self-contained) with jigs, templates
Trial prostheses, total ankle prostheses, and specific instrumentation
Pulsed lavage suction irrigator and tip, e.g., Simpulse, MicroAire (optional)

Supplies

Basin set
Tube (or impervious) stockinette
Esmarch bandage
Needle magnet or counter
Blades, (2) #10 and (1) #15
Electrosurgical pencil and cord with holder and scraper
Suction tubing (2) or cojoined suction and irrigation tubing for pulsed lavage (available)
Irrigation solution (lactated Ringer's solution) in 3000-ml bags for pulsed lavage (optional), or graduated pitcher, bulb syringe, antibiotic irrigation (optional)
Antibiotic (optional)
PMMA cement kit
Closed drainage system (e.g., Hemovac)

Special Notes

- Apply **Special Notes** from ***Arthroplasty of the Knee***, p. 613, as indicated.

Repair of Tendo Calcaneus (Achilles Tendon)

Definition

Surgical correction of a disruption of the Achilles tendon.

Discussion

An Achilles tendon injury with complete disruption can occur due to direct trauma (as laceration) or severe forceful stress (jumping from height), but it most often results from multiple lesser stresses over a period of time that do not heal optimally (possibly due to relatively poor blood supply to the distal part of the tendon) and then abrupt mechanical overload with dorsiflexion of the ankle and extension of the knee, which causes the weakened tendon to rupture. Casting with the ankle flexed (equines position) is effective in some cases, but surgical repair gives better results. Complications include infection and the general risks that accompany most surgeries.

Procedure

Numerous techniques for repair have been described. Several common variations will be included.

The patient is placed in the prone position. A pneumatic tourniquet is applied. A 10- to 15-cm posteromedial longitudinal (or S-shaped) incision is made, distally ending above the shoe line. The sural nerve is protected; the tendon sheath is left attached to the subcutaneous tissues (in order to minimize vascular supply injury). The site of the disruption is identified, and heavy (e.g., #1) nonabsorbable encircling tension-relieving suture is placed above and below the separation. The site of injury is repaired with absorbable suture. If elected, employing a tendon stripper, the plantaris tendon is harvested and splayed out and used as "cover" and reinforcement of the repair. Strips of gastrocnemius tendon (1 × 8 cm) may be folded down (leaving the distal attachment) and anchored to the distal segment of the ruptured tendon or to the calcaneus directly. Another modification includes the division of the insertion of the peroneus brevis tendon from the fifth metatarsal. The distal portion of the tendon is used as a loop; it is passed through the stump of the disrupted calcaneal tendon or through a drill hole made transversely in the calcaneus. After hemostasis is achieved, the incision is closed. A short leg cast with the ankle flexed is applied.

A percutaneous technique that may reduce potential wound problems is performed through four small incisions medial and lateral to the tendon above and below the injury site. Repair suture is placed through the tendon, criss-crossed (using double-armed technique), approximating the proximal and distal portions with the suture knot buried within the depths of one incision. A cast is applied as above.

For delayed repair, scar tissue may need to be excised to mobilize the gastrocnemius tendon. A strip from the gastrocnemius tendon is used to reinforce the repair (similar to that described above). To obtain appropriate length of the gastrocnemius tendon, if contraction has occurred since the injury, V-Y advancement of the proximal tendon is performed. A technique using the flexor hallucis longus has been described using its distal tendon as a loop for the repair. To see V-Y repair, see ***scar revision***, p. 690. A cast is applied.

For **Preparation of the Patient, Skin Preparation, Equipment,** and **Supplies,** see ***Open Reduction and Internal Fixation of Fractures of the Ankle***, p. 616.

Instrumentation

Add:

Pulsed lavage suction irrigator and tip, e.g., Simpulse, MicroAire (optional)

Supplies

Add:

Sutures of choice

Special Notes

Apply **Special Notes** from ***Arthroplasty of the Knee***, p. 613, as indicated.

Bunionectomy

Definition

Excision of soft tissue and/or bony mass on the medial aspect of the first metatarsal head.

Discussion

Correction may be achieved by a variety of procedures. Excision of exostosis, realignment of the great toe, or transfer of tendons and/or osteotomy of the first metatarsal shaft may be performed. In minimal-access procedures, excision of the exostosis is eliminated; abrasion with burrs or laser ablation is performed to reduce the exostosis. The most frequently performed bunionectomy procedures are the Keller and the Chevron; others include the McBride and Silvers.

Procedure

Keller Procedure. A curved incision is made dorsally along the medial aspect of the first metatarsophalangeal joint. Care is taken to preserve the cutaneous nerves. The capsule and periosteum at the base of the proximal phalanx are incised and retracted. The metatarsal head is dislocated. The proximal half of the phalanyx is resected. The exostosis and osteophytes are excised. The sesamoids are excised if they are enlarged, deformed, or arthritic. A Kirschner wire is inserted, aligning the toe and the metatarsal head. (The resected joint surfaces may be replaced by Silastic prostheses.) A figure-of-eight suture is placed in the capsule, and periosteum is used to cover the end of the phalanx. The wound is closed. A bulky dressing is usually placed; if fixation pins are used, a splint is applied.

Chevron Procedure. Osteotomy of the first metatarsal shaft is performed; fixation is achieved by placing divergent absorbable pins. In other modifications, the several local tendons (adductor, abductor, and extensors of the great toe) are shortened or relocated to improve alignment and function.

Preparation of the Patient

Antiembolitic stocking is placed on the unaffected extremity, as requested. The patient is supine; arms may be extended on padded armboards. A pillow may be placed under the lumbar spine and/or under the knees to avoid straining back muscles and for comfort. The safety belt is secured with the safety strap placed over the blanket covering the unaffected extremity. Pad all bony prominences and areas vulnerable to skin and neurovascular trauma or pressure. Webril and a tourniquet are applied high on the thigh of the operative leg. Apply electrosurgical dispersive pad.

Skin Preparation

A leg holder may be used. Begin with the great toe; prep the extremity from the tips of the toes to the knee. Include interdigital spaces.

Draping

The leg is elevated and abducted. The foot is grasped with a tube stockinette and covered with it. A large sheet is draped over the end of the table. A split sheet is draped under the leg and fastened above, or an extremity drape with a rubberized fenestration is used. If a drape with a trough for collection of irrigation solution is available, it is used. The tube stockinette is brought over the knee. A folded towel (in thirds, lengthwise) is wrapped around the top of the stockinette and fastened. Proximally, a split sheet is draped over the thigh and fastened underneath. The extremity is passed through a fenestrated sheet (e.g., laparotomy or transverse sheet), or additional drape sheets cover the field.

Equipment

Leg holder (optional)
ESU
Tourniquet and pneumatic insufflator with microprocessor regulator
Power sources for drill and saw
Cast cart

Instrumentation

Minor orthopedic procedures tray
Osteotomes, straight, in rack (small size)
Kirschner wires
Small power drill with cord (or self-contained), chuck, key, and drill bits

Supplies

Antiembolitic stocking (unaffected extremity), as requested
Basin set
Webril (sheet wadding)
Tube stockinette
Esmarch bandage
Blades, (2) #10 and (1) #15
Needle magnet or counter
Graduated pitcher, bulb syringe, and antibiotic solution (optional)
Electrosurgical pencil and cord with holder and scraper
Bulky dressing or splint supplies

Special Notes

- Apply **Special Notes** from ***Abdominal Laparotomy***, p. 134, as they apply (e.g., to all patients in surgery regarding correct identification of the patient, observing *"time out,"* employing comfort measures that make a difference, etc.); see p. 5. All nursing care interventions and outcomes are documented.
- **Reminder:** Be certain that x-rays are in the room prior to the start of the procedure. Verify that the correct x-ray films in the room are for the *correctly identified* patient.
- Circulator notifies x-ray department if surgeon requires x-ray taken at the conclusion of the surgery; all x-ray safety precautions are observed, see p. 52.
- Check gauge to ascertain that there are adequate levels of pressure (gas or compressed air) in the tank when required to operate power equipment or when power equipment uses batteries, check level of battery.
- **Reminder:** Wearing a protective face shield or goggles is recommended to protect those scrubbed from splashing of irrigation and other fluids.

Correction of Hammer Toe Deformity with Interphalangeal Fusion

Definition

Resection and fixation of the proximal interphalangeal joint of a toe.

Discussion

The resection and fixation corrects the deformity and alleviates pain and symptoms associated with bunions, etc. Corns are not disturbed, as they usually resolve following the procedure.

Procedure

A longitudinal incision is made over the dorsum of the proximal interphalangeal joint. The extensor tendon is split and retracted, exposing the joint. The base of the middle phalanx and the head of the proximal phalanx are excised. The remaining parts of the proximal and middle phalanges are affixed with Kirschner wires drilled through the distal phalanx and out through the skin. A dorsal capsulotomy may be performed through a second incision to release a contracture. The wounds are closed. The wires may be capped.

For **Preparation of the Patient, Skin Preparation, Draping, Equipment, Instrumentation, Supplies,** and **Special Notes,** see *Bunionectomy*, p. 625.

Metatarsal Head Resection

Definition

Excision of the metatarsal bone head(s).

Discussion

The procedure is indicated in patients with pain related to the prominence of the metatarsal heads. It is often performed on patients with rheumatoid arthritis and dorsally dislocated toes. In selected cases, metatarsal head arthroplasty is performed with insertion of a silastic jointed prosthesis into the medullary canal of the resected distal metatarsal and proximal phalanx.

Procedure

A longitudinal incision is made in the interspace adjacent to the particular metatarsal head to be excised. The metatarsal head and neck, as well as the articular surface of the proximal phalanges, are freed of soft tissue and resected. Contracted soft tissue (including extensor tendons) is released. The end of the metatarsal is smoothed with a bone rasp. A Kirschner wire is inserted through the medullary canal of the metatarsal stump, aligning and fixing it in proper relation to the appropriate toe. The wound is closed. A bulky pressure dressing is applied. The wire is cut and capped (for safety).

Alternatively, an articulated prosthesis may be inserted to replace the metatarsalphalangeal joint.

For **Preparation of the Patient, Skin Preparation, Draping, Equipment, Instrumentation, Supplies,** and **Special Notes,** see *Bunionectomy*, p. 625.

Supplies

Add Silastic prostheses in selected cases

Procedure for Correction of Scoliosis

Definition

The reduction or relaxation of three-dimensional deformities of the spine (scoliosis) by excision and fusion of intervertebral discs and joint facets and traction maintained by the insertion of various orthopedic hardware devices.

Discussion

Procedure for Correction of Scoliosis is described. Scoliosis is a relatively common disorder, usually asymptomatic, often discovered on school screening exams or incidental x-ray study. Most often idiopathic in origin, scoliosis may be caused by congenital presentation, neuromuscular disorder, Marfan's syndrome, polio, etc. Surgical treatment of scoliosis is performed when musculoskeletal and respiratory functions become compromised, or the procedure may be performed for cosmesis. Scoliosis is frequently noted in adolescence, in significantly greater incidence in females. When bracing (with Milwaukee and thoracolumbosacral orthotic, etc.), exercise, chiropractic, electrical myoneural stimulation, etc., are ultimately ineffective, or when the curvature (deviation) is greater than 40° to 50° (measured by Cobb angle technique), surgery is indicated to prevent musculoskeletal problems, respiratory compromise, and severe cosmetic deformities. Surgical correction is most often performed on adolescents, but also on children and adults (in whom the results are less satisfactory). Total correction is not anticipated; the goals are improvement and prevention of further deformity.

The Harrington rod system has been supplanted by a large variety of specific instrumentation systems developed to treat the different aspects of deformity as they present in scoliosis. Factors guiding the surgeon's choice of instrument system are patient's skeletal age, extent and site (thoracic, thoracolumbar, and lumbar) of the deformity, respiratory compromise requiring thoracoplasty, etc., and experience of the surgeon. Strenuous physical activity is restricted for 3 to 12 months until the spinal fusion is well healed. A cast or brace is infrequently applied postoperatively.

Approaches for the surgical treatment for deformities of the vertebral column include:

1. Posterior approach
2. Open (or video-assisted thoracic surgery [VATS]) procedure employing anterior approach only
3. Open (or VATS) procedure employing anterior approach combined with the posterior approach

For the anterior approach (either open or VATS), the patient is in the lateral position first and later turned to the posterior approach, with the patient in the prone position when a combined procedure is performed. The patient is placed in the lateral position (convex side of the curvature "up"). General anesthesia via double-lumened endotracheal tube (permits unilateral lung deflation for exposure) is administered.

Some procedures or hardware systems that use the **posterior approach** include:

- **Luque** (especially for neuromuscular scoliosis) with L-shaped flexible, contoured rods placed on either side of the spine attached with sublaminar wires at each affected vertebral level. The Luque distributes the corrective forces to vertebral levels rather than to the entire length of the deformity. Osteotomies are sometimes performed in conjunction with the Luque procedure to facilitate the correction.
- The **Cotrel-Dubousset** (C-D) method, employing shorter rods attached by hooks and screws to correct rotational deformity by applying corrective forces to segmental areas of the curvature, as well as the full length of the curvature.
- **Texas Scottish Rite Hospital** (TSRH), in which modification of C-D incorporates cross plates from left to right.

Anterior approach procedures or hardware systems include:

- **Isola** method, with screw fixation into the vertebral bodies with rod insertion after disc excision and bone grafting of the interspaces.
- **The Halm-Zielke and Keneda** anterior scoliosis system (KASS) are similar, using lateral vertebral plates correcting rotational deformities.
- **Dwyer procedure,** performed to correct a thoracolumbar or lumbar deformity, stabilizes the convex curvature with a flexible cable passed through fenestrated heads of screws placed with staples driven into the affected vertebral bodies. Dwyer procedure, using an anterior approach, permits growth (of the child) to diminish the deformity; however, this procedure does not address any rotational deformity. The Dwyer procedure can be performed by anterior approach combined with a posterior approach for placement of hardware and bone grafting.

Numerous additional systems, including **Colorado, Wisconsin segmental spine instrumentation (WSSI), Moss-Miami, CD Horizon,** and others, are employed in different centers according to clinical criteria encountered. Under development for younger patients (in whom fusion is to be avoided) are "growth rods." The "growth rods" are extended every few months as a **vertically expandable prosthetic titanium rib cage implant** (VEPTR) pushes apart the ribs on the concave side of the curvature.

When a bone graft is necessary for posterior lumbar interbody spinal fusion, bone may be obtained from the patient's own rib, rib heads, or iliac crest. Bone (for the graft) can also be obtained from a "bone bank." The most frequent donor site is the patient's own iliac crest (ipsilateral side when patient is in the lateral position). Bone obtained for the graft is kept moist with normal saline prior to its insertion. When the skin is prepped at the surgical site, the donor site is prepped as well. Multi-axial screws facilitate lining up the rods with the pedicle screws. A cell-saver should be available, as there is potential for significant blood loss. During surgery, a wake-up test may be employed (the **Stagnara intraoperative wake-up test)** in which the patient is awakened briefly (with no later recall) to respond to commands to move the lower extremities to ascertain any neurological compromise related to the surgical adjustments.

Procedure

Anterior Approach (Open Procedure). The thorax is entered in the sixth to seventh intercostal space with rib resection; the rib is saved for bone graft, as necessary. The pleura is incised over the involved spinal segments and dissected from the vertebral bodies and rib heads. Care is taken to avoid the local neurovascular structures. Fluoroscopy confirms the level of an inserted K-wire. The annulus of each disc involved is incised by electrosurgery (or similar, e.g., intradiscal thermablation or laser), and the disc is excised. Cobb elevator and Cobb curettes are used to reflect muscular and ligamentous structures from the end plates of the disc. Hemostasis is achieved (with Surgicel™, Gelfoam, etc.) in the disc space. The anterior longitudinal ligament is attenuated so that enough remains to hold bone grafts packed into the disc spaces for fusion. Depending on the levels and the degree of three-dimensional deformity, selected hardware is inserted into the lateral aspect of the vertebral bodies and secured. Penetration of the opposite cortex or pedicles is avoided. Titanium cages may be used to secure bone grafts. Prior to final tightening of the hardware, rib heads and ligaments may be released to permit appropriate mobility for the correction.

If both anterior and posterior approaches are to be performed, the insertion of hardware may be omitted from the anterior approach. The incisions are closed, thoracostomy tubes (e.g., Argyle) and closed suction drains (e.g., Hemovac) are placed, and the patient is turned to prone position.

Anterior Approach (VATS Procedure). Endoscopic ports are established at the 6th interspace and at lower levels. The thoracoscopic procedure is performed as above, employing endoscopic instrumentation, e.g., curettes, pituitary forceps, Kerrison rongeurs, rasps, etc. When performed as a minimal-access procedure, the operating time may be longer and the technical aspects more demanding for the surgeon, but the advantages for the patient include smaller incision, less pain, and shorter hospital stay.

Posterior Approach. The patient is turned to the prone position on the standard OR table, on a specialty table, or in a scoliosis frame placed on a specialty table, e.g., Andrews or Jackson table with or without Wilson frame (with integrated C-arm). The specialty tables are completely radiolucent, permitting fluoroscopy during spinal procedures. Skin prep includes the area over the iliac crests (in anticipation of obtaining a bone graft). A midline incision is made; a Cobb elevator (or similar instrument) is used to deepen the exposure. The transverse processes are decorticated, and facetectomies are performed to enable triplanar reduction of the deformity and placement of the hardware to correct exaggerated lordosis and kyphosis. The selected rods are bent, accordingly, to maintain the corrections. If the procedure is performed without anterior bone fusion, the fusion may be performed directly employing iliac bone or fragments of resected bone. Postoperative cast application is usually not required.

Preparation of the Patient

Correction of a scoliosis deformity can be performed using many different instrument systems. The surgery can be performed on a variety of frames and tables, according to the method of correction, the instrumentation system chosen, and the preference of the surgeon. When any of these tables are employed (for any position), all bony prominences and areas prone to skin and neurovascular pressure or trauma are padded. Apply electrosurgical dispersive pad.

Lateral Position, Anterior Approach for "Open" or VATS Procedure. Antiembolitic hose are applied (adult), when requested. The anesthesia provider may place Swan-Ganz or central venous pressure (CVP) and arterial lines. If the patient does not arrive with a Foley catheter, one should be inserted. The patient, in supine position, receives general anesthesia via double-lumen endotracheal tube (permits unilateral lung deflation for exposure). Following the administration of anesthesia, the patient is turned to the lateral position (convex side of the curvature "up"). A padded head extension is secured to the table to support the head and neck. If the standard OR table is used, a doughnut can be placed under the head for stabilization and to protect the ear. The torso may be stabilized with padded kidney rests (the larger blade in front), pillows, and/or sandbags. The arm on the unaffected side (down) is extended on a padded armboard; a pad may be placed under the arm to avoid pressure injury to brachial neurovascular structures. The arm on the affected side is supported by a Mayo stand, padded with a pillow (or a padded double armboard may be used). The leg on the unaffected side (down) is flexed, and the leg on the affected side (uppermost) is straight or slightly flexed (to stabilize the position) with a pillow placed between the knees; padding is placed around the feet and ankles. Tincture of benzoin is applied to protect the skin if the position is secured by wide adhesive tape at the shoulder and lower thigh anchored to the underside of the table. These same positioning considerations apply when specialty tables are employed; gel-filled positioning aids are integrated in the table (at pressure points). Check with the surgeon regarding insertion of a Foley catheter.

Posterior Approach. The patient is turned to the prone position on the Andrews table, the Jackson table (with or without the Wilson frame), or the OR table (e.g., Ritter). When the OR table is used, the patient is turned to the prone position with arms extended on padded armboards angled toward the head of the table (the hands, pronated). Chest rolls are placed under the thorax and abdomen to facilitate respiration; a roll is placed in front of the ankles to prevent undue pressure on the toes. A sterile, plastic adhesive drape may be used to isolate the anal area from the field prior to the skin prep.

Skin Preparation

Lateral Position. Begin cleansing for a mid-costal incision; extend the prep from the shoulder (include the axilla) to the lower thighs and down to the table in front and back (or to the positioning aids). The prep for the adult patient includes the skin over the ipsilateral iliac crest, in anticipation of possible bone graft taken from that site.

Prone Position. Begin at the midline of the back, extending from the top of the shoulders to mid-thigh and down to the table at the sides.

Draping

Folded towels are placed around the perimeter of the intended incision(s) to include the iliac crest(s).

Sterile, plastic adhesive drapes (2), optional. Four large sheets may be used to drape the foot, sides, and head of the table. A fenestrated sheet (e.g., laparotomy) is placed; it may require enlarging the fenestration to provide access to the iliac crest area to obtain a bone graft.

A drape may be required for the C-arm.

Equipment

Specialty scoliosis tables (e.g., Andrews or Jackson) with or without frame (e.g., Wilson) and required accessory extensions complete with gel pads at points of contact to avoid pressure injury, or headrest extension or padded doughnut placed at head of OR table with adequate padding for prone position, including rolls (two chest, one front of ankles), and pillow (between knees and legs)

Mayo stand padded with a pillow or double-padded armboard

Padded kidney rests (larger in front)

Sequential compression device with disposable leg wraps, when requested

ECG

Temperature probe (esophageal)

CVP manometer and arterial line supplies to anesthesia provider

Extra IV standards

Suctions (2) or cojoined suction and irrigation tubing for pulsed lavage (available)

Scales for weighing sponges (two)

ESU

Power source for drill (as necessary)

Blood pump and warmer, or cell saver (auto-transfusion) cell-saver (auto-transfusion)

Fiber-optic headlight and fiber-optic light source, e.g., Xenon 300 W (when endoscopy not employed)

Laser, e.g., Nd:YAG, optional

Generator for pulsed lavage suction irrigator, e.g., Simpulse, MicroAire, optional

Endoscopic VATS

Monitor

Camera console

Fiber-optic light source, e.g., Xenon 300 W

VCR

Printer

CD burner

Instrumentation

Laminectomy tray

Kerrison rongeurs and pituitary forceps tray

Cell-saver suction, optional

Self-retaining retractors

Bone cutters, rongeurs, rasps, and additional curettes (in addition to those on the tray)

Titanium cage to hold bone chips for graft, optional

Endoscopic

Thoracoscope with camera and cord and associated instrumentation, e.g., ports

Specific distraction device and instrumentation: compression rods, rod clamps, spreader, drivers, wrench, hooks, screws, plates, wires, staples, cables, etc.

Posterior Approach

Spinal fixation device system, e.g., Luque™, Cottrel-Dubousset™, Texas Scottish Rite Hospital (TSRH)™

Anterior Approach

Spinal fixation distraction device system, e.g., Isola, Halm-Zielke and Keneda (KASS), Dwyer

Intradiscal thermablator (e.g., ArthroCare™ or TOPAZ™), coblation handpiece tip, and cord, optional

Laser handpiece, cord, and tip, optional

Pulsed lavage suction irrigator and tip, e.g., Simpulse®, MicroAire® (optional)

Supplies

Antiembolitic hose, optional

CVP manometer and arterial line set ups to anesthesia provider, as requested

Sterile, plastic adhesive drapes (two), optional

Basin set

Blades, (2) #10 and (1) #15

Suction tubing (2)

Electrosurgical pencil (one or two) and cord with holder and scraper

Magnetic instrument pad (optional)

Needle magnet or counter

Surgicel or Gelfoam (usually soaked in thrombin, 1000 units in 10 ml saline)

Cottonoids, assorted sizes

Stainless steel wire, 16- or 18-gauge (optional)

Graduated pitcher, bulb syringes (2), antibiotic irrigation (optional)

Suctions (2) or cojoined suction and irrigation tubing for pulsed lavage (available)

Closed drainage system (e.g., Hemovac)

Chest tube, e.g., Argyle tube, connector, and closed drainage unit, e.g., Pleurevac™

Special Notes

- Apply **Special Notes** from ***Abdominal Laparotomy,*** p. 134, and Abdominal Laparoscopy, p. 140, as they apply to all patients in surgery (e.g., regarding correct identification of the patient, observing ***"time out,"*** etc.); see p. 18. Take extra precautions to correctly identify the pediatric patient.

- Assess patient's physical and emotional needs (assess anxiety). The circulator conveys emotional support to the patient and the patient's parents or legal guardian, as applicable, by explaining that he/she will act as the patient's advocate.
- Documentation in the **Perioperative Record** of nursing care, pertinent observations, interventions, and their outcomes are required for continuity of care of the patient and for medicolegal reasons.
- **Reminder:** Ascertain that the *correct* x-ray films, studies, and reports for the *correctly identified* patient are in the room prior to starting the surgery.
- Before surgery begins, be certain that there are two working suctions in the room (in addition to the suction used by anesthesia provider); have additional suction collection containers ready.
- Circulator ascertains that blood is available as ordered and ready for immediate use. When the surgery is elective, the patient may have given blood in advance for an autoinfusion.
- Ascertain if the cell-saver is required before starting the surgery. If additional (specialized) assistance is necessary, notify the supervisor (or the person in charge or the qualified person), according to hospital policy. The unit should be set up in advance of the surgery.
- When the cell-saver is used, all intraoperative blood is suctioned, filtered, and reinfused into the patient. The scrub person should squeeze the blood out of the sponges following use, before discarding them into the kick bucket. The cell-saver is used only when the blood *is free of contamination*; it cannot be employed once antibiotic irrigation, etc., is used.
- If the cell-saver use is not anticipated, the circulator must anticipate the possibility of blood transfusion(s), obtain items necessary to administer the blood (e.g., tubing set, blood warmer, pressure bag), and assist the anesthesia provider to administer the blood (identify patient and blood type, etc.).
- Circulator obtains necessary equipment and assists anesthesia provider as necessary to administer blood transfusions when indicated.
- Circulator documents blood transfusion and any reaction or lack of reaction to the transfusion.
- Maintain an accurate record of irrigation used and weigh sponges (when indicated) to determine blood loss.

- **Reminder:** *Persons scrubbed should wear a protective plastic face shield or goggles to prevent injury from splashing or spraying of the patient's blood and irrigation fluids that are used.*

Amputation of Lower Extremity

Definition

Severance of a portion of lower extremity.

Discussion

When progressive vascular insufficiency with failed reconstructive procedures, gangrene secondary to diabetes, malignancy, or severe trauma, etc., of the lower extremity results in infection with necrosis, amputation becomes necessary. The level at which amputation is performed depends on tissue viability and the patient's diagnosis, general health, and ability to cooperate with rehabilitation. Major lower-extremity amputations are performed above the knee (AK) or below the knee (BK); a toe or toes are frequently the level of the initial amputation. Amputation of a portion of the foot, e.g., transmetatarsal (TM), or at the ankle (Syme amputation) is infrequently performed, as immediate prosthesis fitting is best done at the BK or AK levels. These patients are prone to healing difficulties, again due to vascular disease or diabetic neuropathy. Great care is taken to achieve hemostasis and prevent infection in these compromised patients.

Procedure

Above-the-knee amputation (AKA) is described. A circular (or V-shaped in the anterior-posterior plane) incision is made above the distal femur and continued through the muscles and fascia down to the bone to create musculocutaneous flaps for coverage of the femoral stump. The distal adductor canal is entered, and the neurovascular bundle (superficial femoral artery, vein, and saphenous nerve) is ligated and divided (each component separately). Muscles are further transected circumferentially. The sciatic nerve is ligated and divided. The femoral periosteum is incised and the bone transected by saw. Bone edges are smoothed with a rasp. The wound is irrigated with copious amounts of normal saline (with or without antibiotics). Following meticulous hemostasis, the wound is closed. A closed suction unit may be employed (e.g., Hemovac). A bulky dressing or a cast can be applied, but a temporary prosthesis used to minimize postoperative edema and prepare the stump for a permanent prosthesis later on is the preferred treatment.

Preparation of the Patient

Preparation described is for AK amputation. An antiembolitic stocking may be applied to the unaffected extremity, particularly in the older adult patient with vascular insufficiency. Spinal, epidural, or a general anesthetic may be employed. Following the administration of anesthesia, the patient is placed in the supine position. Arms may be extended on padded armboards, or one or both arms may be padded and tucked in at the patient's sides. The safety belt is secured over the unaffected extremity. Observe all safety precautions to *be absolutely certain that the safety belt is placed over the correctly identified* (unaffected) extremity, the extremity that will ***not*** be amputated. ***Great care is taken to ensure the correct extremity is exposed for skin preparation.*** At the surgeon's discretion, a septic extremity may be wrapped in a Mayo stand cover, or a large plastic bag may be used to contain the septic portion of the extremity and to protect the OR table from gross contamination prior the skin prep. A sterile, plastic adhesive drape may be used to drape the perineum out of the field. Webril and a tourniquet may be applied on the thigh of the affected extremity at the surgeon's discretion. Pad all bony prominences and areas vulnerable to skin and neurovascular pressure or trauma. Apply electrosurgical dispersive pad.

Skin Preparation

The extremity may need to be isolated from soiling the OR table before the skin prep and from contaminating the sterile field after the prep; a Mayo stand cover may be used to isolate the portion of the extremity to be amputated.

Begin at the level of the umbilicus; extend the prep from beyond the midline of the abdomen to the table on the ipsilateral side and the extremity to include an acceptable margin distal to the level of amputation, but proximal to the isolated portion of the extremity.

Draping

The extremity is abducted and the foot and leg are covered with a double tube stockinette. A large sheet is draped over the end of the table. A drape (or split) sheet is draped under the thigh and clipped at the top of the thigh. A folded towel (in thirds, lengthwise) is wrapped around the top of the stockinette and clipped. A cuffed drape (or split) sheet is draped proximal to the thigh and clipped underneath. The extremity is passed through a fenestrated sheet, or individual drape sheets complete the draping. During the procedure, an extra Mayo cover may be used to hold (and contain) the amputated extremity.

Equipment

Sequential compression device with leg wrap (unaffected extremity), as requested

Forced-air warming blanket, when ordered
Tourniquet and pneumatic insufflator with microprocessor regulator, optional
ESU
Suction
Power source for oscillating saw, optional
Cast cart

Instrumentation

Basic orthopedic procedures tray
Gigli saw, guide, and handles, amputation knife, bone hook
Power saw (oscillating) with blades and cord (optional)

Supplies

Antiembolitic stocking
Sterile, plastic adhesive drape, optional
Tube stockinettes (2)
Basin set
Blades, (2 to 4) #10
Needle magnet or counter
Graduated pitcher, bulb syringe, and normal saline or antibiotic irrigation
Electrosurgical pencil and cord with holder and scraper
Culture tubes, aerobic and anaerobic
Closed suction unit (e.g., Hemovac)
Cast cart

Special Notes

- Apply **Special Notes** from ***Abdominal Laparotomy***, as they apply to all patients in surgery (e.g., regarding identifying the patient, maintain body temperature, etc.); see p. 134.
- **Every precautionary measure must be taken to ensure that the CORRECTLY identified patient will have the correct surgical procedure (according to site and side) and that the CORRECT EXTREMITY IS AMPUTATED. Following the Joint Commission (JC) (formerly the Joint Commission on Accreditation of Healthcare Organizations)** ***Universal Protocol*** **is MANDATORY** (see p. 18) to prevent errors. Amputation of the correct extremity is of extreme importance.
- **N.B.** *As block anesthesia (with the patient awake) is often employed, the circulator and the person scrubbed* **must be**

absolutely certain that the amputated extremity is not visible to the patient.

- Considering the serious nature of this surgery, it is important for the circulator to convey emotional support to the patient; measures such as maintaining eye contact, using touch to convey caring, holding the patient's hand during the administration of anesthesia, offering a warm blanket, etc., are essential.
- Permit the patient to ask questions and answer the questions in a knowledgeable manner or to refer the questions to the surgeon.
- The circulator assures the patient that he/she will act as his/her advocate with an explanation of that role, in an effort to help reduce the patient's anxiety.
- Consult the surgeon regarding his/her preferred method to dress the stump and obtain the necessary supplies prior to the patient's entry to the room; an orthotics technician should be on "standby," according to hospital policy.
- Do not permit preparation solutions to pool under tourniquet, as they excoriate the skin. Document the appearance of the skin preoperatively and immediately postoperatively. Also, pooled prep solutions may be flammable.
- **N.B. Reminder:** The skin prep should begin with work in the cleanest area, working outward toward the dirtiest area (part to be amputated). A sponge used on the "dirtiest" skin surface is **never** taken back over a "cleaner" skin surface.
- The circulator must prepare culture requisitions for aerobic and anaerobic as soon as the need becomes evident or the request is made.
- **Reminder:** every person scrubbed should wear a protective plastic face shield or goggles to prevent injury from splashing or spraying of the patient's blood and irrigation fluids.
- **N.B.** *The circulator prepares the amputated part and sends it to the laboratory or morgue, as per hospital policy.* It must be well wrapped, labeled with the correct identification, and **kept from** the patient's view.

CHAPTER 24
Neurologic Surgery

Craniotomy

Definition

A surgical opening of the cranium.

Discussion

The most basic form of craniotomy is the ***burr hole***, a limited opening through which blood or fluid may be evacuated or instruments inserted to divide neural tracts (as in prefrontal lobotomy). Additional uses of the burr hole include biopsy of an intracranial mass/lesion and aspiration of the contents of an abscess. A ***craniectomy*** refers to the procedure in which a section of the cranium is removed. ***Trephination*** refers to a procedure performed through burr holes that are larger than those usually made to perform limited maneuvers. When applicable, a twist drill is used in lieu of a burr. Computed tomography (CT) scan, magnetic resonance imaging (MRI), angiography or magnetoencephalography, electroencephalogram (EEG) mapping, angiographic stress tests, and ultrasound modalities are employed with tomography and three-dimensional (3D) coordinates to localize a lesion, i.e., stereotactic localization. Image-guided stereotactic burr hole biopsy, employing a CRW3 (or similar) head frame, provides accurate craniocortical entry transit and targeting minimizing craniocerebral trauma.

Approaches employing endoscopy and stereotactic procedures decrease morbidity and mortality; some cranial procedures performed in specialized radiology departments or specially equipped operating rooms are "same-day" noninvasive procedures, such as those employing the Gamma knife. Intracerebral hematomas can be evacuated endoscopically through a burr hole; the cortical incision is approximately 6 mm in diameter. For removal of an intracranial hematoma, the cortical incision is made from a location with the shortest trajectory to the clot. Endoscopic instruments, smaller but similar to standard instruments, used to perform the procedure are inherently less traumatic to the brain. Endoscopic procedures may require more than one burr hole (port).

During craniotomy (or burr hole procedure), intracranial pressure, when elevated, is reduced as a result of entry. In addition, as underlying tissues are manipulated, the location of the previously defined lesion shifts (thereby deviating somewhat from preoperative localization studies). In some institutions, highly sophisticated intraoperative MRI systems are in use. This may be in the form of cylindrical

MRI chamber, a section of which can be advanced for imaging and retracted to continue the surgery. Another system is one in which reference point electronic sensors are placed about the operative field in coordination with a computer to provide interactive localization.

When a limited-access endoscopic procedure is not applicable, burr holes are made and a portion (a "flap") of the cranium is lifted after the bone is cut by craniotome (with periosteum and muscle attached), i.e., craniotomy. When ***decompressive craniotomy*** is performed, bone (with overlying soft tissues dissected away) is excised, i.e., ***craniectomy***, and preserved for later reimplantation. Methods of bone preservation include placing the skull section in the patient's subcutaneous tissue, freezing the bone section (in antibiotic solution), or sterilizing it with ethylene oxide and holding it in a bone/tissue bank for later reimplantation. When the bone fragment cannot be retained, a prosthetic substitute is made. The craniotomy prosthesis can be a plate made of polymethylmethacrylate (PMMA) cement (fashioned over a mesh frame, i.e., template), titanium, or Vitallium®, or various plastics may be used for making the substitute. Burr holes can be repaired with silicone or other materials.

Numerous neurosurgical conditions treated by craniotomy include the following:

Intracranial aneurysm is an arterial dilation secondary to muscular weakness prone to rupture or hemorrhage. Controlling the blood pressure is essential during the repair. The aneurysm is isolated, and clips may be applied, or the aneurysm can be coated with PMMA or cyanoacrylate to strengthen the aneurysm wall and provide external support to the blood vessel. When feasible, endovascular approach (via femoral artery) with placement of embolitic materials, e.g., plastic spheres, muscle fragments, or Guglielmi detachable coils, effectively thrombose the aneurysm; however, collateral channels may develop subsequently, requiring further intervention.

Arteriovenous malformation results from an arteriovenous communication without intervening capillary beds; the veins are prone to rupture. Arteriovenous malformation can be detected by CT scan, spiral CT, scanning MRI, MRI angiography, and digital angiography; in addition, a transcranial Doppler may be employed. These vascular malformations may be mapped using single-photon emission tomography (SPECT) and xenon cerebral blood flow studies. The arterial side of the malformation may be clipped, coagulated, or treated by laser.

Intracranial arterial occlusion may be treated by microsurgical anastomosis; the involved vessel (e.g., middle cerebral artery) is bypassed distal to the point of obstruction. In this instance, the superficial temporal artery is dissected free for an appropriate distance and passed intracranially through a frontotemporal burr hole incision preparatory to anastomosis.

Intracranial tumors include astrocytoma, glioblastoma multiforme, meningioma, oligodendroglioma, medulloblastoma, lesions of neural, vascular, and connective tissue origin, and metastases from other sites. The lesions are treated according to their location, size, degree of malignancy (or nonmalignancy), status of the patient, etc. Chordomas, meningiomas, and others may be treated endoscopically. Treatment of acoustic neuroma and tumors about the pituitary are noted below.

Acoustic neuroma, derived from the neural sheath tissues of the acoustic (VIII cranial) nerve, is potentially life threatening. Removal of the bony superior wall of the auditory canal or direct drilling into the temporal bone with access to the middle or posterior fossa is necessary to expose the tumor. The cranial nerves (auditory, trigeminal, abducens, and facial) are protected, depending on the extent of the tumor. When necessary, a facial nerve branch may be divided for exposure, to be nerve grafted at a later date. A small acoustic neuroma can be fully excised via translabyrinthine approach or endoscopically through a small "keyhole" opening drilled directly behind the ear, via suboccipital retrolabyrinthine approach. A nerve stimulator, microscope, and high-speed power drill are employed. Hearing loss may result from the procedure, influencing the approach. A CO_2 laser may be employed; see safety precautions, p. 94.

Tumors near the pituitary, e.g., optic glioma and craniopharyngioma (suprasellar and parasellar), when resected, are accessed by a frontal or frontotemporal craniotomy approach. A fully endoscopic approach through a nostril may be used to treat craniopharyngiomas. No skin incision is made; total excision is not always possible.

Hydrocephalus results from conditions where the flow cerebrospinal fluid is obstructed by intraventricular lesions or arachnoid or parenchymal cysts, aqueductal or foraminal stenoses, hemorrhages, tumors, and infarctions or when there is an overaccumulation of cerebrospinal fluid (CSF) that collects in the ventricles or the subarachnoid space, causing undue pressure on the brain. Hydrocephalus (with excessive production of CSF) may be congenital and the result of a disease process (such as meningitis) or trauma, etc., that interferes with the secretion/absorption pathways. Hydrocephalus can be managed by shunting or by relieving the underlying obstruction, as applicable. In patients with late-onset hydrocephalus due to aqueduct stenosis, ***third ventriculostomy*** (i.e., opening into the third ventricle with shunt placement) is performed.

Otorrhea or rhinorrhea is the leakage of CSF due to a tear in the dura mater when the cranium is fractured; the subsequent leakage of CSF drains into the ear (otorrhea) or the nose (rhinorrhea). If the leakage does not resolve promptly (>24 hours), the patient is at risk for meningitis and surgery must be performed. The approach for repair of a dural tear with cerebrospinal otorrhea is temporal or bifrontal. A frontal approach is indicated for cerebrospinal rhinorrhea.

Epidural (acute) or subdural hematoma (subacute or chronic) may necessitate the evacuation of blood, clots, and membranes, the elevation and debridement of associated depressed fractures, and the excision of devitalized brain. ***Epidural hematoma***, usually the result of a forceful traumatic injury to the head, can become life threatening within in a short period of time, as significant blood loss (with ensuing elevation of intracranial pressure) leads to loss of consciousness and rapid physical and mental deterioration. The middle meningeal artery on the dura (outermost protective membrane covering the brain, just under the cranium) is most often torn; blood collects between the dura mater and the cranium. In contrast, a ***subdural hematoma*** represents a slow leak of venous blood into the subarachnoid space (between the arachnoid and the pia mater layers of the meninges). The condition may be acute, subacute, or chronic. Endoscopy provides the most efficacious approach to blood clot removal and control of the bleeding.

Neurological disorders include the following:

Parkinson's disease, as it advances with tremor and muscular rigidity, can be improved by various ablative techniques. A cryoprobe, electrosurgical device, or catheter (delivering absolute alcohol) is inserted under stereotactic guidance into the globus pallidus (or thalamus) through a burr hole, destroying the neural pathways.

Trigeminal neuralgia is characterized by severe pain along the distribution of branches of the trigeminal nerve; rhizotomy is performed, or absolute alcohol (or phenol or glycerol) injected. Percutaneous imaging-guided radio-frequency ablation may be considered in lieu of an "open" operative procedure. Additionally, microvascular nerve decompression (including transendoscopic approach) may be performed for this condition, as applicable.

Neuropsychiatric disorders, such as depressive states, anxiety, obsessive-compulsive disorders, etc., refractory to noninterventional treatment, may respond to various frontal lobe nerve pathway interruptions and are currently performed with minimal-access technique. Stimulating electrodes may be implanted as well.

Congenital abnormalities include the following:

Craniosynostosis, a premature closure of the sutures between cranial bone plates, results in various craniofacial deformities and increased intracranial pressure. To avoid brain damage and bone-growth deformities, surgical repair of the cranium should be performed prior to 4 months of age; cosmesis is an additional factor. Disease entities characterized by craniosynostosis include ***Alpert's, Carpenter, Crouzon, Pfeffier, and Saethe-Chotzen syndromes.*** The syndromes are characterized according to which bone plates prematurely close. There are a variety of characteristics for each syndrome that may present requiring correction. The infant may have facial hypoplasia and a variety of skull deformities, shortened and/or webbed digits, widely spaced or crowded teeth (resulting in protrusion), small, deformed ears, or an underdeveloped jaw; the eyes may protrude (*exophthalmos*), and/or the eyelids may droop. Infants with Carpenter syndrome may have heart defects as well. Depending on the particular skull abnormality, craniotomy is performed, sutures are divided, and osteotomies and other revisions are made to the skull as it is remodeled. Various plates and hardware, including biodegradable fixation devices, can be employed. A less-traumatic craniotomy modality (as compared to craniotomy with osteotomies) utilizes an internal craniofacial distraction device (plate and shaft secured by screws) placed after the involved sutures are divided; multiple osteotomies are avoided. Periodic adjustment (distraction) of the distraction post shaft is done, usually weekly (0.5 mm for cranial and 1.0 mm for facial bones), for approximately 2 to 3 months. Following maturation of the callous, the distraction shaft is removed by rotating the device in the opposite direction; no anesthesia is required. Corrections of some presentations of the syndromes are performed as endoscopically assisted procedures. For isolated sagittal synostosis, an incision is made into the prematurely closed suture, with application of polyethylene film over the bone edges to prohibit its regeneration.

Additional congenital cranial abnormalities include the following:

Platybasia, the fusion of the occipital bone and upper cervical vertebrae with encroachment of the vertebral canal and/or posterior fossa.

Persistent parietal foramina, may not require treatment, if asymptomatic.

Lacunar skull associated with *meningomyelocele*; specific procedures are performed according to the clinical findings.

Procedure

A "generic" craniotomy is described. General anesthesia (with endotracheal intubation) is administered. The patient is positioned; extensions, headrests, and/or fixation devices (e.g., Mayfield) are secured to the table to hold (or "fix") the skull in position. The surgeon marks the line of incision prior to the skin prep (a pen with indelible ink, the back of a #15 blade, or the tip of a 15-gauge needle may be used). The surgeon usually injects the scalp with a local anesthetic containing epinephrine to reduce bleeding, or the scalp may be injected with normal saline to create pressure to discourage bleeding. Pressure is applied along both sides of the line of incision as the layers of the scalp are incised; scalp clips (e.g., Raney) are applied. Dandy hemostatic clamps may be applied on the lower edges of the skin incision and secured by a rubber band that is clipped to the drapes. The scalp is reflected; care is taken to protect the temporal artery when presented by the approach to avoid muscle atrophy with difficulties in mastication. The scalp flap is covered with a moist sponge. When a section of the cranium is to be removed (i.e., craniectomy), the cranium is separated from the soft tissues for later reattachment, or it may be saved in a bone bank. Mannitol, furosemide, and intravenous (IV) steroids may be employed to reduce intracranial pressure and decrease cerebral edema before the cortical incision is made. Lumbar drainage of cerebrospinal fluid may be used as well.

Burr holes are made and connected by craniotome (protecting the underlying dura mater) to remove a segment of cranial bone, or when the bone is to be reattached, a bone flap is made (hinged on the adjacent periosteum and musculature) and covered with a moist lap sponge. Bleeding is controlled electrosurgically; when the bone is bleeding, bone wax is employed. If the bone flap is to be reattached at the end of the procedure, drill holes are made in the periphery of the skull and matching holes are drilled in the bone flap. The dura mater is incised; vessels in the dural margins are coagulated (with bipolar electrosurgery) or ligated with clips (e.g., Hemoclips®); the dura mater may be "tacked up" to the pericranium. Moist cottonoids are placed as necessary; the brain is continually moistened by saline irrigation or moist cottonoids are placed to prevent cortical injury caused by drying.

A subcortical mass is approached by the most direct route, except when this is through a vital region such as a motor or speech area. In these cases, the incision is made in a less-important area and continued obliquely. An ultrasonic probe with a special tip, e.g., cavitron ultrasonic surgical aspirator (CUSA), can be utilized. CT scan or MRI may be employed intraoperatively to facilitate defining such subcortical mass. Blood vessels are electrosurgically coagulated or clipped. Moist cottonoids and cotton balls are employed to restrict capillary oozing or to tamponade blood vessels. Arterial walls of aneurysms may be reinforced with PMMA or similar material or preferably clipped with special brain aneurysm clips, e.g., Heifetz, Yasargil, Sundt-Kees, Mayfield, Keer, Olivecrona. The clips may also be used in the treatment of arteriovenous malformation and pituitary tumors. They may be employed during tumor resection to facilitate dissection and exposure. Clips also control the vascular supply to a neoplasm that is then evacuated, or applied to a neoplastic cyst which is aspirated. Tumor removal is performed with curettes, pituitary forceps, and brain spoon; complete excision of some lesions is not always feasible. Following cerebral resection, the wound is irrigated and hemostasis achieved.

The dural flap is closed, making the suture line watertight. If the defect in the dura is too large to be closed, a graft may be inserted (using temporalis fascia, periosteum, and fascia lata or an artificial dura substitute). DuraGenPlus®, a dural substitute composed of collagen matrix, provides a barrier that may be cut to size and sutured over a defect when brain coverage by the dura is inadequate. Dura Seal™ liquid may be applied to a suture line to prevent leakage. The dura mater may be left open after operations in the posterior fossa (when there is adequate closure of the nuchal muscles), beneath simple burr holes, and following subtemporal craniectomy (small burr hole-sized excision of the cranium) for subdural hematoma. In the craniotomy procedure, bone flap is wired back. Burr holes may be covered with silicone rubber buttons or methylmethacrylate or filled with autogenous bone chips. As the scalp is closed, skin clips are removed. The wound is dressed and the head is wrapped in a turban-like gauze bandage.

Pediatric Craniotomy. Minimal discussion is provided here. It must be remembered that pediatric patients are not smaller versions of adult patients; special considerations for the care of the pediatric patient in surgery are found in Pediatric General Information, p. 978. The many varieties of approaches and incisions used for adult craniotomy, depending on the individual presentation, may be employed for pediatric procedures as well. However, since the infant is not as resilient to insult (as surgery) as the adult, and because emergent events occur far more rapidly during pediatric craniotomy, extreme vigilance must be employed to alert caretakers to deleterious, severe, and sometimes fatal conditions, should they present.

Subperiosteal subtemporal approach may be employed to correct cranial bone abnormalities and facial hypoplasia in the infant with craniosynostosis. Blood transfusion is not uncommon during full craniotomy procedures; infant morbidity and mortality are considerably higher for craniotomy than for the revised endoscopic procedure. Complete osteotomy is achieved with a high-speed craniotome (e.g., Midas Rex® with long curved guide and bit). A craniofacial distraction device (of titanium) is inserted intracranially. As stated previously, the metal shaft part of the device is exposed, i.e., extracranially, following the procedure. The shaft is used to rotate the distraction device weekly for 2 to 3 months until the cranial sutures mature. Cranial bone is distracted by 0.5 mm, and the bones of the mid-face are distracted 1 mm weekly using the shaft. A helmet must be worn following the procedure for pediatric craniofacial repair. The shaft part of the distraction device is removed following maturation of the bones; anesthesia is not required.

Correction of craniofacial defects by "distraction osteogenesis" may also be achieved employing a rigid endoscope when the surgery is performed as an endoscopically assisted procedure. CT scans or magnetic resonance imaging provides a guiding system to find the ideal access route.

Hydrocephalus. In addition to the correction of obstructed cerebrospinal fluid (CFS) by craniotomy with the insertion of a shunt (see **Ventricular Shunt,** p. 666), in selected cases, control may be achieved by **third ventriculostomy** via endoscopic approach, thereby eliminating the need for a prosthetic shunt. The infant is placed in supine position with the head, slightly rotated, supported in a padded or gel-type donut or in a horseshoe headrest with built-in gel pad (e.g., Mayfield Infinity Support System). The most important aspect of the surgery is the correct placement of the perforation; the fenestration is made halfway between the infindibular recess and mammillary bodies in the midline, just behind the sellae. Care must be taken to avoid neurovascular structures (to avoid hypothalamic injury, oculomotor palsy, and the basilar artery, i.e., hemorrhage). On occasion, two endoscopes may be employed simultaneously to provide the surgeon with a picture-in-picture video display on a single screen. In aquaductal stenoses, endoscopic aquaductoplasty with or without stenting may be performed.

Neuroendoscopy is employed with the intention of reducing the invasiveness of intracranial procedures, resulting in reduced traumatization of the brain tissue. A prerequisite for safe neuroendoscopy is a clear, unobstructed visualization of the anatomy (a lens-irrigation cleaning feature eliminates the need to withdraw the scope). Indications as hydrocephalus, intraventricular lesions, and space-occupying arachnoid or parynchymal cysts, appropriate correction of craniosynostosis, and even some highly vascularized lesions can be treated endoscopically. Bipolar coagulation probes and appropriate laser devices used for hemostasis help to create optimal conditions under which neuroendoscopy can be performed.

Microneuroendoscopy, procedures employing both endoscope and microscope, can be used to obtain extremely detailed information regarding the anatomical presentation of the anatomy; those tools greatly facilitate safe dissection. In transsphenoidal pituitary surgery, the endonasal approach can avoid the more invasive transseptal dissection. The benefits of a minimal-access neurovascular procedure are less brain retraction and the small burr hole access. Time constraints, the learning curve for performance of neuroendoscopic procedures, and the technical equipment are improving rapidly. Should the endoscopic procedure fail or be aborted, craniotomy is another option. The major limiting factor in neuroendoscopy is the size of the scope (most have working channels no greater than 2.4 mm). That limits the size of the tumor to be excised; excision of most tumors becomes too time-consuming and too tedious.

Additional Approaches. When intracranial lesions are inaccessible by craniotomy or are known to be responsive to radiotherapy, the Gamma knife may be employed. The ***Gamma knife*** is a **stereotactic radiotherapeutic noninvasive modality** used to treat intracranial lesions, including acoustic neuroma, pituitary adenomas, pinealomas, craniopharyngiomas, meningioma, chordomas, chondrosarcomas, glial tumors and metastases, arteriovenous malformations, and neurological conditions (including trigeminal neuralgia, Parkinson's disease, epilepsy, intractable pain, and, recently, psychoneurological dysfunction, such as obsessive-compulsive disorders). This modality is particularly useful when the lesion is deep, small (<3.5 cm), and relatively inaccessible via "open" surgery techniques or in poor-operative-risk patients. Image-guided stereotactic procedures are performed with accuracy to target and destroy intracranial lesions with minimal craniocerebral trauma. The precision of the Gamma knife by means of 3D tomographic imaging supplants the imprecision of brain surgery. Once a brain lesion has been defined by various imaging techniques, the stereotactic Gamma knife head form can be fixed to the patient's cranium with four penetrating conical screws. Two hundred and one beams of ionizing radiation from a cobalt^{60} source are directed from points circumferentially about the "helmet-like" fixation device, focused to simultaneously converge and destroy the localized target lesion. As the beams emanate from different locations around the apparatus, the amount of radiation the surrounding tissues receive is negligible while the exact site of the tumor receives a high dose of radiation. This application can be used to treat tumors deep in the brain, even when located close to blood vessels and vital structures that make the lesion inaccessible by surgical maneuvers. The Gamma knife is useful for treating high-risk patients, as the procedure can be performed with local anesthesia (with or without *conscious sedation*). General anesthesia is employed when the Gamma knife is used to treat children; it may be employed for adults as well. The procedure is performed in special suites of the radiotherapy department or specially equipped operating rooms. When applicable, the lower overall cost (a limited-stay procedure), the absence of postoperative discomfort or a wound, and minimal morbidity are undeniable advantages of this modality.

Preparation of the Patient

Described is a "generic-type" approach. ***Planning is essential*** prior to the surgery; see the *suggested plan* of care, **Patient Care Plan**, p. 9. When planning ahead, in addition to those measures, assessments, and interventions, see the **Special Notes** for **craniotomy** for additional information. The position of the patient depends on the procedure to be performed, the approach, and the location of the lesion (e.g., frontal, parietal, temporal, occipital, or a combination thereof). Equipment for positioning and surgical instrumentation, etc., should be in the room prior to the patient's arrival. A warming mattress, e.g., Multi-Thermia blanket, may be used, or a forced-air warming blanket may be employed. The patient is assisted, as necessary, to move from the gurney to the table. When assistance is required, the circulator is responsible for obtaining adequate number of persons to safely transfer the patient from the gurney to the table. Antiembolitic hose (adult) are applied to the patient's legs (if the patient does not arrive wearing them) to prevent venous stasis. When ordered, a sequential compression device with disposable leg wraps may be placed over antiembolitic hose (if the patient is obese, the leg wraps may be used without the hose underneath). Leads are placed for EEG and electrocardiogram (ECG). An esophageal thermometer, IV, and right atrial (or central venous pressure) line may be inserted. ***Somatosensory evoked potentials (SSEP)*** are monitored. An alteration of these signals from the norm indicates dysfunction along a neural pathway, either peripheral or central, due to excessive pressure from surgical manipulation (e.g., forceful use of retractors) or decreased oxygenation to the tissues; SSEP monitoring indicates that adjustments in the anesthesia mixture may be required to assure adequate brain and systemic oxygenation. Electrodes are placed on the scalp, on the spine, and over peripheral nerves; intrathecal electrodes are in use as well. The anesthesia provider may use SSEP to monitor a specific nerve, such as the optic or auditory nerve to monitor procedures performed about the sella or the posterior fossa, respectively, or for local procedures, and for procedures on the brain stem and other surgeries. An electrosurgical dispersive pad and a Foley catheter are routinely placed; urine output is monitored. All bony prominences and areas vulnerable to skin and neurovascular pressure or trauma are adequately padded.

General anesthesia (with endotracheal intubation) is administered.

Positions

The patient is positioned at the discretion of the anesthesia provider; ***the patient is never moved without the anesthesia provider's permission.*** Special frames, positioning aids, padding, headrests, and/or fixation devices (e.g., Mayfield) are secured to the table to hold (or "fix") the skull in position for the most frequently employed positions; these are mentioned below. The circulator must ensure adequate assistance to position the patient to avoid injury to the patient and the staff.

Supine. An extension may be secured to the table with a headrest device (e.g., Mayfield, Codman Co.). The skull is "fixed" in position by steel pins (sterilized by autoclaving, or sterile, disposable pins are used). As the pins are placed in the headrest device, sterility of the pins should be maintained; the pins are inserted into the cranium. Alternatively, the head may be positioned on either a padded donut (that also protects a padded dependent ear when the head is turned to the side), or a gel-filled horseshoe headrest may be used (the shoulders are positioned at the top of the table). The arms may be extended on padded armboards alongside the patient, or the arms may be padded and tucked in at the patient's sides. A pillow may be placed behind the lumbar spine and/or under the knees (to avoid straining back muscles).

Sitting. In Fowler's position, the top section of the table is removed, and a table extension and a headrest (e.g., Mayfield with pins or horseshoe with pins) are secured to the table to support the patient's head and neck. Sterile pins that were placed in the headrest attachment (with maintenance of sterility) are inserted into the patient's skull. The table is raised from the middle break, and the foot of the table is lowered; the knees are positioned over the lower break of the table. A pillow may be placed behind the legs, and a padded footboard supports the feet. The arms are placed in the patient's lap on a pillow and secured with padded restraints. The safety strap is secured across the thighs. The table may be turned 90°, with the anesthesia provider opposite the operative side (surgeon's side). Extra caution must be taken to avoid injury to the patient's fingers when the foot of the table is raised at the conclusion of the procedure.

Prone. The patient is intubated on the gurney and, at the discretion of the anesthesia provider, carefully rolled over (face down) onto the table. *Obtaining adequate assistance to move and/or position the patient is essential.* The head may be placed in a padded donut, or, more often, the head is placed in a gel-filled horseshoe attachment that replaces the top section of the table. Care is taken to ensure that the patient's eyes are protected from excessive pressure. Chest rolls are placed under the patient's torso, from the acromioclavicular joints to the iliac crests, to facilitate respiration. The arms may be extended on padded armboards (angled toward the head of the table) with the forearms pronated, or the arms may be padded and tucked in at the patient's sides. A roll is placed in front of the ankles to protect the toes. Pillow(s) are placed in front of the legs.

Padding is placed under the elbows, knees, and other points of contact by bony prominences. Female breasts and male genitalia are protected from pressure. The safety strap is secured across the back of the patient's thighs.

Lateral. The patient may be intubated on the gurney and, at the direction of the anesthesia provider, carefully turned (shoulders and hips are turned simultaneously to prevent torsion of the spine) to lateral position onto the table, using coordinated teamwork. The torso may be stabilized with padded kidney rests (the larger blade in front), or a beanbag device that conforms to the patient's body is used. (If the beanbag is used, it is placed on the table prior to moving the patient [the U-shaped end should be at the head of the table]. The head and feet portions of the table are padded with blankets to even out the table and to prevent hyperextension of the body when the patient is returned to supine position. A gel ring is placed beneath the head [with a blanket under the ring] to support the spinal column. Suction is continuously applied to the beanbag throughout the surgery.) ***Use of a heating mattress (e.g., K -Thermia pad) is contraindicated when the beanbag is used, as trapped heat could burn the patient.*** After checking the chart for patient allergies, the position is stabilized with wide adhesive tape (tincture of benzoin protects the skin), or a folded towel or a blanket may be placed under the tape. The arm on the dependent side is extended on a padded armboard. An axillary roll (e.g., 1000-ml fluid bag wrapped in towel) or a small pad is placed to relieve pressure on the brachial plexus. A Mayo stand, padded with a pillow, supports the uppermost arm, or a padded double armboard may be used. The leg on the dependent side is flexed; the upper leg may be straight or slightly flexed (to stabilize the position) with a pillow placed between the legs; padding, foam, or gel pads are placed around the feet and ankles.

Skin Preparation

Most surgeons prefer to cut the hair and shave the scalp. Check with the surgeon regarding the area to be prepped and the solution to be used for the skin prep (by the circulator). Antibiotic ointment (e.g., Polysporin) may be put in the eyes, and eye pads and nonirritating tape may be used to tape lids shut; plastic eye shields are helpful to avoid undue pressure on the eyes. Care is taken to avoid getting prep solution in the eyes. Small cotton pledgets or cotton balls are placed in the ears to prevent prep solution from pooling in the ears (some surgeons prefer removing them with a mosquito forceps before draping). To avoid a fire hazard, prep solutions are not allowed to pool on the drapes. The surgeon usually marks the line of incision before draping. The prepped area must be carefully dried; otherwise, the plastic drape will not stick. Use sterile technique when removing the towel. If a bone grafting is anticipated, the bone graft area is prepped and draped at the same time.

Draping

Surgeons usually prefer to do the draping. Folded towels are placed around the operative site and secured by towel clips, staples, or sutures; the scrub person prepares ahead heavy silk sutures (e.g., #2) on cutting needles, two needle holders, toothed forceps, and suture scissors. A large drape sheet is placed below the head. A craniotomy sheet with an adhesive plastic backing in the fenestration is used, or a sterile, plastic adhesive drape is placed, followed by a drape sheet under the head, and a sheet with an aperture sized for craniotomy exposure is used. The prepped area ***must*** be dry, or the adhesive drape will not stick. An impervious drape (e.g., plastic) with a collection pouch is usually preferred. If an overhead table (e.g., Mayfield) is used, a large drape sheet, fanfolded at the front edge of the table, is used. The fanfolded sheet is brought down to close off the space between the unsterile area under the table and the operative field. The disposable craniotomy sheet will eliminate the need for additional drape sheets; otherwise, a fenestrated sheet and drape sheets, as necessary, are placed to avoid contamination.

Additional draping may be required for the microscope, C-arm, stand, drills and saws, and table with the endoscopes, etc.

For iliac bone graft, add: towels, sterile, plastic adhesive drape, a drape sheet with a medium-sized fenestration, and a towel or sheet to cover the graft site until exposure is necessary.

Equipment

Sequential compression device with disposable leg wraps, if requested
Forced-air warming blanket, hyperthermia mattress, e.g., K-Thermia pad, optional
Table extension for seating the headrest, optional
Headrest device, e.g., Mayfield skull clamp, Crutchfield, Gardner, horseshoe or donut (padded, foam, or gel), optional
Pillows, padding, chest rolls, padded kidney rests, elbow pads, heel cups, gel pads, padded restraints, pad to prevent pressure on the brachial plexus 1000-ml fluid bag wrapped in towel or a rolled towel, etc., depending on position
Overhead instrument table (e.g., Mayfield), optional
Arkive osciloscope ECG, EEG
Temperature-monitoring device, e.g., esophageal thermometer and equipment for atrial line or CVP to anesthesia provider
Fiber-optic headlight, optional
Fiber-optic light sources for retractors and headlight, e.g., Xenon 300 W, as necessary
Magnifying loupes or operating microscope (e.g., Zeiss or Omni)
Doppler console, optional
Power source for power high-speed drill and saw (or self-contained), optional

Blood-warming units and blood pumps (for transfusion), optional
Scales (2) to measure blood loss, optional
Footstools and platforms (several available)
Suctions (2)
Electrosurgical unit (ESU) (2), monopolar and bipolar (e.g., Malis)
Laser (e.g., CO_2, Ho:YAG, or Nd:YAG), optional; see mandatory laser safety precautions, p. 94; optional
CUSA console, optional

Pediatric

Pediatric headrest, e.g., Mayfield Infinity Skull Clamp and the Mayfield Infinity Support System with built-in gel pad; horseshoe with gel pad or as requested

Endoscopic, Add

Monitor(s), VHS VCR, camera console, CD burner, printer, irrigator light fountain (e.g., Malis with foot control), computer-guided navigation system, fiber-optic light source 6000 K, CUSA (Cavitron Ultrasonic Surgical Aspirator)

Instrumentation

Craniotomy tray
Kerrison and Rongeur tray
Raney gun and clip cartridge, Dandy clamps and rubber bands
Budde retractor system with multiple parts (attaches to the Mayfield skull clamp)
Penfield dissector, flexible brain retractors, extra Frazier suctions and stylets, assorted ligating clip appliers (e.g., Hemoclip appliers)
Bayonet bipolar diathermy forceps with "micro" tip and cord
Metal pattie tray, e.g., Anspah for cottonoids, bone wax, etc.
Caliper (to measure graft tissue or substitute, e.g., DuraGenPlus)
Osteotomes and mallet, Raney clips and gun, optional
Micro craniotome (high-power drill), e.g., Stryker®, Hall, or Midas Rex, MicroAire® self-contained (or with cord), chuck, drill sleeve, drill bits and burr
Power saw, cord, blade, chuck, and key
Bipolar bayonet forceps and cord, e.g., Malis
For craniofacial abnormalities, angled lighted rhinoplasty retractor
Doppler probe and cord, optional
Laser, optional, e.g., laser hand piece and tip, Rhoton covered or other nonreflecting instrumentation; observe safety measures (mandatory)
CUSA, optional, hand piece and wand
Graft substitute for dura (e.g., DuraGenPlus), optional

Iliac Bone Graft

Limited procedures tray, Taylor retractors, bone gouge (medium), mallet, Cloward bone grafting instruments, optional

Transphenoidal

Limited procedures tray, add nasal specula (3; long, short, and oronasal), long and short; bayonet smooth forceps; dull Senn's retractors; small dull rakes; Cottle elevator-freer enucleator, and micro instruments, see p. 1142

CSF Shunts

Limited procedures tray

Microsurgical Instruments (Titanium)

Microscope handles (optional), micro forceps, micro scissors (curved, straight), Beaver knife handle, micro needle holders (curved, straight), micro curettes (curved, straight, angled), micro suction tips, micro hooks (90°, semi-sharp, blunt), bayonet bipolar forceps with cord, micro dissectors (small, medium, large, straight), micro elevators (variety of straight and curved), assorted aneurysm clips and clip appliers (e.g., Heifetz, Yasargil, Sundt-Kees, Mayfield, Keer, Olivecrona)

Endoscopic Instruments

Hopkins rigid endoscope (0°, 30°, 70°, and 120°), 2.7 mm, 20 cm with sheath, 6.5- or 4.0-mm "mini" camera and optical bridge, surgical tips attached to telescope, electrosurgical suction-irrigator and coaxial cable, laser fiber and hand piece, 1-mm scissors, 1-mm pituitary forceps, 1-mm grasping forceps

Supplies

Antiembolitic hose
Foley catheter tray
Atrial or CVP line, angiocath, IV tubing
Hair-cutting and scalp-shaving supplies
Marking pen (sterile, indelible) and paper labels
Sterile, plastic adhesive drape or craniotomy sheet with insert
Sterile, plastic adhesive drape (e.g., 3M 1018) for autograft
Local anesthetic with epinephrine (to inject site of incision for hemostasis), paper labels and marking pen
Control syringe and #18 needle
Medications to anesthesia provider: Dilantin, furosemide, or Mannitol, 20% with filter, to reduce intracranial pressure; Dexamethasone/Decadron, a synthetic steroid, to decrease inflammation; sodium nitroprusside/Nipride to induce hypotension. (Note: when mixed in solution for intravenous use, is unstable in light. Cover bottle and tubing with aluminum foil.)
Basin set
Blades, (2) #10, (1) #15, (1) #11
ESU monopolar pencil, and cord with holder and scraper

Needle magnet or counter
Suction tubing
Nerve stimulator (locator)
Graduated pitcher, bulb or asepto syringes (2), antibiotic irrigation
Ringer's lactate solution for irrigation (at 37°C)
Telfa pad for tumor specimens
Cottonoids, assorted (e.g., 1/2″ × 1/2″, 1″ × 1″, 1″ × 3″, 1/2″ × 3″), and cotton balls
Rubber bands for Raney clips (inferior edge of incision), optional
Bone wax packages (2)
Hemostatic agents, e.g., compressed Gelfoam (sponges) soaked in thrombin, spray or powder thrombin, Surgicel™, Fibrillar™, and Avitene™
Bicol™ collagen sponge, optional
Ligating clips, e.g., Hemoclips (small, medium)
Scalp clips (e.g., Raney, Michel)
Syringe, 20 ml, to force-rinse Frazier suction tips
Antibiotic irrigation (optional)
PMMA, e.g., kit or supplies and wire mesh, optional
Dural sealant, e.g., Dura Seal™, optional
Graft for dural patch substitute (e.g., DuraGenPlus™), optional
Dura patch, e.g., DuraGenPlus, optional
Telfa dressing pad for specimens
Closed suction drain, e.g., Hemovac or Jackson-Pratt™
Skin closure, e.g., skin tapes, as Steri-strips™, skin stapler, or skin suture
Bulky dressing, e.g., 4 × 4 sponges, kerlix rolls, tape of choice (e.g., transpore), and tincture of benzoin, optional
Adaptic™ gauze 1/2″ packing (frontal approach)

Special Notes

- Apply **Special Notes** from ***Abdominal Laparotomy,*** p. 134, as they apply to all patients in surgery (e.g., regarding correct identification of the patient, observing ***"time out,"*** etc.). Take extra precautions to correctly identify the pediatric patient.
- ***Planning***, prior to the patient's arrival in the OR, is essential. The perioperative practitioner and the surgical technologist plan ahead to ensure the patient's safety. Considerations include required equipment (in particular, the type of headrest), individualized plan of care to meet that patient's needs, the surgical approach and positioning aids (e.g., padding to avoid pressure injury to heels), instrumentation (standard, microsurgical, and/or endoscopic), supplies, medications, etc.

- The circulator may convey (even more than is usual) emotional support to the patient due to the serious nature of the surgery. Assess and document patient's anxiety level; employing measures such as maintaining eye contact, using touch to convey caring, holding the patient's hand during the administration of anesthesia, offering a warm blanket, etc., is essential.
- The circulator may provide the patient a measure of comfort to reduce anxiety by explaining that he/she will act as the patient's advocate. Documentation of nursing care, pertinent observations, interventions, and their outcome are required for continuity of care of the patient and for medicolegal reasons.
- The circulator is responsible for obtaining adequate assistance (before anesthesia is induced) to safely move the patient and to protect the employees involved in positioning the patient.
- Team members can prevent musculoskeletal injuries by using methods that employ ergodynamic movements when lifting, moving, and positioning the patient.
- *Avoid injury to the patient's fingers by preventing them from being caught in the table mechanism when the table is readjusted following the procedure.*
- **N.B.** *Document the appearance and condition of the skin preoperatively and immediately postoperatively.* Avoid injuries to the patient caused by undue pressure on neurovascular structures and the skin overlying bony prominences; the body should be placed in correct anatomical alignment on a well-padded table.
- **Reminder:** Use safety precautions to identify, label, and dispense medications or solutions and to avoid medication errors; see p. 30. It is mandatory that all medications and solutions on the sterile field be labeled by name and strength. The medication bottle is retained in the room until the procedure has concluded.
- The scalp and underlying tissues may be injected with a vasoconstricting agent such as epinephrine; *advise anesthesia provider accordingly* when they are used.
- When available, a plastic fluid-control drape with a collection pouch should be used to prevent "strike-through" contamination of the sterile field.
- Before surgery begins, the circulator ascertains that there are two ***working*** suctions in the room (in addition to the suction used by anesthesia provider); additional suction collection containers must be readily available.

- ***The circulator checks with the blood bank to verify that blood is available as ordered and ready for immediate use before the surgery is permitted to begin.***
- The circulator obtains needed equipment and assists the anesthesia provider as necessary to administer blood transfusions, etc.
- Circulator documents blood transfusion administration and any reaction or lack of reaction to the transfusions in the **Perioperative Record**.
- When the patient's hair (over the site of the intended incision) is not removed in the OR, the "pre-op" area or postanesthesia care unit (PACU) is often used. The patient's privacy is maintained by screening off a cubical. Hair is not routinely saved unless it is saved per patient's request. *As a courtesy to the patient, the circulator may save the hair, placing it in a plastic bag labeled with the patient's identification. The hair may be given to a waiting family member, or following the surgery the circulator may entrust it to the PACU. Although it is not required, it is better to save the hair unnecessarily than to realize too late that the cut hair is* ***irretrievable***.
- The surgeon usually cuts the patient's hair and shaves the scalp prior to the skin prep (by the circulator). Include scissors, plastic bag with identification label, clippers (battery powered, if available), disposable razors, basin of warm water, scrub prep solution (usually contains iodoform and 4 × 4 gauze sponges), towels, eye ointment (e.g., antibiotic), eye pads or cotton balls (optional), and hypoallergenic tape to cover the eye pads, with or without eye shields.
- ***Headrests (e.g., Mayfield, horseshoe) and two or three pins disposable, sterile) or reusable pins (autoclaved) are brought into the room prior to the patient's entry.*** The headrest, when used, "fixes" the skull (to prevent it from moving). Sterility is maintained as the pins are placed in the device. Prep solution is applied to the scalp areas designated for pin insertions.
- **N.B.** ***Keep the headrest device and the pins from the patient's sight, as seeing them may cause undue anxiety; the items should be placed on the cart/table following removal of shaving equipment.***
- **Reminder:** Ascertain that the *correct* x-ray films, studies, and reports for the *correctly identified* patient are in the room prior to starting the surgery.
- Notify x-ray department when intraoperative fluoroscopy is anticipated. Observe all x-ray safety precautions; see p. 52.

- The circulator takes appropriate measures to maintain patient's body temperature, e.g., use blankets (warmed) and warmed irrigation fluids and adjust room temperature; a K-Thermia pad and/or a forced-air warming blanket may be used, when ordered. Infants are kept warm in addition with overhead heat lamps and/or K-Thermia pad and the extremities, etc.
- The scrub person keeps track of the amount of irrigation used; the circulator records accurately the amount of irrigation used and weighs sponges (when indicated) for determining blood loss.
- The scrub person monitors the temperature of the irrigation (before passing the filled bulb syringes) to the surgeon to avoid burn injury to brain tissue.
- Cotton balls, cottonoids, small parts of instruments (e.g., screws), etc., used during the procedure are included in the count; any small object that could be sequestered in a wound must be counted.
- The scrub person should secure the metal pattie tray (Anspah) to the drapes within view and reach of the surgeon before the bone flap is raised.
- A suggestion for preparing hemostatic agents is to make compressed Gelfoam (sponges) soaked in thrombin (spray or powder thrombin may also be used), Surgicel and Fibrillar cut strips approximately $\frac{3}{4} \times 2''$, also squares slightly smaller than postage stamp size and the Avitene cut approximately $\frac{1}{4} \times \frac{1}{4}''$. Microsurgical endoscopy may require smaller cuts.
- Towels placed around the periphery of the operative site may be secured with towel clips, staples, or suture during draping; the scrub person prepares (in advance) the required items, as heavy sutures (e.g., silk on a cutting needle), needle holders, forceps with teeth, and Mayo straight scissors.
- The back of a #15 knife blade, a needle, or a sterile marking pen (indelible ink) may be used to mark the incision; methylene blue is not used, as the dye causes an inflammatory reaction on nervous tissue.
- *When the laser is employed, all safety precautions must be observed; for safe usage,* *see p. 94.*
- The equipment (ESU, suction, microscope, drills, etc.) is best connected after the "sterile" team members are in position, to prevent tripping accidents. Devices are available for cord and tubing containment. Before the skin incision is made, all necessary equipment should be connected and ready for use.

- Check with surgeon regarding the settings for ESUs; a suggestion for the usual amounts: for the monopolar unit (e.g., BLEND 2, CUT 50, COAG 50), bipolar 45, micro-bipolar 20.
- Care is taken by all team members (the circulator, in particular) to avoid potential burn injuries caused by electrosurgery. The circulator documents the appearance of the patient's skin before and after the procedure.
- Two bulb or asepto syringes are filled (always readily available) with saline or Ringer's lactate to minimize heat to surrounding tissues during the use of bipolar coagulation, during drilling to prevent burns from heat produced by the friction, and to keep the brain tissue moist to prevent cortical injury due to drying.
- Weigh sponges and measure irrigation fluid accurately to determine blood loss replacement.
- When PMMA or cyanoacrylate is used to coat an aneurysm within the cranium, all surrounding brain tissue must be protected by moistened cottonoids.
- Aneurysm clips are applied using the applier that is specific for that type of clip; clips should be discarded after being compressed.
- *In the event of an incorrect count, the floor, shoe soles, under the drapes, etc., should be checked. Before calling for an x-ray to be taken, check the suction canister's contents and filters for cottonoids or any other small object.*
- To facilitate counting, used cottonoids and cotton balls may be placed on a covered Mayo stand (grouped according to type).
- The circulator should pay particular attention to the safe transfer of the patient from the OR table onto the gurney postoperatively; the numerous lines, catheters, tubes, drains, etc., must not be kinked, tangled, or pulled out.
- The circulator accompanies the patient along with the anesthesia provider to PACU or neurology intensive care unit (NICU); he/she gives the PACU or NICU RN all information pertinent to continuity of care.
- Upon the patient's arrival, and at intervals in the PACU or NICU, the perioperative practitioner monitors the patient's vital signs, and continuously assesses the patient's pain level, level of consciousness, and neurological status (i.e., strength and movement of extremities). The dressing is observed for bleeding. All data, interventions, and patient outcomes are documented in the **Perioperative Record** (postoperative section).

Cranioplasty

Definition

Repair of a defect in the skull (cranium).

Discussion

Cranial defects can occur as the result of skull fractures, infections, or surgical procedures such as cranial bone biopsy or ***craniectomy*** or as a congenital deformity. Over the years, many materials have been used as a substitute for creating a synthetic cranial bone section. Problems that resulted were not only technical, i.e., the mechanics, but also, and of greater concern, the rate of infection. There is no perfect substitute for the cranium; even the reimplantation of calvarial bone has had significant infection rates.

Indications for cranioplasty include protection of the brain from external trauma (with the inevitable neurological deficits caused by swelling), the alleviation of pain or seizures, and cosmesis. The substituted portion of the cranium may be autogenous (e.g., iliac bone graft) when the defect is small. The bone grafts taken from the iliac crests are inordinately painful postoperatively, making some physicians avoid taking the autologous graft. Metal (e.g., titanium) may be fashioned to create the missing bone, but it is infrequently employed, as it is difficult to mold. The cranial substitute most often used is an acrylic composed of biocompatible PMMA. PMMA can be "molded" easily and is the preferred material for cranioplasty, particularly when the defect is large. The surgeon fashions a template of wire mesh that is incorporated into the PMMA that is molded to fit over the defect.

Newer substitutes have included a biocomposite material (hydroxyapatite) and an alumina-ceramic with a heavy hydroxyapatite mesh.

The patient's own calvarial bone (when resected) may be saved in the bone bank [e.g., preserved in 100% alcohol at −4°F (−20°C)] and autoclaved before it is reinserted. The bone is secured with titanium clamps. This has been done with pediatric patients, but there is a significant amount of bone resorption.

In the field of bioengineering, custom prostheses for cranioplasty have been developed, employing ***rapid prototyping technology*** to produce models made of biocomposite material (hydroxyapatite) from 3D CT data. Done preoperatively, the prosthesis is manufactured to precisely fit the defect, thus saving considerable time in the OR. This technology is not yet in widespread use.

Cranioplasty may be performed in conjunction with the initial craniectomy or as an interval procedure. The latter is described.

Procedure

Cranioplasty is described. The scalp is incised over the defect. A ledge is formed to seat the prosthetic substitute. If the patient's own cranial bone flap (i.e., craniectomy) was saved, it must be retrieved from the hospital's bone bank.

The following describes the general directions for creating a PMMA acrylic substitute to replace the bone defect. The PMMA bone substitute must be made according to the manufacturer's directions. One volume of liquid monomer is mixed with one volume of powdered polymer (the powder and liquid are premeasured by the manufacturer). The "cement" ingredients are mixed until dough-like. The "dough" is then placed in a polyethylene bag and rolled flat (while in the bag). PMMA is removed from the polyethylene bag; the surgeon then molds the material accordingly to fit the defect. Heavy metal mesh may be incorporated into the PMMA material. (The PMMA mixture becomes very warm after it is mixed and turns hard in 7 minutes.) When cooled, the excess material may be trimmed with rongeurs or a power saw.

A craniotome may be used to smooth rough spots. A high-speed drill is used to place holes in the periphery of the acrylic plate to correspond with holes drilled into the cranium. The substitute plate is placed over the cranial defect and secured by stainless steel wire sutures passed through the holes. The wound is irrigated (usually with an antibiotic solution) and closed.

For **Preparation of the Patient, Skin Preparation,** and **Draping,** see **Craniotomy,** pp. 649, 651–652.

Equipment

Suction
ESU (2); monopolar and bipolar (e.g., Malis)
Power sources (2) for power saw and power drill

Instrumentation

Craniotomy tray (includes wire cutter)
Kerrison, Rongeurs, and pituitary forceps tray
Stainless steel roller
Raney clip applier/remover
Bipolar bayonet forceps with "micro" tip and cord
Power saw or craniotome and cord
High-speed power drill or micro drill and cord with burr, drill bits, drill sleeve, and key

Supplies

Antiembolitic hose, when requested
Marking pen (sterile, indelible ink)
Local anesthetic with epinephrine (to inject site of incision for hemostasis), paper labels and marking pen
Control syringes and needles
Sterile, plastic adhesive drape (if craniotomy sheet with insert is unavailable)

Basin set
Blades, (2) #10
Needle magnet or counter
Electrosurgical pencil and cord with holder and scraper
Suction tubing
Graduated pitcher, bulb syringes (2), antibiotic irrigation (optional)
Bone wax
PMMA and mixing container
Stainless steel wire sutures (reattach cranial prosthesis)
Cottonoids, variety, particularly large (e.g., 1″ × 3″)

Special Notes

- See **Special Notes** from ***Craniotomy***, p. 655, as applicable.
- **N.B.** ***Extra precautions must be taken to correctly identify the pediatric patient.*** In addition to checking identification on the wristband, chart, and addressograph plate, the parent or legal guardian should be asked to corroborate the child's identity and chart information (e.g., allergies).
- PMMA cement must be mixed according to the manufacturer's directions. The materials are sold as a unit with separate packages containing the powder, the liquid, and a mixing container.

Transsphenoidal Hypophysectomy

Definition

Excision or destruction of all (or a portion) of the pituitary gland.

Discussion

Hypophysectomy is performed for endocrine disorders, primary tumors of the pituitary, some presentations of diabetic retinopathy, and hormonally dependent metastatic breast and prostatic carcinoma. Its use in control of other malignancies is controversial (e.g., malignant melanoma, hypernephroma, thyroid cancer). Diabetes insipidus results from hypophysectomy; it can be controlled with Pitressin®/vasopressin (anti-diuretic hormone) replacement. More than 90% removal of the gland is usually necessary to effect the theraputic results. In addition, the several hormones elaborated by the anterior pituitary (tropins) must be compensated for by the administration of exogenous hormones (e.g., thyroid). Radiotherapy to ablate the pituitary by either interstitial radiation (placed by stereotactic approaches) or external beam radiation (including Gamma knife) may provide less than favorable results. Open craniotomy presents greater stress and risk to these patients, who are often fragile.

Stereotactic hypophysectomy employs an integrated computer-controlled system. The patient's head is secured in a stereotactic frame, e.g., CRW-3. Preoperatively the patient undergoes computerized axial tomography, tomographic pneumoencephalography, and vascular angiography. Using coordinates thus established, the surgeon places the patient in the same frame in the OR. The patient is anesthetized and the position checked by computerized fluoroscopic control. A drill is used to perforate the sphenoid sinus and the floor of the sella turcica; the opening is enlarged by rongeurs, as necessary. A cryoprobe is placed in the sella turcica (position predetermined) via cannula.

Cryodestruction of the pituitary is then performed. On removal of the probe, a plug of muscle, fat, or silicone is placed in the sellar opening to prevent cerebrospinal fluid leakage. The approach may be transnasal or sublabial. This procedure may be performed in a specially designed radiology suite or a specially designed OR.

The procedure may be performed as **endoscopic transsphenoidal hypophysectomy.**

Procedure

The transnasal approach is described. General anesthesia is administered by endotracheal tube. When a "plug" of muscle, fascia lata, or fat will be used, it is taken before the transnasal procedure. A patch of fascia lata, fat, or muscle is excised (from the previously prepared thigh) and packed into the empty sella. The tissue plug is kept moist in a solution of normal saline with an antibiotic. The nasal mucosa is infiltrated with a local anesthetic containing epinephrine to minimize blood loss and aid in elevation of the mucosa. An incision is made into the nasal cavity. The mucosa is elevated, and a portion of the cartilaginous septum is excised and saved in a saline-soaked sponge. Using a bivalve nasal speculum, the floor of the sphenoidal sinus is exposed and incised by rongeur. The boundaries of the sella are determined by direct vision with microscope and by fluoroscopy. The sella is entered in the midline; a sphenoidal punch is used to enlarge the opening, exposing the dura of the pituitary fossa. The dura is incised avoiding entry into the pituitary capsule. The gland is dissected extracapsularly, and the stalk is identified. Care is taken not to penetrate the posterior wall of the sella. Again, fluoroscopy confirms the position of the instruments. A sickle knife or scissors may be used to sever the stalk; ligating clips (e.g., Hemoclips) may be used prior to amputation. Further dissection, with a specifically designed blunt dissector, frees the remainder of the gland from its dural attachments, and the gland is delivered intact. Gelfoam soaked in thrombin is used to control oozing.

The previously excised "plug" patch of fascia lata, fat, or muscle is packed into the empty sella. A segment of previously excised cartilaginous nasal septum or sphenoid is used to seal the floor of the sella, "snapping" it into place. Antibiotics may be instilled. Nasal packing may be employed to support the bony fragments. The thigh incision (donor site) is closed.

Endoscopic Approach. The nasal septum is not incised. Following anterior sphenoidotomy, an endoscope is passed transnasally and mounted to an endoscope holder; use of a microscope may not be necessary. The endoscopic instruments are passed and manipulated parallel to the scope (not within, as the scope diameter is 4 to 5 mm, 0° or 30°). A nasal speculum is not needed. The procedure performed is otherwise similar to that described above.

Preparation of the Patient

Antiembolitic hose are applied. The procedure is usually performed under general anesthesia with endotracheal intubation. The patient is supine with the head positioned in a halo head frame with stereotactic cage, the head tilted slightly to the left (when the right nostril or right sublabial area is employed). The arms may be padded and tucked in at the patient's sides, or they may be extended on padded armboards. One thigh (usually the right) is not restrained by the safety belt to provide access to obtain the muscle or fat tissue graft. After the patient is prepped and draped, the nasal cavity is infiltrated with local anesthetic containing epinephrine (notify anesthesia provider when doing so). An electrosurgical dispersive pad is applied.

Skin Preparation

Two prep sets are required. Check with the surgeon for the type of solution to be used and the area to be prepped; the area may include the face and oral and nasal cavities. In addition to the prep set (used for the face), include bayonet forceps, nasal speculum, long cotton-tipped applicators, medicine cup, and hemostat on the tray.

Do not permit the prep solution to run into the eyes; eye ointment, eye pads, and shields may be placed. ***Do not permit*** solution to pool in the ear; a cotton plug is placed in the ear. ***Do not permit*** solution to pool under the patient, as the solution excoriates the skin. In addition, when a flammable solution pools under the patient, it creates a fire hazard.

The second prep set is used for the graft site; the thigh is prepped from the knee to the groin and down to the table at the sides.

Draping

Towels are placed around the periphery of the patient's face and the intended site of incision on the thigh. A sterile plastic adhesive drape is placed over the face and the exposed thigh, taking care not to contaminate either sterile field. A laparotomy sheet may be used when the entire face is to be exposed; the laparotomy sheet covers the upper part of the body. The graft area on the thigh is surrounded with drape sheets. A drape sheet or towel is placed over the face until access is needed.

Drapes are also needed for the C-arm image intensifier and the microscope (when used).

Equipment

Head frame, e.g., halo
Stereotactic cage, e.g., BRW, CRW-3
Suction
ESU (2), bipolar and monopolar
Microscope, e.g., Zeiss or Omni (not for endoscopic procedure)
Image intensifier (with C-arm)
Monitor(s) and VHS VCR
Camera console
Fiber-optic headlight and light source (available)
Laser console, optional

Instrumentation

Limited procedure trays (2)
Nasal instruments tray, optional
Bipolar bayonet forceps with "micro" tip and cord
Bivalve nasal speculum (long blades), sphenoidal punch forceps, small ring curettes (angled), Hardy's enucleator (angled), pituitary spoon (angled), micro scissors (straight, curved, angled), micro dissectors (angled), sickle knife (angled)

Endoscopic

Electrosurgical irrigator/light fountain (e.g., Malis with foot control), computer-guided navigation system, and fiber-optic light source
Rigid neuroendoscopes 4 to 5 mm, 0° or 30° with camera and optical bridge, surgical tips (similar to the above instruments) attached to the tip of the telescope, electrosurgical suction-irrigator and cord, pituitary cupping forceps (1 mm), grasping-type forceps (1 mm), and laser fiber

Supplies

Antiembolitic hose
Sterile plastic drapes (2)
Basin set
Blades, (1) #10, (2) #15, (1) #12
Needle magnet or counter
Electrosurgical pencil and cord with holder and scraper
Suction tubing
Bulb syringes (2) and antibiotic irrigation (optional)

Cottonoids, e.g., ½″ × ½″, ½″ × 1″ (sizes most frequently used)
Syringe (e.g., 10 ml, control), spinal needle, and local anesthetic with epinephrine in small bowl
Paper labels and sterile marking pen
Bone wax
Nasal packing (e.g., ½″ petrolatum-impregnated gauze) and antibiotic powder
Hemostatic agents (e.g., Gelfoam and thrombin, Surgicel, Avitene)

Special Notes

- See **Special Notes** from ***Craniotomy***, p. 655, as applicable.
- **N.B.** *Always take extra precautions to correctly identify the pediatric patient.*
- When fluoroscopy is employed, lead aprons are worn. The scrub person should don a lead vest before scrubbing. Observe all x-ray safety precautions; see p. 52.
- A second tray of instruments and a second Mayo stand may be used for taking the muscle tissue graft.
- Materials should be readily available for aerobic and anaerobic cultures.
- A syringe, 20 ml, may be used to force rinse a Frazier suction tip after a stylet is used to unclog it.

Ventricular Shunts

Definition

Insertion of a catheter and valve system to divert the flow of cerebrospinal fluid (CSF) from the brain's ventricular system and the subarachnoid space to the peritoneal or pleural cavities or the right atrium.

Discussion

Shunting CSF from the ventricles may be performed to treat hydrocephalus (congenital, neoplastic, traumatic, and infectious). The distal end of the shunt is placed in the peritoneal cavity, unless contraindicated. If peritoneal placement cannot be performed, the shunt may be placed intrapleurally via thoracostomy or into the right atrium via the internal jugular vein. The advantages of peritoneal (or pleural) over atrial placement of the distal catheter are avoidance of vascular and cardiopulmonary complications, faster, simpler placement of the distal catheter, and relative ease of revision. The pleural shunt, if intrapleural absorption is reduced, can lead to pulmonary compression with fluid accumulation. Shunts are available with the distal catheter attached, avoiding the problems that occurred previously with disconnection and potential contamination.

Most shunts respond to the different pressures between the ventricle and the cavity into which they drain, e.g., ***pressure differential shunts.*** The modern shunts (e.g., Codman-Hakim programmable shunt and the Medtronic Strata Valve programmable shunt) are made so that the device prevents "over-shunting"; some shunts are programmable by a magnetic field transmitted through the skin.

Some types of late-onset hydrocephalus may be treated by **third ventriculostomy,** in which the need for a shunt is obviated; see third ventriculostomy, p. 647.

Procedure

Ventriculoperitoneal Shunt for Hydrocephalus. Lines are marked for a right-sided shunt incision (several centimeters above and posterior to the ear) and a transverse right-upper-quadrant incision of the abdomen. The scalp is incised and reflected on its base. Bleeding is controlled electrosurgically. Burr holes are made. Bleeding is checked at the burr hole site in the periosteum, and a self-retaining retractor is placed. The dura mater (outer layer covering the brain) is incised. Bipolar electrosurgery is used to seal the dura to the pia and cortex. A straight ventricular catheter is passed into the posterior aspect of the lateral ventricle, the stylet is removed, and the opening pressure is recorded. A premeasured length of catheter is advanced anterior to the foramen of Munro. Fluoroscopy confirms catheter placement. An incision is made through the scalp behind the ear, and a pocket is created to accommodate the valve (and reservoir, if included). A limited abdominal incision is carried down to the anterior rectus sheath. The distal portion of the shunt catheter is passed (tunneled) from the scalp incision subcutaneously via the neck and thorax to the abdominal incision.

The valve/reservoir is attached to the proximal (intraventricular) catheter. The valve mechanism is placed in the subgaleal space behind the ear. If not incorporated into the valve, the distal catheter is attached to the valve. The peritoneum is exposed, seized, and incised to permit passage of the distal end of the catheter. Wounds may be irrigated with antibiotic solution. The abdominal wound is closed. An antibiotic may be injected into the ventricle through the reservoir after compression of the valve. The incision is closed.

Note: A reservoir can be periodically compressed to assure patency of the system. The reservoir is available for percutaneous needle manometry.

Preparation of the Patient

Special consideration is given the pediatric patient; see **Pediatric General Information**, p. 978, for measures to maintain pediatric patient's body temperature, to restrain the extremities, etc. For the adult patient, antiembolitic hose may be applied. The patient is supine with a small pad placed under the right thorax; the arms are extended on padded armboards. For right-side shunt placement, the patient's head is slightly elevated and gently turned to the left; a padded gel donut headrest, Mayfield Infinity skull clamp with Mayfield Infinity Support System horseshoe with gel pad (pediatric), or Mayfield skull clamp (adult) may be used. Fluoroscopy or x-rays confirm the correct placement of the proximal and distal catheters.

Skin Preparation

Two prep sets are used. Check with the surgeon regarding areas to be prepped and the solution to be used. The head is shaved in the OR as close as possible to the time of the skin incision (most often by the surgeon). For shunt placement on the right side, include the right lateral aspect of the scalp and face to the orbital rim, the neck and clavicular area, and down to the table at the sides. Use the second set to continue the prep from the right clavicular area to include the right thorax and abdomen and down to the table at the sides.

Do not permit the prep solution to run into the eyes; eye ointment, eye pads, and shields may be placed. Do not let solution to pool in the ear; a cotton plug is placed in the ear. ***Do not permit*** solution to pool under the patient.

Draping

The surgeon usually does the draping. Folded towels are placed around the two operative sites. A cuffed drape sheet is placed under the right side. Drape sheets are placed about the head and the bottom of the table. The superior tip of the ear may be bent gently forward and sutured to the facial skin (to keep it out of the field). A craniotomy sheet with a plastic adhesive insert is used. A sterile, plastic adhesive drape is placed over the second incision site (abdominal), followed by a drape sheet with a small fenestration. The second site is covered with a sheet or towel until access is needed.

Equipment

Padded gel donut headrest (adult and pediatric), optional
Pediatric headrest, e.g., Mayfield Infinity skull clamp with Mayfield Infinity Support System horseshoe with gel pad, optional
Adult head-fixation device, e.g., Mayfield skull clamp, optional
Body heat maintenance equipment, e.g., heating lamps overhead, for infants, and a warming mattress pad on the table, e.g., K-

Thermia pad or forced-air warming blanket (adult), when ordered. For the many additional considerations regarding the pediatric patient in surgery, see p. 978.

Restraints, soft-padded (pediatric)

Suction

ESU (2); monopolar and biopolar (e.g., Malis)

Power source for high-speed power drill or micro drill

Scale to weigh sponges, optional

Instrumentation

Craniotomy tray

Limited procedure tray (abdominal incision)

Bayonet bipolar forceps and cord (e.g., Malis)

Power drill (e.g., micro Stryker) and cord

Shunt (e.g., Codman-Hakim programmable shunt or Medtronic Strata Valve programmable shunt)

Small bulldog clamps (4)

Uterine packing forceps or a long narrow passing instrument (tunneling)

Supplies

Antiembolitic hose (adult)

Sterile plastic adhesive drape (if craniotomy sheet with insert is unavailable)

Basin set

Blades, (4) #15 (2) for each incision, cranial and reservoir site

Needle magnet or counter

Electrosurgical pencil with needle tip, cord, holder, and scraper

Suction tubing

Plastic syringe (e.g., 3 ml) and blunt needle (e.g., 18 gauge) to pump through shunt reservoir and tubing

Cottonoids, e.g., variety, particularly $1/2'' \times 1/2''$

Hemostatic agents, e.g., compressed Gelfoam (sponges) soaked in thrombin, spray or powder thrombin, Surgicel, Fibrillar, and Avitene

Bone wax

Graduated pitcher, bulb syringes (2), and antibiotic irrigation (optional)

Special Notes

- *Apply* **Special Notes** *from* **Craniotomy,** *p. 655, as applicable.*
- **N.B.** Always take extra precautions to correctly identify the pediatric patient.

- Check with the surgeon and anesthesia provider regarding measures to prevent loss of body heat, such as increasing room temperature, heating lamps, warming mattress, and wrapping extremities. Use warmed solutions.
- Employ measures to protect the skin, such as hypoallergenic tape (to tape eyes shut) and application of tincture of benzoin under adhesive tape used in positioning. Check patient's chart regarding allergies before applying tape; if patient is allergic, document the tape substituted in the **Perioperative Record.**
- Document the appearance of the skin at the sites of tape application preoperatively and immediately postoperatively.
- Do not allow prep solution to pool under the patient, as prep solution may excoriate the skin. Also, pooled prep solution poses a fire threat.
- Notify the x-ray department before the surgery starts regarding the necessity for equipment such as a portable x-ray machine or fluoroscopy unit. Observe x-ray safety precautions; see p. 52.
- Consult the surgeon and anesthesia provider regarding whether sponges are to be weighed; obtain necessary equipment.
- Follow hospital policy for recording insertion of an implant, as some facilities request documentation in a hospital log.
- Check that the valve (in the shunt) is patent with normal saline before use. Use a plastic syringe (3 ml) and blunt needle (e.g., 18 gauge) to pump through shunt reservoir and tubing.
- **N.B.** Flush the shunt with saline or Ringer's solution (surgeon's preference); do *not* allow air into the shunt.
- **N.B.** ***Regarding the shunt unit,*** handle the shunt only as much as absolutely necessary. Avoid contact with lint or other foreign materials; do not place the unit on gauze sponges. Always place the unit in a basin. The valve must be properly oriented to allow one-way passage of fluid only. Antibiotic solution may be used for irrigation.

Laminectomy

Definition

Laminectomy is the removal of one or more vertebral laminae.

Discussion

Indications for laminectomy, hemilaminectomy, and an interlaminar procedure include herniated disc, compression fracture, dislocation, and spinal cord tumor. Patients who have severe spinal pain and myelopathy that may be exhibited by numbness, decreased motor strength, decreased reflexes, and extremity weakness that cannot be controlled by nonoperative measures are candidates for laminectomy. CT scans may be employed to confirm diagnosis. Other procedures may be performed in conjunction with laminectomy, such as **cordotomy,** that is, the division of the anterolateral quadrant of the spinothalamic tract of the spinal cord for intractable pain, and **rhizotomy,** the interruption of spinal (sensory or posterior) nerve roots for relief of intractable pain and the division of motor (anterior) roots for uncontrolled spastic conditions.

Degenerative disc disease (with accompanying disc protrusion, spinal cord stenosis, myelopathy, spondylitis, and osteophyte formation) unresponsive to conservative medical therapies may be treated by discectomy and **spinal bone fusion. Cortical ringbone grafting** (allograft) can be performed using internal fixation; locking plates are employed.

Prior to an open operative approach for **cordotomy** (see p. 686) or **rhizotomy** (see p. 688), imaging-guided percutaneous injection of absolute alcohol, phenol, or glycerol or use of ***radio-frequency ablation*** may be considered. Similarly, for unilateral-level disc herniation, **microdiscectomy** or **percutaneous discectomy** can be performed. Alternative procedures for herniated disc with limited application include the injection of ***chymopapain*** and ***electrothermal ablation*** of the herniated portion of the nucleus pulposis.

An additional modality for treating degenerative lumbar disc disease that can avoid fusion is ***prosthetic disc replacement.*** A synthetic disc is implanted to replace the existing diseased intervertebral disc; original disc space is restored, thereby alleviating subsequent nerve compression. Special user-friendly instrumentation has been developed for use with this new modality. Disc-replacement procedures enhance pain reduction and shock absorption while preserving spinal mobility. The ***Charite® Artificial Disc*** consists of three components, two toothed metal alloy end plates and a biconvex polyethylene spacer that shifts dynamically within the disc space during spinal motion. A similar unit, ***ProDisc®***, that can be used for multi-level diseased discs has Food and Drug Administration approval.

Procedure

Laminectomy for herniated intervertebral disc is described. A midline vertical incision may be used. The wound is deepened with a knife or, more frequently, with an electrosurgical pencil. Self-retaining retractors are placed, and the fascia is incised. The paraspinous muscles and periosteum are reflected (this may be done unilaterally on the side of the involved disc). Sponges are packed along the vertebrae with a periosteal elevator to aid in blunt dissection and effect hemostasis. A larger retractor (e.g., Beckman, Taylor, or Scoville) is placed for exposure. Small portions of the laminae overlying the herniated disc are removed with a Kerrison rongeur; portions of vertebral spines and intervertebral facets may also be excised. Hemostasis is achieved with bone wax. The ligamentum flavum is incised; care is taken to avoid injury to the epidural veins. If the monopolar electrosurgery is employed, the vein is held away from the dura to prevent thermal injury to neural tissues. Moistened cottonoids are placed to protect the dura. Additional ligament or bone may be removed to provide adequate exposure. Nerve roots are cautiously retracted, exposing the herniated disc, which is removed with a pituitary rongeur and curettes; anteriorly, care is exercised to avoid the aorta and vena cava and the branches of the vertebral venous plexus. The wound is irrigated. The area is examined to ensure that all protruding disc has been removed. Hemostasis is achieved (bipolar electrocoagulating forceps). The wound is closed in layers.

Microdiscectomy. The operating microscope may be employed; a limited (<5 cm) vertical (or transverse) incision is made over the appropriate intervertebral space, as confirmed radiographically by fluoroscopy. Hemilaminotomy with incision of the ligamentum flavum is performed. The nerve root is protected and the disc is excised as noted above. The epidural space is explored to make certain that there is no further compression on the nerve root. After hemostasis is achieved, the wound is irrigated and closed.

Percutaneous Discectomy. Several modifications of this technique are performed. The procedure may be performed under local anesthesia with *conscious sedation*, allowing the patient to vocalize pain produced by nerve root contact. Under fluoroscopic guidance (C-arm), a trocar and K-wire is passed into the disc. An incision is made to permit passage of an automated dilator assembly via cannula (e.g., Medtronic) to be passed over the wire or trocar. The L-5 to S-1 space is the most difficult to cannulate; the table may be flexed or extended to facilitate passage of the cannula. An automated cutting and irrigating probe (Nucleotome, Clarus Medical) is passed through the cannula and, after final confirmation of placement, activated, removing disc fragments (15 to 30 minutes). **Endoscopic discectomy** technique employs a rigid endoscope through which disc fragments are removed with fine bone-biting forceps, etc. (see ***Cervical Discectomy and Fusion,*** p. 682). Still another technique employs a **Nd:YAG, Ho:YAG, or KTP laser** fiber that is passed through a 20-cm 18-gauge needle radiologically controlled to ablate the extruded disc material.

Note: These limited-access procedures have a 50% to 80% success rate and the patient is informed of same preoperatively. Conversion to an open disc fusion or another type of disc procedure performed through a standard "open" laminectomy may become necessary.

Preparation of the Patient

Antiembolitic hose (e.g., TED) may be applied to the legs to prevent venous stasis and to help maintain blood pressure. The position of the patient depends on the type of laminectomy to be performed, the approach, and the surgeon's preference. Cervical laminectomy is most frequently performed in the sitting position. Thoracic and lumbar laminectomies are most frequently performed in the prone or a modified knee-chest position. Occasionally, the lateral position is used for thoracic or lumbar laminectomy. General anesthesia is employed with endotracheal intubation. For all patient positions on any table, all bony prominences and areas prone to skin and neurovascular pressure or trauma are padded. Apply electrosurgical dispersive pad.

Sitting. The patient is supine with knees over the lower break of the table. The head of the table is raised from the middle break. The foot of the table is lowered; a padded footboard supports the feet. The arms are placed in the patient's lap on a pillow and secured with padded restraints. The safety strap is secured above the knees. The head of the table is removed and the Mayfield (skull) clamp (or similar) is secured to a table extension (cervical laminectomy).

Prone. While the patient is on the gurney or the hospital bed, the patient is carefully rolled over to the prone position onto the Andrews table, the Jackson table (with or without the Wilson frame), or the standard OR table (e.g., Ritter). The arms are extended on armboards angled toward the head of the table with the forearms pronated. Chest rolls are placed under the thorax and abdomen to facilitate respiration. A pillow or roll is placed in front of the ankles to prevent undue pressure on the toes. Pads are placed under the elbows and knees. Female breasts and male genitalia are protected from pressure. The safety strap is secured across the patient's thighs. A sterile plastic adhesive drape may be placed on the buttocks (to isolate the perianal area from the field) prior to the skin prep.

Modified Knee-Chest. The patient, on the gurney or the hospital bed, is carefully rolled over to the prone position onto the Andrews table, the Jackson table (with or without the Wilson frame), or the standard OR table (e.g., Ritter). When the standard OR table is used, adjust the patient's position so that the hips are over the middle break in the table. Chest rolls are placed under the thorax and abdomen to facilitate respiration. The arms are extended on armboards angled toward the head of the table with the forearms pronated. Pads are placed under the elbows and knees. Female breasts and male genitalia are protected from pressure. The foot of the table is lowered, and a padded footrest extension may be added on, perpendicular to the table. A pillow is placed in front of the legs, and a roll is placed in front of the ankles to prevent undue pressure on the toes. The patient's position is secured with the safety strap across the thighs. If using wide adhesive tape across the thighs, check chart for patient allergies; tincture of benzoin is employed prior to applying tape. A sterile plastic adhesive drape may be placed on the buttocks to isolate the perianal area out of the field. After the patient is positioned, apply electrosurgical dispersive pad.

For ***cervical laminectomy***, hair on the lower portion of the scalp (supra-auricular border) and the neck may be removed in the operating room. Hair on the top of the head need not be removed (for this procedure). Long hair is secured at the top of the head. Hair (in the designated area) is cut off or clipped with electric clippers prior to shaving. The operative site is then shaved with warm water, scrub solution (preferably containing iodofor; check chart for sensitivity or allergy), and disposable razor.

Skin Preparation

Check with the surgeon regarding hair removal and the skin area to be prepped. Hair is usually shaved in the OR by the circulator.

Cervical. Prep solution is applied to the insertion sites of the pins; some hair will probably need to be shaved. Begin cleansing at the midline, extending from the supra-auricular border to the level of the axillae and down to the table at the neck and shoulders.

Thoracic. Begin cleansing at the midline, extending from the base of the skull to the level of the waist and down to the table at the neck, shoulders, and sides.

Lumbar. Begin cleansing at the midline, extending from the shoulders to the coccyx (or the adhesive drape) and down to the table at the sides.

Draping

The surgeon usually prefers to do the draping. Folded towels are placed around the operative site and secured with towel clips, staples, or sutures. (To suture towels, the surgeon uses heavy silk sutures on a cutting needle, needle holder, toothed forceps, and suture scissors.) The field is covered with a sheet with an appropriate-sized fenestration inset with plastic adhesive, or a sterile plastic adhesive drape may be used.

Drapes are required for microscope and portable fluoroscopy unit.

Equipment

Sequential compression device with disposable leg wraps, if requested

Do not use any type of warming mattress

Forced-air warming blanket or temperature regulating blanket

Table extension for seating the headrest and (cervical) headrest device, e.g., Mayfield skull clamp
Pillows, padding, chest rolls, elbow pads, heel cups, gel pads, and/or padded restraints depending on the position and type of table used
Temperature-monitoring device, e.g., esophageal thermometer to anesthesia provider
Fiber-optic light sources for retractors, headlight, endoscopy, e.g., Xenon 300 W Doppler console
High-speed power source for power drill and saw (or self-contained)
Magnifying loupes or operating microscope (e.g., Zeiss or Omni), optional
Suction
ESU (2), monopolar and bipolar, e.g., Malis
Portable fluoroscopy unit (call x-ray department)
Lead aprons for team members
Laser (e.g., CO_2, Ho:YAG, or Nd:YAG), optional; see safety precautions, p. 94
CUSA console, optional

Instrumentation

Laminectomy tray
Kerrison rongeurs and pituitary forceps tray
Nerve hooks (blunt and micro), small angled curettes
Power drill (e.g., micro Stryker), drill bits and burr (5 mm; cervical), drill sleeves, and cord (or self-contained, e.g., battery)
Distraction pins (cervical) and vertebral body distractor (disc fusion)
Locking plates with vertebral screws (cortical bone ring in disc fusion for allograft)
Bipolar electrosurgical forceps (insulated)
Allograft bone (freeze-dried) and allograft bone sizers (disc fusion)

Supplies

Antiembolitic hose
Sterile, plastic adhesive drapes (2); perianal and incision sites
Basin set
Suction tubing
Blades, (2) #10, (1) #15, (1) #11
Needle magnet or counter
Electrosurgical pencil and cord with holder and scraper
Bone wax
Graduated pitcher, bulb or asepto syringes (2), antibiotic irrigation (optional)
Gelfoam in thrombin (e.g., 5000 units), Surgicel

Roller gauze, 2″ (to hold retractor, lumbar)
Cottonoids (variety, e.g., 1/2″ × 1/2″, 1″ × 1″)
Peanut/Kittner dissectors, optional
Antibiotic irrigation (optional)
Closure absorbable sutures and staples or nonabsorbable suture (as desired)

Special Notes

- Apply **Special Notes** from ***Abdominal Laparotomy***, p. 134, as they apply to all patients in surgery (e.g., regarding correct identification of the patient, observing ***"time out,"*** etc.).
- **N.B.** Take extra precautions to correctly identify the pediatric patient; see Pediatric General Information, p. 978.
- The circulator conveys emotional support to the patient. Assess patient's physical and emotional needs (assess anxiety). Employing measures as maintaining eye contact, using touch to convey caring, holding the patient's hand during the administration of anesthesia, offering a warm blanket, etc., is essential.
- Documentation in the **Perioperative Record** of nursing care, pertinent observations, interventions, and their outcomes are required for continuity of care of the patient and for medicolegal reasons.
- The circulator may provide the patient a measure of comfort to help to reduce anxiety by explaining that he/she will act as the patient's advocate.
- The circulator is responsible for obtaining adequate assistance (before anesthesia is induced) to safely move the patient and to protect the employees involved in positioning the patient from injury.
- **Reminder:** Team members can prevent musculoskeletal injuries by using methods that employ ergodynamic movements when lifting, moving, and positioning the patient.
- *Document the appearance and condition of the patient's skin preoperatively and immediately postoperatively.* Avoid injuries to the patient caused by undue pressure on neurovascular structures and the skin overlying bony prominences. The body should be placed in correct anatomical alignment on a well-padded table.
- *Avoid injury to the patient's fingers by preventing them from being caught in the table mechanism when the foot of the table is raised following the procedure.*

- **Reminder:** Use safety precautions to identify, label, and dispense medications or solutions and to avoid medication errors; see p. 30. It is mandatory that all medications and solutions on the sterile field be labeled by name and strength. The medication bottles are retained in the room until the procedure has concluded.
- The skin and underlying tissues may be injected with a vasoconstricting agent such as epinephrine; *advise anesthesia provider accordingly* when they are used.
- **N.B.** *Circulator ascertains that blood is available as ordered and ready for immediate use* ***before*** *the surgery is permitted to begin.*
- The circulator anticipates blood transfusions and obtains items to administer the blood (e.g., tubing set, blood warmer, pressure bag) and assists the anesthesia provider as necessary (to identify patient and blood type, etc.).
- *Circulator documents blood transfusions administered and any reaction or lack of reaction to the transfusions in the* **Perioperative Record.**
- **N.B.** *The Mayfield head clamp is used to "fix" the skull to prevent it from moving; disposable, sterile or reuseable pins (autoclaved) are brought into the room prior to the patient's entry.* Sterility must be maintained as the pins are placed in the device. Prep solution is applied to the scalp areas designated for pin insertion.
- **N.B.** *Keep the headrest device (used for cervical laminectomy) and the pins from the patient's sight, as seeing them may cause undue anxiety.*
- **Reminder:** Ascertain that the *correct* x-ray films, studies, and reports for the *correctly identified* patient are in the room prior to starting the surgery.
- **N.B.** *Surgical team members don lead aprons prior to scrubbing, as fluoroscopy is routinely used.*
- Notify x-ray department when intraoperative fluoroscopy is anticipated. Observe all x-ray safety precautions; see p. 52.
- To avoid contamination when draping, nonpiercing towel clips are used on disposable paper drapes.
- The circulator takes appropriate measures to maintain patient's body temperature, e.g., warmed irrigation fluids and/or a forced-air warming blanket may be used, when ordered.

- The scrub person keeps track of the amount of irrigation used to assist in determining blood loss.
- The scrub person monitors the temperature of the irrigation solution (before passing the filled bulb syringes) to the surgeon to avoid burn injury to the tissues.
- Any items, such as cottonoids and the small parts to instruments (e.g., screws) used during the procedure that could be sequestered in the wound, are included in the count.
- ***When the laser is employed, observe all safety precautions for laser usage; see p. 94.***
- The equipment (ESU, suction, microscope, drills, etc.) is best connected after the "sterile" team members are in position to prevent tripping accidents. Devices are available for cord and tubing containment. Endoscopic procedures require a fiberoptic light source. Before the skin incision is made, all necessary equipment should be connected and ready for use.
- When the Taylor retractor is used during lumbar laminectomy, after it has been appropriately placed, the surgeon wraps the roller gauze around the tail of the retractor and drops the roll to the circulator, who secures it to the table.
- Care is taken by all team members (the circulator, in particular) to avoid potential burn injuries caused by electrosurgery and pressure injuries to skin in areas covering bony prominences. The circulator documents the appearance of the patient's skin before and after the procedure.
- Saline irrigation is used to minimize heat to surrounding tissues with the use of bipolar coagulation and during drilling to prevent burns from heat produced by the friction.
- The circulator accompanies the patient and the anesthesia provider to the PACU or NICU. Special attention is paid to the safe transfer of the patient postoperatively to the gurney in the OR and to the PACU. Care is taken so that the numerous lines, catheters, tubes, drains, etc., are not kinked, tangled, or pulled out as the patient is transferred.
- The circulator employs measures to maintain patient's temperature en route to PACU and sees that the Ambu bag is readily available. He/she gives the perioperative practitioner in the PACU any information pertinent to continuity of care of the patient.

- Upon patient's arrival (and at intervals) in the PACU, the perioperative practitioner monitors and documents the patient's vital signs. He/she assesses pain level, level of consciousness, and neurological status (i.e., strength and movement of extremities). The amount of bleeding on the dressing is also observed and documented.

Percutaneous Vertebroplasty and Kyphoplasty

Definition

Vertebroplasty is the repair of vertebral fractures via minimal access approach by the (percutaneous) injection of bone cement (PMMA with a contrast medium) into the fractures, employing radiographic guidance (fluoroscopy).

Kyphoplasty is a vertebroplasty performed by re-expanding the vertebral body collapse configuration with a balloon catheter and injecting bone cement.

Discussion

Vertebral fractures are common in elderly persons (especially associated with osteoporosis). Many of these fractures are asymptomatic, but when painful and not responsive to medical treatment (e.g., pain medication and a back support), and particularly if kyphosis develops secondary to vertebral body compression, with ensuing loss of mobility and decreased lung capacity, these percutaneous techniques are safe and effective in selected patients.

Vertebroplasty refers to presentations wherein a symptomatic fracture is surgically stabilized by filling the fracture defect.

Kyphoplasty treats the fracture as well, but also by re-expanding the vertebral body collapse configuration with the use of a balloon catheter and injection of cement (usually PMMA).

Ideally this treatment should be done within 8 weeks of the fracture, but as longer periods are often taken for assessment and trial of nonoperative measures, the procedures can be delayed. Partial healing can interfere with the ability to correct the compression; MRI exam may distinguish healing versus local edema. More than a single level can be treated in a single procedure.

Complications of **Percutaneous Vertebroplasty and Kyphoplasty** procedures include:

- Leakage of cement compressing the spinal cord or nerves
- Inadvertent intravascular injection into the vertebral venous plexus with pulmonary embolism (rarely).

These procedures may be performed in the operating room or special procedures radiology suite. Some patients may be discharged the same day as the procedure.

Procedure

Local anesthesia and *conscious sedation* or general anesthesia (e.g., for **kyphoplasty**) is employed. The patient is placed in the prone position. Intravenous antibiotics may be administered. Through a small incision, a thin cannula is passed (employing radiographic guidance) through the pedicle into the body of the involved vertebra or vertebrae to stabilize the fracture; injection of radio-opaque dye confirms placement. **Vertebroplasty** may be performed on both sides of the vertebra; PMMA is injected into the fracture site (requires approximately 10 minutes to harden).

In **kyphoplasty,** a balloon catheter is inserted into the body of the collapsed vertebra. As the balloon is carefully inflated (with radio-opaque contrast dye), the fracture is elevated so that the kyphotic presentation is normalized (correcting the wedging), leaving a space within the vertebral body into which PMMA is injected when the balloon catheter is removed. Two balloon catheters may be used simultaneously if additional force is required to reduce the deformity.

Repair of each level treated takes approximately 1 hour. Unfortunately, even with preoperative assessment to the contrary, the collapsed vertebral fracture may not be able to be reduced.

For **Preparation of the Patient, Skin Preparation,** and **Draping,** see ***Laminectomy***, p. 673.

Equipment

ESU

Instrumentation

Limited procedures tray

Kyphon Kyphoplasty instruments (as suggested by the manufacturer)

KyphX Xpander Inflatable Bone Tamp (Kyphon) and bone needle (for injection of PMMA plus contrast media)

Supplies

Antiembolitic hose, when requested

Sterile plastic adhesive drape

Blades, (2) #15

Control syringe (Luer lok), needle, and local anesthetic

Paper labels and sterile marking pen

Electrosurgical pencil with needle tip and cord with holder and scraper

Kphyx™ HV-R bone cement (PMMA plus contrast media)

Special Notes

- Use **Special Notes** from ***Laminectomy***, p. 676, as applicable.
- The patient is placed in prone position; see prone position for laminectomy, p. 673.
- KyphX® HV-R™ Bone Cement is a commercial product that contains PMMA and radio-opaque barium sulfate, obviating the need for injection of additional contrast dye.
- A kit is available that contains needed items to perform kyphoplasty, such as KyphX Xpander® Inflatable Bone Tamp (Kyphon), and an inflation syringe with a pressure gauge for the expander.
- The PMMA cement is mixed to consistency of thin paste (to be injected under fluoroscopic control). A portable C-arm is used. The surgical team wears lead aprons. Observe all x-ray safety precautions.
- **Reminder:** Use safety precautions to identify, label, and dispense medications or dyes and to avoid medication errors; see p. 30. It is mandatory that all medications and solutions on the sterile field be labeled by name and strength. The medication bottles are retained in the room until the procedure has concluded.

Excision of Cervical Intervertebral Disc with Fusion, Anterior Approach

Definition

The excision of a cervical herniated intervertebral disc and stabilization of the cervical spine.

Discussion

The procedure is indicated when nerve deficits and pain (caused by herniated disc or spondylosis) persist despite conservative medical treatments, such as bed rest and traction. The anterior approach is preferred when spondylotic bars compromise the cord or the nerve root; fluoroscopy identifies the vertebral level (aids in the correct position of the patient on the table). The posterior approach is employed when multiple nerve roots must be decompressed. Fusion is accomplished by the insertion of a bone graft. The bone graft may be taken from the patient's own iliac crest (painful postoperatively); more recently, frozen allografts from the bone donor bank are used.

Degenerative disc disease (with accompanying disc protrusion, spinal stenosis, myelopathy, spondylitis, and osteophyte formation) unresponsive to conservative medical therapies may be treated surgically by **discectomy** and **spinal fusion**. A **cortical ringbone** allograft can be inserted using internal fixation with locking plates. In appropriately selected cases, discectomy and fusion of the cervical spine can be accomplished by anterior endoscopic approach.

Procedure

Excision of Cervical Intervertebral Disc with Fusion, Anterior Approach is described. A transverse incision is made at the level of the cricoid cartilage. The incision is deepened, usually to the right of the midline, retracting the carotid sheath and prevertebral muscles laterally (Weitlaner retractor) and the trachea and esophagus medially to expose the spine. Care is taken to avoid injury to the carotid sheath contents, the vertebral vessels, and the recurrent laryngeal nerve. The anterior longitudinal ligament is incised, exposing the intervertebral disc. The disc level is confirmed by fluoroscopy (using a needle as a marker). After the periosteum has been reflected, a moist sponge is placed in the wound and the wound is covered with a towel while the bone graft is obtained.

A bone autograft from the iliac crest is obtained with an osteotome or a dowel cutter, or an allograft may be obtained from the hospital's bone bank. All bone chips from either site are saved and kept moist for later packing of the fusion site. Fluoroscopy is employed to document the graft site. The iliac crest wound is closed after hemostasis is achieved; a closed-wound drainage system may be placed.

Following closure of the iliac crest wound, the diseased cervical disc is incised and removed piecemeal by rongeurs. Bony spurs compressing the nerve roots may be excised with small rongeurs and/or burrs (5mm). The intervertebral space is packed with the bone graft (and bone chips). A depth gauge or caliper is employed to determine the size required for the bone plug. After hemostasis is achieved, the cervical wound is closed in layers.

The operating microscope or magnifying loupes may be employed.

Endoscopic Discectomy with Fusion, Anterior Approach is described. The patient is in the supine position with a support (IV fluid bag, sandbag, rolled towel, etc.) placed under both shoulders (to best accentuate exposure of the operative level). Radiologic imaging confirms the location of the diseased disc. A limited incision (less than 2 cm) is made between the sternomastoid muscle just to the right of the midline at the chosen level and deepened through the platysma and superficial fascia. Blunt finger dissection protects the carotid sheath contents; the esophagus is medially displaced and the vertebral column palpated. Dilators widen the incision to permit insertion of the endoscope. The fibrous annulus is incised; the disc and any bony spurs are excised with a variety of "biting" instruments (e.g., rongeurs) and high-speed drill. A moist sponge is placed in the wound; the wound is covered with a towel.

The bone graft is harvested from the iliac crest (see above) or banked bone may be obtained. A titanium cage (7–8 mm) is filled with cancellous bone chips and inserted into the disc space. The incision is irrigated and closed. During the healing process, fusion occurs. When performed without surgical problems (as excessive bleeding or dissection, etc.), postoperative morbidity is minimized. Most patients can be treated in "same day" or overnight stay.

Preparation of the Patient

Antiembolitic hose (e.g., TED) are applied to the legs to prevent venous stasis and to help maintain blood pressure. The position of the patient is supine with a support (IV fluid bag, sandbag, rolled towel, etc.) placed under both shoulders (to best accentuate exposure of the operative level) with the head gently turned to the left (usually). The arms are padded and tucked into place with the draw sheet. A piece of wide (adhesive) silk tape may be used to hold the arms and shoulders in place after the shoulders are lightly pushed downward. The tape is applied from the underside of the head of the table (over the shoulders and down the length of the arms) to the underside of the foot of the table to facilitate fluoroscopic viewing of the cervical area. The right hip may be elevated (e.g., with a folded sheet) when the autograft (from the iliac crest) will be taken. General anesthesia is employed with endotracheal intubation. All bony prominences and areas prone to skin and neurovascular pressure or trauma are padded. An electrosurgical dispersive pad is applied.

Note: If cervical laminectomy is to be performed at the completion of the cervical discectomy and fusion procedure, the patient is later repositioned into the sitting position for the posterior approach.

Skin Preparation

For **cervical incision** the entire neck and chest are prepped. Beginning at the neck (midline), extending from the infra-auricular border, the entire neck is prepped to the level of the nipples and down to the table at the sides of the neck and shoulders. Lap pads or towels may be placed at the sides of the neck to prevent prep solution from pooling under the patient. Following the skin prep, they must be removed very carefully.

For **donor site incision** (e.g., iliac crest), begin cleansing the iliac crest area, extending from the midthorax to the upper thigh, down to the table on the donor (usually right) side, and well beyond the midline.

Draping

The patient is draped with folded towels at the neck and folded towels at the hip; towel clips, staples, or suture may be used to secure the towels. A sterile plastic iodine impregnated adhesive drape may be applied.

A craniotomy sheet with a small fenestration may be used for the cervical incision; a sterile, plastic adhesive drape and laparotomy sheet may be used for the donor graft incision. The donor site is covered with a sheet or towel until it is necessary to access the area for the autograft.

Drapes are required for the microscope and the fluoroscopy unit.

Equipment

Suction
ESU (bipolar and monopolar)
Fiber-optic headlight and fiber-optic power source
Power source for high-speed power drill (if not self-contained)
Magnifying loupes or operating microscope (e.g., Zeiss or Omni), optional

Endoscopic, Add

Fiber-optic light source, e.g., Xenon 300 W with remote connection for instruments
Monitor(s)
VCR
Printer
CD burner
Camera console

Instrumentation

Laminectomy tray
Kerrison rongeurs and pituitary forceps tray
Suction punch forceps
Cervical fusion instruments (e.g., Cloward self-retaining retractors, drill guards, drills, dowel cutters, bone graft holder, impactor, vertebral spreaders)
Hudson brace, mallet with nylon heads, trephines 2.5 and 3.5mm, depth gauge, and caliper
High-speed power drill (e.g., Stryker, Midas Rex), small burrs, and cord (optional)
Ligating clip applier, e.g., Hemoclip appliers (short, medium)

Endoscopic

Flexible fiber-optic endoscope with 1.9 mm inner diameter and separate suction and irrigation channels (Karl Storz), adaptor for light, endoscope holder with clamp (attaches to OR table), eyepiece with integrated light, irrigation and suction, ring curette with 45° angle, dilatation sleeve and rod with opening for guide wire, blunt palpation hook with 90° angle, biopsy forceps 1.7 mm, grasping forceps 1.7 mm, cannulas, luer-lock adaptor, puncture needles 1.7 and 1.4 mm with opening for guide wire, and guide wire 1.2 mm.

Note: Most endoscopes require the attachment of a microscope; however, the Karl Storz Smart™ Endoscopic Spinal System contains a built-in camera.

Supplies

Antiembolitic hose
Sterile, plastic adhesive drape (2 if sheets do not have plastic adhesive insets)
Basin set
Suction tubing
Blades, (2) #10, (1) #15, (1) #11
Bayonet bipolar forceps
Spinal needle, 3½″ (inserted into disc space to determine level)
Cassette drape, optional (if x-ray is taken instead of using fluoroscopy)
Graduated pitcher, bulb or asepto syringes (2)
Gelfoam and thrombin (e.g., 5000 units)
Cottonoids variety (e.g., ½″ × ½″)
Ligating clip cartridge, e.g., Hemoclips (small, medium)
Titanium bone cages (7–8 mm)

Endoscopic

Silastic® intravenous (IV) tubing (2) for inflow (irrigation) and outflow (suction)

Special Notes

- Use **Special Notes** from ***Laminectomy,*** p. 676, as applicable.
- Have the correct x-ray films in the room for the correctly identified patient.
- Notify the x-ray department in advance regarding portable films to be taken (e.g., initially to identify the correct position of the patient on the table and at the conclusion to document the bone graft, as stated above).
- Observe x-ray precautions; see p. 52.
- **Reminder:** The site of the donor graft is covered with a towel until the surgeon is ready to take the graft.
- A high-speed power drill with a small burr may be used on the vertebrae to facilitate access to the disc.
- *The cervical incision is covered with a towel while the graft is taken from the donor site (e.g., iliac crest).*
- Some surgeons may employ the *Stagnara Test* ("wake up test") in which at an appropriate time during the excision about the nerve roots, anesthesia is sufficiently lightened to allow the

patient "on command" to move his/her feet (demonstrating that the nerve pathways have not been compromised).

- A more sophisticated means of monitoring is the placement of electrodes to monitor motor evoked potentials and SSEP. The electrodes are placed directly in the epidural space after laminectomy, or they may be placed transcutaneously to measure the effects of transcranial cortical stimulation (or stimulation of the brain stem or cervical cord) to measure the integrity of neural pathways. They can also be placed to compare preoperative and postoperative values. These modalities can be used for other presentations of spinal surgery, such as in repair of scoliosis and in major vascular surgery as for correction of thoracic aortic aneurysm to monitor any suggestion of neurological effect secondary to surgically created ischemia (that can be corrected intraoperatively). Unfortunately, these monitoring modalities can reveal false positive and false negative results and are compromised by certain neurological conditions (e.g., cerebral palsy).

Cordotomy

Definition

The interruption of the lateral spinothalamic tracts of the spinal cord.

Discussion

This procedure is performed for the patient who suffers with intractable pain due to metastatic malignancy, such as when tumor invades the bone and compresses neural plexuses. It is also employed for patients with spinal cord injuries and other forms of neuropathic pain that cannot be controlled by nonoperative modalities, including morphine drip. Since often the pain does not originate from a single level, ***rhizotomy*** (see p. 688) and ***peripheral neurectomy*** are not options for pain relief. Alternative options include ***thalamotomy***, ***cingulotomy***, morphine instilled into the third ventricle, and electrical stimulation of the periventricular gray matter.

Approaches to cordotomy include open and percutaneous; the latter is utilized most often and is usually performed at the cervical level. When performed at the C1 to C2 level, the effect is below C5. For pain related to the lower trunk and lower extremities, selective cordotomy of the posterolateral portion of the tract is done. For pain of the upper torso and upper extremities, the anterolateral portion is targeted, but a bilateral procedure in the latter has a high risk of respiratory compromise due to injury to the ventrolateral reticulospinal tract, and its use is controversial.

Procedure

Open Procedure Cordotomy is described. The patient is placed in prone position. Local anesthesia, e.g., epidural block or general may be employed. A midline incision, as for ***laminectomy*** (see p. 671), is used. The C1 to C2 interlaminar space is developed, and laminar bone fragments are removed, as necessary, exposing the dura. The dura is incised, leaving the denticulate ligaments intact; the anterolateral aspect of the cord is exposed and the tract incised, interrupting the pain-conducting fibers. If local anesthesia is used, the level of analgesia may be assessed and the cordotomy extended accordingly. When a bilateral procedure is performed, respiratory and cardiovascular changes (due to stimulation of adjacent neural structures) must be anticipated; measures are undertaken immediately to counteract cardiovascular consequences. As noted above, injury or interruption of the ventrolateral reticulospinal tract (in proximity to the anterior portion of the spinothalamic tract) can result in sleep apnea, especially if a bilateral procedure is done. After hemostasis is achieved, the wounds are closed.

Percutaneous Cordotomy is described. The procedure is performed in a specialized suite in the radiology department or an OR with appropriate radiographic equipment. The patient is in supine position with special head holding frame to "fix" the skull. Local anesthesia (epidural block with *conscious sedation*) is preferred. Strict attention is paid to the proper positioning of the head. Access to C1 to C2 (or the occiput to C1) is achieved under careful radiologic monitoring. CT control is preferable. A lumbar puncture needle is advanced through the ligamentum flavum and dura until cerebrospinal fluid is encountered. Iodinated oil-based contrast (e.g., Pantopaque®Myodil® [i.e., iophendylate]) is injected (to visualize the local anatomy), and using the denticulate ligament as a marker, an insulated electrode (diameter 0.4 or 0.25 mm) capable of delivering radio-frequency energy (with a bared tip projecting 2 mm) is guided into the cord substance. An electrical impedance monitor that distinguishes the lower impedance of spinal fluid, in contrast to higher level of cord tissue, is employed. Iophendylate can potentially cause arachnoiditis.

If the patient is able to cooperate, neural segment test levels are ascertained. Contractions and tetany of neck muscles are noted. The therapeutic dose for radio-frequency energy is levels of 140°F to 176°F (60°C to 80°C) for 60 seconds. Using the Owl Cordotomy System (Diros Technology) or Radionics Corporation unit (monitors impedance and energy level at various frequencies), the electrode tip temperature is determined and the selected dose is delivered. Sensory levels are retested; parameters of respiratory depression must be monitored.

In bilateral cordotomy, the contralateral procedure is delayed for about 1 week.

For **Preparation of the Patient, Skin Preparation, Draping, Equipment, Instrumentation, Supplies,** and **Special Notes,** see ***Laminectomy***, p. 673, as applicable.

Add to supplies:

Contrast medium (e.g., iophendylate), optional

Rhizotomy

Definition

The interruption of cranial or spinal nerve roots.

Discussion

In general, the dorsal (posterior) nerve roots are pathways for the perception of segmental pain; the division of the pathways by **radio-frequency wave ablation** or **chemical ablation** provides relief from intractable pain, especially pain resulting from a malignancy, post-herpetic neuralgia, etc. However, there is some overlap of pain fibers in the ventral roots that pass through the corresponding dorsal root ganglion. When rhizotomy is performed, two segments above and below the target segment must be ablated to achieve optimal results. Pain in the extremities usually is not treated in this manner, as the limbs function poorly due to the loss of proprioception.

For ***trigeminal neuralgia***, **percutaneous** or **chemical rhizotomy** is performed. The foramen ovale is cannulated entering the trigeminal cistern with injection of various chemicals (e.g., glycerol). When possible, the Gamma knife can be used to treat trigeminal neuralgia noninvasively. Open or endoscopic microvascular nerve decompression, in which vascular structures surrounding and compressing nerve fibers are dissected away and a minute Teflon patch is placed between the nerve and the displaced vessel(s), gives satisfactory results.

Ventral (anterior) rhizotomy, the interruption of motor nerve transmission, is performed to relieve spastic conditions, but **peripheral microneurectomy** (employing microscopic control) is usually preferable, as it avoids risking paralysis of uninvolved muscles.

Dorsal rhizotomy can be performed, but only after other modalities, as **electrical nerve stimulation, hypnosis, acupuncture, biofeedback, Botox injection, and nerve blocks,** are ineffective. Rhizotomy is performed employing an intradural approach with laminectomy or rhizotomy via extradural approach.

Procedure

Cervical level **rhizotomy** is described. The sitting or prone position is employed for cervical rhizotomy; for unilateral procedures, lateral position may be used. The approach is as for laminectomy; see p. 671. Radiologic control is necessary to determine that the correct level is treated. The dissected nerve roots are followed to their origin in the spinal cord. The operating microscope is used to visualize rootlets and radicular vessels. (In the sacral area, placement of a urinary bladder catheter can be used to determine response [e.g., contraction of the bladder] to stimulation of the appropriate roots.) The dura is incised; micro scissors, nerve hooks, and bipolar coagulator are employed to dissect out and divide the roots; ligating clips may be placed. In the extradural approach, laminectomy and the opening of the dura can be avoided, but more extensive paraspinal dissection (with radiographic control) is necessary.

Rhizotomy (percutaneous technique) is used primarily for cervical levels, performed under local anesthesia with *conscious sedation* (p. 71). Fluoroscopic guidance is employed to verify levels and position and electrical nerve stimulator. Radio-frequency energy at 140°F to 176°F (60°C to 80°C) for approximately 60 seconds is used for each site. The results are not as good as in the open procedures.

For ***dorsal root ganglionectomy*** (usually reserved for the thoracic and lumbar regions), laminectomy approach is employed; lumbodorsal fascia is incised, and subperiosteal dissection of paraspinal muscles and intervertebral foramina are identified and confirmed radio-graphically. A microscope is used; the dura is incised and ganglia identified and separated from the sheath. The posterior (dorsal) and anterior (ventral) roots and peripheral nerve are identified. Clips may be employed. Usually, five levels are excised (except when post-disc-removal symptoms persist and only that corresponding level need be removed). The wounds are treated as per laminectomy; see p. 670.

For **Preparation of the Patient, Skin Preparation, Draping, Equipment, Instrumentation, Supplies,** and **Special Notes,** see ***Laminectomy***, p. 673, as applicable.

CHAPTER 25
Plastic Surgery

Scar Revision

Definition

Excision and repair of a scar to effect improved cosmesis or function or both.

Discussion

Skin scars result from trauma (laceration, burns, surgery, etc.), infection, and chronic local irritation. When the scar results in a poor cosmetic appearance, becomes hypertrophic (as in keloid formation), or results in contracture that is not only unsightly but may limit underlying joint and soft-tissue motion, scar revision is indicated. When the scarring involves a large area, such as post-burn or prior tumor excision with resulting deformity, skin grafting or flap transfer may be indicated.

Keloids respond to local injection of steroids, various chemotherapeutic agents, and laser application combined with reexcision; however, recurrence is frequent. Most simple scars can be improved by excision of the scar with step-like transfer of local flaps to reconstruct the wound with less tension and better cosmetic appearance. Numerous configurations of these local flaps are employed, including ***Z-plasty***, ***M-and-W plasty***, ***lazy S-plasty***, ***V-Y plasty***, etc. Common to all of these maneuvers is the undermining of the pre-incision-marked flaps with rotation of the flaps; excessive dissection is avoided to prevent flap necrosis due to compromised local circulation. Another presentation of unsightly scar is the ***"dog-ear" deformity,*** consisting of excessive skin and scar, usually at the extremity of a previous incision in which there was an uncorrected discrepancy of skin on opposing sides of the wound.

Procedure

Z-plasty, V-Y plasty, and correction of dog-ear deformity will be described. The anesthetic may be local, regional, or general.

Z-Plasty is described. The skin is marked, followed by injection of local anesthetic; hyaluronidase/Wydase® may be added to the anesthetic solution to avoid tissue distortion. The projected central limb of the Z is incised, paralleling the skin lines if possible. The angles of the Z limbs are usually 60° (but may be more acute or obtuse depending on the extent of lengthening desired). The Z is incised at the time of scar removal. The triangles of skin created are undermined by sharp and blunt dissection but not to compromise local circulation to the resulting flap. Hemostasis is achieved. The flaps are rotated and sutured in place. If the scar is long, multiple "Z's" are performed along its course. A pressure dressing may be employed.

V-Y Plasty is described. The skin is marked with a V; the base is pointed toward the scar or defect to be closed. After the incision is completed and hemostasis achieved, appropriate undermining of the soft tissues is performed. The base of the V is advanced and sutured closed. The apex of the V incision is distracted to create the linear limb of the Y; the Y is then sutured closed. Dressings are applied.

Dog-Ear Deformity Revision is described. The base of the excessive skin deformity is marked. Excess tissue is excised; hemostasis is achieved. The wound sutured closed. Depending on the presentation of the configuration of the excessive skin, the resulting closure may be directly in line with the prior incision, or the closure may be done at an angle.

Preparation of the Patient

The patient is in supine position with one arm extended on a padded armboard; the other arm is padded and tucked in at the patient's side. A pillow may be placed under the knees to prevent lower back strain, or the table may be flexed for comfort. All bony prominences and areas vulnerable to skin and neurovascular pressure or trauma are padded. An electrosurgical dispersive pad is applied.

Skin Preparation

Begin at the site of the scar; extend the prep outward to an appropriate distance.

Draping

The site is draped according to the location of the scar.

Equipment

Electrosurgical unit (ESU)

Instrumentation

Plastic procedures tray
Skin hooks

Supplies

Indelible marking pen
Control syringes (2) and needles (2), 25 or 27 gauge × 1½″, paper labels

Local anesthetic, medicine cup, paper labels
Wydase/hyaluronidase (enzymatic diffusing agent)
Small basin
Blades, (2) #15
Needle magnet or counter
Electrosurgical pencil with needle tip, cord, holder, and scraper
Nonadherent dressing, e.g., Adaptic®, Xeroform®, Opsite®, and gauze fluffs

Special Notes

- Apply **Special Notes** from ***Abdominal Laparotomy***, p. 134, as applicable.
- If the scar is on an upper extremity, equipment and supplies needed include padded hand table, tourniquet and pneumatic insufflator with microprocessor (regulator), Webril, a tube stockinette, and Esmarch bandage; for the lower extremities, omit the hand table. When a tourniquet is used, apply all safety precautions; see p. 45. Document the location, the length of time, and the appearance of the skin before and immediately after the procedure.
- **Reminder:** *Use safety precautions to identify, label, and dispense medications or solutions and to avoid medication errors; see p. 30.* It is mandatory that all medications and solutions on the sterile field be labeled by name and strength. The medication bottle is retained in the room until the procedure has concluded.
- **Reminder:** *Provide emotional support to the patient regarding feelings of altered body image and give the patient an opportunity to express his/her feelings.*
- When surgery is performed using only local anesthetic, keep movement and conversation in the room to a minimum, as the patient hears all that is said.

Skin Grafting

Definition
The transplantation of skin to cover a defect.

Discussion
Skin grafting is done to transplant skin from a donor site to a recipient site to cover an area where there has been skin loss. There are many terminologies that describe the variety (type) of skin grafts. An ***autograft*** is a graft of skin from one site to another site on the same individual. A

homograft or **allograft** is a graft taken from another individual (or cadaver). A ***heterograft*** is a graft derived from another species (e.g., porcine). In addition, grafts or graft substitutes may come from skin cell cultures or collagen matrices covered by a silicone film, etc.

Full-thickness skin grafts (Wolfe) include all elements of the epithelium and dermis that may be used to graft tissue to the face, hands, over joints, etc. Skin sources include eyelids, post-auricular skin, nasolabial fold, supraclavicular skin, foreskin, groin, etc. ***Split-thickness*** skin grafts (Thiersch) include varying depths of the dermis. Common sources of split-thickness grafts may be taken from the thighs and trunk. ***Free skin grafts*** are those from which the donor tissue is completely separated from its source, as opposed to other sources of skin, such as tubes, flaps, pedicles grafts, etc. Skin grafts are employed to cover areas of skin loss due to infection, burns, excised scar, or surgical loss (e.g., to cover open areas created by rotational flaps, etc.). Successful skin grafting depends on the state of the recipient site, the medical status of the patient, and the operative technique. Some skin grafts are intended to be temporary, such as a cover for large burn surfaces, e.g., with cadaver or porcine skin, used until permanent coverage can be achieved according to donor site availability and the patient's condition. A split-thickness graft may be passed through a ***meshing device*** (Meshgraft dermatome) that creates multiple small slits in the graft; stretching the skin can then provide coverage to several times the area of the graft. Good wound care is necessary for the donor site; the donor site may be needed again (10 to 20 days) for large surfaces that require coverage. Numerous instruments, modification of the instruments, and varying techniques may be employed in skin grafting.

Procedure

Full-Thickness and Split-Thickness Grafting are described. Skin grafting may be done under local, regional, or general anesthesia depending on the extent of the procedure and the patient's condition.

Full-Thickness Graft is described. The recipient site is outlined on a template with a vital dye or a pen with indelible ink. The donor site is marked accordingly with very slight increase in size, as the graft tends to contract when excised. A scalpel and skin hooks are employed as the tissue under the skin is defatted. The graft is sharply excised and sutured to the recipient site. The suture ends may be left long, to cross tie over the graft (on top of dressing pads) as a pressure dressing. The donor site is often closed primarily, or it may require a split-thickness graft.

Split-Thickness Graft is described. A manually operated ***oscillating knife*** (Humby, Blair, multiple other variations) or an ***oscillating handheld dermatome*** can be employed; the donor site is lubricated with mineral oil. An assistant places the skin in front of the knife on stretch using a tongue blade. The surgeon cuts the graft with a to-and-fro motion. Angulation of the knife determines the degree of thickness; the surgeon's technique and experience are important in this procedure. When an adequate amount of skin has been cut, the leading edge is severed from the donor site. A pressure dressing with a nonadherent base pad (Adaptic, Xeroform, Opsite, etc.) is applied to the donor site. Epinephrine or thrombin solution may be applied prior to the dressing to inhibit bleeding. The graft is sutured to the recipient site; slits may be cut in the graft to allow for drainage and prevent accumulation of blood or fluid. Skin staples may be used in some instances. The suture ends about the graft may be left long to cross tie over a pressure dressing.

Alternatively, an electrically or compressed air-powered ***handheld oscillating dermatome*** (Brown, Padgett, etc.) with disposable blades and cord may be used; a more precise thickness can be achieved using a dermatome (8 to 21 thousandths of an inch) by most experienced surgeons. Mineral oil and countertraction are applied to the donor site. An additional instrument may be used to obtain a skin graft. A ***drum dermatome*** (Reese, Padgett-Hood) is a hand-controlled oscillating knife within a hemicircumferential drum. Two-faced adhesive tape is applied to the drum and the skin so that the skin can be lifted during the cutting and rotation of the drum face. The special adhesive permits removal of the cut graft without tearing it. Again, an experienced surgeon is required to apply this technique.

It is extremely important that when the graft is applied, the ***dermis side is down***. When a graft is applied over a joint, splinting may be necessary to avoid undue motion of the graft. A vacuum sponge dressing technique, ***vacuum-assisted closure (VAC),*** may be used; it keeps pressure on the graft while it evacuates excessive local fluids or blood. If the graft is cut into small pieces, sutures may be omitted, and a pressure dressing is relied on to aid in the graft's adherence. ***When the graft is not to be used immediately after it is cut, it should be kept moist with saline or in antibiotic solution.***

Preparation of the Patient

The position of the patient is determined according to the location of the donor skin for grafting and the site (on the recipient) where the skin must be grafted. When the location of the skin to be grafted from is the patient's thigh to the patient's cheek, the head may be placed on a padded or gel headrest (donut) with the cheek on the receiving side turned upward. The dependent ear should be well padded. The ipsilateral arm is padded and tucked in at the patient's side; the opposite arm is extended on a padded armboard. A pillow may be placed under the knees to avoid straining the lower back, or the table may be flexed for comfort. The legs are parted and the thigh opposite the donor site is secured with the safety belt; the (donor) thigh is "free." Bony prominences and areas vulnerable to skin and neurovascular pressure or trauma are padded. Kerlix (sheet wadding) and a tourniquet, when used, are applied high on the donor thigh. An electrosurgical dispersive pad is applied.

Skin Preparation

Skin Graft from Thigh to Cheek. When skin is to be grafted to the patient's cheek, the donor site (skin taken from) is often the inside of the ipsilateral thigh; both the cheek and the thigh must be prepped. Begin at the donor site; extra sponges and prep solution are added to the prep set. The thigh is prepped; begin at the graft site and extend the prep from the tourniquet to below the knee and down to the table on the sides.

The receiving site (e.g., the face) is prepped; extend the prep from the top of the head to the shoulders and down to the table at the sides of the neck.

Draping

Skin Graft from Thigh to Cheek. The patient is draped with a "head drape," two towels and a sheet under the head. The uppermost towel is wrapped around the head and secured. Four towels are placed to border the site on the thigh. The patient's body is covered with a fenestrated sheet (e.g., laparotomy, transverse, or extremity); additional drape sheets are placed to complete the draping, as necessary.

Alternate Draping. A disposable adhesive-backed sheet is placed across the forehead. A split or U drape sheet covers the patient's body.

Equipment

ESU, unipolar or bipolar
Suction, available

Instrumentation

Plastic procedures or limited procedures trays
Oscillating knife (Humby, Blair) or electric handheld oscillating dermatome (Brown, Padgett), optional
Drum dermatome (Reese, Padgett-Hood), optional
Derma carrier (used with meshing device), optional
Skin hooks, ALM retractor (7 or 10 cm self-retaining toothed retractor spread by a turn-knob screw mechanism)

Supplies

Indelible marking pen
Control syringes (2) and needles (2), 25 or 27 gauge × 1½″
Local anesthetic, e.g., lidocaine 0.5% with epinephrine 1:200,000
Wydase/hyaluronidase (enzymatic diffusing agent)
Medicine cup, paper labels

Tube stockinette for extremities, optional
Epinephrine or thrombin solution (vasoconstriction)
Basin set, antibiotic irrigation, and bulb syringe, optional
Mineral oil and tongue depressors (2)
Blade, (1) #15
Electrosurgical pencil with needle tip, cord, holder, and scraper
Needle magnet or counter
Double-faced tape for drum dermatome
Suture and/or staples
Nonadherent dressing pad, e.g., Opsite, Bioclusive™, and gauze fluffs
Vacuum-assisted closure (VAC) for wounds with healing difficulty

Special Notes

- Apply **Special Notes** from ***Scar Revision***, p. 692, as applicable.
- **N.B.** *It is extremely important that when the graft is applied, the* **dermis (cut surface) side is face-down.**
- **Reminder:** Provide emotional support to the patient regarding feelings of altered body image and give the patient an opportunity to express his/her feelings. Answer questions with factual information or refer questions to the surgeon, as necessary.
- **N.B.** *Never immerse an electric dermatome (or any electrical appliance) in water.* An electric dermatome is not to be immersed during the cleaning or sterilization process.
- **N.B.** *When the graft is not to be used immediately after it is cut, it should be spread out on top the surface of a basin and kept moist with saline or antibiotic solution as per surgeon's preference.*

Cleft Lip Repair

Definition

Correction of a congenital deformity due to a fusion failure of the upper lip of the fetus.

Discussion

A cleft lip is a congenital deformity that occurs when there is a failure of the two sides of the upper lip to fuse during the embryonic process in the fetus. There are many presentations and degrees of cleft lip deformity; it can range from a slightly noticeable scar to a complete gap through the nose. Feeding problems are created by the infant's inability to suck.

Children with this congenital deformity will require a multidisciplinary team approach to correct hearing, speech, dental, and psychosocial problems. ***See Cleft Palate Repair,*** p. 701.

Categories include:

1. Unilateral incomplete cleft with nasal deformity
2. Unilateral complete cleft with nasal deformity
3. Bilateral incomplete cleft with or without adequate columella
4. Bilateral complete cleft on one side and incomplete on the other side

The cleft lip can be closed in the neonate, but repair at 3 months of age is preferable, as growth of the tissues facilitates the initial detailed surgery. Many surgeons prefer to wait to minimize the stress of surgery on the infant; they prefer to use the rule of 10s to determine an infant's readiness for surgery. The rule is: the infant is better prepared for surgery when he/she has a hemoglobin of 10 grams, a weight of 10 pounds, and is 10 weeks of age. Still other surgeons prefer to use a medical approach; presurgically, a fabricated, passive, intraoral orthodontal appliance is custom made to maintain the palatal arch to prevent the collapse of the arch. Palatal and alveolar deformities may also be present.

Procedure

General anesthesia is administered, and a noncuffed oro-Rae endotracheal tube is inserted. When indicated, bilateral myringotomy is performed and pressure-equalizing polyethylene tubes are placed. Prior to injecting the anesthetic, the skin is marked for the elevation of flaps. Local anesthetic containing epinephrine is infiltrated locally to aid in vasoconstriction and postoperative pain relief. According to surgeon's preference, instead of local anesthetic, a lip clamp may be used to aid in hemostasis. Simple closure of the defect does not usually suffice but may render subsequent stages easier. Approaches to repair can utilize a rotation advancement of flaps, or two triangular flaps employing a Z-plasty (p. 690) method may be used, in addition to a number of modifications to this method. The approach followed depends on the severity of the deformity and the surgeon's preference. Most often, repair involves the prolabial flap and lip-advancement flaps; the flaps are isolated and advanced. The desired outcome includes the restoration of the "proper" shape to the philtrum and the bow of the lip. The peak of the bow is made 2 to 2.5 mm on either side of the midline. The lateral elements are tailored to reconstruct the nasal sill. The mucosa is turned down to create the labial sulcus. The muscle is divided inferiorly to accompany the vermillion flap. The prolabial skin flap is approximated. The alar and the intranasal incisions are closed. Xeroform bolsters and nasal stents may be placed. The incision is protected with antibiotic ointment, and the cheeks are splinted with a Logan's bow (to counter the effects of crying).

Secondary repairs are performed according to individual situations even months or years later. Similarly, palatal and alveolar deformities are repaired in due time, commensurate with the patient's feeding requirements and tissue growth. Postoperatively, the child's arms are restrained with Velcro® elbow restraints to avoid injury to the repair.

Preparation of the Patient

Special measures must be taken for the pediatric patient to prepare the room, restrain the patient, and maintain the patient's body temperature, etc. To prevent the infant's body heat loss, the room temperature may be raised, adjusted to 80°F to 85°F (27°C to 29°C). In addition, a warming mattress is placed on the table and radiant heat lamps are placed overhead. Refer to **Pediatric General Information**, p. 978, for more considerations.

Following induction of general anesthesia, the table is turned 90°. The surgeon stands or sits at the patient's head, while the anesthesia provider is at the patient's side. The table may be positioned in slight reverse Trendelenburg position. The patient is supine with the head at the top edge of the table, stabilized by a headrest (e.g., padded or gel donut). The infant may be wrapped in a mummy-like wrap; less often, the extremities are padded and secured with padded restraints. Bony prominences and areas vulnerable to skin and neurovascular pressure or trauma are padded. An electrosurgical dispersive pad is not necessary if bipolar electrosurgery is used.

Skin Preparation

The procedure is a "clean-contaminated" procedure. The oral cavity is not prepped. Check with the surgeon regarding prep solution to be used for the face. Begin at the upper lip; prep the face. Extend the prep from the hairline to the shoulders and down to the table at the sides of the neck. Towels or lap sponges may be placed at the sides of the neck to prevent prep solution from pooling under the patient.

Care is taken to avoid getting prep solution in the eyes. The eyes are irrigated with normal saline from inner to outer canthus. Antibiotic ointment is placed in the conjunctival sacs. Small cotton plugs or cotton balls are placed in the ears to prevent prep solution from pooling in the ears (they are removed with a mosquito forceps before draping). Prep solutions are not permitted to pool on the drapes, as the prep solution excoriates the skin. In addition, pooled prep solutions are a fire hazard and should be avoided.

Draping

The patient is usually draped with a "head drape," i.e., drape sheet and two towels under the head with the uppermost towel wrapped around the head and clipped. A split or U drape sheet is draped over the patient's body.

Alternate Draping. A disposable adhesive-backed sheet is placed across the forehead. A split or U drape sheet is draped over the patient's body.

Equipment

Warming mattress (e.g., K-Thermia pad) and radiant heat lamps
Small headrest, e.g., padded or gel donut
Mummy-like wrap or soft padded restraints
Suction
ESU (bipolar)
Fiber-optic headlight (may contain camera) and fiber-optic light source, e.g., Xenon™ 300 W
Camera console, optional
Monitor, optional
Sitting stools (3), optional

Instrumentation

Basic plastic procedures tray
Caliper, ruler, lip clamp, Foment retractor, Beaver knife handle, bipolar bayonet forceps and cord, and Logan's bow

Supplies

Indelible marking pen or methylene blue applied with the wood part of applicator stick
Medicine cups, paper labels
Control syringes (2) and needles (2), 25 or 27 gauge × 1½″
Local anesthetic, e.g., 0.5% lidocaine with epinephrine 1: 200,000
Basin set
Blades, (1) #15, (1) #11
Beaver blades, (1) #64, (1) #65
Needle magnet or counter
Suction tubing
Antibiotic ointment
Velcro elbow restraints

Special Notes

- Apply **Special Notes** from ***Abdominal Laparotomy***, p. 134, and **Pediatric General Information**, p. 978 as applicable to the pediatric patient.
- **N.B. Reminder:** *Use every precaution to correctly identify the pediatric patient for patient safety.* Document methods used to identify the pediatric patient for medicolegal reasons.
- *The circulator should verify infant patient information with the parent(s) or legal guardian(s), such as sensitivi-*

ties and allergies, etc. Document all information that was obtained and noted, interventions performed, and outcomes that resulted for the patient in the **Perioperative Record** *(p. 12).*

- **N.B.** *Remember that* **"the pediatric patient is not a small adult."** Special measures and precautions for the pediatric patient and the neonate, in particular, must be observed. Administering preoperative medication (if any), administering anesthesia, preparing the room, and monitoring body temperature to retain body heat, accurate fluid balance, methods of restraining the patient, etc., are vitally important. Again, to plan and consider all of the special measures that must be taken for the pediatric patient, refer to **Pediatric General Information**, p. 978.
- Transport the neonate or infant patient to and from the operating room (OR) in an isolette to maintain the infant's body temperature.
- Avoid getting prep solution into the patient's eyes. The eyes are irrigated with normal saline from inner to outer canthus and antibiotic ointment is placed in the conjunctival sacs. Observe and document the care given and the appearance of the eyes before and following the skin prep.
- Small cotton plugs are placed to prevent prep solution from pooling in the ears; they are removed before draping. Observe and document that prep solution did not pool in the ears for patient safety and medicolegal reasons.
- Prep solutions must not pool in the drapes, as the prep solution excoriates the skin. Observe and document the condition of the skin preoperatively and postoperatively.
- To avoid fire, prevent prep solutions from pooling in the drapes, as most prep solutions are flammable.
- **Reminder:** *Use safety precautions to identify, label, and dispense medications or solutions and to avoid medication errors; see p. 30.* It is mandatory that all medications and solutions on the sterile field be labeled by name and strength. The medication bottle is retained in the room until the procedure has concluded.
- *Use warmed solutions (prep and irrigation); check the temperature before dispensing.*
- **N.B.** The circulator should obtain Velcro elbow restraints to be applied following the surgery to avoid injury to the repair.

- **Note:** *In the pediatric post-anesthesia care unit (PPACU) or the PACU, the perioperative practitioner must observe and document the observations regarding checking the infant for bleeding and for breathing difficulties (that may be caused by tissues swelling).*

Cleft Palate Repair

Definition

Correction of a congenital defect, split, or opening in the palate due to failure of the hard palate to fuse while the fetus is developing.

Discussion

The defect occurs when there is a lack of embryonic development of elements in the prepalate (face, lips, premaxilla, and incisors) and the palate (hard and soft palate, uvula, and additional maxillary teeth). Multiple combinations and defects may present, and often the infant will have both a cleft lip and palate. The exact reason for the defect is unknown, but heredity, inadequate blood supply, radiation exposure, severe vitamin deficiencies, drugs, and biochemical processes can affect the fetus. In severe defects, the infant feeding/nursing is difficult; the infant may be capable of sucking, but the suction is inadequate. Making certain the infant receives adequate nutrition for necessary weight gain is a major concern. In addition, respiratory problems may be present. The infant may have the cleft palate in conjunction with micrognathia and retrognathia, making him/her particularly prone to airway obstruction.

There are several techniques advocated for the anatomic reconstruction. The repair may involve a simple palatal closure, a palatal closure with palatal lengthening, or both may be performed with palatal muscle approximation. A palatal substitute such as absorbable membranes made of poly-DL-lactic acid may be used to compensate for the defect.

Mobilization of lateral tissue (by undermining it) allows for midline closure. Anterior detachment of the hard and soft palate and "push back" of the whole palate may be the necessary treatment. In addition to the palatal repair, orthodontia is required for these infants as they grow. To minimize speech difficulties, repair is desirable prior to the age of 2 years. Secondary repairs are performed to surgically adjust the facial tissues during ongoing growth, to correct residual fistula and speech problems, and to facilitate dental restoration.

Although controversies exist regarding the timing, surgical technique, and management of the repair, most often a team-based approach allows for an efficient coordination of all aspects of care that involves each specialty. Each specialty develops a plan of care that is individualized for the child according to his/her needs and growth. The team combines the approaches into a protocol that follows the guidelines established by the American Cleft Palate Craniofacial Association.

Procedure

General anesthesia is administered, and a noncuffed oro-Rae endotracheal tube is inserted. One of the several established surgical techniques for repair or a modification of these techniques is performed. Each approach has its advantages and disadvantages. The ultimate goal of the repair is to achieve facial symmetry. A local anesthetic containing epinephrine is infiltrated locally to aid hemostasis. A mouth gag (retractor) and a throat pack are placed; the throat pack prevents blood from trickling down the throat. To repair a complete unilateral (prepalatal and palatal) defect, soft palate margins are incised. Layers for oral mucosa, muscle, and nasal mucosa are developed; the tissues in the midline that are part of the defect are elevated as mucoperiosteal flaps. The concern is to align each of the different layers of tissue (to each other) in the same plane. Nasal mucosal flaps are freed and sutured. The nasal mucosa of the soft palate is sutured. The greater palatine vessels are preserved. Holes may be drilled in the hard palate for suture placement. Bone grafts may be employed. Muscle layers and the oral mucosa are sutured. Palatoplasty is performed, as necessary. If the lip appears vertically short, a small triangular flap is inset into the medial lip just above the vermilion at the vermilion-cutaneous junction. Following the surgery, the child's arms are restrained with Velcro elbow restraints to avoid injury to the repair.

Some deformities will require additional procedures; the repairs are performed in due time, commensurate with the patient's feeding requirements and tissue growth.

For **Preparation of the Patient, Skin Preparation,** and **Draping,** see **Cleft Lip Repair,** p. 698.

N.B. Note: The surgeon may be seated at the head of the table and cradle the infant's head in his/her hands.

Draping

The patient is usually draped with a "head drape," i.e., drape sheet and two towels under the head with the uppermost towel wrapped around the head and clipped. A split or U drape sheet covers the patient's body.

Alternate Draping. A disposable adhesive-backed sheet is placed across the forehead. A split or U drape sheet covers the patient's body.

N.B. Note: with either method of draping, a drape sheet may be fastened to the head of the table and draped across the sitting surgeon's lap. This permits the surgeon to cradle the infant's head in his/her hands while performing the surgery.

Equipment

Warming mattress and radiant heating lamps
Small headrest, e.g., padded or gel donut
Blanket mummy-like wrap or soft padded restraints
Magnifying loupes or fiber-optic headlight (may contain camera) and fiber-optic light source, e.g., Xenon 300 W, optional
Camera console, optional
Monitor, optional
ESU (bipolar)
Suction
Power source for high-speed power drill, optional
Sitting stools (3), optional

Instrumentation

Basic plastic procedures tray
Power drill (e.g., micro Stryker or Midas Rex), cord, and drill bits (fine)
Bipolar bayonet forceps
Skin hooks, Dingman mouth gag with blades, caliper, ruler, palate hook, palate elevators, Foman lower lateral scissors
Palatal substitute, e.g., absorbable membranes made of poly-DL-lactic acid, optional

Supplies

Indelible marking pen or an applicator stick (stick portion) used to apply methylene blue
Control syringes (2) and needles (2), 25 or 27 gauge × 1½″
Local anesthetic (e.g., 0.5% lidocaine with epinephrine 1:200,000), paper labels, and marking pen, as needed
Basin set
Blades, (2) #15, (1) #11, (1) #12
Beaver blade #64 (optional)
Needle magnet or counter
Suction tubing
Throat pack with radiolucent thread
Bunnell needles for mattress suture of the tongue, optional
Velcro elbow restraints

Special Notes

- Apply **Special Notes** from ***Cleft Lip Repair***, p. 699, as indicated.
- **N.B. Reminder:** *Use every precaution to correctly identify the pediatric patient for patient safety.* Document methods used to identify the pediatric patient for medicolegal reasons.

- The throat pack (with radiolucent thread) is inserted into the back of the throat to absorb blood. Prior to its insertion, the pack must be moistened with normal saline.
- The throat pack (with radiolucent thread) is included in the count.
- **N.B. Note:** *A large mattress suture may be placed through the tongue; in case of an airway obstruction, instead of placing an artificial airway and possibly damaging the repair, the tongue suture is pulled to open the airway.* Document the placing of the mattress suture and describe its purpose in the **Perioperative Record.**
- **Note:** *The circulator accompanies the pediatric patient to the PACU (or PPACU) and describes the purpose of the mattress suture to the PACU (or PPACU) perioperative practitioner.* Before leaving the PACU, the circulator documents in the patient's chart that this was done.
- **Note:** *In the PACU, the perioperative practitioner must observe, report, and document the nursing interventions taken regarding checking the infant for bleeding and for breathing difficulties (that may be caused by tissues swelling), as well as the outcomes of the nursing interventions.*

Reduction of a Nasal Fracture

Definition

Realignment and fixation of fractured nasal cartilage, bones, and/or septum.

Discussion

Fractures of the nasal bones, cartilage, septum, and frontal processes of the maxilla due to trauma may occur in multiple combinations. Most often, reduction is accomplished by the closed method. When closed reduction is unsuccessful, open reduction is indicated.

Procedure

When local anesthesia is employed, the surgeon will insert topical anesthetic (cocaine pledgettes or other agents such as pontocaine, lidocaine, etc.) and inject lidocaine with epinephrine; these serve to provide anesthesia and effect some degree of hemostasis. When general anesthesia is employed, the surgeon may elect to apply these same agents to effect hemostasis and provide postoperative analgesia.

A forceps (e.g., Asch) is placed to provide traction under the nasal bones. External digital manipulation reduces the fracture. Nasal packing is inserted, and a nasal splint is applied.

If the results of closed reduction are unsatisfactory, open reduction exposing the septum and portions of the nasal bones is indicated. Modified techniques similar to rhinoplasty may be necessary for realignment of the malpositioned bony and cartilaginous fragments; see ***Rhinoplasty***, p. 721. The fragments may be stabilized with packing or by intranasal sutures. Following the insertion of nasal packing (with antibiotic ointment), an external nasal splint is applied.

Preparation of the Patient

Anesthesia may be local or general. The patient may be in supine or semi-Fowler's ("beach chair") position. A padded or gel headrest may be used. One arm may be extended on a padded armboard and the opposite arm padded and tucked in at the patient's side, or both arms may be padded and secured at the patient's sides with padded restraints. A pillow may be placed under the knees to avoid straining the low back, or the table may be flexed for comfort. Bony prominences and areas vulnerable to skin and neurovascular pressure or trauma are padded. An electrosurgical dispersive pad is applied.

When the **semi-Fowler's ("beach chair")** position is employed, the table is raised from the middle break, and the foot of the table is lowered; the knees are positioned over the lower break of the table. The arms are placed in the patient's lap on a pillow and secured with padded restraints. A pillow may be placed behind the legs. A padded footboard is secured to the table and the heels are padded as necessary to avoid pressure injury. The safety strap is secured across the thighs. The table may be turned 90°, with the anesthesia provider opposite the operative side (surgeon's side). An electrosurgical dispersive pad is applied. ***Extra caution*** must be taken to avoid injury to the patient's fingers when the semi-Fowler's position is employed and the foot of the table is raised at the conclusion of the procedure.

Most surgeons do a preliminary nasal preparation. If an anesthesia provider is not in attendance, a perioperative RN, in addition to the circulator, must be present to monitor the patient and to administer *conscious sedation* at the surgeon's direction; see responsibilities of the perioperative RN monitoring the patient, p. 74.

Preliminary Nasal Preparation (Set Up a "Clean" Tray)

Cotton-tipped applicators (long; wood or metal)
Medicine cups (2), paper labels, marking pen
Topical anesthetic (e.g., 5ml of cocaine 4%) or a decongestant solution
Local anesthetic, e.g., lidocaine 0.5% with epinephrine 1:200,000
Control syringes (2) and needles (2), 25 or 27 gauge × 1½″
Atomizer

Scissors (e.g., straight Mayo), smooth bayonet forceps
Packing (e.g., 1/2″ plain gauze or cotton)

Skin Preparation

Closed Reduction. None is required for closed reduction.

Open Reduction. An interior nasal prep is not done. This is considered a "clean" procedure. Check with the surgeon regarding the type of prep solution to use. Begin at the external nose; prep the face and neck, extending the prep from the hairline to the shoulders and down to the table at the sides of the neck. Lap pads or towels are placed to prevent the prep solution from pooling under the patient; they must be carefully removed to avoid inadvertent contamination of the prepped area.

Care is taken to avoid getting prep solution in the eyes. The eyes are irrigated with normal saline from the inner to outer canthus. Moist cotton pads are placed over the eyes; when general anesthesia is employed, antibiotic ointment is placed in the conjunctival sacs. Small cotton plugs or cotton balls are placed in the ears to prevent prep solution from pooling in the ears (they are removed with a mosquito forceps before draping). Prep solutions are not permitted to pool on the drapes, as the prep solution excoriates the skin. To avoid a fire hazard, prep solutions should not pool in the drapes.

Draping

Closed Reduction. None is required for closed reduction; however, the patient's body may be covered with a drape sheet and the Mayo stand is draped. Instruments are sterilized; however, again note that this is a "clean" procedure, not a sterile one as it involves the respiratory tract. A gown may be worn. Gloves and a facial shield or goggles must be worn.

Open Reduction. The patient is usually draped with a "head drape," i.e., drape sheet and two towels under the head with the uppermost towel wrapped around the head and clipped. A split or U drape sheet covers the patient's body. A gown and gloves are worn.

Alternate Draping. A disposable adhesive-backed sheet is placed across the forehead. A split or U drape sheet covers the patient's body.

Equipment

Padded restraints
Suction
Fiber-optic headlight (may contain camera) and fiber-optic light source, e.g., Xenon 300 W
Camera console
Monitor, optional
ESU, unipolar and/or bipolar

Instrumentation

Preliminary nasal preparation instruments for tray (see above); in addition, add:

Closed

Frazier suction tips, bayonet forceps, Asch forceps (or rubber shod Crile forceps, straight), nasal speculum (one long and one short), ruler, caliper

Open

Nasal procedures tray

Basic Plastic Procedures tray (contains ruler and caliper), Bipolar electrosurgical bayonet forceps and cord

Supplies

Closed

Suction tubing

Small basin

Nasal packing, e.g., 1/4″ plain gauze packing and antibiotic ointment

Nasal splint (external) and 2″ × 2″ gauze for moustache dressing

Open, Add to the Back Table

Topical anesthetic (e.g., 5 ml of cocaine 4%) or a decongestant solution

Local anesthetic, e.g., lidocaine 0.5% with epinephrine 1:200,000

Control syringes (2) and needles (2), 25 or 27 gauge × 1½″, paper labels

Basin set, saline or antibiotic irrigation, and bulb syringe

Blades, (2) #15

Beaver blade (e.g., #64)

Suction tubing

Needle magnet or counter

Electrosurgical pencil with needle tip, cord, holder, and scraper

Nasal packing, e.g., 1/4″ plain gauze packing and antibiotic ointment, optional

Nasal splint and 2″ × 2″ gauze for moustache dressing

Special Notes

- Apply **Special Notes** from ***Abdominal Laparotomy***, p. 134, as applicable.
- **Reminder:** *Use safety precautions to identify, label, and dispense medications or solutions and to avoid medication errors; see p. 30.* It is mandatory that all medications and solutions on the sterile field be labeled by name and strength. The medication bottles are retained in the room until the procedure has concluded.

- Particularly when surgery is performed using only local anesthetic or local and *conscious sedation*, keep movement and conversation in the room to a minimum, as the patient hears all that is said.
- **Reminder:** Assess and document the patient's anxiety regarding the procedure and the unfamiliar environment; provide emotional support, such as maintaining eye contact and holding the patient's hand during the administration of anesthesia, etc., and answer questions in a knowledgeable manner. Document that these measures were done for patient safety regarding continuity of care and for medicolegal reasons.
- **Reminder:** Provide emotional support to the patient regarding feelings of altered body image and give the patient an opportunity to express his/her feelings.
- **N.B.** *When cocaine is used, both the circulator and the scrub person must observe the discarding of any remaining cocaine following the procedure.* Both persons must observe that the cocaine is discarded; the discarding is documented for medicolegal and accountability reasons.
- **N.B. Note:** *In the PACU, the perioperative practitioner must observe, report, and document the actions taken regarding checking for bleeding (e.g., hemorrhage) and for breathing difficulties (i.e., airway obstruction may be caused by tissues swelling) and the outcomes of the interventions in the* **Perioperative Record.**

Reduction of a Mandibular Fracture

Definition

Correction of malocclusion of the jaws resulting from a fracture of the lower jaw.

Discussion

Treatment of facial fractures is done following the treatment of more pressing emergencies, such as establishing an airway, stabilizing hemodynamics, and attending to injuries to the head, chest, skeleton, and orbital globe. Numerous variations of facial fracture may present; all should be reduced and fixed as soon as possible after more serious injuries (if present) are stabilized or corrected. With fractures of the mandibular condyle(s), there is preauricular pain, swelling, and difficulty in opening the mouth or a limited ability to open the mouth. In unilateral fractures of the jaw, diagnosis can be made if the jaw deviates to the injured side when the mouth is opened. Bilateral fractures of the jaw produce an anteriorly opening bite. Panoramic x-rays or computed tomography (CT) scan confirm the diagnosis. When the fracture is in the anterior portion of the jaw with teeth on either side of the fracture, intermaxillary fixation may suffice to restore dental occlusion. When the fracture(s) is posterior to the teeth, both intermaxillary fixation and open reduction of the fracture(s) are necessary to correct the maligned jaw.

Closed reduction is indicated for nondisplaced fractures in:

- Grossly comminuted fractures
- Fractures of the severely atrophic edentulous mandible
- Fractures with a lack of soft tissue overlying the fracture site
- Subcondylar fractures
- Fractures of children with developing dentition
- Fractures where there is limited blood supply and miniplate stabilization is unlikely (e.g., in some patients over age 60). In these patients, splints with intermaxillary fixation may be used to effect closed reduction.

Procedure

Anesthesia may be local or general; however, local anesthetic with epinephrine is usually injected with either type of anesthesia.

Closed Reduction. *Maxillomandibular fixation (MMF)* is the term applied to this methodology. An arch bar is bent to conform to the teeth and the dental arch. Fine wire is used to encircle the necks of the teeth; the bars are attached to the teeth with intermaxillary stainless-steel wires. Maxillary and mandibular arch bars may be placed to set the jaws in occlusion to each other; wire or multiple small latex bands are applied to attach the bars and to produce occlusion of the jaws. When a tooth has been fractured, antibiotic therapy is instituted.

Open Reduction. Open reduction is indicated in displaced and unstable fractures, with associated midface fractures, and when MMF is contraindicated. The line of the jaw may be marked prior to the local injection. One or more incisions are made in the mucosa, below the inferior border of the mandible. The fracture site(s) is exposed and the periosteum reflected. The fracture is reduced by manipulation. ***Arch bars*** (see p. 948) may be applied prior to open reduction and internal fixation (ORIF) to establish occlusion or fixation may be achieved with dynamic compression plates and screws. Holes are drilled for the screws. Holes are drilled into the mandible on both sides of the fracture and stainless steel wires are passed through the holes to maintain alignment. An experienced surgeon may use a lag screw to compress bone on either side of the fracture. In addition, the fracture site may be stabilized with an autologous bone graft or bone chips (fragments). The wound(s) is (are) irrigated and closed in layers. A small drain may be placed. Latex bands are usually placed by the PACU perioperative practitioner after the patient is awake (in the PACU); he/she checks the chart for patient allergy.

Preparation of the Patient

Anesthesia may be local or general with endotracheal intubation; however, general is most often used. The table is usually turned 90° to facilitate the surgeon's access; the anesthesia provider is at the patient's side. The patient may be in **supine position** with the head tilted backwards slightly; a padded or gel headrest may be used. One arm may be extended on a padded armboard and the opposite arm padded and tucked in at the patient's side, or both arms may be padded and secured at the patient's sides with padded restraints. A pillow may be placed under the knees to avoid straining the low back, or the table may be flexed for comfort. Bony prominences and areas vulnerable to skin and neurovascular pressure or trauma are padded. An electrosurgical dispersive pad is applied when monopolar surgery is employed.

The **semi-Fowler's ("beach chair") position** with the head tilted backwards (slightly) may be employed. The table is raised from the middle break and the foot of the table is lowered; the knees are positioned over the lower break of the table. The arms are placed in the patient's lap on a pillow and secured with padded restraints. A pillow may be placed behind the legs. A padded footboard is secured to the table and the heels are padded to avoid pressure injury. The safety strap is secured across the thighs. The table may be turned 90°, with the anesthesia provider opposite the operative side (surgeon's side). An electrosurgical dispersive pad is applied when monopolar surgery is employed. ***Extra caution*** must be taken to avoid injury to the patient's fingers when the foot of the table is raised at the conclusion of the procedure.

Skin Preparation

Closed Reduction. None is required for closed reduction. Some surgeons may request male patients be shaved. Other surgeons may request swabbing the mouth with prep solution or the patient may be requested to brush his/her teeth and rinse the mouth with mouthwash.

Open Reduction. This is a "clean" procedure. If prep is requested, check with the surgeon regarding the type of prep solution to use. Begin with the face; extend the prep from the hairline to the shoulders and down to the table at the sides of the neck. Infrequently the surgeon may prep the inside of the mouth with swabs saturated in prep solution.

Care is taken to avoid getting prep solution in the eyes. The eyes are irrigated with normal saline from inner to outer canthus. Moist cotton pads are placed over the eyes; when general anesthesia is employed, antibiotic ointment is placed in the conjunctival sacs. Small cotton plugs or cotton balls are placed in the ears to prevent prep solution from pooling in the ears (they are removed with a mosquito forceps before draping). Prep solutions are not allowed to pool on the drapes, as the prep solution excoriates the skin. To avoid a fire hazard, prep solutions should not be permitted to pool in the drapes.

Draping

Closed Reduction. None is required for closed reduction; drapes are often placed as for the open reduction. The Mayo stand is draped, and sterilized instruments are placed on it, again to keep the surgery "as clean as possible." Gowns may be worn. Gloves and a facial shield or goggles must be worn.

Open Reduction. The patient is usually draped with a "head drape," i.e., drape sheet and two towels under the head with the uppermost towel wrapped around the head and clipped. A split or U drape sheet covers the patient's body. The procedure is "clean-contaminated" (as it involves the gastrointestinal tract).

Alternate Draping. A disposable adhesive-backed sheet is placed across the forehead. A split or U drape sheet covers the patient's body.

Equipment

Closed Reduction

Padded or gel headrest (e.g., Richards, Shea, doughnut)
Extremity restraints, padded
Suction

Open Reduction

ESU
High-speed power source for power drill
Fiber-optic headlight and fiber-optic light source, e.g., Xenon 300 W

Instrumentation

Closed Reduction and Intermaxillary Wiring

Bite block, Yankauer and Frazier suction tips, bayonet forceps, Weider tongue depressors (large and small), Freer septal elevator, probe, wire cutters, wire twister, Mayo-Haney needle holders, ruler, caliper
Arch bars, latex bands or stainless-steel wire, 24 or 26 gauge
N.B. Wire cutter and disposable wire cutter

Open Reduction

Minor orthopedic procedures tray (contains wire cutter, but disposable wire cutter still needed)
Electrosurgical bipolar bayonet forceps and cord

Bone grafting instruments (include bone dowel and tamp), available
Weider tongue depressors (large and small), bone-holding clamps (2)
High-speed power drill (e.g., Mini Stryker® or Hall II), cord, bits, tap, and drill guide
Depth gauge, caliper, dynamic compression plates (variety sizes) and screws, arch bars, latex bands or stainless-steel wire, 24 or 26 gauge
Nerve stimulator/locator (e.g., Concept), optional
N.B. ***Wire cutter (in addition to the one on the Minor/Basic procedures tray), e.g. disposable wire cutter***

Supplies

Closed Reduction

Marking pen with indelible ink
Local anesthetic (e.g., 0.5% lidocaine with epinephrine 1:200,000), control syringes (2), needles (2), 25 or 27 gauge × 1½″, paper labels
Small basin, saline or antibiotic irrigation, and bulb syringe
Suction tubing
Disposable suction tips, Yankauer and Frazier, assorted sizes, when available

Open Reduction, Add

Basin set
Blades, (2) #15
Electrosurgical pencil and cord, needle tip, holder, and scraper
Needle magnet or counter
Drain (e.g., Penrose ¼″), optional
N.B. ***Remember disposable wire cutter (tape to top of the gurney for emergency)***

Special Notes

- Apply **Special Notes** from ***Reduction of Nasal Fracture***, p. 707, as applicable.
- **Reminder:** Ascertain that the *correct* x-ray films for the *correctly identified* patient are in the room prior to starting the surgery.
- The surgeon may wear a fiber-optic headlight for both a closed and open procedure for better visualization of the wound. The circulator pins the cord from the fiber-optic light to the back of the surgeon's gown to keep it out of the way .
- When arch bars (or other intermaxillary devices) are applied first, another (separate) setup is required for the open reduction (e.g., sterile gowns, gloves drapes, instruments, and supplies are required).

- The surgeon may request the scrub person to irrigate (slow trickle of saline) over the drill point to prevent buildup of heat from the friction of the power drill.
- The circulator must anticipate and request x-ray personnel, as necessary.
- Document the application of the fixation device according to type, size, and serial numbers, etc., in the **Perioperative Record** and hospital log, according to policy.
- **N.B. Reminder:** *Always tape (disposable) wire cutters to the top of the gurney to accompany patient on leaving the operating room in case of emergency.* The wire cutter must be visible at the head of the gurney or bed should the patient vomit or have breathing difficulty due to tissue swelling. Document in the **Perioperative Record** that the wire cutter has been placed at the head of the gurney or bed to accompany the patient. Documentation is done for patient safety and for medicolegal reasons.
- The circulator accompanies the patient to PACU; he/she shows the PACU RN that the wire cutter is taped to the head of the gurney.
- **N.B.** *The PACU perioperative practitioner should check that the wire cutter is visible at the head of the gurney; he/she documents that the wire cutter is visible on the* **PACU Record.**
- The PACU perioperative practitioner applies ice packs, as ordered. The ice pack must be covered with fabric (e.g., pillow case, etc.) to prevent "burn" injury to the skin. The appearance of the skin is documented before ice packs are applied and after they are removed.
- **N.B.** The patient's wound is observed for bright red bleeding and hemorrhage; the PACU perioperative practitioner must observe, report, and document the absence or presence of bleeding in the **PACU Record.** He/she reports to the surgeon when there is a significant amount of bright red bleeding immediately.
- In the PACU, the perioperative practitioner must observe, report, and document the nursing interventions taken regarding checking the patient for breathing difficulty, as swollen tissues may obstruct the airway; the patient outcomes are documented.

Reduction of a Zygomatic Fracture

Definition

Correction of fracture(s) of the cheek bones.

Discussion

Many facial fractures are the result of complex forces applied to the midface, e.g., injuries to the cheek bones are rarely simple. Depressed fractures of the cheek may be fractures of the arch and/or three fractures of the zygoma (sometimes referred to as trimalar fractures). Closed reduction is the treatment of choice for simple zygomatic arch fractures, whenever possible. No anatomical fixation is required. However, when the fracture is severe, as in depressed trimalar fractures, or in comminuted fractures, ORIF is performed; the bones are elevated and secured with pins or wires, or miniplates with miniscrews or microplates with cyanoacrylic cement are required. Controversy exists over the closed reduction treatment of zygomatic complex and depressed zygomatic arch fractures. CT scans are a valuable means of making the diagnosis.

The multiple approaches to fractures of the zygoma, include temporal and supraorbital, gingivobuccal sulcus, transconjunctival, coronal, and endoscopically assisted procedure. Fractures of the zygomatic complex frequently result in infraorbital nerve dysfunction and sensory disturbances.

Procedure

A temporal approach is described to correct fractures of the zygoma. Small access incisions to the fracture fragments are made in the lateral third of the eyebrow and in the infraorbital region. The periosteum is elevated conservatively to prevent devascularization. When there is a gap >5 mm in the bone, bone graft with calvarial bone is indicated. This bone is less resorbed than bone taken from other sources. If the interfragment gap is <5 mm, wires or miniplates and/or microplates with screws are required for the fixation. Antibiotics intravenously and in irrigation solutions may be employed to avoid infection.

The resorbable microplate with cryoacrylate fixation is believed to be adequate in most instances for fixation of the zygoma; the microplate offers a more cosmetic result, but if the repair must be stronger, a miniplate with miniscrews or two microplates may be used. The plate(s) is removed after the bone heals. The position of the bone fragments can also be "fixed" by stainless-steel wires (e.g., Kirshner wires), Steinmann pin, and titanium devices. The device is chosen according to the surgeon's experience, the location of the fracture, and preference of the surgeon. Holes are drilled into the fragments. The fragments are realigned, and the fixation device of choice is applied. The wound is irrigated with saline or antibiotic irrigation, and the incisions are closed.

Preparation of the Patient

Anesthesia may be local or general with endotracheal intubation; however, general is most often used. The table is usually turned 90° to facilitate the surgeon's access; the anesthesia provider is at the patient's side.

The patient may be in supine position with the head supported on a padded or gel headrest. One arm may be extended on a padded armboard and the opposite arm padded and tucked in at the patient's side, or both arms may be padded and tucked in at the patient's side. A pillow may be placed under the knees to avoid straining the low back and/or the table may be flexed for comfort. Bony prominences and areas vulnerable to skin and neurovascular pressure or trauma are padded. An electrosurgical dispersive pad is applied if monopolar electrosurgery is used.

Skin Preparation

Closed Reduction. None is usually required. Check with the surgeon.

Open Reduction. The surgeon may request that the male patients be shaved. Check with the surgeon regarding the type of prep solution to use. Begin the prep on the affected cheek. Prep the face and neck from the hairline to the shoulders and down to the table at the sides. The ear on the affected side is prepped.

Alternate Prep. Rather than prepping the affected side alone, the surgeon may prefer the entire face be prepped, to make it easier to view both sides of the face for symmetry. Begin the prep on the cheeks. Prep the face and neck from the hairline to the shoulders and down to the table at the sides. Prep both ears.

N.B. Note: Care is taken to avoid getting prep solution in the eyes. The eyes are irrigated with normal saline from inner to outer canthus. Moist cotton pads are placed over the eyes; when general anesthesia is employed, antibiotic ointment is placed in the conjunctival sacs. Small cotton plugs or cotton balls are placed in the ears to prevent prep solution from pooling in the ears (they are removed with a mosquito forceps before draping). Prep solutions are not permitted to pool on the drapes, as the prep solution excoriates the skin. Also, to avoid a fire hazard, prep solutions should not pool in the drapes.

Draping

Closed Reduction. No drapes are required, but they may be placed for the closed reduction. The Mayo stand is draped and sterilized instruments are placed on it (to keep the procedure "as clean as possible"). Gowns may be worn. Gloves must be worn.

Open Reduction. The patient is usually draped with a "head drape," i.e., drape sheet and two towels under the head with the uppermost towel wrapped around the head and clipped. A split or U drape sheet covers the patient's body.

Alternate Draping. A disposable adhesive-backed sheet is placed across the forehead. A split or U drape sheet covers the patient's body.

Equipment

Closed Reduction

Padded or gel headrest (e.g., Richards, Shea, doughnut)
Extremity restraints, padded
Suction
Fiber-optic headlight and fiber-optic light source, e.g., Xenon 300 W

Open Reduction, Add

ESU, bipolar or ophthalmic cautery (disposable)
High-speed power source for power drill

Instrumentation

Closed Reduction

Check with the surgeon

Open Reduction

Minor orthopedic procedures tray (wire cutter on tray)
Kerrison rongeurs, jaw bone hook, zygomatic bone hook, retractors, as requested
High-speed power drill (e.g., Mini Stryker or Hall II), cord, bits, tap, drill guide, and depth gauge
Bipolar bayonet forceps and cord
Fixation device, e.g., pins, K wires, stainless-steel wire (e.g., 25, 26, or 28 gauge), miniplates with miniscrews, and/or microplates with cyanoacrylate cement
Nerve stimulator (locator) (e.g., Concept), optional

Supplies

Closed Reduction

Marking pen with indelible ink
Local anesthetic (e.g., 0.5% lidocaine with epinephrine 1:200,000), for vasoconstriction Control syringes (2), and needles (2), 25 or 27 gauge × 1½″
Medicine cup and paper labels
Small basin, saline or antibiotic irrigation, and bulb syringe
Suction tubing
Disposable suction tips, Yankauer and Frazier, assorted sizes, when available
Disposable wire cutter (to accompany the patient following procedure)

Open Reduction, Add

Basin set
Blades, (2) #15
Needle magnet or counter

Ophthalmic cautery
Drain (e.g., Penrose 1/4″), optional
Ophthalmic antibiotic ointment

Special Notes

- Apply **Special Notes** from ***Reduction of Nasal Fracture***, p. 707, as applicable.
- **Reminder:** Ascertain that the *correct* x-ray films for the *correctly identified* patient are in the room prior to starting the surgery.
- The surgeon may wear a fiber-optic headlight for both the closed and open procedure (for better visualization of the wound). The circulator pins the cord from the headlight to the back of the surgeon's shirt.
- **Reminder:** When local anesthesia with epinephrine is administered, the patient may have *increased* feelings of fear and anxiety regarding the surgery and the unfamiliar environment due to the effects of the epinephrine in the anesthetic.
- **Reminder:** Assess and document the patient's anxiety, provide emotional support, such as maintaining eye contact and holding the patient's hand during the administration of anesthesia, etc., and answer questions in a knowledgeable manner. This is done for continuity of patient care and for medicolegal reasons.
- **Reminder:** Provide emotional support to the patient regarding feelings of altered body image and give the patient an opportunity to express his/her feelings.

Open Reduction of Orbital Floor Fracture

Definition

Elevation and restoration of bone integrity supporting the eye and intraorbital contents.

Discussion

Orbital floor fractures often occur in combination with other facial fractures, usually maxillary and/or zygomatic bone fractures. "*Blowout*" *fracture* refers to a fracture due to the direct frontal application of force. The orbital floor is the path of least resistance in blows to the face; the result may be an isolated depressed fracture of the orbital floor with retrograde displacement of the globe. The infraorbital rim may remain intact; however, the orbital contents may protrude into the maxillary sinus. There may be increased intraorbital (intraocular) pressure. Common clinical signs of globe or retinal injury are enophthalmos and monocular diplopia (especially on upward gaze). *Traumatic optic neuropathy* is a true emergency, requiring immediate repair. X-rays or CT scan can confirm the diagnosis.

Procedure

Initially, the fracture site is assessed and debris is removed. An incision is made over the infraorbital rim (avoiding injury medially to the orbicularis oculi muscle) and continued down to the periosteum. The periosteum is incised and reflected over the fracture site. Care is taken not to undermine the tissue excessively, as devascularization will occur. Various structures including the supra and infraorbital nerves, as well as the extra-ocular muscles, must be identified and protected. The difficulty in performing surgery in this area is that the edematous reaction of the tissues locally obscures the identification of the structures. The herniated contents of the orbital cavity are reduced and the defect in the orbital floor may be repaired with synthetic material (e.g., a Teflon® or Silastic® sheet), autogenous cartilage, or autogenous bone. The globe is rotated to test the security of the implant and to make certain there is no entrapment involving the inferior rectus muscle. The periosteum is sutured back to its site of origin, as are the orbicularis oculi muscle and skin. The surgeon usually orders ice packs applied to the area, following the application of an antibiotic ***ophthalmic*** ointment and eye patch.

Preparation of the Patient

Anesthesia may be local or general; general anesthesia with endotracheal intubation is most often used. The table may be turned 90° to facilitate the surgeon's access; the anesthesia provider is at the patient's side. The patient may be in supine position with the head supported on a padded or gel headrest. One arm may be extended on a padded armboard and the opposite arm padded and tucked in at the patient's side, or both arms may be padded and secured at the patient's side with padded restraints. A pillow may be placed under the knees to avoid straining the lower back or the table may be flexed for comfort. Bony prominences and areas vulnerable to skin and neurovascular pressure or trauma are padded

Skin Preparation

Check with the surgeon regarding the type of prep solution to be used. Begin by prepping the operative eyelid (some surgeons may request the entire face be prepped to aid in determining facial symmetry). Prep the face and neck from the hairline to the shoulders and down to the table at the sides; include the ear on the affected side or both ears, according to surgeon's preference. Avoid pooling of the prep solution, see **Reduction of a Nasal Fracture**, p. 706.

Care is taken to avoid getting prep solution in the eyes. The eyes are irrigated with normal saline from inner to outer canthus. Small cotton plugs or cotton balls are placed in the ears to prevent prep solution from pooling in the ears (they are removed with a mosquito forceps before draping).

Draping

A "head drape" is used; see **Reduction of a Nasal Fracture**, p. 706.

Equipment

- Padded or gel headrest (e.g., doughnut)
- ESU (bipolar) and/or ophthalmic cautery (disposable)
- High-speed power source for power drill (optional)
- Suction
- Fiber-optic headlight and fiber-optic light source, e.g., Xenon 300 W (optional)
- Sitting stools (optional)

Instrumentation

- Basic eye procedures tray
- Globe and orbit procedures tray
- Minor orthopedic procedures tray
- Bone grafting instruments (available)
- Bone hook, bipolar bayonet forceps
- High-speed power drill, cord, guide, and drill bits
- Bipolar bayonet forceps and cord

Supplies

- Indelible marking pen
- Local anesthetic, e.g., 0.5% lidocaine with epinephrine (1:200,000 for vasoconstriction) Control syringes (2) and needles (2), 25 or 27 gauge × 1½″, paper labels
- Cotton-tipped applicators or cellulose sponges
- Normal saline eye irrigation, balanced salt solution (BSS)
- Basin set
- Needle magnet or counter
- Blades, (2) #15
- Bulb syringe
- Suction tubing
- Ophthalmic cautery
- Implant (e.g., porous polyethylene sheets Medopor; Porex Surgical Inc, Newnan, GA, Sweden), available
- Antibiotic **ophthalmic** ointment, eye patch, and eye shield
- Ice pack, available

Special Notes

- Apply **Special Notes** from **Reduction of a Nasal Fracture**, p. 707, as indicated.
- The surgeon performing the procedure may be from the plastic surgery, ophthalmology, or otorhinolaryngology discipline. **Equipment, Instrumentation, Supplies,** and **Special Notes** particular to each specialty must be considered when preparing (setting up) for the surgery.
- Donor cartilage may be used or an autogenous graft is harvested, check with the surgeon regarding the donor site. Prep the donor graft site at the time the face is prepped.
- Prep solutions are not permitted to pool on the drapes, as the prep solution excoriates the skin. Document the appearance of the skin prior to and immediately following the surgery.
- To avoid a fire hazard, the prep solution should not pool in the drapes; document in the **Perioperative Record** that prep solution was not permitted to pool in the drapes following the procedure.
- To avoid a medication error, be certain the antibiotic ointment used (in the wound) is **"ophthalmic."**

Rhinoplasty

Definition

Modification of the external appearance of the nose.

Discussion

Rhinoplasty is performed to improve the appearance of the nose and thereby enhance the patient's physical appearance. In addition to cosmetic considerations, this procedure is performed to alleviate nasal airway obstruction due to deviation of the septum and/or nasal trauma not relieved by closed reduction. Goals of rhinoplasty may include tip reshaping, hump removal, narrowing of the nares, and septoplasty (straightening the nasal septum). The rhinoplasty procedure is modified according to each patient's needs. The surgeon must endeavor to obtain a shape, symmetry, and proportion of the nose in proportion to the other components of the patient's face. Before the surgeon performs the surgery, he/she interviews the patient to be assured that the patient's expectations of the outcome of the surgery are realistic. ***Mentoplasty Augmentation*** (see p. 724) is often necessary in conjunction with rhinoplasty to achieve a more balanced appearance to the face.

Procedure

For **Rhinoplasty,** an intercartilaginous incision is made through the nares along the rim of the upper lateral cartilage bilaterally. The incisions are connected, freeing the skin from over the dorsal septum, and the columella anteriorly. Prominent septal, lateral, and alar cartilages are excised and, after reassessment, are retrimmed as necessary. The nasal bones are osteotomized laterally and medially (and horizontally, if necessary) and compressed to infracture the bones, creating a more "normal" contour. Rasping smooths bony irregularities. Alignment of the septum is achieved. The anterior septum and columella are sutured; alar incisions and marginal (rim) incisions of the lower lateral cartilages are sutured as well. Intranasal packing is inserted, and an external splint is applied.

Preparation of the Patient

Anesthesia may be local or general, but local anesthesia with *conscious sedation* is usually preferred, as these patients are often discharged the same day. The patient is in supine position; a padded or gel headrest is often used. One arm may be extended on a padded armboard and the opposite arm padded and tucked in at the patient's side, or both arms may be padded and secured at the patient's sides. A pillow may be placed under the knees to avoid straining the low back, or the table may be flexed for comfort. Bony prominences and areas vulnerable to skin and neurovascular pressure or trauma are padded. An electrosurgical dispersive pad is applied.

The surgeon often does a preliminary nasal preparation before the skin prep. If an anesthesia provider is not in attendance, a perioperative RN, in addition to the circulator, is required to monitor the patient and to administer *conscious sedation* as directed by the surgeon. For a description of the role of the RN monitoring the patient, see p. 74.

Preliminary Nasal Preparation (on a "Clean" Tray)

- Cotton-tipped applicators (long; wood or metal)
- Medicine cups (2), paper labels
- Topical anesthetic (e.g., cocaine 4% or 5%) or a decongestant solution
- Cottonoids, e.g., 1/2″ × 3″
- Local anesthetic, e.g., lidocaine 0.5% with epinephrine 1:200,000
- Control syringes (2) and needles (2), 25 or 27 gauge × 1 1/2″
- Atomizer
- Scissors (e.g., straight Mayo), smooth bayonet forceps

Skin Preparation

An interior nasal prep is not done. This is considered a "clean" procedure. If a prep is requested, check with the surgeon regarding the type of prep solution to use. Begin at the external nose; prep the face and neck, extending the prep from the hairline to the shoulders and down to the table at the sides of the neck.

Care is taken to avoid getting prep solution in the eyes. The eyes are irrigated with normal saline from inner to outer canthus. Moist cotton pads are placed over the eyes; when general anesthesia is employed, antibiotic ointment is placed in the conjunctival sacs. Small cotton plugs or cotton balls are placed in the ears to prevent prep solution from pooling in the ears (they are removed with a mosquito forceps before draping). Prep solutions are not allowed to pool on the drapes, as the prep solution excoriates the skin. To avoid a fire hazard, prep solutions should not pool in the drapes.

Draping

The patient is usually draped with a "head drape," i.e., drape sheet and two towels under the head with the uppermost towel wrapped around the head and clipped. A split or U drape sheet covers the patient's body. A gown and gloves are worn.

Alternate Draping. A disposable adhesive-backed sheet is placed across the forehead. A split or U drape sheet covers the patient's body.

Equipment

Padded or gel headrest (e.g., doughnut, Shea, Richards)
Padded restraints, optional
Suction
Fiber-optic headlight (may contain camera) and fiber-optic light source, e.g., Xenon 300 W
Camera console, optional
Monitor, optional
VCR
CD burner
Printer
ESU, unipolar and/or bipolar

Instrumentation

Atomizer, scissors (e.g., straight Mayo), smooth bayonet forceps
Nasal procedures tray
Basic plastic procedures trays (contain ruler and caliper)
Beaver knife handle, bipolar bayonet forceps

Supplies

Control syringes (2) and needles (2), 25 or 27 gauge × 1½″
Topical anesthetic (e.g., cocaine 4% or 5%) or a decongestant solution
Cottonoids, e.g., ½″ × 3″
Local anesthetic, e.g., lidocaine 0.5% with epinephrine 1:200,000

Control syringes (2) and needles (2), 25 or 27 gauge × 1½″
Cotton-tipped applicators (long; wood or metal)
Medicine cups (2), paper labels
Basin set, saline or antibiotic irrigation, and bulb syringe
Blades, (4) #15
Beaver blade (e.g., #64)
Needle magnet or counter
Electrosurgical pencil with needle tip, cord, holder, and scraper
Suction tubing
Syringe, disposable (for cleaning suction tip), optional
Nasal packing, e.g., ¼″ plain gauze and antibiotic, optional
Nasal splint and 2″ × 2″ gauze for moustache dressing

Special Notes

- Apply **Special Notes** from ***Reduction of Nasal Fracture***, p. 707, as indicated.
- An otorhinolaryngologist or a plastic surgeon usually performs a **rhinoplasty** procedure. When preparations are made for the surgery, consider choosing items from the surgeon's specialty.
- **Reminder:** Assess and document the patient's anxiety regarding the surgery and the unfamiliar environment, provide emotional support, such as maintaining eye contact and holding the patient's hand during the administration of anesthesia, etc., and answer questions in a knowledgeable manner. Documentation is done as a patient care measure and for medicolegal reasons.
- **N.B. Reminder:** *When cocaine is used, both the circulator and the scrub person must observe the discarding of any remaining cocaine following the procedure.* Both persons must observe the cocaine being discarded; discarding the cocaine is documented for medicolegal and accountability reasons.
- **N.B. Note:** *In the PACU, the perioperative practitioner must observe, report, and document nursing interventions regarding observing the wound for bleeding (e.g., in hemorrhage, the pad under the noose is soaked through) and for breathing difficulties (e.g., airway obstruction may be caused by tissues swelling); a negative observation should be documented, as well.*

Mentoplasty (Genioplasty) Augmentation

Definition

Modification of the appearance of the chin with the insertion of a prosthesis.

Discussion

Mentoplasty augmentation is performed to add size and contour to the chin and thereby balance the features of the face. The cosmetic appearance of the face is improved by correcting (reshaping or modifying) the size of the chin by adding an autologous bone graft or an implantable synthetic allograft prosthesis/implant, a device of silicone, Teflon, Dacron, porous polyethylene, mersilene, polymethylmethacrylate, or hydroxyapatite. A simple augmentation mentoplasty is sufficient when the chin recedes to a modest degree and the patient has normal dental occlusion. *Micrognathia* requires osteotomy of the mandible (to project it forward), repositioning the jaw, in addition to augmentation of the chin to reconstruct the facial profile. Mentoplasty augmentation is often performed to follow mandibular reconstruction to further enhance the facial profile by contouring the shape of the chin and giving it dimension. For some patients, apposition of the lips may be required as well. The approach to mentoplasty augmentation can be submental or transoral through the labial sulcus.

Procedure

A line of incision may be drawn with the patient sitting, prior to the instillation of the local anesthetic with epinephrine (for vasoconstriction and postponement of postoperative pain). A short transverse incision is made in the submental region or in the labial sulcus. When the incision is made in the labial sulcus, no scar can be seen, but the oral incision has a greater incidence of infection. A supraperiosteal pocket is developed by undermining the periosteum with a periosteal elevator just enough to accommodate the prosthesis, usually directly over the leading edge of the chin, inferior to the mental nerve. Care must be taken not to undermine the tissue too much or the blood supply to the area may be compromised. Chin bone sizers are employed until the desired choice of shape and size is determined. The implant is positioned over the surface of the chin, aligning it according to the blue line that is found in the midline of most commercially made implants. The implant may be "fixed" or stabilized with a deep mattress suture. The transoral wound is irrigated with saline or antibiotic solution and closed in layers. A bulky pressure dressing is applied. The submental wound is irrigated with saline or an antibiotic solution and closed in layers. The skin closure may be Steri-Strips™, and simple gauze dressing.

Preparation of the Patient

Anesthesia may be local or general, but local is preferred if the patient is discharged the same day. When osteotomy is performed for adjustment of the mandible, general anesthesia employed and the hospital stay is extended. The table may be turned 90° to facilitate the surgeon's access. The patient is in supine position; a padded or gel headrest may be used. One arm may be extended on a padded armboard and the opposite arm padded and tucked in at the patient's side, or both arms may be padded and secured at the patient's sides. A pillow may be placed under the knees to avoid straining the lower back, or the table may be flexed for comfort. Bony prominences and areas vulnerable to skin and neurovascular pressure or trauma are padded. Apply electrosurgical dispersive pad if the monopolar electrosurgery is used.

If an anesthesia provider is not in attendance, a perioperative RN, in addition to the circulator, is required to monitor the patient and to administer *conscious sedation* as directed by the surgeon. For a description of the role of the RN monitoring the patient, see p. 74

Skin Preparation

Check with the surgeon regarding the type of prep solution to be used. When the approach is transoral, the surgeon may have requested the patient use mouthwash for the week prior to the procedure and intraoperatively prior to the skin prep. Begin at the chin and prep the face. Extend the prep from the hairline to the shoulders and down to the table at the side of the neck.

Note: Care is taken to avoid getting prep solution into the eyes. The eyes are irrigated with normal saline from inner to outer canthus. Moist cotton pads are placed over the eyes; when general anesthesia is employed, antibiotic ointment is placed in the conjunctival sacs. Small cotton plugs or cotton balls are placed in the ears to prevent prep solution from pooling in the ears (they are removed with a mosquito forceps before draping). Prep solutions are not permitted to pool on the drapes, as the prep solution will excoriate the skin. To avoid a fire hazard, prep solutions should not pool in the drapes.

Draping

The patient is usually draped with a "head drape," e.g, drape sheet and two towels under the head with the uppermost towel wrapped around the head and clipped. A split or U drape sheet covers the patient's body. A gown and gloves are worn.

Alternate Draping. A disposable adhesive-backed sheet is placed across the forehead. A split or U drape sheet covers the patient's body.

Equipment

Headrest (e.g., doughnut, Shea, Richards), optional
Padded restraints, optional
Suction
ESU, monopolar or bipolar
Fiber-optic headlight and fiber-optic light source, e.g., Xenon 300 W

Instrumentation

Basic plastic procedures tray
Bipolar bayonet forceps
Chin prosthesis, e.g., Medpor®, Proplast I and II

Supplies

Indelible marking pen
Local anesthetic, e.g., lidocaine 0.5% with epinephrine 1:200,000
Control syringes (2) and needles (2), 25 or 27 gauge × 1½″
Medicine cups (2), paper labels
Small basin, saline or antibiotic irrigation, and bulb syringe
Blades, (4) #15
Electrosurgical pencil with needle tip or bipolar bayonet forceps
Needle magnet or counter
Dressing, e.g., telfa, gauze fluffs, and Elastoplast®, for submental approach (check the chart for patient allergy to rubber products before placing Elastoplast)

Special Notes

- Apply **Special Notes** from ***Reduction of Nasal Fracture***, p. 707, as indicated.
- An otorhinolaryngologist or a plastic surgeon may perform the rhinoplasty. When preparing for the surgery, consider choosing items from the surgeon's specialty.
- **Reminder:** Provide emotional support to the patient regarding feelings of altered body image, and give the patient an opportunity to express his/her feelings. Answer questions with factual information or refer questions to the surgeon.
- The surgeon may wear a fiber-optic headlight to improve visualization. The circulator pins the cord from the headlight to the back of the surgeon's gown to keep it out of the way.
- **Reminder:** *Use safety precautions to identify, label, and dispense medications or solutions and to avoid medication errors; see p. 30.* It is mandatory that all medications and solutions on the sterile field be labeled by name and strength. Medication bottles are retained in the room until the procedure has concluded.
- **Reminder:** Assess and document the patient's anxiety regarding the surgery and the unfamiliar environment, provide emotional support, such as maintaining eye contact and holding the patient's hand during the administration of anesthesia, etc., and

answer questions in a knowledgeable manner. Documentation is done for medicolegal reasons.

- Before the circulator applies a pressure dressing using Elastoplast, he/she should check the patient's chart regarding allergy to rubber products.

Blepharoplasty

Definition

Excision of redundant muscle and skin of the eyelids to enhance one's physical appearance.

Discussion

The eyelids of the mature adult are one of the first areas to show progressive permanent changes due to aging and genetics. The tissues surrounding the orbit loose their elasticity, resulting in the appearance of "baggy" eyelids. **Blepharoplasty** is designed to negate this aspect of the aging process. For many years, blepharoplasty meant the transcutaneous or transconjunctival excision of the pseudoherniated fat pad and correction of muscle and skin laxity in the lower eyelids. In the mid-1990s, the plastic surgeon's approach to blepharoplasty was revised. The fat pad of the lower lids is no longer excised but instead preserved and repositioned over the orbital rim to correct the groove over the nasojugal fold. Excessive muscle is transected, and after redraping, the excessive skin is excised from the lower eyelids transcutaneously. The amount of muscle and skin that is resected depends on the severity of the deformity, i.e., the amount of redundant muscle and skin and the age of the patient.

When the upper lids are redundant so as to interfere with vision, correction is regarded as a medical necessity rather than cosmetic procedure; health insurance may cover a portion of the expenses incurred for the surgery. The cosmetic procedure is distinguished from ***blepharoptosis*** (drooping eyelid due to paralysis), see p. 881.

Procedure

Transcutaneous Approach to Blepharoplasty of the Upper Lid is described.

An elliptical incision is made in the recess of the orbitopalpebral fold of the upper lid according to previously placed markings. The orbicularis oculi muscle is incised parallel to its fibers at the apex of the bulge. The fat protrudes through the incision and is excised. The upper-lid incisions may be covered with moist saline sponges while resection of a portion of the lower lids is done. The skin is undermined. The orbicularis oculi muscle is split. Fat compartments are isolated; the fat is repositioned, the skin is redraped, and the redundant skin is resected. The upper lids are checked for bleeding; hemostasis is obtained. Incisions in the upper lids are closed with fine interrupted sutures. The procedure is repeated for the lower lids. An occlusive (not pressure) dressing is applied. A consideration encountered when performing the blepharoplasty of the lower lids **transconjunctively** is that while the procedure is performed through a "hidden" incision, the excess tissue must be excised transcutaneously. The second incision for the excision of the redundant skin may show just as much as if the entire procedure were performed via transcutaneous approach.

Preparation of the Patient

Local anesthesia is usually preferred. The table may be turned 90° to facilitate the surgeon's access. The patient is in supine position; a padded or gel headrest may be used. One arm may be extended on a padded armboard and the opposite arm padded and tucked in at the patient's side, or both arms may be padded and secured at the patient's sides. A pillow may be placed under the knees to avoid straining the low back, or the table may be flexed for comfort. Bony prominences and areas vulnerable to skin and neurovascular pressure or trauma are padded. An electrosurgical dispersive pad is not required when bipolar electrosurgery is used.

If an anesthesia provider is not in attendance, a perioperative RN, in addition to the circulator, is required to monitor the patient and to administer *conscious sedation* as directed by the surgeon. For a description of the role of the RN monitoring the patient, see p. 74.

Skin Preparation

Check with the surgeon regarding the type of prep solution to be used. Begin at the eyelids and prep the face; extend the prep from the hairline to the shoulders and down to the table at the side of the neck.

Care is taken to avoid getting prep solution in the eyes. The eyes are irrigated with normal saline from inner to outer canthus. Moist cotton pads are placed over the eyes; when general anesthesia is employed, antibiotic ointment is placed in the conjunctival sacs. Small cotton plugs or cotton balls are placed in the ears to prevent prep solution from pooling in the ears (they are removed with a mosquito forceps before draping). Prep solutions are not allowed to pool on the drapes, as the prep solution excoriates the skin. To avoid a fire hazard, prep solutions should not pool in the drapes.

Draping

The patient is draped with a "head drape," i.e., drape sheet and two towels under the head with the uppermost towel wrapped around the head and clipped. A split or U drape sheet covers the patient's body.

Alternate Draping. A disposable adhesive-backed sheet is placed across the forehead. A split or U drape sheet covers the patient's body.

Equipment

ESU (bipolar)
Sitting stools (2), surgeon and scrub person
Fiber-optic headlight and fiber-optic light source, e.g., Xenon 300 W, available

Instrumentation

Basic plastic procedures tray
Bipolar bayonet forceps

Supplies

Indelible marking pen
Local anesthetic, e.g., lidocaine 0.5% with epinephrine 1:200,000
Control syringes (2) and needles (2), 25 or 27 gauge × 1½″
Medicine cups (2), paper labels
Small basin, saline or antibiotic irrigation, and bulb syringe
Blades, (2) #15
Needle magnet or counter
Ophthalmic cautery, optional

Special Notes

- Apply **Special Notes** from ***Reduction of Nasal Fracture***, p. 707, as applicable.

Rhytidectomy

Definition

Excision of redundant facial skin and subcutaneous tissue to minimize wrinkles and rejuvenate the appearance of the face.

Discussion

Rhytidectomy ("face-lift") is performed to minimize the appearance of wrinkles and restore a youthful contour to facial skin. The procedure may include a lift of the forehead, neck and the central facial zone; excess skin in these areas is excised. ***Blepharoplasty***, p. 727, is often combined with **rhytidectomy**. Numerous nonsurgical modalities have been developed to augment or postpone rhytidectomy. Examples include the injection of various "fillers" such as collagen and synthetics, autologous fat, Botox injection, laser application, chemical irritants ("peel"), ***dermabrasion*** (see p. 732), and use of innumerable nonprescription "cosmetic" creams. An endoscopic approach to rhytidectomy permits lifting the tissues selectively, without extensive incisions. Rhytidectomy combined with blepharoplasty is the standard; patients often require a second procedure within several years to maintain the result. The extensive procedure includes meticulous hemostasis and may take several hours. Preoperative consultation is comprehensive, explaining various technicalities and review of "before and after" photos of other patients. No guarantee of "acceptable" result is given; preoperative photos are taken and included in the patient's record. Many of these procedures are performed in a surgeon's private operatorium.

Procedure

The incision follows previously made markings that follow the anterior contour of the ear, extending superiorly into the scalp, inferiorly curving about the posterior aspect of the ear, and extending posteriorly to the scalp. The skin and subcutaneous tissue are mobilized by undermining. Dissection of tissues under the platysma muscle, referred to as the submuscular aponeurotic system (SMAS) procedure, minimizes the amount of skin that must be undermined. Care is taken to avoid injury to nerves (e.g., the facial nerve branches and the greater auricular nerve). After hemostasis is secured, plication sutures are placed in the musculofascial tissues. Tension is placed on the flap, directing it superiorly and posteriorly as anchoring sutures are placed. Excess skin is trimmed. Wound closure is completed with fine interrupted sutures. Care is exerted not to distort the ear. A closed suction drainage unit may be placed. A pressure dressing is applied, taking care to pad the ears. Ice compresses are applied immediately following the procedure.

Preparation of the Patient

Anesthesia may be local or general, but local anesthesia with *conscious sedation* is usually preferred, as these patients are usually discharged on the same day. The table may be turned 90° to facilitate the surgeon's access. The surgeon usually marks the face prior to skin preparation and injects the local anesthetic. The patient is in supine position with the back slightly elevated; a padded or gel headrest may be used. One arm may be extended on a padded armboard and the opposite arm padded and tucked in at the patient's side, or both arms may be padded and secured at the patient's sides. A pillow may be placed under the knees to avoid straining the low back, or the table may be flexed for comfort. Bony prominences and areas vulnerable to skin and neurovascular pressure or trauma are padded. An electrosurgical dispersive pad is not usually applied as bipolar electrosurgery is used.

When the procedure is performed under local anesthesia, in the absence of an anesthesia provider, a perioperative RN, in addition to the circulator, is required to monitor the patient and administer *conscious sedation*, as directed by the surgeon; see p. 74 for the responsibilities of the perioperative RN monitoring the patient. Hair is rarely shaved, but the surgeon may request that hair around the hairline be secured.

Skin Preparation

Check with the surgeon regarding the type of prep solution to be used. Secure hair around the hairline in small rubber bands away from the face. Begin at the eyelids and prep the face; extend the prep from the hairline to the shoulders and down to the table at the side of the neck.

Care is taken to avoid getting prep solution in the eyes. The eyes are irrigated with normal saline from inner to outer canthus. Moist cotton pads are placed over the eyes; when general anesthesia is employed, antibiotic ointment is placed in the conjunctival sacs. Small cotton plugs or cotton balls are placed in the ears to prevent prep solution from pooling in the ears (they are removed with a mosquito forceps before draping). Prep solutions are not allowed to pool on the drapes, as the prep solution excoriates the skin. To avoid a fire hazard, prep solutions should not pool in the drapes.

Draping

The patient is usually draped with a "head drape," i.e., drape sheet and two towels under the head with the uppermost towel wrapped around the head and clipped. A split or U drape sheet covers the patient's body.

Alternate Draping. A disposable adhesive-backed sheet is placed across the forehead. A split or U drape sheet covers the patient's body.

Equipment

Padded or gel headrest (e.g., doughnut, Shea, Richards), optional
Restraints, padded
ESU (bipolar)
Sitting stools, 2 (surgeon and scrub person)

Instrumentation

Basic plastic procedures tray
Facelift scissors, Deaver retractors (2) 1″, bipolar bayonet forceps

Supplies

Marking pen with indelible ink
Local anesthetic, e.g., lidocaine 0.5% with epinephrine 1:200,000
Control syringes (2) and needles (2), 25 or 27 gauge × 1½″
Medicine cups (2), paper labels
Small basin, saline or antibiotic irrigation, and bulb syringe
Blades, (4 to 6) #15
Needle magnet or counter

Cotton-tipped applicators
Drain (e.g., Hemovac™, Jackson-Pratt™), optional
Nonadherent dressing, e.g., Adaptic, Owen's, Xeroform, Opsite, antibiotic ointment, and gauze fluffs

Special Notes

- Apply **Special Notes** from ***Reduction of Nasal Fracture***, p. 707, as applicable.
- In the PACU, the perioperative practitioner observes the patient for signs of excessive bleeding or hematoma formation; observations, nursing interventions, and the appearance of the face are documented for medicolegal reasons.
- In the PACU, the perioperative practitioner checks that head of the patient's bed is elevated and ice packs are applied. Both measures serve to reduce any postoperative swelling.

Dermabrasion

Definition

Sanding the skin to smooth scars and resurface irregularities in the skin.

Discussion

Dermabrasion serves to help the body to generate a new layer of skin. Cutaneous lasers seem to have replaced dermabrasion, or at least lessened the frequency of its use; however, **dermabrasion** may still be the treatment of choice in some instances. Like the CO_2 laser, Nd:YAG laser (e.g., Orion™ laser system), and the ultra pulsed laser, dermabrasion is performed to remove or minimize the appearance of scars (e.g., from facial acne vulgaris and chicken pox), remove tattoos, and remove or minimize fine wrinkling around the mouth by planing the skin with a dermatome or laser. Wrinkle eradication is temporary; as with aging, the wrinkling eventually returns. **Dermabrasion** may be performed in conjunction with ***rhytidectomy*** or other plastic surgeries; the procedure is often performed in a surgeon's office operatorium.

Possible complications include uneven changes in skin tone, scarring, and infection. Patients are advised to stay out of the sun as much as possible, and when they are out of doors, they must wear sunscreen.

The advantages of using dermabrasion versus laser are:

- It is easy to learn and perform
- It does not require expensive equipment
- The equipment does not take up much floor space
- It does not require specialized assistants or equipment

- It does not require special safety equipment
- It is significantly less expensive than incisional or laser modalities

Procedure

Dermabrasion may be performed using a local anesthetic, but when the entire face is dermabraded, general anesthesia is recommended. The skin is marked prior to the injection of the anesthetic (that may alter the appearance of scars). The skin is stretched by hand and held taunt as the surgeon abrades the epidermis using a motor-driven sanding cylinder and/or a wire brush. When a laser is employed (e.g., CO_2 laser, Nd:YAG laser [e.g., Orion laser system], and the ultra-pulsed laser) to resurface the skin, all laser safety measures must be employed. The advantage of using the ultra-pulsed laser is that it generates a minimal amount of heat that does not damage surrounding tissues. The area is irrigated copiously with saline during (and following) the procedure. The wound may be dressed with nonadherent gauze and gauze sponges moistened with saline. A compression bandage may be applied.

Preparation of the Patient

The surgeon marks the scars prior to the skin prep. Local anesthesia is usually employed, but as stated above, when the entire face is dermabraded general anesthesia is most often used. The table may be turned 90° to facilitate the surgeon's access. When the scar(s) is (are) on the face, the patient is supine with the head positioned on a padded or gel headrest (affected side up) to stabilize it and the dependent ear well padded. The ipsilateral arm is padded and tucked in at the patient's side and the arm on the unaffected side may be extended on a padded armboard, or both arms may be padded and secured at the patient's sides. A pillow may be placed under the knees to avoid straining the lower back, or the table may be flexed for comfort. Bony prominences and areas vulnerable to skin and neurovascular pressure or trauma are padded.

For special considerations for the pediatric patient, see **Pediatric General Information,** p. 978.

Skin Preparation

Check with the surgeon regarding the type of prep solution to be used. Begin at the location of the scar; if the scar is on the cheek, begin at the cheek. Extend the prep from the hairline to the shoulders and down to the table at the sides of the neck.

A perioperative RN, in addition to the circulator, is required to monitor the patient (receiving local anesthetic) and administer *conscious sedation*, as directed by the surgeon; see p. 74 for the responsibilities of the perioperative RN monitoring the patient. Hair is rarely shaved, but the surgeon may request that hair around the hairline be secured.

Draping

The patient is usually draped with a "head drape," i.e., drape sheet and two towels under the head with the uppermost towel wrapped around the head and clipped. A split or U drape sheet covers the patient's body.

Alternate Draping. A disposable adhesive-backed sheet is placed across the forehead. A split or U drape sheet covers the patient's body.

Equipment

Padded or gel headrest (e.g., doughnut, Shea, Richards), optional
Restraints, padded
Dermabrader power unit, unless electrical
Laser (e.g. CO_2, Nd:YAG [e.g. Orion laser system], or the ultra pulsed laser), optional

Instrumentation

Limited procedures tray
Dermabrader and cord (e.g., Stryker), wire brush, and sanding cylinder

Supplies

Indelible marking pen
Local anesthetic, e.g., lidocaine 0.5% with epinephrine 1:200,000
Control syringes (2) and needles (2), 25 or 27 gauge × 1½″
Medicine cup, paper labels
Small basin, saline or antibiotic irrigation, and bulb syringe
Nonadherent dressing (e.g., Adaptic, Owen's, Xeroform, Opsite, Tegaderm™, Bioclusive™, or Second Skin™), gauze fluffs, kerlix (for headwrap)

Special Notes

- Apply **Special Notes** from ***Reduction of Nasal Fracture***, p. 707, as applicable.
- As this procedure requires concentration, keep distractions in the room to a minimum. Distractions could cause the surgeon to divert his/her attention, causing a gouge in the skin or worse scarring defect.
- **Reminder:** *Use safety precautions to identify, label, and dispense medications or solutions and to avoid medication errors;* *see p. 30.* It is mandatory that all medications and solutions on the sterile field be labeled by name and strength. Medication bottles are retained in the room until the procedure has concluded.

- **N.B.** *The scrub person should avoid leaving loose sponges near the dermabrader, as they may get caught in the mechanism; this could inadvertently result in scarring the patient.*

Otoplasty

Definition

Otoplasty involves reshaping, remodeling, and/or reforming the external ear.

Discussion

Otoplasty is performed to correct congenital deformities of the ear(s), as microtia (i.e., small, often misshapen ears) and anotia (i.e., absence of the external ear), as well as "lop" ears (i.e., prominent ears that protrude unduly from the sides of the head). Patients with microtia may also have aurel atresia (absence of ear canal) in addition to other facial abnormalities, such as hemi microsomia (first and second branchial arch syndrome), other mandibular syndromes, and Treacher Collins syndrome. The latter occurs bilaterally and tends to be an inherited trait. The patient or the patient's parents have three options; choices include no treatment, prefabricated prosthesis, or ear reconstruction. Planning is essential in every step of the prefabricated prosthesis placement or the ear reconstruction procedure.

Reconstruction of the ear can be performed in one of three ways:

1. With prosthetic replacement
2. With prosthetic framework
3. With autologous tissue (flap may be necessary) and prosthetic framework

Complications include poor healing and infection.

The prefabricated prosthetic replacement requires placement of titanium posts into the temporal bone to secure the artificial ear; the ear needs to be changed approximately twice a year. Care is taken to avoid injury to the facial nerve. A bone graft may be required for sufficient bone to place posts. The bone graft may be secured with a lag screw or micro plate and micro screws. Matching the color of the skin is often difficult. The complications most frequently encountered with the prefabricated prosthesis are erosion and exposure.

Formerly, if microtia was unilateral, the procedure was performed when the child was about 6 years old, just before starting school. By the age of 6, the ears have "almost" developed to their adult size; however, most experienced surgeons prefer to wait until the child is 10 years old. Waiting for reconstruction permits the child's cartilage from the ribs (sixth to ninth) to better develop, and the surgery is more successful. The age at which the reconstruction is actually performed is somewhere between 4 to 10 years old. The surgeon must balance the psychological impact of the defect versus having adequate tissue to perform the surgery. If microtia occurs bilaterally, the surgery is performed at about 4 years old, giving the child an opportunity to hear and thereby learn how to speak (with an acceptable speech pattern) before entering school. For the child with ears that are too small, even though both ears may appear small, they are less noticeable than asymmetric ears. The ideal time for the correction of "lop ears" is about 4 years old (prior to school-age). Significant technical advances are being made in the field of microtia reconstruction. The surgeons find insuring symmetry and positioning are the most difficult aspects to achieve with any procedure chosen. In addition to the psychological issues for the child with microtia, another important factor to consider is the child's ability to hear. When internal ear reconstruction is necessary, the surgeon must be highly specialized with extensive experience in this aspect of ear reconstruction. Some patients will require a functioning ear canal. The ear must function by directing sound waves into the auditory canal and by maintaining the proper environment for the inner ear membrane. The surgeon performing this aspect of surgery must have complete knowledge of the transmission of sound. When the external ear is reconstructed, the surgeon must possess complete understanding of the three-dimensional anatomy of the ear and knowledge of the principles of tissue transfer. Hearing without hearing aids is the goal. Total ear reconstruction requires three to four surgical procedures (one every few months). The sixth and seventh synchondroses are used to form the base of the "new" ear. The eighth rib is used to form the rim or helix. In addition, an ear canal must be drilled for some patients. When necessary, skin may be grafted from the buttocks to cover the frame constructed from the rib. Some surgeon specialists are using a "tissue-engineered autologous cartilage" composed of autologous chondrocytes that are seeded into an ear-shaped mesh instead of the rib. When hearing cannot be reconstructed, a bone anchoring hearing aid (BAHA) must be worn.

Procedure

The more common **"lop ear" surgery** is described. A planned skin excision is marked behind the ear. A new antihelical fold is marked. Several diagonal lines are marked on corresponding sides of the elliptical incision. An incision is made on the distal side and a flap is undermined, taking care not to compromise the circulation. The anterior surface of the cartilage is exposed and abraded with a rasp to reduce the perichondrium; thereby subsequently reducing forward curling of the ear. A predetermined wedge may be excised. Mattress sutures are inserted through the previously made markings. Overlapping skin is excised. The ear skin is sutured with nonabsorbable interrupted sutures (4-0 or 5-0). A compression dressing is applied.

For microtia, a version of the several varied procedures for **ear reconstruction** is described; the steps for the surgery vary with the surgeon and the type of procedure chosen. Two teams may participate in this arduous surgery. One surgeon brings or draws two templates on x-ray film; one demonstrates the position of the ear in relation to the rest of the face, and the other delineates the shape of the ear framework. The template is flash autoclaved for use during the procedure. The surgeon marks the skin with indelible ink about the ear and at levels on the chest wall indicating the sixth through ninth ribs. He/she infiltrates the sites with local anesthetic with epinephrine (e.g., lidocaine 0.5% with epinephrine 1:200,000). An incision is made on the chest wall; segments of the ribs are obtained. Care is taken not to injure the perichondrium. Saline irrigation is employed to test the integrity of the pleural cavity. Should bubbles appear, a chest tube is inserted and later connected to a closed chest drainage system. When there is a question regarding the pleura's integrity, an x-ray may be taken. The chest incision may be injected with the local anesthetic for postoperative analgesia and to reduce bleeding. The chest wound is closed. When there are two teams, one team closes the chest as the other team carves the ribs according to the template; 4–6mm gouges (Buxton) may be used to refine the carving. The cartilage is shaped to reproduce the ear prototype; fine stainless steel wire is used in construction of the ear framework. At the completion of the framework construction, a section of unused cartilage is placed at the donor for harvest at the second procedure. An incision is made about the ear depending on where there is skin available to be used to the best advantage. A transtemporal fascial flap or a postauricular flap is developed. The vascularity of the graft is determined using a doppler and sterile conduction gel. The cartilage remnant is excised, freeing the maximum amount of skin to drape over the ear framework. The skin flap is elevated and additional skin is freed for a tension-free closure of the reconstructed ear. Meticulous hemostasis is obtained before the framework is secured. Particular care is paid to ensure the symmetry and level of the placement of the ear. Suction drains and a nonadherent dressing pad and cotton fluffs are placed; a headwrap secures the dressing.

Three or four months later, the second stage refines the reconstruction. Following this antibiotic, ointment may be applied to the repair and a nonadherent dressing and cotton fluffs are placed, and a headwrap secures the dressing.

If the inner ear is to be reconstructed, it is done as a third stage at a later date.

Preparation of the Patient

The patient may be an adult (usually male) or a child; **otoplasty** for the adult patient is described, as well as ear reconstruction. The table may be turned 90° to facilitate the surgeon's access. The surgeon marks the skin prior to skin preparation. Local anesthesia is usually employed. The patient is supine with head on a padded or gel headrest; the surgeon will position the head as necessary in order to see both ears at the same time. The ipsilateral arm is padded and tucked in at the patient's side and the arm on the unaffected side may be extended on a padded armboard, or both arms may be padded and secured at the patient's sides. A pillow may be placed under the knees to avoid straining the low back, or the table may be flexed for comfort. Bony prominences and areas vulnerable to skin and neurovascular pressure or trauma are padded. An electrosurgical dispersive pad is applied when unipolar electrosurgery is used. For the special considerations concerning the pediatric patient, see **Pediatric General Information**, p. 978.

Skin Preparation

Check with the surgeon regarding the type of prep solution to be used. Usually both ears are prepped so to surgeon can assess symmetry and level. Begin by placing a small cotton ball in each ear to prevent the solution from pooling in the ears; prep each external ear; extend prep from the hairline to the shoulders and down to the table at the sides.

Draping

The patient is draped with a "head drape" with both ears exposed (drape sheet and two towels under the head with the uppermost towel wrapped around the head and clipped). A split (or drape) sheet covers the body. An additional drape sheet may be needed to cover the foot of the table.

Equipment

Padded or gel headrest (e.g., Shea, doughnut), optional
Padded restraints, optional
ESU, unipolar and/or bipolar

Instrumentation

Basic plastic procedures tray (contains caliper, calibrated knife handle, Freer elevator)
Small rasp, small periosteal elevator (on tray), small bone cutter, small bone rongeur, and bipolar bayonet forceps

Prefabricated Prosthetic Replacement, Add

Minor orthopedic procedures tray
Prefabricated prosthethesis

Titanium posts
Lag screw or micro plate and micro screws

Ear Reconstruction, Add
Minor orthopedic procedures tray
Doppler probe and sterile gel
Buxton gouges 4–6mm, caliper and depth gauge (ruler on tray), ALM self-retaining retractor, and fine stainless steel wire

Supplies

Indelible marking pen
Small cotton balls (2) for ear during skin prep
Local anesthetic, e.g., lidocaine 0.5% with epinephrine 1:200,000
Control syringes (2) and needles (2), 25 or 27 gauge × 1½″
Medicine cup, paper labels
Small basin, saline or antibiotic irrigation, and bulb syringe
Blades, (2) #15
Needle magnet or counter
Cotton-tipped applicators
Electrosurgical pencil with needle tip and cord, holder, and scraper
Bunnell needles (2)
Suction drain, e.g., Hemovac
Nonadherent dressing, e.g., Adaptic, Owen's, Xeroform, Opsite, gauze fluffs, and roller gauze (for a headwrap)

Special Notes

- Apply **Special Notes** from ***Reduction of Nasal Fracture***, p. 707, as applicable for the adult patient and as applicable. For the pediatric patient, see the special considerations in the **Pediatric General Information** p. 978.
- **N.B. Reminder:** *Use every precaution to correctly identify the pediatric patient for patient safety.* Document methods used to identify the pediatric patient for medicolegal reasons.
- **N.B. Reminder:** Assess and document the patient's anxiety regarding the procedure and the unfamiliar environment; provide emotional support such as maintaining eye contact and holding the patient's hand during the administration of anesthesia, etc., and answer patients' or parents' questions in a knowledgeable manner. Document that these measures were done for medicolegal reasons.
- **N.B.** Provide emotional support to the pediatric patient's parents. During the lengthy ear reconstruction procedure, the cir-

culator may offer periodic updates regarding the surgery to help to decrease parental anxiety.

- **N.B. Reminder:** Provide emotional support to the patient regarding feelings of altered body image and give the adult patient an opportunity to express his/her feelings.
- When ear reconstruction is performed, the surgeon may draw templates on x-ray film. These templates can be flash sterilized (autoclaved) for use during the surgery.
- Extreme care is taken to avoid contamination of the graft site and the prosthetic ear or the reconstructed ear.

Repair of Syndactyly

Definition

Separation and reconstructive repair of webbed or fused digits.

Discussion

Syndactyly most often occurs in the hand; the middle and ring finger are the most frequently webbed. Repair is advised according to the severity of the fusion; repair is most often performed between the ages of 6 months to 2 years. Toe syndactyly does not always require surgical intervention because the movement of the toes individually is not necessary for walking. Syndactyly may exist with only skin involvement (simple), or the webbing may involve other soft tissues (e.g., nerves, blood vessels, and tendons), but it can also involve fused bones. In addition, syndactyly may occur with other digital anomalies. The repair may require full-thickness grafting; when webbing involves many digits, full-thickness skin grafts *must* be done. When syndactyly is noted in the newborn male, circumcision may be delayed so that the foreskin can be used for the full-thickness graft; this obviates the need to obtain skin for the graft from an additional area. In other instances, skin can be obtained from the groin, buttocks, or the medial aspect of the arm or the thigh.

Procedure

The pediatric patient is supine on the table. The lower segment of the table may be removed to permit closer access to the pediatric patient. Skin areas are marked prior to the skin prep. A pediatric pneumatic tourniquet may be used. Z-plasty type incisions are made in the webbing to create flaps at the sides of the fingers for the web-spacing reconstruction; this avoids later contracture. The neurovascular bundles are protected. Bony and ligamentous defects, if present, are corrected. The flaps are rotated and sutured into position. If there are areas where the skin is absent, full-thickness grafts are obtained to close the defects. The incisions are closed. Stents may be sutured over the grafts. If a tourniquet was used, it is deflated. A bulky dressing and splint are applied to immobilize the hand.

Preparation of the Patient

Special measures must be taken for the pediatric patient to prepare the room, restrain the patient, and maintain the patient's body temperature, etc. To prevent body heat loss, the room temperature may be raised and a warming mattress may be placed on the table.

Anesthesia may be general, regional, or local; general anesthesia is employed for children. For the special considerations concerning the pediatric patient, see **Pediatric General Information**, p. 978. The table may be turned 90° to facilitate the surgeon's access.

For syndactyly of the fingers, the patient is supine; the patient is brought as close to the ipsilateral edge of the table as possible. The arm on the affected side may be extended on a padded hand table, or a padded armboard may be used; the unaffected hand is secured with a padded restraint. Webril (sheet wadding) and a pediatric tourniquet are applied to the arm on the affected side. Bony prominences and areas vulnerable to skin and neurovascular pressure or trauma are padded. An electrosurgical dispersive pad is not applied as bipolar electrosurgery is used.

Skin Preparation

For syndactyly of the fingers, begin with the fingers at the area of syndactyly and prep the hand (including interdigital spaces). Extend the prep from the fingertips to the level of the tourniquet on the affected arm (includes the elbow).

Draping

For syndactyly of the fingers, the hand is grasped, abducted, and elevated with a tube stockinette as a sheet is draped over the hand table. A split sheet is draped under the arm. A towel is folded (in thirds, longitudinally), wrapped around the top of the arm (over the tube stockinette), and clipped. A split sheet is draped over the arm and shoulder and clipped under the arm. The arm is passed through an extremity drape (fenestrated sheet), and individual drape sheets complete the draping, as necessary.

Equipment

Padded hand table

Pneumatic tourniquet (pediatric, when indicated) and pneumatic insufflator with microprocessor regulator

ESU, unipolar or bipolar

Sitting stools, 2 to 3 (surgeon, scrub person, assistant surgeon)
Cast cart

Instrumentation

Minor orthopedic procedures tray or
Plastic procedures tray or
Vascular shunt tray
Skin hooks (on tray), bipolar bayonet forceps and cord

Supplies

Indelible marking pen
Webril (sheet wadding)
Small tube stockinette
Small Esmarch bandage
Blades, (2) #15
Electrosurgical pencil with needle tip, cord, holder, and scraper, optional
Needle magnet or counter
Small basin, saline or antibiotic irrigation, bulb syringe
Stents, optional
Nonadherent dressing, e.g., Adaptic, Owen's, Xeroform, Opsite, and gauze fluffs
Splint supplies, optional

Special Notes

- Apply **Special Notes** from ***Abdominal Laparotomy***, p. 134, as applicable. Special considerations for care of the pediatric patient are necessary; see **Pediatric General Information,** p. 978.
- **N.B. Reminder:** *Use every precaution to correctly identify the pediatric patient.* Document methods used to identify the pediatric patient for medicolegal reasons.
- **N.B.** *The circulator should verify infant patient information with the parent(s) or legal guardian(s), regarding sensitivities and allergies, etc.* Document all information that was obtained and noted, nursing interventions, and patient outcomes in the **Perioperative Record** (p. 12).
- **N.B.** *Remember that* **"the pediatric patient is not a small adult."** Special measures and precautions for the pediatric patient and the neonate, in particular, must be observed. Administering preoperative medication (rarely), administering of anesthesia, preparing the room, and monitoring body temperature to

retain body heat, accurate fluid balance, methods of restraining the patient, etc., are vitally important. Again, to plan and consider all the special measures that must be taken for the pediatric patient, refer to **Pediatric General Information**, p. 978.

- **Reminder:** Ascertain that the *correct* x-ray films for the *correctly identified* patient are in the room prior to starting the surgery.
- When a tourniquet is used, document the location, the length of time, and the appearance of the skin before and immediately after the procedure medicolegal reasons. Remember, children require much lower tourniquet pressure; apply all safety precautions; see p. 45.
- Check with the surgeon regarding whether a graft is needed and the location of the donor site when a graft will be taken.
- **N.B. Note:** It is extremely important that when a graft is applied, one must be sure the graft is ***dermis side down***.
- **N.B. Reminder:** *All safety precautions regarding the safe use of the tourniquet must be observed and documented; see p. 45.* The appearance of the extremity must be documented before and after the surgery for medicolegal reasons.

Digital Flexor Tendon Repair

Definition

Approximation of severed ends of a tendon caused by injury or a failed previous tendon repair.

Discussion

Free grafts are obtained to repair the ends of a damaged digital flexor tendon. When a large defect exists, the palmaris longus tendon is most frequently used for the repair. Tendons to the digits may be severed from the forearm to the base of the distal phalanx. Injuries between the distal palmar crease, and proximal interphalangeal joint should be repaired initially and treated by a tendon graft at a later time. Tension must be adequate but not excessive; during surgery, the elimination of bowstringing without restricting tendon excursion (through excessive friction) is necessary. Avoidance of excessive tension, meticulous handling of tissue, good hemostasis, fine nonreactive sutures, and dynamic immobilization are important factors for a successful repair.

Procedure

The incision is made according to the site of the injury. Midlateral digital incisions are often employed. Care is taken to avoid injury to neurovascular bundles. Pulleys are preserved when possible. The proximal tendon end is retrieved; intrasynovial donor tendons provide the best gliding characteristics. If length is not sufficient, a graft (e.g., from the palmaris longus tendon) is prepared. The tendon ends are approximated. If the tendon insertion is involved, suture to the bone may be facilitated using fine drill holes. The suture fixing the tendon graft to the insertion is tied over a button on the dorsum of the distal phalanx to prevent soft tissue necrosis. The wound is closed. A splint is applied.

Preparation of the Patient

Anesthesia may be general, regional, or local. The patient is supine; the arm on the affected side is extended on a padded hand table, while the arm on the unaffected side may be extended on a padded armboard. Webril (sheet wadding) and a tourniquet are applied high on the affected arm. A pillow may be placed under the knees to avoid straining the lower back, or the table may be flexed for comfort. Bony prominences and areas vulnerable to skin and neurovascular pressure or trauma are padded. An electrosurgical dispersive pad is not applied as bipolar electrosurgery is used.

Skin Preparation

Begin at the repair site; prep the hand (including interdigital spaces). Extend the prep from the fingertips to the level of the tourniquet. This prep includes the area from which the palmaris longus donor graft is obtained from the forearm.

Draping

The extremity is abducted, elevated, and grasped in a tube stockinette as a sheet is draped over the end of the hand table. A split sheet is draped under the arm. A towel is folded (in thirds, longitudinally), wrapped around the top of the arm (over the tube stockinette), and clipped. A split sheet is draped over the shoulder and clipped under the arm. The arm is passed through a fenestrated sheet (e.g., extremity drape), and individual drape sheets complete the draping.

When a microscope is used, a microscope drape is necessary.

Equipment

Padded hand table
Tourniquet and pneumatic insufflator with microprocessor regulator
ESU bipolar
Loupes or microscope (available)
Sitting stools, 2 to 3 (surgeon, scrub person, assistant surgeon)
Cast cart

Instrumentation

Minor orthopedic procedures tray or
Plastic procedures tray
Bipolar bayonet forceps, optional
Skin hooks, hand drill, chuck, key, and fine drill points, optional
Microinstrumentation; see Peripheral Nerve Repair, p. 747.
ALM self-retaining retractor

Supplies

Indelible marking pen
Tube stockinette
Webril (sheet wadding)
Esmarch bandage
Blades (2) #15
Electrosurgical pencil with needle tip, cord, holder, and scraper, optional
Needle magnet or counter
Small basin, saline or antibiotic irrigation, bulb syringe
Bunnell needles (2) and sterile button
Nonadherent dressing, e.g., Adaptic, Owen's, Xeroform, Opsite, and gauze fluffs
Splint (dynamic splint, optional)

Special Notes

- Apply **Special Notes** from ***Repair of Syndactyly*** p. 742, as applicable.
- When a tourniquet is used, see p. 45 for safety precautions. Document the location, the length of time the tourniquet is up, and the appearance of the extremity before and after the procedure for medicolegal reasons.

Peripheral Nerve Repair

Definition

The complete or partial anastomosis of a transected or otherwise injured peripheral nerve.

Discussion

Peripheral nerves may be completely or partially divided by trauma, such as acts of violence, burns, or crush injury, or during the course of surgery (accidental or by intent), particularly with excision of malignant tumors. According to the patient's general condition and the condition of the site of injury, it is determined whether primary or secondary repair is appropriate. If a significant length of nerve has been damaged, several methods can be employed to achieve tension-free repair, including additional mobilization (avoiding injury to local blood supply), positioning adjacent joints accordingly, transposition, nerve grafting, and, less often, bone resection. When interpositional nerve grafting is necessary, cutaneous nerves (e.g., lateral antebrachial or sural) are used. A segment of the sural nerve is harvested from the posterolateral calf and sectioned into smaller lengths that are used to connect individual fascicles (perineural repair, see below).

Different nerves exhibit different fascicular patterns; these patterns are taken into consideration during the repair. When nerve repair is delayed, areas of fibrosis or neuroma occur and must be excised (with microscissors or diamond knife); when feasible, direct anastomosis should be effected with anatomical alignment of fascicles to improve ultimate function. The operating microscope and nerve stimulator are employed.

Procedure

For upper- or lower-extremity procedures, general, regional, or local anesthesia may be employed. Most often a pneumatic tourniquet is utilized. Wound cleansing and trimming of bone ends, if applicable, are done. The course of the involved nerve is marked on the skin, and an incision extending beyond the anticipated site of mobilization is made. The uninvolved nerve proximal and distal to the site of injury is carefully mobilized prior to dissecting and trimming the involved segment. To preserve alignment, longitudinal epineurial vessels are identified or marking sutures are placed. Care is taken to avoid injury to the local nerve branches. When necessary, endoneurolysis (dissection of the nerve trunk) is performed, while disturbing uninvolved neural tissues as little as possible. Anastomosis is achieved after fascicles are rotationally aligned and approximated, employing fine nylon sutures (8-0 to 10-0 monofilament).

Three basic techniques are used for nerve repair:

- **Epineural**: the fascicles are aligned tension free, the epineurium is circumferentially approximated.
- **Perineural**: the epineurium is trimmed or reflected to expose the individual fascicles that are directly approximated.
- **Epiperineural**: the central fascicles are approximated directly and epineural sutures align the peripheral fascicles.

Hemostatic agents, such as Gelfoam and thrombin, may be employed. The wounds are closed and splinting is applied as necessary. During the surgery, a nerve stimulator is used to identify whether nervous tissue is functioning.

Preparation of the Patient

For **upper-extremity peripheral nerve repair,** the patient is supine; the arm on the affected side may be extended on a padded hand table and the arm on the unaffected side may be extended on a padded armboard or padded and tucked in at the patient's side. Webril (sheet wadding) and a tourniquet are applied to the arm on the affected side.

For **lower-extremity peripheral nerve repair,** the patient is supine. Sheet wadding and a tourniquet are applied to the affected extremity, and the safety strap is secured over the thigh of the unaffected extremity.

The table may be flexed for the patient's comfort. Bony prominences and areas vulnerable to skin and neurovascular pressure or trauma are padded. An electrosurgical dispersive pad is not applied as bipolar electrosurgery is used.

Skin Preparation

Upper-Extremity Peripheral Nerve Repair. Begin at the repair site; prep the hand (including interdigital spaces). Extend the prep from the fingertips to the level of the tourniquet.

Lower Extremity Peripheral Nerve Repair. Begin at the repair site; prep the foot. Extend the prep from the toes to the level of the tourniquet.

Draping

See **Digital Flexor Tendon Repair**, p. 744.

When a microscope is used, a drape is required.

Equipment

Padded hand table (upper-extremity repair)
Tourniquet and pneumatic insufflator with microprocessor regulator
ESU, bipolar
Suction, optional
Cast cart
Nerve stimulator console, e.g., Concept
Loupes or microscope (available)

Instrumentation

Basic plastic procedures tray
Bipolar bayonet forceps
Nerve stimulator probe (locator), e.g., Concept

Microinstruments

Von Graefe muscle hook, jewelers' forceps (2), micro elevator, microdissector, micro electrosurgical suction, diamond knife, Castroviejo-Vannas scissors, Castroviejo needle holder without lock, Castroviejo needle holder with lock

Supplies

Indelible marking pen
Tube stockinette

Webril (sheet wadding)
Esmarch bandage
Blades, (2) #15, (1) diamond
Gelfoam and thrombin
Needle magnet or counter
Small basin, saline or antibiotic irrigation, bulb syringe
Suture for repair (e.g., monofilament nylon 8-0 to 10-0)
Nonadherent dressing, e.g., Adaptic, Owen's, Xeroform, Opsite, and gauze fluffs
Splint, optional

Special Notes

- Apply **Special Notes** from ***Digital Flexor Tendon Repair***, p. 745, as applicable.
- Have the correct x-ray films in the room for the correctly identified patient before bringing the patient into the room.
- Check with the surgeon regarding the donor site (of graft, when taken) before starting to prep. If another site is used for the nerve graft, that extremity may have a tourniquet, and the extremity must be prepped and draped.
- **N.B. Reminder:** *All safety precautions regarding the safe use of the tourniquet must be observed and documented; see p. 45.* The appearance of the extremity must be documented before and immediately after the surgery for medicolegal reasons.
- **Reminder:** The donor graft site is covered with a towel until the surgeon is ready to take the graft.

Microsurgical Vascular Repair

Definition

The repair or reconstruction of vascular structures under magnification.

Discussion

When arteries and veins are traumatized by transection, complete or partial, or suffer crush injury, or when vascular anastomoses are necessary, such as in interpositional grafting or in replantation procedures, magnification and the use of microsurgical techniques are necessary for optimal results when smaller vessels are involved. This modality is also used when myocutaneous or muscular flaps are transposed. Prior to definitive repair or anastomosis, the involved structures are debrided and trimmed to remove devitalized tissue. Mobilization (with sacrifice of lesser side branches) is done in order to provide adequate length to achieve a tension-free repair. When adequate length cannot be obtained, grafting is necessary. Vascular grafts may be harvested from local or remote site arteries or veins or vascular prostheses. Loupes or the operating microscope, microsurgical instruments, and the use of fine suture material, as well as a stabile operative field, is inherent is this application.

Procedure

Microsurgical Vascular Repair of an Artery is described. When an extremity is involved, a pneumatic tourniquet is employed. The surgeon may choose to wear magnifying loupes, but more often a microscope is employed. Following appropriate skin prep and draping, the principal local artery is identified and mobilized from surrounding supportive tissues. Ligation or coagulation of side branches with micro bipolar electrosurgical forceps is necessary to obtain adequate length for a tension-free anastomosis. As necessary, a noncritical venous segment may be harvested for an interpositional arterial graft, making certain to identify proximal and distal ends, as to be used in reversed direction. When used for venous repair, the anatomical direction is maintained.

Heparinized Ringer's solution, diluted to surgeon's preference, is used to irrigate the vessels. Lidocaine or topically applied papaverine solution can be used to overcome vasospasm. With the tourniquet inflated, microvascular clamps are applied. The anastomosis is done under appropriate magnification using interrupted sutures often initially placed at the 90° or 120° positions around the circumference. These sutures are used to create tension for placing the intervening sutures. Dilators and probes may be used to assure adequate patency. End-to-end or end-to-side (45° angle) anastomoses are performed. The tourniquet and microvascular clamps are released to check for bleeding. As indicated, a Doppler probe can be employed to test blood flow. Two local veins are repaired with similar techniques. Repair of other structures may be done (or delayed); the wound may be irrigated with saline or an antibiotic solution, closed, and bulky dressings and splint(s) applied.

Preparation of the Patient

Microsurgical Vascular Repair of an Artery (e.g., in the Forearm). The patient is in supine position with the affected arm extended on a padded hand table. The unaffected arm may be extended on a padded armboard, or the arm is padded and tucked in at the patient's side. A pillow may be placed under the knees to prevent lower back strain, or the table may be flexed for comfort. Webril and a tourniquet are applied to the affected extremity. All bony prominences and areas vulnerable to skin and neurovascular pressure or trauma are padded. An electrosurgical dispersive pad is not applied as bipolar electrosurgery is employed.

Skin Preparation

Begin at the site of the repair; extend the prep outward to an acceptable distance, e.g., begin prepping the forearm. Prep the forearm, the hand (including interdigital spaces), and the arm. Extend the prep from the fingertips to the level of the tourniquet.

Draping

The site is draped according to the location of the repair, e.g., forearm. The extremity is elevated in a tube stockinette as a sheet is draped over the end of the hand table. A split sheet is draped under the arm. A towel is folded (in thirds, longitudinally), wrapped around the top of the arm (over the tube stockinette), and clipped. A split sheet is draped over the shoulder and clipped under the arm. The arm is passed through a fenestrated sheet (e.g., extremity drape), and individual drape sheets complete the draping.

If a microscope is used, a drape is necessary.

Equipment

Padded hand table, optional
Tourniquet and pneumatic insufflator with microprocessor regulator
ESU, bipolar (e.g., Malis)
Suction, optional
Loupes or microscope
Sitting stools, 2 to 3 (surgeon, scrub person, assistant surgeon)
Cast cart

Instrumentation

Shunt tray
Micro bipolar bayonet forceps and cord
Skin hooks, ALM self-retaining retractor
Doppler and probe, optional

Microinstruments

Von Graefe muscle hook, jewelers' forceps (2), micro elevator, microdissector, micro electrosurgical suction, diamond knife, Castroviejo-Vannas scissors, Castroviejo needle holder without lock, Castroviejo needle holder with lock

Supplies

Indelible marking pen and sterile labels
Control syringes (2) and needles (2), 25 or 27 gauge × 1½″
Local anesthetic, medicine cup, paper labels
Small basin, antibiotic solution, bulb syringe
Heparinized lactated Ringer's solution
Lidocaine or topical papaverine

Blades, (1) #15, (1) diamond blade
Microvascular suture
Needle magnet or counter
Nonadherent, dressing, e.g., Adaptic, Owen's, Xeroform, Opsite, and gauze fluffs
Splint

Special Notes

- Apply **Special Notes** from ***Digital Flexor Tendon Repair***, p. 745, as applicable.
- **N.B. Reminder:** *All safety precautions regarding safe use of the tourniquet must be observed and documented; see p. 45.* The appearance of the extremity must be documented before and after the surgery for medicolegal reasons.
- **Reminder:** *Use safety precautions to identify, label, and dispense medications or solutions and to avoid medication errors; see p. 30.* It is mandatory that all medications and solutions on the sterile field be labeled by name and strength. Medication bottles are retained in the room until the procedure has concluded.

Palmar Fasciectomy

Definition

Excision of the fascia (partial or total) of the palm.

Discussion

Dupuytren's contracture is a hereditary condition caused by a benign thickening of fibrous connective tissue in the palmar subcutaneous tissues with nodules fixed to the palmar fascia (located closer to the wrist). Subsequent contracture results in deformity with contractures of the dermis and/or digits. The condition may also affect the plantar surface of the foot, commonly referred to as lederhosen disease. The extent of this process is variable and does not always require surgical intervention.

Procedure

For less-involved presentations, a short longitudinal palmar incision is made adjacent to the restrictive band; the restrictive band is resected. For more extensive disease, a longer incision with Z-plasty configuration (see p. 690) is made to create flaps and lengthen the scar to avoid contracture. The palmar fascia is resected distally. Care is taken to avoid injury to digital nerves and flexor tendons. A more extensive presentation of fascia requires excision of more tissue. Wound closure may be done by primary suture using Z-plasty closure, or full-thickness free skin graft may be necessary (e.g., from the medial aspect of the ipsilateral arm). An anterior splint is applied.

For **Preparation of the Patient, Skin Preparation, Draping,** and **Equipment,** see *Digital Flexor Tendon Repair,* p. 744.

Instrumentation

Basic plastic procedures tray
Skin hooks (on tray) and ALM self-retaining retractor

Supplies

Indelible marking pen
Webril (sheet wadding)
Tube stockinette
Esmarch bandage
Electrosurgical pencil with needle tip, cord, holder, scraper
Blades, (2) #15
Needle magnet or counter
Nonadherent dressing, e.g., Adaptic, Owen's, Xeroform, Opsite, and gauze fluffs
Splint, optional

Special Notes

- Apply **Special Notes** from ***Digital Flexor Tendon Repair***, p. 745, as applicable.
- When a skin graft is to be taken, check with the surgeon regarding donor site before starting the skin prep.
- This procedure is generally performed with the patient receiving local anesthesia (e.g., nerve block) with or without *conscious sedation*. Remember that the patient is awake and can hear all that is said; limiting conversation is advised.

Reduction Mammoplasty/Mammaplasty

Definition

Excision of breast tissue hyperplasia with recontouring of the breasts.

Discussion

Excessive breast tissue may be referred to as breast hyperplasia or *macromastia*, and where there is extreme virginal hypertrophy of the breast, it may be referred to as *gigantomastia*. The excessively large and pendulous breasts cause symptoms of back, neck, and shoulder pain and can result in kyphosis due to the strain placed on the spine caused by the weight (greater than 0.45 kg or approximately 1 pound), in addition other symptoms including bra strap grooving, mammary intertrigo, and headache.

The principle indication for reduction mammoplasty is to alleviate the painful symptoms associated with excessive breast weight. Women also request the procedure seeking a more aesthetic appearance. Prior to surgery, the surgeon counsels the patient regarding scar appearance, the possible inability to breastfeed, the possible partial or complete loss of nipple sensation, and the possibility of nipple necrosis. The techniques employed for correction of the condition are determined by the shape and size of the breasts, the surgeon's experience and preference for a certain technique, and the patient's choice (following consultation with the surgeon). Proper symmetry, including nipple and areolar position, is most important.

Approaches include:

- **Lateralizing procedure**, which leaves no obvious scar; scar is along natural skin lines in the axilla.
- **Inverted T procedure**, which employs a vertical infraareolar and a transverse inframammary fold incision (with corresponding scar formation). Two variations include:
  - **Lassus reduction modification:** the nipple is on a superiorly based pedicle; there is no skin undermining, and vertical incisions are employed. The patient may receive collagen treatments to rehydrate and firm the skin and calm swollen tissue.
  - **Lejour reduction modification:** liposuction, skin undermining, and short vertical incision (above the inframammary fold). A complication that may occur as a result of liposuction is skin retraction secondary to scarring.

For patients with extremely large breasts, the nipple is transplanted on a pedicle to preserve its neurovascularization whenever possible, or the nipple may be excised (with the areola) and reapplied as a free graft.

Reduction of gynecomastia is the removal of hypertrophic breast tissue, a commonly occurring condition in males, most often around the time of puberty or after the age of 40. Generally, excess subcutaneous tissue is excised through a circumareolar incision. Liposuction, via a small circumareolar incision, is another approach option to reduce male breast size. Skin, glandular, and subcutaneous tissues may require removal in extreme presentations of gynecomastia. The procedure may be performed using general or local anesthesia with or without *conscious sedation*.

Breast reduction mammoplasty and **reduction of gynecomastia** may be performed as an endoscopic-assisted procedure.

Procedure

Inverted T Breast Reduction is described. The incisions have usually been marked with indelible ink preoperatively; the marks are checked for accurate assessment of symmetry and level prior to the skin prep (with the patient in the sitting position). The tissues are infiltrated with local anesthetic with epinephrine to reduce bleeding. An incision circumscribes the areola, which is left attached to underlying tissue as a pedicle graft with its neurovascular attachments; a Freeman areola marker may be used. The skin above the areola is undermined to create "thick" skin flaps (to avoid skin necrosis), using a knife, a CO_2 laser, or a Harmonic® ultrasonic scalpel. A wedge of excessive breast skin and glandular and adipose tissues are excised inferiorly, taking care to preserve the skin's vascularity, where needed. Liposuction may be employed to reduce the volume of fat to be excised. The procedure may also be performed as an endoscopic-assisted procedure, and liposuction can be employed as well (preserving the retroareolar area). As breast tissue is highly vascular, the coagulating effects and sealing properties of the laser or ultrasonic modalities are effective. A fiber-optic lighted retractor is particularly useful to achieve hemostasis. The new sites for nipple replacement are carefully cut out of the skin; a Freeman areola marker may be employed. The nipple on the pedicle is brought through the new opening. The breast is reconstructed by approximating the medial and lateral breast tissue with the skin flaps inferior to the "new" nipple site and transversely in the IMF, creating an inverted T. Drainage tubing may be inserted into the vertical incision. The procedure is repeated on the contralateral breast. Drainage tubing, when used, is connected with a Y connector and attached to a closed-suction device. A bulky dressing and a surgical bra for firm support are applied.

Preparation of the Patient

General anesthesia is employed. The patient is placed "symmetrically" on the table in supine position with arms placed on padded armboards, abducted, and secured (using padded arm restraints). Following induction of general anesthesia, the patient may be briefly paced in sitting position (by changing the position of the table from flat to achieve the sitting position) to assess the position of the breasts (to aid in ensuring symmetry). A padded footrest may be secured to the table for use when the table is repositioned to the sitting position. Later during the procedure the sitting position is employed to assess the breasts according to size, shape, and symmetry. Antiembolitic hose may be applied, as per request. The surgeon may request a sequential compression device with disposable leg wraps; they can be applied over the antiembolitic hose, or the leg wraps may be used alone (i.e., without hose). A pillow may be placed under the knees to prevent lower back strain, or the table may be flexed for comfort. All bony prominences and areas vulnerable to skin and neurovascular pressure or trauma are padded. An electrosurgical dispersive pad is applied.

Skin Preparation

Prep both breasts beginning at the nipples; extend preparation from the neckline to the level of the iliac crests and down to the table at the sides. Include the axilla in the prep. For extremely large pendulous breasts, the prep may be extended to the symphysis pubis.

Draping

Folded towels and a disposable transverse sheet and/or individual drape sheets may complete the draping.

The advantage of using disposable drapes is the adhesive backing on the underside of the fenestration that permits the drape to be secured around the perimeter of the surgical field.

Equipment

Sequential compression device with leg wraps, as requested
Padded footrest (for position change intraoperatively, to sitting position)
ESU, unipolar and/or bipolar
Scale (weigh each breast tissue specimen separately)
Fiber-optic headlight (may contain camera)
Fiber-optic light source, e.g., Xenon 300 W (may be used for fiber-optic headlight and fiber-optic lighted retractor or rigid fiber-optic endoscope)
CO_2 laser console, optional
Harmonic scalpel (ultrasound) generator and foot pedal, optional
Liposuction high-pressure vacuum unit, e.g., LySonix® ultrasonic liposuction
Video monitor, optional
Camera console, optional

Instrumentation

Basic/Minor procedures tray
Freeman areola marker, caliper, ruler, bipolar bayonet forceps
Fiber-optic lighted retractor with sleeve, blades, and cord, optional
Hopkins rigid endoscope and cord, electrosurgical suction-irrigator, optional
CO_2 laser handpiece and cord, optional (Note: obey all laser safety precautions; see p. 94)
Harmonic scalpel handpiece with scissors or blade tip (variety types) and cord, optional
Liposuction hand piece blunt suction cannulas (e.g., 4 mm preferred)

Supplies

Antiembolitic hose
Indelible marking pen
OR table sheet, absorbent impervious (HK Surgical™)
Control syringes (2) and needles, (2) 25 or 27 gauge, (2) 22 gauge, and spinal

Local anesthetic, e.g., 0.5% lidocaine with epinephrine 1:200,000 for vasoconstriction Wydase/hyaluronidase (agent that assists spreading of the anesthetic solution in the tissues and may limit postoperative edema), infrequent, optional
Medicine cups, paper labels
Basin set
Blades, (4 to 6) #10, (1) #15
Cojoined irrigation-suction tubing for ultrasound (Harmonic scalpel)
Electrosurgical pencil, extender, needle tip, cord, holder, and scraper
Suction tubing
Needle magnet or counter
Drainage unit, Y connector and tubing, e.g., Hemovac (optional)
Nonadherent dressing, e.g., Adaptic, Xeroform, Opsite, gauze fluffs, and a supportive surgical bra

Special Notes

- Apply **Special Notes** from ***Abdominal Laparotomy***, p. 134, as applicable.
- The circulator should assess hemodynamic factors. Apply antiembolitic hose (per surgeon's request) when the patient arrives in the room before positioning the patient.
- A sequential compression device with leg wraps may be applied (when ordered) to prevent deep vein thrombosis. The leg wraps may be worn without the hose.
- All nursing care must be documented in the **Perioperative Record** for patient safety in regard to continuity of care and for medicolegal reasons.
- **Note:** *when the patient has extremely large breasts and a good deal of bleeding is anticipated or when tumescent liposuctioning will be performed, an OR table sheet (HK Surgical Co.) may be placed on the table to absorb the copious drainage.* It has an impermeable backing to maintain sterility intraoperatively.
- To help to alleviate some degree of the patient's anxiety, the circulator conveys to the patient that he/she will act as the patient's advocate while the patient is in surgery.
- Provide emotional support regarding feelings of altered body image and give the patient an opportunity to express his/her feelings. Provide factual answers to the patient's questions or refer the question to the surgeon, as necessary.

- **N.B.** *When a laser is employed, all safety precautions must be observed; see p. 94.* The room should be prepared for the laser portion of the procedure before starting the surgery, e.g., warning signs, eyewear for all participants in the room, special instruments (e.g., ebonized finish), etc.
- **N.B.** *A scale is used to weigh the breast tissue; keep tissue removed from each breast in a separate container.* Send specimens to pathology correctly labeled, right and left, accordingly. Infrequently, the specimen may contain a malignancy necessitating treatment.
- Record amount of tissue taken from each breast separately in the **Perioperative Record**.
- **Reminder:** *Circulator confirms with blood bank that the patient's blood is readily available.*
- **N.B.** *The procedure usually requires several knife blades changes due to the type and amount of tissue that is cut; the scrub person must always tell the surgeon verbally when the blade has been changed for a* **"new knife."**
- Prior to closure, the patient may be placed in a semi-sitting position to assess size, shape, and symmetry of the breasts; be prepared to make this transition. *Avoid injury to the patient's fingers by preventing them from being caught in the table mechanism when the position of the table is changed from sitting and the lower section of the table is raised.*
- A surgical bra is applied over the dressing; the nipples may be left undressed (if they were transplanted) for observation of nipple viability.
- In the PACU, dressings are checked for fresh blood; excessive bleeding is reported to the surgeon immediately. The amount of bleeding is documented in the **Perioperative Record.**
- In the PACU the color of the nipples is noted. If the nipple(s) change color (e.g., from pinkish brown to dusky blue) the surgeon is notified immediately. This may indicate loss of circulation to the nipple. The color change is documented in the postoperative section of the **Perioperative Record**.

Augmentation Mammoplasty

Definition

Implantation of breast prostheses to enhance the appearance of the breasts.

Discussion

In augmentation mammoplasty (mammaplasty), the breast tissue is supplemented with prostheses/implants to make the breasts appear larger and/or more symmetrical, to improve breast shape, or to supplement or recreate the breast following surgery (e.g., lumpectomy or mastectomy, respectively). Indications for this procedure include micromastia (unilateral or bilateral), postpartum involution of the breasts, ptosis, postsurgical deformity, and/or simply the desire to improve the cosmetic appearance of the breasts. Prior to surgery, the surgeon and patient select the shape, texture, and volume (size). The thickness of the mammary skin and the degree of breast ptosis (if any) are factors in determining the best placement (position) of the prosthesis (implant), either submuscularly (pectoralis) or subglandularly. The approaches to prosthesis insertion are **inframammary, periareolar, transaxillary,** or **transumbilical (TUBA).** Each position for placement and approach has advantages and disadvantages.

Breast implants are composed of an outer silicone shell; they can be filled following insertion (saline, only), or they may be prefilled with silicone gel. The Food and Drug Administration (FDA) has approved the use of prefilled silicone gel implants; once temporarily restricted, they have been reapproved for use. The advantage of using saline-filled prostheses is that a larger size can be placed while employing a smaller incision. Gel-filled implants feel and look more "natural"; they can be placed endoscopically, but not through the endoscope. The prosthesis is inserted and pushed along the previously made tunnel with the scope.

Procedure

The line of the incision is marked for all approaches. When the implant is to be placed submuscularly, epinephrine solution 1:10,000 may be injected into the pectoralis muscle; however, care must be taken to avoid penetration of the chest wall. Final adjustment in the placement of the prostheses may be made after placing the patient in a sitting position to assess size, contour, and symmetry.

Inframammary. A 3- to 4-cm incision is placed just above the inframammary crease. A flap is developed inferiorly to the pectoralis fascia. A plane is developed between the pectoralis fascia and the posterior capsule of the breast (subglandular approach). A pocket is created by blunt dissection to accommodate the implant. Care is taken to avoid intercostal nerve damage. Meticulous hemostasis is obtained prior to implant insertion. A fiberoptic lighted retractor may be employed. The implant is inserted, and the subcutaneous flap is approximated. The process is repeated bilaterally. The patient may be placed in a sitting position following insertion of the implants to assess the size and symmetry of the augmentation. The skin may be closed using a running subcuticular closure.

Periareolar. The line of the incision is marked hemi-circumferentially. The incision is made along the inferior border of the areola. The subcutaneous tissue is dissected to the inferior border of the breast. The retromammary space is enlarged by blunt dissection to accommodate the prosthesis. Hemo stasis is accomplished; a fiber-optic lighted retractor may be employed for better visualization. The prosthesis is inserted. The inferior border of the breast tissue is sutured to the pectoralis fascia. The process is repeated bilaterally. The patient may be placed in a sitting position following insertion of the implants to assess the size and symmetry of the augmentation. The periareolar incision may be closed with a subcuticular suture.

Transaxillary. The line of the incision is marked in the axilla. The vertical or oblique incision is carried down through the subcutaneous tissue. The pectoralis major fascia is incised and a submuscular plane developed by blunt dissection (including finger dissection). A Hopkins rod (rigid) endoscope may be inserted through the sleeve of a fiber-optic retractor. A pocket to accommodate the prosthesis is made under direct vision (endoscopic). Hemostasis is achieved with endoscopic electrosurgery. External palpation (with observance of the endoscopic light percutaneously) helps to guide the scope. An inflatable trial prosthesis or an "expander" may be inserted, noting the volume of saline required to create the desired pocket size. Excessive dissection superiorly or inferiorly is avoided. The expander is removed and the selected prosthesis is inserted and pushed by the end of the scope via the tunnel and filled (via the self-sealing port). The process is repeated bilaterally. The patient may be placed in a sitting position following insertion of the implants to assess the size and symmetry of the augmentation. Wound closure is performed.

Transumbilical. An incision is made in the superior half of the umbilicus and a subcutaneous plane of dissection developed. Both sides will be approached from this incision. If the implant is to be placed submuscularly, a solution of local anesthetic with epinephrine (and hyaluronidase) is usually injected percutaneously beneath the pectoralis muscle fascia. A subcutaneous tunnel is developed toward the desired placement site for the implant underlying either breast using an endotube dissector (e.g., Johnson tube™ per Dr. Gerald Johnson). An endoscope is inserted, and under direct vision, the pocket is completed using an "expander." (Initially, an expander is introduced into the pocket and overinflated, noting the amount of saline required to achieve the desired pocket dimensions.) Hemostasis is achieved. External pressure may be employed to better position the expander. The expander is removed and replaced with the prosthesis. The process is repeated bilaterally. The patient may be placed in a sitting position following insertion of the implants to assess the size and symmetry of the augmentation. The umbilical incision is closed.

Preparation of the Patient

Anesthesia may be either general or local with *conscious sedation*. The patient is placed "symmetrically" on the table in supine position with arms extended, abducted, and secured in position on padded armboards at approximately an 80° angle using padded restraints. During the procedure, the patient will be placed in sitting position to assess breast size and symmetry (without distortion, as breast distortion could appear in the supine position). A pillow may be placed under the knees to prevent lower back strain, or the table may be flexed for comfort. All bony prominences and areas vulnerable to skin and neurovascular pressure or trauma are padded. An electrosurgical dispersive pad is applied.

Skin Preparation

Prep both breasts beginning at the sites of incision (periareolar, transaxillary, inframammary, or transumbilical). Extend prep from the neckline to below the umbilicus, using extra care to prep the axilla well; for extremely large breasts, prep extends down to the pubis. Continue the prep down to the table at the sides.

Draping

Folded towels and a disposable transverse sheet may be used for all of the approaches, except for transumbilical, for which a laparotomy sheet is preferred. The advantage of the adhesive backing on the underside of the fenestration is eliminated.

The advantage of using disposable drapes is the adhesive backing on the underside of a fenestration that permits the drape to be secured around the perimeter of the surgical field.

Equipment

Padded restraints for the arms
ESU, unipolar and/or bipolar
Suction
Fiber-optic lighted retractor, optional
Fiber-optic light sources (2), e.g., Xenon 300 W (for retractor or for endoscope), optional
Monitor, optional
Camera console, optional

Instrumentation

Basic/Minor procedures tray
Bipolar bayonet electrosurgical forceps and cord, optional
Fiber-optic lighted retractor, blades, and cord (optional)

Transaxillary and Transumbilical, Add

Johnson endotube, Hopkins rigid endoscope with sleeve, cord, camera coupler, electrosurgical suction-aspirator, and cord

Supplies

Antiembolitic hose
Indelible marking pen
Control syringes (2) and needles (2), 25- or 27-gauge spinal × 1½″, and a spinal needle (3½″), optional
Ephedrine solution 1:10,000 or local anesthetic, e.g., 0.5% lidocaine with epinephrine 1:200,000 (for pectoralis intramuscular injection to promote vasoconstriction) for vasoconstriction
Wydase/hyaluronidase (enzymatic spreading agent), optional
Medicine cup, paper labels
Basin set
Blades, (2) #15
Electrosurgical pencil, extended tip, cord, holder, and scraper, optional
Suction tubing
Needle magnet or counter
Saline or antibiotic solution for irrigation and bulb syringe
Breast prostheses (implant with filling tubes, syringes, etc., for injection of saline or prefilled silicone implant)
Closed-suction drainage unit (e.g., Hemovac) with tubing and Y connector, optional
Nonadherent dressing, e.g., Adaptic, Xeroform, Opsite, and gauze fluffs
Wound closure for skin (e.g., Steri-Strips) or subcuticular suture (optional)
Surgical bra

Special Notes

- Apply **Special Notes** from ***Abdominal Laparotomy***, p. 134, as applicable.
- The circulator must ascertain that the breast implants are in the room for the correct patient before bringing the patient into the room.
- The circulator should not open the prostheses until the surgeon makes a final decision regarding type and size.
- *Documentation regarding the date, patient's name, brand name, type, size, and serial numbers of the implanted prostheses is made in the* **Perioperative Record** *and in the hospital's log (for insertion of an implant), according to facility policy.*
- Whereas the patient will be supine, Fowler's or sitting position may be requested toward the latter part of the procedure to assess size and symmetry of the breasts.
- *Avoid injury to the patient's fingers by preventing them from being caught in the table mechanism when the lower section of the table is brought up to its original position.*

Abdominoplasty/Abdominal Lipectomy

Definition

The repair of a lax, redundant abdominal wall.

Discussion

Abdominoplasty is also referred to as **abdominal lipectomy** and is often performed in conjunction with **panniculectomy,** the excision of a redundant apron of subcutaneous tissue (and skin). Techniques employed to perform abdominoplasty are varied; lax, redundant subcutaneous fat (and the overlying abdominal skin) are excised and the abdominal musculature is tightened. **Abdominoplasty** is performed to lessen the discomfort associated with performing daily tasks and concerns regarding personal hygiene, and for cosmesis. The surgeon determines the approach according to fat distribution, amount of abdominal wall weakness or presence of a frank ventral hernia, size of the panniculus, and his/her experience and preference.

In addition to the excision of involved tissues, **tumescent liposuction** (see p. 766) is often employed to assist in removal of the excess fat; the abdomen is simultaneously contoured. **Tumescent liposuction** may be combined with an endoscopic-assisted approach that enables placement of musculofascial sutures employing limited incisions. For extensive presentations, a transverse or transverse curvilinear incision extends from iliac crest to iliac crest. When a large panniculus is excised, a double incision is made, a "lazy" M superiorly and a U inferiorly, the lower extent of which is at the pubis (this has largely supplanted the W incision). The length of the M is made to equal the length of the U so that with wound closure there will be no discrepancy. Generally, lesser plastic procedures performed to remove redundant tissue from below the umbilicus are referred to as a **"tummy-tuck."** The excess lax skin and subcutaneous tissue are excised and a limited muscle plication is performed through a "bikini" incision. The surgeon marks the skin prior to the skin prep.

Procedure

A U-M Incisional Repair is described. General anesthesia is usually employed. The M incision is made above the umbilicus and the U incision is made with its center just above the pubis symphysis, the lateral extent of which meets with the M incision bilaterally. The umbilicus on a pedicle may be incised in a diamond shape, preserving its support and blood supply for later replacement under the flap. Dissection is begun at the lower portion of the U incision and progresses upward bilaterally; a fine layer of areolar tissue over the fascia is retained. Similar dissection is done superiorly with the M incision. The amount of intervening skin and adipose tissue to be excised is carefully estimated before removal so that the defect can be closed with moderate tension. Diastasis of the rectus abdominis muscle, if present, is plicated. A ventral hernia, if present, is repaired (large ventral hernia repair will require synthetic mesh). The umbilicus is brought through an appropriately located position in the superior wound flap and sutured. The wound is closed with heavy absorbable suture; the skin may be closed with a subcuticular running suture. Drains may be employed.

Preparation of the Patient

General anesthesia is usually employed. An HK OR sheet is placed on the table (see ***Liposuction and Tumescent Liposuction / Suction-Assisted Lipectomy,* Preparation of the Patient, p. 768**). Antiembolitic hose are applied, as requested. The surgeon may request a sequential compression device with disposable leg wraps; they can be applied over the antiembolitic hose, or the wraps may be used without the hose. The patient is supine with arms extended on padded armboards. A pillow may be placed under the knees to prevent lower back strain, or the table may be flexed for comfort. All bony prominences and areas vulnerable to skin and neurovascular pressure or trauma are padded. An electrosurgical dispersive pad is applied.

Skin Preparation

Begin prepping below the umbilicus, extending from the midthorax to the knees and down to the table at the sides.

Draping

Folded towels and a transverse sheet and/or individual drape sheets complete the draping.

Equipment

- Additional OR table (for extremely obese patient)
- Sequential compression device with disposable leg wraps, when requested
- ESU, monopolar and/or bipolar
- Scale for weighing specimen
- Monitor, optional
- Camera console, optional
- Liposuction high-pressure vacuum aspirator unit (for liposuction, if employed) (Cosmetech SSB I, MD Engineering LS 1000 Liposuction unit), optional
- LySonix® for ultrasonic liposuction (UAL), optional
- High-pressure infusion pump for tumescent liposuction, e.g., Cabot or Klein (with foot pedal), optional
- Fiber-optic headlight and cord (may contain camera), optional
- Fiber-optic light sources (3), for Xenon 300 W (for fiber-optic headlight, lighted retractor, or endoscope), optional
- Power-assisted liposuction (PAL) device (e.g., MicroAire®), optional

Instrumentation

Basic/Minor procedures tray

Extra Crile and Kocher forceps (or similar), bipolar electrosurgical forceps and cord, ruler and/or caliper

Handpiece and cannulas (e.g., Mercedes) for liposuction, optional

Endoscopic, Add

Fiber-optic retractor with blades and cord, optional

Hopkins rigid endoscope and cord, electrosurgical suction-irrigator, optional

Dissector, scissors, electrosurgical scissors, suturing devices (e.g. Endo Stitch™), knot pusher (e.g., Clark Reich), electrosurgical suction, Allis clamps (2), etc.

Supplies

Antiembolitic hose

Indelible marking pen

OR table sheet, sterile, absorbent with impervious backing (HK Surgical Co.)

Local anesthetic, e.g., lidocaine and solution of epinephrine 1:200,000 (in lactated Ringer's solution)

Control syringes 30 ml (2), and needles (2), 22 gauge × 1½", or small cannulas (special to be used with infusion pump)

Medicine cups, paper labels

Basin set

Blades (4 to 6) #10 (depends on amount and toughness of tissue)

Needle magnet or counter

Electrosurgical pencil with extender tip, cord, holder, and scraper

Plication suture, optional

Suction tubing

Liposuction flexible noncollapsing tubing for infusion of tumescent fluid, e.g., Cabot or Klein

Synthetic mesh for large hernia repair, e.g., Marlex™, Gor-Tex™ or Mersilene mesh, for large hernias

Closed-suction drainage unit (e.g., Hemovac, Jackson-Pratt)

Additional HK OR table sheet (for gurney at the conclusion of the surgery)

Special Notes

- Apply **Special Notes** from ***Abdominal Laparotomy***, p. 134, as applicable.
- Assess hemodynamic factors, e.g., keep patient's legs uncrossed; apply antiembolitic hose before positioning patient,

when requested. Antiembolitic hose should be applied when the patient arrives in the room. A sequential compression device with leg wraps may be applied over the antiembolitic hose, when ordered, to prevent deep vein thrombosis.

- If the patient has an extremely large panniculus, the surgeon usually devises a method of supporting the panniculus that enables the circulator to prep the skin area under the panniculus adequately.
- Check with the surgeon regarding the type of mesh to be used for the ventral hernia repair; several types of synthetic mesh should be in the room.
- *When synthetic mesh is employed, documentation regarding the date, patient's name, brand name, type, size, and serial numbers is made in the Perioperative Record.*
- When closing the wound, the surgeon may request that the table be flexed to facilitate wound closure. The scrub person should check that the patient's toes have cleared the Mayo stand tray to avoid injury to the patient.
- *Avoid injury to the patient's fingers by preventing them from being caught in the table mechanism when the position of the table is changed.*
- At the conclusion of the procedure, an HK OR table sheet (sterile and absorbent with impervious backing) is placed on the gurney prior to transferring the patient, as it is effective in containing the continuous drainage from the incisions.
- Following placement of the dressing, a pressure garment is opened up on the gurney on top of the HK sheet. Placing the garment on the gurney facilitates application of the pressure garment.

Liposuction and Tumescent Liposuction/ Suction-Assisted Lipectomy

Definition

Removal of localized deposits of excessive subcutaneous fat by suctioning.

Discussion

Liposuction is the percutaneous insertion of perforated suction cannulae to mechanically disrupt adipose tissue and aspirate the loosened fat. The procedure is not employed for weight reduction, but for cosmesis; it may also be employed to remove lipomas, treat gynecomastia, and evacuate organized hematomas and as an adjunct (limited) in breast reduction procedures, etc. Liposuction modalities can be combined with other procedures, such as for **panniculectomy** (see p. 762). When performed in morbidly obese patients, **megaliposuction** is highly controversial, as there is increased risk of complications and mortality due to the extremely large volume of fluid shifts that occur. Liposuction can be performed simply, using a needle (or cannula) and syringe to create suction, or more often a high-pressure vacuum unit is used. The cannula size varies from 1 to 10 mm. As the cannulae are deliberately moved in a fan-shaped pattern around the area being treated, fibrous bands are broken, facilitating fat aspiration. Numerous sites can be treated, from minimal volume sites, such as eyelids and other facial areas, to larger areas, such as the extremities, torso, abdomen, etc.

Liposuction may be performed using a diluted amount of anesthetic agent in IV solution (e.g., Lactated Ringers). Liposuction is referred to as **"dry," "wet," "superwet,"** or **"tumescent,"** referring to the amount of very dilute anesthetic with epinephrine (e.g., 1:200,000 lactated Ringer's solution) injected. "Dry" technique does not employ injection of fluid; this method is little used. If the fluid injected is less than the amount of fat to be removed, it is referred to as **"wet."** If the fluid injected is equal to the amount of fat to be removed, it is referred to as **"superwet."** If the amount of fluid is twice the amount of fat to be removed, it is referred to as "tumescent." The solution is injected via cannula into subcutaneous tissues to the point of turgidity. A high-pressure infusion pump may be employed to infuse the tumescent solution. Suction cannulae attached to high-powered suction apparatus are deployed to reduce and contour the targeted sites. The lidocaine dosage (in dilute solution) should not exceed 35 mg/kg, which, if given undiluted, would be toxic. This extremely diluted solution has demonstrated that it is "avidly" bound to the tissues and only slowly released systemically; Wydase (previously used) is unnecessary when these "wet" solutions are used. Toxic plasma levels are not reached. Generally, there is more blood loss with the lesser amounts of fluid injected. Transfusion, although infrequently used, must be available for considerably extensive procedures. Patients may receive an autologous transfusion, obtained and reserved in advance for this purpose. An ultrasonic wave generator may be attached to the suction handpiece enhancing liquification of the fatty tissues (ultrasound assisted liposuction, UAL). This technique requires a lower level of suction with a lesser degree of bleeding. More efficient is power-assisted liposuction (PAL), which employs an oscillating suction cannula that facilitates easier removal of the fatty tissues, is less physically demanding on the surgeon, and employs smaller diameter cannulae with resulting smaller incisional scars. Additionally, radio-frequency energy can be coordinated with the reciprocating power cannulae to achieve some degree of hemostasis; there is a lesser risk of local burn than with UAL. The resulting lipid solution (an emulsion of excess fat and a limited amount of blood inherent in the local trauma) is removed by suction, i.e., **suction-assisted lipectomy (SAL).** The fluid in the suction canister is layered, an upper layer, *supranatant,* of fat and oil and a lower layer, *infranatant,* of blood and other fluids.

The 3LT™ laser, a handheld low-level light (1-mW), 635-nm helium-neon diode (Erchonia Medical Co.), may be used for areas on the face, as well as larger surfaces. The transcutaneous laser energy loosens the fat; the fat can be suctioned via smaller cannulae than the cannulae required when laser is not employed. The laser is passed over the tissues, externally, for 6 to 12 minutes, usually after the tumescent fluid injection.

Additionally, **ultrasonic-assisted liposuction (UAL)** delivers ultrasonic energy causing (bloodless) cavitation of fat into an oily emulsion; its use has been curtailed amid safety issues. Extreme care must be exercised to avoid burning overlying skin.

Possible risks and complications of **abdominoplasty** include, but are not limited to:

- Bleeding, hemorrhage
- Seroma, hematoma formation
- Scarring, hypertrophic scars, keloids
- Deep vein thrombosis, phlebitis
- Pulmonary edema, fat emboli, pulmonary emboli
- Skin necrosis
- Burns, especially from UAL
- Unfavorable or unsatisfactory results

Procedure

Tumescent Liposuction is described. The targeted areas are infused with large amounts of extremely dilute, buffered lidocaine with epinephrine in lactated Ringer's solution until the site appears turgid. Through many small incisions made with a #11 blade, blunt suction-tipped cannulae are inserted and tunneled under the skin, separating it from underlying subcutaneous and connective tissues. Excess subcutaneous fat is suctioned from the pretunneled areas using a high-pressure vacuum. Smaller cannulae are used around the periphery of the site to transitionally mold and contour the targeted areas. An electric, compressed-air, or compressed nitrogen-powered **power-assisted liposuction** device (PAL) may be used to produce a rapid in-and-out or rotary motion or oscillations of the cannula, relieving some of the physical effort for the surgeon, as explained above. The incisions may be closed with a subcuticular stitch. A compression dressing is applied on the extremities, and a compression garment is applied for the torso.

Preparation of the Patient

A general anesthetic may be employed; regional or a local anesthetic may be used in conjunction with *conscious sedation*. The patient is positioned as for any other surgery performed on that particular part of the body. Antiembolitic hose may be applied, as per request, when the thighs, calves, and ankles are not to be liposuctioned. Prior to positioning, the surgeon may have the patient stand for the targeted areas to be marked. When the torso, hips, and thighs are targeted, the patient may stand for the skin prep and later positioned on sterile sheets [e.g., HK OR sheet, sterile, absorbent with impervious backing (see **Supplies,** this procedure)]. The patient may be placed in supine position with arms extended on padded armboards (or the prone position may be employed; see p. 25). A pillow may be placed under the knees to prevent lower back strain, or the table may be flexed for comfort. All bony prominences and areas vulnerable to skin and neurovascular pressure or trauma are padded. An electrosurgical dispersive pad may be applied; consult the surgeon regarding whether monopolar electrosurgery will be used.

As a large volume of fluid is used for tumescent liposuction, an anesthesia provider is required to monitor the patient to avoid or treat any fluid shifts that might occur.

Skin Preparation

For Liposuction of the Abdomen, Hips, and Thighs. Begin the prep at the site of the most central incision and extend the prep an appropriate distance. Ideally, two people are needed when the targeted areas are on the lower extremities to elevate, abduct, and adduct them as necessary, in order to ensure that the areas around and under each thigh and hip are adequately prepared. Sterile drape sheets may be placed under each hip after it is prepped. When the pubic area is to receive liposuction, it is prepped last. When the pubic area will not receive liposuction, it may be covered by a small sterile plastic adhesive drape that is applied to the perineum.

When extensive areas or several areas require prepping, the surgeon may have the patient stand as the body is prepped. The patient is then helped onto the sterile covered operating table and placed in the desired position.

Note: An orthostatic table may be employed to "stand" the patient following the procedure to assess the results (rarely).

Draping

For Liposuction of the Abdomen, Hips, and Thighs. The legs are elevated and abducted as each foot is grasped in a tube stockinette. Each stockinette is brought up over the leg, up to the knee. A sheet is draped over the end of the table. A towel may be folded as necessary, placed over the pubic area, and secured with a sterile, plastic adhesive drape. Cuffed drape sheets are tucked in at the patient's sides. An additional sheet is draped under the legs and thighs. The legs are lowered onto the table. Drape sheets cover areas that will not be treated.

As the patient's position is changed to permit liposuctioning of an area, additional drape sheets or towels are required.

Disposable drape sheets with adhesive-backed fenestrations or edges have the advantage of adhering to the sites in desired areas.

Equipment

Sequential compression device with leg wraps
Suction
High-pressure liposuction vacuum unit, e.g., Cosmetech SSB I, MD Engineering
Low level light laser beam (3LT®, Erchonia Medical), optional
Ultrasound generator and foot pedal, Misonix, LySonix, Mentor Contour, unit
High-pressure pump, tumescent fluid infusion, e.g., Cabot, Klein
Power-assisted liposuction (PAL) device (e.g., MicroAire®)

Instrumentation

Limited procedure tray
Fiber-optic retractor, blades, and cord

Liposuction

Blunt suction cannulas, e.g., triple-holed, multi-holed, holes on one side, holes around the tip, and/or Mercedes tip
Ultrasound handpiece and probe, e.g., Misonix unit, LySonix, Mentor Contour
Nitrogen or air tank to power liposuction

Supplies

Antiembolitic hose
Marking pen with indelible ink
OR table sheet, sterile, absorbent with impervious backing (HK Surgical Co.)
Control syringes (2), 30 ml, and needles (2), 22 gauge × 1½″, Medicine cup, paper labels
Local anesthetic, e.g., lidocaine with epinephrine 1:200,000 in lactated Ringer's solution
Wydase/hyaluronidase (enzymatic diffusing agent), optional
Basin set
Blade, (2) #11
Needle pad or magnet

Liposuction tubing (flexible, noncollapsing)
Surgical pad and island dressing (super absorbent), Opsite, Bioclusive, optional
Compression garment, type depends on area

Special Notes

- Apply **Special Notes** from ***Abdominoplasty***, p. 764, as applicable.
- Assess hemodynamic factors; apply antiembolitic hose before positioning the patient. Antiembolitic hose should be applied when the patient arrives in the room.
- A sequential compression device with leg wraps may be applied over the antiembolitic hose or the leg wraps may be worn without hose to prevent deep vein thrombosis if the lower extremities are not receiving liposuction.
- **N.B.** The circulator reviews the patient's medication list, as certain drugs interfere with the metabolism of lidocaine, such as cimetidine, beta blockers, anxiolytics, etc. Review the list with the anesthesia provider.
- **Reminder:** Use safety precautions to identify, label, and dispense medications and solutions to avoid medication errors; see p. 30. It is mandatory that all medications and solutions on the sterile field be labeled by name and strength. The medication bottle is retained in the room until the procedure has concluded.
- Scrub person needs to prepare and keep available two 30-ml syringes (with 22-gauge needles) filled with the solution containing the local anesthetic.
- Scrub person needs to keep an accurate record of the total amount of solution that has been injected or infused (tumescent).
- A special compression garment that covers the abdomen, hips, thighs, and buttocks should be put on the patient (when those areas have had liposuction) immediately after the wounds are dressed. The garment is opened on the gurney and the patient is lifted onto it; the garment is then closed. See **Special Notes** in ***Abdominoplasty***, p. 764.
- Make certain blood is readily available, as ordered; ascertain if patient previously donated blood in anticipation of surgery.

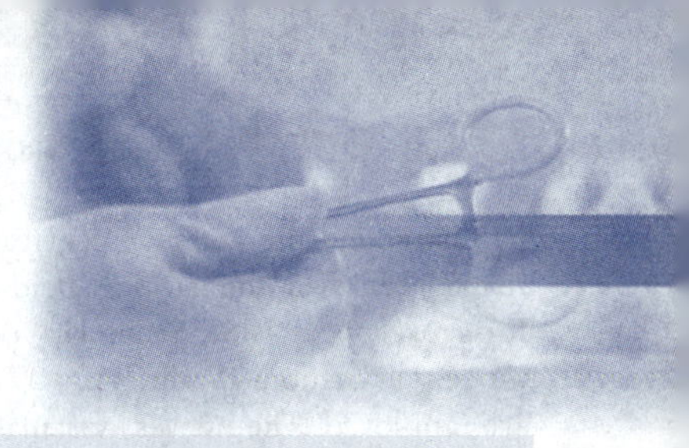

CHAPTER 26
Neck Surgery

Thyroidectomy

Definition

Removal of all or a portion (lobe) of the thyroid gland.

Discussion

Thyroidectomy is performed to treat patients with hyperthyroidism or a thyroid (mass) lesion. Hyperthyroidism is characterized by increased metabolism with resulting weight loss and fatigue, hyperexcitability and emotional lability, heat intolerance, cardiac symptoms such as tachycardia and palpitations, and impaired swallowing due to mechanical obstruction (secondary to compression of the esophagus by the enlarged gland). These characteristics must be taken into account in preparing the individualized plan of care; see the **Patient Care Plan,** p. 9). The most common complications of thyroidectomy are laryngeal nerve injury (recurrent and superior), postoperative bleeding with airway compromise, and, later, hypothyroidism. The patient must be observed postoperatively for symptoms of hypocalcemia, the result of inadvertent excision of the parathyroid glands.

The thyroid is a highly vascular gland composed of two lobes connected by a narrow bridge (isthmus). It is located on the anterior aspect of the trachea adjacent to the second, third, and fourth rings. Thyroid lobectomy is performed for the treatment of some thyroid nodules and localized carcinomas. Various medical regimens and radioactive iodine (RAI) are employed to obviate surgery in certain presentations or used in conjunction with surgery postoperatively. Total thyroidectomy is indicated for certain carcinomas and to relieve tracheal or esophageal compression. When preoperative evaluation, including physical exam, scanning (computed tomography [CT], magnetic resonance imaging [MRI], positron emission tomography [PET], ultrasound), and ultrasound-guided fine-needle aspiration, or intraoperative findings indicate that a thyroid carcinoma has spread, various modifications of radical neck dissection (p. 857) may be performed. Infrequently, thyroid tissue may be located substernally or lingually (base of the tongue), necessitating a more extensive surgery than the usual cervical approach. When the Harmonic Scalpel® (ultrasonic) is employed the surgery is referred to as "bloodless" and "sutureless."

Endoscopic thyroid surgery (video-assisted neck surgery [VANS]) may be performed using an infraclavicular, lateral cervical, transaxillary approach, or areola (of the breast). Visualization is enhanced by distracting the anterior cervical skin with wires attached to an L-shaped bar over the surgical field (similar to the principle of ***gasless laparoscopy***, p. 138). Secondary ports are made; an ultrasound dissector (e.g., Harmonic Scalpel, p. 109) and various endoscopic instruments are employed. The nerves, vasculature, and parathyroids are visualized and avoided to prevent injury. The endoscopic approach is employed for thyroid nodule excision and lobectomy; more extensive surgery requires an open approach due to the limited size of the endoscope's lumen. An adjunct to VANS, robotics (da Vinci system) may be employed to perform thyroid surgery. For this modality to be routinely used, the surgeon must be experienced in endoscopy, VANS, and the use of robotics to limit operative time.

Procedure

General anesthesia with endotracheal intubation is most often employed; local anesthetics infiltration of subcutaneous tissue or field (regional) block with epinephrine 1:100,000 may be used by some surgeons. A marking pen is used to indicate the transverse curvilinear line for the skin incision, made above the sternal notch, in a natural skin crease. Skin flaps are developed as the platysma muscle is incised and retracted. The exterior jugular veins are ligated only when they limit exposure. The strap muscles are separated or divided. Blunt and sharp dissection is employed until the cricoid cartilage and the thyroid isthmus are exposed. The recurrent and superior laryngeal nerves are identified and protected and the parathyroid glands are avoided. The larger vessels and supporting tissues (including Berry's ligament that attaches the thyroid to the trachea) should not be divided prior to identifying these structures, particularly the branches of the recurrent laryngeal nerve. Care is taken to disturb the gland and the vasculature as little as possible. The gland is mobilized. All or a portion of the gland (lobe) is removed. Meticulous hemostasis is obtained. If a parathyroid gland has been excised, it may be transplanted back into the sternomastoid muscle or a forearm muscle. The divided strap muscles are repaired; the wound may be irrigated, and a drain may be inserted. The incision is closed in layers by interrupted stitches. The skin is often closed with Steri-Strips™ for a more cosmetic-appearing scar.

Endoscopic thyroidectomy is performed for selected cases such as hemithyroidectomy, excision of a single nodule <6 cm, multinodular goiter all in one lobe, and papillary carcinoma <1 cm.

Preparation of the Patient

When general anesthesia is employed, a specialized endotracheal tube (NIM™ electromyographic [EMG] endotracheal tube) that incorporates a sensor ring with attached sensor wires (above the balloon cuff) is positioned at the level of the larynx to continuously record EMG tracing of the vocal cords. When deviations in the tracing are noted, indicating manipulation or other disturbance of the recurrent laryngeal nerve, the surgeon is alerted. This cuffed tube, when employed, is an adjunct to prevent potential injury to the laryngeal nerves. Following induction of general anesthesia, the patient is placed in supine position, with the head stabilized on a padded or gel donut headrest and a shoulder roll or small sandbag placed between the scapulae, extending the neck to optimize exposure. Arms may be extended on padded armboards. A pillow may be placed under the knees to avoid straining back muscles, or the table may be flexed for comfort. The table is positioned in reverse Trendelenburg. A padded footboard is secured to the table. All bony prominences and areas vulnerable to skin and neurovascular trauma or pressure are padded. An electrosurgical dispersive pad is applied.

Skin Preparation

Begin at the anterior neck; extend the prep from just below the level of the infra-auricular border and the lower lip to a level just above the nipples and down to the table at the sides of the neck and around the shoulders. Folded towels are placed at the sides of the neck to prevent prep solution from pooling under the patient.

Draping

Folded towels and a sheet with a small fenestration (with a clear plastic adhesive insert) are used; individual drape sheets complete the draping. A sterile sponge may be placed on either side of the neck to prevent blood from pooling under the neck.

Equipment

Headrest, e.g., padded or gel donut
Roll, IV bag, or small sandbag for extending the neck
Sequential compression device with disposable leg wraps, e.g., Jobst athrombic pump, if requested
Footboard table extension (padded)
ESU, monopolar and bipolar
Suction
Harmonic Scalpel (ultrasound) generator and foot pedal, optional
Fiber-optic headlight (may contain camera) with fiber-optic light source, e.g., Xenon™ 300 W

Endoscopic, Add:

Fiber-optic light source for endoscope, e.g., Xenon 300 W (for headlight and endoscope)
Monitor
VCR
Printer

CD burner
Camera console

Instrumentation

Thyroid procedures tray
Tracheostomy tray (available)
Spring retractor, right-angle clamps with fine points (2), Lahey clamps (extra available)
Bipolar forceps and cord
Harmonic Scalpel handpiece with scissors tip and cord, optional

Endoscopic, Add

Limited procedures tray
Endoscopes, 2 and 5 mm; 30° and 45°, cord, camera and optical bridge (adaptor)
Trocars (short, dull, cannulas), grasping instruments, electrosurgical suction-irrigator and coaxial cable, camera and optical bridge, dissector, electrosurgical dissector, scissors, electrosurgical scissors and cord, and Harmonic Scalpel

Supplies

Antiembolitic hose
Indelible marking pen to mark line of incision
Basin set
Blades, (2) #10, (1) #15
Needle magnet or counter
Magnetic instrument pad
Suction tubing
Electrosurgical pencil with needle tip and cord with holder and scraper
Peanuts/kittners/bullets for dissection
Bulb syringe
Small drain (e.g., 1/4″ Penrose)
Skin closure, e.g., Steri-Strips or subcuticular running suture
Ice packs available, optional

Special Notes

- Apply **Special Notes** from ***Abdominal Laparotomy***, p. 134, as applicable.
- Prior to bringing the patient into the room, the thyroid scans performed preoperatively should be brought into the room for the *correctly identified* patient.
- **Reminder:** Antiembolitic hose are applied when the patient arrives in the room, before the patient is positioned, when requested. A sequential compression device with leg wraps may

be applied when ordered to prevent deep vein thrombosis. The leg wraps may be worn without the hose.

- **Reminder:** The circulator conveys to the patient that he/she will act as the advocate for him/her while he/she is in surgery.
- **Reminder:** The circulator provides emotional support regarding feelings of altered body image regarding the resulting scar and gives the patient an opportunity to express his/her feelings.
- To provide a measure of emotional support to the patient, answer the patient's questions in a knowledgeable manner whenever possible and refer questions to the surgeon as necessary.
- **Reminder:** *Assess and document the patient's anxiety, provide emotional support, such as maintaining eye contact and holding the patient's hand during the administration of anesthesia, etc.*
- **Reminder:** All nursing care must be documented in the **Perioperative Record** for patient safety regarding continuity of care and for medicolegal reasons.
- During positioning, extra care is taken to pad all bony prominences, as patients with hyperthyroidism have lost weight, making these areas more vulnerable to pressure injuries. Injuries can be avoided by using positioning aids such as elbow and heel cups.
- **Reminder:** Prep solutions are not permitted to pool under the patient, as the prep solution will excoriate the skin. In addition, pooled prep solutions are not permitted to pool on the drapes, as this constitutes a fire hazard that should be avoided.
- The surgeon may prefer to clamp and cut many times before ligating vessels or structures; the scrub person should be prepared with extra mosquito clamps (readily available).
- When the Harmonic Scalpel is employed, the need for clamps and sutures is virtually eliminated.
- During the procedure, multiple biopsies of the thyroid gland, surrounding tissue, and suspect lymph nodes, etc., may be obtained for frozen section; the circulator needs to partially prepare the requisitions in advance. That way, the specimen is ready for immediate dispatch.
- It is important for the circulator to identify and document on the requisition the exact location from which the specimen was obtained.

- When the patient receives local anesthesia, the circulator must indicate prominently (in bold letters) **"patient is awake"** on the requisition slip; this alerts the pathologist **not** to announce findings aloud over the room intercom.
- Remembering that the patient may be emotionally labile (a characteristic of hyperthyroidism), keep conversation to a minimum to avoid causing the patient anxiety. When the patient receives local anesthesia, he/she can hear all that is said.
- **N.B.** *The scrub person should remain sterile and the back table kept sterile until the patient is extubated, breathing satisfactorily on his/her own, and taken from the room.*
- **N.B.** *The scrub person should be prepared for a* ***tracheostomy*** *(**see p. 843**) to be performed if the patient's airway becomes compromised or obstructed.*
- In many institutions, a tracheostomy tray accompanies the patient to the postanesthesia care unit (PACU) and later to the patient's room until the risk of airway obstruction, e.g., secondary to edema of the glottis or the surrounding tissues or hematoma formation, has passed.
- In the PACU, the perioperative practitioner observes the patient for signs and symptoms of respiratory difficulty due to airway obstruction. He or she immediately notifies the anesthesia provider and the surgeon, employs an ambu bag, and documents nursing interventions and patient outcomes.
- The PACU perioperative practitioner assesses the patient's voice for hoarseness (as this usually indicates injury to the laryngeal nerve) and documents findings in the **Postoperative Record** section of the **Perioperative Record**. This is done for medicolegal reasons.

Parathyroidectomy

Definition

Removal of one or more of the four parathyroid glands.

Discussion

Hyperparathyroid symptoms may be subtle or undetectable; the condition is often discovered when routine blood tests reveal high calcium blood levels. The nonspecific symptoms include feelings of depression and/or aches and pains. Loss of appetite, nausea, confusion, and thirst may occur. Bone loss with fractures and kidney stones may be seen in association with peptic ulcer, hypertension, and pancreatitis in more advanced presentations.

Parathyroidectomy is performed to excise adenomas, carcinomas, and hyperplasia; normal or atrophic glands are usually left intact. In cases of hyperplasia, where all four glands appear to be involved (less than 5%), three and a half of the glands are excised or all are excised and a portion of one is transplanted into the musculature of the forearm (however, one third of these do not function, requiring indefinite hormone replacement therapy [HRT]). When there is no malignancy, a portion of at least one gland is usually not resected to prevent hypocalcemia. A residual gland may require later treatment if excessive hormone production occurs. Total excision of all parathyroid glandular tissue, unrecognized and untreated, results in tetany and death. Postoperatively, appropriate chemistries (calcium, phosphate, etc.) are closely monitored. When the gland is located in the mediastinum, excision will require a different approach, e.g., open surgery or mediastinoscopy (see p. 451).

The use of *sestamibi radioactive scanning (99mTc-sestamibi)* to identify parathyroid hyperactivity has revolutionized parathyroid surgery. Minimally invasive radio-guided parathyroid (MIRP) surgery works by making the overproductive parathyroid gland radioactive, differentiating it from all other structures in the neck (the thyroid pick up is relatively minimal). Other techniques, such as CT, ultrasound, and subtraction scans are usually not necessary. The single-proton emission computerized tomography (SPECT) scan may be useful when the sestamibi scan alone does not provide adequate information. For hyperparathyroidism, the sestamibi scan will most often identify a single adenoma; excision endoscopically is achieved with intraoperative guidance, employing a handheld gamma probe. The radiopharmaceutical (sestamibi) is given intravenously shortly prior to surgery (radioactivity lasts for 2 to 4 hours). When the scans cannot identify the location of the pathology, an "open" exploration for the four glands must be done. For the rarely encountered parathyroid malignancy, an open procedure with modified neck dissection (see p. 778) is performed accordingly. The approach to parathyroidectomy may be endoscopic, or an "open" standard (traditional) approach may be employed.

An additional adjunct to parathyroid surgery is the *intraoperative assay* of parathyroid hormone (level may drop as much as 50% from the preoperative level following excision of the affected gland[s]).

Procedure

Endoscopic Approach/Minimally Invasive Radioguided Parathyroidectomy (MIRP). Employing local anesthesia with *conscious sedation* (or additional cervical plexus block or general anesthesia), a 1-inch incision is made above the suprasternal notch; a more exact location can be determined by placing the (plastic-protected) radioactivity detection probe, the Neoprobe, over the neck. The endoscope and the Neoprobe (protected by a sterile plastic sleeve) are inserted through the incision. The audible signal leads to the location of the enlarged gland; it is carefully dissected from surrounding structures. Its artery and vein are clipped, being certain that no nervous structure is jeopardized, and the lesion is removed. The excised specimen is then scanned, and if the radioactive signal is commensurate with the preoperative level, no further excision or exploration is indicated. If otherwise parathyroid hormone assay is done and is still inconclusive regarding whether pathological glandular tissue remains, the other glands must be explored (with an open procedure, as necessary). Hemostasis is assured and the wound closed.

Standard (Open) Approach. The approach is as for ***Thyroidectomy*** (p. 772). The thyroid gland is mobilized and rotated to either side of the neck. Care is taken, as in thyroidectomy, to identify and protect the recurrent and superior laryngeal nerves. The NIM endotracheal tube may be employed (see ***Thyroidectomy***, p. 772). Once parathyroid glands are identified, they are isolated and excised, as indicated according to the pathology. As stated above, when all four glands are uniform, a portion of one may remain in situ. Hemostasis is achieved, the wound may be irrigated, and a drain may be inserted. The incision is closed in layers by interrupted stitches.

For **Preparation of the Patient, Skin Preparation, Draping, Equipment, Instrumentation,** and **Supplies,** see ***Thyroidectomy,*** pp. 772–774.

Equipment, Add

Neoprobe™ portable radioisotope detector console (US Surgical)

Instrumentation, Add

Neoprobe (handheld) and cord (for radioisotope detector)

Special Notes

- Apply **Special Notes** from ***Thyroidectomy,*** p. 774, as applicable.
- When a portion of the parathyroid gland is transplanted to the forearm (or other muscular location), the forearm is prepped and draped at the same time as the neck. The forearm site is covered with a towel until the surgeon is ready to transplant the resected portion of the parathyroid gland.
- **N.B. Reminder:** *The scrub person should remain sterile and the back table kept sterile until the patient is extu-*

bated, breathing satisfactorily on his/her own, and taken from the room.

- **N.B.** A tracheostomy tray is brought into the room; it is opened if the patient shows signs of airway obstruction. Following surgery, the circulator should bring the tracheostomy tray to the PACU. The tray may also accompany the patient to his/her hospital room.
- **N.B.** In the PACU the perioperative practitioner observes the patient's breathing; should the patient show signs of airway obstruction, he/she immediately notifies the anesthesia provider and the surgeon, employs an ambu bag, and documents nursing interventions and patient outcomes.

Thyroglossal Duct Cystectomy

Definition

Excision of thyroglossal duct cyst and duct in continuity with the mid-portion of the hyoid bone to the foramen cecum.

Discussion

The thyroglossal duct is an embryological remnant that extends from the foramen cecum at the base of the tongue, through the hyoid bone to the thyroid gland. Remnants of this embryonic duct may form a cyst. When a ductal sinus or cyst is present, it is usually found inferior to the hyoid bone. Although most patients with thyroglossal duct cyst are children, patients with thyroglossal duct cyst can even be elderly. Rarely, ectopic thyroid tissue (including papillary carcinoma) may be encountered along the tract; squamous cell carcinoma, likewise, is a rare finding.

A Tracheostomy tray should be available in the room, the PACU, and sometimes brought up to the patient's hospital room, as the surgery is proximate to the airway.

Procedure

The Sistrunk Operation is described. An incision is made between the hyoid bone and thyroid cartilage, along natural skin lines. A superior flap is raised to the level of the hyoid bone. An inferior flap is raised until the inferior aspect of the cyst is identified. The platysma muscle is incised and retracted. Strap muscles are separated and/or divided. Sharp and blunt dissection are employed to mobilize the cyst and duct. A central portion of the hyoid bone is removed to prevent recurrence, and the cephalad portion of the duct is ligated or preferably dissected to the foramen cecum. The specimen is excised (with a 5- to 10-mm core of muscle at the base of the tongue, when applicable). The anesthesia provider can facilitate exposure of the operative field by applying digital pressure on the base of the tongue intraorally, or the surgeon's assistant can use a curved retractor. A drain may be inserted. The wound is closed with interrupted stitches.

Preparation of the Patient

For children, see the special considerations in **Pediatric General Information**, p. 978. The patient is placed in supine position with a folded sheet, IV bag, or small sandbag (adult), or a towel (child), placed between the scapulae to extend the neck; the shoulders are lowered (to provide better exposure). Arms may be extended on padded armboards (adult), or padded restraints may be used on extremities (for the pediatric patient). A pillow may be placed under the knees to prevent lower back strain, or the table may be flexed for comfort. All bony prominences and areas vulnerable to skin and neurovascular pressure or trauma are padded. An electrosurgical dispersive pad is applied.

For **Skin Preparation, Draping,** and **Equipment,** see ***Thyroidectomy***, p. 773.

Instrumentation

- Thyroidectomy tray (adult)
- Minor orthopedic procedures tray, available
- Tracheostomy tray (available)
- Basic pediatric procedures tray (child)
- Right-angle clamps with fine points (2)

Supplies

- Antiembolitic hose (adult), optional
- Indelible marking pen, optional
- Basin set
- Blades, adults (2) #10, (1) #15; children (2) #15
- Suction tubing
- Needle magnet or counter
- Magnetic instrument pad
- Electrosurgical pencil, needle tip, cord, holder, and scraper
- Medicine cup and labels
- Control syringe, methylene blue dye, and needle, optional
- Skin closure, e.g., Steri-Strips or subcuticular running suture
- Drain, e.g., ¼″ Penrose or closed suction drain Hemovac™

Special Notes

- Apply **Special Notes** from ***Thyroidectomy,*** p. 774, as applicable.
- Bone cutters, rongeurs, and periosteal elevator from Minor orthopedic procedures tray may be needed to remove a portion of the hyoid bone.
- Identification of the duct tract may be determined by injecting the duct with a solution of methylene blue.
- A curved retractor may be placed intraorally to exert counter-pressure on the tongue, facilitating exposure for dissection, when needed.
- *Remember, "the pediatric patient is not a small adult."* Special measures and precautions for the pediatric patient must be observed. Administering preoperative medication (if any), administration of anesthesia, preparing the room, monitoring body temperature to retain body heat, maintenance of accurate fluid balance, methods used to restrain the patient, etc., are vitally important. To plan and consider all the special measures that must be taken for the pediatric patient, refer to **Pediatric General Information**, p. 978.
- **Reminder:** *Use every precaution to correctly identify the pediatric patient.* Document methods used to identify the pediatric patient for medicolegal reasons.
- *The circulator should verify information about the pediatric patient with the parent(s) or legal guardian(s) including sensitivities and allergies, etc.* Document all information obtained, nursing interventions employed (with respect to the information obtained), and patient outcomes in the **Perioperative Record** (p. 12).
- **N.B. Reminder:** The scrub person should remain sterile and the back table should be kept sterile until the patient is extubated, breathing satisfactorily on his/her own, and taken from the room.
- **N.B. Reminder:** In the PACU, the perioperative practitioner observes the patient's breathing; should the patient have signs of airway obstruction, he/she immediately notifies the anesthesia provider and the surgeon, employs an ambu bag, and documents observations, nursing interventions, and patient outcomes.

Excision of Pharyngoesophageal (Zenker's) Diverticulum

Definition

Resection or functional elimination of an out-pouching (or weakening) of the wall of the hypopharynx and proximal esophagus.

Discussion

A Zenker's diverticulum collects food (in the out-pouching of the esophagus), causing an uncomfortable feeling of fullness in the throat. A variety of diverticula are seen in the hypopharynx and proximal esophagus; they are classified according to anatomical zone, pulsion versus traction, and, rarely, congenital. The most common is the pulsion-type pharyngoesophageal (Zenker's) diverticulum. This entity presents more often in males, after age 60. Its location is usually protruding through the fibers of the inferior pharyngeal constrictor muscle (posteriorly) just superior to the cricopharyngeus muscle. A less often-encountered Killian-Jamieson diverticulum presents more inferiorly and laterally, adjacent to the recurrent laryngeal nerve.

Symptoms of these diverticula may include the inability to swallow easily and, in neglected cases, malnutrition, dehydration, and pulmonary problems due to aspiration, necessitating surgical treatment. Larger diverticula are excised. Smaller lesions or, in high-risk patients, ***cricopharyngeal myotomy*** (with or without division of the septum between the esophagus and the diverticulum), while not excising the diverticulum, is performed. This decreases the pressure about the orifice of the diverticulum, permitting the protrusion aspect to be minimized, with relief of symptoms. ***Myotomy*** can also be combined with excision by open surgery or by endoscopic excision (***Dohlman procedure***). Numerous techniques may be employed.

Procedure

Excision of Pharyngoesophageal (Zenker's) diverticulum is described. General or local anesthesia can be employed. The table may be positioned in reverse Trendelenburg (20°). Precautions are taken to avoid aspiration of the contents of the diverticulum. An oblique incision is made paralleling the anterior border of the left sternomastoid muscle. The platysma is incised, as are the various layers of the cervical fascia. The sternomastoid and carotid sheath are retracted laterally, and the thyroid gland and trachea medially (protecting the recurrent laryngeal nerve). The esophagus and diverticulum are identified and the latter dissected free from the surrounding structures (sometimes associated with dense adhesions if an inflammatory reaction had been present). The diverticulum is excised, and the esophagus sutured closed in layers (or, alternatively, a transverse stapler may be used). The wound is closed; a simple drain may be employed.

Excision of Zenker's diverticulum may be performed endoscopically (transorally); this approach may be employed for the high-risk patient, in particular, who cannot tolerate open surgery. It involves the division of the diverticular wall with an endoscopic stapler. A double-bladed rigid endoscope is positioned with one blade in the esophagus and the other in the diverticulum. A roticulating endoscopic linear stapler is employed, resulting in an opening of the pouch and a division of the cricopharyngeus muscle. The pouch wall becomes incorporated as a wall of the esophagus. A drain may be placed.

Preparation of the Patient

Anesthesia may be general or local with *conscious sedation*. The patient is placed in supine position, with the head on a padded or gel donut headrest turned to the side; the dependent ear is padded to prevent pressure injury. The table may be positioned in reverse Trendelenburg; a padded footboard is secured to the table. A shoulder roll or small sandbag is placed between the scapulae, extending the neck, to optimize exposure. Arms may be extended on padded armboards. A pillow may be placed under the knees to avoid straining back muscles, or the table may be flexed for comfort. All bony prominences and areas vulnerable to skin and neurovascular trauma or pressure are padded. An electrosurgical dispersive pad is applied.

For **Skin Preparation** and **Draping,** see *Thyroidectomy,* p. 773.

Equipment

Headrest, e.g., padded or gel donut, extra padding for dependent ear
Padded footboard (for reverse Trendelenburg)
Roll or small sandbag for extending the neck
Sequential compression device with disposable leg wraps, e.g., Jobst athrombic pump, if requested
ESU, monoplolar and/or bipolar
Suction
Fiber-optic headlight with fiber-optic light source, e.g., Xenon 300 W

Endoscopic, Add

Fiber-optic light source for fiber-optic endoscope, e.g., Xenon 300 W
Monitor
VCR
Printer
CD burner
Camera console

Instrumentation

Thyroid procedures tray
Tracheostomy tray (available)
Pennington clamps
Bipolar forceps and cord

Endoscopic, Add

Double-bladed rigid diverticuloscope (Weerda-Collard, Holinger-Benjamin), cord, and camera with coupler, grasping instruments, electrosurgical suction-irrigator and cord
Roticulating endoscopic linear stapler (US Surgical); variety of staple sizes

Supplies

Antiembolitic hose
Basin set
Blades, (2) #10, (1) #15
Needle magnet or counter
Magnetic instrument pad
Suction tubing
Electrosurgical pencil with needle tip and cord with holder and scraper
Peanuts/kittners/bullets for dissection
Bulb syringe
Small drain (e.g., 1/4″ Penrose)
Skin closure, e.g., Steri-Strips or subcuticular running suture

Special Notes

- Apply **Special Notes** from *Thyroidectomy*, p. 774, as applicable.
- **Reminder:** Apply antiembolitic hose when the patient arrives in the room, before positioning the patient, when requested. A sequential compression device with leg wraps to prevent deep vein thrombosis may be applied when ordered. The leg wraps may be worn without the hose.

CHAPTER 27

Otorhinolaryngological (ENT) Surgery

Myringotomy

Definition

Incision of the tympanic membrane.

Discussion

When myringotomy (myringocentesis) is performed, fluid is aspirated from the tympanum; polyethylene (PE) tubes may be placed. Myringotomy is performed to treat otitis media, an infection of the middle ear. Otitis media results when the fluid (effusion or exudate) collects and becomes infected. The fluid is under pressure due to a blocked eustachian tube, causing pain. The potential danger presented by otitis media is hearing loss. Middle-ear effusions can resolve spontaneously. When the infection persists, medical treatment may include antibiotics, steroids, antihistamines, decongestants, and/or analgesics. Myringotomy is indicated in both acute and chronic otitis media following unsuccessful medical treatment. Myringotomy is usually performed bilaterally. Myringotomy tubes (e.g., PE tubes) may be implanted to equalize pressure, facilitate drainage, maintain patency, and aid in ventilation. Long-term ventilation of the inner ear is necessary for the mucous membranes to "dry" (i.e., return to proper tissue turgor). Incision of the tympanic membrane relieves the pain and restores hearing immediately.

Myringotomy is often performed with a fiber-optic otoscope. The CO_2 laser may be used as an alternative to placement of PE tubes. The myringotomy incision appears to be bloodless. Some surgeons prefer a laser-made myringotomy incision, believing the technique permits better visualization than those made with a "cold" myringotomy knife.

Procedure

A standard procedure is described. The microscope is employed to visualize middle- and inner-ear structures. An aural speculum is inserted in the ear canal, and cerumen, if present, is removed by wire curette. For acute and some chronic infections, the inferior posterior portion of the tympanic membrane is incised with a (disposable) myringotomy knife. The incision of the tympanic membrane immediately relieves the pressure, and the serous fluid and/or pus exudate is suctioned. For chronic otitis media, the incision may be made in additional positions on the tympanic membrane. Aerobic and anaerobic cultures are taken of the exudate. A PE myringotomy drainage tube may be inserted. The tube is grasped and passed to the surgeon using alligator forceps. The use of antibiotic eardrops is controversial. A small amount of cotton is placed in the ear canal. The procedure is repeated on the other side.

Following surgery when the PE tube falls out, the incision quickly heals.

The CO_2 laser may be employed to make the incision in the tympanic membrane. The power on the CO_2 laser console is set at 0.3 to 1.0 watts for 0.1 seconds to create a tympanic membrane aperture (2 mm). The aperture remains patent longer when made by laser, about 4 to 6 weeks, as opposed to only a few days when made by myringotomy knife.

Preparation of the Patient

The patient is most often a child. Special measures must be taken for the safe care of the pediatric patient in surgery, e.g., to prepare the room, restrain the patient, maintain the patient's body temperature, etc. Refer to **Pediatric General Information**, p. 978, for additional considerations.

Myringotomy is performed employing general anesthesia for children and some adults, or the adult patient may receive a local anesthetic topically. In the operating room (OR), a microscope is used (versus an otoscope in the physician's office). Most often myringotomy is performed bilaterally. The table may be rotated 90° or the table may be reversed with the patient's head at the foot of the table to facilitate the surgeon's access to the patient; in addition, when the patient is a small child, the lower section of the table is removed. The patient is supine, positioned at the top edge of the table with the head on a padded, foam, or gel headrest, turned to the side, with the dependent ear well padded to avoid pressure injury. The arms are padded and may be restrained using softly padded restraints secured to the table, or one arm is restrained using a softly padded restraint and the contralateral arm is extended on a padded armboard and secured. A pillow may be placed under the knees to avoid straining back muscles, or the table may be flexed for comfort (adult). All bony prominences and areas vulnerable to skin and neurovascular trauma or pressure are padded. When the procedure is bilateral, the patient's head is repositioned, (the contralateral ear may be prepped), and surgery is repeated.

Skin Preparation

Myringotomy is a "clean" (i.e., not "sterile") procedure. Check with the surgeon regarding the prep; most surgeons do not require the skin prep. When the skin is to be prepped, the ear on the first side is prepped. Following surgery on the first side, the skin on the contralateral side is prepped and the patient may be draped again (infrequently).

Begin the prep by placing a small cotton ball in the ear to prevent the prep solution from pooling in the ear (it can be removed with a mosquito forceps before draping). Begin by prepping the auricle, working outward to include the periauricular skin. Lap sponges, placed at the sides of the neck, prevent the prep solution from pooling under the patient. Prep solutions are not permitted to pool on the drapes, as they excoriate the skin. In addition, pooled prep solutions are a fire hazard and should be avoided.

Care is taken to avoid getting prep solution in the eyes; antibiotic ointment may be placed in the conjunctival sacs to protect the eyes.

Draping

Draping is optional, according to the surgeon's preference; usually gloves only are worn. Three folded towels may be placed around the ear, and a drape (U or split) sheet may be used to cover the body.

A microscope drape is not necessary; sterile handles may be used with the microscope.

Equipment

- Padded, foam, or gel headrest, e.g., donut
- Padded upper-extremity restraints
- Suction
- Fiber-optic otoscope, or fiber-optic operating microscope, e.g., Zeiss
- CO_2 laser console, optional (observe all laser safety precautions)
- Laser adaptor/attachment to the microscope, e.g., micromanipulator, optional
- Sitting stools

Instrumentation

- Myringotomy tray
- Handgrips for the microscope
- CO_2 laser handpiece, cord, and tip

Supplies

- Topical anesthetic, e.g., Otowick with 8% tetracaine (Xomed), optional
- Small basin, warm saline, and bulb syringe (antibiotic and/or steroid solution, optional)
- Suction tubing
- Myringotomy knife (2), disposable or disposable blade on Beaver folding knife
- Culture tubes (aerobic and anaerobic), optional
- Myringotomy tubes, disposable (e.g., Pepparella, Sheppard), in assorted sizes, 0.045 grommet most frequently used
- Cotton ball(s)

Special Notes

- Apply **Special Notes** from ***Abdominal Laparotomy***, p. 134, as applicable.
- **N.B. Reminder:** *Use every precaution to correctly identify the pediatric patient.* Document methods used to identify the pediatric patient for safety and medicolegal reasons.
- **N.B.** *Remember that "the pediatric patient is not a small adult."* Special measures and precautions for the safety of the pediatric patient in surgery must be observed, e.g., preparing the room, assisting the anesthesia provider, using appropriate restraints, monitoring pediatric patient's temperature to retain body heat, maintaining an accurate fluid balance, etc. To plan and consider the special measures for the pediatric patient, refer to **Pediatric General Information,** p. 978.
- *The circulator must verify information regarding the pediatric patient with the parent(s) or legal guardian(s) and the chart, e.g., regarding sensitivities, allergies, etc.*
- All information obtained regarding the pediatric patient, substitutions made (when the patient is allergic), nursing interventions employed, and patient outcomes are documented in the **Perioperative Record,** p. 12.
- When the procedure is performed on an adult local anesthetic may be employed; the patient is advised that any movement could prove injurious, resulting in hearing loss.
- The operating microscope is set up by the surgeon or by the scrub person according to the surgeon's preference (consult preference card) before the surgery. Adjustments to be set include balance, focus, correct bend in the arm, and oculars (i.e., eyepiece, lenses).
- The most frequently used lens has 12.5 magnification set at a focal length (f) of 250 or 300 mm, or the focal length may be adjustable. An adjustable focal length permits the surgeon to change the distance from 200 to 400 mm (f) without changing lenses.
- The microscope should not be moved or disturbed once the surgery has begun; the scrub person should not lean on it or use it as a footrest. Any movement could cause serious injury and result in the patient's loss of hearing.
- The scrub person checks the lens prior to the surgery to ensure it is lint free, unsoiled, and undamaged.

- When the microscope is used, the scrub person guides instrumentation, e.g., the suction tip, alligator forceps, etc., into the speculum as necessary to enable the surgeon to concentrate on his/her field of vision.
- When a PE tube (myringotomy ear drainage tube) is passed to the surgeon, the scrub person grasps the tube with an alligator forceps and passes it to the surgeon without touching the tube; he/she directs the forceps into the speculum.
- Delicate micro-instrumentation for ear surgery requires extra care when being handled. The scrub person should remove cerumen from the wire curettes etc., gently using a moistened microwipe.
- **Reminder:** *When the laser is employed, all laser safety precautions must be observed for safe usage, e.g., using ebonized instruments or instruments completely covered by (wrapping with) black tape, wearing protective eyewear, posting warning signs on the doors, etc.; see p. 94.* Document observance of safety precautions in the **Perioperative Record**. Safety precautions are observed to prevent injury to the patient and staff, as well as to prevent fire.
- Insertion of prosthesis (or prostheses) is documented in the **Perioperative Record.** In some facilities, insertion of prosthesis (or prostheses) is also documented in a hospital log.
- The perioperative practitioner in the postanesthesia care unit (PACU) instructs the patient or the parent(s) or legal guardian(s) to prevent the patient's ears (i.e., PE tubes) from getting wet (or from getting water in them) after he/she returns home. Some surgeons reccommend that patients wear earplugs when swimming or bathing.
- Following use of the microscope, it is wiped clean and a protective cover is placed over it before it is stored away to prevent it from becoming dusty.

Tympanoplasty

Definition

Repair of the tympanic membrane with reestablishment of the ossicular continuity.

Discussion

A variety of inner ear reconstructive procedures, including procedures on the tympanic membrane and the ossicles (middle-ear structures) may be performed.

Tympanoplasty restores or improves hearing in patients with a conductive-type hearing loss. A perforated tympanic membrane (eardrum) is usually due to trauma and will heal spontaneously on its own. **Tympanoplasty** may be performed to reconstruct or replace the perforated tympanic membrane when it does not heal spontaneously. Replacement is made by graft; an autograft of postauricular fascia is the most commonly used grafting material. Allografts from cadavers, once abandoned due to fear regarding transmission of viral infection, are again being used as well. The fear of human immunodeficiency virus (HIV) transmission has been resolved, as the fixation process used for allografts inactivates the virus. Materials used for synthetic prostheses include stainless steel, platinum, tantalum, polyethylene, Plastipore, Fluoroplastic, and hydroxlapatite.

Tympanoplasty is performed to repair ossicular discontinuity, for the treatment of chronic otitis media, adhesive otitis, and tympanosclerosis, and to excise cholesteatoma (in conjunction with ***mastoidectomy***, p. 801), as necessitated by the disease process. Cholesteatoma is a benign cyst-like tumor of keratinized epithelium that erodes bone as it grows. Often a flap of atrophic epithelium (from the cholesteatoma) has retracted into the middle ear; it must be excised, along with any infected or questionably infected tissue. Approach to tympanoplasty, without mastoidectomy, may be endaural or postauricular. When both ears are involved, only one ear is operated upon; the ear with the worst hearing is selected for the first repair procedure. This leaves the patient with the better-hearing ear uninjured, should the procedure be unsuccessful.

Tympanoplasty is classified according to the condition of the ossicles.

Types

I Malleus, incus, and stapes are intact and mobile.
II Malleus is eroded.
III Malleus and incus are absent; stapes is intact and mobile.
IV All ossicles are absent, except a mobile stapes footplate.
V All ossicles are absent, except an immobile stapes footplate.

Infection, a rare complication of tympanoplasty, must be treated immediately to prevent sensorineural hearing loss and meningitis. An additional complication, a delayed reaction (6 weeks postoperative), is the formation of a granuloma over the oval window. The granuloma appears as a gray mass and results in sudden hearing loss.

Procedure

When tympanoplasty involves repair of the ossicles, it is usually performed using general anesthesia, but local anesthetic with *conscious sedation* may also be employed. When using either type of anesthesia, local anesthetic injection is employed as well. In the endaural approach, the ear canal is injected with lidocaine with epinephrine 1:100,000 (to eliminate pain and effect vasoconstriction); in the postauricular approach, the postauricular tissues are injected prior to placing the ear speculum. The canal skin is elevated or removed; ***canalplasty*** may be necessary to provide better exposure. The tympanic membrane, if not widely perforated, is incised and reflected. When repair is required, the edges of the perforation are separated and later prepared for a graft, e.g., temporalis fascia graft. To harvest the autograft, a duckbill elevator is used and lidocaine is injected under the fascia to separate it from the temporalis muscle. The graft is excised as micro-suction is employed. The graft is trimmed and laid flat or molded, or pressed (with a House Gelfoam® press) and set aside to dry. A micro dissector, such as a Rosen needle, may be used to assess the pathology within with regard to the mobility of the ossicles. Diseased tissues, including atrophic epithelium, fibrotic tissue, and damaged ossicles or any portions thereof, are excised using microcup forceps, etc. A synthetic prosthesis, e.g., titanium gold angled prosthesis for type II tympanoplasty, may be used to replace an eroded malleus. Any part of the ossicular chain that is diseased must be reconstructed or replaced individually with homografts (ossicular bone fragments) or by synthetic replacement: with a **partial or total ossicular replacement by prosthesis (PORP** or **TORP)**. Following ossicular reconstruction or by replacement, some surgeons pack the area around the ossicles with Gelfoam pledgets to provide support.

Myringoplasty is performed utilizing the previously harvested temporalis fascia graft (as mentioned above) or other tissue, such as perichondrium, vein, or periosteum. The tympanic membrane is prepared to accept the graft. The graft material is placed on the drum remnant employing either underlay fashion (e.g., medial to the eardrum) or overlay (lateral to the eardrum) technique; a Rosen needle may be used in positioning. A sheet of silicone is placed over the graft, and Gelfoam is placed beneath it to hold the graft in place. The middle ear is filled with gelatin sponge fragments combined with blood that support and nourish the graft. Skin flaps in the canal, if employed, are sutured. A protective pressure dressing is applied.

Preparation of the Patient

General anesthesia is most often employed via endotracheal tube. The table may be rotated 90° or the table may be reversed with the patient's head at the foot of the table to facilitate the surgeon's access to the patient. The patient is supine with the head at the top edge of the table, positioned on a padded, foam, or gel donut or a Shea headrest, and turned to the side; the dependent ear is well padded. The ipsilateral arm is padded and secured in at the patient's side and the contralateral arm may be secured on a padded armboard, or both arms may be padded and secured at the patient's sides. A pillow may be placed under the knees (adults) to avoid straining low back muscles, or the table may be flexed for comfort. All bony prominences and areas vulnerable to skin and neurovascular trauma or pressure are padded. The hair is secured out of the field, e.g., using rubber bands. An electrosurgical dispersive pad is applied if monopolar electrosurgery is used.

Skin Preparation

Begin prepping the auricle working outward, including the periauricular area behind the ear. Extend the prep from the hairline to the shoulder and well beyond midline of the face. A lap sponge may be placed at the sides of the neck to prevent prep solution from pooling under the patient. A small cotton ball is placed in the ear to prevent prep solution from pooling in the ear (it can be removed with a mosquito forceps before draping). Prep solution should not touch a perforated eardrum (painful). The prepped area may be blotted dry; care is taken not to contaminate the operative site. Prep solution is not permitted to pool on the drapes, as it excoriates the skin. In addition, pooled prep solutions are a fire hazard and should be avoided.

Care is taken to avoid getting prep solution in the eyes; antibiotic ointment may be placed in the conjunctival sac for protection; the circulator must advise the patient that his/her vision will seem blurry following the application of the ointment.

Draping

When the operating microscope is used, the surgeon usually adjusts the microscope before scrubbing. The scrub person drapes the microscope with a sterile cover.

Three or four towels are placed around the ear, followed by a sterile, plastic adhesive drape (optional), or a drape with a small fenestration with a plastic adhesive insert is placed. The head is draped with a disposable sheet, placing the adhesive strip at the forehead. Two folded towels (V-shape) are draped at the patient's neck, and the body is covered with a U or split drape sheet.

If disposable drapes are unavailable, the patient may be draped with a "head drape" (drape sheet and two towels under the head with the uppermost towel wrapped around the head and clipped). Three towels are draped around the ear followed by a sterile, plastic adhesive drape (optional), or a fenestrated sheet with a plastic adhesive inset is used. Two folded towels are draped at the patient's neck, and the body is covered with a (split or U) drape sheet.

Note: Following the skin prep, the circulator, scrub person, or surgeon's assistant folds the ear forward as the surgeon places the sterile, plastic adhesive drape to better seal the perimeter around the ear. The prepped area must be dry or the adhesive drape will not stick.

Equipment

Padded, foam, or gel headrest (e.g., Shea, donut)
Padded upper-extremity restraints
Sterile, plastic adhesive drape or small-aperture drape with plastic adhesive inset, optional
Suction
Electrosurgical unit (ESU), optional
Power source for high-speed drill
Fiber-optic operating microscope, e.g., Zeiss
CO_2 laser console and foot pedal, optional (observe all laser safety precautions)
Video and/or laser adaptor/attachment to the microscope, e.g., micromanipulator, optional
Heat lamp for drying graft, optional
Sitting stools
Monitor, optional
Camera console, optional
VCR, optional
CD burner, optional
Printer, optional

Instrumentation

Ear procedures tray (includes sharp inner ear instruments and speculum holder)
Myringotomy tray
Limited procedures tray
Speculum holder, Buckingham mirror, Senn retractors (2) for canalplasty
High-speed power micro drill (e.g., micro Stryker®), with cord, micro drill bits, and micro burrs
Laser handpiece and tip, optional
Kartush tympanic membrane patcher (protective cover for perforations)

Prosthesis

Instrumentation particular to each type of prosthesis for implantation including bone or synthetic ossicular prosthesis (e.g., titanium gold angled prosthesis) for type II tympanoplasty or partial ossicular replacement prostheses (PORP) or total ossicular replacement prostheses (TORP) is needed.

Supplies

Antiembolitic hose (adult)
Antibiotic ophthalmic ointment

Sterile, plastic adhesive drape (or small-aperture drape with plastic adhesive inset), optional
Control syringes, 1 ml (1) and 3 or 5 ml (1); needles, 27 gauge (1½″) and 27-gauge spinal needle
Local anesthetic, e.g., lidocaine with epinephrine 1:100,000
Basin set
Blades, (3) #15
Needle magnet or counter
Suction tubing (latex preferred for flexibility)
Gelfoam (cut approximately 1 × 1 mm) soaked in thrombin
Antibiotic-soaked Gelfoam (e.g., bacitracin) to pack middle ear, optional
Bulb syringe, antibiotic irrigation (e.g., bacitracin), optional
Heat lamp to dry temporalis fascia graft, available
Tongue blade (to smooth graft over small basin), optional
Synthetic prosthesis, e.g., titanium gold™ angled for type II tympanoplasty (when malleus is eroded)
PORP or TORP
Silicone sheeting to place over graft, e.g., EpiFilm®, Lamina
Packing, e.g., Gelfoam soaked with cortisporin and Merocel® pack for outer ear, optional
Protective dressing, e.g., fluffs and Kerlix™

Special Notes

- Apply **Special Notes** from ***Myringotomy***, p. 788, as indicatd.
- The circulator should verify that the correct preoperative x-ray studies or scans are in the room for the correctly identified patient prior to bringing the patient into the room.
- The involved ear is marked preoperatively to avoid operating on the wrong side. The circulator confirms the ear to be operated on (side) with the patient or the parent (or legal guardian) and the signed surgical permit. Method used to determine confirmation of the side to operate is documented in the **Perioperative Record** for safety, medicolegal, and accountability reasons.
- Identification of the operative ear is made again during the "*time out*" taken prior to starting the procedure. Documentation is made regarding whether or not discrepancies were found regarding the ear to be operated in the **Perioperative Record** for patient safety, medicolegal, and accountability reasons.
- When there are discrepancies found regarding the ear to be operated, an **Incident Report** is completed for medicolegal and accountability reasons.

- **Reminder:** *Use safety precautions to identify, label, and dispense medications or solutions and to avoid medication errors; see p. 30.* It is mandatory that all medications and solutions on the sterile field be labeled by name and strength. Medication bottles are retained in the room until the procedure has concluded as a safety measure.
- **Reminder:** The operating microscope is set up by the surgeon or by the scrub person according to the surgeon's preference (consult preference card or surgeon when card is unavailable) before bringing the patient into the room.
- Adjustments to the microscope include balance, focus, use of laser attachment, bend in the arm, and setting the oculars (e.g., set at –2).
- **N.B. Reminder:** *When a microscope drape is used, care is taken to avoid covering the built-in fan that cools the microscope's light source to prevent overheating and the possibility of fire.*
- Care is exercised when removing the microscope drape to avoid dislodging the lens and dropping and/or damaging it.
- **Reminder:** *When the laser is employed, all safety precautions regarding laser use must be observed for safe usage, e.g., using ebonized instruments or instruments completely covered by (wrapping with) black tape, wearing protective eyewear, posting warning signs on the doors, etc.; see p. 94.* Safety precautions are observed to prevent injury to patient and staff, as well as to prevent fire.
- **N.B.** *New knife blades are used when cutting a graft for the tympanic membrane, e.g., temporalis fascia.* **The scrub person must advise the surgeon that the blade is new.**
- When the temporalis fascia graft is harvested, the area is first irrigated with an antibiotic solution; the scrub person needs to prepare the bulb syringe prior to obtaining the graft.
- The scrub person prepares the temporalis fascia graft by smoothing it over a flat surface, such as an overturned small basin; it is fragile and must be handled with care.
- **N.B.** *The scrub person handles the graft and all grafting items (e.g., sponges) used with forceps; it is not touched by hand. The graft is set aside to dry under a heat lamp (for approximately 5 minutes).*
- When a ***canalplasty*** is performed, the surgeon may request a suture packet to fashion a protector for the mastoid air cells.

- The circulator records the name, type, and size of prosthesis that is implanted in the **Perioperative Record** and documents this information in the prosthetic log (or similar), according to the policy of the facility.

Stapedectomy

Definition

Excision of the third ossicle, the stapes.

Discussion

Partial or total stapedectomy or **stapedotomy** may be performed to treat otosclerosis. In otosclerosis, an overgrowth of bone around the stapes eventually immobilizes it, resulting in hearing loss. The prevalence of otosclerosis is highest in young women; it is made worse by pregnancy or birth control pills. Otosclerosis is less common today, as drinking water contains fluoride that inhibits the disease process. The stapes is the third bone (ossicle) in the ossicular chain required for sound transmission. It sets the inner ear fluids in motion, stimulating the auditory nerve to transmit sound-induced electrical impulses to the brain. Otosclerosis can occur unilaterally or bilaterally. As fixation of the stapes advances, acoustic reflexes in both ears are affected, even if the disease is unilateral. Treatment for otosclerosis includes **partial or total stapedectomy** or **stapedotomy** (including **endoscopic** approach) with insertion of a prosthesis. When the disease is bilateral, the ear with the worst hearing is selected for the first repair procedure. This leaves the patient with the better hearing ear uninjured, should the procedure be unsuccessful. The second procedure can be performed 4 months later.

Complications that may result following total stapedectomy include:

- Hearing loss
- Vertigo
- Tinnitus
- Numbness on the side of the tongue and taste disturbance
- Rarely, facial paralysis or meningitis.

In **stapedotomy**, only a portion of the proximal immobilized bone is excised and an aperture (0.6 mm) is made in the retained footplate, into which a piston-like prosthesis is inserted and secured to the incus. In **partial or total stapedectomy**, the stapes footplate, anchored to the oval window, is partially or totally excised, requiring an autologous graft for placement over the oval window. The stapedius tendon (which protects against loud noises) is sectioned in stapedectomy procedures but is undisturbed in stapedotomy. Both **stapedectomy** and **stapedotomy** require the placement of a prosthesis to reconstruct the chain of sound transmission between the incus and the oval window. Materials used for prostheses include carved autogenous bone, such as the crus of the stapes, or synthetic materials, such as stainless steel or platinum wire, Teflon®, e.g., the Fluoroplastic piston type (Teflon) and the Schucknecht-type piston prosthesis (wire and Teflon).

Laser-assisted endoscopic technique and **laser-assisted robotic endoscopic technique** may be employed to perform both stapedectomy and stapedotomy; however, extensive practice to perfect the technique is required. The benefit of these additional modalities (to the surgical outcome) is controversial. In *laser-assisted robotic endoscopic technique*, the surgeon controls endoscopic instrumentation with his/her voice. Robotics can be employed to create the aperture (0.6 mm) for stapedotomy with the laser and for crimping a synthetic prosthesis to the incus.

Procedure

General anesthesia is employed for children and adults; local anesthesia with *conscious sedation* may be employed for select adult patients. The operating microscope, microinstrumentation, and CO_2, KTP, or Er:YAG laser may be used for the open procedure.

Stapedectomy using microsurgical technique is described. The external auditory canal is cleaned of cerumen and debris. A graft for the oval window (e.g., vein, mucous membrane, connective tissue, fat, perichondrium, or collagen) may be harvested initially. Hearing will be affected by the choice of tissue used, according to the physical qualities of the transplanted tissue. The skin of the ear canal is injected with local anesthetic containing epinephrine. An aural speculum is placed, and an incision is made with a sickle knife (e.g., House) in the posterior and superior auditory canal wall above the annulus, creating a tympanomeatal flap. The tympanic membrane is reflected with an elevator; care is taken to avoid injury to the chorda tympani nerve. The extent of the pathologic process is assessed to determine the extent of the stapes excision. The ossicles can be separated, as necessary, by knife with microsuction using epinephrine-soaked Gelfoam pledgets for hemostasis or by laser (e.g., CO_2, KTP, or Er:YAG), which simultaneously promotes hemostasis. The CO_2 laser beam provides the most reliable results (without direct contact). A high-speed micro drill or curettes may be used to remove excess bone for visualization of the oval window. The stapedius tendon is sectioned. The incus-stapes joint is disarticulated. The crura of the stapes are transected, and the footplate is removed (totally or partially) with alligator forceps. In total stapedectomy, after the stapes is separated from the incus and removed, the oval window graft is placed. The prosthesis may be attached by wire to the long process of the incus using footplate hooks and an alligator crimper forceps (depending on the type of prosthesis chosen). Extreme care must be taken to crimp the prosthesis; too much pressure causes necrosis, too little causes the prosthesis to fall off. Antibiotic irrigation and systemic antibiotics may be used. A dry field is secured with suction and epinephrine-soaked Gelfoam sponges, as necessary. The tympanomeatal flap is replaced; Gelfoam sponges may be placed over the flap, and cotton is placed in the canal.

Stapedotomy or Endoscopic Stapedotomy is the preferred procedure, as it is the least invasive; it does not require sectioning of the stapedius tendon and as the stapes footplate is not excised, obviating the need for an oval window graft. An aperture (0.6 mm) is made in the crus of the stapes by CO_2 laser beam; the beam is guided via a hinged mirror to the micromanipulator to create a "single-shot" perforation through which the prosthesis is secured. Some surgeons performing endoscopic stapedotomy have abandoned use of Gelfoam sponges, as they believe the sponges result in an increased incidence of sensorineural hearing loss and vertigo.

For **Preparation of the Patient, Skin Preparation,** and **Draping,** see **Tympanoplasty**, pp. 791–792.

Equipment

Padded, foam, or gel headrest (e.g., Shea, donut)
Padded upper-extremity restraints, optional
Suction
ESU, monopolar, optional
Power source for high-speed power micro drill
Sitting stools
Fiber-optic operating microscope, e.g., Zeiss, optional
Video and/or laser attachment to the microscope, e.g., micromanipulator, optional
Laser unit, e.g., CO_2, KTP, or Er:YAG, optional
Stapes SurgiTouch™ scanner

For Laser-assisted Endoscopic or Laser-assisted Robotic Endoscopic Technique, Add

Console for CO_2 laser (Lumenis™), optional fiber-optic light source for the endoscope, e.g., Xenon™ 300 W
Hydrodissector console, optional
Monitor
VCR
CD burner
Printer
Camera consoleRobotic console (e.g., Steady Hand™), optional

Instrumentation

Basic ear procedures tray (includes middle-ear sharp instruments with ear speculum holder and alligator crimper forceps for prosthesis)
High-speed power micro drill (e.g., micro Stryker), micro drill bits, micro burrs, and cord

Micro Instruments

Micro-electrosurgical suction tip and cord, micro curettes, micro alligator forceps, Austin strut caliper and measuring gauge, attic hook, House strut hook, House oval window hook, and Schucknecht roller knife
Laser handpiece, optional

Endoscopic Instruments

Rigid endoscopes 0° and 30° angle with optional port for laser, camera, coupler, cord, and robot (can be voice-directed), optional; micro instrumentation similar to the middle-ear sharp instruments on the basic ear tray (e.g., Rosen needle, micro dissector) that are used with the micro elevators, micro suctions with side opening for varying the amount of suction, micro curettes, right angle pick, micro pick, micro alligator forceps, Austin strut caliper and measuring gauge, attic hook, House strut hook, House oval window hook, Schucknecht roller knife, prosthesis footplate hooks, and McGee crimper
Prostheses, e.g., Robinson stapes prosthesis, House wire type, or Teflon and stainless steel or platinum wire may be used, e.g., the Fluoroplastic piston type (Teflon) or the Schucknecht type piston prosthesis (wire and Teflon)

Supplies

Antiembolitic hose (adult), optional
Sterile, plastic adhesive drape or small-aperture drape with plastic adhesive inset, optional
Local anesthetic with epinephrine, e.g., lidocaine with epinephrine 1:100,000
Control syringes, 1 ml (1) and 3 or 5 ml (1); needles, 27 gauge (1½″) and 27-gauge spinal needle
Basin set
Blade, (1) #15
Suction tubing (latex preferred for flexibility)
Gelfoam (cut approximately 1 × 1 mm) soaked in epinephrine 1:1000, optional
Bulb syringe and antibiotic irrigation (e.g., bacitracin), optional

Syringe (to flush suction tips)
Protective dressing, e.g., gauze fluffs and Kerlix

Special Notes

- Apply **Special Notes** from ***Myringotomy***, p. 788, as applicable.
- When positioning the patient, the surgeon may tape the patient's head (in the desired position) to the headrest to prevent it from moving during drilling. The circulator checks (and documents) the tightness of the tape to avoid pressure injury to the patient's scalp.
- Documentation regarding placement of the tape is included in the **Perioperative Record** for medicolegal reasons.
- The circulator sees that tincture of benzoin and a gauze sponge are applied under the tape (after checking the chart for allergy to adhesive tape). The appearance of the skin is documented preoperatively and immediately postoperatively for medicolegal reasons.
- The circulator consults with the surgeon regarding the donor site for harvesting the graft (to cover the oval window). The skin at this site is usually prepped at the same time as the involved ear.
- The circulator shows the surgeon the variety of prostheses available before surgery begins. To reduce costs of unnecessary repackaging (when possible), the prosthesis packaging is not opened until the surgeon definitely determines the type and size that will be used.
- Gelfoam sponges may be employed to aid in vasoconstriction and reduce bleeding; when used, the Gelfoam is cut into pieces approximately 1 × 1 mm and moistened with epinephrine, e.g., 1:1000.
- The circulator and the scrub person should be familiar with each type of laser used for this procedure (e.g., CO_2, KTP, or Er:YAG), and its particular properties, uses, and safety precautions. According to the type of laser used, appropriate attachments and specialized instrumentation should be obtained and prepared for use. Equipment and instrumentation must be in working order; they must be checked for completeness prior to the surgical procedure.
- **Reminder:** *When the laser is employed, all safety precautions must be observed for safe usage, e.g., using ebonized instruments or instruments that are completely covered (by wrapping with black tape), wearing protective eyewear,*

posting warning signs on the doors, etc.; *see p. 94.* Laser safety precautions are observed to prevent injury to patient and staff and to prevent fire. Observance of laser safety precautions is documented in the **Perioperative Record**.

- When the CO_2 laser (e.g., SurgiTouch™ unit) is used to make the stapedotomy aperture, coagulation may be set at 0.3 to 1 watt for 0.1 seconds; when cutting mode is employed, a 0.2-mm hole is made. When coagulation mode is used, it makes a 0.6-mm hole.
- When the KTP laser is used, the setting may be made at 1.6 watts for 0.6 seconds.
- **N.B.** Any smoke plume made by the laser should be suctioned away to avoid the health hazard of noxious smoke and fumes resulting from thermal destruction.
- **Do not set up the Stapes SurgiTouch scanner until after the laser has been used** *to sever the stapedius tendon and excise the crus (crura).* To operate, press "last set-up" on the monitor. Set it at 28 watts for a 0.6-mm sized aperture (usually). The power and size of the hole are adjusted according to the surgeon's preference.
- The circulator records in the **Perioperative Record** the name, type, and size of prosthesis that is implanted and also documents this information in the prosthetic log (or similar) according to the policy of the facility.
- In the PACU, the perioperative practitioner instructs the patient to keep his/her head elevated to reduce perilymphatic pressure in the vestibule.
- The PACU perioperative practitioner gives the patient discharge instructions that include the following: avoid lifting heavy objects, keep the ear dry, and avoid straining when defecating (by using stool softeners). He/she documents that postoperative instructions were given and records the patient's perceived understanding of the information and the patient's responses.

Mastoidectomy

Definition

Removal of bony partitions that form the air cells in the mastoid process of the temporal bone.

Discussion

Prior to the introduction of antibiotics, mastoidectomy was routinely performed to treat infections in the mastoid bone (process) and the mastoid air cells (located throughout the mastoid bone). The air cells are connected to a cavity in the superior aspect of the bone, which connects to the middle ear. As a result, infections in the middle ear can easily spread through the mastoid bone. **Mastoidectomy** is performed to obtain an aseptic dry ear; until this is achieved, procedures to restore hearing, e.g., ***tympanoplasty*** (p. 789), are not likely to succeed.

Currently, mastoidectomy is less frequently performed to treat mastoiditis, as antibiotics can effectively eradicate the infection. **Mastoidectomy** is performed to treat and prevent recurrence of cholesteatoma. *Cholesteatoma,* congenital or acquired, is a benign tumor composed of layers of inflamed keratinized skin cells (squamous-cell epithelium) and associated infected debris; it erodes bone as it grows. Often a flap of atrophic epithelium (from the cholesteatoma) that has retracted into the middle ear must be excised, along with any infected or questionably infected tissue. Mastoidectomy is performed to treat complications of otitis media, such as paralysis related to facial nerve branches, or used as the surgical approach for cochlear implantation. Preoperatively, the surgeon warns the patient regarding postoperative deformity in the area where the bone was drilled.

Types of Mastoidectomy

Simple. Removal of the air cells in the mastoid bone only.

Modified Radical. Removal of the air cells in the mastoid and the posterior external auditory canal wall. The stapes is retained; the middle ear is not disturbed.

Radical. Removal of the air cells in the mastoid, tympanic membrane, malleus, incus, tensor tympani muscle, and mucoperiosteal lining of the mastoid bone.

Potential risks of mastoidectomy include hearing loss, tinnitus, dizziness, facial paralysis, and loss of or an altered sense of taste. Particular care is taken to avoid lint on the drapes and instruments, as these particles have a tendency to induce formation of granulomata. During drilling, the bone is continuously irrigated and suctioned to reduce dust particles and minimize heat to the tissues.

In **mastoidoscopy,** the incision is smaller and operative time is reduced, thereby affording a safe alternative to second-look surgery techniques that provides similar results. Via this technique, biopsies and acoustic neuromas can be dissected from the lateral auditory canal. Limited access to the mesotympanum, eustachian tube, and sinus tympani can be achieved for excision of the incus and the head of the maleus to facilitate inspection of the middle ear.

Procedure

In **simple mastoidectomy,** a postauricular skin incision is made and deepened to the level of the mastoid bone; a periosteal elevator may be used to expose the cortex. Care is taken to identify and protect the temporalis muscle and the facial nerve; a nerve monitor may be employed. Blood vessels are ligated or sealed with diathermy. Subperiosteal abscesses, when encountered, are opened and drained. Once inside the mastoid bone, any granulation tissue and swollen mucosa that blocks the antrum is removed to gain access to the middle ear. The mastoid cells are exenterated using a high-speed drill with a diamond burr. The wound is continuously irrigated with a warmed antibiotic solution and suctioned. ***Myringotomy*** (p. 785) may be performed. At one time, cochlear implants were not placed until several weeks postoperatively (when there were no signs of infection); however, today, due to the effective use of antibiotics to prevent infection, hearing devices may be implanted immediately following mastoidectomy. ***Tympanoplasty*** (p. 789) is performed, involving the reconstruction of the tympanic membrane and the sound conducting mechanisms of the middle ear, and the hearing device is implanted; see ***Cochlear Implant***, p. 809.

In **modified radical mastoidectomy,** the posterior and superior walls of the auditory canal are resected; the middle ear, the attic, and the mastoid cavity are combined into a single space. Micro drills and micro burrs are employed to eradicate the bone. Care is taken to avoid injury to the facial nerve and canal skin as well as the adjacent sigmoid sinus and inner-ear structures. A tympanomeatal flap is created and draped over the ossicles to partially line the mastoid cavity. A gelatin sponge may be used to pack the cavity. The incision may be closed and the wound dressed; however, more often, following the reconstruction of the middle ear, a cochlear implant is inserted.

Radical mastoidectomy includes the excision of the malleus, incus, tympanic membranes, tensor tympani muscle, and mucosa of the middle ear. A strip of temporalis muscle may be used to fill the cavity or it may be left to heal by secondary intention. The wound is packed and dressed. Postoperatively, no attempt will be made to reconstruct the hearing mechanism of the middle ear.

Mastoidoscopy may be performed employing local or general anesthesia, depending on the procedure. The patient is placed in supine position as described above. The external auditory canal is cleaned of cerumen and debris. Topical phenol is applied to the posterior inferior quadrant of the tympanic membrane. The posterior canal skin is injected with local anesthetic with epinephrine (this is not done for perilymphatic fistulae). When perilymphatic fistulae are suspected, a 2-mm radial myringotomy incision is made along the anesthetized area. The surgeon watches the monitor screen to direct the endoscope through the myringotomy site into the middle ear. The patient is asked to perform the Valsalva maneuver during direct visualization of the fistula ante fenestram and the round window. A Teflon patch is placed on the myringotomy site at the conclusion of the procedure. Possible risks include discomfort due to excessive heat from the light source.

Mastoidoscopy, when performed for second-look procedures for residual cholesteatoma, is done using *McKennan's method*. General anesthesia with endotracheal intubation is employed. A 1-cm stab incision is made in the postauricular region, and an aural speculum is placed. When bony regrowth is present, a hole is drilled into the mastoid for passage of the endoscope. Rigid endoscopes with 0° and 30° angles are employed to view the mastoid cavity. When cholosteotoma is found, the procedure is converted to an open procedure. Possible risks include damage to the ossicular chain and the tympanic membrane.

Preparation of the Patient

General anesthesia is administered via endotracheal intubation. The table may be rotated 90° or the table may be reversed with the patient's head at the foot of the table to facilitate the surgeon's access to the patient. The patient is supine with the head at the top edge of the table, positioned on a padded or gel donut or a Shea headrest and turned to the side; the dependent ear is well padded. The surgeon may tape the patient's head to the headrest, placed at a shallow 45° angle with the chin down; pressure injury to the scalp is avoided by not applying tape too tightly. A facial nerve monitor may be placed (to be monitored by anesthesia provider). The ipsilateral arm is padded and tucked in at the patient's side and the opposite arm may be extended on a padded armboard, or both arms may be padded and secured at the patient's sides. A pillow may be placed under the knees of adults to avoid straining back muscles, or the table may be flexed for comfort. All bony prominences and areas vulnerable to skin and neurovascular trauma or pressure are padded. The hair is secured out of the field, e.g., using rubber bands (check chart for latex allergy). An electrosurgical dispersive pad is applied if monopolar electrosurgery is used.

Skin Preparation

Begin at the external ear, prepping outward; particular attention is given to the periauricular area behind the ear. Extend the prep from the hairline to the shoulder and well beyond midline of the face. Lap sponges placed at the sides of the neck prevent prep solution from pooling under the patient. A small cotton ball is placed in the ear to prevent prep solution from pooling in the ear (cotton ball can be removed with a mosquito forceps before draping). Prep solution should not touch a perforated eardrum (painful). The prepped area may be blotted dry, as the adhesive-backed drape will not stick to wet skin; care is taken not to contaminate the operative site. Prep solutions are not permitted to pool on the drapes, as they excoriate the skin. In addition, pooled prep solutions are a fire hazard and should be avoided.

Care is taken to avoid getting prep solution in the eyes; the eyes may be irrigated with normal saline, as necessary. Antibiotic ointment is placed in the conjunctival sacs.

Draping

When the operating microscope is used, the surgeon usually adjusts the microscope before scrubbing. The scrub person covers the microscope with a special microscope drape.

Three or four towels are placed around the ear followed by a sterile, plastic adhesive drape (optional) and a drape with a small fenestration. Alternatively, the head is draped with a disposable sheet, placing the adhesive strip at the forehead. Two folded towels (V-shape) are draped at the neck. The body is covered with a split or U drape sheet.

If disposable drapes are unavailable, a head drape may be used (drape sheet and two towels under the head with the uppermost towel wrapped around the head and clipped). Three towels are draped around the ear followed by a sterile, plastic adhesive drape (optional), or a fenestrated sheet with a plastic adhesive insert is used. Two folded towels are draped at the neck, and the body is covered with a drape sheet.

Note: Following the skin prep, the circulator, scrub person, or surgeon's assistant folds the ear forward as the surgeon places the sterile, plastic adhesive drape, securing it, to better seal the perimeter around the ear.

Equipment

Padded, foam, or gel headrest (e.g., Shea, donut)
Padded restraints, optional
Suction
ESU, monopolar
Diathermy unit, bipolar
Power source for high-speed micro power drill
Nerve stimulator/locator monitor (e.g., Concept), detects possible nerve injury; unit faces anesthesia provider, optional
Fiber-optic operating microscope, e.g., Zeiss
Video attachment to the microscope, optional
Sitting stools

For Mastoidoscopy, Add

Fiber-optic light source for the fiber-optic endoscope, e.g., Xenon 300 W

Monitor, optional
Camera console, optional
VCR, optional
CD burner, optional
Printer, optional

Instrumentation

Limited procedure tray
Basic ear procedures tray
Video adaptor/attachment to the endoscope
High-speed power micro drill (e.g., micro Stryker), cord, micro drill bits and micro burrs (for mastoidectomy), diamond burr (for smoothing), ossicle holder (if ossicle remnants will be reshaped and reused for autograft)
Diathermy forceps and cord
Stimulator/locator wires (2) and electrodes attach to Concept unit
Cochlear implant and insertion tool
Sterile telemetry device for impedance testing

Mastoidoscopy

Rigid endoscopes and cord, 1.2 mm × 0° and × 30° angle, myringotomy knife, auricular knife blade, high-speed power micro drill with cord, micro drill bits and micro burrs, and micro suction

Supplies

Antiembolitic hose (adult), optional
Sterile, plastic adhesive drape or drape with a small fenestration and a plastic adhesive inset, optional
Local anesthetic, e.g., lidocaine/xylocaine with epinephrine
Control syringes, (2) 5-ml needles, e.g., (1) 27 gauge × 1½″, 1 25 gauge × 1½″; (1) 27-gauge spinal needle
Basin set
Blades, (2) #15
Needle magnet or counter
Electrosurgical pencil and cord with holder and scraper, optional
Suction tubing (2) for irrigation and suction (latex preferred because of flexibility)
Gelfoam (cut approximately1 × 1 mm) used dry and soaked in epinephrine 1:1000 for hemostasis
Bone wax, optional
Bulb syringe, warm saline (or steroid solution) with antibiotic
Cotton for the ear, protective pressure dressing, e.g., fluffs and Elastoplast® (after checking the chart for allergy to latex)

Mastoidoscopy

Topical anesthetic, phenol

Local anesthetic, lidocaine 1% with epinephrine 1:100,000
Teflon patch
Blade, (1) #11

Special Notes

- Apply **Special Notes** from ***Myringotomy***, p. 788, as applicable.
- **Note:** The table may be rotated 90° or the table may be reversed to facilitate the surgeon's access to the operative field.
- Hair near the surgical site may be secured with a rubber band. The circulator should check with the surgeon regarding the necessity for shaving any hair around the ear (in the adult patient). Check the chart for allergy to the latex in rubberbands and make substitution, as necessary. Documentation of the acknowledging that the patient is allergic to rubber, the nursing intervention employed (e.g., product substituted), and the patient's outcome (e.g., patient's skin remained free of irritation, etc.).
- When periauricular hair is shaved (about two finger-breaths), the stray hairs are removed with tape to prevent them from later contaminating the sterile field.
- The surgeon may request use of a facial nerve monitor, e.g., Concept; it is set at 100 microvolts and requires two grounding electrodes. The circulator needs to be certain that the screen faces the anesthesia provider.
- The surgeon may use continuous irrigation and suction. Equipment needed includes irrigating solution (e.g., warm normal saline, lactated Ringer's, or Physiosol), irrigation set, and suction tubing, or small Y-connector, straight polyethylene (e.g., intravenous [IV] tubing), and suction tubing.
- The surgeon may follow use of the micro drill (with diamond burr) with bone wax to halt bleeding in the bone.
- **Reminder:** *The scrub person checks the lens eyepiece to ensure that it is lint free, unsoiled, and unmarred before use in the surgical procedure.*
- **N.B. Reminder:** *When a microscope drape is used, care is taken to avoid covering the fan for the light source to prevent overheating and the possibility of fire.*
- Care is exercised when removing the microscope drape to avoid dislodging and dropping and/or damaging the lens.
- *When a cochlear implant is employed, the circulator records the name, type, and size of prosthesis that is implanted in the* **Perioperative Record** *and documents this information in the prosthetic log (or similar), according to the policy of the facility.*

- **N.B.** *Before placing the pressure dressing, e.g., Elastoplast, the circulator checks the chart for patient allergy to rubber (contained in Elastoplast).* If the patient is not allergic, that fact is noted and documented in the **Perioperative Record**. Knowledge of the patient's allergy to rubber, the nursing intervention [product substituted (e.g., Guardflex LF™)], and the patient's outcome (e.g., patient's skin remained free of irritation, etc.) is documented in the **Perioperative Record**.
- *The circulator documents the appearance of the skin before the Elastoplast or the substitute tape is placed for the pressure dressing; tincture of benzoin may be applied to protect the skin.*
- In the PACU, in addition to monitoring vital signs and checking the dressing for bleeding, etc., the perioperative practitioner checks the condition of the skin where the Elastoplast or similar tape has been placed. All information regarding the tape is documented in the **Postoperative Record** section of the **Perioperative Record**.
- **Reminder:** Following use of the microscope in surgery, it is wiped clean and a protective cover is placed over it to prevent it from becoming dusty before it is stored away.

Cochlear Implant

Definition

Placement of an audiologic electronic device with electrodes introduced into (or adjacent to) the cochlea to directly stimulate the auditory nerve to effect sound perception.

Discussion

The implant may be referred to as the "bionic" ear. In most cases of deafness or severe hearing loss in children or adults not amenable to improvement with a hearing aid, some residual function of the auditory nerve persists. For these patients, a **cochlear implant** system comprised of a microphone, signal processor, signal coupler (transmitter and receiver), and implantable electrodes may provide the answer. The microphone collects sound (mechanical energy), which the processor filters according to frequencies (e.g., of consonants and vowels), and selects and codes signals, transmitting these useful speech-coded sound signals to the receiver, which converts them to electrical energy sent to the electrodes. When hearing loss is due to inner-ear dysfunction of the cochlear hair cells, it prevents the physiologic conversion of sound when the auditory nerve is electrically stimulated, as in neurosensory loss. The implanted electrodes bypass this pathway, directly stimulating the auditory nerve, as in an **auditory brainstem implant (ABI),** in which the electrodes directly stimulate the cochlear nucleus of the brainstem. The "normal" sounds are not provided by this system, but with intensive postoperative auditory training, the patient obtains limited hearing ability. Patients may be discharged from same-day surgery to meet later that day with the audiology team.

The surgeon determines the side of implantation in consultation with the patient. Although it is recommended that the "better ear" not receive the implant (in case of implant failure), some patients prefer to have the implant received by the ear that hears better. The patient who wears a hearing aid is permitted to wear it into surgery; the hearing aid is removed following the induction of anesthesia. The side to receive the implant is marked prior to the patient's entry into surgery. The circulator confirms the side marked with the patient (or parent or legal guardian) and verifies the side detailed on the signed operative permit preoperatively; during the "*time out*" before the skin incision is made, the side to be operated is once again confirmed. Antibiotics are administered intravenously, and a facial nerve monitor may be employed for patient safety and for medicolegal reasons.

There are several varieties of implantable cochlear devices available with various permutations; the electrodes are placed either within or adjacent to the cochlea. The Food and Drug Administration (FDA) has granted approval for the following devices: Clarion, Nucleus 22, Nucleus 24, PULSARCI^{100}, TEMPO + BTE processor, and COMBI 40 + implant. The DUET is the first device worldwide to integrate both the cochlear implant with speech processing and hearing aid technology.

Cochlear implants have been placed in children as young as 5 months old (Germany 2004), and investigations are ongoing regarding the benefit of cochlear implant placement in even younger infants. Prior to any consideration for cochlear implant surgery, the patient must undergo extensive medical and otologic physical examination and radiologic scanning procedures to note evidence of infection or excessive sclerotic changes; auditory and psychological evaluations must be done as well. The results of this surgery vary widely according to the degree of intact auditory nerve fibers, prior speech and hearing ability, psychological and intelligence factors, etc.

Procedure

General anesthesia with endotracheal intubation is employed. Antibiotics are administered. The postauricular crease is infiltrated with lidocaine with epinephrine 1:100,000. The retroauricular area for placement of the implant is determined and marked. An incision is made posterior to the tip of the mastoid, extending as a flap superiorly and posteriorly (includes temporalis muscle). A subperiosteal pocket is created in the temporal bone, within which the implant induction coil/receiver/stimulator is placed, under a periosteal flap, secured by suture. When ***mastoidectomy*** (p. 801) or ***partial mastoidectomy*** is performed, the mastoid cortex is removed by high-speed drill or by curette. Most of the diseased air cells are opened. Any granulation tissue and swollen polypoid mucosa that blocks the antrum is removed, providing access to the middle ear. The horizontal semicircular canal and incus are identified. The facial recess (bordered by fossa incudis and chorda tympani and facial nerve trunk) is opened. ***Cochleostomy*** is performed with a diamond burr anterior and inferior to the round window, and the electrodes (or split electrodes) are placed within or (adjacent to) the cochlea. The site is packed with a (previously obtained) temporalis fascia graft. Cerebrospinal fluid (CSF) leakage is avoided; additional bone may have to be removed if ossification due to prior infection is present. Four dural tie-down holes are created using a small burr and a brain retractor to protect the dura. Nonabsorbent suture is placed through the holes. The wound is irrigated and hemostasis is achieved. The prosthesis is introduced with the technique particular to that device.

At one time, the auditory device was placed several weeks postoperative; however, as antibiotics are effectively employed, a cochlear device can be placed immediately following the mastoidectomy. Intraoperative impedance testing using a sterile telemetry device is performed to test for implant integrity. The periosteal flap is closed over the mastoidectomy site. The wound may be closed with a running subcuticular stitch, followed by tincture of benzoin, Steri-Strips™, and a pressure dressing. The surgeon may request x-rays be taken to confirm the intracochlear placement of the electrodes.

The external component of the transmitter/receiver (which is held in place transcutaneously over the internal component by a magnet) is placed. Sound is transmitted by radio-frequency signal to the internal component. The microphone (worn behind the ear) and signal processor (worn about the waist, in a pocket, or in another location) are connected to one another. The transmitter, a smaller-sized processor, may be incorporated with the microphone as a unit and worn behind the ear. An intensive sound-interpretation program (with the aid of speech pathologist and audiologist) is begun.

For **Preparation of the Patient, Skin Preparation, Draping, Equipment, Instrumentation, Supplies,** and **Special Notes,** see ***Mastoidectomy***, pp. 804–807.

Add to Instrumentation

Cochlear implant and inserter tool

Sterile telemetry device

Special Notes

- Add **Special Notes** from ***Mastoidectomy***, p. 807, as indicated.
- **Reminder:** *The circulator records the name, type, and size of prosthesis that is implanted in the* **Perioperative**

Record *and documents this information in the prosthetic log (or similar), according to the policy of the facility.*

- The circulator can facilitate patient comfort by providing the patient with a small writing board for communication. The circulator should discuss use of the writing board or similar device with the patient prior to the induction of anesthesia.
- The patient who wears a hearing aid is permitted to wear it into surgery; the hearing aid is removed following the induction of anesthesia.
- The circulator places the hearing aid in a bag labeled with the patient's identification and makes certain that the hearing aid is given to the perioperative practitioner in the PACU or a waiting member of the patient's family. Disposition of the device is entered into the **Perioperative Record,** including the name and the relationship of the patient to the person receiving the hearing aid.
- At the conclusion of the surgery, the surgeon may request that the circulator notify the x-ray department that x-ray is needed to verify placement of the cochlear device's electrodes.
- In the PACU, the perioperative practitioner should be alert to the patient's need for nausea medication.

Submucous Resection (SMR) of the Nasal Septum

Definition

Resection of the nasal mucosa, with extensive excision of the nasal septum, the vomer, and the perpendicular plate of the ethmoid.

Discussion

Submucous resection (SMR) is performed to relieve nasal obstruction. The approach to SMR may be external or endoscopic. For the endoscopic approach, apply information from ***Sinus Endoscopy***, p. 815, as applicable. ***Septoplasty***, the straightening of a deviated nasal septum, is often performed to relieve nasal obstruction in conjunction with the external approach to SMR. The **SMR** procedure involves an extensive resection of cartilage and bone, in contrast to ***septoplasty***, in which a conservative amount of cartilage and bone are excised. Numerous anatomic configurations of the intranasal structure can cause the obstructive airway. Each individual's surgery is modified, accordingly, to provide a clear airway that establishes an adequate partition between the left and right nasal cavity. Both cartilaginous and osseous portions of the nasal septum, a portion of the vomer, and part of the ethmoid are excised, leaving a 1-cm caudal and dorsal strut in place to support the exterior nasal structure. The procedure is frequently combined with

rhinoplasty (p. 720), a plastic procedure, performed to improve the external appearance of the nose. Preoperatively, patients are advised **not** to take medications that prolong bleeding time, prevent platelet adhesion, or delay blood coagulation (e.g., aspirin, ibuprofen, etc.).

Postoperative risks of SMR include possible need for additional revision procedure, in addition to septal hematoma, sinus infection, breathing unimproved or made worse, septal perforation, nasal deformity, toxic shock syndrome, and CSF leak.

Procedure

An external nasal procedure for SMR is described. Most surgeons do a preliminary nasal preparation. An incision is made anteriorly over the septum, through mucous membrane; the subperichondrial space is developed employing avascular dissection to create the mucoperichondrial flaps. The flaps are reflected with elevators beyond the septal area to be resected. The cartilaginous and/or osseous portions of the nasal septum are excised carefully, avoiding penetration of the opposite mucoperichondrium. The elevated mucoperichondrium of the opposite side is developed to be noncontiguous with the first side (to avoid later communication that may result in fistula). A punch, rongeur, and/or cutting forceps is used to excise portions of the ethmoid and the deviated vomer; a gouge and mallet may be required to extract the vomer, as well. ***Septoplasty*** and modified rhinoplastic techniques may be necessary to realign malpositioned cartilage and bone. Although the cartilage is extensively excised, excessive excision is avoided to prevent postoperative deformity. Occasionally, a cartilaginous graft may be placed within the flaps. Intranasal incisions are sutured to support the cartilaginous revisions. A petrolatum gauze packing or nasal packing (with antibiotic ointment) is inserted to exert pressure on the tissues in the midline to promote healing and aid in hemostasis. An external splint is applied. A moustache dressing of 2 × 2 gauze may be placed under the nose.

The preliminary nasal preparation is done prior to the skin prep. If an anesthesia provider is not in attendance, a perioperative RN, in addition to the circulator, is required to monitor the patient and to administer *conscious sedation,* as directed by the surgeon. For a description of the role of the RN monitoring the patient, see p. 74.

Preliminary Nasal Preparation (Set Up a "Clean" Tray)

Nasal speculum, smooth bayonet forceps, atomizer
Cotton-tipped applicators (long; wood or metal)
Medicine cups (2), paper labels, marking pen (for labels)
Topical anesthetic (e.g., 5 ml cocaine 4%) or a decongestant solution substitute
Cottonoids, e.g., ½″ × 3″
Local anesthetic, e.g., lidocaine 0.5% with epinephrine 1:200,000 or 1% lidocaine with epinephrine1:100,000

Control syringes (2) and needles, e.g., 27 gauge × 1½", and spinal needle, e.g., 27 gauge

Preparation of the Patient

Local anesthesia is usually employed. The patient is supine with the head at the top edge of the table, positioned on a padded or gel headrest. The table may be rotated 90° or it may be reversed with the patient's head at the foot of the table to facilitate the surgeon's access to the patient. The ipsilateral arm is padded and secured at the patient's side and the contralateral arm may be secured on a padded armboard, or both arms may be padded and secured at the patient's sides. A pillow may be placed under the knees of adults to avoid straining back muscles, or the table may bê flexed for comfort. All bony prominences and areas vulnerable to skin and neurovascular trauma or pressure are padded. An electrosurgical dispersive pad is applied if monopolar electrosurgery is used.

Skin Preparation

Submucous resection (SMR) of the nasal septum, as with other nasal procedures, is considered a "clean" procedure. The interior of the nose is not prepped. The best technique possible is used.

Check with the surgeon regarding the type of prep solution to be used. Begin at the external nose and prep the face; extend the prep from the hairline to the shoulders and down to the table at the sides of the neck. (A lap sponge may be placed at either side of the neck to prevent the prep solution from pooling under the patient.)

Care is taken to avoid getting prep solution in the eyes. The eyes may be irrigated with normal saline from inner to outer canthus, as necessary. Antibiotic ointment may be placed in the conjunctival sacs. Small cotton plugs or cotton balls are placed in the ears to prevent prep solution from pooling in the ears (they can be removed with a mosquito forceps before draping). Prep solutions are not permitted to pool on the drapes, as the prep solution excoriates the skin. In addition, pooled prep solutions are a fire hazard and should be avoided.

For **Draping, Equipment, Instrumentation,** and **Supplies,** see ***Rhinoplasty,*** p. 722.

Special Notes

- Apply **Special Notes** from ***Rhinoplasty***, p. 723, as applicable.
- **N.B. Reminder:** *In the preliminary nasal prep, one 5-ml vial of 4% cocaine is needed for the adult patient (to soak the cottonoids).*
- **N.B. Reminder:** *Both the circulator and the scrub person* **must** *witness the discarding of unused cocaine; witnessing*

the discarding of the cocaine is documented in the **Perioperative Record** *for safety, medicolegal, and accountability reasons; both team members must sign the* **Perioperative Record.**

- **N.B. Reminder:** The procedure may be performed under local anesthetic; to help to allay anxiety and offer a measure of emotional comfort, advise the patient regarding the perioperative events to be expected during the procedure.
- The circulator advises the patient to remain still to avoid injury during the procedure.
- When surgery is performed using only local anesthetic, keep movement and conversation in the room to a minimum, as the patient hears all that is said. Any personal personnel conversation overheard may be misconstrued by the patient, causing undue anxiety.
- **Note:** *In the PACU, the perioperative practitioner must observe, report, and document the nursing interventions regarding bleeding from the wound, as applicable (e.g., hemorrhage, pad soaked through) and the patient outcome.*
- **N.B.** *In the PACU, the perioperative practitioner must observe, report, and document the nursing interventions regarding breathing difficulties (i.e., airway obstruction may be caused by swollen tissues) and the patient outcome.* The observation that the patient had no breathing difficulties should be documented as well.

Functional Endoscopic Sinus Surgery (FESS)

Definition

Direct examination and treatment of conditions of the paranasal sinuses via endoscopy.

Discussion

Infections of the paranasal sinuses often result from a deviated or deformed nasal septum that prevents nasal drainage. When bacterial buildup occurs, the infection is easily spread, as the mucous membrane that lines the nose and the paranasal sinuses is continuous. Candidates for **functional endoscopic sinus surgery (FESS)** have had a history of chronic sinusitis or recurrent sinusitis. Prior to surgery, in addition to physical examination, the surgeon performs a preliminary sinus endoscopy (an office procedure) to establish the diagnosis by directly visualizing paranasal sinuses and lateral nasal walls. The goal of surgical sinus endoscopy is to reestablish drainage; some mucosa must be retained because the cilia are necessary to maintain flow of secretions. Diagnosis may be made with sinus computed tomography (CT) scan (without contrast), nasal physiology, smell, and blood tests, as appropriate. CT scan may be employed to locate the site of the obstruction. An emergent problem for patients with these recurring infections is antibiotic resistance.

FESS is employed in the treatment of chronic sinusitis unresponsive to medical therapy (e.g., antibiotics). In **FESS**, abnormal and obstructive tissue is removed entirely through the nose; nasal polyps and antrochoanal polyps, sinus mucoceles, nasal masses, and certain tumors can be excised, and cerebrospinal fluid (CSF) leak, conditions of the orbit or optic nerve requiring decompression, dacryocystitis, and choanal atresia can be treated. **FESS** is also employed for foreign body removal and epistaxis control. When available, radiologic guidance may be employed. During FESS, excision of the ethmoidal tissues and partial or total resection of the middle turbinate can be performed, as well as more radical procedures, such as total sphenoethmoidectomy, although the more radical procedures are avoided whenever possible. The endoscopic approach is used more often today because it is safer, as the sinuses are viewed directly. The *microdebrider* (similar to the shaver used in arthroscopic surgery) has greatly enhanced endoscopic sinus surgery because it is less traumatic to the tissue. ***Maxillary antrostomy*** can be performed to promote sinus drainage by the enlargement of the natural ostia, which, if not done, may lead to failure of the procedure. When more extensive lesions necessitate en bloc tumor excision, an external approach via ***lateral rhinotomy*** is performed.

Image-Guided Surgery (IGS) provides the surgeon with valuable information when working close to the optic nerve, eyes, and/or brain. A preoperative CT scan is taken. Then, intraoperatively, the patient's head position is registered into the computer. Data from the preoperative CT scan is integrated into an image that appears on the computer screen in the OR. Localizers (sensors) are attached to the working end of the instruments showing the surgeon (in three dimensions on a monitor screen) the location in which he/she is working. IGS is performed in the radiology department or in an OR equipped an IGS system, e.g., with the Landmark Element that provides autorecognition of instruments and autoprogression of tasks.

Procedure

Functional sinus surgical endoscopy (**FESS**) is usually performed under general anesthesia, but it may be performed under local anesthesia with *conscious sedation*. The surgeon performs a preliminary nasal preparation; 4% cocaine soaked cottonoids are inserted into the nares (nostrils). Prior to the injection of local anesthetic with epinephrine into the ethmoidal prechambers, bilaterally, excess cocaine is squeezed out of the cottonoids (into the nares). A small-gauge spinal needle is used for the injections. After several minutes, the cocaine-soaked cottonoids are removed and the endoscope is inserted through either nostril to complete the procedure successively.

The procedure performed depends on the pathology encountered. When **IGS** is used, the head position is set in a special head frame. A throat pack may be placed, or the stomach is suctioned following the procedure. ***Septoplasty*** (p. 811) may be necessary to correct a deviated septum, thereby relieving nasal obstruction. Employing an external approach, rhinoplastic techniques may be necessary to realign malpositioned nasal bone and cartilage; see ***Rhinoplasty***, p. 720. The ethmoidal prechambers are examined, tissue may be excised, and ethmoidectomy may be performed; infrequently, total ***sphenoethmoidectomy*** may be done. The microdebrider may be employed to excise diseased bone, cartilage, and infected hypertrophic mucosa; the inferior turbinates are often swollen, and turbinate reduction may be necessary. The uncinate processes may be excised. Maxillary sinus ostia may be enlarged to promote drainage. When the frontal sinus is blocked, endoscopy is performed employing a rigid sinuscope with 45° and/or 70° angle(s). A fog-eliminating device is placed within the surgeon's view on the sterile field (for the convenience of the surgeon); a film of FRED® or ELVIS™ may be left on the lens and should not be wiped off. Once dissection is complete and hemostasis is achieved, nasal packing, such as 1/4″ telfa dressing with antibiotic ointment (e.g., Bactroban or bacitracin), and topical anesthetic with epinephrine may be placed. The packing is removed at the conclusion of the procedure. Some surgeons also place Gelfilm® (Upjohn) within the middle meatus; the Gelfilm is removed at the first postoperative visit. Alternative packing options are Merocel Injectable Bioresorbable Nasal gel dressing or MeroPack™ (see **Special Notes**). Nasal packing acts as a stent to prevent bleeding, septal hematoma, CSF leak, and epistaxis. Not all surgeons use packing for uncomplicated nasal procedures, as many patients complain of discomfort. MeroPack may be the most often used, as it is less uncomfortable than most packing and is resorbed within 2 weeks or can be removed during the first postoperative visit.

Note: An emergent complication, hematoma/postoperative proptosis (e.g., exophthalmos) requires immediate removal of nasal packing and immediate ophthalmologic consultation. An emergency canthotomy is performed.

Preparation of the Patient

The patient most often receives general anesthesia with endotracheal intubation (a Rae tube may be employed) in addition to the preliminary supplementary topical and local anesthetic preparations. The table may be reversed or rotated 90° with the patient's head at the foot of the table to facilitate the surgeon's access. The table may be positioned in slight reverse Trendelenburg; the surgeon may be seated. The patient is supine, positioned with the head at the top edge of the table, turned to the side, gently tilted backward, and stabilized on a padded, foam, or gel headrest; the operative ear is uppermost, and the dependent ear is well padded. Extra care is taken to assure that excessive pressure is not placed on the scalp or dependent ear. When IGS is performed (in a specially equipped OR), the patient's head is secured in the head frame following the injections of local anesthetic. The ipsilateral arm may be padded and secured at the patient's side and the contralateral arm may be secured on a padded armboard, or both arms may be padded and secured at the patient's sides. A pillow may be placed under the knees of adults to avoid straining low back muscles, or the table may be flexed for comfort. All bony prominences and areas vulnerable to skin and neurovascular trauma or pressure are padded. An electrosurgical dispersive pad is applied.

Preliminary Nasal Preparation (Considered a "Clean" Procedure; Set Up Is on a Tray or Separate Table)

Nasal speculum, atomizer, and smooth bayonet forceps
Cotton-tipped applicators (long; wood or metal)
Medicine cups (2), paper labels, marking pen (for labels)
Topical anesthetic (e.g., 5 ml cocaine 4%) or a decongestant solution
Cottonoids, e.g., ½″ × 3″
Local anesthetic, e.g., lidocaine 0.5% with epinephrine 1:200,000 or lidocaine 1% with epinephrine 1:100,000
Control syringes, 3 and 5 ml; needles, e.g., 27 gauge × 1½″, and spinal needle, e.g., 27 gauge (surgeon may bend needle)

Skin Preparation

Check with the surgeon regarding prep solution. The internal nose is not usually prepped. Prep the external nose and face; extend the prep from the hairline to the shoulders and down to the table at the sides of the neck. A lap sponge may be placed at either side of the neck to prevent the prep solution from pooling under the patient. Small cotton balls may be placed in the ears to prevent prep solution from pooling in the ears; they can be removed with a mosquito forceps before draping, as necessary. Prep solution is not permitted to pool on the drapes, as the solution excoriates the skin. In addition, pooled prep solutions are a fire hazard and should be avoided.

Care is taken to avoid getting prep solution in the eyes. The eyes may be irrigated with normal saline from inner to outer canthus, if necessary. The eyes may be protected with antibiotic ointment and eye patches placed prior to draping.

Draping

Three towels are placed around the head, followed by a disposable drape sheet, placing the adhesive strip across the forehead. A split or U drape sheet covers the body.

Alternative Draping

A "head drape" may be used, e.g., a drape sheet and two towels under the head with the uppermost towel wrapped around the head and clipped. A split or U drape sheet covers the patient's body.

Equipment

Padded, foam, or gel headrest (e.g., Shea, donut) or head frame for IGS
Padded upper-extremity restraints
Fiber-optic headlight (to administer local anesthetic) and fiber-optic light source (e.g., Xenon 300 W), optional
Suction
ESU, unipolar and/or bipolar fiber-optic Xenon light source 300 W for fiber-optic endoscopes (e.g., OES CLK-4 [Olympus®])
Microdebrider generator, e.g., Viaso (Xomed®), Gateway® (Johnson & Johnson), or XPS 3000 (Medtronics Xomed®) with shaver, or power source for high-speed power micro drill
Video monitor(s), optional
Camera console, optional
VCR, optional
CD burner, optional
Printer, optional
Sitting stools

Instrumentation

Nasal procedures tray
High-speed power microdrill, cord, and microburrs, or microdebrider handpiece, cannula with serrated shaver tip, and cord
Micro instruments similar to endoscopic instruments

Endoscopic

Rigid sinuscopes, e.g., OES CLK-4 (Olympus) 2.4 and 4 mm with 0°, 30°, 45°, and 70° viewing angle(s) and 4 mm with 115°angle; camera, coupler, and cord, Endosheath™ and Endoscrub®, biting forceps and Grundwald forceps, Sickle scalpels, angled and calibrated suction tips (with side hole to adjust the force of olive-tipped suction), right-angle forceps (e.g., with a variety of sizes and shapes, straight and flexed) with regulating suction (e.g., Blakesley), various biopsy forceps (including alligator, some delicate), optical biopsy forceps, Freer elevator, backward biting forceps, Kerrison rongeur, J-shaped curette, nasal bone-cutting forceps, variety of scissors (straight, angled, curved), mushroom punch forceps, and optical biopsy forceps

Supplies

Topical anesthetic and decongestant, e.g., cocaine 4% (5-ml vial may be diluted 50%) for adults; and for children, neosynephrine 0.5% nasal spray

Cottonoids, e.g., ½″ × 3″

Local anesthetic, e.g., lidocaine 0.5% with epinephrine 1:200,000 or 1% lidocaine with epinephrine 1:100,000

Medicine cup, paper labels, and marking pen

Control syringes, 3 and 5 ml; needles, e.g., 27 gauge × 1½″ and spinal needle, e.g., 27 gauge × 3½″

Culture tubes, (aerobic, anaerobic, and fungal)

Dual tubing for microdebrider irrigation and suction, or polyethylene IV tubing, irrigation solution (e.g., Physiosol), and suction tubing

Basin set, saline or antibiotic irrigation, and bulb syringe

Fog reduction-elimination device (FRED, ELVIS), optional

Syringe, disposable (for cleaning suction tips), optional

Sinus packing, optional

Ice pack, available at the conclusion of the procedure, optional

Special Notes

- Apply **Special Notes** from ***Submucous Resection***, p. 813, as applicable.
- The circulator should verify x-rays or CT scan for the correctly identified patient are in the room, available for reference during the surgery.
- **N.B. Reminder:** *When 4% cocaine is used in the preliminary nasal prep, one 5-ml vial of cocaine is used to soak the cottonoids (for an adult patient).*
- **N.B.** Remember that both the circulator and the scrub person must witness the discarding of cocaine that is not used; discarding the cocaine is documented for medicolegal and accountability reasons.
- When positioning the patient, the circulator **gently** tilts the head backwards, avoiding overextension of the neck. The posi-

tioning aids used and the appearance of the neck preoperatively and immediately postoperatively is documented in the **Perioperative Record** for medicolegal reasons.

- Micro instrumentation must be available before starting the surgery, [e.g., MicroFrance™ (Medtronics Xomed)] that utilizes rigid fiber-optic scopes with light cords and adaptors. Sinuscopes include Sharpsite by Medtronic Xomed; Innovative Endoscopy Components, LLC; and Trueview II™ by Olympus.
- The most frequently used sinuscopes are rigid fiber-optic 4 mm scopes with 0° and 30° viewing angles.
- An Endosheath device can be placed on the end of the telescope during nasal advancement to prevent blood from obscuring the lens.
- An Endoscrub sheath (device) can be placed over the end of the telescope to provide irrigation. Endosheath and Endoscrub cannot be used simultaneously.
- A camera system may be integrated into the sinuscope; the unit can be held in one hand.
- **Reminder:** All fiber-optic instruments and light cables must be handled with great care to avoid breaking the tiny light fibers.
- **N.B.** Most rigid fiber-optic sinuscopes are **not** autoclavable. Always check with the manufacturer's recommendations for sterilization before autoclaving.
- An alternative to sterilization, Slide-On™ Sensory Sheath (Xomed), provides a sterile, protective barrier between the scope and the patient.
- **N.B. Reminder:** When the microscope or an endoscope is used, the scrub person must guide instrumentation, e.g., the suction tip, alligator forceps, etc., into the scope, as necessary, to enable the surgeon to concentrate on his/her field of vision.
- The circulator prepares laboratory requisitions in advance for specimens, when possible; specimens must be correctly identified and labeled according to the area from which the tissue was obtained, e.g., right and left turbinate bones and right and left ethmoid bones (for a total of four specimen labels).
- In FESS, the microdebrider is similar to the shaver used in arthroscopy; it provides power for the high-speed micro shaving device. The console connects to the handpiece and cannula that has two lateral ports: an outer blunt tip protects vital structures, as only soft tissue is extracted, and an inner cannula with shaver blade cuts and extracts tissue, simultaneously suctioned through a side port.

- The microdebrider connects to irrigation with coolant and suction; the motor is activated by foot pedal that the circulator places next to the surgeon's foot.
- Dressing of choice and/or sinus packing may include telfa with antibiotic ointment (e.g., Bactroban or bacitracin) in combination with topical anesthetic with epinephrine. Gelfilm may be placed at the conclusion of the procedure.
- More often, Merocel Injectable Bioresorbable Nasal Dressing (contains the largest amount of hyaluronic acid) is preferred. The gel (available in a kit complete with filled syringe and flexible catheter) can be injected into otherwise inaccessible areas, acting to physically separate the tissues.
- MeroPack (80% hyaluronic acid, 20% collagen to control bleeding) is another option that can be used; it is biocompatible and acts as a resorbable stent as it expands, promoting cell regeneration.
- The circulator should prepare an icepack for immediate application at the conclusion of the procedure, as it is often ordered.
- The PACU perioperative practitioner employs nursing interventions, as he/she elevates the head of the bed, monitors the patient's vital signs, checks the site for bleeding, and continues to apply an ice pack to the operative area. These interventions are documented in the **Postoperative Record** portion of the **Perioperative Record** for continuity of patient care and patient safety and for medicolegal reasons.
- The PACU perioperative practitioner sets up a humidifier to keep mucous membranes moist.
- *In the PACU, the perioperative practitioner must observe and document his/her nursing care interventions regarding checking for bleeding or hemorrhage and observing for breathing difficulties (i.e., airway obstruction may be caused by tissues swelling) in the* **Postoperative Record** *portion of the* **Perioperative Record** When postoperative complications do not occur, the absence of these symptoms is documented in the **Postoperative Record** portion of the **Perioperative Record** for patient safety and for medicolegal reasons.
- In the PACU, the perioperative practitioner reviews postoperative instructions with the patient prior to discharge, e.g., to breathe through the mouth, to try not to sneeze with force, to use normal saline nasal spray, and when to contact the surgeon immediately, e.g., temperature 101°F (38°C) or greater, excessive bright red bleeding, or pain that cannot be relieved with medication.

- The perioperative practitioner documents in the **Postoperative Record** portion of the **Perioperative Record** that postoperative discharge instructions were given to the patient and/or family member(s), as appropriate; he/she includes the instructions given and documents the patient outcome, as a result of the teaching, e.g., perceived patient's understanding.

Intranasal Antrostomy/Intranasal Fenestration of the Nasoantral Wall

Definition

An opening made in the maxillary sinus though the nasoantral wall.

Discussion

Conservative medical treatment of purulent maxillary sinusitis includes antibiotics, steroids, saline washes, nasal decongestant, and a mucolytic agent (guaifenesin). Evaluation may be made by nasal endoscopic examination in the surgeon's office; in addition, a vision test and *acoustic rhinometry* are suggested. When the confirmed diagnosis of chronic purulent maxillary sinusitis is not responsive to medical therapy, as documented in patient's history, the suggested physical examination findings, and CT scan, **intranasal antrostomy** is indicated. Surgical treatment includes perioperative antibiotics and drainage of the sinus to reestablish mucociliary clearance.

Many surgeons prefer the minimally invasive endoscopic approach versus an "open" approach, in that it is less traumatic, with faster recovery. Additionally, further ***FESS*** (p. 814) with mucosal sparing techniques may be performed if disease is present in the ethmoid, sphenoid, and/or frontal sinuses. Infrequently, for treatment of severe fungal sinusitis or when adequate drainage cannot be accomplished, a ***Caldwell-Luc procedure*** (p. 824) must be performed.

Procedure

Open Approach. Most surgeons do a preliminary nasal preparation (see **Preparation of the Patient**) to follow use of a decongestant preoperatively. Although an open approach may be employed, direct endoscopic visualization of the anatomy is safest. If ***septoplasty*** is required, it is performed at this point or at the end of the procedure. A mucosal incision is made over the inferior turbinate; a flap is elevated superiorly with a periosteal elevator. The nasoantral wall and the area beneath the inferior turbinate are fenestrated; the opening is enlarged with a rongeur. When present, polyps and diseased mucosa are excised. The sinus may be irrigated with saline (to which antibiotics have been added) and suctioned.

When the disease process cannot be completely addressed, a ***Caldwell-Luc procedure*** (p. 824) is performed. Intranasal packing is indicated only for hemostasis, as necessary. A moustache dressing may be placed.

Endoscopic Approach. Most surgeons do a preliminary nasal preparation (see **Preparation of the Patient**) to follow use of a decongestant preoperatively. An *image-guided system (IGS)* to establish three-dimensional reference points may be employed but is not usually necessary; see ***FESS***, p. 814. If ***septoplasty*** (p. 811) is required, it is performed at this point or at the end of the procedure. **Intranasal antrostomy** is performed to correct the underlying pathology in the paranasal sinuses and to reestablish drainage with normal mucociliary clearance. A 4-mm sinuscope with 0°, 30°, 70°, and/or 120° angles may be employed. With various biting forceps, the uncinate process is excised; the ostium to the maxillary sinus is identified and enlarged with cutting forceps. Care is taken to avoid injury to the turbinates, lamina papyracea, and underlying sphenopalatine artery. Excision of polyps (if present) is performed; the area may be irrigated with an antibiotic solution. As above, if drainage is inadequate or excision of inflammatory tissue or polyps cannot be accomplished, a ***Caldwell-Luc procedure*** (p. 824) is performed. Sinus packing (e.g., Merocel or rolled Gelfilm) may be used, if bleeding occurs.

Preparation of the Patient

The procedure can be performed using local anesthesia with *conscious sedation* or general anesthesia; however, preliminary nasal preparation is performed prior to both types of anesthetic. The table may be rotated 90° or the table may be reversed with the patient's head at the foot of the table to facilitate the surgeon's access; the surgeon may be seated. The patient is supine. The ipsilateral arm is padded and secured at the patient's side and the contralateral arm may be secured on a padded armboard, or both arms may be padded and secured at the patient's sides. A pillow may be placed under the knees of adults to avoid straining low back muscles, or the table may be flexed for comfort. All bony prominences and areas vulnerable to skin and neurovascular trauma or pressure are padded. An electrosurgical dispersive pad is applied.

An anesthesia provider is preferred to administer *conscious sedation* when the procedure is performed under local anesthetic. Oxymetazoline nasal spray and/or cocaine is administered intranasally. The tissues (nasal mucosa, turbinate, and uncinate processes) are infiltrated with lidocaine 1% with epinephrine 1:100,000.

Preliminary Nasal Preparation (on a Clean Mayo Stand)

Nasal speculum, smooth bayonet forceps, and atomizer
Cotton-tipped applicators (long; wood or metal)
Medicine cups (2), paper labels, and indelible marking pen

Topical anesthetic, e.g., 5 ml cocaine 4% or decongestant, e.g., oxymetazoline spray
Cottonoids, e.g., ½″ × 3″
Local anesthetic, e.g., lidocaine 1% with epinephrine 1:100,000
Control syringes (2) and needles, e.g., 27 gauge × 1½″ and spinal needle, e.g., 27 gauge

For **Skin Preparation, Draping, Equipment, Supplies,** and **Special Notes,** see *Functional Endoscopic Sinus Surgery (FESS),* pp. 817–818 and 819.

Instrumentation

Nasal procedures tray
Limited procedures tray
Metal tongue depressor, polyp forceps, and tonsil snare with wires

Endoscopic

Rigid sinuscopes, 4.0 and 2.7 mm with 0°, 30°, 70°, or 120°
Microdebrider handpiece with tip (hollow shaver blade or burr and sheath) or handheld power shaver, 3.5 and 5.5 mm
Add ***FESS*** endoscopic instruments, p. 818

Caldwell-Luc Procedure (Radical Drainage of the Maxillary Sinuses)

Definition

Creation of an intraoral opening in the antrum of the maxillary sinus through the canine fossa.

Discussion

A **Caldwell-Luc procedure,** the radical drainage of the maxillary sinuses, is performed to relieve chronic sinusitis by the evacuation of diseased tissues and the excision of sinus scar tissue; the connection of the maxillary sinus with the nose is done to achieve satisfactory drainage when ***intranasal antrostomy*** (p. 822) alone is inadequate. The procedure is most often performed under direct visualization afforded by endoscopy, with decreased patient morbidity.

Procedure

Most surgeons do a preliminary preparation of the nasal mucosa and also infiltrate the maxillary sinus area; see p. 817 to prepare tray. Adequate time is given to allow for the anesthetic and hemostatic effect of the topical and local medications. General anesthesia with endotracheal intubation is preferred but is not a requirement for the patient with comorbidities.

An incision is made above the canine tooth and the first premolar, leaving adequate gingiva intact to facilitate closure. To improve drainage, a window is created connecting the maxillary sinus with the nose. Employing electrosurgery, the incision is extended down to the bone. The periosteum is widely elevated from the anterior wall of the maxilla. The infraorbital nerve is identified and protected. The anterior wall of the maxillary sinus is fenestrated with mallet and osteotome, or a drill and burr are employed; the opening is enlarged by rongeur. The pathologic process is assessed. The nasoantral wall in the inferior meatus is perforated with a trocar. Diseased mucosa, cysts, polyps, etc., are excised. Pus, when found in the maxillary cavity, is cultured and suctioned. The opening is enlarged under direct vision from the antral incision. The wound is irrigated with saline (to which antibiotics have been added). The gingival incision is closed with 3-0 or 4-0 absorbable suture. Intranasal packing is used for hemostasis only, as necessary. An ice pack is applied to the cheek.

For **Preparation of the Patient, Preliminary Nasal Preparation, Skin Preparation, Draping, Equipment, Instrumentation, Supplies,** and **Special Notes,** see ***Functional Endoscopic Sinus Surgery (FESS)***, pp. 816–819.

Add to **Special Notes:**

- **N.B. Reminder:** *An ice pack is placed at the conclusion of the procedure.*

Nasal Polypectomy

Definition

Excision of a hypertrophic, edematous mucosal lesion of the nasal cavity or paranasal sinuses.

Discussion

Nasal polyps located in the lining of the middle meatus of the nose are often the result of an inflammatory process (e.g., sinusitis); they may occur singly or in multiples, pedunculated or sessile. The antrochoanal polyp arises from the mucosal lining of the maxillary sinus near the posterior sinus wall; these polyps may grow large enough to obstruct the entire nasopharynx. The antrochoanal polyp may recur unless complete excision is done. When ***intranasal antrostomy*** alone is inadequate to accomplish satisfactory drainage, radical drainage of the maxillary sinuses, a ***Caldwell-Luc procedure*** (p. 824), may be necessary to permit evacuation of the diseased tissues. An open approach employing the operating microscope or an endoscopic approach employing a sinuscope may be used. A CT scan is helpful in identifying the complete anatomy of the polyp prior to surgery.

An *image-guided surgery system (IGS)* (Medtronic Landmarx®) can provide the surgeon with valuable information when working close to the optic nerve, eyes, and/or brain (when more extensive procedure is done). The patient has a preoperative CT scan. Then, intraoperatively, the patient's head position is registered into the computer. Data, from the preoperative CT scan, is integrated into an image that appears on the computer screen in the OR. Localizers (sensors) are attached to the working end of the instruments to show the surgeon the location in which he/she is working on a monitor screen, in three dimensions. IGS is performed in the radiology department or in an OR equipped with an IGS system, e.g., with the Landmark Element that provides autorecognition of instruments and autoprogression of tasks.

Procedure

General anesthesia with endotracheal intubation is employed. The operating microscope or a sinoscope is used. A preliminary nasal preparation with topical and local anesthesia is done. Time is given for the medications to take effect as the surgeon scrubs. The snare wire is passed into the nasal cavity and into the nasopharynx and looped around the polyp. The polyp is grasped with forceps that are introduced through the oropharynx and amputated with the snare (using electrosurgical, ultrasound, or laser energy modality). Each polyp is individually encircled with the wire of the nasal polyp snare, grasped with forceps, and amputated. The nasal cavity may be packed with a petrolatum-impregnated gauze, or Merocel packing or injectable MeroGel® bioabsorbable gel dressing may be used to lessen postoperative scarring (for description of the packing, see **Special Notes** from ***FESS***, p. 819).

Equipment

Padded, foam, or gel headrest (e.g., Shea, donut) or head frame for IGS, e.g., Medtronic Landmarx
Padded upper-extremity restraints
Fiber-optic headlight (to administer local) and fiber-optic light source (e.g., Xenon 300 W), optional
Suction
ESU, monopolar and/or bipolar
Operating fiber-optic microscope, e.g., Zeiss, optional
Fiber-optic light source for fiber-optic rhinoscope, optional
Laser console, optional
Harmonic Scalpel® (Ethicon) generator, optional
Video monitor(s), optional
Camera console, optional
VCR, optional
CD burner, optional

Printer, optional
Sitting stools

Instrumentation

Nasal procedures tray
Limited procedure tray
Metal tongue depressor, polyp forceps, and nasal snare with wires
Laser handpiece and tip, optional
Harmonic Scalpel handpiece and shaver tip, optional
Add FESS endoscopic instruments, p. 818, nasal snare, and wire

For **Preparation of the Patient, Preliminary Nasal Preparation, Skin Preparation, Draping, Supplies,** and **Special Notes** see *FESS*, p. 816–818 and 819.

Drainage of the Frontal Sinus

Definition

Incision made into the frontal sinus to permit drainage.

Discussion

The chronically infected sinus not responsive to antibiotics or antihistamines and for conditions where there is spreading of acute infection, **drainage of the frontal sinus** by any of several approaches is indicated. Methods for treating fractures of the frontal sinus are controversial, as the method can lead to infection. Nondisplaced or minimally displaced frontal sinus fractures should receive local wound care and analgesics. If an infection ensues, drainage is directed externally; open reduction and internal fixation, with obliteration and exenteration of the sinus cavity, are performed. Silicone stents may be placed in the sinus cavity, exiting within the nasal passage; they remain from 2 weeks to several months to permit drainage and avoid premature closure of the infected sinus cavity. Patients are taught to irrigate the sinus to maintain patency.

While not applicable for cases in which the inflammatory tissues are in remote positions, **endoscopic drainage** avoids the scarring and deformities associated with any of several external incisions. In cases where the sinus is to be obliterated to prevent recurring infection, an "osteoplastic" flap of local tissue or Gelfoam, fat, silastic sponge, or cartilage may be employed.

Procedure

General anesthesia is employed. A preliminary nasal preparation is performed.

Modified Lynch approach is described; as much mucosa as possible will be preserved, especially in the frontal recess to prevent stenosis. Other approaches are similar. The operating microscope is employed. An incision is made along the inferior margin of the eyebrow to the anterolateral aspect of the nasal bone. The periosteum is reflected. The anterior ethmoidal artery is controlled by ligation-employing clips, suture, or electrosurgery. The lacrimal crest is identified. Additional ethmoidal vessels are controlled; the ethmoid sinus is entered, and the frontal sinus is then likewise entered after bone is rongeured, removing the floor of the sinus. Diseased mucous membrane is excised using curettes, periosteal elevators, and pituitary forceps. Care is taken to remove all involved membrane to avoid later mucocele formation and recurrent infection. Additional ethmoidal cells may be removed. By removing a portion of the middle turbinate, a nasofrontal passage is made. In bilateral disease, the bony septum between the left and right sinuses may be excised to provide additional drainage. Packing, e.g., Merocel packing, injectable MeroGel bioabsorbable gel dressing, rolled sheet of silicone, or other material, may be used as a stent for several weeks to maintain patency, or a drain is placed to maintain the passage. The external wound is closed and dressed.

Endoscopic approach to drain the frontal sinus is more difficult; however, it has advantages over the open approach, as it is more cosmetic (no external scar), bony supports are preserved without the possibility of soft tissue collapse, and opening the anterior ethmoid and agger nasi region may relieve the obstruction, obviating the need for opening of the frontal sinus. Telescopes, such as 4-mm sinuscopes with 0°, 30°, 45°, or 70° viewing angle, are employed. The area between the middle turbinate and uncinate process is identified. A rongeur, Kerrison forceps, and/or micro drill is used to excise the uncinate process. The anterior ethmoid sinus wall is entered. Portions of the middle turbinate and nasal septum may be removed. The contralateral sinus is entered. As much as possible, normal mucosa is left intact. Nasal packing may be inserted to act as a stent.

Preparation of the Patient

Oxymetazoline nasal spray may be used in the preliminary nasal preparation prior to the administration of either general or local anesthesia. General anesthesia with endotracheal intubation is most often used. The table may be rotated 90° or reversed with the patient's head at the foot of the table to facilitate the surgeon's access. The patient is supine. The ipsilateral arm is padded and secured in at the patient's side and the contralateral arm may be secured on a padded armboard, or both arms may be padded and secured at the patient's sides. A pillow may be placed under the knees of adults to avoid straining low back muscles, or the table may be flexed for comfort. All bony prominences and areas vulnerable to skin and neurovascular trauma or pressure are padded. An electrosurgical dispersive pad is applied.

An anesthesia provider is preferred to administer *conscious sedation* when the procedure is performed under local anesthetic.

Preliminary Nasal Preparation (on a Clean Mayo Stand)

Topical anesthetic, e.g., 5 ml cocaine 4% or decongestant, oxymetazoline spray
Cottonoids, e.g., 1/2″ × 3″
Nasal speculum, smooth bayonet forceps, and atomizer
Cotton-tipped applicators (long; wood or metal)
Medicine cups (2), paper labels, and indelible marking pen
Local anesthetic, e.g., lidocaine 1% with epinephrine 1:100,000
Control syringes (2) and needles, e.g., 27 gauge × 1 1/2″ and spinal needle, e.g., 27 gauge

Skin Preparation

Check with the surgeon regarding choice of prep solution. The internal nose is not usually prepped. Begin at the external nose and prep the face; extend the prep from the hairline to the shoulders and down to the table at the sides of the neck. (A lap sponge may be placed at either side of the neck to prevent the prep solution from pooling under the patient.) Small cotton balls may be placed in the ears to prevent prep solution from pooling in the ears; they can be removed with a mosquito forceps before draping, as necessary. Prep solution is not permitted to pool on the drapes, as the solution excoriates the skin. In addition, pooled prep solutions are a fire hazard and should be avoided.

Care is taken to avoid getting prep solution in the eyes. The eyes may be irrigated with normal saline from inner to outer canthus, if necessary. The eyes may be protected with antibiotic ointment and eye patches placed prior to draping.

Draping

Three towels are placed around the head, followed by a disposable drape sheet, placing the adhesive strip across the forehead. A split or U drape sheet covers the body.

Alternative Draping

A "head drape" may be used, e.g., a drape sheet and two towels under the head with the uppermost towel wrapped around the head and clipped. A split or U drape sheet covers the patient's body.

Equipment

Padded, foam, or gel headrest (e.g., Shea, donut)
Padded upper-extremity restraints, optional
Fiber-optic headlight (to administer local) and fiber-optic light source, optional
Suction

ESU, monopolar and/or bipolar
Operating fiber-optic microscope, e.g., Zeiss, and/or video attachment to the microscope
Fiber-optic light source for fiber-optic rhinoscopes (e.g., Olympus, OES CLK-4), optional
Power source for micro saw
Harmonic Scalpel generator, optional
Video monitor(s), optional
Camera console, optional
VCR, optional
CD burner, optional
Printer, optional
Sitting stools, optional

Instrumentation

Nasal procedures tray
Limited procedure tray
Self-retaining retractor, e.g., Weitlaner
High-speed power micro saw with oscillating blade and cord
Harmonic Scalpel and cord, hand piece, scissors, optional

Endoscopic

Sinuscopes, e.g., 2.4 and 4 mm with 0°, 30°, 45°, and 70° viewing angle and 4 mm with 115° angle; camera, coupler, and cord, electrosurgical suction and cord, various biopsy forceps (including alligator, some delicate), optical biopsy forceps, Freer elevator, backward biting forceps, Kerrison rongeur, J-shaped curette, nasal bone cutting forceps, variety of scissors (straight, angled, curved), multifire ligating clip appliers and optical biopsy forceps

Supplies

Topical anesthetic and decongestant, e.g., cocaine 4% (5-ml vial may be diluted to 50% strength) or Neosynephrine® 0.5% nasal spray
Cottonoids, e.g., ½″ × 3″
Local anesthetic, e.g., lidocaine 1% with epinephrine 1:100,000
Medicine cup, paper labels, and marking pen
Control syringes, 3 ml; needles, e.g., 27 gauge × 1½″ and spinal needle, e.g., 27 gauge
Culture tubes aerobic, anaerobic, fungal
Basin set, saline or antibiotic irrigation, and bulb syringe
Fog reduction device (e.g., FRED, ELVIS), optional
Syringe, disposable (for cleaning suction tips), optional
Blades, (2) #15

Needle magnet or counter
Electrosurgical pencil and cord, holder, and scraper
Stents, 5 mm (packing), optional, e.g., Merocel packing, injectable MeroGel bioabsorbable gel dressing, silicone (rolled)
Drain, e.g., 1/4″ Penrose
Ice pack, available at the conclusion of the procedure, optional
For **Special Notes,** see ***FESS***, p. 819, as indicated.

Tonsillectomy and Adenoidectomy (T & A)

Definition

Excision of the faucial (palatine) and nasopharyngeal tonsils (adenoids).

Discussion

T & A is routinely performed to excise chronically infected tonsils and adnoids. The faucial tonsils and the nasopharyngeal tonsils are aggregates of lymphoid tissue in the posterior pharyrnx and nasopharynx; the tissue hypertrophies secondary to infection (usually). In children, **tonsillectomy** is relatively simple, whereas in adults, because of chronic infections and the resultant long-standing fibrosis, the procedure is more difficult. The adenoids are usually atrophied by age 15; hence, **adenoidectomy** in adults is uncommon. Whereas the use of antibiotics has reduced the number of tonsillectomies performed for infection-related indications, **T & A** are also performed to relieve pediatric snoring and sleep apnea secondary to airway obstruction. Special preoperative teaching and orientation (video) is provided by many facilities for the pediatric patient anticipating T & A; this often results in reduced anxiety and increased cooperation of the pediatric patient.

Traditional T & A technique may use a cold knife (scalpel), scissors, or wire snare excision of tonsils, alone or in combination with low-energy monopolar electrosurgery, bipolar diathermy, or laser (CO_2, KTP, or Nd:YAG) for the extracapsular tonsillar excision (all tonsillar tissue is excised, including the capsule). When monopolar electrosurgery is employed, the tissue is dessicated to effect cauterization, causing increased postoperative pain. The laser is less injurious to surrounding tissues than electrosurgery, as the size of the area and the amount of energy used can be better controlled. Either of these extracapsular techniques exposes throat muscles, large blood vessels, and nerves to bacterial toxins that increase pain and swelling.

Intracapsular T & A uses the microdebrider, radio-frequency (RF) coblation, or the Harmonic Scalpel to excise tissues more precisely. When each of these techniques is employed, the result is decreased pain and morbidity postoperatively; the patient returns to his/her usual activities sooner. The surgeon considers the cost, the amount of postoperative pain, the possibility of complications, and his/her familiarity with the technology and instrumentation.

Complications of **T & A** include swallowing difficulties, vomiting, fever, ear and throat pain, and hemorrhage.

Procedure

Traditional cold knife T & A is described. The operating microscope may be employed. The mouth is retracted and held open with a self-retaining mouth gag. The tongue is depressed with a tongue blade. A soft catheter (e.g., Foley) may be passed via the nose into the nasopharynx and grasped orally to retract the soft palate and enhance exposure. **Adenoidectomy** is performed with an adenotome, adenoid curette, or punch; a dental-type mirror aids visualization. In **tonsillectomy,** the tonsil is grasped, and the mucosa is dissected free, preserving the posterior tonsil pillar. The capsule of the tonsil is separated from its bed. A forceps is passed through the loop of the snare, and the tonsil is seized. The snare loop is passed over the free portion of the tonsil, and the tonsil is amputated.

During any of the approaches, great care is taken during intraoperative suctioning not to dislodge the endotracheal tube, while preventing blood from being aspirated or from entering the stomach. The tonsillar fossa is usually packed with a tonsil sponge. Bleeding may be controlled with electrosurgery, ties (slip knot), and/or by suture ligature. The procedure is repeated on the contralateral tonsil.

Alternate Approaches

Laser T & A may be performed utilizing a contact CO_2 or the Nd:YAG laser, [e.g., SLT Contact Laser™ system (Surgical Laser Technologies)]; tissue is vaporized. The laser may be handheld, or a laser beam or fiber may be directed through a microscope or endoscope.

T & A by micro debrider, a powered rotary shaving device [e.g., Straightshot® M4 (Medtronic)] that uses interchangeable outer cutting tubes, and special blade (e.g., RADenoid®) with continuous suction; better visualization of the operative area is permitted.

Harmonic Scalpel T & A utilizes high-frequency ultrasonic vibration (e.g., ultrasound power for oscillating vibration) of the titanium blades to simultaneously cut and coagulate tissue, thereby reducing blood loss. The Harmonic Scalpel offers precise cutting with minimal thermal damage.

(RF) coblation T & A uses bipolar radio frequency low-level l energy delivered by probe; the probe is applied to the tonsillar tissue in a saline medium. This method shrinks the tissues in the nasopharynx, improving airway patency. Multiple treatments may be required to achieve the desired results. RF coblation causes shrinking of tonsillar tissue using low-level heat (140° to 185°F, 60° to 85°C) from radio-frequency energy. After 8 to 12 weeks, the residual tissue is reabsorbed. As bipolar RF coblation reduces tonsillar tissue size utilizing a lower output of energy; there is no open wound and the patient has less discomfort. This modality is being used with increasing frequency.

Transoral or transnasal endoscopic adnoidectomy may be performed in conjunction with electrosurgical, laser, or microdebrider instrumentation. The endoscopic approach is preferred over cold knife adnoidectomy, as it more completely enables elimination of adenoidal tissues that may obstruct the eustachian tubes.

Preparation of the Patient

The patient may be a child or an adult; however, children do not receive a local anesthetic. For adults, the position of the patient usually depends on the type of anesthesia administered. Most adults receive local anesthesia while children receive general anesthesia. When local anesthetic is employed, the patient is placed in a semi-Fowler's (sitting) position for the local injections and may stay in this position or may be placed in supine position for the surgery. For semi-Fowler's (sitting) position, the patient is supine with knees over the lower break of the table. The head of the table is raised from the middle break. The foot of the table is lowered; a padded footboard supports the feet. The arms may be placed on the patient's lap on a pillow and secured with softly padded restraints. The safety strap is secured over a blanket above the knees.

For the special nursing interventions to consider regarding the child as patient, see **Pediatric General Information**, p. 978. When general anesthesia with endotracheal intubation is administered (to all children and some adults), the patient is supine, positioned at the top edge of the table; the head may be placed on a padded, foam, or gel headrest. A rolled towel is placed under the shoulders to *gently* extend the neck. The arms may be restrained using softly padded restraints secured to the table for either the adult or child (depending on the size of the child), or one arm is padded and restrained and the contralateral arm is secured on a padded armboard. A pillow may be placed under the knees to avoid straining low back muscles, or the table may be flexed for comfort (adults).

For both positions [i.e., semi-Fowler's (sitting) and supine] all bony prominences and areas vulnerable to skin and neurovascular trauma or pressure are padded. When monopolar electrosugery is employed an electrosurgical dispersive pad is placed (e.g., under the shoulder).

Skin Preparation

T & A is considered a "clean" procedure, and there is no skin prep. The best possible technique is employed to prevent infection.

Draping

A sheet is draped over the patient's body. Use of a head drape is optional; for head drape, see **Draping**, ***Submucous Resection of the Nasal Septum***, p. 813.

When the operating fiber-optic microscope is used, it is not draped.

Equipment

Padded, foam, or gel headrest, e.g., donut, optional
Padded upper-extremity restraints and additional padding (e.g., foam padded cups on elbows and heels), as necessary to avoid pressure injury
Shoulder roll, e.g., rolled towel, optional
Padded footboard and pillow (sitting position, adults)
Suction
Blade, (1) #12
ESU, monopolar or bipolar (monopolar for electrosurgical suction), optional
Diathermy unit for bipolar bayonet forceps, optional
Fiber-optic headlight (may contain camera) and fiber-optic light source (e.g., Xenon 300 W)
Operating fiber-optic microscope, e.g., Zeiss, optional
Laser, CO_2 or SLT Contact Laser system and laser adaptor for microscope **(use all laser safety precautions)**
Sitting stools (when microscope is used)
Fiber-optic light source (e.g., Xenon 300 W) for fiber-optic endoscope, optional
Monitor, optional
Camera console, optional
VCR, optional
CD burner, optional
Printer, optional
Video attachment to the microscope
Microdebrider console with foot pedal, e.g., Medtronic XPS 3000, optional
Harmonic Scalpel generator with foot pedal (or hand activation), optional
RF coblation generator, optional

Instrumentation

Tonsillectomy and Adenoidectomy tray
Electrosurgical suction (with side port) and cord (optional), Beckman adenotomes, Guggenheim forceps, Luc's forceps, and pilar retractor
Diathermy bipolar bayonet forceps and cord, optional
RF coblation probe and cord (radio frequency)

Alternate technology uses adapted instrumentation similar to that used in the open procedure

Laser

Adaptor for endoscope, laser (e.g., Nd:YAG) fiber, cord, and special instrumentation

Microdebrider (shaver)

Handpiece, oscillating blade set with removable interchangeable 12° and 40° blades, outer cutting tubes, and an RADenoid blade (4.5-mm blade for adults and 4.0-mm blade for children), Hurd dissector (7 mm), pilar retractor (11 mm), and left and right stabilizers

RF Coblation

Radio-frequency probe and cord

Harmonic Scalpel (Ultrasonic)

Cord, handpiece, and open or endoscopic instrumentation

Endoscopic

Video coupler and laser adaptor, rigid Hopkins 0° and 30° angled, ebonized rhinoscope and cord, and special instrumentation for that approach

Supplies

Medicine cups (2), paper labels, and indelible marking pen
Local anesthetic, e.g., lidocaine/xylocaine 1% with epinephrine 1:100,000
Control syringes (2) and needles, e.g., 27 gauge × 1½″ and spinal needle, e.g., 27 gauge
Basin set
Suction tubing
Blade, (1) #12
Needle magnet
Electrosurgical pencil with extender, cord, holder, and scraper
Foley catheter for retraction
Tonsil sponges
Plain suture (usually), 2–0 ties or 2–0 swaged on tonsil needle
Microdebrider dual tubing for irrigation and suction, or polyethylene IV tubing connected to bag of irrigation solution and suction tubing

Special Notes

- Apply **Special Notes** from *Myringotomy*, p. 788, as applicable.
- **Reminder:** *Use every precaution to correctly identify the pediatric patient.* Document methods used to identify the pediatric patient for safety and medicolegal reasons.

- **Reminder** *that "the pediatric patient is not a small adult."* Special measures and precautions for the safety of the pediatric patient in surgery must be observed, e.g., preparing the room, assisting the anesthesia provider, using appropriate restraints, monitoring pediatric patient's temperature to retain body heat, maintaining an accurate fluid balance, etc. To plan and consider the special measures for the pediatric patient, refer to **Pediatric General Information**, p. 978.
- *Before bringing the patient into the room, the circulator must verify that there are two working suctions in the room, in addition to the one used by the anesthesia provider.*
- When Jennings mouth gag is used, the anesthesia provider disconnects the oxygen circuit for the insertion of the retractor and then reconnects the tubing. During the surgery, care is taken not to dislodge the endotracheal tube.
- The table may be rotated 90° to facilitate the surgeon's access. Small children are placed close to the side of the table where the surgeon stands.
- **Reminder:** *Use safety precautions to identify, label, and dispense medications or solutions and to avoid medication errors; see p. 30.* It is mandatory that all medications and solutions on the sterile field be labeled by name and strength. Medication bottles are retained in the room until the procedure has concluded, as a safety measure.
- **Reminder:** *When the laser is employed, all safety precautions must be observed for safe usage, e.g., using ebonized instruments or instruments completely covered by (wrapping with) black tape, wearing protective eyewear, posting warning signs on the doors, etc.; see p. 94.*
- **N.B. Reminder:** When the microscope or endoscope is used, the scrub person guides instrumentation, e.g., the suction tip, into the speculum or scope as necessary to enable the surgeon to concentrate on his field of vision. Care is taken not to dislodge the endotracheal tube.
- **N.B.** *When electrosurgery or the laser is employed, the plume should be suctioned away or a smoke evacuator should be employed to remove (the harmful effects of) the plume.*
- When the microscope is used, the scrub person checks the lens prior to the surgery to ensure it is lint free, unsoiled, and undamaged.

- **N.B.** When the scrub person will be holding the retractor during the procedure (open), he/she places the needed instruments and supplies on the Mayo stand within reach of the surgeon.
- The scrub person prepares ties (e.g., 2–0 plain) mounted on a tonsil clamp in advance.
- When the snare will be used, the scrub person loads the wire on the snare in advance (prior to beginning the procedure).
- In the cold knife approach to tonsillectomy, tonsil sponges and ties are mounted on a tonsil forceps before they are passed to the surgeon.
- According to institutional policy, tonsil specimens are placed in separate containers, identified as right and left tonsil.
- The patient's face is cleaned following the procedure, and the patient is moved to the gurney, placed on his/her side, before he/she is taken from the room. If the patient vomits, this position reduces the chance that vomitus will be aspirated.
- **N.B.** *The suction and instruments are not dismantled or removed from the room until the patient is taken from the room, as they must be available in case of sudden bleeding.*
- In the PACU, the perioperative practitioner observes the patient for airway obstruction and excessive bleeding. He/she elevates the head of the gurney to reduce postoperative swelling. The observations, nursing interventions, and patient outcomes are documented in the **Postoperative Record** section of the **Perioperative Record**.
- In PACU, the perioperative practitioner provides the patient with ice chips as ordered, as a comfort measure and to reduce postoperative swelling.
- The PACU perioperative practitioner reviews written patient discharge instructions with the patient and/or parent(s) or legal guardian. Their perceived comprehension of the instructions (patient outcome) is documented in the Postoperative Record section of the **Perioperative Record** for patient safety and for medicolegal reasons.

Uvulopalatopharyngoplasty

Definition

Excision of the uvula, adenoids and faucial tonsils, and partial excision of the hard and soft palate and contiguous structures.

Discussion

The primary purpose of **uvulopalatopharyngoplasty (UPPP)** is to increase the size of the pharyngeal airway. It is performed most often for intractable snoring and obstructive sleep apnea not responsive to nonsurgical treatment. The uvula, portions of the soft palate, tonsils, and redundant pharyngeal mucous membranes are removed. Depending on the site of obstruction, portions of the hard palate, palatoglossus muscle, and base of the tongue may be excised and maxillomandibular osteotomy with fixation may be required.

It is essential for the perioperative practitioner to plan perioperative nursing care in advance. He/she should obtain adequate positioning aids prior to bringing the patient into the room. Particular care must be taken to properly reposition the patient (from semi-Fowler's position to supine) in good body alignment following local preliminary preparation. The circulator should secure adequate assistance or bring a means of lifting or moving the obese patient. An assortment of tracheostomy tubes should be made available to the anesthesia practitioner that are long enough when the patient is obese, as well as longer surgical instrumentation.

In obese and other poor-risk patients, ***tracheostomy*** is performed initially. Note that ***tracheostomy*** (p. 844) may be necessary for all patients in the immediate postoperative period due to postoperative edema. An unopened tracheostomy tray should accompany the patient to the PACU. A CO_2 laser or radio-frequency (RF) probe may be employed to coblate the involved tissues. ***Somnoplasty*** employs a modality that is a variation of coblation, often performed in an outpatient or office setting, involves the application of radio-frequency (RF) energy to the soft palate (and less often to the base of the tongue) under local anesthesia over several sessions. This method results in the "shrinking" of the affected tissues with relief of symptoms in selected cases. In the surgeon's office preoperative endoscopic visualization of the pharyngeal structures and airway with the patient awake trying to simulate snoring is helpful in identifying the most affected anatomical sites responsible for the problem.

Procedure

The surgeon administers a preliminary preparation to include local field block of the area with the patient in the semi-Fowler's (sitting) position. Following the local anesthetic, care is taken in repositioning the patient to maintain proper body alignment. Preliminary tracheostomy and tonsillectomy may be performed; in the obese patient tracheostomy is performed routinely. A mouth gag is placed and the tissues to be excised are marked with indelible ink prior to their resection (perhaps during the preliminary preparation). Standard instrumentation may be employed; special instrumentation is required when the CO_2 laser (e.g. Swiftlase™) is employed. The tissues may also be smoothed with Swiftlase™. When it is necessary to shrink the tissues RF coblation may be used. Excision of posterior portions of the hard palate may be done, requiring small bone cutting instruments. Hemostasis is achieved with electrosurgery, laser, or direct ligation of larger pharyngeal and palatine vessels by sutures or clips. Wounds are closed with runs of absorbable suture. The oral cavity and pharynx are cleansed of clots and tissue debris prior to completion of the procedure.

For **Preparation of the Patient, Skin Preparation, Draping, Supplies,** and **Special Notes,** see *Tonsillectomy and Adnoidectomy (T & A),* pp. 833–834 and 835, and *Tracheostomy*, pp. 844–846, as indicated.

Add to Equipment

Padded upper-extremity restraints
Fiber-optic headlight (to administer local anesthetic) and fiber-optic light source (e.g., Xenon 300 W, optional
Footstool for patient
Operating fiber-optic microscope, e.g., Zeiss, with 400-mm lens
CO_2 laser unit (e.g., Swiftlase), optional
RF coblator, optional

Add to InstrumentationTracheostomy Tray

T & A tray
Small bone cutters and rongeurs, electrosurgical suction (e.g. Cameron-Miller), CO_2 laser, RF coblation probe, optional

Add to Supplies

Indelible marking pen (on preliminary preparation tray), optional
Magnetic instrument pad, optional

Add to Special Notes:

- Apply **Special Notes** from ***T & A,*** p. 835, and ***Tracheostomy***, p. 846, as applicable
- **N.B.** *Special note should be made that tracheostomy may be necessary for all patients in the immediate postoperative period.* The circulator should be certain that a Tracheostomy tray accompanies the patient to the PACU. This should be documented in the **Perioperative Record** and noted in the circulator's report to the perioperative practitioner in the PACU.
- If there is a possibility that a portion of the hard palate is to be excised, small bone-cutting instruments should be included on the instrument setup.

- **N.B. Reminder:** When the microscope is used, the scrub person must place instrumentation (e.g., the suction tip, alligator forceps, etc.), in the surgeon's hand, to enable the surgeon to concentrate on his/her field of vision.
- **N.B. Reminder:** Prevent a fire hazard by making sure that the microscope fan is not obstructed by the disposable drapes.

Laryngoscopy

Definition

Direct visual examination of the larynx and hypopharynx with an endoscope.

Discussion

Indirect laryngoscopy, usually performed as a diagnostic office examination, utilizes a dental-type mirror that the surgeon holds in the posterior pharynx with a headlamp or head mirror as a light source. **Direct laryngoscopy** may employ a variety of rigid and flexible scopes with which diagnosis, biopsy, and/or treatment of laryngeal lesions, aspiration of secretions, assessment of laryngeal trauma, or removal of a foreign body is performed. Use of a microscope facilitates visualization. In **suspension laryngoscopy**, a self-retaining laryngoscope holder gives the surgeon bimanual freedom.

Microlaryngoscopy, with a CO_2 laser (observe all laser safety precautions, p. 94), may be used to remove benign lesions and early malignant tumors of the larynx. The advantages of using the CO_2 laser are that excision is facilitated, hemostasis is quickly achieved, and there is rapid wound healing with a minimum of postoperative pain and swelling. Lesions removed by laser energy are vaporized by intense heat, leaving a small crater; this means that the vaporized tissues are unavailable for histologic examination (except in circumstances when the laser is used to transect the stalk of a pedunculated lesion, the remainder of which is retrieved as a specimen). **Flexible scope laryngoscopy** may be performed using topical anesthetic; since the scope is very small, it is primarily for diagnostic exam and limited procedures, such as biopsy, aspiration of fluids, destruction of smaller lesions, or retrieval of small foreign objects.

Procedure

Rigid laryngeal endoscopy (laryngoscopy) is described. Under general anesthesia without intubation, the patient's head is tipped back and the laryngoscope is inserted. The oropharynx and the larynx are inspected; the scope is lifted as necessary. Care is taken not to use the teeth as a fulcrum; a bite block may be used. A self-retaining laryngoscope holder can be employed to let the surgeon operate with both hands. The microscope may be used. Lesions may be biopsied, secretions may be aspirated, etc. For **CO_2 laser microlaryngoscopy,** a micromanipulator, used to direct the laser beam, is coupled to a standard microscope. Stainless steel mirrors (built in) reflect the beam to inaccessible areas. A special vocal cord retractor with suction attachments is used to clear smoke resulting from tissue vaporization. Two suctions are employed when performing cancer surgery for rapid clearing of the plume or a plume evacuator may be used.

Flexible laryngoscopy is used to evaluate the upper airway when the patient gags and cannot tolerate the rigid endoscope or when a more clear view of laryngeal structures is needed for diagnostic evaluation of laryngeal structures.

Preparation of the Patient

Anesthesia may be general or topical. The table is rotated 90° so that the surgeon is at the head of the table. All bony prominences and areas vulnerable to skin and neurovascular trauma or pressure are padded. An electrosurgical dispersive pad is applied when monopolar electrosurgery is anticipated.

General anesthesia is required for microlaryngoscopy. When general anesthesia (employing a small endotracheal tube) is administered, the patient is supine, positioned at the top edge of the table; use of a headrest is optional. To facilitate passage of the laryngoscope, the patient's head is gently tilted backward, the neck may be supported with a roll or small sandbag. The arms may be restrained using padded restraints secured to the table, or one arm is restrained and the opposite arm is extended on a padded armboard. A pillow may be placed under the knees to avoid straining back muscles, or the table may be flexed for comfort.

In the preliminary preparation, injections of local anesthetic (adults), with the patient in the sitting position is used. Following the injections, the patient may be returned to supine position, or he/she may stay in the sitting position for the procedure, according to surgeon's preference. For the sitting position, the patient is supine with knees over the lower break of the table. The head of the table is raised from the middle break. The foot of the table is lowered; a padded footboard supports the feet. The arms may be placed on the patient's lap on a pillow and secured with padded restraints. The safety strap is secured above the knees.

Topical Anesthesia Preparation (on a Clean Mayo Stand)

Laryngeal spatulas and mirror
Small basin with very warm water (for mirror)
Topical anesthetic spray (e.g., Cetacaine)
Gauze sponges (not raytex)

Jackson-Krause right angle forceps (for holding gauze pads with anesthetic)
Laryngeal syringe with straight and curved cannulas
Medication cup
Topical anesthetic (e.g., cocaine 4%)
Cotton-tipped applicators
Tissues

Skin Preparation

Laryngoscopy is considered a "clean" procedure; there is no prep. The best possible technique is employed to prevent infection.

Draping

Towels may be placed around the operative site. The patient may be covered with a drape sheet. The back table is covered with a drape sheet. Folded towels are used to stabilize the laryngoscope holder. Gloves, masks, and protective goggles are worn.

Equipment

Padded headrest, optional
Small roll or sandbag
Fiber-optic headlight and fiber-optic light source for laryngoscope (e.g., Xenon 300 W)
Suction
Footstool for patient
Operating fiber-optic microscope, e.g., Zeiss, with 400-mm lens (microlaryngoscopy)
CO_2 laser, optional (**observe all laser safety precautions**)

Instrumentation and Supplies

Medicine cup
Bite block
Laryngoscope and cord (e.g., Jackson)
Self-retaining laryngoscope holder (e.g., Lewy)
Laser adaptor for microscope, optional
Magnetic instrument pad, optional
Suction tubing
Aspiration/specimen tubes (2) (e.g., Lukens)
Biopsy forceps (assorted), suction tip and tubing, sponge carriers (2, preload)
Telfa and needle, 25 gauge (for specimen removal)
Small basin with saline
Toluidine blue, 1 ml (stain to detect carcinoma), optional

Add for Microlaryngoscopy

Double-barrel scope (e.g., Dedo, Jako) and cord (use with laryngoscope holder)

Microlaryngeal forceps (assorted), micro scissors, micro knife, hook, micro aspiration tube, vocal cord retractor (with suction attachments)

Special Notes

- Apply **Special Notes** from ***Functional Endoscopic Sinus Surgery***, p. 819, as applicable.
- The circulator takes care to verify the location of any loose teeth, bridges, caps, etc. and reports findings to the anesthesia provider and the surgeon and documents this in the **Perioperative Record.**
- **N.B.** Patients who arrive in the OR with false teeth must remove them prior to the procedure; the circulator puts the false teeth in a plastic bag with the patient's identification and gives the bag to a waiting family member. The circulator documents who the teeth were given to and his/her relationship to the patient. When there is no waiting family member, the circulator attaches the bag to the patient's chart and later gives the bag to the perioperative practitioner in the PACU following surgery.
- The scrub person works directly from the back table without the Mayo stand.
- **N.B. Reminder:** *The circulator and the scrub person **must** witness the discarding of any cocaine that is not used; discarding the cocaine is documented in the **Perioperative Record** for safety, medicolegal, and accountability reasons; both team members must sign the **Perioperative Record.***
- **Reminder:** When the microscope or an endoscope is used, the scrub person must guide instrumentation, e.g., the suction tip, alligator forceps, etc., into the scope, as necessary, to enable the surgeon to concentrate on his/her field of vision.
- **Reminder:** When the microscope is used, the scrub person must pass biopsy forceps with tip closed.
- The scrub person can remove the biopsy specimen from forceps with a needle to avoid crushing the specimen; the specimen is placed on telfa or similar product with nonsticking surface.

Tracheostomy

Definition

Opening made in the trachea to facilitate breathing.

Discussion

Tracheostomy is often done as an emergency, but it is also performed electively to maintain a patent airway. Any of several techniques may be used; numerous endotracheal cannulas are available, including those adapted for administering anesthesia or for use with a respirator. Cannulas may be stainless steel or plastic, cuffed or non-cuffed, in graded sizes, including those used in pediatrics. A *phonate valve* permits speech without having to manipulate or occlude the tracheostomy tube.

Tracheostomy is not usually performed in the OR unless it is done in conjunction with another procedure. Crudely, an ordinary knife and a hollow tube (as the barrel of a ballpoint pen) can be effective for establishing an airway in a dire emergency. ***Cricothyrotomy,*** a similar procedure, is performed in the OR; in cricothyrotomy, an airway is established via the cricothryroid membrane. Numerous commercial kits for ***percutaneous cricothyrotomy*** are available.

For the tracheostomy patient for whom prolonged ventilator assistance is anticipated, the *Hi-Lo Evac tube* is recommended, as it includes a channel for suctioning secretions that accumulate above the inflated cuff, thus lessening the occurrence of aspiration pneumonia. An additional recommended modification is to include the *Lanz® pressure-regulating valve* with the tube; the valve regulates cuff pressure (not to exceed 25 to 30 cm H_2O) to avoid ischemia to the tracheal mucosa. This tube and valve are also used when an *oroendotracheal tube* is placed, intraoperatively or otherwise, in patients who are on a ventilator for an extended period.

Procedure

A transverse (or longitudinal) incision is made overlying the proximal trachea. The platysma and deep fascia are incised; the thyroid isthmus is retracted superiorly, and the superior tracheal rings are exposed. An anterior disc of the second and third tracheal rings is excised. Stay sutures are placed to mark the stoma; they are also used for retraction, should the cannula need replacement. Hemostasis is achieved. Several sutures approximate the skin. The tracheostomy tube is held in place with umbilical tapes tied in a square knot behind the neck. A gauze dressing, split around the tube (customary dressing), is applied to the wound.

Preparation of the Patient

Tracheostomy may be performed under local or general anesthesia (or in urgent circumstances, no anesthesia, as any delay might result in irreversible hypoxic sequelae). When the surgery is elective, the patient is supine with a folded sheet under the shoulders to extend the neck. The table may be rotated 90° to facilitate the surgeon's access. The ipsilateral arm is padded and secured at the patient's side and the contralateral arm may be secured on a padded armboard, or both arms may be padded and secured at the patient's sides. A pillow may be placed under the knees of adults to avoid straining low back muscles, or the table may be flexed for comfort. All bony prominences and areas vulnerable to skin and neurovascular trauma or pressure are padded. An electrosurgical dispersive pad is applied.

Skin Preparation

Begin at the neck; prep the neck, extending from the infra-auricular border to the axillae and down to the table at the neck and shoulders. A lap sponge may be placed at either side of the neck to prevent the prep solution from pooling under the patient. Prep solution is not permitted to pool in the eyes or ears or on the drapes (as the solution excoriates the skin). In addition, pooled prep solutions are a fire hazard and should be avoided.

Draping

Folded towels and a sheet with a small fenestration; for emergency tracheostomy no drapes are used, thereby avoiding loss of time.

Equipment

Suction
ESU

Instrumentation

Tracheostomy tray

Supplies

Indelible marking pen, optional
Local anesthetic (e.g., lidocaine 1% with epinephrine)
Small basin
Suction tubing
Blades, (1) #10, (2) #15, and (1) #11
Portex Flex tracheostomy disposable inner cannula (D.I.C.) tubes with Soft-Seal™ cuff, adult sizes #6 to # 10, with snap in obturator, syringe (10 ml) to inflate cuff, and velcro tracheostomy tube holder, optional
Catheters (2) for suctioning tracheostomy tube (e.g., Robinson 14 Fr or 16 Fr)
Electrosurgical pencil and cord with holder and scraper
Umbilical tapes

Special Notes

- Apply **Special Notes** from ***Laryngoscopy***, p. 843, as applicable.
- The circulator makes certain the cardiac arrest cart is nearby before the surgery is begun.
- Before passing the tracheostomy tube, the scrub person tests the tube cuff for air leakage.
- *When* ***tracheostomy*** *is performed under general anesthesia, an endotracheal tube is inserted. As the tracheostomy tube is placed, the endotracheal tube is withdrawn.*
- **N.B.** *The obturator for the tracheostomy tube must accompany the patient. The obturator is taped to the top of the gurney. It will be needed to reinsert the tube if it becomes dislodged.*

Excision of Submandibular (Submaxillary) Gland

Definition

Excision of a salivary gland.

Discussion

The submandibular (second largest), the parotid (largest), and the sublingual glands comprise the major salivary glands. Tumors of the submandibular gland, including malignancy, are infrequently encountered (less frequently than tumors of the parotid). Most often, medical and supportive treatment is indicated for infectious or inflammatory disease, including the use of antibiotics, hydration, massage, and transductal cannulation with stone removal. Abscesses of the submandibular gland necessitate incision and drainage.

Submandibular gland excision is performed when symptomatic treatment is refractory, most often for benign disease, such as *chronic sialadenitis* (involving gland enlargement without erythema), *sialolithiasis* (linked to reduced salivary flow and stasis), or ductal stricture following transductal cannulation (of Wharton's duct). Malignant lesion diagnosis can be made by fine-needle biopsy. Open dissection with wide tumor margins is performed for malignancies. When malignancy presents with evidence of extraglandular spread, ***radical neck dissection*** (p. 857) may be performed on an immediate basis, or as a staged procedure, with or without adjunctive radiation therapy, e.g., brachytherapy.

Endoscopic diagnosis and treatment of certain submandibular gland disease may be performed. Extracorporeal **ultrasonic lithotripsy** is an alternative modality for treatment of sialolithiasis with stones 2 to 10 mm in the proximal duct, particularly in children.

Procedure

Open submandibular gland excision is described. A transverse incision is made over the mastoid process, approaching the midline; the gland is below the lower edge of and parallel to the mandible. The fascia is incised, as is the platysma muscle, leaving muscle attached to the skin as a thick musculocutaneous flap. The dissection begins at the level of the hyoid bone and the lower aspect of the gland. Structures to be protected during dissection are the mandibular branch of the facial nerve, the lingual nerve, and hypoglossal nerve, unless there is direct tumor involvement; a nerve stimulator/locator may be employed. The facial (external maxillary) artery is ligated and divided (or retracted). The anterior facial vein is divided and the fascial envelope about the gland incised. The gland is dissected free of surrounding tissues; intracapsular dissection is preferred, when possible. Electrosurgical modalities, including bipolar scissors, may be used. If only a portion of the gland is to be removed, the Harmonic Scalpel may be used. The mylohyoid muscle is retracted and the lingual nerve is visualized. Blood supply to the gland is ligated. The pedicle of the gland is ligated; care is taken to avoid injury to the lingual nerve. Wharton's duct is identified adjacent to the lingual nerve, ligated, and divided. The wound is closed in layers with a cosmetic closure, often employing a closed-suction drain to ensure hemostasis.

Preparation of the Patient

Antiembolitic hose may be applied. General anesthesia via endotracheal intubation is employed. The table may be rotated 90° to facilitate the surgeon's access to the patient. The patient is supine with the head turned to the side, placed on a padded, foam, or gel donut (or other head support) with the face and neck on the operative side uppermost. The dependent ear is well padded to prevent pressure injury. A folded sheet may be placed under the shoulders to facilitate access to the operative area. The arm on the operative side may be padded and secured at the patient's side; the contralateral arm may be secured on a padded armboard. A pillow may be placed under the knees to prevent low back strain, or the table may be flexed for comfort. All bony prominences and areas vulnerable to skin and neurovascular pressure or trauma are padded. An electrosurgical dispersive pad is applied.

Skin Preparation

Check with the surgeon regarding choice of prep solution. The inside of the mouth is not usually prepped. Begin under the chin; extend the prep from the infra-auricular border (well beyond the midline) include the ear, the area around the neck and shoulder, down to the axillae. A lap sponge may be placed at the sides of the neck to prevent prep solution from pooling under the patient. A small cotton ball may be placed in the ear to prevent prep solution from pooling in the ear (it can be removed with a mosquito forceps before draping). The prepped area may be blotted dry; care is taken not to contaminate the operative site while doing this. Prep solution is not permitted to pool on the drapes, as it excoriates the skin. In addition, pooled prep solutions are a fire hazard and should be avoided.

Care is taken to avoid getting prep solution in the eyes; antibiotic ointment may be placed in the conjunctival sac.

Draping

The neck is draped with folded towels secured with a sterile, plastic adhesive drape, sutures, or staples applied to the skin or a sheet with a small fenestration and plastic inset. The patient's body is covered with a sheet; a split or U drape sheet.

Alternate Draping

Disposable drapes: towels are draped around the neck. A sterile, plastic adhesive drape, sutures, or staples secure the towels to the skin. The edge of an adhesive-backed drape sheet covers the top of the head and an adhesive-backed split or U drape sheet covers the body.

Equipment

Padded, foam, or gel headrest (e.g., donut or Richards), optional
Suction
ESU, monopolar and/or bipolar
Harmonic Scalpel system generator with foot pedal activation, optional
Fiber-optic headlight (may contain video camera) and fiber-optic light source (e.g., Xenon 300 W), optional, or fiber-optic operating microscope, e.g., Zeiss, available (when nerve graft is taken)
Video adaptor/attachment to the microscope, optional
Video monitor, optional
Camera console, optional
VCR, optional
CD burner, optional
Printer, optional
Nerve stimulator/locator unit (e.g., Concept™)

Instrumentation

Basic plastic procedures tray
Extra mosquito clamps, lacrimal duct probes (available for submaxillary duct exploration)

Bipolar electrosurgical scissors and cord
Harmonic Scalpel handpiece, scissors, and cord, optional

Supplies

Antiembolitic hose
Sterile, plastic adhesive drape, optional
Indelible marking pen, optional
Magnetic instrument pad, optional
Basin set
Blades, (1) #10, (2) #15
Needle magnet or counter
Suction tubing
Electrosurgical pencil and cord, holder, scraper, and needle tip (available)
Dissectors (e.g., peanuts or Kittners)
Umbilical tape, vessel loops (for nerve traction/protection), optional
Sterile wires (2) with needle electrodes (attach to the Concept unit)
Bulb syringe and antibiotic irrigation for inflammatory disease, optional
Closed suction drain, e.g., Hemovac™

Special Notes

- Apply **Special Notes** from ***Abdominal Laparotomy,*** p. 134, as applicable.
- The circulator checks with the surgeon regarding the area to be prepped and the choice of prep solution, as a nerve graft may be necessitated during the procedure.
- When a nerve graft is harvested during the procedure, the surgeon may request a headlight or microscope, according to preference.
- When a nerve stimulator/locator is employed (e.g., Concept), the screen should face the anesthesia provider.
- When intracapsular dissection of the submandibular gland is performed, bipolar electrosurgical scissors may be employed to reduce blood loss during dissection.
- The circulator arranges for the operating microscope to be available for possible nerve grafting prior to bringing the patient into the room.
- For partial intracapsular dissection of the submandibular gland, the ***Harmonic Scalpel*** (high-frequency vibration, e.g., ultrasound power) may be used to simultaneously cut precisely and coagulate tissue with minimal thermal damage and reduced blood loss.

- In the PACU, the perioperative practitioner observes the patient for airway obstruction. He/she elevates the head of the gurney to reduce postoperative swelling (leads to obstructed airway). All nursing interventions are documented in the **Postoperative Record** section of the **Perioperative Record**.
- The PACU perioperative practitioner reviews written patient discharge instructions with the patient and/or parent(s) or legal guardian (nursing care intervention). He/she answers the patient's [or parent(s) or legal guardian's] questions, if any, and documents his/her perception of the patient's or parent's understanding (outcome of the teaching session). This is documented in the **Postoperative Record** section of the **Perioperative Record**.

Parotidectomy

Definition

Partial or total excision of the parotid gland.

Discussion

Parotidectomy is performed to treat inflammatory disease and benign and malignant tumors of the parotid, a major salivary gland. Diagnosis may be made with *fine-needle aspiration, ultrasonography, CT scan, magnetic resonance imaging (MRI), sialogram, or radionuclide imaging.* Inflammatory disease receives conservative medical treatment, according to the underlying etiology; chronic inflammation may be treated surgically on an individual basis regarding frequency of occurrence and type of symptoms. Benign tumors may require superficial (partial) parotidectomy or complete excision of the gland. Surgery involves protection of the facial nerve, a major concern, when dividing the larger superficial portion from the deeper portion of the gland. **Parotidectomy** with complete excision is done for some types of benign disease or tumor and for malignant tumors, according to size and histology, and to minimize the possibility of tumor cell spillage and recurrence. Preoperatively, the surgeon discusses with the patient the possibility of sacrificing the facial nerve in direct tumor involvement, with immediate grafting; he/she also discusses possible need for ***cervical lymphadenectomy*** and ***mandibulectomy,*** p. 858. In malignant neoplasms when suspicious lymph nodes are encountered, a ***radical neck dissection*** (p. 857) and/or ***dissection of the skull base*** or mandible may be indicated in addition to parotidectomy.

Procedure

An incision is made in the preauricular region and continued inferiorly around the earlobe, anteriorly to parallel the angle of the jaw. Sharp dissection is performed as the superficial parotid fascia is incised. The skin flap is sutured and retracted from the field. Careful exposure of the facial nerve is necessary, unless there is direct tumor involvement; a nerve stimulator is used to test and confirm the integrity of the facial nerve branches. When a major nerve branch courses through the tumor, it is sacrificed and a nerve graft substituted. The graft may be obtained from the great auricular nerve or superficial branches of the cervical plexus. The superficial portion of the gland may be resected after blunt and sharp dissection; removal of the deeper portion may be necessary, as mentioned above. The gland is exposed anteriorly along the anterior border of the sternocleidomastoid muscle, exposing the auricular nerve that carries sensation to the ear lobe; it is the best option for nerve grafting, if needed. The wound is closed in layers with a cosmetic closure.

Preparation of the Patient

Antiembolitic hose may be applied. General anesthesia via endotracheal intubation is employed. The table may be turned and a folded sheet may be placed under the shoulders to facilitate the surgeon's access. The patient is supine with the head turned to the side, on a padded, foam, or gel donut (or other head support) with the face and neck on the operative side uppermost. The dependent ear is well padded to prevent pressure injury. The arm on the operative side may be padded and tucked in at the patient's side, and the contralateral arm may be extended on a padded armboard. A pillow may be placed under the knees to prevent low back strain, or the table may be flexed for comfort. All bony prominences and areas vulnerable to skin and neurovascular pressure or trauma are padded. An electrosurgical dispersive pad is applied.

Skin Preparation

Check with the surgeon regarding choice of prep solution. The inside of the mouth is not usually prepped. Begin the prep on the affected cheek; extend the prep from the hairline to the axilla (include the entire side of the face well beyond the midline, including the ear). A lap sponge may be placed at the sides of the neck to prevent prep solution from pooling under the patient. A small cotton ball may be placed in the ear to prevent prep solution from pooling in the ear (it can be removed with a mosquito forceps before draping). The prepped area may be blotted dry; care is taken not to contaminate the operative site. Prep solution is not permitted to pool on the drapes, as it excoriates the skin. In addition, pooled prep solutions are a fire hazard and should be avoided.

Care is taken to avoid getting prep solution in the eyes; antibiotic ointment may be placed in the conjunctival sac.

Draping

The patient may be draped with a drape sheet and two towels under the head with the uppermost towel wrapped around the head and clipped; this head drape may not be used. The neck is draped with folded towels secured with a sterile, plastic adhesive drape or sutured or stapled to the skin. The operative field is covered with a sheet, with a small fenestration and plastic inset; the body is covered with a U or split drape sheet.

Alternate Draping

The patient may be draped with disposable drapes. An adhesive-backed sheet is placed across the forehead, and towels are draped around the head and neck. A plastic adhesive drape may be used. The body is covered with an adhesive-backed split or U drape sheet (draped around the neck to secure the perimeter of the operative area).

Equipment

Padded, foam, or gel headrest, e.g., donut or Richards, optional
Suction
ESU, monopolar
Nerve stimulator/locator (e.g., Concept)
Fiber-optic headlight (may contain video camera) and fiber-optic light source (e.g., Xenon 300 W), optional
Operating fiber-optic microscope, e.g., Zeiss, available (when nerve graft is done)
Video adaptor/attachment to the microscope, optional
Video monitor, optional
Camera console, optional
VCR, optional
CD burner, optional
Printer, optional

Instrumentation

Basic/Minor procedures tray
Thyroid tray
Tracheostomy tray (available)
Right-angle clamps, finely pointed (4), small Yankauer suction, nerve hook, and skin hooks (2)
Sterile wires (2) with needle electrodes (attach to the Concept unit)

Supplies

Antiembolitic hose, optional
Sterile, plastic adhesive drape, optional
Indelible marking pen
Magnetic instrument pad, optional

Basin set
Blades, (1) #10, (3) #15
Suction tubing
Electrosurgical pencil and cord, holder, scraper, and needle tip (available)
Dissectors (e.g., peanuts or kittners)
Umbilical tape, vessel loops (for nerve traction/protection), optional
Bulb syringe with saline (or antibiotic irrigation for inflammatory disease)

Special Notes

- Apply **Special Notes** from Excision of ***Submandibular Gland***, p. 849, as applicable.
- **Reminder:** The circulator checks with the surgeon regarding the area to be prepped, as a nerve graft may be chosen from an additional site. The area from which the nerve graft is taken must be prepped; whenever possible, the nerve graft site is prepped at the same time.
- Nerve grafting usually requires a microscope, instead of a headlight, according to the surgeon's preference.
- When the nerve stimulator/locator (Concept) is used, it may first be tested on local skeletal muscle prior to the procedure. The most frequently used setting is 0.5 mA. The unit is turned to face the anesthesia provider.
- The circulator needs to have the operating fiber-optic microscope available for possible nerve grafting. In the PACU, the perioperative practitioner observes the patient for airway obstruction and elevates the head of the gurney to reduce postoperative swelling. Nursing interventions are documented in the postoperative section of the **Perioperative Record**.
- The PACU perioperative practitioner reviews written patient discharge instructions with the patient (and/or parent(s) or legal guardian). His/her perception of patient's understanding (outcome) is documented in the postoperative section of the **Perioperative Record**.

Laryngectomy

Definition

Partial or total removal of the larynx.

Discussion

Laryngectomy is performed for malignancy. Numerous presentations may occur, from small unilateral lesions to those that are extensive and widely invading with cervical lymph node metastasis. Associated with these cancers are those of the hypopharynx and pyriform sinus. Treatment modalities include laser treatments (primarily used for limited lesions), radiation, surgery, laser surgery, and palliative measures and chemotherapy in advanced stages of malignant lesions. **Hemilaryngectomy, partial** or **total laryngectomy**, local lesion excision, or adjunctive **radical neck dissection** will be determined by the clinical extent of the malignancy and the patient's general status. The thyroid gland (or a portion) may be excised, when involved. When less than total laryngectomy (e.g., partial laryngectomy, all or part of one vocal cord, or just the epiglottis) is required, normal or modified speech can be preserved and a laryngeal stoma is temporary.

Cancers of the larynx are classified according to anatomic position:

- **Supraglottic:** From the epiglottis to and including the false cords
- **Glottic:** Floor of the ventricle to below the glottis including the true cords
- **Infraglottic:** From below the true vocal cords to the cricoid cartilage
- **Transglottic:** Lesions that extend from above the ventricle to true and false cords and subglottically.

For more extensive lesions involving both true and false cords, transglottic lesions, or when laryngeal cartilages are involved, **total laryngectomy** is done.

Postoperative complications include hemorrhage, airway obstruction, infection, and nerve damage.

At the time of laryngectomy or subsequently, the patient undergoes swallowing function rehabilitation and speech therapy. Modalities by which the patient can speak include esophageal speech ("belching" of ingested air), placement of an implanted prosthesis, or use of an external instrument (e.g., **electrolarynx). Tracheoesophageal puncture** is required for modified esophageal speech; a one-way shunt valve is placed between the trachea and esophagus (e.g., *Blom-Singer prosthesis*). The electrolarynx (Ultravoice, Optivox, or Servox Inton, etc.), a handheld battery-powered instrument, is another option for speech; it is placed at the corner of the mouth or below the mandible to produce a humming noise that, with training, can produce intelligible speech.

Procedure

Total laryngectomy is described. A curvilinear incision is made above the suprasternal notch. The strap muscles are divided, as is the isthmus of the thyroid gland. The trachea may be divided between rings 2 and 3, and the endotracheal tube is replaced or repositioned in the distal trachea. Packing is placed in the infraglottic area to prevent secretions from filling the wound or entering the airway. Some surgeons perform tracheostomy prior to making the operative incision (and inferior to same so that the tracheostoma presents via a separate wound). Skin flaps are elevated. The larynx is sutured closed inferiorly. The superior cornua of the thyroid cartilage and hyoid bone are freed from strap and supraglottic muscles (which may also be excised). The superior laryngeal vessels and nerves are ligated and divided. A portion of the thyroid may be excised in continuity, or the gland separated from the larynx. The inferior constrictor muscles are divided posterolaterally and separated from the thyroid cartilage. The hyoid bone and cricoid cartilage are included in the specimen. Dissection continues to the base of the tongue with separation of the esophagus employing traction on the epiglottis and the severed end of the trachea, completing the dissection. The pharynx and any esophageal defect are closed. A nasogastric tube is placed. The strap muscles are approximated to the inferior constrictor muscle (to obliterate "dead space" created by the resected structures). The tracheostomy stoma is matured to the surrounding skin. A tracheostomy tube (e.g., Hi-Lo) is inserted in the tracheal stoma until the edema subsides (about 48 hours). The wound flaps are approximated over a closed suction catheter. A moderate pressure dressing is placed.

Preparation of the Patient

Antiembolitic hose are applied. The surgeon may request a sequential compression device with disposable leg wraps; they can be applied over the antiembolitic hose, or the wraps may be used alone. General anesthesia is employed via endotracheal intubation. The patient is supine with arms extended on padded armboards, or arms may be tucked in at the patient's sides. A folded sheet may be placed under the shoulders to facilitate exposure. A pillow may be placed under the knees to prevent lower back strain, or the table may be flexed for comfort. All bony prominences and areas vulnerable to skin and neurovascular pressure or trauma are padded. An electrosurgical dispersive pad is applied.

Skin Preparation

Begin at the anterior neck; extend the prep from the inferior auricular border and the lower lip to the level of the axilla and down to the table at the sides of the neck and around the shoulders. Lap sponges, placed at the side of the sides of the neck, prevent the prep solution from pooling under the patient. Prep solutions are not permitted to pool on the drapes, as they excoriate the skin. In addition, pooled prep solutions are a fire hazard and should be avoided.

Draping

Folded towels and sheet with a small fenestration with clear plastic adhesive insert (or a sterile, plastic adhesive drape and a sheet with a small fenestration, e.g., thyroid sheet) and individual drape sheets complete the draping. A sterile sponge may be placed on either side of the neck to prevent blood from pooling under the neck.

Equipment

Padded, foam, or gel headrest, e.g., donut
Folded sheet, roll, or small sandbag for extending the neck
Sequential compression device with disposable leg wraps, e.g., Jobst athrombic pump, optional
Forced-air warming blanket, hyperthermia mattress, e.g., K-Thermia pad, optional
Suction
ESU, monopolar
Fiber-optic headlight (on a headband, may have loupes attached and may contain camera), optional
Fiber-optic light source, e.g., Xenon 300 W
Monitor, VCR, printer, and CD burner, optional
Camera console, optional

Instrumentation

Basic/Minor procedures
Thyroid tray
Tracheostomy tray (available)
Right-angle clamps (finely pointed), small Yankauer suction

Supplies

Antiembolitic hose
Sterile plastic adhesive drape, optional
Marking pen with indelible ink
Magnetic instrument pad, optional
Basin set
Blades, (2) #10, (3) #15
Needle magnet or counter
ESU with needle tip, cord, holder, and scraper
Suction tubing
Dissectors (e.g., peanut, Kittners)
Umbilical tape
Open-ended catheters, flexible (2) for suctioning tracheostomy tube
Tracheostomy tubes, Hi-Lo (assorted sizes)
Closed suction drain, e.g., Hemovac or Jackson-Pratt™

Special Notes

- Apply Special Notes from **Uvulopalatopharyngoplasty**, p. 839.
- The circulator may remind the patient of general postoperative information:
  - He/she will receive O_2 by mask, over the tracheal stoma, until the edema subsides
  - That the head of the bed will be elevated to reduce postoperative swelling
  - He/she needs to move his/her legs while in bed to encourage and increase circulation
  - **N.B.** Call button and a message board, such as Magic Slate, will be provided in the PACU and on the nursing unit
  - The first feeding is by IV or feeding tube, progressing to soft foods
  - He/she reminds the patient not to move or lift heavy items.
- The circulator checks that a message board is available for postoperative communication and orders the board, if necessary. He/she assures the patient regarding call button and message board postoperatively. This is documented in the **Perioperative Record**.
- In the PACU, the perioperative practitioner elevates the head of the patient's bed (high Fowler's position) to decrease postoperative swelling, attaches O_2 via oxygen mask over the tracheal stoma, secures call button near patient's hand, and ensures that a message board is nearby (nursing interventions).
- In the PACU, the perioperative practitioner reviews important postoperative information with the patient (when the patient is alert enough to comprehend) and caregivers, e.g., explains the method for suctioning, intermittent positive pressure breathing (IPPB) equipment, and when it is important to contact the surgeon.
- In the PACU, the perioperative practitioner provides measure for pain management, e.g., applies warm compresses to relieve pain. On the nursing unit, use of analgesics is encouraged (least-strong medications, as applicable), advises patient to avoid strain, and teaches and encourages self-care. Nursing interventions and their outcomes are documented in the **Perioperative Record.**

Radical Neck Dissection

Definition`

Excision of cervical lymph node-bearing tissue and the adjacent muscular and vascular structures.

Discussion

Radical Neck Dissection is performed for malignancies, e.g., metastatic squamous cell carcinoma in the head and neck region; it is usually done unilaterally. The dissection may be performed as an independent procedure or in conjunction with primary tumor resection of local structures whose lymphatics drain to the cervical lymph nodes, such as intraoral lesions, thyroid, larynx, and jaw. Radical neck dissection may necessitate ***mandibulectomy***. When combined with more extensive resections about the pharynx and larynx, a ***tracheostomy*** (p. 843) is performed as well. Radiation therapy may be recommended in conjunction with this procedure. Physical examination, x-ray scans [CT, MRI, ultrasound, positron emission tomography, (PET)], as well as the intraoperative findings aid in determining the extent of any metastases and lymph node involvement. The defect caused by this extensive procedure necessitates an immediate composite graft procedure, intensive critical care postoperatively, and considerable psychological support of the surgeon, nursing staff, and the patient's family.

In lesser presentations, **modified neck dissection** sparing the sternomastoid muscle, internal jugular vein, and spinal accessory nerve (in any combination) is done. When indicated, a bilateral procedure is performed with preservation of one internal jugular vein (unless grossly involved with tumor or is thrombosed or obliterated). Prior radiation therapy makes the dissection more difficult.

Procedure

Radical neck dissection is described. The operative area may be injected with local anesthetic with epinephrine for vasoconstriction. A ***tracheostomy or laryngostoma*** may have been established previously (or may be done in conjunction with the neck dissection and primary tumor resection, accordingly). An incision (Y, double Y, T, parallel-transverse, Z) is marked and made in the lateral neck usually from beneath the jaw to the supraclavicular region. Skin flaps (including the platysma) are mobilized. The external jugular vein is divided, the deep cervical fascia is incised (including some cutaneous nerve branches), and the sternoclavicular origins of the sternomastoid muscle are divided. The internal jugular vein is isolated and divided (protecting the carotid artery and vagus nerve). The omohyoid muscle is transected. Fatty tissues bearing lymph nodes are dissected from underlying structures in continuity with other transected structures. The operating microscope is used to view delicate structures, as necessary.

The insertion of the sternomastoid muscle is divided, as is the lower pole of the parotid gland, avoiding injury to branches of the facial nerve; the nervous structures are identified, stimulated, and monitored intermittently for patient safety and medicolegal reasons.

The facial artery and vein are divided; retracting the mylohyoid muscle, the marginal mandibular nerve is protected after incising the capsule of the submandibular gland. The submandibular gland is excised and proximal end of the internal jugular vein is divided, following dissection of additional fatty node bearing tissues from under the jaw. Segments of muscle may be excised, depending on local findings. In the posterior triangle, the phrenic nerve and brachial plexus are protected. The en bloc specimen is then removed; the surgeon indicates and marks by suture various aspects of the specimen to orient the pathologist. Frozen section is requested for the specimens; the pathologist informs the surgeon regarding adequate specimen margins. The accessory nerve may be preserved, and the thoracic duct (left side) is protected. The flaps are closed over closed-suction drains. Meticulous attention is paid to the approximation of the wound edges. Hemostasis is obtained. Irrigation is employed to remove clots and debris. The circulator checks the patient's chart for allergy or sensitivity to latex products before applying a moderate-pressure dressing, following the application of tincture of benzoin to protect the skin.

Preparation of the Patient

Antiembolitic hose are applied and a sequential compression device with disposable leg wraps is used, when ordered. A forced-air or warming blanket may be requested to maintain the patient's body temperature. General anesthesia via endotracheal intubation is employed (with subsequent replacement directly via the tracheostomy when performed, or initially, if a tracheostomy had already been established). The patient is supine; the head may be placed on a padded, foam, or gel donut or other head support with the face and neck turned to the side and the operative side uppermost. The dependent ear is well padded to prevent pressure injury. A folded sheet may be placed under the shoulders to facilitate access; the head of the table may be elevated 30°. The arm on the operative side may be padded and tucked in at the patient's side, and the contralateral arm may be extended on a padded armboard. A pillow may be placed under the knees to prevent low back strain, or the table may be flexed for comfort. All bony prominences and areas vulnerable to skin and neurovascular pressure or trauma are padded. A Foley catheter may be inserted. An electrosurgical dispersive pad is applied.

Skin Preparation

Check with the surgeon regarding choice of prep solution. Begin cleansing the neck and face; extend the prep from the hairline to the nipples and down to the table at the sides. A lap sponge may be placed at either side of the neck to prevent the prep solutions from pooling under the patient, as they excoriate the skin.

Care is taken to avoid getting prep solution in the eyes. Antibiotic ointment may be placed in the conjunctival sacs. Prep solutions are not permitted to pool on the drapes, as they are a fire hazard.

Draping

The patient may be draped with a head drape (drape sheet and two towels under the head with the uppermost towel wrapped around the head and clipped). The neck is draped with folded towels secured with a sterile, plastic adhesive drape or suture or they may be stapled to the skin. The patient is covered with a fenestrated sheet (e.g., laparotomy).

Alternate Draping

Disposable drapes: adhesive-backed sheet is placed across the forehead and towels are draped around the neck. An adhesive-backed split or U drape sheet is draped around the neck and covers the body.

Equipment

Sequential compression device with disposable leg wraps, e.g., Jobst athrombic pump, as requested
Forced-air blanket or hyperthermia mattress (e.g., Bair Hugger™ or K-Thermia pad, respectively), when ordered
Suction
ESU
Fiber-optic headlight (may contain camera) and fiber-optic light source (e.g., Xenon 300 W or fiber-optic operating microscope (e.g., Zeiss),
Power source for high-speed power micro drill and saw, if they are not self-contained units (battery), optional
Scales to weigh sponges (2)
Blood pump, blood administration set and blood warmer, additional IV stands to hang blood, optional
Nerve stimulator (locator), e.g., Concept
Video monitor, optional
Camera console, optional
VCR, optional
CD burner, optional
Printer, optional

Instrumentation

Basic/Minor procedures tray
Thyroidectomy tray
Tracheostomy, Vascular procedures, Basic/Minor orthopedic procedures, and Dental instruments trays (available in the room)
Additional mosquito clamps (e.g., 24), towel clips (e.g., 8), finely pointed right-angle clamps (4), Andrew's suction tip, and skin hooks, optional

High-speed power micro drill and cord with drill tips and burrs, power micro saw, optional
Sterile magnetic instrument pad, optional

Supplies

Antiembolitic hose
Foley catheter and urimeter/urometer
Indelible marking pen
Portex Flex tracheostomy disposable inner cannula (D.I.C.) tubes with Soft-Seal™ cuff, adult sizes #6 to #10, with snap in obturator, syringe, 10 ml (to inflate cuff), and velcro tracheostomy tube holder, optional

If Tracheostomy Is Performed

Local anesthetic with epinephrine, 5-ml control syringes, and needles, e.g., 27 gauge × 1½″, and spinal needle, e.g., 27 gauge × 3½″ and medicine cups and paper labels
Basin set
Suction tubing
Electrosurgical pencil and cord, holder, and scraper (with needle tip, available)
Blades, (2) #10, (3) #15
Needle magnet or counter
Graduate and bulb syringes (2)
Dissectors (e.g., peanuts or kittners)
Umbilical tapes, vessel loops
Sterile wires (2) with needle electrodes (attach to Concept)
Bone wax
Blood administration set, optional
Closed-suction drainage unit, e.g., Hemovac(s) or Jackson-Pratt

Special Notes

- Apply **Special Notes** from ***Abdominal Laparotomy***, p. 134, as indicated.
- **N.B.** The circulator may convey (even more than is usual) emotional support to the patient due to the serious nature of the surgery. Assess and document the patient's anxiety level and employ measures, such as maintaining eye contact, using touch to convey caring, holding the patient's hand during the administration of anesthesia, offering a warm blanket, etc.
- The circulator may provide the patient a measure of comfort to reduce anxiety by explaining that he/she will act as the patient's advocate. Documentation of nursing care interventions, pertinent observations, and patient outcome are

required for continuity of care for patient safety and for medicolegal reasons.

- **N.B.** Before surgery begins, the circulator ascertains that there are two ***working*** suctions in the room (in addition to the suction used by anesthesia provider).
- **Reminder:** A protective face shield is suggested for those scrubbed to avoid inadvertent splashing of contaminated fluids onto mucous membranes and eyes.
- **N.B.** *Before surgery begins, the cardiac-arrest cart should be brought immediately outside or nearby the room for use in an emergency.*
- If tracheostomy is done, the skin and underlying tissues may be injected with a vasoconstricting agent (as epinephrine) in conjunction with a local anesthetic, even though general anesthesia is employed; *advise anesthesia provider accordingly* when used.
- **N.B.** Before the scrub person passes the tracheostomy tube (with cuff) to the surgeon, the cuff must be tested for leaks.
- **N.B.** *Tape the tracheostomy tube obturator to the top of the gurney when patient is transferred to the PACU; it will be needed to reinsert the tube if the tube should become dislodged. The circulator documents that this has been done in the Perioperative Record and specifically reports that the obturator is taped to the top of the gurney upon arrival in the PACU.*
- *Circulator verifies with the blood bank that blood is available as ordered and ready for immediate use* ***before*** *the surgery is permitted to begin.*
- The circulator must anticipate possible blood transfusion(s); transfusion is not routinely administered. He/she and the anesthesia provider verify the patient's identity and compare the blood type and identification number on the unit and with the patient's blood type, etc. The circulator obtains equipment to administer the blood (e.g., tubing set, blood warmer, pressure bag) and assists the anesthesia provider in its administration.
- **N.B.** *Circulator documents blood transfusions (when administered) and any reaction or lack of reaction to the transfusions.*
- **N.B.** A nerve stimulator/locator (e.g., Concept) may be employed to locate and/or stimulate a nerve (e.g., facial) to determine viability or injury. The unit is positioned to face the anesthesia provider.
- The scrub person keeps track of the amount of irrigation used; the circulator records accurately the amount of irrigation used.

- The circulator weighs sponges to assist in determining accurate assessment of blood loss for replacement.
- To weigh sponges, two scales are used, one for raytec sponges and one for lap pads. To weigh sponges, calculate the weight of the dry sponge and set the scale to 0 after weight adjustment.
- The scrub person may use a sterile magnetic instrument pad to prevent instruments from sliding off the operative field.
- **N.B.** The scrub person must pay particular attention to account for the instruments from the numerous trays to achieve a correct instrument count.
- **N.B. Reminder:** Umbilical tapes and dissector sponges (e.g., peanuts, Kittner) are included in the sponge count.
- The circulator notes on the laboratory requisition that the specimen is oriented and labeled accordingly, and/or the pathologist may be called to consult with the surgeon in the OR.
- **Reminder:** The circulator and anesthesia provider accompany the patient to the PACU; he/she gives the perioperative practitioner a detailed report regarding the course of intraoperative events for continuity of care and the patient's safety
- The circulator employs measures to maintain patient's temperature (e.g., normothermia) en route from the OR to the PACU.
- Upon patient's arrival in the PACU and at intervals, the perioperative practitioner monitors the patient's vital signs. He/she continuously assesses the patient's pain level, level of consciousness, and respiratory status. Patient data is documented in the **Postoperative Record** portion of the **Perioperative Record.**
- In the PACU, the perioperative practitioner observes the amount of blood on the dressing pad. Excessive bleeding (e.g., if dressing becomes saturated within a relatively short period of time) is reported to the surgeon immediately; a description of the amount of blood on the dressing is documented in the **Postoperative Record** portion of the **Perioperative Record.**

Excision of Lesions of the Oral Cavity (Partial Glossectomy with Marginal Resection of the Mandible)

Definition

Excision of intraoral malignant lesions, including portions of the tongue and mandible, and the lymphoid-bearing tissues of the ipsilateral neck.

Discussion

Malignancy of the tongue, the most frequently encountered cancer of the oral cavity, represents one of the greatest management challenges for the head and neck oncologist because of the adverse effects of treatment on oral and pharyngeal function, the eventual quality of life, and the poor prognosis of advanced disease. The unique behavior of these tumors also requires aggressive management to minimize the risk of locoregional spread. Oral cavity malignancies are aggressive and spread rapidly. Leukoplakia, human papillomavirus, squamous cell cancer and other malignant tumors of the tongue, and the many oral cavity cancers, etc., require extensive tissue excision. Tumor cells in lymph channels (that drain the tongue and floor of the mouth into the cervical glands) may be carried directly into the periosteum and cortex of the mandible. Excision of the lesions involves excising lymphoid-bearing tissues as well as a portion of the mandible. Depending on the size, stage, extent, and cell type of the tumor, multiple permutations of the definitive procedure are performed. The procedure may include local tumor excision, excision of the mandible or maxilla or portions of same, if any, and variations of neck dissection, depending on the findings. When the procedure is performed for advanced presentations, e.g., large fungating, painful, noncurative tumors, alleviation of local symptoms, accordingly, is appropriate.

Extensive oral and pharyngeal surgery adversely affects the patient's quality of life. In addition, prognosis most often is poor. In potentially curative procedures (i.e., if the tumor occupies a well-defined, limited, and circumscribed area), the extent of the procedure supersedes the considerations of reconstruction. If inadequate tissue remains for closure, split-thickness skin grafts are applied, or a flap may be transposed (e.g., from the forehead, deltopectoral area, rectus abdominis muscle, radial forearm, or temporalis muscle), which, in addition to wound coverage, allows some degree of mobility for the remaining tongue and cheek. Microvascular anastomosis of flaps of bone, periosteum, muscle, and skin (usually from the iliac region) may be utilized. In absence of mandibular periosteal involvement of tumor, excision of the mandible may be omitted or the outer cortex retained. The mandible may be transected to provide exposure (even without excision) and later repaired with stainless steel wire. Grafts of fibula or iliac crest or cancellous bone chips (contained in a vitalium or titanium tray) may be employed to reconstruct the mandible. Definitive reconstruction of soft tissues and bone is performed primarily, or as a secondary (delayed) procedure. If bilateral neck dissection is indicated, the contralateral side is done a few weeks after the initial procedure. Postoperatively radiation therapy and/or chemotherapy may be administered.

Procedure

A ***tracheostomy*** (p. 843) may be performed under local anesthesia or following induction of general anesthesia. A radical neck dissection (p. 857) is done in conjunction with the oral cavity tumor excision. The lower lip is transected in the midline. The submental region is dissected, excising adipose tissue and lymph nodes. The outer cortex of the mandible is exposed and transected, and if it is to be excised (with a Gigli saw or high-speed power micro saw), the condylar portion is retained, when possible. Alternatively, employing a power saw, the inner cortex of the mandible, including the alveolar ridge, is separated from the outer cortex, preserving the latter. The tongue is split in the midline to the posterior third and a cheek flap is mobilized behind the last molar. Excised soft tissue should include 5- to 10-mm margins when other oral lesions are treated. The intrinsic muscles of the tongue and muscles attached to the hyoid bone are further transected in continuity with the remainder of the specimen. The anterior and posterior bellies of the digastric muscle, submaxillary gland, and hypoglossal and lingual nerves are included in the specimen.

Reconstruction is begun with a short Kirschner wire centrally placed. The remaining mandible is stabilized with additional stainless steel wires that are passed through drill holes and tightened. Various grafting techniques (as noted in the discussion above) may be employed. Soft tissues are approximated from the tongue to tissue above the hyoid bone and platysma, tying the sutures over the mandible. Additional tissue coverage may be obtained from mobilization of the forehead or a deltopectoral flap. The remaining portion of the exposed mandible can be covered by tissues of the floor of the mouth and by skin. The mucosal sutures complete the repair of the floor of the mouth. The lip must be repaired in layers, snugly, to prevent excessive drooling. The neck incisions are closed over suction drains. A nasogastric tube may be placed for postoperative feeding.

An alternate treatment dependent on findings is to combine glossectomy with ***brachytherapy***, p. 403. Following excision of the lesion with adequate margins, brachytherapy needles are placed. Approximately 2 days later, radioactive seeds are placed for up to 72 hours.

Preparation of the Patient

Antiembolitic hose and disposable leg wraps (applied over the hose) are connected to a sequential compression device (e.g., Jobst athrombic pump), when ordered. A forced-air warming blanket or hyperthermia mattress, e.g., Bair Hugger and K-Thermia pad, respectively, may be requested to maintain the patient's body temperature at normothermia. General anesthesia with endotracheal intubation is employed (noting the endotracheal tube will be replaced with a tracheostomy tube or anesthesia is administered via a pre-established tracheostomy). The patient is supine; the head may be placed on a padded, foam, or gel donut with the face and neck on the operative side uppermost, turned to the side. The dependent ear is well padded to prevent pressure injury. A folded sheet may be placed under the shoulders to facilitate access; the head of the table may be elevated 30°. Usually both arms are padded and tucked in at the patient's sides. A pillow may be placed under the knees to avoid straining back muscles, or the table may be flexed for comfort. All bony prominences and areas vulnerable to skin and neurovascular trauma or pressure are padded. A Foley catheter is inserted. An electrosurgical dispersive pad is applied.

Skin Preparation

Check with the surgeon regarding Foley catheter insertion, choice of prep solution, and the extent of the area to be prepped, particularly regarding the mouth. The Foley catheter is inserted, when necessary.

Prep the entire face and neck; extend prep from the hairline to nipples and down to the table at the sides around the neck and shoulders. A lap sponge may be placed at the sides of the neck to prevent prep solution from pooling under the patient. The inside of the mouth may be painted with swabs. The prepped area may be blotted dry; care is taken not to contaminate the operative site. Prep solution is not permitted to pool on the drapes, as it excoriates the skin. In addition, pooled prep solutions are a fire hazard and should be avoided.

Care is taken to avoid getting prep solution in the eyes; antibiotic ointment may be placed in the conjunctival sac for protection.

Draping

The patient may be draped with a head drape (drape sheet and two towels under the head with uppermost towel wrapped around the head and clipped). The neck is draped with folded towels that are secured by staples or sutures and/or a sterile, plastic adhesive drape. The patient's body is covered with a fenestrated sheet.

Alternate Draping

Disposable drapes: adhesive-backed sheet is placed across the forehead, and towels are draped around the neck. An adhesive-backed split or U drape sheet is draped around the neck and covers the body.

Equipment

Sequential compression device with disposable leg wraps, as requested
Forced-air warming blanket, when ordered
Headrest (e.g., padded, foam, or gel donut) and padding for dependent ear

Fiber-optic headlight (may contain camera) and fiber-optic light source (e.g., Xenon 300 W) or fiber-optic microscope, optional
Suctions (2), in addition to one for the anesthesia provider
Power sources for high-speed power micro drill and high-speed power micro saw, optional
Scales to weigh sponges (2)
Blood pump and blood warmer, additional IV stands
Video monitor, optional
Camera console, optional
VCR, optional
CD burner, optional
Printer, optional

Instrumentation

Tracheostomy tray
Basic/Minor procedures tray
Thyroid tray
Minor orthopedic procedures (wire cutter included on tray)
Vascular procedures, Tonsillectomy and Adenoidectomy (T & A), and Dental Instruments Trays (available, but not opened, until need determined)
Gigli saw with handles (2), nerve hook, Andrew's suction tip, and Kirschner wires
Additional finely pointed right-angle clamps (2) and tonsil clamps (4)
High-speed power micro drill and cord with drill tips and burrs, power micro saw and blades, optional
Sterile magnetic instrument pad, optional
Vitalium or titanium tray for containing bone fragments, if bone graft required, optional

Apply **Supplies** and **Special Notes** from ***Radical Neck Dissection***, p. 857, as applicable.

Add to Supplies
Stainless steel wire

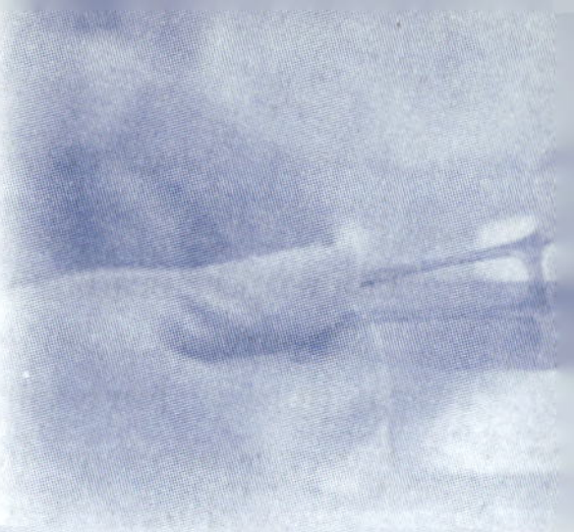

CHAPTER 28
Ophthalmic Surgery

General Information

Numerous conditions and diseases affect the eyes. The ophthalmologist takes a health history and performs a physical examination, followed by an in-depth optical examination of both eyes. The data that are gathered may provide the surgeon with valuable information for diagnosis that will help to determine needed medical and/or surgical treatment, as a wide variety of systemic diseases have ophthalmologic manifestations. The physical exam must be thorough enough to provide personal patient data to facilitate perioperative patient care in case of emergency.

The perioperative practitioner gathers pertinent information from the patient's history and physical and ocular examinations, in addition to the results of laboratory and x-ray studies, as applicable, to formulate a *nursing assessment* of the patient. The suggested **Surgical Assessment and Perioperative Checklist** and the **Patient Care Plan,** p. 9, are used to plan the best nursing care for the individual patient perioperatively. These documents may be further utilized to create a discharge plan, including home care management best suited to meet the needs of the individual patient. In the operating room (OR), the circulator, a perioperative practitioner, begins by determining the patient's understanding of his/her eye condition and the proposed surgical procedure. Patient education is of prime importance regarding optimal patient outcomes, particularly for the ophthalmic surgical patient.

Additional considerations for the plan of care for the ophthalmic patient in the OR and afterward include the following:

- Description of the general appearance of the globe(s) and eyelids, including mobility, amount of irritation, and the presence of drainage or discharge, if any
- Level of pain prior to and following the ophthalmic surgery
- Ability to see prior to and following the ophthalmic surgery
- Ability to care for himself/herself postoperatively, with particular consideration to physical limitations and age-limiting factors.

Risk factors must be addressed in the plan of care, as well as the expected and/or desired patient outcomes identified for the individual patient. Perioperative care of the patient anticipating ophthalmic surgery requires the circulator to employ the *universal protocol* (as in other surgeries) suggested by the Joint Commission (JC) (formerly the Joint Commission on Accreditation of Healthcare Organizations) to identify the patient, the type of procedure, and the site and/or side for the surgery. All other measures to ensure patient safety, such as "*time-out*," p. 18, must also be included.

Perioperative Considerations

Ophthalmic surgery requires close attention to detail; a minor breach in aseptic technique could lead to partial or complete loss of vision. Preparation and protection of the operative site, maintenance of aseptic technique throughout the surgical procedure, and prevention of infection are of paramount importance. In order to avoid undue repetition, the following information will apply to all ophthalmic surgical procedures in this section, unless otherwise stated.

Anesthesia

The anesthetic employed for ophthalmic surgery may require **akinesia** (immobility of the globe and lids), anesthesia of the globe and adnexa, control of intraocular pressure (IOP), general relaxation of the patient, and prevention of retching, coughing, and blood pressure fluctuations, even after the procedure is completed. The choice of anesthetic depends on the nature of the procedure, the surgeon's (and patient's) preference, the patient's general health status, and the patient's level of anxiety.

Topical anesthesia is effected by the instillation of an agent (e.g., tetracaine 0.5%) into the conjunctival sac. This method may suffice for superficial procedures (e.g., excision of a pterygium) or may precede the administration of local anesthetic injection.

Infiltration anesthesia is the direct injection of an agent into the surgical site (as in surgery of the lids). For more involved procedures, a regional block of cranial nerve branches can be employed. For procedures requiring immobilization of the globe, a *retrobulbar block* and an O'Brien and/or Van Lint block (or their modifications) are performed to provide akinesia of the lids and extraocular muscles. In a *retrobulbar block,* the anesthetic agent is injected into the muscle cone (behind the globe) blocking cranial nerves III, IV, and VI to immobilize the extraocular muscles and to produce anesthesia of the conjunctiva, cornea, and uvea by blocking the ciliary nerve branches. The *O'Brien block* deposits the anesthetic about branches of the facial nerve (over the condyle of the mandible, inferior to the posterior zygomatic process) to paralyze the orbicularis oculi muscle. The *Van Lint block* similarly produces paralysis of the orbicularis muscle, anesthetizing facial nerve branches over the periosteum just lateral to the orbital rim. Combining these blocks ensures complete akinesia. Any of the aforementioned methods to effect conduction anesthesia may be preferred and/or combined with general anesthesia or heavy sedation.

Preparation of the Patient

The table may be turned 90° or the table may be reversed with the patient's head at the foot of the table to facilitate the surgeon's access to the patient. In addition, when the patient is a small child, the lower section of the table is removed. The patient is in supine position; a padded, foam, or gel donut headrest may be employed, with the head turned (affected side up). One arm may be extended on a padded armboard and the contralateral arm is padded and tucked in at the patient's side, or both arms may be padded and extended or secured at the patient's sides. A pillow may be placed under the knees to avoid straining low back muscles, or the table may be flexed for comfort. All bony prominences and areas vulnerable to skin and neurovascular pressure or trauma are padded to avoid injury.

Skin Preparation

Unilateral. Initially, eye drops containing a povidone-iodine-type solution may be instilled into the conjunctiva of the eye. The eyelid of the affected eye is cleansed with the antimicrobial solution of choice; include the lid margin eyelashes and eyebrows on the correct side of the face. Use applicator sticks when carefully cleansing the lid margins. Extend the prep from the hairline to the inferior border of the mandible and from the anterior auricular border to well beyond the midline. Irrigate the eye from the inner to outer canthus using a bulb syringe containing normal saline; an absorbent towel or pad may be applied to the side of the face to prevent the saline from pooling on the drapes.

Bilateral. Use similar technique and prep both eyes simultaneously. Extend the prep from the hairline to the inferior border of the mandible, working outward in concentric circles until the entire face is prepped. Use applicator sticks to carefully cleanse the lid margins. Irrigate the eyes from the inner to outer canthus using a bulb syringe containing normal saline; an absorbent towel or pad may be applied to either side of the face to prevent the saline from pooling on the drapes.

Do not allow preparation solution to pool in or around the eye(s). Prep solutions are not permitted to pool on the drapes or under the patient, as they excoriate the skin. In addition, pooling of certain prep solutions are a fire hazard and care should be taken to avoid this.

Draping

Disposable drapes are preferred by most ophthalmic surgeons to minimize the amount of lint on the surgical field.

Unilateral. The adhesive-backed strip of a drape sheet is placed on the forehead. A split sheet is then draped so that the operative eye and the surrounding area fits into the split (V) of the drape; the adhesive-backed tails of the split sheet are secured at the top of the head and the remainder of the split sheet is draped over the patient's body. A sterile, plastic adhesive drape is placed over the operative eye and the surrounding field.

Bilateral. The adhesive-backed strip of a drape sheet is placed on the forehead. A split sheet is then draped so that the bridge of the nose fits into the split (V) of the drape; the adhesive-backed tails of the split sheet are secured at the top of the head, and the remainder of the split sheet is draped over the patient's body. A sterile, plastic adhesive drape is placed over both eyes and the surrounding field.

Special Notes

- Apply **Special Notes** from ***Abdominal Laparotomy***, p. 134, as applicable. Especially important are implementation of the *universal protocol*, "*time-out*," and measures of comfort and safety; see suggested **Patient Care Plan** (p. 9) and consult the **Special Notes** listed following each ophthalmic surgery when adapting and implementing perioperative care for the individual patient.
- The circulator, must provide emotional support to assure the patient during the administration of anesthesia and throughout the procedure. Because many ophthalmic surgical procedures are often performed employing local anesthesia by infiltration or block, reassuring the patient is particularly important.
- **N.B.** Reaction to increased urinary bladder pressure can cause an increase in IOP; therefore, the circulator should offer use of a bedpan to the patient, as necessary, before transferring him/her to the operating room (OR) table. The offer may be especially necessary for geriatric patients taking diuretics. Increased IOP may jeopardize the surgical results, possibly causing a loss of vision.
- ***Note:*** *Eyelashes are not routinely clipped; when lashes are trimmed, it is done prior to the skin prep.* The scissors are coated with a thin layer of petrolatum so that the severed lashes adhere to the scissors, preventing them from falling into the eye.
- When eyes are irrigated, they are *always* irrigated from inner to outer canthus to avoid possible foreign body from entering or blocking the tear duct.
- Loupes or an operating microscope are necessary for most ophthalmic surgical procedures. The oculars (eyepieces) fit into the binoculars, and the two eyepieces provide the magnified stereoscopic view that is three-dimensional. The magnification usually requires a 12.5× eyepiece.

- The objective lens is attached to the telescope by screw thread. The distance between the objective lens and the operative field is the *focal length*. Ophthalmic procedures usually require a 175- or 200-mm objective lens.
- The microscopes most frequently used are illuminated by a fiber-optic light source that is transmitted (or directed) to the field by fiber-optic cable, providing *cold light*, as opposed to the incandescent bulb that generates heat.
- The degree of magnification can be changed using a control that can be operated by the surgeon using an integrated foot control (most often).
- When a portable floor-model microscope is used, it is brought over the patient on the side opposite the operative eye.
- The operating microscope is usually draped with a drape specifically made for the microscope; it is draped prior to draping the operative field.
- Disposable drapes and ("powderless") gloves are preferred to limit the amount of lint within the operative field and to minimize the possibility of "foreign" material in the wound. Precautions are taken to keep lint off the instruments and to limit the use of linen (e.g., towels, cloth drapes, etc.) on the surgical field.
- A sterile, plastic adhesive drape is usually placed over the eye and the immediate surrounding field to diminish or limit the amount of lint in the sterile field, particularly when cloth towels are used in draping.
- Patients may be transferred to and from the OR table using a "lift" sheet, or the pad of a mechanical lifting device (e.g., Hoyer) is placed on the table before the patient is positioned. The patient should move to the table himself/herself to avoid possible increase in IOP.
- A padded, gel, or foam headrest (e.g., donut) is used to stabilize the head; this helps to avoid movement intraoperatively and potentially prevents possible loss of vision.
- Hemodynamic factors must be assessed, e.g., keep patient's legs uncrossed. All measures necessary to assist venous return are observed, as obstruction of venous return may increase IOP.
- To help patients avoid the feeling of claustrophobia, drapes may be placed over a Mayo stand or clipped to intravenous (IV) standards (poles).
- Cotton-tipped applicator sticks may be used when some superficial eye procedures are performed; however, cellulose

sponges, e.g., Weck, are preferred for more involved eye procedures, such as ***correction of strabismus***, p. 894.

- **N.B.** The patient is often awake during the ophthalmic procedure. Talking and movement in the room must be kept to a minimum, as they could be distracting and/or interfere with the surgeon's concentration and performance. Excessive or loud talking could also cause the patient to move during the procedure, possibly causing a loss of vision.
- When the scrub person and the circulator are able to anticipate the surgeon's needs, conversation in the room can be limited, thus the surgical environment may seem more tranquil and secure to the patient.
- **N.B. Note:** *A corneal protector is used to protect the patient during most ophthalmic procedures while oxygen is being administered, as a flash burn could result in injury to the patient.*
- For procedures in which local anesthesia is used without the presence of an anesthesia provider, a perioperative RN, in addition to the circulator, must be present to monitor the patient and to administer *conscious sedation* at the direction of the surgeon; see monitoring responsibilities of the perioperative RN, p. 74.
- See safety precautions that must be used to identify, label, and dispense medications or solutions to avoid medication errors, p. 30. It is mandatory that all medications and solutions on the sterile field be labeled by name and strength. All medication bottles or containers ***must be retained*** in the room until the surgery is completed.
- Local anesthesia (infiltration or block) may be administered prior to the final skin preparation and draping.
- Hyaluronidase/ Wydase™ may be added to the local anesthetic solution to enhance its absorption and aid in the dispersion of the anesthetic agent.
- Bleeding intraoperatively may be controlled with cellulose sponges, extremely fine suture material, hemostatic/vasoconstricting agents (e.g., epinephrine), coagulating substances (e.g., thrombin), heat (e.g., bipolar wet-field coagulation), laser, and/or freezing (e.g., Frigitonics®).
- The scrub person as first assistant views the operative area through the assistant's ocular and may be required to irrigate the patient's eye frequently to keep the cornea moist and clear; the eye is irrigated from the inner to outer canthus.

- Caffeine intake should be limited or omitted by the surgeon and the first assistant to promote steady hand movements when the operating microscope is used.
- Extreme care is taken to examine, clean, and protect and prevent damage to the delicate microsurgical eye instruments; particular care is taken to guard the tips and cutting surfaces of sharp instruments.
- Ophthalmic drops are applied topically over the surface of the globe, as the eyelids are held open (without touching the mucous membrane). Ophthalmic ointment is instilled into the conjunctival sac.
- Irrigating solutions for ocular use should be administered through a micropore filter.
- Ophthalmic instruments are usually placed on the Mayo stand in the order of their use; this should be listed on the surgeon's preference card.
- Often a single-use wet-field bipolar ophthalmic diathermy, e.g., Solan® (Xomed), or a nondisposable Solan bipolar wet-field Hemostatic Coagulator provides hemostasis during intrascleral and intraocular procedures; the precisely controlled diathermy provides hemostasis with reduced peripheral tissue damage. No electrosurgical dispersive pad is necessary, as the unit is bipolar.
- **Reminder:** When the fiber-optic operating microscope (e.g., Zeiss) is used, the scrub person should guide instrumentation (e.g., the suction tip, alligator forceps, etc.) into the speculum as necessary to enable the surgeon to concentrate on his/her field of vision.
- **Reminder:** The scrub person must check the microscope lens prior to the surgery to ensure that it is lint free, unsoiled, and undamaged.
- **Reminder:** The microscope should not be moved or disturbed once the surgery has begun; it must not be leaned on or used as a footrest. Any movement could cause serious injury and result in the loss of vision.
- **Reminder:** *For procedures in which the laser is employed, all safety precautions must be observed; for safe usage, see p. 94.* The safety precautions are observed, as documented in the **Perioperative Record,** to avoid injury to patient and staff as well as to prevent fire.
- The microscope is wiped clean so that it is "dust-free" prior to use. Following surgery when the microscope has been used, it

is wiped clean, and a protective cover is placed over it (to prevent it from becoming dusty) before it is stored.

- All nursing care interventions are employed, safety measures are observed, and any procedures performed, etc., are documented in the **Perioperative Record** for patient safety regarding continuity of care and for medicolegal purposes.
- **Reminder:** In the postanesthesia care unit (PACU), the perioperative practitioner explains to patients not to get out of bed alone to avoid falls, to avoid bending over from the waist, and not to lift heavy objects, as these movements may result in increased IOP. IOP may jeopardize the surgical results.

Excision of Chalazion

Definition

Incision and curettage of a granulomatous swelling due to blocked meibomian gland(s).

Discussion

A **chalazion** can occur as a single, painful, slowly enlarging nodule, or there may be multiple nodules that occur on the eyelid margin, as the result of blocked meibomian gland(s) found between the tarsal plate and conjunctivae. The chalazion is usually sterile; it may subside spontaneously. Medical treatment includes warm compresses applied for 10 to 12 minutes a few times per day, the application of antibiotic eye drops or ophthalmic ointment (if infection is suspected), and the possible injection of a steroid to decrease swelling. When medical treatment is ineffective, surgical curettage and/or excision may be indicated. The approach can be conjunctival or transcutaneous. Recurrence is not uncommon.

Procedure

A conjunctival approach is employed for a chalazion pointing through the conjunctiva. The chalazion is centered in a chalazion clamp, and the lid is everted. Employing a vertical incision, the chalazion is incised at right angles to the lid margin. Contents of the meibomian gland are often evacuated with a curette; the cyst lining is also removed. Chalazion may occur in multiples; larger chalazia may require dissection. Injury to the lid margin is avoided. The clamp is slowly removed when hemostasis has been effected.

For the **transcutaneous approach,** the chalazion is centered in the chalazion clamp. An incision is made parallel to the lid. The orbicularis oculi muscle is incised, exposing the meibomian gland. The gland is incised and its contents thoroughly curetted. The wound is approximated. Antibiotic ophthalmic ointment may be instilled in the conjuctival sac, and an eye pad is applied.

Preparation of the Patient

The table may be turned 90° or the table may be reversed with the patient's head at the foot of the table to facilitate the surgeon's access. The patient is in supine position; a padded, foam, or gel headrest (e.g., donut) may be employed, with the head turned (affected side up). The arm on the affected side may be secured on a padded armboard and the contralateral arm may be padded and secured at the patient's side, or both arms may be padded and secured at the patient's sides. A pillow may be placed under the knees to avoid straining low back muscles, or the table may be flexed for comfort. All bony prominences and areas vulnerable to skin and neurovascular pressure or trauma are padded to avoid injury.

Local anesthesia is usually preferred (and most often employed). Topical anesthetic eye drops may be instilled. When an anesthesia provider is not in attendance, a perioperative RN, in addition to the circulator, is required to monitor the patient and to administer *conscious sedation,* as directed by the surgeon. For a description of the role of the RN monitoring the patient, see p. 74.

Equipment

Padded, foam, or gel headrest, e.g., donut
Magnifying loupes
Sitting stools

Instrumentation

Basic eye procedures tray
Eyelid and conjunctival procedures tray

Supplies

Topical anesthetic ophthalmic drops, e.g., tetracaine, optional
Sterile, plastic adhesive drape
Local anesthetic, e.g., lidocaine (Xylocaine) 0.5 to 2% with epinephrine, local syringes, needles, medicine cup, labels, and marking pen
Basin set
Cotton-tipped applicators or cellulose sponges
Balanced salt solution (BSS), tear substitute
Blade, (1) #15 or (1) #11
Wet-field bipolar ophthalmic diathermy (e.g., Solan), disposable
Antibiotic ophthalmic ointment, optional
Dressing, e.g., eye pad and shield

Special Notes

- Apply **Special Notes** from ***Abdominal Laparotomy,*** p. 134 as they apply to most surgical procedures. Also refer to ***Ophthalmic Surgery, Perioperative Considerations***, p. 869.

Canthotomy

Definition

Incision of the canthus.

Discussion

The procedure is indicated when there is an adhesion of the eyelids or when exposure to the globe is inadequate. **Canthotomy** may be performed prior to cataract extraction or in conjunction with other procedures. **Canthotomy** is also employed to relieve elevated intraorbital pressure following orbital trauma; incision of the lateral canthal tendon (*cantholysis*) is done.

Procedure

A straight mosquito hemostat is clamped over the outer canthus for at least 60 seconds to effect hemostasis. The skin and conjunctiva are incised. Antibiotic ophthalmic ointment may be instilled, and an eye patch is applied. For **cantholysis**, Stevens' scissors may be used.

For **Preparation of the Patient, Equipment, Instrumentation, Supplies,** and **Special Notes,** see ***Excision of Chalazion,*** pp. 876–877.

Tarsorrhaphy/Canthorrhaphy

Definition

Tarsorrhaphy is the approximation of the margins of the eyelids.

Canthorrhaphy is the approximation of the lid margins, with partial excision of the lateral or medial canthus.

Discussion

Tarsorrhaphy and **canthorrhaphy** are employed when there is a chronic corneal ulceration, when a prosthesis is not utilized following the removal of the globe, when the palpebral fissure is abnormally widened, as in facial nerve palsy (e.g., Bell's palsy or secondary to surgery or trauma), in ptosis secondary to Horner's syndrome when the lids cannot adequately protect the cornea and prevent undue drying of the conjunctival membranes, or with a retrobulbar hematoma due to acute orbital trauma. **Tar-**

sorrhaphy is indicated when the condition is either temporary or permanent and can be reversed with a minimal procedure. Permanent reduction of the palpebral fissure is achieved by lateral (and less often medial) **canthorrhaphy**. Numerous modifications and alternative procedures have been described, including ***tarsoconjunctival flap rotation*** from the upper lid to the lower lid and the implantation of a gold weight beneath the orbicularis oculi muscle, use of spring wire implants, etc.

Procedure

Tarsorrhaphy is described. Topical anesthetic drops are instilled in the conjunctival sac and the lids are infiltrated with a local anesthetic. The lids are grasped and manipulated to determine the extent of closure necessary. The lateral (or medial) lid margins are approximated by placement of mattress sutures passed through the lid margins, avoiding the eyelash-bearing surfaces. If any tension is created, the sutures are tied over silicone pegs (or other stent material). For a more permanent union, a section of conjunctiva is excised prior to suture placement. For reversal (if the underlying condition necessitating the procedure is corrected or resolved), the **tarsorrhaphy** is incised and the wound surfaces are sutured to prevent readhesion.

Canthorrhaphy is described. After anesthesia is instituted, the extent of the **canthorrhaphy** is determined (and marked). The lid margin is split to the canthal angle, and a segment is excised including the lash follicles; the adjacent mucosa is abraded. Sutures approximate the lid margins and are tied over stents (e.g., silicone pegs). When performed medially, the caruncle canaliculi are preserved. If further support is required, the canthal tendon (palpebral ligament) is shortened and/or sutured to adjacent orbital periosteum.

For **Preparation of the Patient, Equipment, Instrumentation, Supplies,** and **Special Notes,** see *Excision of Chalazion*, pp. 876–877.

Add to Supplies
Silicone pegs or other stent material, optional

Ectropion Repair

Definition

Correction of abnormal eversion of the eyelid margin away from the globe.

Discussion

Ectropion usually involves the lower lid and usually occurs concurrently with horizontal lid laxity. In the most common type of **ectropion,** involution occurs as the result of aging; there is relaxation of the orbicular muscle. The lack of normal lid globe opposition results in corneal exposure, tearing, and keratinization of the palpebral conjunctiva. A loss of vision may result. Ectropion may be *congenital* or *acquired* and usually occurs bilaterally. Types of acquired ectropion include involutional, paralytic, cicatricial (as the result of scarring due to trauma), and mechanical (e.g., tumors of the lid).

Congenital ectropion is the result of an elongation of the lower lid, associated with Down's syndrome, orbital cysts, blepharophimosis syndrome, micropthalmos, buphthalmos, and ichthyosis (collodion baby). Occasionally, congenital ectropion is due to paralysis.

Acquired (or paralytic) ectropion is caused by cranial nerve VII paralysis; the orbicularis oculi has lost its tone, as associated with Bell's palsy, cerebellopontine tumors, herpes zoster oticus, and parotid gland lesions.

The correction employed depends on the type and severity of the deformity. Medical treatment includes various methods of lubrication; in patients with seventh nerve paralysis, weights matched to the patient's skin color may be used. The use of steroids is controversial; however, acyclovir in conjunction with prednisone taken by mouth has benefited some patient's with Bell's palsy. Surgical treatment depends on the etiology.

Various presentations may require a **lateral tarsal strip** to correct horizontal laxity or a **z-plasty or v-y plasty repair** (p. 690) with bolsters (to prevent hematoma formation), and a superior traction suture may be performed. In patients with extreme paralytic ectropion, a fascia lata or Gortex™ sling may be employed. Gold weights (spring wire) may be implanted in patients with *lagophthalmos*; in time, the implant is often extruded.

Procedure

The Kuhnt-Szymanowski (Modification of Byron Smith) is described. A skin incision is made below the lower lid margin, extending from the punctum to just beyond the lateral canthus. A lacrimal duct probe may be utilized to delineate the local anatomy. A second incision (an extension of the first) is made in the direction of the earlobe. A skin-muscle flap is developed and elevated across the lower lid; Wescott scissors are usually employed. A vertical incision is made through the tarsus (in the lateral third of the eyelid) and angled into the inferior cul-de-sac ("lazy T" procedure). The two free edges of the lid are overlapped until tight, and the redundant portion is excised. The two lid edges are approximated. The orbicularis oculi muscle is approximated. The skin is pulled laterally; redundant skin is resected. The skin is approximated. In younger patients, if the punctum is still everted, a tarsal-conjunctival resection may be necessary. Antibiotic ophthalmic ointment may be instilled and an eye pad placed.

Preparation of the Patient

The table may be turned 90° to facilitate the surgeon's access. The patient is in supine position; a padded or gel donut headrest may be employed, with the head turned (affected side up). The arm on the affected side is padded and secured in at the patient's side and the contralateral arm may be secured on a padded armboard, or both arms may be padded and secured at the patient's sides. A pillow may be placed under the knees to avoid straining low back muscles, or the table may be flexed for comfort. All bony prominences and areas vulnerable to skin and neurovascular pressure or trauma are padded to avoid injury.

The procedure is usually performed bilaterally, employing topical anesthesia with tetracaine ophthalmic drops and a supplemental infraorbital block and subconjunctival injections of lidocaine/xylocaine 0.5 to 2% with epinephrine.

For **Skin Preparation, Draping, Equipment, Instrumentation, Supplies,** and **Special Notes,** see *Excision of Chalazion,* pp. 876–877.

Add to Draping
Microscope drape

Add to Equipment
Operating fiber-optic microscope, e.g., Zeiss

Add to Instrumentation
Basic eye microscope tray

Add to Supplies
Cellulose sponges, e.g., Weck
Topical anesthetic, e.g., tetracaine ophthalmic drops

Entropion Repair

Definition

Correction of inversion of the lid margins and lashes.

Discussion

Entropion results in ocular surface irritation and damage that usually affects the lower lid; corneal abrasions and scarring may occur. Entropion may be congenital, acute spastic, involutional, or cicatricial.

Types

Congenital. May be due to dysgenesis of the lower lid retractors; instability of the lid follows, with entropion resulting. Due to hypertrophy of the marginal and pretarsal orbicularis oculi muscle and a paucity of tissue, the eyelid margin is pushed up and against the globe.

Acute Spastic. Due to spastic closure of the obicularis oculi muscle, often occurs with involutional type.

Involutional (Most Common). May result due to horizontal laxity of the medial or lateral canthal tendons, or it may occur as the result of weakness of the retractor muscles of the lower lid when canthal tendons retain their rigidity but the apposition of the lid to the globe is changed (e.g., from senile atrophy of orbital fat), resulting in the inversion of the eyelid.

Entropion must be distinguished from lid retraction or epiblepharon, in which the pretarsal obicularis muscle and the skin of the lid override the lid margins and push the lashes inwards. Epiblepharon usually resolves as the child's face matures. The treatment of entropion depends on the etiology.

Procedure

Internal Tarsal-Orbicularis Resection is described. The lower lid is everted with a chalazion clamp. The line of incision may be marked inside the eyelid. A base-down triangle of skin, orbicularis oculi muscle, and tarsus is excised. The edges are sutured together, and the "dog ear" edge of remaining tissue is excised.

In an alternate method, **skin-tarsal fixation**, the orbicular muscle is divided and sutured to the lower border of the tarsus. If significant scarring (from chronic irritation) is present, a graft of oral mucous membrane may be used. Immobility of the graft is maintained by placing stents.

For further **Preparation of the Patient, Equipment, Instrumentation, Supplies,** and **Special Notes,** see *Excision of Chalazion,* pp. 876–877.

Blepharoptosis Repair/Blepharoplasty

Definition

Correction of ptosis of the upper eyelid.

Discussion

In **blepharoptosis repair,** a correction is made to the upper lid that is abnormally low-lying when the eye is in the primary gaze. Blepharoptosis may occur unilaterally or bilaterally. The most common cause of congenital myogenic ptosis is due to improper levator muscle development.

Causes of Blepharoptosis

Congenital. Can be mild to severe (eyelid droops 1.5 to 4 mm or more).

Acquired. Cause may be neurogenic or myogenic; defects are in aponeurosis and muscle.

Traumatic. May result from an accident, from use of contact lenses, or as a result of ocular surgery.

Mechanical. May be caused by *blepharochalasis* or *enophthalmos*. Any one of a number of techniques may be employed as treatment, depending on the type and severity of the deformity. **External levator resection** is indicated in patients with moderate to severe ptosis and fair to poor levator function.

Blepharoplasty is not usually covered by most medical insurance plans. Unless interference with vision is determined and documented preoperatively, the corrective procedure is regarded as cosmetic surgery.

Procedure

External Levator Resection is described. A traction suture is placed in the lid to permit downward traction. An incision is made from canthus to canthus and carried through the orbicularis oculi to the superior border of the tarsus. The upper half of the tarsus is exposed. The upper skin edge is grasped, and the orbicularis is separated from the orbital septum. The fat is retracted posteriorly, and the levator aponeurosis is excised. The eyelid is everted, and the conjunctiva is incised. The aponeurosis may be buttonholed at its medial and lateral border; a straight hemostat is placed across it, and Müller's muscle and the tissues are transected. The conjunctiva is reapproximated. Müller's muscle and the levator are sutured to the tarsus. The excess levator is excised. Lid crease skin sutures are placed. The lower lid is pulled up over the globe by sutures placed in the lower lid through silicone pegs or bolsters that are taped to the forehead. These sutures are removed the next day.

For **Preparation of the Patient, Skin Preparation, Draping, Instrumentation, Equipment,** and **Supplies,** see *Excision of Chalazion,* p. 876.

Special Notes

- Apply **Special Notes** from **Ophthalmic Surgery General Information**, pp. 871–875.
- This procedure is performed employing local anesthesia; the circulator must advise the patient that he/she may be asked to open and close his/her eyes as requested during the surgery.
- Serrefines (small bulldog clamps) are usually used to tag traction sutures.

Excision of Eyelid Lesion

Definition

Excision of skin lesions of the eyelid.

Discussion

An **excision of an eyelid lesion** should include the lid margin; when both benign and malignant tumors are excised, cosmetic and functional repair of the wound is done. Various benign skin lesions of the eyelid, such as cysts, nevi, infections, tumors, etc., may require simple excision with orientation of the incision according to natural skin lines to diminish the appearance of the scar. Skin lesions of the eyelid that are malignant include basal cell carcinoma, squamous cell carcinoma, and melanoma; basal cell carcinoma is the most common malignant lesion that may affect the eyelid.

Treatment as *radiation therapy* may be employed to ablate neoplastic lesions of the eyelid, but the side effects of radiation therapy include dermatitis, keratitis, and scarring. The *CO_2 laser* may be used to excise lesions, as well as *photodynamic therapy (PDT);* PDT is effective for patients with recurrent lesions or poor-risk patients. *Moh's micrographic chemosurgery* is effective, but depending on the size of the lesion, surgical reconstruction may be required. Repair of any wounds following excision includes orientation of the tissue according to skin lines; the closure must be done without tension for adequate wound healing. For additional information, see the previous entry, ***Blepharoptosis Repair/Blepharoplasty***, p. 881, and ***Blepharoplasty*** in ***Plastic Surgery***, p. 727.

Procedure

In excision of lesions of the eyelid and lid margin, the incision is often *pentagon-shaped*; the base of the pentagon is positioned at the lid margin and the apex points upward, away from the lid margin. Care must be taken to include adequate tumor margins. *Lateral canthotomy* may be done to effect closure without undue traction. A variety of types of tarsal/conjunctival flaps may be used, as *Tenzel* (semicircular is lateral-based) or *Cutler-Beard* (flap of the opposing lid is passed under the lid margin to cover the defect in the affected lid, which requires closure of the lid with loss of vision for 6 to 8 weeks); this is inappropriate for patients with limited vision or absence of vision in the other eye. In reconstruction, the lid margins are approximated first. The tarsal plate is closed separately with absorbable sutures. The skin is closed with nonabsorbable suture, as is the canthus.

Preparation of the Patient

Excision of an eyelid lesion may be performed employing topical, local, and/or general anesthesia.

For further **Preparation of the Patient, Equipment, Instrumentation, Supplies,** and **Special Notes,** see *Excision of Chalazion,* pp. 876–877.

Add to Special Notes

- **Reminder:** When a laser is employed, all safety precautions are mandatory, e.g., protective goggles, special laser-safe instrumentation (e.g., ebonized), etc.; see laser safety precautions, p. 94.

Eyelid Laceration Repair

Definition

Repair of a torn eyelid.

Discussion

Eyelid laceration repair may be performed in response to any traumatic eyelid laceration to restore the integrity of the lid. The defects are classified according to size and location; they may involve the lid, lid margins, and canthus. The major causes of the eyelid defect are trauma and tumors; basal cell carcinoma is the second most common cause. The skin surfaces (only) of the wound may be approximated with cyanoacrylate tissue adhesive, e.g., Dermabond®. Cyanoacrylates should not be used in the treatment of human or animal bites, puncture wounds, and stellate lacerations. Deep sutures should be placed (on eye muscles and facial areas) to relieve the stress on the wound closure as necessary for wound healing.

When the *canaliculus* is not involved, a defect through the lid margin is repaired employing direct closure, as in ***Excision of an Eyelid Lesion***, p. 883. Care is taken to avoid injury to the canaliculus. The *medial canthal tendon* is repaired, as applicable.

Ice compress dressings rather than tight pressure dressings should be used following the procedure to ensure that visual acuity does not deteriorate.

Procedure

When **eyelid laceration repair** is performed, if the canaliculus is injured (especially in children), as in dog bites and claw injuries, a *Veirs*™ *stainless steel rod* may be placed through the cut end of the laceration, inserted into the upper and/or lower lid canalicula. A nonabsorbable suture (e.g., 10–0 nylon) is used to reapproximate the canaliculus around the rod. The subcutaneous tissue and skin are closed. Dermabond may be employed for skin closure, as it works as a barrier against bacteria. To prevent hematoma formation, meticulous hemostasis must be achieved using an ophthalmic diathermy and ice compress dressings postoperatively, rather than tight pressure dressings.

Alternatively, lacrimal duct probes may be passed (with a *silicone tube* at each end) through the upper canaliculus and the cut end of the lower canaliculus. The silicon tubes are then passed down into the nose (with the tubes untied). The lacrimal duct probes are removed.

Instrumentation

Basic eye microscope procedures tray
Basic eye muscle and dacryocystorinostomy trays, available
Lacrimal duct-probing instruments, p. 886 (optional, depending on presentation)
Silicone tubes/stents, e.g., *Quickert-Dryden*™, *Crawford*™, *Jones*™/*Lester-Jones*™, or *Veirs stainless steel rod,* available

For **Preparation of the Patient, Equipment, Supplies,** and **Special Notes,** see ***Excision of Chalazion***, pp. 876–877.

Add to Supplies

Tissue adhesive 2-Octyl cyanoacrylate, e.g., Dermabond (works as a barrier against bacteria), optional
Culture tubes (aerobic and anaerobic), optional

Add to Special Notes

- The circulator is often requested to send a traumatized tissue specimen to the laboratory for aerobic and anaerobic culture and sensitivity studies; this is documented in the Perioperative Record for continuity of care (to advise others that this has been done) and for medicolegal reasons.
- The *Quickert-Dryden stent* silicone tubing includes a swaged-on lacrimal duct probe.
- The *Veirs*™ *stainless steel rod* includes attached "pull-out" sutures.
- Ice pack dressings are placed at the conclusion of surgery; the circulator accompanies the patient to the PACU and explains the need for the icepacks postoperatively to the PACU perioperative practitioner.
- The PACU perioperative practitioner observes and documents the appearance of the wound and nursing care (interventions) in the **Postoperative Record** portion of the **Perioperative Record** for patient safety and medicolegal reasons.

Lacrimal Duct Probing

Definition

Opening and enlargement of the nasolacrimal duct to correct epiphora.

Discussion

Epiphora, an abnormal overflow of tears, indicates a problem in the lacrimal drainage system. When medical management of the lacrimal duct obstruction is unsuccessful, probing is indicated. **Lacrimal duct probing** must be done to prevent acute infection due to the obstruction. Probing of the ductal system is corrective in the majority of presentations; balloon dilatation may be employed as well. When there is severe scarring, a graft from oral mucous membrane may be used. Anomalies of the puncta, canaliculi, or lacrimal sac may be encountered and are corrected as indicated (e.g., in cases of punctal agenesis, insertion of a Lester-Jones tube is done). When repeated probings are technically successful but have otherwise failed, ***dacryocystorhinostomy,*** p. 888, may be performed.

Procedure

In **lacrimal duct probing,** the upper canaliculus is dilated and a lacrimal probe (e.g., size 000) is inserted and passed through the imperforate duct opening into the nose. The procedure may be repeated with the next-larger size lacrimal dilator and probe, serially, as necessary. A lacrimal cannula is used for irrigation (through the upper canaliculus into the nose). Antibiotic ophthalmic drops may be instilled.

Preparation of the Patient

Lacrimal duct probing is usually performed using topical and local anesthesia.

For the special considerations in preparation of the room and special measures taken for care of the pediatric patient, see **Pediatric General Information**, p. 978. The head and foot of the table may be removed to provide closer access to the child patient. The extremities are restrained using softly padded restraints.

In *infants 6 months of age and younger*, the lacrimal duct probing may be performed using a topical anesthetic, e.g., tetracaine. A mummy-like wrap is used; care is taken to avoid pressure injury to bony prominences and areas vulnerable to skin and neurovascular pressure or trauma.

In *children over 6 months of age,* the procedure is usually performed employing general anesthesia. The child is placed in supine position; care is taken to avoid pressure injury to bony prominences and areas vulnerable to skin and neurovascular pressure or trauma.

For **Skin Preparation,** see **Ophthalmic Surgery General Information**, p. 870.

Draping

Draping is not always used. Usual draping for ophthalmic surgery (see **Ophthalmic Surgery General Information**, p. 870.) may be done, or absorbent (disposable) towels may be folded and placed around the eye; a drape sheet to cover the body is used infrequently.

Equipment

Padded, foam, or gel headrest, e.g., donut
Magnifying loupes or operating microscope
Mummy wrap or restraints, softly padded

Instrumentation

Basic eye procedures or basic eye microscope procedures tray
Infant punctal dilator, Heath punctal dilator, Castroviejo lacrimal dilator (double-ended), Wilder lacrimal dilator, Ziegler lacrimal dilator, double ended, curved
Lacrimal duct probes, e.g., Bowman 0000-000, 00-0
Jones punctual dilators with sharp tips, 1–2
Bowman lacrimal probes, 5–6 and 7–8
Lacrimal cannula
Lester-Jones prosthesis (scarring or absence of duct), optional

Supplies

Topical anesthetic ophthalmic drops, e.g., tetracaine
Local anesthetic, e.g., lidocaine with epinephrine, control syringe, hypodermic needle, medicine cups, labels, and marking pen
Small basin
BSS, tear substitute
Cotton-tipped applicators or cellulose sponges
Fluorescein dye, optional
Antibiotic ophthalmic drops, optional
Dressing, e.g., eye pad

Special Notes

- Apply **Special Notes** from **Ophthalmic Surgery General Information**, p. 871, as indicated.
- **Reminder:** *Use every precaution to correctly identify the pediatric patient.* Document methods used to identify the pediatric patient for patient safety and medicolegal reasons.
- *The circulator should verify infant patient information with the parent(s) or legal guardian(s), as sensitivities and allergies, etc. All information obtained and noted, interventions performed, and patient outcomes are documented in the* **Perioperative Record** *(p. 12).*

- *Remember that* ***"the pediatric patient is not a small adult."*** Special measures and precautions for the pediatric patient and the neonate, in particular, must be observed. Administering preoperative medication (if any), administering anesthesia, preparing the room, monitoring body temperature to retain body heat, maintaining accurate fluid balance, methods of restraining the patient, etc., are vitally important. Plan and consider the special measures that must be taken for the pediatric patient; for further considerations refer to **Pediatric General Information**, p. 978.
- Transport the neonate or infant patient to and from surgery in an isolette to maintain the patient's body temperature.
- Local anesthesia with epinephrine may be administered during the procedure to aid in hemostasis.
- The use of drapes is optional; gloves are worn.
- Fluorescein dye may be used to test the patency of the duct.

Dacryocystorhinostomy

Definition

Reestablishment of the channel between the lacrimal duct and the nasal cavity for the drainage of tears.

Discussion

Epiphora is a condition characterized by abnormal tearing that occurs due to blockage in the lacrimal drainage system. Etiology may be congenital or acquired; this condition has been noted in the fetus when the blockage results in formation of a bluish cyst-like mass. *Dacrocystostenosis* occurs in the neonate when the extreme end of the nasolacrimal duct fails to complete its canalization, but this condition may also occur in the adult. When tears are blocked, stagnation occurs, and recurrent infections result in *chronic dacryocystitis*. In patients who have not responded to conservative treatment, such as probing, irrigation, balloon dilatation, silicone intubation, etc., **dacryocystorhinostomy** is indicated. **Dacrocystorhinostomy** establishes an alternate channel for tear drainage. Fluorescein dye studies are often employed to determine ductal patency. CT and MRI scan may be helpful for delineating the local anatomy. Care is taken during the procedure to avoid injury to the intraorbital vessels and the optic nerve.

The **endoscopic transnasal approach** is the preferred approach to reestablish the channel; it replaces the long-time standard "open" (external) approach, although either approach can be equally successful. The Ellman Surgitron™ radiosurgery unit is used in the endoscopic approach; the electrosurgical unit (ESU) is used in the open approach. Using the Surgitron unit results in decreased inflammation, edema, and postoperative pain.

Advantages of endoscopic transnasal approach include:

- More esthetic result; no scar
- Employs one stage that addresses the probable cause, i.e., nasolacrimal blockage
- Avoids injury to medial canthus by scarring
- Obicularis oculi muscle (pumping action) is preserved
- Active infection is not a contraindication
- It is less bloody, and perioperative time is shorter.

The disadvantages to the endoscopic approach are that the surgeon may require extra training, there may be excessive bleeding that could cause the procedure to be abandoned, and there are added costs for the instrumentation and equipment.

Procedure

Dacryocystorhinostomy. General or local anesthesia may be employed. Most surgeons prefer local anesthesia; however, general anesthesia may be given to an infant (according to his/her temperament) and select older patients following the topical/local preliminary nasal preparation with an anesthetic. The anesthetic is used to saturate nasal packing; the packing is left in place for 10 minutes to achieve its effect. The middle turbinate is infiltrated (injected) with a local anesthetic solution with epinephrine (see below). Following the preliminary nasal preparation, either endoscopic or "open" (i.e., external) approach may be employed.

Endoscopic Approach. An endoscope, 4-mm diameter 30° viewing angle, is used, and a fiber-optic light probe, e.g., Endo-Illuminator™ (20 gauge) is passed via the upper or lower canaliculus into the lacrimal sac. Through the endoscope, an incision (1 cm) is made over the transilluminated lacrimal sac. The light from the endoscope may require dimming to visualize the light of the illuminator probe at the posterior end of the lacrimal sac (overlying the lacrimal bone). After removing the illuminator, an Ellman Surgitron radiosurgery unit is employed to achieve hemostasis in the mucosa and a drill or Ho:YAG laser is used to incise the lacrimal bone (part of the uncinate process may be removed). The lacrimal sac is entered with 45° cutting forceps, used to create an opening that is enlarged to a 1-cm opening. Further hemostasis may be achieved with the radiosurgery unit. A siliconized tubing with metal stents may be passed through the upper and lower canaliculus in the inferior direction into the nasal cavity, retrieved with Blakesley forceps, and cut. The tubing may be secured to provide a continous loop [with a knot or by threading a 16 gauge needle (Becton-Dickenson Autoguard) across 23 gauge tubing (2) around the canaliculi] forming an alternate path for tear drainage. Care is taken so that the tenting is neither too loose nor too tight. This approach is abandoned when there is uncontrollable bleeding.

Open (External) Approach to Dacryocystorhinostomy. An incision is made along the side of the nose 1 cm from the canthus to the level just above the alar cartilages. Traction is placed on the skin so that the deeper incision does not lie directly under the skin incision, thus avoiding a direct cutaneous-osseous scar. The periosteum is incised and separated from the bone with a periosteal elevator. The sac is separated from the fossa, and the superior punctum is probed to identify its location. An H-incision is made in the sac, which is retracted laterally as a power drill is used to remove the lacrimal crest. The nasal packing (from the preliminary nasal preparation) is removed. The nasal mucosa is exposed, and a Kerrison rongeur is employed to enlarge the opening. Care is taken to protect the corneas (corneal shields). An H-incision is made in the nasal mucosa. The flaps of the lacrimal sac and the flaps of the nasal mucosa are reapproximated. Hemostasis is achieved with electrosurgery. The nose is packed with thrombin-soaked Gelfoam pledgets or gauze packing (e.g., Adaptic®, iodoform, or petrolatum-impregnated gauze). The subcutaneous and skin layers are closed. A catheter may be passed through the nasolacrimal duct for postoperative irrigation. A folded eye pad (only) may be placed over the incision.

Another modification includes the use of the Pawar Intracystic Implant™ passed from the opened lacrimal sac into the nasal cavity.

Preparation of the Patient

Dacryocystorhinostomy is performed employing general (or local) anesthesia; the table may be turned 90° or the table may be reversed with the patient's head at the foot of the table to facilitate the surgeon's access to the patient. When the patient is a small child, the lower section of the table is removed. The patient is in supine position with the head turned to the side (affected side up) and stabilized with a padded, foam, or gel headrest (e.g., donut); the dependent ear is well padded. The head of the table is elevated; a padded footboard is secured to the table. The arm on the affected side is padded and secured at the patient's side and the contralateral arm may be secured on a padded armboard, or both arms may be padded and secured at the patient's sides. A pillow may be placed under the knees to avoid straining lower back muscles, or the table may be flexed for comfort. All bony prominences and areas vulnerable to skin and neurovascular pressure or trauma are padded to avoid injury. If monopolar electrosurgery is employed, apply an electrosurgical dispersive pad to ground the patient.

The surgeon usually does a preliminary nasal preparation prior to the skin prep to deliver topical anesthetics and hemostatic agents. The local anesthetic, lidocaine 1% with epinephrine, is injected into the middle turbinate; it may also be administered during the procedure as the local anesthetic. The advantage of employing only topical and local anesthetics is lesser morbidity.

Preliminary Nasal Preparation (on a "Clean" Mayo Tray)

Medicine cups (2), paper labels, and marking pen Nasal speculum and bayonet forceps
Control syringes (2) and needles (2), 25 or 27gauge × 1½″
Topical agent, e.g., lidocaine 4% added to (2 ml) of epinephrine 1:1000 or 2 ml of lidocaine 2% and cocaine 4%, may be used to saturate the packing (left in place 10 minutes). Local injection: lidocaine 1% with epinephrine 1:100,000
Packing material, e.g., ¼″ gauze and Adaptic dressing

For **Skin Preparation,** see **Ophthalmic Surgery, Perioperative Considerations**, p. 869. Prep as for a unilateral or bilateral ophthalmic procedure, but include the external nose.

Draping

The adhesive-backed strip of a drape sheet is placed across the forehead. A split sheet is then draped so that the bridge of the nose fits into the split (V) of the drape; the operative eye and the nose are draped within the operative field. The adhesive-backed tails of the split sheet are secured at the top of the head, and the remainder of the split sheet is draped over the patient's body. A sterile, plastic adhesive drape is placed over the eye, nose, and immediate surrounding field.

Equipment

Padded, foam, or gel headrest, e.g., donut, optional
Padding (for dependent ear)
Operating fiber-optic microscope, e.g., Zeiss
Footboard, padded (adult)
Suction
Sitting stools

Endoscopic

Fiber-optic light source for fiber-optic endoscope, e.g., Xenon™ 300W
Video monitor, optional
VCR

Printer
CD burner
Camera console
Radiosurgery unit, e.g., Ellman Surgitron, with footswitch controls, optional
High-power micro drill power source, e.g., Surgitron, optional
Laser console, e.g., Ho:YAG, optional

Open
ESU
Power source for micro drill, e.g., Stryker® micro drill, unless the drill is self-contained (i.e., battery)
Radio-frequency (RF) bipolar wet-field diathermy unit, e.g., Solan

Instrumentation

Basic eye procedures microscope tray

Endoscopic
Endoscope, 4-mm diameter, 30° viewing angle
Specific endoscopic instrumentation (similar to external approach), including cutting forceps (45°), camera coupler, fiber-optic Endo-Illuminator (e.g., 20 gauge) and cord
Radiosurgical hand piece IEC for Surgitron with Varitip™ (wire electrode) and cord, optional
Drill, e.g., Surgitron, burr, and cord, optional
Laser hand piece (Ho:YAG), tip, cord, and specific instrumentation [for use with the laser (see mandatory laser safety precautions, p. 94)]

Open, Add
Limited procedure tray
Dacryocystorhinostomy tray
Kerrison rongeurs, sphenoidal punches, Senn retractors (2), self-retaining spring retractor
Bipolar wet-field diathermy forceps and cord, e.g., Malis
Power micro drill (e.g., micro Stryker) with micro burr and cord or drill may be self-contained (e.g., battery)

Supplies

Supplies for preliminary nasal preparation as noted above
Bulb syringe (for prep)
Basin set
BSS, tear substitute
Cellulose sponges, e.g., Weck
Suction tubing
Corneal shield

Endoscopic

Siliconized stent prosthesis (intubation set), silastic, IV tubing, 23Fr and 16Fr Becton-Dickenson Autoguard needle, or Insyte™ needle, O'Donaghue DCR set, optional

Open

Blades, (1) #15, (1) #11

Needle magnet or counter

Gelfoam (cut into pledgets approximately 2 × 1 cm) soaked in Thrombin, e.g., 5000 units

Gauze packing (e.g., Adaptic, iodoform, or petrolatum-impregnated gauze)

Pawar Intracystic Implant (silicone duct tubing with metal stents), O'Donaghue DCR set or butterfly IV tubing, 16Fr and 16Fr Becton-Dickenson Autoguard needle

Dressing, e.g., folded eye pad (only, no shield), moustache dressing, optional

Special Notes

- Add to **Special Notes** in ***Excision of Chalazion***, p. 877, as applicable.
- When **dacryocystorhinostomy** is performed using the open or external approach, the procedure may be long and tedious (until hemostasis is achieved); special attention must be given to ensure the maintenance of the patient's circulation and to avoid pressure injury. Hemodynamic factors must be assessed by the circulator during the procedure, e.g., keep patient's legs uncrossed. Pad elbows and heels to avoid pressure injury.
- **Reminder:** All measures necessary to assist venous return are observed, as obstruction of venous return may increase IOP. Antiembolitic hose (e.g., TED hose) should be applied when requested, before positioning patient. A sequential compression device with leg wraps may be applied over the antiembolitic hose, when ordered, to prevent deep vein thrombosis. The leg wraps may also be applied alone without the antiembolitic hose.
- **Reminder:** When the laser is used, all mandatory laser safety precautions must be enforced; see p. 94.
- To minimize friction and buildup of heat, the area being drilled is lightly irrigated with saline; saline and bone fragments are suctioned.
- **N.B. Reminder**: Wearing a protective face shield or goggles is required to protect those scrubbed from the splashing of irrigation fluid, blood, and bone chips, etc.

- In the endoscopic approach, the setting for the Ellman Surgitron radiosurgery unit is usually begun at 2 MHz; it may be increased by increments of 0.5 MHz, usually up to the level of 3.8 MHz. The unit produces a filtered radiowave that cuts soft tissue with minimal heat spread and minimal tissue alteration.
- **N.B.** The Ellman Surgitron RF unit should not be used with the patient who has a pacemaker. The circulator must verify and document that the patient does or does not wear a pacemaker in the **Perioperative Record** for patient safety (to alert other caregivers) and for medicolegal purposes.
- The sphenoidal punch (open approach) must be wiped clean of debris after each use.
- A moustache dressing may be placed under the nose.

Correction of Strabismus

Definition

Alignment of the visual axes of the eyes.

Discussion

Correction of strabismus, a condition usually seen in infants or young children, is first treated medically with glasses, patching, and fusion exercises, Botox injections, etc. When these treatments fail to align the axes of the eyes, surgical treatment is indicated. Complete restoration to normal alignment cannot always be achieved.

Types of Corrections

Lateral rectus resection is the shortening of this extraocular muscle by removing a portion of it and then reanastomosing the cut ends.

Medial rectus recession is the lengthening of this extraocular muscle by detaching it from its original insertion and reattaching it more posteriorly on the sclera.

The term "transposition" refers to the division of muscle and reattachment to a site other than its original insertion, such as when the inferior oblique muscle is used. When a muscle is divided near its insertion at the tendinous portion, the term "tenotomy" is used.

Procedure

Correction of strabismus is performed using general anesthesia in addition to local (retrobulbar block) anesthesia. When the correction (i.e., alignment) is not optimal, 24 hours after surgery, lesser adjustments in the muscle tension are done as a secondary procedure. To facilitate the same, an "adjustable" suture is used that can be tightened or loosened the next day; topical anesthesia is employed.

Lateral Rectus Resection is described. An eye speculum is inserted. An incision is made in the conjunctiva at the limbus to expose the lateral rectus muscle. The eye is rotated medially as far as possible. Two traction sutures are placed in the conjunctiva. The conjunctiva is freed from underlying tissue. A muscle hook is passed under the muscle insertion. The amount of muscle to be resected is measured with a caliper (previously adjusted). A muscle clamp is clamped over the muscle of the eyelid and the measured portion (specimen) is excised. The end of the muscle is reattached to the original point of insertion. Hemostasis is achieved. The conjunctiva is closed. Antibiotic ophthalmic ointment may be instilled, and an eye pad is applied.

Medial Rectus Recession is described. An eye speculum is inserted. An incision is made in the conjunctiva at the limbus; the conjunctiva is undermined. The distance from the original point of insertion to the new one is measured with a caliper (previously adjusted). The new point of insertion may be marked. Two absorbable sutures are placed in the end of the muscle (and left untied with the needles attached). A straight mosquito hemostat is clamped across the muscle (between the sutures and the insertion) in order to compress small blood vessels and discourage oozing. The clamp is removed, and a muscle hook is passed under the muscle. The muscle is incised, and the eye diathermy (disposable) is employed as necessary to achieve hemostasis. The muscle is reattached at the new point of insertion further back on the globe with the previously placed sutures. The conjunctiva is closed. Antibiotic ophthalmic ointment is instilled, and an eye pad is applied.

Preparation of the Patient

Correction of strabismus is usually performed on infants and children using general anesthesia, although the procedure may be performed on adults; the table may be turned 90° to facilitate the surgeon's access. A retrobulbar injection (see p. 902) may be administered prior to the skin preparation (adults). For the special considerations for preparing the room and for care of the pediatric patient, see **Pediatric General Information**, p. 978. The head and foot of the table may be removed to provide closer access to the small child patient. The extremities are secured using softly padded restraints.

In *infants 6 months of age and younger,* a mummy-like wrap is used; care is taken to avoid pressure injury to bony prominences and areas vulnerable to skin and neurovascular pressure or trauma.

For the child over 6 months of age, the child is placed in supine position; care is taken to support the joints and to avoid pressure injury to bony prominences and areas vulnerable to skin and neurovascular pressure or trauma. The patient is supine; the arm on the side of the affected eye may be secured at the patient's side, and the contralateral arm may be secured on a padded armboard.

For **Skin Preparation, Draping,** and **Special Notes,** see *Ophthalmic Surgery, Perioperative Considerations*, pp. 870–871.

Note in **Skin Preparation and Draping** that the procedure is usually bilateral.

Equipment

Mummy wrap (small child) or extremity restraints (child or adult), softly padded
Padded, foam, or gel headrest, e.g., donut
Padding (for dependent ear)
Magnifying loupes or operating fiber-optic microscope, e.g., Zeiss
Sitting stools

Instrumentation

Basic eye procedures tray or basic eye microscope procedures tray
Basic eye muscle procedures tray

Supplies

Local anesthetic for retrobulbar block, e.g., lidocaine, control syringe, and hypodermic needles (adult)
Medicine cups, paper labels, and marking pen
Basin set
Cellulose sponges, e.g., Weck
BSS, tear substitute
Needle magnet or counter
Antibiotic ophthalmic ointment
Dressing, e.g., eye pads and shields

Special Notes

- Apply **Special Notes** from *Excision of Chalazion,* p. 877, as applicable.
- **Reminder:** For the special considerations for preparing the room and for care of the pediatric patient, see **Pediatric General Information,** p. 978.

Evisceration of the Eye

Definition

Removal of the contents of the globe within the scleral shell.

Discussion

When **evisceration of the eye** is performed, a cosmetic prosthesis is placed. The sclera and muscles attached to the sclera remain intact to accommodate the prosthesis and provide the means for mobility. Indications for **evisceration** include a hopelessly traumatized eye in a young person with no history of previous eye disease or a blind painful eye. The cosmetic result is superior when compared to the result of enucleation, as the extraocular muscles still attached to the scleral shell result in a moveable prosthesis. Prostheses may be composed of aluminum oxide, mesh-wrapped bioceramic material, hydroxyapatite (porous, encourages ingrowth), which may be wrapped in human sclera or Silastic sheeting, or porous polyethylene (permits direct suturing of the rectus muscle, eliminating the wrapping). Intraorbital fat grafts may be employed to enhance the appearance of fullness. A conformer, vented or nonvented, is placed to fill the cul-de-sac. The cosmetic prosthesis is placed in the postoperative period; a magnetic peg and sleeve system inserted into the prosthesis may be used to help secure it.

Procedure

For **evisceration of the eye**, a peritomy is made superiorly from the 3 o'clock to 9 o'clock position. An incision of the same length is made in the exposed sclera through to the uvea. The entire uvea is separated from the sclera using an evisceration spoon and is removed. The remaining uvea may be removed with a gauze sponge on a hemostat rotated within the scleral shell or with a chalazion curette. A 95% alcohol swab may be used to remove pigment within the scleral envelope. The wound is irrigated. Hemostasis is achieved. Scleral edges are held open by tagged sutures while a "sized" implant/or prosthesis is inserted into the space using a sphere introducer. The posterior surface of the cornea is removed to reduce its sensitivity. The sclera is closed with interrupted sutures. The conjunctiva is approximated with interrupted sutures. A socket conformer is placed in the cul-de-sac space. Antibiotic ophthalmic ointment is instilled; an eye patch is applied.

Preparation of the Patient

Evisceration of the eye is performed employing general anesthesia; the table may be turned 90° to facilitate the surgeon's access. The patient is in supine position with the head turned to the side (affected side up) and stabilized with a padded, foam, or gel headrest (e.g., donut). The head of the table is elevated; a padded footboard is secured. The arm on the affected side is padded and secured at the patient's side and the contralateral arm may be secured on a padded armboard, or both arms may be padded and secured or extended and secured at the patient's sides. A pillow may be placed under the knees to avoid straining lower back muscles, or the table may be flexed for comfort. All bony prominences and areas vulnerable to skin and neurovascular pressure or trauma are padded to avoid injury.

For **Skin Preparation and Draping,** see **Ophthalmic Surgery, Perioperative Considerations,** p. 869.

Equipment

Padded, foam, or gel headrest, e.g., donut
Operating fiber-optic microscope, e.g., Zeiss
Bipolar wet-field diathermy unit, e.g., Solan
Suction
Sitting stools

Instrumentation

Basic eye procedures or basic eye microscope procedures tray
Globe and orbit procedures tray
Curettes, bipolar bayonet forceps and cord, skin hooks
Sphere sizers (in sets of four, polyoxymethylene), and sphere introducer
Sphere implant/prosthesis (correctly determined size) and conformer
Bipolar wet-field diathermy forceps, cord, and holder

Supplies

Basin set
BSS, tear substitute
Cellulose sponges, e.g., Weck
Blade, (1) #11
Suction tubing
Antibiotic ophthalmic ointment
Eye-pad pressure dressing

Special Notes

- Apply **Special Notes** from ***Dacryocystorhinostomy,*** p. 893, as applicable.
- The patient will understandably have feelings of anxiety regarding the loss of the eye. The perioperative practitioner, as circulator, must provide emotional support to the patient throughout the procedure, e.g., convey to the patient that he/she will act as the patient's advocate by speaking for him/her while the patient is in surgery, maintain eye contact and hold the patient's hand during the administration of anesthesia, help the patient regarding discomfort in the unfamiliar environment by explaining perioperative interventions before they are done, and answer

questions in a knowledgeable manner or refer questions to the surgeon, as necessary.

- The circulator provides emotional support to the patient regarding feelings of altered body image by offering the patient an opportunity to express his/her feelings in a nonjudgemental environment.
- The sphere sizers and the sphere introducer should be sterilized prior to starting the surgery. A variety of sterile sphere implants/prostheses and conformers should also be available in the room before surgery is begun.
- Prior to their insertion, implants are soaked in antibiotic solution.
- Documentation regarding the date, patient's name, brand name, type, size, and serial numbers of the implanted prosthesis and the conformer are made in the **Perioperative Record** and in the hospital's log (for insertion of an implant), according to hospital policy.
- The circulator must complete the manufacturer's forms for the prosthesis and the conformer; duplicate information may be provided to the patient as a source of reference.
- **Reminder:** *Tincture of benzoin may be used to protect the skin when a pressure dressing is placed (e.g., made with Elastoplast tape).* The circulator must check with the patient and the chart regarding an allergy to latex (composition of the tape) before applying the pressure tape. Record of the verification is noted in the **Perioperative Record** for patient safety (to inform other caretakers) and for medicolegal reasons.
- In the PACU, the perioperative practitioner will observe the patient for signs of hemorrhage; the appearance and amount of bright red bleeding on the dressing, increased pulse, etc., is reported to the surgeon immediately and documentation is made that includes the action (nursing intervention) taken and the patient outcome.

Enucleation of the Globe

Definition

Excision of the globe of the eye.

Discussion

In **enucleation**, the globe of the eye is removed, leaving the eye muscles and the remaining orbital contents. **Enucleation of the globe** is indicated in certain instances of severe trauma, intraocular malignancy (e.g., melanoma, involving the iris or retinoblastoma, involving the retina), intolerable pain, and unsightly appearance. Most often, a plastic, hydroxyapatite, or silicone sphere is placed within Tenon's capsule. A conformer is placed over the sphere. The conformer is replaced with an artificial eye 8 weeks postoperatively.

Procedure

Under general anesthesia, a peritomy is made at the limbus, circumferentially separating the conjunctiva and Tenon's capsule from the globe. The superior oblique tendon is grasped with a muscle hook and divided. The inferior oblique muscle and four rectus muscles are double-clamped with hemostats for hemostasis; the muscles are divided after being marked with sutures to reattach to the implant or donor sclera. Hemostats are released after several minutes. All attachments to the globe are separated, permitting the globe to move freely. The eye is held steady by the medial rectus insertion. The location of the optic nerve is identified. The optic nerve is transected, the globe is delivered, and the remaining attachments are separated. Hemostasis is achieved. A sphere implant may be sutured into Tenon's capsule. The remaining palpebral conjunctiva is approximated. A conformer is placed over the sphere in the cul-de-sac. An intermarginal suture is placed to produce a mild pressure effect. Antibiotic ointment may be instilled, an eye pad is placed, and a pressure dressing is applied.

For **Preparation of the Patient, Equipment, Instrumentation, Supplies,** and **Special Notes,** see ***Evisceration of the Eye***, pp. 897–898.

Orbital Exenteration

Definition

Removal of the entire contents of the orbit and a significant portion of the surrounding orbital tissues.

Discussion

In **orbital exenteration,** the tissues removed beyond the globe depends on the origin and extent of the disease process. Some malignant tumors may require excision of the periosteum surrounding the orbit. Some malignancies will require excision of the eyelids as well. Although orbital exenteration is usually performed for malignant tumors; it may also be performed for benign disease, such as *phycomycosis*.

Types of exenteration include:

1. **Subtotal:** Eye and epibulbar tissues excised
2. **Total** (with or without eyelid skin): Removal of all tissues within the bony orbit, including periorbita

3. **Radical:** Removal of one or more bony orbital walls in addition to soft tissues and periosteum.

The **subtotal procedure** is performed to remove tumors involving the anterior portion of the eye and the conjunctiva. The **total procedure** is indicated when intraocular tumor (e.g., melanoma) extends into the orbit. Malignant tumors not involving bone that do not respond to radiation may require **total exenteration. Radical exenteration** is indicated when a malignant sinus tumor invades the orbit or when a malignant skin tumor involves the orbital bones (portions of which may be excised). After the wound has healed, the cavity may be covered with a black patch or a cosmetic plastic prosthesis (individually crafted from varying plastic materials to occupy the surgically created deformity).

Procedure

For **total exenteration**, with preservation of eyelid skin, an incision is made circumferentially around the palpebral fissure. The skin is dissected to the orbital rim. Orbicularis muscle may be incised with the cutting blade of an electrosurgical pencil. The periosteum is separated from the orbital rim and walls; care is taken to avoid perforation of bony walls. The eye and soft tissues within the orbit are removed. The skin is undermined and closed over the lateral orbital rim. A split-thickness skin graft may be used to cover denuded orbital walls. Alternatively, the bone surfaces may be permitted to heal by spontaneous granulation. The orbital cavity is packed with gauze impregnated with antibiotic ointment, and a moderate pressure dressing is applied.

For **Preparation of the Patient,** see *Evisceration of the Eye*, p. 897.

Add to Preparation of the Patient

Apply electrosurgical dispersive pad.

Equipment

Padded, foam, or gel headrest, e.g., donut
Suction
Bipolar wet-field diathermy unit, e.g., Solan
ESU, monopolar
Sitting stools
Power unit for dermatome, optional

Instrumentation

Limited procedure tray
Basic eye procedures tray
Globe and orbit procedures tray
Dermatome and blades (disposable), optional (e.g., Brown)

Supplies

Basin set
BSS, tear substitute
Bipolar wet-field diathermy forceps, e.g., Solan and cord
Electrosurgical pencil and cord, holder, and scraper
Cellulose sponges, e.g., Weck
Needle magnet or counter
Bone wax
Suction tubing
Mineral oil and tongue blades (2), if dermatome is used, optional
Packing, e.g., 1/4″ gauze and antibiotic ophthalmic ointment
Eye-pad pressure dressing

Special Notes

- Apply **Special Notes** from ***Evisceration of the Eye***, p. 898.
- The circulator should confer with the surgeon to determine if a skin graft is to be obtained and if a (Brown) determatome is needed.
- When the Brown determatome is used, new blades should be used, as the new blades are always sharp, and to avoid the transmission of blood-borne diseases.
- The donor site is prepped and draped at the same time as the operative eye (and the area surrounding the eye).
- During the exenteration, the donor site is draped and covered with a towel until the skin graft is needed to avoid contaminating the area.
- **N.B. Reminder:** ***Tincture of benzoin may be used to protect the skin when a pressure dressing is placed (e.g., made with Elastoplast tape).*** The circulator must check (preoperatively) with the patient and the chart regarding an allergy to latex (consider composition of the tape) before applying the pressure dressing. Record verification of allergy in the **Perioperative Record** for patient safety (to inform other perioperative practitioners) and for medicolegal reasons.

Corneal Transplant/Keratoplasty

Definition

The grafting of corneal tissue from the eye of one person to another.

Discussion

Corneal transplant/keratoplasty is indicated when corneal injury or disease has resulted in opacification of the cornea, to improve the patient's vision; the retina and optic nerve must be functioning properly to merit doing the surgery. Once corneal transplant/keratoplasty is performed, light passes uninhibited through the clear donor cornea. The most frequent indication is **pseudophakic bullous keratopathy**, following cataract surgery; physical or chemical trauma, scarring related to infection, keratonconus, and congenital opacities are additional indications for performing the procedure.

The donor cornea is obtained from an eye bank (facility that procures corneas for transplantation); donor eyes are removed within several hours after death according to guidelines established by The Eye Bank Association of America. The immunological considerations for a corneal transplant are minimal (as the tissue is avascular) compared to other forms of tissue or organ transplantation, although blood serum tests for hepatitis B and human immunodeficiency viruses are performed on the donor. In many instances, the procedure is performed as an outpatient procedure. Vision usually improves immediately, but optimal results may take 6 to 12 months to be realized. **Corneal transplant/keratoplasty** is the most successful type of organ/tissue transplant surgery.

Types

Lamellar: Replacement of a partial thickness of the cornea
Penetrating: Replacement of a full thickness of the cornea
Total: Replacement of the entire corneal area (limbus to limbus)

Lamellar and total keratoplasty are rarely performed. **Penetrating keratoplasty** may be performed as an emergency procedure.

Descemet's Stripping Automated Endothelial Keratoplasty (DSAEK) involves, in selected cases, the removal or stripping of a disc of Descemet's membrane and the endothelium from the posterior aspect of the cornea via a small supralimbic incision and replaced with a similar disc (8 to 9 mm) harvested from the donor eye. A micro keratotome is employed to separate the posterior 20% of the cornea (the remaining portion may be used for anterior lamellar transplantation in another patient). During the procedure, a maintainer prevents the anterior chamber from collapsing, in addition to the instillation of physiologic fluid or air to hold the graft in place. The graft is introduced in a folded state via a small incision and positioned within the anterior chamber. The major portion of the cornea is undisturbed; sutures are placed at the periphery of the scleral incision and healing is rapid.

For superficial opacities and corneal dystrophies, in selected cases, the excimer laser can be employed to ablate the opacity and smooth (and reshape) the corneal surface; this procedure is referred to as **phototherapeutic keratectomy (PTK).**

An intraocular lens (IOL) is usually implanted prior to placing the donor button.

Procedure

Corneal Transplant/Penetrating Keratoplasty is described. Local anesthesia with *conscious sedation* is used for most adults; general anesthesia is used for children or anxious adult patients. The operating microscope is used. The eye is "supported" by a ring sewn peripherally to the ocular surface. A trephine size is chosen, and the donor corneal button is prepared. If the donor button has been prepared by the excision of a cornea with scleral rim (corneoscleral button), it is placed into a Teflon block and the button is punched from behind (on the endothelial surface). The trephine used for the donor button should be approximately 0.5 mm larger than the host trephine. A single nonabsorbable suture is placed through the cut edge of the excised button. The excised button is placed epithelial-side down in a culture dish with a solution of Likerol®, Likerol DX®, Inosol®, Exosol®, or Optisol GS®. The fluid must cover the entire surface of the button to prevent drying.

The host cornea is removed by trephining it to a depth of 0.4 mm. The anterior chamber is entered with a sharp knife (stab incision). Care is taken to remove any adventitious tissue from the host site. Lens extraction, vitrectomy, or any other necessary procedures are performed. The donor button (graft) is placed into the host, and the previously placed suture is tied at 12 o'clock. The graft is fixed at the 6 o'clock, 3 o'clock, and 9 o'clock positions employing fine (e.g., 10-0) nylon sutures. The graft (donor button) is secured with additional sutures. Before the last suture is tied, the anterior chamber is reformed to normal depth with BSS. Fluid is expressed and any leaks are repaired. Steroids, as well as antibiotics, may be applied topically.

Preparation of the Patient

Tetracaine drops are usually instilled. The eyelashes may be clipped; check with the surgeon. **Corneal transplant/penetrating keratoplasty** is performed employing local anesthesia. A retrobulbar anesthetic injection may be administered prior to the skin preparation. The patient is in supine position with the head turned to the side (operative side up) stabilized on a padded, foam, or gel headrest (e.g., donut); the dependent ear is well padded to prevent pressure injury. The table may be turned 90° to facilitate the surgeon's access. The arm on the affected side is padded and secured at the patient's side and the contralateral arm may be secured on a padded armboard, or both arms may be padded and secured at the patient's sides. A pillow may be placed under the knees to avoid straining lower back muscles, or the table may be flexed for comfort. All bony prominences and areas vulnerable to skin and neurovascular pressure or trauma are padded to avoid injury.

For **Skin Preparation and Draping,** see **Ophthalmic Surgery General Information,** p. 870.

Equipment

Padded, foam, or gel headrest, e.g., donut
Lift sheet or pad for Hoyer lifting device (placed on operating table)
Operating fiber-optic microscope, e.g., Zeiss
Bipolar wet-field diathermy unit, e.g., Solan, optional
Autoref® topography autorefractor, e.g., RT 6000 (TOMEY)
Sitting stools

Instrumentation

Basic eye microscope procedures tray
Corneal procedures tray
Caliper, micro keratome, and Flieringa fixation ring, optional
Bipolar wet-field diathermy forceps Solan and cord or disposable diathermy

Supplies

Sterile, plastic adhesive drape
Basin set
BSS, tear substitute
Cellulose sponges, e.g., Weck
Culture dishes (to hold corneal donor button)
Medium for holding the corneal donor button, e.g., Likerol, Likerol DX, Inosol, Exosol, or Optisol GS
Blades, (1) #15, (1) #64 Beaver, and 1 superblade 30°
Needle magnet or counter
Fluorescein strip (topical agent used to temporarily stain denuded corneal epithelial surface of the donor button)
Control syringes, hypodermic needles, medicine cups, labels, and marking pen
Celestone Soluspan®/betamethasone (anti-inflammatory agent, reduces inflammation)
Miochol-E 1%/acetylcholine chloride with mannitol (miotic intraocular solution used to irrigate and rapidly constrict the pupil after delivery of the lens); see **Special Notes** below for directions to reconsitute
Eye-pad dressing

Special Notes

- Apply **Special Notes** from ***Excision of Chalazion***, p. 877, as applicable.
- **Reminder:** *A lift sheet or Hoyer pad for a mechanical lift is placed on the table before the patient is positioned on the table; either may be used to transfer the patient from*

the table to the gurney postoperatively. The patient is ***not*** permitted to assist in the transfer to the gurney, as the action may increase IOP.

- **N.B.** *The circulator and the scrub person should confirm that the donor cornea is in the operating room suite and is ready for placement in the host before bringing the patient into the room.*
- **Reminder:** When a portable floor-model microscope is used, it is brought over the patient on the side opposite the operative eye.
- A separate sterile table may be requested to prepare (cut out with a trephine) the donor button for transplantation.
- An antibiotic solution is used to cleanse donor button, preparing it for placement in the host.
- **N.B.** *Once the donor button has been prepared (i.e., cut to size by trephining), it is placed in a culture dish filled with medium solution, e.g., Likerol, Likerol DX, Inosol, Exosol, or Optisol GS.* The medium solution must cover the surface of the corneal button to preserve its clarity.
- **N.B.** If the donor solution is cloudy (sign of possible infection), the donor cornea must be returned. The circulator must notify the eye bank regarding the return and request a new corneal transplant. This is documented in the **Perioperative Record** for patient safety (to alert others to the problem) and for medicolegal reasons.
- **N.B.** Donor button tissue should be handled as little as possible to avoid crushing, damaging, or contaminating it and to avoid introducing foreign material.
- **N.B.** A Charlie forceps that coapts only at the distal tip may be used to hold the folded donor button at its periphery during placement in the host, as it prevents crushing the tissue.
- **N.B.** A Sinskey reverse hook may be used in positioning for the endothelial side of the donor button during placement in the host.
- **N.B** The surgeon may request that sutures be "wet" before they are used to aid in their smooth passage through the tissue.
- When BSS is injected into the anterior chamber following suturing of the graft, a fine cannula (e.g., 30 gauge) is used. Instillation of the fluid is done to assure that the closure is "water-tight."

- **N.B. Reminder:** *The scrub person should reconstitute/ Miochol-E/acetylcholine chloride (and mannitol) immediately before use; it is amioticintraocular agent used to irrigate and rapidly constrict the pupil.* To reconstitute it, mix the lyophilized powder with an ampule of diluent. The blister pack includes the powder, diluent, syringe, and a luer-lok type filter hub (5 μ) that must be used for administration. After mixing, the syringe with the luer-lok filter hub is passed to the surgeon.

Cataract Extraction

Definition

Removal of an opaque ocular lens.

Discussion

When the ocular lens becomes opacified, vision becomes cloudy, and it is referred to as a cataract. The cataract may be congenital, or it may be the result of trauma, metabolic effects (such as diabetes), or drug side effects, but it is most often due to aging (with the resultant excessive exposure to sunlight). **Cataract extraction** surgery is indicated at an appropriate time in the maturation of the cataract when there is sufficient loss of vision.

Methods

Intracapsular. Removal of the opaque lens and the capsule. A cryoprobe is applied to the cataract and the lens capsule; both are removed by gentle pressure. This modality is seldom used in current practice.

Extracapsular. Removal of the opaque lens using an irrigation and expression (aspiration) technique; the posterior capsule is left in situ.

Phacoemulsification. A variation of the irrigation-aspiration technique; the contents of the lens capsule are fragmented by ultrasonic energy as the lens material is simultaneously irrigated and aspirated.

INFINITI™ fluidics management system (FMS) produces a state-of-the-art method to perform cataract extractions. An irrigation pressure sensor is a safety feature. It may be used for phacoemulsification employing three different types of energy delivery: ultrasound waves, **AquaLase**™ liquefaction, and **NeoSonix**® linear ultrasonic motion (with oscillatory sonic motion).

AquaLase liquefaction is a variation of the irrigation-aspiration technique, using a vibrating probe at ultrasound frequency to soften and break apart the contents of the lens capsule. The AquaLase liquefaction device uses an AquaLase hand piece and (polymer) tip. Instead of ultrasound energy, an applied vacuum is used to crack the cataract; jets of warmed BSS pulverize the cataract fragments that are then aspirated. The AquaLase softer tip is purported to be less traumatic that the ultrasound tip. This method for **clear cornea cataract extraction** may reduce thermal burns; however, it is ***not*** preferred for dense cataracts.

Another variation, **NeoSonix** (also by Alcon INFINITI Vision System), uses both ultrasound and mechanical oscillation to break up the cataract faster; this method is thought to give the surgeon greater control of the lens contents.

An artificial intraocular lens (IOL) is commonly implanted after the cataract has been removed. The IOL is made of inert material (silicone or acrylic) that does not trigger a rejection response. The surgeon selects the lens prosthesis prior to surgery; measurements are taken and used to select a lens power that may reduce or eliminate the patient's need for corrective eyewear. Examples of Food and Drug Administration (FDA)-approved IOL include AcrySof IQ™, AcrySof ReStor™, AcrySof Natural™ (Alcon), and ReZoom™ (Advanced Medical Optics). These newer lenses provide greater than monofocal refraction, often enabling the patient to see without the need of corrective eyeglasses or contact lenses. The Crystalens™ has hinges on either side, permitting a degree of focusing by ciliary muscle movement. Postoperatively, the posterior lens capsule may opacify; this usually responds to YAG laser treatment performed as an office procedure. All laser safety precautions must be observed whenever the laser is employed; see p. 94.

While not related to cataract extraction per se, phakic intraocular lenses are implanted without natural lens removal to correct nearsightedness (myopia) to reduce the patient's need for corrective glasses or contact lenses; see ***Secondary Lens Implant***, p. 913).

Procedure

Intracapsular Cataract Extraction is described. A lid speculum is placed. Traction sutures are placed in the sclera. The conjunctiva is reflected from the corneal superior hemicircumference. Bleeders are cauterized. The anterior chamber is entered. An iridotomy is performed as the cornea is retracted by suture traction. Alphachymotrypsin (Zolyse) is instilled into the anterior chamber (to dissolve the zonules suspending the lens). After 3 minutes, a cryoextractor is applied to the lens, which adheres to it, and the lens is withdrawn from the eye. The corneal incision is closed. Traction sutures are removed, and the conjunctival flap is approximated. Ophthalmic ointment may be instilled, and an eye pad is applied.

Extracapsular Cataract Extraction is described. The lens is opened with a tiny incision using a cystotome and capsule forceps. The lens cortex is removed using expression and a lens loop of a coaxial cannula system.

Cycloplegic agents (e.g., atropine) may be employed. The corneal incision is closed. The wound is closed as for the intraocular procedure.

An extracapsular IOL may be placed more commonly in the posterior chamber behind the iris. Posterior lenses can be implanted only where the cataract was removed by extracapsular lens extraction. This is the most physiologic position for the artificial lens, which has led to a return to extracapsular lens extraction. Anterior chamber lenses are used following intracapsular lens extraction and for ***secondary lens implantation*** (p. 913).

Phacoemulsification is described. The anterior lens capsule is excised, the lens nucleus is prolapsed into the anterior chamber, and the ultrasonic probe (with capabilities of irrigation and aspiration as well as delivery of ultrasonic energy) is inserted into the capsule. The remaining lens substance (cortex) in the posterior capsule is partially excised or "polished" with a moist cellulose sponge (to remove any fragments). **Healon®**, **Discovisc™**, or **Duovisc™** may be injected into the anterior chamber to prevent collapse (until aqueous humor content is reestablished). Phacoemulsification permits use of a smaller (more cosmetic) wound. The incision may be closed with fine suture(s), or it may be self-sealing, requiring "no stitch." The need for suture is decided on an individual basis at the time of surgery. An IOL is usually placed in the capsular "bag." The lens is folded during placement, allowing it to pass through a limited incision. The Healon is aspirated and a miotic agent (e.g., Miochol-E 1%) is instilled to constrict the iris and aid in holding the lens in place (see below to reconstitute the Miochol-E).

INFINITI FMS System (Alcon Laboratories) AquaLase Liquefaction is described. Use of a topical anesthetic ophthalmic drop (e.g., tetracaine 0.5%) placed into the operative eye before the patient enters the room eliminates the retrobulbar block. The patient must be able to hear and follow directions. A stab incision (2.6 mm) is made into the anterior chamber. Capsulorrhexis of anterior capsule of the lens is performed. The lens is loosened and fragmented by hydrodissection using microimpulses of fluid (e.g., BSS) with delamination and emulsification without disruption of the lens capsule, employing the **AquaLase** polymer tip. **AquaLase** liquefaction instrumentation also provides irrigation/aspiration (I/A). The IOL is folded and placed in the capsular "bag."

Preparation of the Patient

The patient is in supine position with the head turned to the side (eye to be operated is up and the dependent ear is well padded) stabilized in a padded, foam, or gel headrest (e.g., donut); the table may be turned 90° to facilitate the surgeon's access. The arm on the affected side is padded and secured in at the patient's side and the contralateral arm may be secureded on a padded armboard, or both arms may be padded and secured at the patient's sides. A pillow may be placed under the knees to avoid straining lower back muscles, or the table may be flexed for comfort. All bony prominences and areas vulnerable to skin and neurovascular pressure or trauma are padded to avoid injury. Tetracaine drops (may replace the retrobulbar block anesthetic) may be instilled in both eyes followed by the application of a Honan IOP reducer cuff for 10 to 15 minutes. The lashes may be trimmed (infrequently).

For **Skin Preparation and Draping,** see **Ophthalmic Surgery, General Information,** p. 870.

Add to Draping

Barrier drape for phacoemulsification unit, as necessary

Equipment

Padded, foam, or gel headrest, e.g., donut
Fiber-optic operating microscope, e.g., Zeiss
Honan IOP-reducing cuff
Lift sheet or Hoyer pad placed on the operating table
Sitting stools

Intracapsular

Cryoextractor (e.g., Frigitonics), not often in current use

Extracapsular Phacoemulsification

Irrigtion/aspiration I/A units (e.g., Cavitron® and INFINITI FMS lens-removal systems)

Instrumentation

Basic eye microscope procedures tray,
Cataract extraction and lens procedure tray
Specific instruments according to manufacturer
Calipur
McIntyre infusion set with connector and coaxial I/A system, optional phacoemulsification tray, as indicated, by brand of the I/A unit (e.g., Cavitron) Phacoemulsifier unit with AVIT ultrasonic hand piece with irrigation cystotome [e.g., INFINITI FMS ultrasound hand piece; INFINITI FMS AquaLase liquefaction hand piece with polymer AquaLase tip and (disposable) micro smooth infusion-irrigation sleeve; INFINITI FMS NeoSonix hand piece (with linear ultrasonic motion with oscillatory sonic motion)]
IOL implant, e.g., AcrySof IQ, AcrySof ReSTOR, AcrySof Natural

Supplies

Basin set
Sterile, plastic adhesive drape
BSS, 500 ml
I/A (specific type) pack for phacoemulsification tubing system
Cellulose sponges, e.g., Weck

Wet-field bipolar ophthalmic diathermy (e.g., Solan), disposable
Beaver blade, #69, Super blade 30°, or diamond knife
Control syringes, hypodermic needles, medicine cups, labels, and marking pen
Tubercular syringe and 30-gauge cannula (for local block anesthetic when replacing retrobulbar injection)
Dressing: eye pad and shield

Medications (available)
Topical anesthesia, e.g., tetracaine ophthalmic drops
Retrobulbar block anesthesia, e.g., Xylocaine/lidocaine 2% with epinephrine or Marcaine/bupivacaine 0.5% with epinephrine
Local block into the anterior chamber (replacing retrobulbar block), e.g., lidocaine 2% (without preservatives)
Betinosol 0.1%/betametasone ophthalmic drops is a corticosteroid and anti-inflammatory agent
Celestone Soluspan (betametasone sodium phosphate) is a glucocorticoid and anti-inflammatory agent
Wydase/hyaluronidase is an enzyme used to increase absorption and dispersion of other drugs
Miochol-E 1%/acetylcholine chloride is a miotic intraocular agent used to irrigate and rapidly constrict the pupil. It must be reconstituted *immediately* before use. See **Special Notes** below.
Healon/sodium hyaluronate is a viscoelastic vitreous humor substitute (also, the agent can act as a tamponade)
Discovisc ophthalmic viscosurgical device, Duovisc viscoelastic system

Special Notes

- Apply **Special Notes** from ***Excision of Chalazion***, p. 877, as applicable.
- A Honan cuff is placed over the affected eye prior to surgery; the cuff is used to reduce IOP preoperatively.
- **N.B. Reminder:** *A lift sheet or Hoyer pad (for this mechanical lift) is placed on the table before the patient is positioned on the table; either may be used to transfer the patient from the table to the gurney postoperatively.* The patient is ***not*** permitted to assist in the transfer to the gurney, as the action may increase IOP.
- **N.B. Reminder:** The circulator is responsible for obtaining adequate assistance to safely transfer the patient. Some hospitals employ special lift teams that must be notified in advance.
- Personnel who do the lifting need to employ ergonomic body mechanics to lift the patient in unison while bending their

knees and using their leg muscles to provide strength; lifting the patient in unison is done not only to avoid muscle-strain injuries to personnel, but to avoid patient injury as well.

- **Reminder:** During the transfer, care is taken to protect the patient by preventing all catheters and tubings from becoming tangled or pulled out (e.g., Foley catheter, intravenous lines, Swan Gans lines, etc.).
- **Reminder:** When a portable (floor-model) microscope is used, it is brought over the patient on the side opposite the affected eye.
- **N.B.** *Prior to the procedure, the circulator and scrub person must be thoroughly familiar with the specialty equipment used in ophthalmic* **cataract extraction** *surgery [e.g., Honan intraocular cuff, Frigitonics cryosurgery unit (intraocular extraction infrequently performed), Cavitron phaecoemulsifier (Alcon Surgical), INFINITI FMS ultrasound, AquaLase, or NeoSonix lens-removal system, etc.].*
- The working order of equipment (e.g., Cavitron or INFINITI lens-removal system) must be thoroughly checked by the scrub person and the circulator (as well as the surgeon) prior to the procedure. Also, the surgeon is responsible for checking the amount of vacuum control of the hand piece prior to using it.
- **N.B.** When local anesthetic is used to replace the retrobulbar injection, lidocaine (*without preservative*) is used; it is injected into the anterior chamber with a tubercular syringe and a 30-gauge cannula.
- **N.B. Reminder:** *The scrub person should reconstitute acetylcholine chloride/Miochol-E 1% (with mannitol) immediately before use.* It is reconstituted from a lyophilized sterile powder mixed with an ampule of diluent. A luer-lok filter hub (5 μ) is required for administration. All components (powder, diluent, syringe, and filter) are provided in a blister pack. After reconstituting the solution, the scrub person passes the syringe with the filter to the surgeon.
- **Reminder:** Wearing a protective face shield or goggles is required to protect those persons scrubbed from the splashing of irrigation fluid, blood, etc.
- **Reminder:** Documentation by the circulator regarding the date, patient's name, brand name, type, size, and serial numbers of the IOL are recorded in the **Perioperative Record** and in the hospital's log (for insertion of an implant), according to hospital policy.
- It is the circulator's responsibility to complete the manufacturer's forms for the IOL.

Secondary Lens Implant

Definition

Placement of an intraocular lens (IOL) implanted in an eye previously underwent cataract surgery without lens implantation or when an implantable contact lens (ICL) is inserted in the patient, retaining the natural crystalline lens.

Discussion

Aphakia (absence of a lens) may be corrected with aphakic glasses (only for binocular aphakia) or with corrective ICL for monocular aphakia or preferably with a **secondary lens implant**, e.g., IOL implant. When patients have a refractive error severe enough not to be correctible by external lenses, an aphakic ocular lens may be placed in the anterior or posterior chamber. The crystalline lens is not removed so that the patient retains any preexisting ability to focus.

Procedure

Pilocarpine drops are instilled to constrict the pupil, open the drainage canal, and increase the rate of fluid exiting the eye; this also reduces IOP. The conjunctiva is exposed at the limbus with a 5- to 6.5-mm incision into the corneal scleral junction with a keratome. Healon or other viscoelastic vitreous substitute and Miochol-E 1%/acetylcholine chloride (with mannitol) are placed in the anterior chamber lens (see below for directions to reconstitute Miochol-E). The implant, a folded contact lens, e.g., STAAR Vision ICL (phakic IOL), is slid into position between the iris and the crystalline lens with forceps (e.g., Charlie) and/or hook (e.g., Sinskey). The corneal wound is closed as in ***cataract extraction*** surgery (see p. 907). An IOL can be placed in the posterior chamber via a small incision (3.2 mm) by employing a corneal tunnel approach.

For **Preparation of the Patient, Skin Preparation, Draping, and Instrumentation,** see ***Cataract Extraction,*** pp. 909–910.

Equipment

Lift sheet or Hoyer pad placed on the operating table
Padded, foam, or gel headrest, e.g., donut
Fiber-optic operating microscope, e.g., Zeiss
Sitting stools

Add to Instrumentation

Caliper, ICL (e.g., STAAR Vision)

Supplies

Basin set
Sterile, plastic adhesive drape

Cellulose sponges
Wet-field bipolar ophthalmic diathermy (e.g., Solan), disposable
Beaver blade, #69, Super blade 30°, or diamond knife
BSS
Control syringes, hypodermic needles, medicine cups, labels, and marking pen
Tubercular syringe and 30-gauge cannula (for local block anesthetic when replacing retrobulbar injection)
Dressing: eye pad and shield

Medications

Xylocaine/lidocaine 2% with epinephrine or Marcaine/bupivacaine 0.5% with epinephrine for retrobulbar block, control syringe, and hypodermic needle, or Xylocaine/lidocaine 2% (without preservatives) for local block anesthetic when replacing retrobulbar injection (use tubercular syringe, and 30-gauge cannula)
Betinosol/betametasone 0.1% ophthalmic drops is a corticosteroid, anti-inflammatory agent
Celestone Soluspan/betametasone sodium phosphate is a glucocorticoid, anti-inflammatory agent
Wydase/hyaluronidase is an enzyme used to increase absorption and dispersion of other drugs
Miochol-E 1%/acetylcholine chloride (with mannitol), a miotic agent used to irrigate and rapidly constrict the pupil, must be reconstituted *immediately* before use. It is reconstituted by mixing a lyophilized sterile powder with the ampule of diluent; a luer-lok type filter hub (5μ) is required for administration. The blister pack contains the powder, diluent, syringe, and hub filter.
Healon 1% /sodium hyaluronate, viscoelastic vitreous substitute that can act as a tamponade (supplied in sterile syringe), administered with 27 gauge cannula
Discovisc or DisCoVisc is a viscoelastic system
Sodium chondroitin sulfate and sodium hyaluronate, viscosurgical agent, (supplied in 1 ml syringe)

Special Notes

- Apply **Special Notes** from ***Cataract Extraction***, p. 911, as applicable.
- **N.B. Reminder:** *A lift sheet or Hoyer pad for a mechanical lift is placed on the table before the patient is positioned on the table; either may be used to transfer the*

patient from the table to the gurney postoperatively. The patient is ***not*** permitted to assist in the transfer to the gurney, as the action may increase IOP.

- When local anesthetic is used to replace the retrobulbar injection, e.g., lidocaine (**without preservative**) is used; it is injected into the anterior chamber with a tubercular syringe and a 30-gauge cannula.
- **N.B. Reminder:** *The scrub person should reconstitute Miochol-E 1%/acetylcholine chloride immediately before use; it must be administered through a (5 μ) filter; see above for directions to reconstitute.*
- **Reminder:** Wearing a protective face shield or goggles is required to protect those persons scrubbed from the splashing of irrigation fluid, blood, etc.
- **Reminder:** *All safety precautions for laser must be enforced, e.g., protective goggles, special laser-safe instrumentation, etc.* Safety precautions are documented in the **Perioperative Record** for patient safety and medicolegal reasons.
- **Reminder:** Documentation by the circulator regarding the date, patient's name, brand name, type, size, and serial numbers of the IOL is recorded in the **Perioperative Record** and in the hospital's log (for insertion of an implant), according to hospital policy.
- It is the circulator's responsibility to complete the manufacturer's forms for the IOL.

Extraction of an Intraocular Foreign Body

Definition

Removal of a foreign material from the eye.

Discussion

Extraction of an intraocular foreign body is often related to an on-the-job injury. Foreign bodies within the eye should be identified, localized, and removed whenever possible. Particles of iron or copper are usually removed to prevent later disorganization of ocular tissues by degenerative changes (e.g., siderosis from iron; chalcosis and uveitis from dissolution of copper). Particles of glass or porcelain may be tolerated indefinitely and are usually better left alone. Vegetable matter such as wood and cloth are far more dangerous, as they can potentially result in endophthalmitis. Cultures must be obtained. Documentation of the procedure, including the particular handling and disposition of the foreign body, must be made. Following extraction of the foreign body, visual testing of both eyes should be performed and documented. Tetanus prophylaxis must be considered. When the lens is damaged, removal and replacement are indicated (the latter as a delayed procedure, as necessary).

Several different methods may be used to localize intraocular foreign bodies, including ultrasonography and coronal CT scan of the orbits. The Berman metal locator, an electronic instrument, is useful in pinpointing an intraocular foreign body. The wand of the instrument can be sterilized and passed over the eye during surgery; it is particularly useful in locating nonmagnetic foreign bodies.

Note: The MRI is contraindicated for localization of metallic foreign bodies, as during scanning MRI produces a magnetic field in which the magnetized metallic foreign bodies can become high-velocity intraocular projectiles (with catastrophic results).

Procedure

When **extraction of an intraocular foreign body** is performed, the foreign body is not removed via the entry wound to avoid "redamaging" surrounding tissues. The anterior chamber is filled with BSS or a viscoelastic solution, e.g., Healon (see medications list below). Rare-earth metal foreign bodies are extracted with a metallic magnet 20-gauge needle. Nonmetallic foreign bodies are removed using intraocular forceps; care is taken not to "redamage" surrounding tissues. The specimen should be sent to the laboratory for culture and sensitivity.

If the foreign body is located anterior to the lens zonules, it is removed through a limbal incision placed in the anterior chamber at the limbus. A "lasso" procedure may be effective; a loop of suture (7-0 polypropylene) is passed through a cannula (22 gauge) to seize the foreign body fragment. If the foreign body is located behind the lens, anterior to the equator, it is removed through the area of pars plana nearest to the foreign body (less retinal damage is caused). If the foreign body is located posterior to the equator, it is removed through the pars plana by ***vitrectomy*** (p. 930) using intraocular forceps to avoid major choroidal hemorrhages from incisions into the posterior wall of the eyeball. This method may be used for both magnetic and nonmagnetic foreign bodies. Special forceps are available for grasping spherical pellets.

If the lens is damaged, it is removed; implantation of the lens will be delayed. When the foreign body is large or vitreal, the retina is protected. Should any area of the retina be damaged, it is treated with diathermy, photocoagulation, or endolaser coagulation to prevent retinal detachment. When the laser is employed, following laser safety precautions is mandatory; see p. 94.

A new approach employs diagnostic *x-ray spectrometry*. Nonmagnetic copper foreign bodies do not necessarily require removal; however, if there is any evidence of copper dissolution (disintegration) on serial examinations, the (copper) foreign bodies require removal.

For **Preparation of the Patient, Skin Preparation,** and **Draping,** see **Ophthalmic Surgery, General Information,** p. 870.

Equipment

Lift sheet or pad for Hoyer lifting device (placed on operating table)
Padded, foam, or gel headrest, e.g., donut
Magnifying loupes or slit lamp
Ophthalmoscope, direct and indirect
Bipolar wet-field diathermy unit, e.g., Solan, optional
Sitting stools
Berman metal locator console/unit, available
Argon laser, available

Instrumentation

Basic eye procedures tray
Cataract extraction and lens procedures tray, available
Bipolar wet-field diathermy forceps, e.g., Solan (or disposable)
Berman metal locator wand, available
Specialty forceps for grasping spherical pellets, available
Special magnets (e.g., electromagnet, rare-earth metal magnet), available

Supplies

Basin set
Sterile, plastic adhesive drape
BSS
Cellulose sponges, e.g., Weck
Beaver blade (ask regarding type/number)
Wet-field bipolar ophthalmic diathermy (e.g., Solan), disposable
Control syringes, hypodermic needles, medicine cups, labels, and marking pen

Medications (available)

Xylocaine/lidocaine 2% with epinephrine or Marcaine/bupivacaine 0.5% with epinephrine anesthetic for retrobulbar block
Celestone/betamethasone drops, corticosteroid, anti-inflammatory agent
Miochol-E 1%/acetylcholine chloride (with mannitol), a miotic agent used to irrigate and rapidly constrict the pupil, must be reconstituted *immediately* before use. To reconstitute, mix the lyophilized sterile powder with an ampule of diluent; a luer-lok type filter hub (5 μ) is required for administration (all components are supplied in a prepackaged blister pack)
Wydase/hyaluronidase, an enzyme used to increase absorption and dispersion of other drugs
Healon/sodium hyaluronate, a viscoelastic agent that acts as a tamponade; also may be used as a vitreous substitute

Antibiotic of choice, e.g., ophthalmic drops and/or intravenous administration

Dressing: eye pad and shield

Special Notes

- Apply **Special Notes** from ***Cataract Extraction***, p. 911, as applicable.
- **Reminder:** A lift sheet or a pad for the Hoyer mechanical lift is placed on the table before the patient is positioned on the table; either may be used to transfer the patient from the table to the gurney postoperatively. The patient is ***not*** permitted to assist in the transfer to the gurney, as the action may increase IOP.
- **Reminder:** *The scrub person should reconstitute acetylcholine chloride/Miochol-E 1% immediately before use; it must be administered through a 5μ filter. See above for directions to reconstitute.*
- **N.B.** The circulator should determine the type or category of the ocular foreign object (e.g., metal would require a magnet for extraction); he/she should ask the surgeon about the necessary extraction equipment, necessary laboratory tests to be performed on the foreign object, and deposition of the foreign object (e.g., dry or in formalin) and sent to pathology.
- **N.B.** The circulator must document that the foreign body was retrieved and sent to pathology for verification; identification of the object is documented in the **Perioperative Record** for patient safety (notifies others regarding identification and retrieval) and for medicolegal reasons.
- The scrub person and the circulator must be prepared to assist the surgeon in other ophthalmic procedures as necessary during the course of the surgical procedure, e.g., ***vitrectomy***, p. 930.
- **Reminder:** Applying all safety precautions when a laser is used is mandatory, e.g., wearing protective goggles and using ebonized instruments, etc. Documentation that all safety precautions were observed is recorded in the **Perioperative Record** for patient safety and medicolegal reasons.

Trabeculectomy

Definition

Establishment of an aqueous humor fistula between the anterior chamber and the subconjunctival space, employing a partial-thickness, limbal-based scleral flap with segmental removal of the trabecular meshwork to allow aqueous drainage.

Discussion

When glaucoma is present, increased IOP can damage the optic nerve and reduce the size of the field of vision, compromising vision. Glaucoma can be controlled medically by the instillation of various ophthalmic drops. In **trabeculectomy**, a "filtration" procedure, clogged channels of the trabecular network are bypassed; it is usually performed for narrow-angle and "open" wide-angle glaucoma (chronic) not adequately treated by medical management. A small portion of the "angle" area of the eye is removed, allowing aqueous humor to drain and flow into the subconjunctival space (forming a bleb) that can be absorbed systemically. Additional indications for **trabeculectomy** include posttraumatic angle recession glaucoma, post-keratoplasty glaucoma-induced obstruction (of the channels of the trabecular meshwork), and infantile glaucoma. **Trabeculectomy** may be performed in conjunction with ***cataract extraction*** (p. 907) and lens-replacement surgery (***secondary lens implant,*** p. 913). In certain cases, the ***iridectomy*** may be extended to allow the aqueous humor to flow into the vitreous body. These modalities are instituted to reduce IOP.

Laser trabeculoplasty may be performed in select cases to treat acute (angle-closure) glaucoma and open-angle glaucoma using an Argon or Nd:YAG laser. The laser beam is used to open the "angle" area of the eye to decrease IOP.

In selected cases, **laser trabeculectomy** using Nd:YAG, Ho:YAG, or Argon laser beam may remove scarified obstructing trabecular meshwork. A sponge containing 0.02% solution of mitomycin C (antimetabolite) may be applied between the sclera and the conjunctiva (for 5 minutes); any residual is well irrigated with BSS. Mitomycin C may act to suppress postoperative fibrosis and vascular in-growth that would compromise drainage; however, serious complications, such as endophthalmitis or hypotony have resulted from this modality. Similarly, the use of 5 FU (antimetabolite) has also been used as an adjunct to surgery. Observe special precautions for disposal of a metabolite (see directions below).

On October 13, 2005 the JC issued a statement to hospitals and health-care facilities regarding **General Policy (25493)** on medical management and handling of hazardous drug/waste spills, storage, and disposal. Upon an employee's hiring at a health-care facility, he/she is given information regarding hazardous waste, e.g., what constitutes hazardous waste, education regarding its disposal, measures to take for compliance-monitoring enforcement, and the exemptions to the policy. This policy elaborates how hospitals and health-care facilities must maintain reasonable precautions to protect employees and the public when it disposes of hazardous waste products. When an antimetabolite (hazardous waste) is used, special precautions regarding its disposal are observed.

- The circulator is required to wear gloves to draw-up the antimetabolite drug.
- All disposable items used in conjunction with the antimetabolite must be disposed of as hazardous waste.
- All instruments that come into contact with the antimetabolite must be isolated from the other instruments and washed separately.

As an alternative to **trabeculectomy**, a variety of tubal prostheses (valve implant) that drain the anterior chamber into the subconjunctival space have been used [e.g., the Ahmed glaucoma device that is pressure sensitive with unidirectional valve for IOP greater than 8 mm Hg, and, more recently, the Ex-PRESS® R50 glaucoma shunt (Optonol), a one-piece stainless steel translimbal implant].

Procedure

Trabeculectomy is described. Measures are taken to bring excessively high IOP into the satisfactory range, e.g., a pressure valve implant may be placed. A superior rectus bridle suture is placed. A limbal-based conjunctival flap is developed, under which a mitomycin C-containing sponge, if used, is placed; the area is irrigated after placement of the sponge for 3 to 5 minutes. Episcleral tissue is cleaned anteriorly, up to and including the corneoscleral sulcus. A caliper is used to measure the width of the flap on the globe. The scleral incision is outlined with a blade and then incised two-thirds its thickness. Atropine eye drops may be administered to dilate the pupil. The edge of the flap is developed with a blade (e.g., Beaver); care is taken not to penetrate the base of the flap. The flap is continued to the anterior junction of the conjunctiva and the cornea. A paracentesis track is placed with a sharp-tipped knife into the cornea (1 mm anterior to the limbus). An incision is made through the sclera, through which the iris will prolapse. ***Iridotomy*** is performed. (***Iridectomy*** is performed adjunctively as necessary.) The ophthalmic diathermy is applied for hemostasis. The scleral flap is sutured in place with fine sutures (e.g., 10-0 nonabsorbable). After two sutures are placed, the anterior chamber is filled with BSS or Healon (vitreous substitute) through the paracentesis track, as the IOP is monitored. As filtration is desired postoperatively, a subconjunctival filtering bleb is developed. A valve implant may be inserted. Antibiotic and steroid drops or ointment may be instilled, and an eye patch is placed.

For **Preparation of the Patient, Skin Preparation** and **Draping,** see **Cataract Extraction,** pp. 909–910.

Add to Preparation of the Patient

Ophthaine or tetracaine ophthalmic drops may be instilled. Facial and retrobulbar blocks may be administered. Lashes may be trimmed; check with the surgeon.

Equipment

Lift sheet or pad for Hoyer lifting device (placed on operating table)
Padded, foam, or gel headrest, e.g., donut
Bipolar wet-field diathermy unit, e.g., Solan, optional
Fiber-optic operating microscope, e.g., Zeiss, optional Laser slit-lamp (**laser trabeculectomy**), optional
Laser console unit, e.g., Nd:YAG, Ho:YAG, or Argon, e.g., Lumenis Selecta II®
Glaucoma Laser System, optional
Sitting stools

Instrumentation

Basic eye microscope procedures tray
Glaucoma procedures tray
Tonometer, caliper, retrieval instruments according to type of foreign object, e.g., magnets, optional
Glaucoma implant device for shunting aqueous, e.g., Ahmed glaucoma device or *Ex-PRESS R50 implant* or Bi Directional Glaucoma Implant (GMP Vision Solutions) with inserter, optional
Laser (Nd:YAG, Ho:YAG, or Argon) hand piece, cord, and tip

Supplies

Sterile, plastic adhesive drape
Topical anesthetic ophthalmic drops, e.g., tetracaine or Ophthaine/proparacaine
Local anesthetic, e.g., Marcaine/bupivacaine 0.5% with epinephrine, for facial and retrobulbar blocks
Control syringes, hypodermic needles, medicine cups, labels, and marking pen
Basin set
BSS, tears substitute
Cellulose sponges, e.g., Weck
Blades (e.g., #57 Beaver, 15° Super blade)
Bipolar wet-field diathermy forceps and cord, e.g., Solan or disposable unit
Dressing: eye pad and shield

Additional Medications

Mitomycin C or 5 FU, an antimetabolite contained in a sponge, optional; see **Special Notes** for directions to dispose of an antimetabolite, i.e., hazardous waste disposal. Healon/sodium hyaluronate is a viscoelastic agent that acts as a tamponade; also may be used as a **vitreous** substitute

Atropine ophthalmic drops, an anticholinergic agent that causes the pupil to dilate
Antibiotic ophthalmic drops or ointment

Special Notes

- Apply to **Special Notes** from ***Cataract Extraction***, p. 911, as applicable.
- **N.B. Reminder:** *A lift sheet or Hoyer pad for a mechanical lift is placed on the table before the patient is positioned on the table; either may be used to transfer the patient from the table to the gurney postoperatively.* The patient is ***not*** permitted to assist in the transfer to the gurney, as the action may increase IOP.
- **Note:** *Mitomycin C is an antimetabolite that prevents the conjunctiva from healing onto the sclera, thereby reducing the risk of surgery failure.* An adverse side effect is the increased risk of cataracts.
- **N.B.** *When an antimetabolite is used, special precautions regarding the disposal of hazardous waste material are mandatory; see* **laser trabeculectomy** *above in* **Discussion.**
- **Reminder:** All safety precautions are mandatory when a laser is used, e.g., wearing protective goggles, using special laser instruments that are ebonized, etc. Safety precautions are documented (as observed) in the **Perioperative Record** for patient safety and medicolegal reasons.

Excision of Pterygium

Definition

Removal of elevated, superficial (usually fibrovascular) external ocular mass that extends from the perilimbal conjunctiva onto the peripheral corneal surface.

Discussion

True pterygia are located in the interpalpebral zone, particularly on the medial aspect of the globe. Pterygia often occur bilaterally; they occur twice as often in males as females. Pterygium excision is usually postponed until the growth encroaches upon the visual axis (line of vision). Related tests include *visual acuity,* tested reading the Snellen eye chart; *keratotomy*, in which a keratometer is used to measure corneal curvature; *corneal topography*, in which a computer is used for corneal curvature analysis; *manifest refraction* procedure, in which refraction is determined, indicating the need for corrective lenses; a *phoropter* is used to evaluate each eye with retinoscopy; and testing with the *slit lamp,* a device with a moveable light and binocular microscope used to evaluate the anterior segment of the eye (and the posterior segment with additional special lenses). Indications for removal of pterygia include the following:

1. Inflammation of the eye that does not respond to topical medication
2. Growth of a pterygium so that it interferes with vision
3. A change in corneal contour associated with the growth of the pterygium
4. Cosmetic reasons, i.e., cosmesis.

Several different techniques are advocated for excision. Any lesion that is suspect is first biopsied; the tissue is sent to the laboratory for frozen section. Pterygia are frequently recurrent; different modalities may be employed to prevent or delay their formation, e.g., simple elliptical excision, excision with the placement of a sliding flap of conjunctiva or excision with the placement of a free graft of lamellar autologous conjunctiva, or excision with the placement of banked amniotic membrane grafts that may be transplanted to the denuded area and secured by fibrin tissue glue/adhesive (e.g., Tisseel Duo Quick®) or sutures. When the sclera is not covered, there is a greater chance for regrowth.

Postoperatively, preferably within 3 days, beta radiation (in fractional dosages up to a total of 30Gy or 3000 rad) may be administered. A subconjunctival injection of either metabolite mitomycin C or doxorubicin (0.1 ml of 0.15 mg/ml) may be administered to inhibit fibroblast proliferation 4 weeks prior to surgery. See ***trabeculectomy***, p. 919, for precautions regarding disposal of hazardous waste when an antimetabolite is used.

Procedure

Excision of Pterygium is described. A speculum is inserted. The head of the pterygium may be sharply dissected from the cornea and undermined toward the sclera by superficial stripping (or from sclera to cornea). Alternatively, an incision may be made above or below the pterygium, and a suture is passed under the body of the pterygium. With a sawing motion of the suture, the pterygium is stripped from the cornea as the suture is pulled medially. The corneoscleral limbus is made smooth with a Beaver or #15 blade. The pterygium can also be removed using an Argon laser beam. Hemostasis is achieved with the bipolar wet-field diathermy. With recurrent or large pterygia, every effort is made to carefully excise this tissue and to completely cover the bare sclera to prevent recurrence. If the denuded area is relatively large, direct suture repair of the conjunctiva is done, or grafting with an excised segment of conjunctiva or banked amniotic membrane may be required, as noted above. The graft is secured with stitches or with a fibrin tissue adhesive, according to the surgeon's preference.

Preparation of the Patient

Excision of pterygium may be performed with a topical anesthetic solution of cocaine 10%, subconjunctival injection of lidocaine, or retrobulbar injection of lidocaine, or a similar agent. See perioperative RN responsibilities regarding monitoring the patient receiving local anesthesia and providing *conscious sedation*, as directed by the surgeon, p. 74.

For further **Preparation of the Patient, Skin Preparation,** and **Draping,** see **Ophthalmic Surgery, General Information,** p. 870.

Equipment

Padded, foam, or gel headrest, e.g., donut
Fiber-optic operating microscope, e.g., Zeiss, optional
Laser slit lamp (binocular microscope), optional
Laser console, e.g., Argon, optional
Autoref topography autorefractor, e.g., RT 6000 (TOMEY)
Sitting stools

Instrumentation

Basic eye microscope procedures tray
Keratometer, phoropter
Laser hand piece, for Argon beam, coupler, and cord, optional

Supplies

Sterile, plastic adhesive drape
Topical anesthetic ophthalmic drops, e.g., tetracaine Xylocaine/lidocaine, a local anesthetic used for subconjunctival and retrobulbar blocks
Control syringes, hypodermic needles, medicine cups, labels, and marking pen
Basin set
BSS, tear substitute
Sterile, plastic adhesive drape
Blades, (1) #15, and Beaver, (1) #57 or (1) #64
Cellulose sponges, e.g., Weck
Bipolar wet-field diathermy (disposable), e.g., Solan
Fibrin tissue glue used to seal the transplant (e.g., Tisseel Duo Quick), optional
Hydrocortisone ophthalmic ointment
Eye pad dressing and shield

Medications include

TheraTears Liquid gel and TheraTears Nutrition, with flaxseed oil, etc., used as optic lubricating agents

Xylocaine/lidocaine, anesthetic agent (local injection)
Cocaine 10%, anesthetic agent (topical)
Prednisolone acetate 1% drops, a topical corticosteroid suspension used to reduce significant inflammation, not relieved by topical lubricants
Mitomycin C or doxorubicin, antimetabolites used to inhibit fibroblast proliferation
Hydrocortisone ophthalmic ointment, an anti-inflammatory agent, optional

Special Notes

- Apply **Special Notes** from *Trabeculectomy*, p. 922, as applicable.
- The circulator should ask the surgeon in advance whether banked amniotic membrane is needed for grafting; he/she is responsible for obtaining the graft material.
- The graft may be secured with sutures or fibrin tissue glue may be used (e.g., Tisseel Duo Quick). When not specified on the doctor's card, Tisseel or similar agent should be available in the room.
- **N.B. Reminder:** *When antimetabolite (e.g., mitomycin C or doxorubicin) is used, special precautions regarding the disposal of hazardous waste material are mandatory; see* ***Special Notes*** *from* ***trabeculectomy,*** *p. 922, for directions.*
- **Reminder:** All safety precautions are mandatory when a laser is used, e.g., wearing protective goggles, using special laser instruments that are ebonized, etc. Safety precautions are documented (as observed) in the **Perioperative Record** for patient safety and medicolegal reasons.

Repair of Retinal Detachment/Scleral Buckling

Definition

Compression of the globe and buckling the sclera to seal or repair a linear defect in the retina by inciting an inflammatory reaction adjacent to the defect.

Discussion

Repair of retinal detachment by means of scleral buckling is necessary when the neural retinal layer becomes detached from its underlying pigmented layer, either because of a defect in the retina or by accumulation of fluid behind the retina; serious visual disturbance results (primarily due to deprivation of local blood supply). The major symptom of retinal detachment is the sudden appearance of "flashing lights." Inciting events that will cause retinal detachment are tumor of the choroid, trauma to the retina, and degeneration of the retina.

Vitreous humor, blood, or tissue may accumulate between the retinal and the choroid layers. Treatment consists of repositioning the retina at the site of the detachment, sealing the retinal defect, and draining the subretinal fluid. Repair of the retinal detachment is made by sealing the defect (detachment); it is an emergency surgery because the retina gets most of its blood supply from blood vessels in the wall of the eye and when detached, the cells in the retina begin to die. Early diagnosis and repair are urgent, as greater visual improvement occurs before the macula becomes devascularized.

Several different modalities may be employed to effect closure of the defect(s), e.g., the application of a cryoprobe to the sclera overlying the retinal defect creates an inflammatory reaction that seals the defect. Similarly, the heat from a laser (Ho:YAG or Tm:YAG) can be used to create an inflammatory reaction, sealing the defects. If holes in the retina are discovered before detachment occurs, the holes can be sealed in a noninvasive laser procedure. If detachment has recently begun, a repair procedure, **pneumatic retinopexy,** may be possible. To achieve reattachment of the retina, the globe is encircled with a band of silicone that is sutured to maintain the buckle of the sclera. The **scleral buckle** acts to decrease the potential space in which unwanted fluids can accumulate. In **pneumatic retinopexy**, a bubble of air, or inert colorless, odorless, nontoxic expandable gas [e.g., sulfur hexafluoride (SF_6) or perfluoropropane (C_3F_8) or silicone oil (e.g. ADATO SIL-ol 5000™)] is injected into vitreous body; the air bubble is positioned by rotating the eye (or the patient) to apply local tamponade effect over the detachment. After the insertion of one of the previously noted agents, a laser or cryoprobe can be used to seal the defect, following removal of any fluid accumulation. Air or the gases, as noted, are absorbed; silicone oil usually is removed up to a year following the procedure. Silicone oil should ***not*** be used if a silicone IOL is placed. This modality may suffice alone or be used in combination with ***scleral buckling*** (and ***vitrectomy***, p. 930).

Procedure

Repair of Retinal Detachment is described.

Photocoagulation laser application with an Argon laser may be used to seal a discrete retinal defect that is not surrounded by a retinal detachment; this treatment may be performed in the "eye laboratory" rather than the OR. The defect is exposed under direct visualization with an indirect ophthalmoscope, and a cryoprobe may be applied on the preoperatively mapped-out section of the globe overlying the defect. The conjunctiva and Tenon's capsule are incised. A cryoprobe is applied to the area to create adhesions to seal the defect. The surgeon controls this maneuver as the eye is viewed through a head-mounted ophthalmoscope, while the assistant (or the surgeon) depresses the sclera with the cryoprobe applied against the defect. An incision is made to evacuate the subretinal fluid accumulations, and a preplaced suture is tied at the site of the incision.

The **scleral buckling** is achieved by incising a groove around the equator of the globe, undermining the edges of the groove, and placing a Silastic band in the groove. The band may be secured with multiple mattress sutures or other Silastic components (see instrumentation below) that also close the groove. The Silastic band is then tightened around the globe to effect the buckling to maintain the retinal layers in apposition. A silicone tire wedge may be used under the band to exert additional pressure to assure the proper degree of buckling of the sclera; air or replacement fluids may be inserted after the subretinal fluid is drained. On occasion, one (or more) of the extraocular muscles must be retracted (or transiently detached) to provide adequate exposure. Partial, rather than circumferential, buckling is done for limited presentations. The conjunctiva is closed. An antibiotic may be injected subconjunctivally; antibiotic ophthalmic drops or ointment may be instilled. An eye-pad dressing is placed. When the vitreous contains opacities, hemorrhagic debris, etc., ***vitrectomy*** (p. 930) is usually done prior to the **scleral buckling** phase of the procedure.

Preparation of the Patient

General anesthesia is most often employed; local block with monitored *conscious sedation* administered by an anesthesia provider may be used in selected patients.

For further **Preparation of the Patient, Skin Preparation,** and **Draping,** see **Ophthalmic Surgery, General Information**, p. 870.

Add to Draping

Additional drapes for the microscope and the cryosurgical unit (and any other equipment, as necessary

Equipment

- Padded, foam, or gel headrest, e.g., donut
- Fiber-optic operating microscope, e.g., Zeiss
- Bipolar wet-field diathermy unit, e.g., Solan, optional
- Cryosurgical unit, Frigitonics, optional
- Laser console for Ho:YAG, Tm:YAG, Argon, or photodynamic system, optional
- Sitting stools

Instrumentation

- Basic eye microscope procedures tray
- Retinal procedures tray
- Tonometer and weights
- Bipolar wet-field diathermy forceps, e.g., Solan, optional

Cryosurgical retinal probes (Frigitonics), curved and straight with rubber covering, and cords

Lens (handheld)

Laser (Ho:YAG or Tm:YAG, Argon, or photodynamic) hand piece, probe, and cord

Scleral buckling implant/prostheses, e.g., Silastic bands, boats, sleeves, tantalum clips, radial wedges, flat strips, tires, meridionals, and/or Silicone sponges (Mira®) and other accessories should be readily available for immediate use, as needed

Supplies

Basin set

Sterile, plastic adhesive drape

BSS, tear substitute

Cellulose sponges, e.g., Weck

Bipolar wet-field diathermy, disposable, optional

Beaver blade,(1) #69 or (1) #59

Medications

Betinosol/betametasone 0.1% ophthalmic drops is a corticosteroid, anti-inflammatory agent

Celestone/Soluspan/betametasone sodium phosphate is a glucocorticoid, anti-inflammatory agent

Wydase/hyaluronidase is an enzyme used to increase absorption and dispersion of other drugs

Miochol-E 1%/acetylcholine chloride (with mannitol), a miotic agent used to irrigate and rapidly constrict the pupil, must be reconstituted *immediately* before use. It is reconstituted by mixing a lyophilized powder with an ampule of diluent and administered in a syringe with a luer-lock 5μ filter hub. All components (powder, diluent, syringe, and filter) are included in a blister pack.

Healon/sodium hyaluronate is viscoelastic vitreous humor substitute (the agent can act as a tamponade)

Discovisc ophthalmic viscosurgical device, or Duovisc viscoelastic system

Antibiotic subcutaneous injection, optional

Antibiotic and steroid ophthalmic drops or ointment, optional

Eye-pad dressing

Special Notes

- Apply **Special Notes** from ***Trabeculectomy***, p. 922, as applicable.
- **N. B.** The circulator should consult the surgeon regarding the type of laser (Ho:YAG, Tm:YAG, Argon, or photodynamic system) to be used.

- The surgeon chooses the implant/prostheses, e.g., Silastic band, scleral sponge, and accessories, etc., that will be used prior to the procedure. Before the surgeon scrubs, he/she chooses the necessary components; a variety of components should be available in the room prior to bringing the patient into the room.
- The ophthalmoscope lens may be soaked in Steris® 20 solution for 12 minutes to achieve sterilization. To sterilize the lens, it must be totally submerged; the solution must be prepared in the container available from the manufacturer, according to directions. Refer to techniques for sterilization, p. 43.
- The implants/prostheses (e.g., scleral buckles, etc.) are usually soaked in antibiotic solution after being flash-autoclaved.
- Any optical equipment (e.g., cryosurgical unit, etc.) is checked to ensure working order prior to the procedure. Both the scrub person and the circulator should know how to use the special optical equipment prior to participating in the surgery.
- **N.B.** The surgeon may request the anesthesia provider to administer acetazolamide/Diamox to reduce IOP; the circulator should have the drug in the room prior to the surgery.
- **N.B.** The ophthalmoscope may be handled using a sterile plastic barrier covering made specifically for the purpose.
- Sterile back vests can be used to aid in maintaining sterility of the field for those persons whose back may be facing the sterile field.
- The scrub person must mix the Michol-E 1% solution *immediately* before use; to prepare the solution see directions above.
- **Reminder:** When any of the lasers is used during the procedure (e.g., Endo Optiks® E2 Compact Microprobe Laser and Endoscopy System), all laser safety precautions are mandatory, such as wearing protective goggles, using special laser-safe instruments, etc.; see p. 94. Laser safety precautions are documented (as observed) in the **Perioperative Record** to assure patient safety and for medicolegal reasons.
- **N.B.** When a sulfur hexafluoride (SF_6) or perfluoropropane (C_3F_8) bubble has been placed, special precautions must be observed. The patient must wear a wristband indicating that he/she has had this specific treatment; if the patient requires surgery, he/she must inform the anesthesia provider, as the gas mixes with nitrous oxide to expand it, causing IOP.
- The scrub person should be prepared for culture and sensitivity to be done prior to closure; the circulator prepares the requisition for culture and sensitivity, stating the exact location from which the culture was taken.

Vitrectomy

Definition

Partial or total removal of vitreous humor.

Discussion

The vitreous humor is a clear gel body. In certain eye conditions in which the vitreous has become opacified, **vitrectomy**, once thought inoperable, is performed. When the gel of the vitreous humor becomes opaque, vision is decreased. The examining surgeon is unable to view the retina to adequately assess abnormalities. The vitreous humor may opacify secondary to retinal hemorrhage, as in diabetes or endophthalmitis; other etiologies include a foreign body lodged in the eye, trauma, and the formation of preretinal membranes. Opacification may also occur as a result of band formation following anterior chamber surgery (e.g., ***cataract extraction***); **vitrectomy** is performed to remove organized hemorrhagic areas or foreign matter to restore a clear visual pathway to the retina; restoring vision and correcting retinal disease.

The argon or YAG lasers may be used to lyse bands noninvasively, when applicable; see mandatory laser safety precautions, p. 94.

In the pars plana approach, three ports are established to accommodate an endoilluminator (light pipe), an infusion irrigator/aspirator, and a vitrector. A wide variety of microinstruments can be inserted via the vitrector cannula including an automated guillotine cutter, rotary cutter, vertical cutting scissors, laser fiber, cryoprobe, membrane pick, horizontal cutting scissors, endocoagulator, etc. A paralimbal incision may be used as well. An operating microscope is used in conjunction with an applied or sewn-on contact lens. If the view via the microscope is compromised, an endoscope with illuminator and camera (with the view projected on a monitor) is placed in lieu of the endoilluminator.

The Ocutome II has largely been replaced by Bausch and Lomb SV25, 2nd generation, DORC (Dutch Ophthalmic Research Center) system, and the Eckardt 23 gauge vitrectomy system. The 23 gauge system may be preferred over the 20 or 25 gauge diameters.

Procedure

A trans-pars plana vitrectomy (TPPV) employs three incisions (using a scleral plug cutter) in the pars plana (anterior to the attachment of the retina). The irrigator aspirator cannula may be secured with a 5-0 suture. The lens, if not already absent, is usually removed. Vitreous humor, if displaced into the anterior chamber during prior cataract extraction, is removed. Employing a variety of cutting, irrigating, and aspirating maneuvers, clearing of the diseased vitreous with its membranous bands and other opacities is accomplished. If a retinal tear is present, it is treated with a cryoprobe or endolaser, and/or a scleral buckle. A fibrin patch may be used to seal a "macular hole." During the procedure, BSS, sodium hyaluronate (Healon), a gas, e.g., sulfur hexafluoride (SE_6), or perfluoropropane (C_3E_8) is infused by catheter to replace vitreous volume loss and maintain tonicity to the globe. When tamponade is required for the associated retinal detachment, air, SE_6, C_3E_8, or silicone oil may be injected (see **Scleral Buckling,** p.925. Depending upon the size of instrumentation, the incisions may not require closure, or may be closed with 9-0 suture or scleral plugs. Antibiotics may be injected subconjunctivally. Antibiotic and steroid drops or ointment are instilled; an eye patch may be employed. The various phases of this procedure often takes two to three hours to complete.

Preparation of the Patient

Antiembolic hose are applied, as requested. The table may be turned 90° to facilitate the surgeon's access. The patient is in supine position with the table placed in slight reverse Trendelenburg; a padded, foam, or gel donut headrest may be employed, with the head turned to the side (affected side up) and the dependent ear well padded. A padded footrest may be secured to the table. One arm may be secured on a padded armboard and the contralateral arm padded and secured in at the patient's side, or both arms may be padded and secured at the patient's sides. A pillow may be placed under the knees to avoid straining lower back muscles, or the table may be flexed for comfort. All bony prominences and areas vulnerable to skin and neurovascular pressure or trauma are padded to avoid injury.

For **Skin Preparation** and **Draping,** see **Ophthalmic Surgery, General Information,** p. 870.

Add to Draping

Drape for the Vitrector console, microscope, and other equipment, as necessary. Small ophthalmic incise drape with fluid collecting pouch, e.g., 3 M 1023.

Equipment

Padded, foam, or gel headrest, e.g., donut

Fiber-optic operating microscope with zoom lens and fine focus capability, e.g., Zeiss (high resolution) with XY coupling (motorized), optional **Binocular Indirect Ophthalmo Microscope (BIOM®),** a noncontact wide-angle panoramic viewing system attaches to the microscope, optional

Photocoagulator (laser) system

Directional endophoto coagulator laser console

Cryosurgical unit, CryoStar 1500 III with phacopump vitrectomy system console

Endoilluminator fiber-optic light source, e.g., Xenon 75 W or DORC Brightstar system
Vitrectomy console (e.g., Eckardt 23 ga Vitrectomy System)
Sitting stools
Video monitor
VCR
Printer, CD burner, and camera console optional

Instrumentation

Basic eye procedures microscope tray
Retinal procedures tray
Basic eye procedures microscope tray
Retinal procedures tray
Precalibrated disposable knife, lens forceps, scleral plug removal forceps, caliper, vitreous cutters as horizontal scissors, automated guillotine and rotary cutters, vertical scissors, membrane pick, foreign body forceps
Laser probe 23 gauge (e.g., Alcon), and laser fiber and cable
CryoStar probe and cord
Self-blocking sutureless infusion cannula, 23 ga cannula tip
Vitrectomy lenses, e.g., planoconcave, flat, self-stabilizing, silicone, wide field panoramic, and lens occluder, available
Vitrectomy ring systems, variety of, e.g., 4 post or tall notched, optional
Sew-on lens with viscoelastic cushion
Endocoagulator and cord
Endoilluminator and cord
(Some instruments are disposable)

Supplies

Antiembolitic hose, optional
Basin set
Sterile, plastic adhesive drape
Cellulose sponges, e.g., Weck
I/A tubing pack
BSS, tear substitute
Eye pad dressing

Medications

Healon/sodium hyaluronate viscoelastic agent and physiologic buffer acts as a tamponade and **vitreous** substitute (supplied in glass syringe)
Acetylcholine chloride/Miochol-E 1% (with mannitol), used to constrict pupil; see **Special Notes** to reconstitute
Mydriacaine #2, to dilate pupil

Antibiotic subconjunctival injection, optional
Antibiotic and steroid ophthalmic drops or ointment, optional

Special Notes

- Apply **Special Notes** from *Excision of* **Chalazion**, p. 877, as applicable.
- **N.B.** *Prior to the procedure, the circulator and scrub person must be thoroughly familiar with the specialty equipment used for vitrectomy.*
- The working order of equipment (according to brand) that is necessary to perform the vitrectomy must be thoroughly checked by the scrub person and the circulator prior to the procedure.
- Most microscope lenses can be autoclaved.
- **N.B.** The infusion cannula is primed with the surgeon's choice of solution; air bubbles are removed.
- **N.B.** Rates (cutting, infusion, and aspiration) are adjusted on the vitrectomy console unit according to the surgeon's preference.
- **N.B.** Culture of the vitreous washings may be done; the scrub person should be prepared with a sterile container (e.g., capped test tube).
- **Reminder:** Wearing a protective face shield is required to protect those persons scrubbed from the splashing of irrigation fluid, blood, etc.
- **N.B. Reminder:** The scrub person should reconstitute acetylcholine chloride/Miochol-E 1% (with mannitol) *immediately* before use. It is reconstituted by mixing the lyophilized powder with an ampule of diluent; it must be administered through the 5μ filter hub. A blister pack includes the powder, diluent, syringe, and filter hub.

Refractive Keratoplasty Procedures

Definition

Procedures that reshape the cornea to alter its refractive power.

Discussion

The prevalence of **Photo-Refractive Keratectomy** and similar laser procedures, although usually performed in the surgeon's office, requires a limited presentation of information for the perioperative RN and the surgical technologist. These procedures require the patient's cooperation as he or she focuses his or her gaze while being observed through the operating microscope. Topical and local anesthetics may be employed; *conscious sedation* is used infrequently.

Photo-Refractive Keratectomy (PRK) refers to excimer laser procedures to correct or improve conditions of vision, such as myopia, hyperopia, astigmatism, aphakia, and keratoconus. Excimer lasers (second- and third-generation) produce a "cool" light beam that does not damage surrounding tissue; high-energy photons break the molecular bonds a few layers at a time. In *myopia or "nearsightedness"* (inherited), the cornea is too curved or the globe is too long; light focuses on the front of the cornea, making distance vision blurry. In *hyperopia or "farsightedness"* (inherited or occurring due to aging), the cornea is too flat in relation to the globe; light focuses at a point beyond the retina, making close vision blurry. In *astigmatism* (inherited or acquired, e.g., conditions such as lid swelling, corneal scars, or *keratoconus*), the cornea is curved more in one direction; light focuses in more than one point on the retina, resulting in distorted and blurry vision at all distances. Astigmatism often occurs with myopia and hyperopia. In *presbyopia*, there is unequal curvature of the surfaces of the cornea; the lens has lost its flexibility and it is difficult to focus on close objects and to adjust the focus of vision. **Radial keratotomy (RK)** has been performed to correct myopia. The center of the cornea is flattened by microscopic incisions (employing a diamond knife) made outside the central optical zone. The outer perimeter of the cornea is weakened, causing it to flatten; the point of focus is moved from in front of the retina to a position on the retina. The excimer laser has largely replaced RK with its greater accuracy. Following PRK, in addition to optical medications, a clear contact lens is placed as part of the postoperative dressing.

LASIK (laser in-situ keratomileusis) removes tissue within the cornea to treat low to high levels of "nearsightedness" (myopia), "farsightedness" (hyperopia), presbyopia, and "astigmatism." LASIK uses the excimer laser to reshape the curvature of the cornea to eliminate refractive errors by cutting a corneal tissue flap beneath the surface of the cornea.

An automated micro-keratome is used to ablate the stromal bed under the created hinged flap to correct optical aberrations. *Wavefront mapping technology* is used as a guide, as light is bounced off the retina to provide an accurate, three-dimensional image of the retina. Considerations include the following: patient selection has limitations, the risk of cornea ectasia (distension), and the wavefront sensor may have intrinsic errors.

LASEK (laser-assisted subepithelial keratectomy) combines elements of PRK and LASIK and may have advantages over both. Instead of removing tissue, the corneal epithelium is loosened with an alcohol solution prior and moved aside. The surface under the epithelial layer is ablated by laser (photoablation), and the epithelium is returned to the original position. Compared to PRK, corneal ectasia is reduced, but local pain and recovery are longer than compared to LASIK, and chance of corneal haze is greater.

Conductive keratoplasty (CK) uses controlled release of radio-frequency energy into the stroma (third layer of the cornea). The temperature of the corneal tissue is increased, making the cornea steeper, strengthening the focusing power to treat presbyopia. It is safer than LASIK because no laser is used and no tissue is removed. In "*monovision*," one eye (usually most dominant) is corrected for clear distance vision and the other for clear near vision. "*Monovision*" can be achieved with contact lenses or by a corrective procedure. The brain filters out the vision from either eye that is not clear. Not everyone is able to do this. In contrast, only one eye is corrected with CK for "*blended vision*"; both eyes see at all distances together. Although only one eye is multi-focal, the result is the ability to see things near better. Most people can adjust to "*blended vision*" better than "*monovision*." It is used to treat age-related hyperopia and presbyopia.

Laser Thermal Keratoplasty (LTK) is done with a noncontact laser to change the shape of the cornea, making it steeper. The steeper curvature increases the cornea's focusing power; images are brought into better focus on the retina. LTK can reduce or eliminate hyperopia.

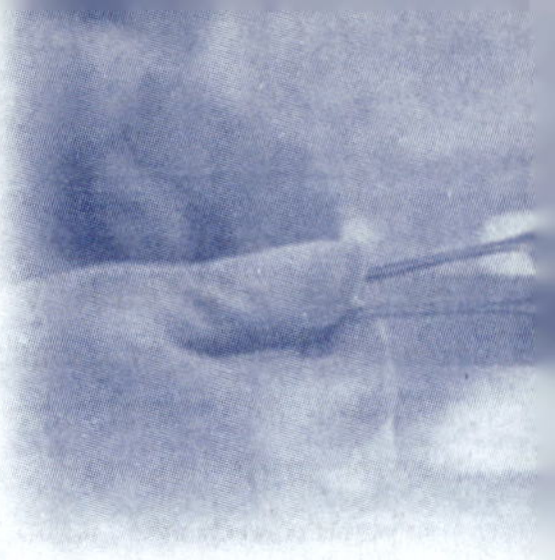

CHAPTER 29
Dental Surgery

Dental Extraction/Odontectomy

Definition
Removal of a tooth or teeth.

Discussion
Dental Extraction/Odontectomy is indicated when a tooth cannot be restored or when it interferes with proper occlusion. Tooth extraction may also be indicated if the tooth is impacted, fractured/broken, or irreversibly diseased. An *impacted tooth* is one that has failed to erupt through the gingival line due to its position or the position of other teeth. Gingivitis usually results from excessive dental caries due to poor oral hygiene or trauma and/or laceration of the gingiva. Diagnosis is made following visual and digital oral examination as well as with panoramic x-rays.

While dental extraction is most often performed in a dental office, the oral surgeon may prefer to bring the patient to the operating room (OR) when there is extensive degeneration of the tooth that extends to include involvement of the gingiva and periodontal ligaments; when the patient has a bleeding problem (e.g., hemophilia or other blood dyscrasia); when the patient is extremely frightened, agitated, or uncooperative; or when general anesthesia is required. An additional reason to perform the extraction in surgery is when the patient presents with a large locally invasive oral lesion surrounding the tooth that must also be excised.

Some oral surgeons prefer to bring their own dental supplies, equipment, and dental assistant to the OR.

Procedure
Dental Extraction is described. Local anesthesia with *conscious sedation* or general endotracheal anesthesia may be employed. A bite block is inserted and a saline-moistened throat pack placed. Exposure is achieved with retractors, as necessary. The gum is injected with a local anesthetic containing epinephrine to relieve postoperative pain (even when general anesthesia is employed) and to decrease blood loss. A graduated probe is placed on the gingival (gum) line to evaluate the amount and degree of gingival damage. An elevator is used to push the gingiva away from the tooth. Mobility of the tooth is tested in a side-to-side and back-and-forth motion. Additional movements and instru-

mentation are used until the tooth is ready to be extracted from its tooth (alveolar) socket with extraction forceps. Following extraction, the alveolar socket is packed with 2 × 2 gauze. When necessary, the base may be drilled to remove any portion of the tooth that remains in the bone. The tooth may require removal in sections, alternately using the drill, curettes, rongeurs, or osteotomes. If the tooth is impacted, the gingiva is incised and the soft tissue is dissected down to a level below the gingival line; pockets of plaque, calculus formation, debris, and inflamed soft tissue are also excised. The alveolar socket is irrigated and suctioned to remove any remaining debris. Direct pressure with gauze packing and/or Gelfoam® may be applied to the tooth socket to control bleeding; a nonasorbable suture may be necessary to achieve hemostasis. The oropharynx is suctioned, the throat pack is removed, and the patient is extubated. Prior to leaving the OR, the patient's face is washed free of blood.

An icepack may be ordered.

Preparation of the Patient

Dental Extraction may be performed using local anesthetic block, general anesthesia with endotracheal intubation supplemented by local injection, or local anesthetic supplemented with *conscious sedation*. The local anesthetic solution contains epinephrine to reduce bleeding; it is also effective for immediate postoperative pain control (as per above).

The table may be turned 90° or the table may be reversed with the patient's head at the foot of the table to facilitate the surgeon's access to the patient. The patient is in supine position; a padded, foam, or gel donut headrest may be employed to stabilize the head. A roll may be placed under the shoulders to facilitate tilting the head upward. One arm may be extended on a padded armboard and the contralateral arm is padded and tucked in at the patient's side, or both arms may be padded and tucked in at the patient's sides. When local anesthesia alone (with or without *conscious sedation*) is administered, the patient's arms are padded and secured with restraints to keep the patient's hands off the surgical field while maintaining good circulation of the extremities. A pillow may be placed under the knees to avoid straining lower back muscles, or the table may be flexed for comfort. All bony prominences and areas vulnerable to skin and neurovascular pressure or trauma are padded to avoid injury. Apply electrosurgical dispersive pad if dental ESU or monopolar ESU will be used.

Skin Preparation

No prep is usually required. Procedures involving the oral cavity are considered "clean"; they are not sterile, as the oral cavity is part of the gastrointestinal tract. The best aseptic technique possible is observed.

While in the preoperative area, the oral surgeon may request a patient brush his/her teeth and gingiva and rinse the mouth with an oral antiseptic (e.g., Peridex®). When local anesthesia alone (with or without conscious sedation) is employed, the patient may be requested to rinse his/her mouth with the oral antiseptic (e.g., Peridex) in the OR. Antibiotic optical ointment may be instilled in the patient's eyelids to keep the eyes moist (only when general anesthesia is employed). Vaseline® may be applied to the patient's lips to prevent their drying.

Draping

Draping is optional, according to the surgeon's preference. Gloves are worn.

The patient may be draped with a "head drape" (drape sheet and two towels under the head, with the uppermost towel wrapped around the head and clipped). The body is covered with a drape sheet.

Optional Draping

Disposable drapes: the head is draped with a disposable sheet, placing the adhesive strip at the forehead. Two folded towels (V-shape) are placed at the patient's neck, and the body is covered with a U or split drape sheet.

Equipment

Padded, foam, or gel headrest (e.g., doughnut)
Extremity restraints, padded (local anesthesia)
Power source for high-speed dental drill, optional, infrequent
Fiber-optic headlight and fiber-optic light source, e.g., Xenon 300™ W, optional
Dental irrigation system with fiber-optic light source, e.g., Dyna-Surg I or Dyna-Surg II (Intl Dental), optional
Suction source (separate)
ESU, monopolar, infrequent
Dental ESU, e.g., Rotex® or Radiosurg® with foot pedal activation (most often used) with an electrosurgical dispersive (grounding) pad

Instrumentation

Dental instruments for extractions tray
Limited procedures tray, available, unopened
Tracheostomy tray and various-sized tracheostomy tubes in the room, unopened
Dental drill (high-speed) handpiece with diamond coated drills, burrs, and cord
Monopolar electrosurgical pencil (disposable) or dental electrosurgical handpiece, tip, and cord (nondisposable), optional

Supplies

Antiseptic mouthwash, e.g., Peridex
Ophthalmic ointment (e.g., antibiotic) to keep eyes moist (general anesthesia only)
Lubrication for the lips, e.g., Vaseline
Local anesthetic, e.g., lidocaine with epinephrine for dental block and to decrease bleeding
Control syringe and hypodermic needle(s) or Vibra-ject® with shield, medicine cups, labels, and marking pen
Small basins (2)
Throat pack (gauze, with radio-opaque thread)
Tubing (2) for suction and irrigation or dual suction and irrigation tubing (prepackaged)
Irrigating solution, e.g., for Dyna–Surg I or DynaSurg II (sterile water)
Bulb syringe and normal saline, optional
Blade, #15
Needle magnet or counter
Sponges, e.g., gauze 2 × 2
Cotton dental rolls or dental pellets
Defogger for dental mirror, e.g., FRED®, Defog®, or ELVIS®
Bone wax, optional
Electrosurgical pencil (disposable), cord, scraper, and holder, optional (infrequent)
Gelfoam and/or packing, e.g., ¼″ gauze may be used for hemostasis
Suture (nonabsorbable) for hemostasis

Special Notes

- Apply **Special Notes** from Excision of ***Submandibular Gland***, p. 849, as applicable.
- **N.B. Reminder:** It is important for *Universal Protocol* and "*time-out*" to be implemented prior to the start of the surgery. The patient must be correctly identified and the correctly identified tooth (must be marked prior to surgery).
- **Reminder:** Ascertain that the *correct* x-ray films for the *correctly identified* patient are in the room prior to starting the surgery, or the surgeon may bring the patient's films.
- **N.B.** As the surgery can be painful, the circulator may convey (even more than is usual) emotional support to the patient. Nursing assessment and documentation is made in the **Perioperative Record** regarding the patient's anxiety level, the nursing meas-

ures employed, such as maintaining eye contact, using touch to convey caring, etc. (interventions), and the expected outcomes.

- **Reminder:** If an anesthesia provider is not in attendance, a perioperative RN, in addition to the circulator, must be present to monitor the patient and to administer *conscious sedation* at the surgeon's direction; see responsibilities of the perioperative RN monitoring the patient, p. 74.
- When the table is not reversed, the anesthesia provider may move the anesthesia machine and equipment to the side of the table to provide the surgeon with comfortable access to the patient's head.
- **N.B.** *Care must be taken by those scrubbed to protect the patient's face and eyes from injury when instruments are handled and/or passed.* A towel may be placed across the patient's eyes when local anesthesia is employed.
- **N.B.** Protective eye goggles may be placed on the patient to avoid getting a foreign object in the eye and to deflect the light.
- The circulator should be certain that there are two working suction sources in the room before the patient enters the room.
- The oral surgeon often will bring his/her instruments that require autoclaving (steam sterilization under pressure) or other methods of sterilization to the OR; see sterilization techniques, p. 41.
- **N.B. Reminder:** *A protective face shield or goggles should be worn by those scrubbed to prevent the patient's secretions from spraying into the eyes, nose, or mouth of team members.*
- The scrub person and the circulator should be familiar with the names of the dental instruments on the dental instrument tray at their hospital, or they may refer to the suggested dental instruments, p. 1176.
- The scrub person and the circulator should count the dental instruments together before the procedure; the instruments (and their intrinsic parts) must be included in the final count.
- The scrub person and the circulator should check that the dental drill and irrigator/aspirator are in good working order before starting the procedure, e.g., how to operate the high-speed drill and the suction-irrigation and aspiration system.
- Usually, during drilling, the alveolar socket is simultaneously irrigated and aspirated. The scrub person may be requested to assist the oral surgeon during the procedure. Care is taken to direct the water (irrigation) onto the area being drilled (to avoid

a build up of heat) while it is simultaneously suctioned, if the drill does not have a port for water.

- **N.B.** When possible, the scrub person should place the instruments on the tray in the order they will be used. Consult the surgeon's preference card for this information.
- To prevent the dental mirror from fogging up, the scrub person wipes the mirror with FRED, Defog, ELVIS, etc.
- **N.B. Reminder:** The throat pack, a dry gauze pad with radio-opaque thread, should be moistened with normal saline before it is placed in the throat to avoid injury to the mucous membranes.
- The scrub person and the circulator are required to include the throat pack in the sponge count.
- **Reminder:** *The throat pack must be removed before the patient is extubated to prevent its aspiration.*
- *The OR team may need a reminder to remember to remove the throat pack at the end of the procedure, e.g., a hemostat swinging from the corner of the Mayo stand is often used to serve that purpose.*

Dental Restoration with Implants

Definition

Dental restoration with implants involves the removal of a damaged or diseased tooth (or teeth) and the insertion of an implant (device) into alveolar bone, to which a dental prosthesis is secured on an immediate or delayed venue.

Discussion

The results of oral visual, digital, panoramic x-ray, and computerized topography are all necessary for complete diagnostic examination to evaluate the extent of dental damage and to determine the possibility of **dental restoration with dental implants.** The purpose of the implant is to provide for support and retention of the prosthesis; the dental fixture (restoration) is placed for function as well as cosmesis. The dental fixture actually helps to preserve the remaining bone and prevent further deterioration that occurs with missing teeth. For patients with healthy gums (gingiva) and adequate bone availability in the mandible or maxilla, a stabilized dental implant can be placed by directly fusing the implant into the bone. No longer is a series of treatments over an extended period of 4 to 6 months necessarily required for the completed restoration to be achieved. Some treatment protocols have drastically reduced or eliminated the amount of time necessary for *osseointegration* between implant placement and restoration.

Individual teeth, several teeth, or a bridge can be secured by this technique. The type of implant to be used is determined according to how the implant will be secured, e.g., *endosseous* (fuses directly into the bone), *transosseous* (for edentulous maxilla), *subperiosteal* (for edentulous maxilla without much bone), and the ramus frame (for the edentulous areas of the wisdom teeth and chin area). Major companies that supply dental implants are Zimmer, Stryker, and Tetra Dynamics®.

Implants may be placed immediately after tooth extraction following inspection of the alveolar socket, or they may be placed after a period of time that allows for healing when the implantation follows resolution of an infection or following osteotomy and bone grafting. Usually, sufficient healing of the soft tissues is required after osteotomy (when necessary for subperiosteal alveolar ridge bone graft). A trap-like apparatus may be added to the suction tubing to salvage bone particles from the blood that are later used for bone-grafting material. When a delay of 4 to 6 months is required, a "healing cap" is placed. The healing cap is placed in the center of the implant to prevent healing within the shaft where the dental fixture or restoration will be placed. A time delay must also be considered for the second stage for tissue ingrowth or osseointegration for patients who have had radiotherapy as a cancer treatment. When the prognosis regarding the cancer is favorable, the patient is a candidate for implantation. When an adequate time allowance is given for vascular regrowth and osseointegration of the implant, healing is usually successful. In cancer patients requiring osteotomy, successful results have been obtained using porous implants that may be filled with salvaged autologous bone chips or a mixture of venous blood and *porous algae-derived hydroxyapatite*. Specially processed lamb-bone grafts have been employed. Some patients have had problems with bone resorption of the alveolar ridge. When the alveolar bone is insufficient to allow good purchase of the implant, a plate is placed on the inferior aspect of the mandible with through-and-through pins that exit the gingival tissues, to which the implant is secured (*transosseous implantation*). An additional technique used when the bone is less than optimal is to secure a nonintegrating metallic frame to the mandible, to which the prostheses are attached (*subperiosteal implantation*). These latter two modalities are not in frequent use. A titanium lapping tool and lap guide are used with a diamond paste to polish and refine fittings.

Note: There is an additional technique for atraumatic bone ridge expansion done in conjunction with evolutionary implant designs using motor-driven instruments at low speeds.

Note: The oral surgeon may bring his/her own dental assistant, dental instruments, equipment, and supplies.

Procedure

Dental Restoration with Osseointegration of a Titanium Dental Implant is described (Endosseous Implant Technique). While dental implantation with placement of a dental fixture or prosthesis is usually performed in a dental office, the oral surgeon may choose to perform dental restoration and implantation of a prosthetic device in the operating room. In the operating room, dental restoration with implantation of a prosthesis can be performed employing general anesthesia concomitantly with injection of a local anesthetic with epinephrine, or the procedure may be performed using local anesthetic block with epinephrine, in addition to the administration of *conscious sedation*.

The mouth is held open with a self-retaining retractor, or a bite block is placed and individual retractors are positioned, as needed. A moistened throat pack is placed. The diseased tooth/teeth are extracted; in addition to dental extraction instruments, a high-speed dental drill may be required. Dissection of the gingiva down to the bone in the maxilla or the mandible is performed, and the bone is prepared for the implant(s). The oral mucosa is incised (with a #15 or #12B blade), and a mucoperiosteal flap is formed. A periosteal elevator is used to expose the bone; the implant site is prepared with the dental drill. The implant may be immediately secured (fused) to the bone. For the patient who requires a waiting period before the dental fixture/prosthesis will be secured to the implant, a cover screw/healing screw/"healing cap" is utilized to prevent scar tissue from forming in the hollow of the implant. When the dental prosthesis is not placed immediately, the site may be left undisturbed following bone preparation for 4 to 6 months.

Endosseous implants may be screw-in or press-fit; all have a standard internal hex screw. In *"H" bridge reconstruction*, the implant attaches to an abutment. Impressions (molds) are made, preoperatively, for making the temporary tooth dentures in the dental laboratory.

The dental implants most often used are *osseointegrated titanium dental implants*; they are made of titanium and have threaded screws that are implanted or fused into the maxilla or mandible. The metal framework of the implant allows for a "fitting" of the dental prosthesis prior to its final implantation by *"H"* tissue extension. Standardization of the implants from different companies has been done for the implants, their parts, and their tools/instrumentation; all have a standard 2.5mm internal hex screw. Restorative components may go directly onto the implants or indirectly to an immediate tissue extension. Following implantation, the oral mucosa is closed with absorbable suture. The porous implants (e.g., titanium) designed for osseointegration may be placed immediately in the patient without complications. Particularly when a single implant is done, it is usually secured into the fresh alveolar socket by threaded screws immediately, unless more healing time is required; healing may require up to 40 days following the day the osteotomy was first performed.

Previously, patients always had to wear temporary dentures during the healing process. Approximately 3 to 6 months were required for osseointegration to have occurred; the implant was then uncovered, and the correct abutment was connected to the implant, followed by closure of the area. Prior to insertion or fusion, the metal framework of the implant is seated to ensure proper fit; it is then removed and sent to the lab with the dental impressions to make the permanent dental fixture/prosthesis that will top the implant. In the final phase, the patient returns for placement of the permanent dental fixture/prosthesis.

Preparation of the Patient

When only local anesthesia will be used, the patient may also be given Motrin® 800 mg by mouth and requested to rinse his/her mouth with an oral antiseptic (e.g., Peridex) for 30 seconds upon his/her arrival in the preoperative area. Dental restoration with implant(s) insertion is most often performed using local anesthetic block. When sedation is necessary due to extenuating circumstances regarding the extraction or the implant insertion procedure, general anesthesia with endotracheal intubation supplemented by local anesthetic injection with epinephrine or local anesthetic injection with epinephrine supplemented with *conscious sedation* may be administered. The epinephrine contained in the local anesthetic solution reduces bleeding; the anesthetic is effective for immediate postoperative pain control. If an anesthesia provider is not in attendance, a perioperative RN, in addition to the circulator, must be present to monitor the patient and to administer *conscious sedation* at the surgeon's direction; see responsibilities of the perioperative RN monitoring the patient, p. 74.

The table may be turned 90° or the table may be reversed with the patient's head at the foot to ensure adequate space for the surgeon's legs and to facilitate the surgeon's access to the patient. The patient is in supine position; a padded, foam, or gel headrest, e.g., donut, may be employed to stabilize the head. A roll may be placed under the neck or shoulders to facilitate tilting the head upward. When local anesthetic and *conscious sedation* are employed, one arm may be extended and secured on a padded armboard and the contralateral arm padded and secured at the patient's side, or both arms may be padded and secured at the patient's sides. A pillow may be placed under the knees to avoid straining lower back muscles, or the table may be flexed for comfort. All bony prominences and areas vulnerable to skin and neurovascular pressure or trauma are padded to avoid injury. An electrosurgical dispersive pad is required, as monopolar ESU or dental ESU will be used.

Second-Stage Implant Exposure

As mentioned above, dental implant surgery may require 4 to 6 months of healing. Most often, the patient's implants are exposed and the dental fixtures are placed, in the oral surgeon's office. The patient may return to the OR for this; upon arrival in the preoperative area, the patient is directed to use antiseptic mouthwash and rinse the mouth for 30 seconds.

Skin Preparation

In the OR, the patient may be asked to rinse his/her mouth with antiseptic mouthwash (e.g., Peridex) for 30 seconds.

Draping, see ***Dental Extraction/Odontectomy***, p. 938.

Equipment

Padded, foam, or gel headrest, e.g., donut, optional
Padded restraints for patients having local anesthesia (with or without *conscious sedation*)
Dental irrigation system with fiber-optic light source, e.g., Dyna-Surg I or Dyna-Surg II (Intl Dental), that may be used with any of 3 hand pieces (electric power source) with "intel-chip" technology
Suction source (separate)
ESU, monopolar (infrequent, only with general anesthetic) or dental ESU (e.g., Rotex or Radiosurg with foot pedal activation) and electrosurgical (grounding) pad

Instrumentation

Dental instruments for extractions tray

Add

Dental restoration
Instrumentation for the specific implant
Minor orthopedic procedures tray
Tracheostomy tray and various-sized tracheostomy tubes (available in the room), available
Dental drill, fiber-optic (*high-speed* with motor in hand pieces), e.g., with 3 hand pieces: HS Canister®, Push Button®, or Quick disconnect® have "intel-chip" technology
Dental drill (*low-speed* with motor in hand pieces) with Merus® electric irrigation latch (used only on implants) with 3 contra-angle hand pieces may be used (this particular company's dental drill set includes a wrench, internal and external irrigation tubing, Y-tube connector, needle, and additional extra tubing)
A cover screw/healing cap (for the implant when second stage is delayed) to prevent scar formation within the screw area where the tooth will be placed
Implant (e.g., osseointegrated titanium dental implant) and screws

Standard UMA Implant Instrument Components

Standard 2.5mm internal hex screw, root elevator, dental pliers, dental extraction forceps, hex wrenches, tissue punch, paralleling pin, depth gauge, implant retractor, implant seating tool, hand mallet, rachet, hex driver for ratchet, threaded hand tap, hand tap wheel, impression pin implant analogue, bar post analogue, series of O rings, series of O ring abutments, heating collar, bar post screw, series bar post abutments, retrievable crown post abutment, simple crown, post screw, and a healing cap

For Implant, Instrument Components for Bio-Vent® Bio-torque®

Left and right wrenches and taps, DDS slot screwdriver, lab driver, DDS hex driver, torque implant hex, left and right drivers, left and right insertion drivers, left and right latch tips, reamer abutment, carbide pin vise for lapping tool, carbide reamers for lapping tool, and guide pin hex driver

For Implant, UCLA Restorative Abutment System Instrument Components (most widely used restoration for a single tooth)

UCLA abutment, retaining bar, CV-UCLA abutment cylinder screw, left and right wrenches, drill tips (e.g., pilot drill, spade drill, and drill extender tip)

Osseointegrated titanium dental implants include: Core-Vent®, Screw-Vent®, Bio-Vent, Micro-Vent®, and Taper-Lock® or CV UCLA Abutment Cylinder Screw and Plug®

Any of the implants are topped or covered with an alloplastic or ceramic dental fixture/prosthesis/implant.

Dental Fixture/Prosthesis/Implant. *PureForm®* ceramic fixtures (that fit atop the threaded hex titanium screw implant) is provided with *Hadereds Bar* master kit for use with UMA standardized prostheses, includes standard drivers, B-T wrenches and left and right reamers, pit vise (used to seat the head of the screw) depth probe, and stabilizing wrench.

Supplies

Antibiotic ophthalmic ointment to keep eyes moist (general anesthesia only)

Lubrication for the lips, e.g., Vaseline

Local anesthetic, e.g., lidocaine with epinephrine is used for the dental block; its purpose is also to promote hemostasis and provide postoperative pain control

Control syringe and hypodermic needle(s) or Vibra-ject with shield

Medicine cups, methylene blue or indelible marker, and labels

Dental impression material, e.g., Permadyne™

Impression coping for UMA or TSi (to take impression of the implant body)

Articulating papers
Small basin set
Throat pack (gauze, with radio-opaque thread)
Dual tubing, prepackaged kit as supplied for suction/irrigation, e.g., tubing with irrigation needles and irrigation clips
Sterile water, irrigating solution for Dyna-Surg I or II
Bulb syringe and normal saline, optional
Blades, (1) #15 or (1) #12B
Gauze sponges 2 × 2
Suture (nonabsorbable) for hemostasis
Cotton dental rolls or dental pellets
Defogger for dental mirror, e.g., FRED, Defog, or ELVIS
Bone wax, optional
Electrosurgical pencil (disposable), cord, scraper, and holder, optional (infrequent)
Gelfoam and/or packing, e.g., 1/4″ gauze packing for hemostasis, optional

Special Notes

- Apply **Special Notes** from ***Dental Extraction/Odontectomy,*** p. 939, as applicable.
- **N.B. Reminder:** It is important for the *Universal Protocol* and "time-out" to be implemented prior to the start of dental surgery. The correctly identified patient and the correctly identified tooth/teeth must be marked prior to surgery.
- **Reminder:** The circulator should ascertain that the *correct* x-ray films for the *correctly identified* patient are in the room prior to starting the surgery.
- **N.B. Reminder:** ***The throat pack is moistened to prevent trauma to the oral mucosa; it must be removed before the patient is extubated to prevent its aspiration.***
- **Reminder:** Scrub person should be prepared with cut Gelfoam sponges that may be employed to aid in hemostasis, thereby reducing bleeding.
- **Reminder:** Care must be taken to protect the patient's face and eyes when passing instruments. When dental procedures are performed using local anesthetic alone, a towel may be placed over the patient's eyes.
- **Reminder:** The circulator must record the date, type, serial number, and size of the implant (dental prosthesis/fixture, as applicable) in the **Perioperative Record.**

- The circulator must follow hospital policy for the recording of insertion of a dental prosthesis or prostheses in the hospital log.
- **Reminder:** *When the OR team needs a reminder to remember to remove the throat pack at the end of the procedure, e.g., a hemostat swinging from the corner of the Mayo stand may be used to serve that purpose.*

Arch Bar Application

Definition

The placing of thin, malleable stainless steel metal strips and interdental wiring applied to the teeth to stabilize and immobilize the jaw following maxillary and/or mandibular fracture.

Discussion

When an external force is strong enough to fracture the maxilla or the mandible, the fracture is often accompanied by one or more other injuries. The person should be checked for injury to the cervical spine, spinal cord injuries, and breathing difficulties. Ideally, treatment of the jaw fracture should begin within 7 days. The **arch bar application** is placed for occlusion; this part of the procedure may be performed prior to (most often) or following open reduction of the jaw. A separate table and another set-up of instruments, gowns, gloves, etc. are required.

Fractures that occur in the region of the teeth are often compound fractures. The wires are placed in the interdigital spaces around each individual tooth. If the patient is edentulous, the fracture(s) are reduced and the jaw is fixed with wiring that is placed circumferentially over dentures or specially made intraoral splints (or screws and bars). For proper fixation, the arch bar placed on the upper jaw must have the hooks pointing upward, and the bar on the lower jaw must have the hooks pointing downward. When the fracture is in the anterior portion of the jaw with teeth on either side of the fracture, *intermaxillary fixation* may suffice to restore dental occlusion. When the fracture(s) is posterior to the teeth, both open reduction of the fracture(s) and intermaxillary fixation, are necessary to correct the maligned jaw, see ***Reduction of a Mandibular Fracture***, p. 708.

Procedure

Usually local anesthetic block injection containing epinephrine (for hemostasis and immediate postoperative pain relief) is employed, whether the anesthesia is to be local, local with *conscious sedation*, or general. A bite block is inserted into the mouth and retractors are positioned, as needed. The arch bar is measured, sized, and cut (with wire cutters) to fit. The arch bars are attached to the maxilla using a precut, stretched 25 or 26 gauge wire. The wire is seated into position with a probe or freer and secured around the neck of each tooth with wire twisters. (The wire is twisted in a clockwise direction). The wire cutter is used to cut the twisted wires the appropriate length. Then needle-nosed pliers are used to bend the sharp edges of the wire downward. This maneuver prevents additional trauma to the gingiva from exposed wire edges. The second arch bar is secured to the mandible using the same technique. The oral cavity is irrigated and suctioned to remove blood, fluid, and any debris. The maxilla and mandible are stabilized with additional wires or elastic bands over the hooks, as necessary. The patient's face is cleaned.

A disposable wire cutter is always taped to the top of the gurney to accompany the patient; in case of emergency, the wires can be cut.

If the patient is edentulous, the arch bars may be attached to dentures or specifically designed dental appliances. The arch bars are anchored by wire placed around the mandible and through the nasal spine and zygomatic arch.

For **Preparation of the Patient, Skin Preparation, Draping** and **Special Notes**, see ***Open Reduction of a Mandibular Fracture,*** pp. 710–712. Also refer to ***Dental Extraction / Odontectomy,*** p. 937.

Equipment

Padded, foam, or gel headrest (e.g., donut)
Extremity restraints, padded
Fiber-optic headlight and fiber-optic power source, optional
Suction source (separate)
ESU, monopolar (infrequent, only with general anesthetic)
Dental ESU (e.g., Rotex or Radiosurg with foot pedal activation) and electrosurgical dispersive (grounding) pad

Instrumentation

Minor orthopedic procedures tray
Tracheostomy tray and various-sized tracheostomy tubes (available, in the room), unopened
Dental instruments for extractions tray and arch bar application instruments: bite block, Yankauer and Frazier suction tips, bayonet forceps, Weider tongue depressors (large and small), Freer septal elevator, probe, wire cutters, wire twister, Mayo-Haney needle holders, ruler, caliper, wire twister, needle-nosed pliers, and suture scissors
Arch bars (cut to appropriate sizes), latex bands/retention bolsters and stainless steel wire 25 or 26 gauge

High-speed power dental drill with drill tips, burrs, and cord (with foot pedal control)

Note: A wire cutter (on dental instruments for extractions tray) and the disposable wire cutter are needed. The disposable wire cutter must be taped to the top of the gurney to accompany the patient, for use in case of emergency.

Supplies

Antiseptic mouthwash, e.g., Peridex, optional
Antibiotic ophthalmic ointment to keep eyes moist (general anesthesia only)
Lubrication for the lips, e.g., Vaseline
Local anesthetic, e.g., lidocaine with epinephrine for hemostasis and to assist in pain control
Control syringe and hypodermic needle(s) or Vibra-ject with shield
Medicine cups, methylene blue or sterile indelible marker, and labels
Cotton rolls or dental pellets
Throat pack (gauze, with radio-opaque thread)
Coil of arch bars (stainless steel) and stainless steel wire, 25 or 26 gauge
Latex bands (if used, check with the patient and the chart regarding patient allergy)
Articulating papers, available
Small basins (2), normal saline and bulb syringe, optional
Electrosurgical pencil with a guarded tip, cord, holder, scraper, optional (infrequent)
Suction tubing
Dual tubing for suction/irrigation (prepackaged with irrigation clips, (2) and irrigation needle
Sterile water
Irrigating solution for Dyna–Surg I or II
Blade, (1) #15
Needle magnet or counter
Note: extra wire cutter (disposable)
Yankauer suction tip (disposable), optional
Sponges, e.g., gauze 2 × 2
Defogger for dental mirror, e.g., FRED, Defog, or ELVIS, optional

Special Notes

- Apply **Special Notes** from ***Open Reduction of a Mandibular Fracture***, p. 712, and ***Dental Extraction/Odontectomy***, p. 939, as applicable.

- **Reminder:** Care must be taken to protect the patient's face and eyes when handling and passing instruments.
- **Reminder:** Oral procedures are considered "clean," not sterile. However, the best aseptic technique possible should be observed.
- **N.B.** The scrub person should stretch out the wire and precut it before passing it to the surgeon for application. To stretch, cut wire segment slightly longer than required, place wire twisters on ends, twist a half turn and pull, stretching; wire is twisted clockwise. Several should be prepared in advance.
- **N.B.** The scrub person and the surgeon must observe extreme care to avoid contaminating the wire or themselves. The sharp ends of the wire can puncture gloves, gown, and skin.
- **Reminder:** The circulator should ask the patient and confirm with the chart any known allergies or the absence of an allergy, particularly to rubber/latex products, as elastic bands may be used. The elastic bands will be cut from retention bolsters with suture scissors.
- The circulator should document in the **Perioperative Record** the appearance of the skin around the mouth and the oral mucosa prior to placement of the elastic bands and following their placement. The allergy information is verified and documented for patient safety and for medicolegal reasons.
- **N.B. Note:** As the circulator accompanies the patient and anesthesia provider to the PACU, he/she must be certain to bring a disposable wire cutter. He/she should document that a wire cutter was taped to the head of the gurney, in case of emergency.
- The circulator points out the wire cutter to the perioperative practitioner in the PACU; he/she must see and document that the disposable wire cutter is indeed taped to the head of the gurney and emphasizes to the patient the importance of having a disposable wire cutter with him/her at all times. These exchanges of information are documented in the **Postoperative Record** section of the **Perioperative Record** for patient safety and for medicolegal reasons.

Total Temporomandibular Joint (TMJ) Replacement Surgery

Definition

The functional reconstruction and/or replacement of the diseased or damaged temporomandibular joint by prosthetic replacement.

Discussion

Temporomandibular Joint (TMJ) Syndrome is a painful condition of the joints of the jaw; it is often stress-related and may be associated with bruxism, malocclusion, and various arthritic conditions. The changes in the joints of the jaw (bilateral) are usually due to degeneration and/or trauma, with resulting pain and decreased mobility. When the condition is unresponsive to conservative treatment, such as soft diet, hot/cold packs, mouth splints, physiotherapy, anti-inflammatories, muscle relaxants, analgesics, and dental treatment (adjustment, restoration, and/or orthodontics), stress management (e.g., biofeedback), or transcutaneous electrical nerve stimulation, arthroscopy and/or condyloplasty may be indicated. Arthroscopy of the temporomandibular joints is performed primarily for diagnosis; correction of some limited conditions, such as lysis of adhesions due to scarring or mechanical debridement, synovectomy, or menisectomy can be performed to bring some relief of symptoms; a rotary shaver similar to the one used in knee surgery can be used to resurface parts of the joints, or the holmium:YAG (Ho:YAG) laser may be employed to simultaneously resect, cauterize, and/or vaporize cartilaginous tissues. The disc between each of the mandibular condyles and the glenoid fossas can be resected. Other open arthroplasty procedures may be performed to improve the shape and contour of the joint components as well. Some procedures using autologous bone grafts to reconstruct the joint may be performed. Total joint replacement is performed only when there is a *mechanical* problem with the jaw.

The **total temporomandibular joint replacement** by prostheses is performed when the mandibular condyles and the glenoid fossas are diseased/damaged. The procedure, when successful, increases the function of the joint while decreasing the amount of pain. Total replacement of the TMJ is indicated for arthritic conditions, ankylosis, and revision procedures for treatment failures. The total prosthesis may also be used when there is avascular necrosis, multiple operated joints, certain fractures, functional deformity, post-tumor excision of malignant and some benign tumors, degenerated or resorbed joints with anatomic discrepancies, and developmental abnormalities. Due to the TMJ difficulty, the patient may have associated jaw and facial deformities that may be corrected when the prostheses is placed.

As the human skull can vary greatly from person to person, total TMJ replacements must be highly customized to fit the individual patient; the customization is very costly. The patient is usually able to recover at least partial function of the artificial joint; although complete relief of jaw pain may not always be achieved, adequate pain relief can usually be obtained.

Making the model for the new joints requires several steps. First the patient undergoes a computed tomography (CT) scan to obtain a precise stereolithographic model, using lasers and epoxy resin. The surgeon performs "surgery" on the model. The adjusted model is sent for specific digitalized, computerized customization (from which the prostheses will be made). The surgeon working with an engineer makes any necessary changes on the newly designed model. When they are satisfied with the product, the prostheses is created and returned to the surgeon to perform the surgery.

Procedure

The TMJ is approached by an endaural/periauricular incision and a submandibular incision is used for the mandibular ramus. The position of the facial nerve necessitates this double approach. Condylectomy, debridement, and bone contouring are performed (just as was done on the model previously). Intermaxillary fixation (wiring of the jaws together) with an intermediate splint is accomplished. The fossa component of the prosthesis is inserted through the endaural/periauricular incision. Three or four 2-mm screws are used to stabilize and secure it to the zygomatic arch; see Reduction of a Zygomatic Fracture, p. 713. The mandibular prosthesis is inserted through the submandibular incision and fixed to the lateral surface of the ramus with 8 to 10 screws, 2 mm. An autogenous fat graft may be harvested (using fat from the abdomen or buttocks); it is positioned around the joint prosthesis to prevent postsurgical fibrosis and reactive bone formation. (The fat pad also "fills-out" the cheek, thereby improving the appearance of the face.) Additional orthognathic/maxillofacial surgical procedures may be performed (p. 957) as necessary. At the conclusion of the surgery, the intermaxillary fixation is removed. Postoperatively, prolonged physical therapy is necessary to achieve and maintain postoperative functional rehabilitation.

Preparation of the Patient

Total temporomandibular joint replacement surgery is performed using general anesthesia with nasotracheal intubation. The table may be turned 90°. The patient is in supine position; a padded, foam, or gel headrest (e.g., donut) may be employed to stabilize the head; the head is turned with the affected side up and the dependent ear well padded. A roll may be placed under the shoulders to facilitate tilting the head upward. One arm may be extended on a padded armboard and the contralateral arm padded and tucked in at the patient's side, or both arms may be padded and tucked in at the patient's sides. A pillow may be placed under the knees to avoid straining lower back muscles, or the table may be flexed for comfort. All bony prominences and areas vulnerable to skin and neurovascular pressure or trauma are padded to avoid injury. Apply electrosurgical dispersive pad, as dental ESU or monopolar ESU will be used.

Skin Preparation

Procedures involving the oral cavity are considered "clean"; they are not sterile, as the oral cavity is part of the gastrointestinal tract. The best aseptic technique possible is observed. Male patients may require a shave unless that was done immediately preoperatively. Hair may need to be removed around the ears; the hair around the face may be secured with rubber bands (use latex allergy precautions, p. 32). The circulator should check with the surgeon regarding the necessity for shaving any hair, the area to be prepped, and the type of prep solution(s) to use. The surgeon may request the mouth be swabbed with an oral antiseptic, e.g., Peridex. The entire face should be prepped. Extend the prep from the hairline to the base of the neck. Begin at the area of the jaws, working outward; include the auricles and both sides of the neck. A lap sponge may be placed at the sides of the neck to prevent prep solution from pooling under the patient. Care is taken to avoid getting prep solution in the eyes; the eyes may be irrigated with saline from inner to outer canthus to avoid possible foreign body from entering or blocking the tear duct. Antibiotic ointment may be placed in the conjunctival sac to provide moisture and protection. A small cotton ball is placed in the ear to prevent prep solution from pooling in the ear (it can be removed with a mosquito forceps before draping). The prepped area may be blotted dry; care is taken not to contaminate the operative site. Prep solution is not permitted to pool on the drapes, as it excoriates the skin. In addition, pooled prep solutions are a fire hazard and should be avoided.

Draping

The patient may be draped with a "head drape" (drape sheet and two towels under the head with the uppermost towel wrapped around the head and clipped). The body is covered with a drape sheet.

Optional Draping

Disposable drapes: the head is draped with a disposable sheet, placing the adhesive strip across the forehead. Two folded towels (V-shape) are draped at the patient's neck, and the body is covered with a U or split drape sheet.

Equipment

- Padded, foam, or gel headrest (e.g., donut)
- Extremity restraints, padded (used with local anesthesia administration)
- Suction (separate source) and irrigation and suction systems

Dental irrigation system with fiber-optic light source, e.g., Dyna-Surg I or Dyna Surg II (Intl Dental), optional
Dental ESU (e.g., Rotex or Radiosurg with foot pedal activation); electrosurgical (grounding) pad required
Fiber-optic headlight and fiber-optic light source, e.g., Xenon 300 W, optional
ESU, monopolar and grounding or electrosurgical dispersive pad, infrequent
Dental ESU (e.g., Rotex® or Radiosurg® with foot pedal activation) and electrodispersive (grounding) pad
Laser (e.g., Ho:YAG), optional

Instrumentation

Dental procedures and extractions tray
Temporomandibular joint (TMJ) instrument tray
Nasal procedures tray, available
Minor orthopedic procedures tray, available
Tracheostomy tray and various-sized tracheostomy tubes (available, as needed)
Implant and specific instrumentation, according to type of prostheses (implant)
Handpiece for suction/irrigation, e.g., DynaSurg I or DynaSurg II
Osteotomes and chisels, 2 sets, (1) curved and (1) straight, mallet, bone clamp, ramus flap retractor, suction/irrigation tips
High-speed dental drill handpiece with port for irrigation, cord, diamond-coated drills, twist drills, round burrs, cortical screws, and rasp, drill guide, screwdriver or fixation screw kit containing these or similar instruments (available from drill manufacturer)
Saw (reciprocating, saggital, or oscillating), handpiece with port for irrigation, assorted blades, tubing, and wrench
Alignment rods, plate, and rod cutter, optional
Maxillofacial fixation plating system, screw set, and instrumentation, optional

Specific Instrumentation for Lorenz Prosthesis

TMJ double-ended drill guide, drill tips, diamond rasp, diamond burrs (coarse, medium, short coarse, short medium), retractors (PDQ zygoma, coronoid, condylar, and posterior), condyle stripper, Dingman bone forceps (light), Dunn-Dautry osteotome, plate-holding forceps, Beuse plate-holding forceps, and screwdriver for cross (Phillips-type screws)

Supplies

Antiseptic mouthwash, e.g., Peridex
Antibiotic ophthalmic ointment (e.g., general anesthesia only)

Lubrication for the lips, e.g., Vaseline
Cotton rolls or dental pellets
Dental sponges 2 × 2″
Throat pack (gauze, with radio-opaque thread)
Small basins (2), bulb syringe, and normal saline, optional
Electrosurgical pencil with a guarded tip, cord, holder, scraper, optional
Dual tubing prepackaged for suction/irrigation with tubing clips (2) and irrigation needle
Sterile water for irrigating solution, e.g., for Dyna-Surg I or II (Intl Dental)
Blades, (1) #10, (2) #15
Needle magnet or counter
Stainless steel wire, 25 or 26 gauge
Retention bolsters, optional
Defogger for dental mirror, e.g., FRED, Defog, or ELVIS
Bone wax, optional
Gelfoam and/or packing, e.g., 1/4″ gauze may be used for hemostasis

Special Notes

- Apply **Special Notes** from ***Dental Extraction***, p. 939, as applicable.
- **N.B.** The prostheses should be handled as little as possible. The scrub person should exercise great care to ***avoid*** depositing any foreign material on the prostheses. Talc-free gloves should be worn, and lint-free raytec sponges should be used.
- **Reminder:** Care must be taken to protect the patient's face and eyes when handling and passing instruments.
- Usually, each brand ofTMJ prostheses (e.g., Lorenz) has its own additional instruments that are specifically used for their prostheses for insertion.
- Usually the dental ESU (e.g., Rotex® or Radiosurg® with foot pedal activation) and electrodispersive (grounding) pad is used; keep the tip of the handpiece free of debris and eschar.
- If a laser (e.g., Ho:YAG) is employed, all laser safety precautions must be followed.
- **N.B.** The scrub person may want to use a small amount of bone wax to help hold the maxillofacial screw head on the screwdriver during application.
- Note that the surgeon may bring the prefabricated model into surgery.
- **Reminder:** Throat pack is included in sponge count; it should be removed prior to extubating the patient to prevent its aspiration.

- **Note Reminder:** *When a reminder to remove the throat pack is necessary, a hemostat may be placed swinging from the corner of the Mayo stand to remind the OR team to remove the throat pack at the end of the procedure.*

Orthognathic/Maxillofacial Surgery

Definition

Correction of deformities, malposition, and/or malocclusion of the jaws and teeth.

Discussion

Orthognathic/maxillofacial surgery combines orthodontia and surgery on the maxilla and the mandible to correct or establish a balance between the teeth, jaws, and facial structures. Malposition and malocclusion of the jaws adversely affects one's appearance; patients with maxillofacial defects are affected socially as well as psychologically.

Corrective orthognathic/maxillofacial surgery can dramatically change one's appearance and therefore dramatically affect the individual's quality of life.

In *prognathism*, one or both jaws project forward beyond normal facial alignment. In *retrognathism,* one or both jaws are positioned posterior to normal facial alignment. Orthognathic/maxillofacial surgery straightens the teeth (orthodontia) and realigns the jaws and may also correct cranio-orbital deformities. Patients with maxillofacial imbalance may have eating difficulties, distorted speech, chronic temporomandibular (TMJ) pain syndrome, and breathing problems. Dentofacial abnormalities can be congenital, developmental, or acquired but usually occur as a result of a differential in the rate of growth of the maxilla and mandible.

Genetic predisposition from conditions such as Apert and Crouzon syndromes may also result in facial clefts and abnormalities in growth and development. Causes of dentofacial abnormalities include trauma that disturbs the normal skeleton in adults and abnormal skeletal growth in children, neoplasms, and iatrogenic radiation. Correction requires careful analysis of the soft tissues and bony skeleton using photographs, visual, digital, skeletal examination, and dental evaluation (with study dental casts) to achieve proper alignment.

Whereas each patient situation is unique, most presentations are treated by established or somewhat modified established techniques. When the maxillae are involved, osteotomy procedures (LeFort type) are employed to advance or widen the maxilla; the techniques may be modified, as necessary. The correction may be stabilized with maxillofacial plating. Alloplastic chin implants are used to correct minimal saggital chin deficiencies, or chin defects may be corrected with osteotomies. Representatives from several surgical specialties are usually involved, collaborating on a preplanned course of preoperative, surgical, and postoperative treatments that will best serve the individual patient. The goal is to achieve a successful patient outcome; a series of procedures is often required.

A distracter system, comprised of screwed-in footplates, trimmed and bent accordingly at the time of surgery, attached to a distracter rod or resorbable plates may be used. The activation screw is adjusted postoperatively (twice daily) by a technician (or trained family member) to achieve gradual separation of the osteotomized fragments, sometimes for as long as 6 to 8 weeks. Special cortical screws, plates, drill bits, alignment rods, and plate and rod cutters are available for this technique, depending on the type of plates used. A fabricated model is created preoperatively; it is important to continually compare the patient to the fabricated model to ensure postoperative stability. Depending on the extent of the deformities, the combined dentosurgical treatment may be divided into five phases:

1. Preorthodontic preparatory phase
2. Presurgical orthodontic treatment
3. Surgery
4. Postsurgery orthodontics
5. Postorthodontic treatment.

The goal is to restore orthognathic form to the face; ultimately, the aesthetic appearance depends on consideration of the patient's request for his/her "ideal facial esthetics."

Procedure

A Maxillofacial Procedure is described Using a Modified LeFort I Osteotomy Procedure. The LeFort I procedure is directed primarily at occlusion; the repositioning affects the upper-lip position, nasal tip and alar base region, and the columellarlabial angle without altering the orbitozygomatic region.

Maxillary Osteotomy is described. Antibiotics are administered; general anesthesia with nasotracheal intubation is preferred. Local anesthetic with epinephrine is injected into the soft tissues around the maxillae bilaterally to reduce bleeding and assist with pain control postoperatively. An intraoral incision is made over the maxilla approximately 1 cm superior to the mucogingival junction. The mucoperiosteal flap is elevated to the superior aspect of the incision from the piriform rim posteriorly to the pterygoid plates. The horizontal osteotomy is made (with a burr or reciprocating saggital saw) extending from the piriform rim posteriorly to just past the second molar. The contralateral maxilla is similarly treated. The entire nasal mucoperiosteum is freed from the superior surface of the maxilla with an elevator. If bone grafting is needed, the anterior nasal spine is removed (using a burr and osteotomes) and set aside for later use. Additional bone or bonelike grafting materials may be used, including hydroxyapatite cement. The nasal septum is separated from the superior surface of the maxilla (using a guarded osteotome and mallet). The lateral nasal walls are transected. The pterygoid plates are separated from the maxillary tuberosities (using a curved osteotome and mallet). The maxilla is "down-fractured." Bone is trimmed as necessary to allow advancement, retraction of the maxilla, or superior repositioning, without interference. The inferior turbinates are "out-fractured." The maxilla is positioned as determined preoperatively and temporary fixation is accomplished with stainless steel wires. A maxillofacial plating system is used to stabilize the bone. Following fixation, any temporary fixation is removed and jaw occlusion is checked for accuracy. The wound is irrigated with normal saline to remove blood and debris. The oral mucosa is closed bilaterally with absorbable suture. The pharynx may be carefully irrigated and aspirated. The throat pack is removed and the patient extubated.

Mandibular Reconstruction is described. The mouth is retracted open or a bite block may be placed; a throat pack is also placed. Local anesthetic with epinephrine may be injected into the soft tissues around the mandible bilaterally, to reduce bleeding and assist with postoperative pain control. An intraoral incision is made into the gingiva from first molar, leaving an adequate mucosal edge to facilitate closure, and continued down onto one mandibular ramus, as care is taken to preserve the neurovascular structures (including the inferior alveolar and lingual nerves). At this stage, the procedure is modified according to the individual's needs. A mucoperiosteal flap is elevated with a periosteal elevator. A horizontal osteotomy is cut (using a drill and burr or saggital saw) from just posterior to the lingual area (where the inferior alveolar nerve, artery, and vein enter the mandible) to the anterior border of the mandibular ramus through the medial cortical plate. A second osteotomy is made vertically from the mid-portion of the second molar down to the area of the inferior border of the mandible, through the lateral cortical plate. A third osteotomy joins the horizontal and vertical cuts to initiate separation of the bone segments. A curved osteotome is driven through the inferior border of the mandible and twisted laterally to secure separation of the segments. The proximal segment is dissected free of the neurovascular bundle. The neurovascular bundle is preserved intact and left with the distal bone segment; the bone may be trimmed with a burr to minimize trauma to the nerve. If the mandible is to be set back, ligaments are stripped from the mandible with a periosteal elevator from the medial aspect of the proximal segment, down and around the mandibular angle to prevent the proximal segment from being rotated posteriorly.

Contralateral mandibular ramus is exposed, and osteotomies are performed, as described above. The mandible is set back or brought forward to the appropriate position, as determined preoperatively. Temporary fixation is accomplished using stainless steel wires. Bone is trimmed, as necessary, to allow the segments to align.

The segments are repositioned (they may be temporarily stabilized with a bone clamp). Rigid internal fixation is achieved with a maxillofacial plating system. Bone grafts may be employed, as applicable. Any temporary fixation is removed; jaw occlusion is checked for accuracy. The wound is irrigated with normal saline to remove blood and debris. The oral mucosa is closed bilaterally with absorbable suture. The pharynx is carefully irrigated and aspirated. When ***mentoplasty*** (see p. 723) is indicated for protrusion, the mental symphysis may be divided and excessive bone resected, followed by rigid fixation. Augmentation mentoplasty with placement of an alloplastic implant may be performed if the chin is receding.

For **Preparation of the Patient, Skin Preparation,** and **Draping,** see ***Dental Extraction Odontectomy*****, pp. 937–938.**

Equipment

Padded, foam, or gel headrest (e.g., donut)
Fiber-optic headlight and fiber-optic light source, e.g., Xenon 300W, optional
Dental irrigation system with fiber-optic light source, e.g., Dyna-Surg I or Dyna-Surg II (Intl Dental) with 3 hand pieces (electric power source) with "intel-chip" technology
Suction source (separate)
ESU, monopolar, or dental ESU (e.g., Rotex or Radiosurg with foot pedal activation) and grounding pad

Instrumentation

Dental instruments for extraction tray

Add

Orthognathic/maxillofacial procedures instrument tray
Nasal procedures tray, available
Minor orthopedic procedures tray, available
Tracheostomy tray and various-sized tracheostomy tubes (available in the room)
Osteotomes and chisels, curved and straight, mallet, bone clamp
High-speed dental drill handpiece, cord, diamond-coated drills, burrs, cortical screws
High-speed power saw (reciprocating, saggital, or oscillating) hand piece with assorted blades
Alignment rods and plate and rod cutters

Maxillofacial fixation plating system, screw set, and instrumentation, optional
Resorbable plates, optional
Distracter system, e.g., footplates, distracter rod, activation screw
Titanium bar for UCLA restoration needs Hader-eds Bar Master Kit: implant insertion drivers, stands, drivers, B-T wrenches (left and right), left and right reamers, internal driver to refine slat at head of (implant) screw, and pit vise
Alloplastic chin implant, optional

Supplies

Antiseptic mouthwash, e.g., Peridex
Antibiotic ophthalmic ointment to keep eyes moist (general anesthesia only)
Lubrication for the lips, e.g., Vaseline
Local anesthetic, e.g., lidocaine with epinephrine for dental block
Control syringe and hypodermic needle(s) or Vibra-ject with shield
Medicine cups, labels, and indelible pen
Topical decongestant nasal spray, e.g., neosynephrine 0.5%, optional
Cottonoids, ½″ × 3″
Methylene blue or indelible pen
Cotton rolls or dental pellets
Throat pack (gauze, with radio-opaque thread)
Articulating papers
Small basins (2), bulb syringe, normal saline
Electrosurgical pencil with a guarded tip, cord, holder, scraper, optional, infrequent
Suction tubing and IV tubing, for suction/irrigation
Dual tubing for suction/irrigation with needles and irrigation clips (2), prepackaged unit
Sterile water, irrigating solution for Dyna-SurgI or II
Blades, (1) #15 or (1) #12B
Needle magnet or counter
Hydroxyapatite cement, optional
Yankauer suction tip (disposable, 2 pieces)
Stainless steel wire, 25 or 26 gauge
Retention bolsters, optional
Gauze sponges, 2 × 2
Suture (nonabsorbable) for hemostasis
Defogger, e.g., FRED, Defog, or ELVIS
Bone wax, optional
Gelfoam and/or packing, e.g., ¼″ gauze packing may be used for hemostasis

Special Notes

- Apply **Special Notes** from **Dental Extraction/Odontectomy,** p. 939.
- Cottonoids may be saturated with nasal spray solution (e.g., neosynephrine) for decongestion; the cottonoids are used to pack the nose preoperatively.
- **Reminder:** Care must be taken to protect the patient's face and eyes when handling or passing instruments.
- **N.B. Reminder:** Protective eye goggles may be placed on the patient to avoid getting a foreign object in the eye and to deflect the light.
- **N.B. Reminder:** Throat pack is included in sponge count; it should be removed prior to extubating the patient.
- **N.B.** The scrub person may want to use a small amount of bone wax to help hold the maxillofacial screw head on the screwdriver during application.
- The surgeon brings a fabricated model into surgery for demonstration of how to place the bone sections while working to ensure postoperative stability.
- The scrub person and the circulator should be aware that different distraction systems may be employed, but all have a standardized universal 2.5 mm central hex screw.
- Arch bar application (p. 948) may be required to stabilize the teeth during healing.

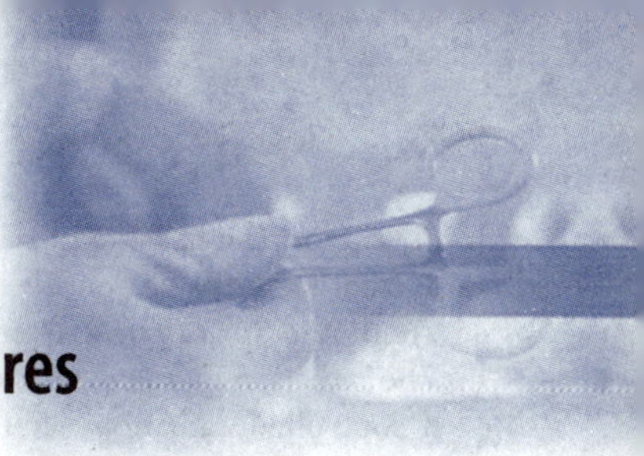

CHAPTER 30 Radiation Therapy/ Radiotherapy Procedures

Introduction to Radiation Therapy Procedures in Surgery

Radiation therapy/radiotherapy procedures in the operating room (OR) are generally limited surgical procedures. This treatment modality may be employed as a distinct procedure or as an adjunct to another surgical procedure. Due to the serious nature of handling radioactive material, discussion regarding radiation safety for OR personnel, physicians, and patients is included here and in Chapter 3, p. 52. Radiation therapy (radiotherapy) is primarily directed to the treatment of malignancies, either as primary therapy or in conjunction with ablative surgery and/or chemotherapy; however, it can be employed to treat benign diseases as well. The cells of the targeted tissues and adjacent tissues are killed or damaged by ionizing radiation and replaced by fibrous (scar) tissue.

Physicians who practice the discipline of radiation therapy (also referred to as **radiation oncology**) have undergone special residency training in this field and utilize the assistance of physicists and technicians and other physicians or surgeons.

Definition

Employment of ionizing radiation to treat a variety of disease entities.

Discussion

An example of a benign condition treated by radiotherapy includes selected presentations of hyperthyroidism in which **radioactive iodine (I^{131})** is administered to the patient. This same treatment measure is also used in different dosages for certain histological types of thyroid malignancy. The sensitivity of tissue to the effects of radiation varies, relating to the amount and type of radiation being administered. A major factor in determining the type and delivery of the radiation is dependent on ensuring that adjacent normal tissue remains (relatively) unharmed. Calculating the dosage is dependent on the distance from the source of radiation, as well as the duration of exposure and the number of times the tissue is exposed.

Radiotherapeutic agents may be implanted directly in tissue, or they may be focused as an external beam that passes through the body to the tumor. The half-life of the particular radiation source is another important factor to be considered prior to its use.

Radiotherapy can be delivered in multiple clinical settings, including the radiation therapy clinic (or radiation therapy hospital suite), in well-controlled, radiation-safe facilities using the **linear accelerator** (a specialized source of x-ray energy) or other sources, such as **radioactive isotopes (e.g., Co^{60})**. After the physicians involved perform a thorough clinical assessment of the patient, **external beam radiation therapy (EBRT)** may be employed; a physicist assists in calculating the dosage and determining the type of radiation source to be used. Certain applications of chemotherapeutic agents may sensitize the targeted tissue to the effects of radiation, sometimes with a lesser dose (of radiation) required. Prior or interactive scanning procedures, such as magnetic resonance imaging (MRI), computed tomography (CT), and ultrasound, and radio-opaque markers placed in the affected tissues by the radiation therapist or surgical specialist provide guidance to the targeted tissue prior to the actual delivery of the radiation modality.

In **brachytherapy,** radioactive isotopes, also referred to as radionuclides, contained in seeds, needles, and other devices can be placed directly into the affected tissues, or they may be after-loaded via specially placed catheters. This latter technique is often performed in the OR with an anesthesia provider and surgical specialist. When the after-loading modality is employed, the radioactive agents are placed later that day or the following day (or days) in appropriately protected areas away from the OR.

Note: The Atomic Energy Commission has set controls for obtaining and using radionuclides; individuals are required to receive special training and licensure before being permitted to use them. All sources of radiation must be accounted for prior to and following the procedure. A complete record of the radiation modality used becomes part of the patient's permanent medical record. Signs attesting to use of radiation must be conspicuously posted outside the room and on the patient's bed.

Specific types of **brachytherapy applications** are included to follow. In addition to the more commonly treated anatomical areas, **direct percutaneous placement of radioactive isotopes** is done for selected lung, brain, and other malignancies. A tenet of this therapy is related to the effect of the ionizing particles diminishing by the square of the distance from the source so that the tissues in contact with the isotopic material receive the preponderance of the doses. In addition, the half-life of the isotope used is a factor in determining whether the radioisotope is permanently implanted or is removed at a predetermined time, having achieved its desired effective dosage (without causing undue injury to adjacent tissues). Brachytherapy may be combined with external beam irradiation accordingly. **Extracorporeal radiation** can be delivered to a patient's bone marrow; the blood elements are extracted from the patient, treated, and reinfused.

Advances in computer technology have led to **"intensity-modulated radiation therapy" (IMRT)** that delivers multiple computer directed beams to affected tissues to maximize the tumoricidal effect of the radiotherapeutic agent with minimal exposure to surrounding tissues. This is particularly of value in prostatic cancer to avoid rectal and bladder injury; it is also employed in head and neck cancer to avoid salivary gland, oral, and dental injury. Similarly, **stereotactic radiosurgery** (see **Gamma Knife**, p. 648) is employed for the treatment of various intracranial malignant and benign lesions. **Proton beam therapy** is a treatment that likewise provides intense local therapy (e.g., prostatic cancer) while sparing surrounding tissues. **Intraoperative radiotherapy (IORT)** is a type of **directed external beam radiation** that spares (relatively) adjacent tissues. In surgical procedures (e.g., recurrent colorectal and other pelvic malignancies), after gross tumor is surgically resected, lap pads or mesh is used to displace local unaffected tissues and organs that are mobilized and placed temporarily out of the path of the intended radiation delivery. A single dose of radiation is given either in a designated "radiation safe" OR, or the anesthetized patient is transported (with the open operative wound protected) to the radiation suite, where radiation is administered, the protected structures are released, the surgery is otherwise completed, and the wound is closed. At present, these modalities, requiring very expensive equipment and appropriately trained ancillary personnel, are limited to some university hospitals and specialty clinic facilities.

Special Notes

- Apply **Special Notes** from ***Abdominal Laparotomy,*** p. 134, as they apply in general to the individual the patient in surgery.
- **N.B.** *For safety precautions regarding* ***radiation therapy,*** *see p. 52 and p. 964.* It is important to note that radiotherapy has the potential, in due time, to promote **malignant transformation in normal tissues** that were exposed during prior treatment of the original malignancy. Similarly, attending personnel may exhibit these adverse tissue responses long-term if safety protocol measures to minimize exposure to radiation are not followed.
- The circulator may convey (even more than is usual) emotional support to the patient due to the serious nature of any of the following surgical procedures. He/she takes an assessment of

the patient's anxiety level and employs measures such as maintaining eye contact, using touch to convey caring, holding the patient's hand during the administration of anesthesia, offering a warm blanket, etc. All nursing care measures (interventions) performed and the patient's perceived outcome are documented in the **Perioperative Record** for continuity of care for patient safety and for medicolegal reasons.

- The circulator may provide the patient an additional measure of comfort to reduce anxiety by explaining that he/she will act as the patient's advocate.
- **N.B. Note:** *Radiotherapeutic procedures are often performed under regional anesthesia and, though sedated, the patient may be awake and misinterpret overheard conversation; therefore, discussions regarding severity or anatomical extent of the patient's pathology and any other comments should be restricted to that necessary for conduction of the procedure.*

Radiation Therapy for Head and Neck Tumors

Definition

The administration of or preparation for the administration of radiotherapeutic modalities for treatment of tumors of the head and neck.

Discussion

Malignant neoplasms of the head and neck region are designated by anatomical site as base of the tongue, tonsillar fossa, gingiva, nasal sinus, larynx, etc. Each area demonstrates its own rapidity of growth and ultimate spread to the cervical lymph nodes. Local versus radical surgery, including **cervical lymph node dissection**, radiotherapy, or a combination of modalities, with or without chemotherapy, is considered according to well-established criteria, noting the site and extent of the tumor, evidence of metastatic disease, the patient's medical status, and, when possible, the patient's (informed) choice. In the head and neck, perhaps more than in other anatomical sites, radiotherapy alone or combined with other modalities may provide functional and cosmetic benefits versus surgery alone.

In the OR, **radioactive isotope seeds** or needles may be placed directly in affected tissues or catheters and needles are placed for use with after-loading modalities. **Higher dose irradiation** is not administered in the OR; instead, as noted, after-loading catheters or needles are inserted in the OR and the actual radiotherapy is administered postoperatively. **Lower-dose therapy** by implantation of seeds is now done infrequently in deference to the higher precisely directed dosage after-loading techniques. **Brachytherapy** may be used in conjunction with surgery or if recurrence appears. Subsequent external beam irradiation may be administered as well.

Prior to therapy, patient assessment, including routine clinical and laboratory studies, dental evaluation, examination under anesthesia, pertinent endoscopies, and any combinations of CT, MRI, positron emission tomography (PET), radionuclide scans, angiography, panorex views, chest x-ray, etc. is done.

Procedure

General anesthesia is most often employed. Depending on the site involved, either as an independent surgical procedure or as a procedure combined with resective surgery, needles are inserted into the tumor (for after-loading). Alternatively, **permanent low-dose seed implants (Cs^{137}, Au^{198})** may be permanently placed in the targeted area in surgery.

Frequently, the radiation oncologist brings his/her own instruments, as well as the (protected) radioactive materials to the OR. Most often, a Limited procedures tray (see p. 1095) will suffice for a simple procedure; during the course of resectional surgery, the radiation oncologist may intervene. For **maxillary sinus adenocarcinoma,** a **V-B-H (Vogele-Bale-Hohner) frame** with three-dimensional CT scan imaging guidance is employed for insertion of after-loading needles; drill holes are made in the skull for the needles' insertion. Treatment of intraocular lesions involves placing **"plaque" (I^{125})** in the eye; it is left in for the calculated dose and then removed. Intraluminal balloon catheters may be inserted under imaging guidance for lesions of the larynx, bronchi, and esophagus (for after-loading).

Preparation of the Patient (including patient positioning), **Skin Preparation, Draping, Equipment,** and **Instrumentation** depend on the anatomic site, the particular procedure in conjunction with the ablative surgery (if any), and the requirements of the radiation oncologist.

Special Notes

- Apply all **Special Notes** in this chapter, **Radiation Therapy/Radiotherapy,** as applicable for any surgical procedure.
- Perioperative care of the patient anticipating radiotherapeutic surgery requires the circulator to employ an attitude of empathetic sensitivity. ***Universal protocol*** (p. 18,) is employed (as in all other surgeries) to identify the patient, the type of procedure, and the site and/or side for the surgery or radiotherapy procedure. All measures to ensure patient safety throughout the

surgical procedure must be included. Every precaution is taken to verify that the correctly identified patient receives the correct radiotherapy treatment.

- Nursing care measures (interventions) performed throughout the intraoperative radiotherapy procedure and the perceived outcome for the patient are documented in the **Perioperative Record** for patient safety (as it applies to continuity of care) and for medicolegal reasons.
- All radiotherapy procedures, particularly those performed intraoperatively, are recorded in the patient's **Perioperative Record** and becomes a permanent document in the patient's chart.
- Radiation safety protocol must be observed when radioactive materials are employed in the conduction of a surgery in the OR (e.g., when seed implantation is performed); see Chapter 3, p. 52. **Note:** OR personnel are not at risk when preparation for after-loading techniques is employed, as the actual loading of radionuclides is done after the patient leaves the OR.
- The circulator must document in the **Perioperative Record** that all radiation safety precautions were observed during the course of the patient's surgery when intraoperative radiotherapy was performed.
- **N.B.** Each site treated requires individual consideration for the use of special instruments and necessary equipment.
- N.B. Radionuclides are never touched by hand; they may be applied to tissue through the use of an applicator or insertion device (e.g., seed applicator).
- The circulator must confer with the radiation therapist and be familiar with his/her routine to plan and prepare for the patient's care during the proposed intraoperative procedure.
- When salivary glands (especially parotid) are involved, **amifostinel/Ethyol**™ 200 mg is infused intravenously for 30 minutes preoperatively, to protect the glands from the effect of radiation or certain chemotherapeutic agents (by biochemical processes), thereby preventing or lessening *xerostomia, ("cotton mouth")*.
- **Reminder:** *Use safety precautions to identify, label, and dispense medications or solutions and to avoid medication errors; see p. 30.* It is mandatory that all medications and solutions on the sterile field be labeled by name and strength.

Radiation Therapy for Tumors of the Breast

Definition

The delivery of or preparation for delivery of ionizing radiation to malignant tumors of the breast.

Discussion

Breast cancer, the most common malignancy in females (found also in smaller numbers in males), is primarily treated surgically (see Chapter 15, p. 124). However, in appropriately selected cases, **adjunctive radiation therapy** (with chemotherapy) may be used to limit the amount of breast tissue excised. This breast conservation technique may be performed, and adjacent lymph node-bearing tissues are treated with results comparable to radical surgery. Palliative treatment for metastatic disease not amenable to surgery is also treated with radiotherapy. All patients are evaluated clinically according to histologic data of excised biopsy specimens, including **sentinel node and axillary dissection** (see p. 124), for evidence of metastatic disease. In addition, patients are advised of treatment alternatives (informed consent) and participate in the selection of their type of treatment; in some states, informed consent (of the patient) regarding the alternatives to breast surgery is mandated by law.

Ongoing revision of protocols for **external beam radiation** with intensity modulated radiotherapy **(IMRT)** can deliver calculated dosages, sparing uninvolved tissues (as ribs and other chest structures); imaging by MRI and CT scan further aids in identifying target tissues. These treatments may be combined with **brachytherapy** and performed in several different treatment settings. Outpatient insertion of interstitial catheters (for after-loading Ir^{192}) guided by imaging scans and a template can be done under local anesthesia in the radiotherapy clinic or, when general anesthesia is required, in the OR. To reduce the dose of external beam irradiation and to reduce the exposure of noninvolved tissues, **accelerated partial-breast irradiation (APBI)** technique is used in the OR, as in conjunction with **"lumpectomy"** (see p. 124).

A **MammoSite™ balloon catheter device** is placed in the lumpectomy wound for after-loading postoperatively. Ir^{192} may be given in twice-daily sessions for 5 days to an approximate dose of 34Gy, or other variations of dosing can be used, after which the catheter is removed. On occasion, this device can be placed up to 6 weeks after surgery under ultrasound guidance, pending final pathology reports. Due to various anatomical considerations, such as breast size, volume of the lumpectomy cavity, etc., some patients are not candidates for this modality.

Under investigation is the **Interbeam™ Targeted Intraoperative Therapy device,** which delivers low-energy x-rays over a period of 20 to 40 minutes in a "shielded" OR. The device is placed directly into the wound, which is closed loosely about the device, until the treatment is completed. Safety precautions to avoid skin injury and placement of the device close to the target in an irregular wound are limitations of this modality. Generally, the total dose of radiotherapy for breast cancer including external beam is approximately 46 to 50Gy, with a booster dose of 10 to 20Gy in ensuing weeks. Each patient's ultimate dosage and means of delivery is individualized.

Procedure

Placement of a MammoSite Catheter is described. A **lumpectomy**, with or without sentinel node biopsy and/or axillary dissection (see p. 124), is performed. Prior to wound closure, the MammoSite catheter with an inflation channel to a silicone balloon tip and a channel for the subsequent passage of the radioactive agent is placed in the wound with the therapy channel close to the (excised) tumor site. The balloon is inflated with saline to fill the defect in the lumpectomy wound. The wound is then closed over the catheter by either the surgeon or radiotherapist. The catheter is protected and dressings, as requested, are applied.

Preparation of the Patient, Skin Preparation, Draping, Equipment, Instrumentation, and **Supplies** are performed as for a ***Lumpectomy (of the breast) procedure*** (p. 127).

Special Notes

- Apply the **Special Notes** in Chapter 15, **Breast Surgery,** p. 128, as indicated.
- All the **Special Notes** in this chapter, **Radiation Therapy/Radiotherapy,** apply to any procedure in which radiotherapy is employed.
- ***Universal Protocol,*** p. 18, (as in other surgeries) is employed to identify the patient, the type of procedure, and the site and/or side for the intraoperative radiotherapy procedure. Documentation of all measures to ensure patient safety throughout the procedure must be included in the **Perioperative Record.**
- The circulator must provide even more emotional support than is usual (e.g., maintain eye contact, use touch to convey caring) to assure the patient during the administration of anesthesia and throughout the radiotherapeutic procedure. He/she should provide factual answers to patient questions in a confident manner whenever possible; questions can be redirected to the physician when necessary.

- The circulator should confer with the radiotherapist to plan the intraoperative radiotherapy procedure in regard to desired supplies, such as sutures, syringes, and wound dressing considerations. Most often the radiotherapist will supply the MammoSite catheter.
- **N.B.** All sources of radiotherapeutic agents must be conspicuously marked when brought to the OR.
- When an x-ray is taken or radiotherapeutic agents are used, everyone in the room must observe x-ray precautions, such as wearing a lead apron or stepping behind a lead screen or out of the room.
- The scrub person or anyone scrubbed staying in the room when x-rays are taken or when the image intensifier is used should don a lead apron before scrubbing.
- **Reminder:** The circulator gives a detailed intraoperative report of the patient's status, noting the presence of the MammoSite catheter, the nursing care implemented, and the patient outcomes achieved in the **Perioperative Record,** for patient safety regarding continuity of care and for medicolegal purposes.

Radiation Therapy for Gynecologic Tumors

Definition

The delivery of or preparation for delivery of ionizing radiation in the treatment of gynecologic tumors.

Discussion

Malignant tumors of the vulva, vagina (and vaginal cuff), uterine cervix, and corpus can be treated by radiotherapy in conjunction with surgery and chemotherapy. **Brachytherapy** is employed in the OR with the direct implantation of **radioactive seeds (Cs^{137}) in lower-dose therapy**, or various devices may be applied for the **after-loading modality (Ir^{192}) for high-dose therapy**. **Inert gold seeds** may be implanted as markers for **external beam therapy**. Total dose of radiotherapy (brachytherapy and external beam) is approximately 65Gy for most presentations (to 85Gy when pelvic nodes are included). In selected institutions, laparoscopic placement of intra-abdominal interstitial catheters (for after-loading) may be employed at sites that are suspect for local nonresectable metastases. Administering preoperative versus postoperative radiotherapy (dosage, method of delivery, use of chemotherapy, etc.) depends on multiple factors, including medical status of the patient, physician's preference, and extent and staging of the tumor. Elaboration of these considerations is beyond the scope of this text. **Radioablation of**

the ovaries, as may be necessary for treatment of some breast cancers and other hormonal based conditions, is performed by **external beam irradiation** (not done in the OR).

Endometrial and cervical cancer can be treated according to those considerations stated above. After hysterectomy, if residual tumor or potential for recurrent tumor is suspect, radiotherapy is employed. Certain presentations of vaginal cancer are treated as for cervical cancer. **Brachytherapy (Cs^{137} seed implants)** may be used for selected presentations of vulvar cancer. After hysterectomy, a vaginal cylinder containing seven channels is placed; doses are calculated and radioactive material placed strategically in five to seven of the channels, according to calculations based on clinical and anatomical presentation. Radiotherapy is utilized for palliation in selected presentations of advanced symptomatic disease using **external beam or interstitially implanted catheters** passed via a perineal template (under anesthesia) with radiologic guidance, such as CT scanning; two days of treatment may be employed before the catheters are removed. The treatment may be repeated in one week.

Procedure

Treatment for Cervical Cancer is described. Employing heavy sedation or epidural, spinal, or general anesthesia, the patient is placed in modified lithotomy position (see p. 23). The radiotherapist marks the cervical os with **gold seeds**. A Foley catheter and rectal tube containing radio-opaque dye are placed. A **Smitt sleeve** is passed into the uterus and sutured to the cervix to maintain patency of the cervix until the treatment protocol is complete. Under radiologic guidance (e.g., CT scan), two vaginal **ovoids** containing elements to shield the rectum and bladder and a transcervical cylinder **(tandem)** are placed and padded, accordingly, to prevent their movement and displacement; two catheters that accept the **radioactive pellets (Ir^{192}, Cs^{137})** are placed at either side of the external os. Depending on the dose of radiation calculated, the catheters are after-loaded postoperatively, and if multiple treatments are required, the appliances are removed and reinserted at dose-calculated intervals. After the final treatment, the Smitt sleeve is removed.

Preparation of the Patient, Skin Preparation, Draping, Equipment, Instrumentation, and **Supplies** are in use in conjunction with the gynecologic procedure in progress, or the back table is prepared as for *Conization of the Uterine Cervix*, p. 281.

For **Supplies,** add Foley catheter and rectal tube, as requested.

Special Notes

- Apply all of the **Special Notes** in this chapter, in particular, to *Radiation Therapy/Radiotherapy* safety measures, as applicable.

- **N.B.** The radiotherapist usually brings the special instruments, such as Smitt sleeve, ovoids, and tandem; he/she also brings applicators for insertion of pellets (inert gold or radioactive elements). The radioactive elements are never touched; they are inserted by means of an applicator.
- If, in addition to preparation for the after-loading technique, implantation of radioactive pellets is to be done in the OR, all radiation safety measures must be observed and documented in the **Perioperative Record**, see p. 12.
- The circulator is responsible for obtaining adequate assistance when the patient, on the OR table, is moved. He/she can help to prevent musculoskeletal injuries to team members by asking those involved to employ ergodynamic measures when positioning the patient. These include lifting by bending the knees, positioning one's body under the load, and then straightening the legs to allow the lower extremity muscles to do the lifting.
- **N.B.** The circulator prevents the risk of a positioning injury to the patient by using stirrups that are adequately padded and positioned correctly, to avoid skin and neurovascular pressure or trauma. The appearance and condition of the skin (in the areas where the stirrups touch the feet) is documented preoperatively and immediately postoperatively.
- **N.B.** The circulator lifts both legs at the same time when putting the patient's legs in stirrups to prevent postoperative lumbosacral strain. Ideally, two people are best able to do this; however one person can lift both legs by placing one leg on his/her shoulder while placing the other leg in a stirrup.
- When an x-ray is taken or the image intensifier is used, everyone in the room should observe x-ray precautions such as wearing a lead apron or stepping behind a lead screen or out of the room.
- **N.B.** The scrub person or anyone scrubbed staying in the room when x-rays are taken or when the image intensifier is used should don a lead apron before scrubbing.
- **N.B.** Raise and lower legs slowly to avoid cardiovascular disturbances, e.g., rapid alterations in venous return.
- **N.B.** *Avoid injury to the patient's fingers by preventing them from being caught in the table mechanism when the foot of the table is raised following the procedure.*
- Place the perineal pad dressing on the patient before removing the drapes to avoid bringing contaminants into the area of the surgical site.

Radiation Therapy for Carcinoma of the Prostate

Definition

The delivery and application of modalities of ionizing radiation to treat carcinoma of the prostate.

Discussion

Carcinoma of the prostate gland, the most common malignancy in the male, can be treated with a wide range of therapeutic protocols, from ***radical prostatectomy including pelvic lymph node dissection*** (p. 407) to simply observing the tumor without definitive treatment (in older asymptomatic patients). In appropriate cases, radiation therapy can offer results equal to radical surgery without the risks of surgery but with its own inherent risks, including radiation-induced cystitis and proctitis and the absence of a specimen (other than biopsy fragments). **External beam radiotherapy** may be combined with surgery, brachytherapy, and/or chemotherapy. Inert gold seeds may be placed in the prostate prior to the administration of **external beam therapy** as markers. External beam therapy may be delivered by intensity-modulated radiotherapy **(IMRT)** and **conformal radiotherapy techniques (CRT)** that deliver the appropriate dose, relatively sparing nonaffected local tissues.

In the OR, **brachytherapy** is performed by permanent insertion by means of a **MICK™ applicator or with needles preloaded** with seeds or a string of radioactive seeds (I^{125}, Pd^{103}, and, less often, Au^{198} and Yb^{169}), as lower dose therapy and with after-loading techniques, high dose Ir^{192}. These applications depend on multiple factors such as the size of the prostate and position and extent of the tumor as determined by various imaging scans, clinical exam, biopsy, etc. Great care is taken to assure exact placement of the element to avoid injury to the surrounding tissues. **Brachytherapy** is delivered in the range of 15 to 26Gy, with added **external beam therapy** to a total of 60 to 70Gy extending to the pelvic lymph node fields. Prophylactic antibiotics are administered.

Procedure

An Example of Preparation for the After-Loading Technique is described.

Following induction of epidural, spinal, or general anesthesia, the patient is placed in a modified lithotomy position (dorsal recumbent position may also be used). A genital and perineal prep is performed, and an *O'Connor plastic drape* is placed to cover the anus. A three-way Foley catheter (18Fr) is placed, and **radio-opaque dye** is instilled into the balloon. An **ultrasound probe** is placed in the rectum (through the plastic drape). An ultrasound technologist from the radiotherapy department is usually present to assist the radiotherapist. A

template (Syed-Neblett) is suture fastened to the perineal skin. Employing ultrasound guidance, approximately 14 (12 to 22) 17 gauge 20 cm long needles are passed transperineally into the prostate, periprostatic tissues, and seminal vesicles, avoiding the urethra and rectum (and other needles). The needles may be "lubricated" with alcohol. A pad is placed between the template and the perineal skin. On occasion, x-ray or CT guidance control may be required (with a change in the patient's position to the supine position).

Postoperatively, an epidural catheter may be left for pain control. After-loading treatments with $\mathbf{Ir}^{192}$ are begun after the patient's condition has stabilized and the patient has been returned to a protected room; the treatment is bi-daily sessions for two days.

Preparation of the Patient, Skin Preparation, Draping, Equipment, Instrumentation, and **Supplies** are as for a simple genitourinary procedure, e.g., with a Limited procedures tray (p. 1095) and a set up for cystoscopy, see ***Cystoscopy***, p. 391.

Add to Equipment
Padded stirrups, e.g., Allen (for modified lithotomy position)

Add to Instrumentation
Ultrasonic probe (x-ray department or radiotherapist)

Add to Draping
O'Connor plastic drape (or similar)

Add to Supplies
Perineal pad

Special Notes

- Apply all **Special Notes** in this chapter, **Radiation Therapy/Radiotherapy,** as applicable.
- Supplies that are added to the back table in addition to those brought by the radiotherapist include: a three-way Foley catheter (18Fr), radio-opaque dye, medicine cups, labels, a marking pen, and a perineal pad. Alcohol should be available to "lubricate" the needles.
- If, in addition to preparation for the after-loading technique, implantation of radioactive pellets is to be done in the OR, a template is suture secured to the perineal skin. The scrub person prepares the sutures for the template in advance of need.
- **Reminder:** When an x-ray is taken or radiotherapy is employed, everyone in the room must observe x-ray precautions by wearing a lead apron or stepping behind a lead screen or out of the room.

- The circulator should advise the x-ray department in advance that an ultrasound technologist is requested (unless the radiotherapist has made other arrangements for this service).

Radiation Therapy for Rectal Tumors

Definition

The application and delivery of ionizing radiation to tumors of the rectum.

Discussion

The standard treatment of rectal tumors, benign and malignant, is surgical excision. However, radiotherapy protocols for treatment of a malignancy are numerous; a primary and sole treatment modality may be applied to the lesion, or the lesion may be "downstaged" prior to surgery or "salvage procedures" may be employed to treat the disease (palliation).

Whether to employ radiotherapy as neoadjuvant (with or without chemotherapy) preoperatively or postoperatively, the dosage, time intervals before and after surgery, required to "protect" a rectal anastomosis performed with irradiated bowel (by means of a proximal temporary stoma), etc. are under ongoing investigations. A comprehensive discussion of this subject (or the use of radiotherapy for prevention or treatment of local metastatic disease) is beyond the purview of this text. In general, the specific lesion and its extent, position, general status of the patient, etc., contribute to any decision made in a particular patient situation. In selected cases in patients who cannot tolerate extensive surgery or electively when established criteria are met, **external beam radiation alone (50 to 60Gy)** is the primary treatment, as noted above; these treatments are performed in radiotherapy facilities.

In the OR or special procedures room in the radiology department, an anesthesia provider administers general anesthesia to the patient unless the patient cannot tolerate it; then, regional anesthesia with *conscious sedation* is employed when various local rectal radiotherapeutic procedures are done. A noncircumferential rectal cancer below 10 cm from the anus and without obvious local extension may be treated by **endocavitary radiotherapy (Papillon technique),** employing *conscious sedation,* usually performed in the radiotherapy suite, by a radiotherapist or surgeon. He/she employs a specialized sigmoidoscope-like applicator that delivers **external beam radiation (9 to 15Gy)** directly to the tumor over a course of several sessions. Infrequently, **radioactive iodine (I^{125}) seeds** may be implanted directly into the tumor.

In another modality employing the after-loading technique, the tumor is marked by (ligating) clips, and under radiographic control, an eight-channel rectal probe is positioned at the level of the tumor. **Ir^{192}** is administered, usually over a course of several sessions (6.5Gy daily × 4 for a total dose of 26Gy), and followed by resectional surgery several weeks later. **IORT** (see p. 965) with the abdominal laparotomy wound open (protected), is available in a limited number of facilities.

Preparation of the Patient, Skin Preparation, Draping, Equipment, Instrumentation, and **Supplies** as are in use in conjunction with the ongoing rectal (transanal) procedure; endocavitary radiation requires a preparation as for sigmoidoscopy (see ***Sigmoidoscopy***, p. 186).

Add to Equipment
Padded stirrups, e.g., Allen

Add to Instrumentation
Ligating clip applier (e.g., Hemoclip® applier)

Add to Supplies
Ligating clips (e.g., Hemoclips) to mark the tumor site

Special Notes

- Apply all **Special Notes** in this chapter, **Radiation Therapy/Radiotherapy**, as indicated.
- The scrub person should prepare the ligating clips (e.g., Hemoclips) in advance; they will be used to mark the tumor.

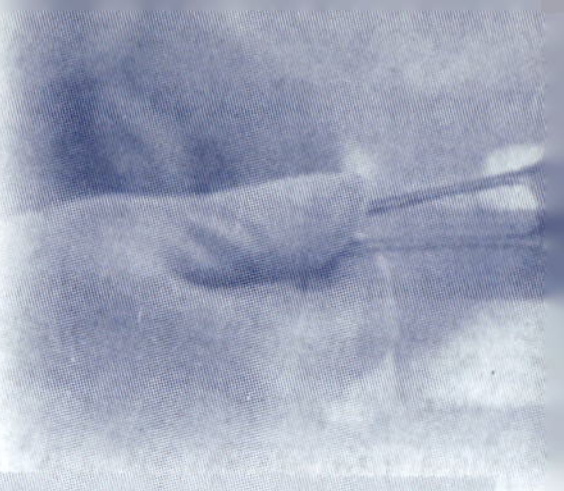

CHAPTER 31
Pediatric Surgery

Pediatric General Information

Whether the child is a neonate (newborn to 4 weeks), an infant (1 month to 12 months), a toddler (1 to 3 years), a preschooler (3 to 6 years), school age (6 to 12 years), or adolescent/teenager, perioperative care of the pediatric patient mandates attention to numerous details and considerations not ordinarily required for the adult population. The need for appropriately sized smaller instruments, equipment, drapes, supplies, etc., is obvious; however, other very important intrinsic factors must be taken into consideration. It is in this context that the propriety of the phrase the *"pediatric patient is not a small adult"* is particularly evident.

There are important concerns regarding the pediatric patient in every hospital department; concerns seem even greater when a child enters the perioperative environment. Special measures must be considered to maintain the child's safety while providing comprehensive care. The perioperative registered nurse practitioner must be familiar with what is "age-appropriate" for children at each stage of development in order to recognize deviations.

In the perioperative environment, the circulator may have precious little time to become familiar with the child and/or parents (guardians or legal representatives) to learn about the particular needs of the child. Ever present is the knowledge that every child requires special precautions that are assumed from the moment the child (patient) enters the perioperative environment.

Some facts hold true for all children, modified by their age, weight, and level of development. Some general information:

- The pediatric patient may be transported by isolette, crib, or gurney to the operating room (OR).
- The child should never be left unattended in the OR.
- When speaking to the pediatric patient, use vocabulary that is (developmentally) age appropriate.
- Pediatric patients, especially adolescents and teens, should be permitted to maintain their privacy as much as possible, as privacy is very important at that stage. Some facilities may permit the adolescent or teenager to wear underwear until he/she is asleep. Keep the patient well covered throughout the induction of anesthesia.
- Nursing interventions that may be perceived as personal or "private" are undertaken after the child is anesthetized (e.g., skin prep, insertion of a urinary catheter, and/or hair removal).

- Unfamiliar, threatening-looking instruments and equipment should be kept out of the child's sight as much as possible. This is true for any patient population.

When medications are administered preoperatively, intraoperatively, and postoperatively, the perioperative practitioner should be aware that children are generally more sensitive to the effects of drugs and their responses are more rapid and sometimes paradoxical. As anesthesia is administered, the anatomical differences between the adult and the child become more evident (e.g., child's airway). Physically, the child has a relatively larger head and tongue, the larynx is more anterior and cephalad, the epiglottis is relatively long, and the neck and trachea are shorter. The cricoid cartilage in the child is the narrowest site in the airway. A seemingly insignificant upper respiratory infection (URI) can become a potential anesthetic hazard, as any increase in congestion or local edema proportionately decreases the lumen of the airway. When a child who is receiving anesthesia has a cold, laryngospasm, bronchospasm, and consequent oxygen desaturation and its sequelae may result.

Children have a relatively higher cardiac output (with higher pulse rate). Their oxygen consumption and respiratory rates are greater than an adult's. They have lower blood pressure, necessitating particular attention to ensure stable blood pressure and vital signs. Additional important influences regarding care of the child are age, weight, nutritional status, degree of hydration, and general medical/physical condition.

Maintaining the child's body temperature and fluid balance is vital. To maintain normothermia, the amount of warmed fluids administered depends on potential preoperative deficits and the length of the proposed procedure. The *microdrip system* is a necessity to accurately administer intravenous fluids. Great care is taken to avoid even small air bubbles in fluid lines. When the child has a patent foramen ovale, intravenous air bubbles present the dire threat of brain embolism. Blood loss is less well tolerated in children than adults. The loss of blood can quickly result in lower blood pressure that potentially triggers dire consequences, as events happen so rapidly there leaves no margin for error with the pediatric patient.

Pediatric Patient Identification, Admission to the OR, and Plan of Care in the Perioperative Environment

In ideal circumstances, the perioperative practitioner has the opportunity to meet and interview the child and his/her parents during the child's preoperative visit to the hospital or on the nursing unit when the child is an inpatient. At the very least, they should meet the day before surgery. However, most often as a result of today's harried way of life, the perioperative practitioner, the person designated as the circulator during the child's surgery, makes contact with the child for the first time in the surgical holding area. At times, the circulator may not be afforded even this much opportunity, such as when another perioperative practitioner assisting in the circulator duties identifies the (child) patient and brings him/her into the room.

As infants and young children are unable to communicate effectively, their lack of ability to communicate is the very reason the parent, guardian, or legal representative must be present preoperatively and throughout the child's hospitalization to provide important personal information about the child. When the perioperative practitioner acknowledges that the parent's role is vital to ensuring the child's safety, he/she may want to assure the parent that he/she will act as the child patient's advocate during the surgical procedure in the operating room. In some facilities such as children's hospitals, after doning hospital garb, the parent may be permitted to accompany the child into the operating room until he/she is asleep.

When the child enters the surgical suite, the circulator implements the Joint Commission's (JC) (formerly the Joint Commission on Accreditation of Healthcare Organizations) 2004 *Universal Protocol* procedure to identify the child patient. The circulator begins by asking the parent(s), guardian, or legal representative, and the child, when appropriate, to state the child's name. The child's date of birth, the admitting doctor or surgeon, the proposed surgical procedure, and the patient hospital number must be identical to the patient data on the chart and the (child) patient's hospital armband. In this text, it is understood that when referring to the parent(s), reference is also made to the guardian(s) and the legal representative(s) and reference to the child in this chapter refers to the patient. The circulator reviews the **Surgical Assessment and Perioperative Checklist** with the parent and initials each item as the information is confirmed with the parent (and child, depending on the child's age). The personal information provided by the parent(s) is utilized by the perioperative practitioner to create the personalized plan of care in the **Perioperative Record** (p. 12) that is referred to throughout the child's perioperative experiencience.

As a safety measure when bringing the pediatric patient to the operating room, perioperative personnel should check the front of the patient's chart for a list of the patient's allergies and a list of the patient's current medications before leaving the pediatric floor or preoperative holding unit. When those lists are not on the front of the chart (as the list is not mandatory), perioperative personnel may request the lists from the person in charge when identification of the pediatric patient is made (prior to transporting the pediatric patient to the OR). The list of patient's allergies and current medications on the front of the child's chart helps not only to ensure the patient's safety, but may become important for medicolegal reasons as well.

Whenever possible, in preparing the pediatric patient anticipating surgery (e.g., some toddlers, preschoolers, and older school-age children), a preoperative visit to the OR with a parent(s), legal guardian, or legal representative may prove most helpful (at facilities where this is permitted).

In some facilities, preoperative assessment of the child may be made by the anesthesia provider and the perioperative practitioner during the preoperative visit a day or two prior to surgery. The visit to the OR may serve to limit the amount of preoperative medication required to calm the child, or it may eliminate the need for preoperative medication entirely. Once in the OR, as time permits, the perioperative events are explained in a nonthreatening manner to the child as they occur using age-appropriate language. When possible, the child may be permitted to make choices, as this permits him or her a sense of autonomy (e.g., choosing which facemask is used when two appropriate choices are offered).

When entering the OR, a child may be crying, appear anxious, and/or express fear (according to the child's developmental level) as he/she is separated from his/her family members. Fear of the unfamiliar uniformed strangers and the OR environment, fear of the unknown, and fear of being hurt are all frightening circumstances that may seem overwhelming to a child. To counteract the fear, the child may be permitted to bring a favorite toy for "security" into surgery (if the OR policy permits).

As the child enters the OR, he/she is greeted by name by perioperative personnel who try to create a "friendly," less-threatening atmosphere than might be anticipated. In responding to the child's questions, perioperative personnel should answer with calm, truthful, and reassuring answers that are age appropriate.

Psychological Preparation and Support of the Pediatric Patient

Psychological (emotional) support is conveyed to a child when holding the infant or small child, using a gentle touch, speaking in a gentle, nonthreatening voice, and using caring gestures, such as smiling or touching the patient's shoulder (older child). When older children ask for information regarding their surgery, the perioperative practitioner should answer as truthfully as possible in a calm and reassuring manner. If the child inquires about a body part that is to be removed, the child should be assured that he/she will be fine without the part and that he/she will feel better. The perioperative practitioner may want to assure the child that he/she will take good care of him/her and that he/she is there to help. In certain situations, a parent's presence in the OR may be permitted until the child is asleep.

The perioperative practitioner, as circulator, may convey support to the child's parent(s), legal guardian, or legal representative by giving them the explanation that he/she will act as the child patient's advocate, just as the parent would. The circulator may also relay information to the parent(s), legal guardian, or legal representative during lengthy surgeries, as appropriate, when directed by the surgeon.

Responding to the Pediatric Patient's Pain

The perioperative practitioner in the preoperative area may be required to assess the pediatric patient's level of pain. Children old enough to understand should be told that they will be given medicine if they hurt after surgery. The perioperative practitioner assesses the child's pain most appropriately by communicating with the child on his/her level. The child may indicate pain by crying, guarding a body part, grimacing, and/or pointing to the area that hurts. In the Faces, Legs, Activity, Cry, Consolability (FLACC) Scale, the level of pain is described according to the patient's behavior (for children from 3 months to 7 years). It is particularly helpful when the child is unable to communicate how he/she feels. A variety of "pain scales" (e.g., numeric scale with 10 the worst, color scale with red describing the most, Wong-Baker Faces Scale with facial expressions, etc.) may be employed to determine the pediatric patient's level of pain. Whenever possible, the child is consulted because "the child is the authority on his/her pain." He/she has the right to expect a rapid and effective response.

Plan of Care for the Pediatric Patient in the Perioperative Environment

The perioperative practitioner may choose to adapt the suggested **Patient Care Plan** (p. 9) to assess the ongoing needs of the individual child in surgery. In the plan of care, the ***foci*** represent the patient's perioperative needs, particularly the intraoperative needs, while ***interventions*** describe the nursing care by the perioperative practitioner (circulator) and others, as necessary, e.g., Nursing Focus I is the observation that the patient appears fearful and begins to cry. *The interventions* might include holding the infant and speaking softly to him/her. The *desired outcome* is demonstrated by the infant calming down enough for the anesthesia provider to place a mask near the infant on the OR table to initiate anesthesia. That the child's needs were met is demonstrated by noting the calm baby on the OR table.

All care (including treatments) is documented in the **Perioperative Record** (p. 12) to provide a written record of the events that occurred during that patient's periooprative experience. In that regard, the **Perioperative Record** becomes a record of contiuity of care, a measure of safety for the patient.

The perioperative practitioner, as the circulator, reviews the current standing orders (as stated on the surgeon's card) and any newly requested measures (with the surgical technologist, as necessary). They work together cooperatively to provide the measures necessary for quality comprehensive care of the child (patient) in the perioperative environment.

Maintenance and Regulation of the Pediatric Patient's Temperature

Measures are instituted to prevent body heat loss or hypothermia during the transportation of pediatric patients. In particular, transporting neonates and infants to the OR through cool hospital corridors can cause a rapid loss of body heat; the heated isolette helps to maintain an infant's body temperature. The child who is larger in stature may be transported to the OR in a crib or on a gurney; he/she should be covered with warm blankets, as necessary. As there is relatively more body surface exposed per area per kilogram of weight in children compared to adults, the child requires more stringent measures to maintain his/her body temperature. Body temperature should be maintained at approximately 98.6°F. Prior to the pediatric patient's arrival in the OR, the circulator and the scrub person prepare the room. The room temperature is raised to help maintain the pediatric patient's body temperature during the surgical procedure. The room temperature is regulated by adjusting the thermostat; the child patient is brought into the room when the room temperature reaches:

26° to 27°C (80° to 85°F) for infants under 11 kg (25 pounds)
23° to 24°C (75° to 80°F) for older children

Another method to help maintain the child's body temperature is the application of radiant heat lamps that are placed over the OR table; lamps should be placed approximately 27″ from the table to prevent overheating or burning the child (patient).

The exposure of a large expanse of body surface (relatively) and/or exposure of an open wound during surgery may cause hypothermia; the radiant heat lamps are placed to help minimize hypothermia in the patient (especially neonates, infants, and small children) to maintain normothermia.

Prior to the child's arrival in the room, a mattress/pad (e.g., K-Thermia® pad) may be placed on the table, or a forced-air warming blanket (e.g., Bair Hugger®) may be placed over the larger child. The temperature of the warming blanket or mattress/pad is kept at approximately 35° to 37.7°C (95° to 100°F); it is closely regulated to avoid burn injury. A warming pad and a forced-air warming blanket are ***never*** used together, as the potential for burning the child (patient) is too great.

The head of neonates and small infants may be covered (e.g., with tube stockinette cap) to prevent loss of body heat; their extremities may also be covered (e.g., with bias stockinette or Webril and plastic wrap). All solutions, such as intravenous (IV) fluids, blood, blood products, etc., are warmed prior to use (with a blood and fluid warmer, e.g., Thermal Angel®) to maintain the child's body temperature during the administration of fluids to avoid hypothermia.

Skin prep solutions are warmed immediately before use. Prep solutions are not permitted to pool under the patient because the body is cooled as the prep solution evaporates, thereby lowering body temperature (resulting in hypothermia); see other skin-care concerns regarding pooled prep solution precautions below. Irrigation fluid is warmed to body temperature prior to use. The circulator may want to wait until just before the irrigation solution is needed to pour it. The scrub person must always check the temperature of the irrigation solution before passing the bulb syringe to the surgeon. Overwarming due to excessive draping is avoided because, as it causes the patient to sweat; evaporation of the sweat can chill the patient and result in hypothermia. At the conclusion of the surgical procedure prior to transporting the patient from the OR to the postanesthesia care unit (PACU), the pediatric patient's normal body temperature is maintained either by placing the infant in an isolette or for the larger child by using warmed blankets (secured from a thermal blanket warmer), to avoid hypothermia.

Anesthesia Considerations for the Pediatric Patient

The circulator is responsible for assisting the anesthesia provider in all ways necessary during the administration of local and general anesthesia to the pediatric patient. He/she should know the names and the effects of medications used for the pediatric population; he/she should also be aware of the untoward effects of the medications. The circulator, as well as the anesthesia provider, must closely observe the child intraoperatively for any untoward reactions to medication.

Although sedatives are infrequently used for the pediatric patient, when sedation is desired, Versed™ (midazolam) is the most-often-used preoperative sedative for children. Versed may be administered orally, intranasally, rectally, intramuscularly (IM), or intravenously (IV); scopolamine hydrobromide may be added for its sedative and amnesic amnestic effect. Alternatively for sedation, fentanyl and ketamine may be used. For information regarding the medications used in general anesthesia, see Table 4–1 in Chapter 4, p. 63. Equipment necessary for use in general anesthesia may be found in Chapter 5, p. 80. During the delivery of general anesthesia, anesthetic gases must be warmed prior to their administration. Children most often receive oxygen, halothane, and nitrous oxide gas that flows from a facemask placed near the child's face, until the child becomes drowsy. At the onset of administration, the mask is not placed directly on the child's face, as that is generally too frightening for children. Once the child is receiving anesthetic agents such as nitrous oxide, oxygen, and halothane combination, delivered by mask, an intravenous line is started to provide intravenous access and to supplement inhalation agents with additional agents during general anesthesia. Postoperative analgesia will be necessary immediately upon arousal when the halothane is discontinued, as the sensation of pain returns.

In anticipation of starting an IV line with prewarmed fluids, EMLA (2.5% lidocaine, 2.5% prilocaine) or LMX4™ (4% lidocaine) anesthetic cream may be applied to a small area on the child's arm (at a potential venipuncture site) about 1 hour preoperatively. The perioperative RN may cover the area with a Tegoderm™ dressing, or a premade disc containing EMLA cream may be applied. Similarly, this may be done 1 hour preoperatively by a parent at home (when given instructions) prior to admission when the child is an outpatient. The anesthetic effect of the EMLA cream occurs when the skin area appears either blanched or reddened; the effect may last up to 4 hours. Excessive use of the cream causes drug toxicity; therefore, following the manufacturer's guidelines closely is mandatory.

Pediatric surgery must be performed early in the day whenever possible so that the child patient does not have "nothing by mouth" (NPO) status for an excessive period of time, as dehydration and its ensuing sequelae may occur rapidly (unless intravenous fluids are administered).

For infants, a guide to the NPO preoperative interval is:

Clear liquids up to 2 hours preoperatively
Breast milk up to 4 hours preoperatively
Cow's milk or solids up to 6 hours preoperatively

The room and anesthesia cart should be prepared in advance for the arrival of the pediatric patient. Pediatric inductions (of general anesthesia), as noted above, are frequently performed through a mask; the mask should be gently applied to avoid local swelling postoperatively. Warmed nitrous oxide (N_2O) and oxygen (O_2) are administered, after which an IV catheter is inserted, and the additional anesthetic gases are administered, as previously mentioned. For older children, IV induction may be employed.

Prior to the child's arrival, all the equipment necessary to administer general anesthesia must be readily available, e.g., assorted types and sizes of intravenous catheters, a pediatric anesthesia circuit, a pediatric rebreathing bag, a humidifier, small suction catheters, and appropriately sized endotracheal tubes.

Recommended endotracheal tube sizes:

2.5 to 3.0 mm (8 to 9Fr) newborn
3.5 to 4.5 mm (10 to 14Fr) infant
5.0 mm (15Fr) small child
7.0 to 7.5 mm (21Fr) most adolescents/teens

When pediatric patients are intubated, straight blades are most often used (on the laryngoscope). Because the pediatric airway is narrow, especially at the cricoid cartilage (as noted above), endotracheal tubes are uncuffed (until approximately age 8); if there is no air leak at a higher pressure (>25 cm H_2O), the tube may be too wide, and potential postoperative edema and airway problems may result. Laryngospasm may result when halothane is delivered too rapidly. Laryngospasm is treated with positive pressure employing oxygen, succinylcholine, and atropine delivered by mask. As suctioning becomes necessary, the suction tube lumen should not exceed 5 to 10Fr. The circulator should verify that two room suction units are in good working order and ready for use prior to the child's entry. In the event that the suction on anesthesia cart does not function properly, the room suctions must be immediately substituted. Pediatric electrodes are necessary for electrocardiogram (EKG/ECG) monitoring. Regional block anesthetic may be instituted following the general anesthesia induction, but it is used primarily for postoperative pain relief.

Malignant Hyperthermia

Malignant hyperthermia (MH), a grave consequence of general anesthesia administration, may result from the use of a combination of succinylcholine with anesthetic gases, such as halothane. Family history may provide essential clues to identifying children who are at high risk for MH. As the succinylcholine and anesthetic gas agents are thought to precipitate MH, they are not used in children when there is a known family predisposition to MH, nor are they used in children with neuromuscular disorders (may be more susceptible to MH). The anesthesia provider and the circulator must be ever alert to a rapid rise in the pediatric patient's temperature. Prompt corrective measures must be undertaken for management of an ***"MH crisis"*** (pp. 68–69) to prevent death.

The circulator must know the location of the MH cart before bringing the child patient into the room.

Should an MH crisis occur, the circulator should immediately summon assistance.

An MH crisis is recorded in the **Perioperative Record;** in addition, an **Incident Report** recording the intraoperative proceedings should be filed. An **Incident Report** must be filed whenever an untoward patient event/reaction occurs; the unusual reaction or circumstance and its resolution or outcome must be fully described.

Fluid Balance Maintenance

An IV line is placed to help maintain the pediatric patient's fluid balance; to administer medications, blood, blood products, and blood substitutes; to prevent hypovolemia; and to keep open a direct line to the patient's vascular system. The circulator assists the anesthesia provider in establishing the IV line. The equipment used to establish an IV line should be preassembled and placed on the anesthesia cart before the child enters the room. Occasionally a cut-down or a venous catheter may be necessary. An IV line is inserted (usually in the upper extremity); following placement of the IV, the upper extremity may be secured to a padded board by padded restraint. The IV route is maintained throughout the surgery and immediately postoperative or longer, as necessary. The amounts and specific composition of the prewarmed fluids administered are recorded; a pediatric-sized IV system with "microdrip" ensures accuracy when administering IV fluids. An accurate measurement of IV fluid intake intraoperatively is documented in the **Perioperative Record**.

Blood Volume Maintenance

As a child's blood volume is proportionately less than an adult's, it is important to replace the loss (IV fluid, blood, or blood products) as soon as possible. Before surgery begins, the circulator should ascertain that blood has been typed and screened (or cross-matched), as ordered; the blood or blood products must be immediately available upon demand. The circulator may obtain the blood administration set and blood warmer to assist the anesthesia provider in administering the blood or blood products. The circulator should assist the anesthesia provider comparing the identifying numbers on the blood (or blood products) and the patient identity number to verify that the correct blood type is being administered to the correctly identified patient. The circulator documents the identification numbers on the unit of blood or blood products administered on the **Perioperative Record.** Sponges must be weighed when significant blood loss is anticipated.

The circulator measures blood loss to assist the anesthesia provider in determining an accurate fluid balance to prevent hypovolemia. The immediate weighing of sponges reduces the "evaporation factor," making the blood loss estimate more accurate. The circulator should use metric (gram) scales to weigh each type of dry sponge. The scale should be set to reflect the weight of the dry sponge by setting this weight as a negative below "point 0." Both raytec and lap sponges are weighed. Using this method, the weight of the dry sponge is automatically subtracted from the weight of the used (wet) sponge. Irrigation solutions must be accurately measured to provide an accurate estimate of fluid lost by the child. To determine the amount of blood in the irrigation fluid recovered, the volume of irrigation utilized is subtracted. Urinary drainage must be accurately measured with a urimeter/urometer or similarly calibrated device marked with small volume increments (e.g., milliliters). Fluid output is measured from all sources. The circulator records the estimated fluid loss in the **Perioperative Record**.

Skin Care Precautions

The condition of skin should be documented in the **Perioperative Record** before beginning the skin prep and following completion of the prep. When the skin is prepped, pooling of prep solutions is avoided to prevent skin maceration and/or chemical irritation; this is especially true for the delicate skin of children. Also, the pooling of prep solutions is not permitted, as most are flammable and a fire hazard. The circulator should describe the skin, noting any reaction to the prep solution. If a reaction occurs, the circulator should discontinue the prep, report the reaction to the surgeon, and ask the surgeon for further directions or measures to take. The circulator documents any untoward skin reaction to the prep solution or the lack of a reaction to the prep solution in the **Perioperative Record**. When an untoward reaction occurs, an **Incident Report** must also be filed; the reaction and its resolution or outcome are fully described.

The direct application of adhesive tape to the skin is avoided, as adhesive tape is irritating; also the patient may be allergic to adhesive tape. Alternate types of tape should be in the room and substituted for adhesive tape whenever possible, e.g., paper, plastic, and nonallergic tape (e.g., Durapore®, Transpore®, Micropore®, Microfoam®). If adhesive tape must be used, the skin is first protected with tincture of benzoin. Tape (any type) should not be placed on skin areas that appear irritated. The circulator should document the condition of the skin in the **Perioperative Record** before the tape is applied and when the tape is removed.

In addition, when positioning the patient, pressure points (e.g., elbows, heels, knees, ankles, and sacrum) must be well padded to avoid skin breakdown and nerve injuries, especially in lengthy surgeries; see positioning considerations below.

Positioning Considerations

To facilitate access to the pediatric patient, the head and the foot of the OR table may be removed. The table may be reversed if the surgeon performs the surgery when seated; this allows room for the surgeon's legs. When positioning the pediatric patient, hyperextension and/or hyperflexion of the joints is avoided to prevent nerve traction-type injuries (e.g., to the brachial plexus). Bony prominences are padded to avoid nerve, vascular, and skin injury. Particular attention should be paid to using padding, especially in lengthy procedures, as a child's skin is fragile and may easily break down. The circulator should document the appearance of the skin in regard to positioning in the **Perioperative Record** prior to starting the surgery and immediately postoperatively.

A mummy-like wrap (sometimes in conjunction with a "papoose" board) may be used to restrain and protect newborns, small infants, and even certain small children when the procedure is performed under local anesthesia. Otherwise, when the child is restrained, soft, padded, nonconstricting extremity restraints are used. The circulator should document the type of restraints used and the appearance of the skin at the points of restraint in the **Perioperative Record** prior to placing the restraints and when the restraints are removed.

Conclusion of Intraoperative Care of the Pediatric Patient

At the conclusion of the surgical procedure, the circulator accompanies the pediatric patient and the anesthesia provider to the PACU where care of the patient is transferred to the PACU perioperative practitioner, who then becomes the child's advocate. During transportation of the pediatric patient, the circulator provides the necessary measures required to maintain the child's body temperature to avoid hypothermia (e.g., using an isolette or warmed blankets in the crib). In addition to the orders given to the perioperative practitioner by the anesthesia provider, the circulator gives a full intraoperative report regarding the patient's status for continuity of care (patient safety and for medicolegal reasons).

The perioperative practitioner and the surgical technologist should consider all of the aforementioned measures of patient care regarding the pediatric patient in the perioperative environment, as applicable.

Pediatric Tracheostomy

Definition

Insertion of a cannula into an opening made in the trachea to facilitate breathing.

Discussion

Pediatric tracheostomy may be indicated when the upper airway is obstructed due to anatomic or neuromuscular conditions, excessive nasal or oral secretions, bronchopulmonary dysplasia (requiring prolonged assisted ventilation), foreign body aspiration, sleep apnea, etc. Today, medical management of upper (and lower) respiratory infections (URI) has diminished the need for this procedure. The long-term presence of a tracheostomy is often associated with speech problems. In infants, the trachea is relatively shorter, and the cartilaginous structures are soft and more difficult to palpate than in adults. The thyroid may be situated lower than in the adult, and a pretracheal fat pad may contain substantial blood vessels.

In acute respiratory emergencies, the cricothyroid membrane may be incised and a trocar or any available hollow tube inserted.

Procedure

Pediatric tracheostomy is most often performed under general anesthesia. The procedure is similar to adult **Tracheostomy**, p. 843, except that segments of the tracheal rings are not excised. A vertical midline incision approximately 1.5″ may be used when landmarks are not readily palpable; in infants and small children there is less bleeding than with a transverse incision, but a more prominent scar results. When the more cosmetic horizontal incision is used for older children, the transverse incision is placed in a skin crease midway between the cricoid and the suprasternal notch. Bleeding is best treated with monopolar electrosurgery. Blunt dissection is carried out through the subcuticular planes until the trachea is reached. The thyroid isthmus is freed from the underlying trachea and retracted superiorly or inferiorly for exposure of the relevant tracheal rings; some surgeons cut through the isthmus.

In infants, a vertical incision through the second, third, and fourth tracheal rings results in less stenosis and less airway resistance. Care is taken not to injure the larynx or the inominate artery. The incision is made from below upwards to avoid injury to the mediastinal contents. The endotracheal tube is withdrawn just proximal to the incision. The stoma is created and a tracheostomy tube that is two-thirds to three-quarters of the tracheal diameter is inserted under direct vision. The tracheostomy tube is placed and both lungs are inflated as the endotracheal tube is completely withdrawn. Tight wound closure is avoided to prevent subcutaneous emphysema, especially when assisted ventilation is employed. Sutures may be used to hold the flanges of the tube to the neck skin. The tube is held in place either with a Velcro band or umbilical tape. All manipulations are done with the neck still slightly flexed to prevent accidental decannulation.

Preparation of the Patient

The room temperature is adjusted prior to the child's arrival. A warming mattress/pad (e.g., K-Thermia pad) may be placed on the table, radiant heat lamps may be positioned over the table, and the head and extremities may be covered to maintain extremities normothermia depending on the size/weight/age of the child (see Pediatric General Information). The foot and/or head sections of the OR table may be removed. For a neonate, infant, or small child, he/she may be placed in a mummy-like wrap until completely anesthetized. Following induction of general anesthesia, the child is placed in supine position with the neck gently extended; a small roll may be placed under the shoulders to extend the neck to optimize exposure. Small sandbags may be placed at the sides of the head for stabilization. An IV line is inserted, and warmed IV solution is administered; the extremity is secured to a padded board while the other extremities are padded and restrained as necessary, using nonconstricting padded restraints, placed after the child is anesthetized. All bony prominences and areas vulnerable to skin and neurovascular trauma or pressure are padded. A pediatric electrosurgical dispersive pad is placed.

Skin Preparation

Using warm prep solutions only, begin cleansing the neck; extend the prep from the level of the infra-auricular border to the axillae and down to the table around the neck to the level of the shoulders. Lap pads may be placed at the sides of the neck to avoid pooling of the prep solution. Care should be taken in removing the pads not to contaminate the prepped surgical field.

Draping

Folded towels and a sheet with a small fenestration

Equipment

Overhead radiant heat lamps
Mattress/pad (K-Thermia pad)
Small roll (placed under the shoulders)
Small sandbags (2, to stabilize the position of the head)
Covering for the head (e.g., tube stockinette and plastic wrap) and covering for the extremities (e.g., bias stockinette or kerlix and plastic wrap), depending on the size/weight/age of the child, optional
Padded board (e.g., to support arm) where IV line placed
Padded extremity restraints
ESU (electrosurgical unit), monopolar (most often) or bipolar
Suction

Instrumentation

Tracheostomy tray
Pediatric minor procedures tray
Tracheostomy tubes, assorted, pediatric-sized (e.g., 2.5 to 3 mm for newborn, up to 7.0 to 7.5 mm for the adolescent/teenager)
Bipolar electrosurgical forceps and cord, optional

Supplies

Basin set
Blades, (2) #15 and (1) #11
Needle magnet or counter
Suction tubing
Umbilical tape or Velcro band for holding tracheostomy tube in place
Electrosurgical pencil (with needle tip) and cord, optional

Special Notes

- Apply **Special Notes** from Abdominal Laparotomy, p. 134, and measures from the **Pediatric General Information**, p. 978, as applicable.
- Prior to the child's arrival, the circulator adjusts the room temperature as follows: 26° to 27°C (80° to 85°F) for infants under 11 kg (25 pounds) and 23° to 24°C (75° to 80°F) for older children.
- **Reminder:** The circulator employs the ***Universal Protocol*** to verify the child's identity. He/she checks the chart and armband and, according to the patient's age, he/she asks the child, as appropriate. In the preoperative area, data was confirmed with the parent.
- The circulator checks the chart for patient sensitivities and allergies. The circulator confirms the child's sensitivities and allergies or the lack of same to avoid potential allergic reactions. In the preoperative area, data was confirmed with the parent.
- The circulator alerts the surgeon and ansthesia provider to any allergy not previously noted and confers with them measures necessary to avoid the child's allergic reaction.
- The circulator documents the noted allergy and the alternative product used in the **Perioperative Record**.
- The circulator documents the appearance of the skin preoperatively and immediately postoperatively with respect to any sensitivity or allergic reaction.
- The circulator may place a warming mattress/pad on the OR table to maintain normothermia and to avoid hypothermia.
- When warming heat lamps are placed over the table, they are placed 27″ from the table to avoid burning the patient.
- The scrub person should be ready in advance with Velcro bands or umbilical tapes (to tie behind the neck) to hold the tracheostomy tube in place.
- Catheters obtained for suctioning should have an external diameter less than one half the internal diameter of the tracheostomy tube to avoid hypoxia or a collapsed lung.
- The surgeon may use a nonadherent pad and a gauze dressing pad is split halfway up the middle and placed around the tube (after the tube is connected to the ventilation equipment) to provide protection and avoid injury to the skin.

- **N.B.** *The circulator ascertains that* **the obturator is taped to the top of the isolette or crib,** *making it easy to find in an emergency.* Should the tracheostomy tube become dislodged, the obturator must be replaced and the tube immediately reinserted.
- **Reminder:** In transit to the PACU, measures to maintain the child's body temperature are instituted, e.g., an isolette or warmed blankets in the crib.
- **Reminder:** The circulator gives a report to the PACU perioperative practitioner regarding the patient's status, the intraoperative care implemented, and the desired patient outcomes for continuity of care (patient safety) and for medicolegal reasons.
- **N.B.** In the PACU, a humidifier is used to prevent drying of mucous membranes and secretions; the ultrasonic type humidifier is preferred.
- In the PACU, the child (patient) is suctioned as needed. To avoid injury to the mucous membranes, the suction catheter is inserted without suction and negative pressure is exerted as the catheter is withdrawn.
- In the PACU, the perioperative practitioner should be alert to signs of acute respiratory emergency, subcutaneous emphysema, or pneumothorax postoperatively. A description of the patient's respirations is documented in the **Perioperative Record.**
- In the PACU, if the peristomal area appears irritated, an order for a barrier cream is requested, if one has not been ordered.

Branchial Cleft Sinusectomy

Definition

Excision of a tract resulting from the nonclosure of an embryologic branchial cleft.

Discussion

Branchial Cleft Sinuses are congenital anomalies that are most often noted in later childhood, but they may be seen in infants. Remnants of embryonic development, first and second branchial clefts are the most common. The first branchial cleft sinus extends from the auditory canal to just below the midpoint of the mandible. The second branchial cleft sinus extends from the tonsillar fossae to the lower anterior border of the sternocleidomastoid muscle. The lesion may present as a chronically draining sinus or an abscess (in which case, the definitive procedure is delayed until after drainage).

Procedure

First Branchial Cleft Sinusectomy in a Small Child is described. A transverse elliptical incision is made around the external sinus opening (usually in the submandibular or upper neck region). The tract is dissected, and the incision is extended posteriorly toward the angle of the mandible and lower portion of the auditory canal. Care is taken to avoid injury to the marginal mandibular (and other) branches of the facial nerve. The tract is divided at the external auditory canal and ligated. The wound is closed in layers, usually over a small drain.

Preparation of the Patient

The room temperature is adjusted in advance of the patient's arrival, a warming mattress/pad may be placed on the table, radient heat lamps may be placed over the table, and other measures may be instituted to maintain normothermia, depending on the size/weight/age of the child (see **Pediatric General Information**). The head and foot sections of the table may be removed. General anesthesia with endotracheal intubation is administered with the child in supine position. The head is turned to the side with the affected side uppermost and the dependent ear well padded. A roll may be placed under the shoulders to gently extend the neck to optimize exposure. Following induction of general anesthesia, an IV line is inserted and the extremity is secured to a padded board. The extremities are restrained using nonconstricting padded restraints, placed after the child is anesthetized. All bony prominences and areas vulnerable to skin and neurovascular trauma or pressure are padded. A pediatric electrosurgical dispersive pad is placed (with monopolar electrosurgery).

Skin Preparation

Using warm prep solutions only, begin prepping the neck; extend the prep from the infra-auricular border to the nipples and down to the table at the sides of the neck and the shoulders. Lap pads may be placed at the sides of the neck to avoid pooling of the prep solution under the patient. Care should be taken not to contaminate the prepped surgical area when the lap pads are removed.

If the sinus is draining (pus), a sponge saturated in prep solution is placed over the opening and the isolated sinus area is prepped last. The area around the sinus opening is prepped from outward in; each sponge used to prep the opening is discarded following use.

Draping

Folded towels and a sheet with a small fenestration

Equipment

Overhead radiant heat lamps,optional
Mattress/pad (e.g., K-Thermia pad); **do not use both at the same time**
Small roll placed between shoulders, optional
Padded extremity restraints, as needed
Padded board (e.g., for upper extremity) to support forearm with IV line
Suction
ESU, monopolar or bipolar
Nerve stimulator/locator/monitor, e.g., Concept® (avoids or detects possible nerve injury; unit should face the anesthesia provider), optional

Instrumentation

Pediatric minor procedures tray
Weitlaner retractor, small
Bipolar electrosurgical forceps and cord, optional

Supplies

Basin set
Blades, (2) #15
Needle magnet or counter
Electrosurgical pencil (with needle point) and cord, optional
Suction tubing
Dissector sponges (e.g., peanuts, Kittners), optional
Drain (e.g., rubber band or 1/4″ Penrose), optional; check chart for latex allergy

Special Notes

- Apply **Special Notes** from ***Pediatric Tracheostomy,*** p.992, and measures from **Pediatric General Information**, p. 978, as applicable.
- Document any allergy noted, the alternative product used, and the appearance of the skin preoperatively and immediately postoperatively in the **Perioperative Record**.
- Dissector sponges (e.g., peanuts or kittners) are included in the sponge count.
- Bipolar ESU may be preferred over monopolar, as less injury is caused to the tissues in the immediately surrounding area. With bipolar ESU, an electrosurgical dispersive pad is ***not*** placed.

- **N.B.** A *nerve monitor* (e.g., Concept) may be requested to avoid injury to the facial nerve branch. The circulator consults the surgeon regarding the settings on the monitor; the screen should face the anesthesia provider during the surgical procedure.
- **N.B.** *The patient's chart is checked for latex allergy before a rubber band or Penrose drain is placed in the wound.* Any untoward reaction to latex or lack of reaction is documented in the **Perioperative Record**.
- If the patient has a sensitivity or allergy to latex, the drain should be composed of a different material (e.g., polyethylene). Document the item used as a substitute.
- Document the appearance of the skin in regard to any sensitivity or allergic reaction preoperatively and immediately postoperatively, as necessary.
- In many institutions, an **Incident Report** must also be filed when the patient has an allergic response.
- A stitch or a small safety pin should be available in advance to secure the drain at the conclusion of the surgical procedure.

Correction of Congenital Dislocation of the Hip

Definition

Restoration of the hip joint in any of several presentations of congenital hip dysplasia with dislocation.

Discussion

When **correction of congenital dislocation of the hip** is performed, the corrective procedure depends on the age of the patient and the degree of dislocation. In females more than males, dysplastic abnormalities of the acetabulum and adjacent tissues, may lead to varying degrees of subluxation and dislocation of the hip. Ensuing soft-tissue contractures may preclude nonoperative reduction. Other conditions such as *coxa vera* in which the angle of the femoral neck and shaft is reduced or distortions in local pelvic angulation (associated with ***exstrophy of the bladder,*** p.1009) may require similar approach procedures for correction. Early lesser presentations of hip dislocation may respond to splinting (e.g., Pavlik harness) or to closed reduction with application of spica cast as well as traction and muscle tenotomies.

Numerous surgical procedures and approaches to the local structures have been devised related to the specific abnormality. Related procedures include derotational osteotomies and shortening of the femur. Complete joint replacement (see ***Total Hip Joint Replacement,*** p. 589) may be required.

Procedure

Treatment of Congenital Dislocation of the Hip by Open Reduction with Salter Innominate Osteotomy is described. The child is placed in supine position (for open reduction) with a radiolucent "sandbag" placed under the thorax so the affected side is elevated, or the child may be placed in the lateral position (for osteotomies) with the lower extremity draped into the field to enable manipulation. An incision is made from the mid iliac crest inferiorly to the anterosuperior iliac spine, continuing to the middle of the inguinal ligament. Adductor tenotomy may be performed. Adjacent muscles are displaced to expose the anterosuperior spine; the heads of the rectus femoris muscle are released from the joint capsule and acetabulum. The periosteum is reflected from the iliac crest to the acetabulum, and posteriorly to the greater sciatic notch. Adhesions are freed about the joint capsule.

When the femoral head cannot be reduced, the joint capsule is opened and redundant soft tissue is excised. If reduction is still not possible, **innominate osteotomy** will be necessary. The hip is fully dislocated and the medial surface of the ilium is exposed. The iliopsoas tendon is detached and by retracting additional soft tissues; a Gigli saw may be passed about the ilium from the sciatic notch to the anteroinferior spine and sawn through. A wedge of iliac crest is removed for a graft. Using towel clips or bone forceps for traction, the ilium is manipulated to restore the angulation of the acetabulum, and the previously cut (iliac crest) wedge is inserted to maintain the position of the ilial segments, fixed by two Steinmann pins or K (Kirschner) wires. The femoral head is reduced, placed in position for appropriate rotation, flexion, and abduction. Capsulorraphy is performed, and divided muscular segments reattached. During the course of surgery with manipulation of the femur, caution is taken to protect the lateral femoral cutaneous, sciatic, obturator, and femoral nerves from direct injury or undue traction. The K wires are trimmed to fit in the subcutaneous adipose tissue, and the wound is closed. A spica cast is applied.

Preparation of the Patient

The room temperature is adjusted prior to the arrival of the child, radiant heat lamps may be positioned over the table, the head and extremities may be covered (see **Pediatric General Information)**, a forced-air warming blanket (e.g., Bair Hugger) or a prewarmed blanket may be placed over the patient to maintain normothermia, according to the weight/age/and size of the patient. ***(Note: a warming mattress pad is not used, as the pad interferes with taking x-rays.)*** Following induction of general anesthesia, the child is placed in supine position with the thorax on the affected side up, elevated by a radiolucent "sandbag," or the patient may be placed in the lateral position (see lateral position, p. 26) with the lower extremity abducted and draped into the field to enable manipulation. An IV line is inserted and the extremity, secured on a padded board. The other extremities are restrained using nonconstricting padded restraints placed after the child is anesthetized. All bony prominences and areas vulnerable to skin and neurovascular trauma or pressure are padded. A pediatric electrosurgical dispersive pad is placed.

Skin Preparation

A plastic adhesive drape (Steridrape™) may be placed to drape the perineum out of the field before the skin prep. Using warm prep solution only, begin over the greater trochanter on the affected side, extending the prep from the nipple to below the knee. Prep beyond the midline of the abdomen (or to the plastic adhesive drape) and down to the table on the affected side.

Draping

For either supine or lateral position, the leg on the affected side is abducted and the foot grasped in a doubled tube stockinette. A drape sheet is placed over the end of the table. The outer tube stockinette is brought up to the top of the thigh (the inner tube covers the foot only). A split sheet is draped under the thigh, and the adhesive-backed tails are draped around the borders of the (intended) incision. Towels may be secured around the (intended) incision site. A sterile, plastic adhesive drape may be placed over the site of the (intended) incision. A sheet may be draped proximal to the incision. The leg is passed through the opening of a pediatric laparotomy or transverse sheet. A drape is required for the C-arm (x-ray).

Equipment

- Radiant heat lamps
- Covering for the head and extremities, and/or
- Warming blanket (e.g., Bair Hugger), depending on the weight/age/size of the child (see **Pediatric General Information)**, optional
- Radiolucent sandbag (for positioning, small), optional
- Padded board to support the extremity (IV line), optional
- Padded extremity restraints, as needed, optional
- EKG/ECG monitor and pediatric leads (anesthesia provider)
- ESU, monopolar or bipolar
- Suctions
- Scales, metric (gram), optional
- Power sources for saw and/or drill, if used, optional
- Cast cart

Fluoroscopy with C-arm (portable x-ray)
Pulsed lavage console (e.g., Impulse™, Simpulse™), optional

Instrumentation

Minor orthopedic procedures tray
Pediatric major procedures tray
Small hand saw (e.g., Gigli saw handles and wire blade; add extra wire blade) or mini power saw with blades, chuck, key, and cord, optional
Small hand drill, chuck, and key or mini power drill with chuck, key, and cord unless self-contained (e.g., battery), optional
Steinmann pins or K (Kirschner) wires (for fixation) and pin cutter
Guide wires (e.g., K wires), include extra
Bone plate and screws or compression plate and screws, optional
Stainless steel wire, heavy gauge (osteotomies), optional
Pulsed lavage suction irrigator and tip, e.g., Impulse, Simpulse, optional
Ligating clip appliers (e.g., Hemoclip® appliers), short and medium
Bipolar electrosurgical forceps and cord, optional

Total Hip, Add

Total hip prosthesis and its specific instrumentation (e.g., acetabular reamer, acetabular knife, extractor, etc.), optional

Supplies

Tube stockinettes, (2) small (4″), optional
Sterile, plastic adhesive drapes (2) for perineum and operative site, optional
Basin set
Suction tubing
Electrosurgical pencil with needlepoint tip and cord, optional
Blades, (2) #15 and (2) #10
Needle magnet or counter
Ligating clips (e.g., Hemoclips), small and medium
Suction tubing (2) for irrigation and suction, cojoined suction and irrigation tubing for pulsed lavage unit, optional
Irrigation solution (lactated Ringer's or antibiotic) for pulsed lavage or graduated pitcher and asepto syringes (2) with antibiotic irrigation
Cast cart (supplies for spica cast)

For Total Hip, Add

Gelfoam, thrombin, and cotton pledgets (available) to dry canal, optional
Polymethylmethacrylate (PMMA), optional
Closed drainage unit (e.g., Hemovac), optional
Abduction pillow

Special Notes

- Apply **Special Notes** for ***Pediatric Tracheostomy,*** p. 992, and **measures** from **Pediatric General Information,** p. 978, as applicable.
- **N.B. Reminder:** *A warming mattress/pad is* **never** *placed on the OR table when x-rays will be taken.*
- The surgeon (particularly orthopedic) may request that the procedure be performed in the OR equipped with *laminar air flow*.
- **Reminder:** The circulator should be certain that the correct x-ray films for the *correctly identified* patient are in the room prior to the start of the procedure. This should be confirmed again during ***"time-out."***
- When indicated, the circulator should notify the x-ray department that x-rays will be needed. Fluoroscopy may be employed (or individual x-rays may be taken) to provide (anteroposterior [AP] and lateral view) guidance for the correct placement of guide wires or pins.
- When an x-ray is taken or the image intensifier is used, everyone in the room must observe x-ray precautions, e.g., by wearing a lead apron or by stepping out of the room, etc. (see p. 52).
- **N.B.** The scrub person (and all persons scrubbed) staying in the room while x-rays are taken or the image intensifier is used should don a lead apron **before** scrubbing.
- **N.B.** *When total hip prosthesis will be performed, prior to bringing the patient into the room, the surgeon is shown a variety of implants and chooses the type he/she prefers.* ***Do not*** start any procedure unless the implant and insertion instrumentation are in the room, ready to be used; they should be sterile or ready to be sterilized by autoclaving. This should be confirmed during "*time out.*"
- **N.B.** The prosthesis (implant) in the requested size as well as implants a size larger and a size smaller (for a total of 3 implants) and the insertion instrumentation required for the specific type of prosthesis must be sterilized.
- **N.B.** The circulator should be certain that an adequate level of pressure (gas or compressed air) is in the tank when power equipment is to be used, unless the equipment is self-contained (e.g., battery).
- **N.B.** *Prior to bringing the patient into the room when a total hip will be performed, the circulator should consult*

the blood bank regarding whether blood or blood products are available as ordered (complete blood count).

- The circulator assists the anesthesia provider in comparing identifiers to ascertain that the correct blood or blood product to be used is for the correctly identified patient (according to identity number and blood type).
- **N.B.** The circulator should document any untoward reaction to transfused blood (or blood products) or lack of reaction in the **Perioperative Record**.
- **N.B.** An **Incident Report** complete with all the facts must be filed when the patient has an untoward reaction to a blood transfusion; additional information is documentated in the **Perioperative Record**.
- **N.B.** The circulator weighs the sponges (when indicated) to assist in determining blood loss. He/she should weigh the sponges immediately to avoid the "evaporation factor." To weigh sponges, see **Pediatric General Information**, p. 978.
- *The scrub person measures accurately irrigation fluid used to assist in determining fluid loss replacement.*
- The circulator maintains an accurate record of the amount of irrigation used to assist in determining fluid replacement.
- **N.B.** Cotton pledgets must be included in the count. Cotton pledgets should be individually pointed out when first counted and should be individually counted again at the beginning of wound closure.
- A pulsed lavage irrigator, e.g., Simpulse, may be used to irrigate and debride the wound prior to closure; follow safety precautions regarding its use; see Chapter 2, p. 46.
- *The scrub person must monitor the temperature of the irrigation solution as it leaves the pulsed lavage outflow tubing (or in the bulb syringe) before passing the solution to the surgeon to avoid burning or chilling the patient.*
- **N.B.** *If* **total hip joint replacement** *is performed, the scrub person provides a moist lap sponge to protect the surface of the implant as the driver is used to seat it.*
- *When* **total hip joint replacement** *(p. 589) is performed, the circulator should document the date, patient's name, brand name, type, size, and serial numbers of the implanted prostheses (2 parts) in the* **Perioperative Record.**

- In addition to documentation in the **Perioperative Record,** prosthesis information is recorded in the hospital's log (for insertion of an implant), according to policy.
- The circulator should have the cast cart available at the conclusion of the surgery, as a spica cast may be applied.
- **Reminder:** When transporting a child to the PACU, an isolette or warmed blankets in a crib are required to maintain normothermia (to avoid hypothermia).
- **Reminder:** The circulator gives an intraoperative report to the PACU perioperative practitioner with the patient's status, the care measures implemented, and the desired patient outcomes included for continuity of care and for medicolegal reasons.

Repair of Congenital Diaphragmatic Hernia

Definition

Repair of an opening in the diaphragm through which the abdominal viscera protrude into the thoracic cavity.

Discussion

Several types of **congenital diaphragmatic hernias** are seen in the newborn. These hernias may require prompt repair to prevent life-threatening cardiorespiratory and obstructive phenomena. Preferably, in the newborn, unless severe respiratory compromise is present, the repair is delayed for several days until thorough medical evaluation is done, including pulmonary and cardiac studies, renal and brain scans, etc. If respiratory distress is present, extra-corporeal membrane oxygenation (ECMO) may be employed preoperatively and postoperatively.

The most common of the congenital diaphragmatic hernias presents through the pleuroperitoneal canal (Bochdalek's hernia). A sac is not usually present; the abdominal viscera enter the pleural space. Hernias that present through the anterior diaphragm at the sternocostal junction (foramen of Morgagni) are usually small, have a true sac, and are closed by thoracic or abdominal approach. Eventration of the diaphragm (an attenuation, not a true hernia) is treated by plication of the diaphragm transthoracically. Esophageal hiatal hernia is repaired by transthoracic approach. The diagnosis is not often suspected in the newborn; treatment of esophageal hiatal hernia is less urgent. Congenital absence of a portion of the diaphragm is rarely encountered. When a portion of the diaphragm is absent, it may be repaired by mobilizing the remaining portions or by employing a prosthetic device (e.g., Silastic® sheeting or Gore-Tex® patch). In all of these patients, additional congenital abnormalities may be present. While not considered a standard of care, when these anomalies are detected ante partum, some centers are prepared to perform in-utero corrective surgery.

The most dangerous postoperative complications of congenital diaphragmatic hernia include surgical-site hemorrhage, pulmonary hypertension, deterioration of respiratory mechanics, and intracranial hemorrhage. Less commonly observed complications include disruption of the suture line, leakage of peritoneal fluid with blood into the thorax, and ipsilateral hydrothorax. Late complications include small bowel obstruction secondary to adhesions or volvulus with recurrence of the diaphragmatic hernia.

Thoracoscopic repair of congenital diaphragmatic hernia is currently being performed in the neonate at specialized centers. Due to longer operating times and increased complication rates, the minimal-access approach is not generally utilized. Patient selection seems to be a decisive factor. In the future, the thoracoscopic approach may prove to be appropriate, particularly for patients who require minimal ventilatory support or whose stomach is intra-abdominal.

Procedure

Abdominal approach is usually used to repair congenital diaphragmatic hernia; however, the transthoracic approach is sometimes used.

The Abdominal Approach Employed for Repair of Bochdalek's Hernia is described. A left paramedian or left subcostal incision is made. Air is introduced intrapleurally to assist with the delivery of the viscera out of the pleural space. The hernia is reduced; the hernia sac, if present, is excised. The hernia is repaired with interrupted nonabsorbable sutures.

Air is aspirated from the pleural space as the compressed lung is inflated, prior to tying the final sutures. If the lung is hypoplastic, an indwelling thoracostomy tube (connected to a sealed drainage unit) may be placed. Additionally, before the abdomen is closed, the viscera are inspected for other abnormalities, especially malrotation, adhesive bands, and intestinal atresia. A ***gastrostomy*** (p. 1035) may be performed, as needed. At times, if the abdomen accommodates the viscera poorly, only skin is closed over the incision in order to avoid respiratory embarrassment with a closure that is too tight. Approximately 2 weeks later, as the abdominal wall stretches, peritoneal and fascial closure may be effected. Alternatively, when the defect is large enough to preclude primary closure, closure may be effected by the insertion of Silastic sheeting, a Gore-Tex patch, Marlex® mesh, rotational muscle flaps, or fascial tissue flaps.

A gastrostomy tube is usually placed.

Preparation of the Patient

The room temperature is adjusted prior to the patient's arrival. The head and foot sections of the table are removed, a warming mattress/pad is placed on the table, radiant heat lamps are positioned over the table, and the infant's head and the extremities are covered to maintain normothermia, as most often the patient is a newborn (see **Pediatric General Information**). EKG/ECG is employed and pediatric leads are placed. General anesthesia with endotracheal intubation is administered with the infant in supine position. The infant may be placed in a mummy-like wrap until completely anesthetized. An IV line is inserted, and the extremity is secured to a padded board. The extremities are restrained using nonconstricting padded restraints, placed after the infant is anesthetized. A Foley catheter is inserted into the bladder; the tubing is connected to a urine collection device (e.g., urimeter or urometer) for accurate urine measurement. All bony prominences and areas vulnerable to skin and neurovascular trauma or pressure are padded. A pediatric electrosurgical dispersive pad is placed.

Skin Preparation

Using warm prep solutions only, prep the entire abdomen. Begin as for a left paramedian or left subcostal incision, extending the prep from the suprasternal notch to the pubic symphysis and down to the table at the sides.

Draping

Folded towels and a pediatric laparotomy sheet

Equipment

Radiant heat lamps
Mattress/pad (e.g., K-Thermia pad)
Covering for the head and extremities (see ***Pediatric Tracheostomy,*** p. 990), optional
Padded board for extremities, support of the upper extremity (IV line placement)
Padded extremity restraints, as needed
EKG/ECG monitor and pediatric leads (to anesthesia provider)
ESU, monopolar or bipolar
Suction
Scales, metric (gram), optional

Instrumentation

Pediatric major procedures tray
Ligating clip appliers (e.g., Hemoclip appliers), short, medium
Bipolar electrosurgical forceps and cord, optional

Supplies

Nasogastric tube (to anesthesia provider)
Pediatric Foley catheter tray U (with urimeter/urometer)

Basin set
Blades, (2) #15
Needle magnet or counter
Electrosurgical pencil with needle tip, and cord, optional
Suction tubing
Normal saline irrigation (warm)
Syringe, 60 ml (for accurate irrigation measurement)
Dissectors (e.g., peanuts, Kittners), optional
Vessel loops or umbilical tapes, 1/4″ (for retraction)
Ligating clips (e.g., Hemoclips,), small and medium
Gastrostomy tube, e.g., Foley, Malecot®, or Pezzar® catheter, optional
Catheter plug for gastrostomy tube
Infant chest drainage unit (e.g., Pleurevac®), optional
Chest tube, e.g., Argyle® (10Fr) and straight connector, optional
Silastic sheeting, Gore-Tex patch, or Marlex mesh (for defect repair), optional
Topical thrombin applied to skin-closure sutures, optional

Special Notes

- Apply measures from the **Pediatric General Information**, p. 978, and **Special Notes** from ***Congenital Dislocation of the Hip***, p. 1000, as applicable.
- **N.B.** Before a gastrostomy tube is placed, the patient's chart is checked for allergy to latex. When the patient is allergc to latex, another type of tube is used for gastrostomy.
- **N.B.** A plug is inserted in the gastrostomy tube to prevent spillage of gastric contents.
- **N.B.** The skin is observed for reaction to latex; the appearance of the skin is documented preoperatively and immediately post-operatively.
- **N.B.** When the patient has an allergic reaction to latex (or any substance), an **Incident Report** must be filed documenting the details.
- Bipolar ESU is usually preferred, as there is less injury to the tissues in the immediately surrounding area than when monopolar ESU is employed.
- **Reminder:** *The circulator assists the anesthesia provider by obtaining necessary equipment and comparing identifiers to ascertain that the correct blood or blood product is available for the correctly identified patient.*
- **Reminder:** The circulator should document any untoward reaction to the blood (or blood products) or lack of reaction in

the **Perioperative Record**. The appearance of the skin preoperatively and immediately postoperatively is documented for continuity of care (patient safety) and for medicolegal purposes.

- **Reminder:** An **Incident Report** complete with the details of the incident is filed when the patient has an untoward reaction to a transfusion.
- **Reminder:** Dissector sponges and any small item that could potentially be sequestered in the wound is included in the count.
- **N.B.** A chest tube (e.g., Argyle tube) may be placed in the chest cavity connected to an underwater sealed drainage unit (e.g., Pleurevac). The Pleurevac is placed (hung) below the level of the chest to prevent the backflow of water from entering the chest.

Omphalocele Repair

Definition

Correction of a defect of the umbilicus through which the abdominal viscera protrude outside the abdominal cavity.

Discussion

In neonates presenting with **omphalocele**, there has been a failure of central fusion at the umbilical ring, causing an incomplete closure of the abdominal wall with persistent herniation of the midgut. Neonates with an omphalocele are not usually in distress, unless pulmonary hypoplasia is present. The omphalocele, a congenital defect, is evident at birth (and may be evident on prenatal scans). The repair depends on the size and extent of the omphalocele; it may vary from one containing the greater portion of the intra-abdominal viscera, including the spleen and liver, to one containing only a small loop of intestine.

There is no skin covering the defect but rather amnion or peritoneum, which may rupture at birth, exposing the patient to increased risk of infection. The viscera involved have not undergone the usual rotation and posterior fixation; the blood supply may be under tension and torsion, leading to edema and/or circulatory compromise. Additional congenital abnormalities are present in approximately half of these newborns. The above presentation considerations and the ability of the abdominal cavity to safely contain the contents of the omphalocele will determine whether a single or a staged-repair will be necessary. Hyperalimentation is usually required to assure adequate nutrition. Respiratory assistance may be required until the abdominal cavity adjusts to the replaced viscera. Maintaining the child's temperature and prevention of infection are of prime importance.

Procedure

Repair of omphalocele is delayed when the omphalocele sac is intact and the child is in no particular immediate distress. Small omphaloceles may be repaired immediately.

Single-stage Repair is described. General anesthesia with endotracheal intubation is instituted; however, nitrous oxide is not used, as it causes increased gas in the intestines, making reduction more difficult. To prevent distention of the bowel, the anesthesia provider passes a nasogastric tube. Antibiotic IV therapy is instituted. The omphalocele is covered with warm saline-moistened laparotomy pads. An incision is made separating the skin from the borders of the sac. The umbilical vessels are ligated. The sac and the rim of the defect are excised. A gastrostomy (***Pediatric Gastrostomy***, p. 1035) may be performed or the nasogastric tube is left in place. The viscera are reduced within the abdomen and inspected for any signs of vascular compromise. The abdomen is inspected for additional anomalies. The abdomen is closed in layers.

Multiple-staged Repair is described. In the larger omphalocele, when the defect cannot be closed and/or the abdominal cavity is too limited to contain the contents of the sac, an attempt is made to mobilize surrounding skin to cover the protruding viscera. When this is not possible, the sac is excised and a synthetic material such as Silastic sheeting or a silicone mesh tent (silo) is sutured around the periphery over the viscera. The silo is covered to prevent heat loss and infection; the silo is suspended from the top of an open isolette. The infant may be transported to the neonatal intensive care unit (where available), and the contents of the omphlocele are reduced a little more each day until the contents are completely reduced. The infant is returned to the OR for skin closure. In time, as growth permits, from between 6 weeks and 24 months, complete repair of the defect may be achieved in one or more procedures (including muscle repair). Prevention of hypothermia and infection are of major medical and nursing concern.

For **Preparation of the Patient,** see ***Repair of Diaphragmatic Hernia***, p. 1003.

Skin Preparation

N.B. ***Note:*** **The surgeon usually prefers to do skin prep.**

If the circulator performs skin prep, full instructions must be obtained from the surgeon regarding treatment of the omphalocele. Using warm prep solutions only, *gently* prep the omphalocele according to the surgeon's directions, taking care not to rupture the amniotic membrane. Prep the remaining portions of the abdomen; extend the prep from the axillae to midthighs and down to the table at the sides.

Draping

Folded towels and a pediatric laparotomy sheet

Equipment

Radiant heat lamps
Coverings for the head and extremities may be placed
A mattress/pad (e.g., K-Thermia pad) may be placed on the table
Padded board to support extremity (for IV placement), optional
Padded extremity restraints, as needed
ESU, monopolar or bipolar
Suction
EKG/ECG monitor and pediatric leads
Metric scales (2), to weigh sponges
Closed isolette is exchanged for an open isolette, as necessary

Instrumentation

Pediatric major procedures tray
Ligating clip appliers (e.g., Hemoclip appliers), short, medium
Bipolar electrosurgical forceps and cord, optional

Supplies

Nasogastric tube to decompress stomach (to anesthesia provider)
Pediatric Foley catheter tray (with urimeter/urometer)
Basin set
Blades, (2) #15
Needle magnet or counter
Electrosurgical pencil (with needle tip) and cord, optional
Warm normal saline irrigation
Syringe, 60 ml (for accurate irrigation measurement), optional
Suction tubing
Dissectors (e.g., peanuts, kittners), optional
Vessel loops or umbilical tapes, 1/4″ (for retraction), optional
Ligating clips (e.g., Hemoclips,), small and medium, optional
Silastic sheeting or silicone mesh tent (silo) to repair defect, available

Special Notes

- Apply **Special Notes** from ***Repair of Diaphragmatic Hernia***, p. 1005, as applicable.
- **N.B.** *Prior to bringing the patient into the room, the circulator should obtain the equipment and supplies for intravenous cutdown and a hyperalimentation line, as either may be inserted following induction of anesthesia.*

- **N.B. Note:** *The surgeon usually preps the abdomen.* **The circulator should not begin the (skin) prep without specific instructions from the surgeon.** If the circulator does the prep, it is done gently with extreme care taken not to disrupt the amniotic sac.
- Observing all measures to maintain normothermia is extremely important, as is the maintenance of the child's fluid balance.
- **N.B.** *Strict aseptic technique must be employed during the surgery to avoid an intraoperative wound infection in the child.*
- **N.B. Reminder:** *The circulator must confirm that blood or blood products, as ordered, have been typed and screened (or cross-matched) and are readily available.*
- **N.B. Reminder:** *The circulator assists the anesthesia provider in comparing identifiers to ascertain that the correct blood or blood product has been obtained for the correctly identified patient.*
- **N.B**. The circulator must consult the surgeon regarding who will prep the abdomen. If the circulator is to prep the abdomen, he/she should obtain explicit directions regarding how it is to be done.
- **Reminder:** At the conclusion of the surgery, en route to the PACU, measures are carefully employed to assure that this patient's body temperature is maintained, as the patient is more susceptible to hypothermia due to his/her physical condition.
- The circulator reports the patient's intraoperative physical status, implemented patient care measures, and the desired patient outcomes to the PACU perioperative practitioner to assure continuity of care (for patient safety) and for medicolegal reasons.

Repair of Exstrophy of the Urinary Bladder

Definition

Correction of congenital anomaly in which a portion of the lower abdominal wall and the anterior urinary bladder wall are absent with the eversion of the posterior wall of the bladder through the defect.

Discussion

Exstrophy of the urinary bladder is also referred to as **ectopia vesicae**. A more severe presentation in which there is externalization of the lower urinary tract, distal gastrointestinal tract involvement, and involvement of the central nervous system is referred to as **cloacal exstrophy**. Gender conversion may be necessitated in these patients; both the child and parents will require psychiatric therapy. The congenital anomalies are thought to be due to the same embryological defect. Correction involves repair of the abdominal wall defect and the exposed and everted urinary bladder, urethral epispadias, and additional associated abnormalities.

Exstrophy of the bladder (in addition to infraumbilical abdominal wall defects, the unfused and exposed urinary bladder and varying degrees of urethral epispadias) may be accompanied by asymmetry of the pelvic bones with rotational effects and separation of the symphysis pubis, pelvic floor defects, shortening and nonfusion of genitalia, inguinal herniae, undescended testes, persistence of a cloaca, anorectal abnormalities, and infrequent upper urinary tract anomalies. These defects may occur in any combination and degree of severity but most often involve the bladder, urethra, abdominal wall, and separation of the pubic symphysis. The incidence is probably greater in males. If the diagnosis is made by prenatal ultrasound scan, the obstetrical delivery should be performed at a center that offers comprehensive care of the problem; the parents often require supportive counseling.

In lesser presentations, combined bladder closure and epispadias repair with pelvic osteotomy and abdominal wall repair may be performed shortly after birth. Often, however, staged procedures even until adolescence may be required for complete correction. In some instances, the bladder tissue is insufficient and ultimately a **urinary conduit** (see ***Ileal Conduit***, p. 425 or colonic conduit in ***Cystectomy***, p. 399) is needed.

In the OR, full latex precautions (p. 32) are instituted to avoid anaphalactic reaction due to the high incidence of latex sensitivity and allergy in these patients (who in the course of treatment have numerous exposures to latex gloves and other latex items). Repair of extensive epispadias is usually delayed. Goals of surgical treatment include restoration of urinary continence, preservation of renal function, and the reconstruction of functional genitalia that are cosmetically acceptable. Creation of a neoumbilicus is usually also desirable. Prevention of hypothermia and infection are of major medical and nursing concern. The more complex presentations are best treated in a comprehensive pediatric surgery center.

Procedure

Surgery for a Less-severe Presentation of Exstrophy of the Exposed and Everted Urinary Bladder with a Single-staged Procedure is described. Antibiotic IV therapy is instituted. Latex precautions are usually instituted (see discussion). General anesthesia via endotracheal intubation is administered with the patient in supine position with the legs apart and the exposed urinary bladder protected by lap sponges moistened with warm normal saline. The pelvis is exposed, the periosteum is reflected locally, and innominate and vertical osteotomies are performed. Halfway between the anterior superior and anterior inferior iliac spines, using a Gigli saw, osteotomies are performed bilaterally and external fixation pins are placed. (Postoperatively, external fixation is applied.) If necessary, the posterior ilium is incised to correct the rotational deformity. The wounds are closed and protected.

The field is changed to expose the bladder area. The bladder is dissected from the abdominal wall, rectus fascia, urogenital diaphragm, peritoneum, and pubic symphysis. The urethral tissues are mobilized and the bladder is repaired vertically in two layers employing absorbable suture. Prior to closure, a suprapubic catheter is positioned, as may be ureteral stents, to exit on the abdominal wall. Male penile lengthening is achieved, when possible, by freeing the corpora cavernosa and incising the suspensory ligaments with relief of any chordee, as necessary. The urethra is then closed as much as possible using nonhair-bearing local skin flaps over a catheter to preserve the diameter; closure is with fine absorbable interrupted sutures. The suprapubic catheter is removed. ***Epispadias repair*** (p. 358) is achieved when sufficient tissue is available; a subsequent procedure may be needed (see p. 353). The pubic rami are approximated and held with heavy nonabsorbable suture (e.g., #2 nylon) or #0 polydiaxonone about the symphysis. The abdominal defect is closed.

Preparation of the Patient

The **Preparation of the Patient** is the same as for ***Congenital Diaphragmatic Hernia,*** p. 1003, with exception that a Foley catheter is not placed. A specially constructed padded board that facilitates exposure of the genitalia while restraining the infant may be used. An electrosurgical dispersive pad is also placed in this procedure.

Skin Preparation

N.B. Note: The surgeon may prefer to do skin prep.

If the circulator performs skin prep, instructions should be obtained from the surgeon regarding treatment of the exposed and everted urinary bladder; great care is employed.

Using warm prep solutions only, gently prep the exposed urinary bladder according to the surgeon's directions. Prep the remainder of the abdomen; extend the prep from the axillae to just above the knees, including the genitalia, and down to the table at the sides. Care is taken to avoid pooling the prep solution under the infant; the barrier drape placed under the buttocks is carefully removed to avoid contaminating the sterile field.

Draping

A towel is folded (to protect the hands), as it is tucked under the buttocks.

Folded towels around the periphery and a pediatric laparotomy sheet are placed.

Equipment

Radiant heat lamps
Coverings for the head and extremities
Mattress/pad (e.g., K-Thermia pad) may be placed on the table
Padded board (specially constructed, facilitates optimal exposure of the genitalia while restraining the infant)
Padded board to support extremity (IV line placement), optional
Padded extremity restraints, as needed
ESU, monopolar or bipolar
Suction
EKG/ECG monitor and pediatric leads
Scales, metric to weigh sponges

Instrumentation

Pediatric major procedures
Minor orthopedic procedures tray
Gigli saw (2 handles and wire blade) and extra wire blades, and internal fixation pins (for osteotomy), optional
Hand drill or small power drill for pin insertion, optional
Ruler, caliper, and caliper skin hooks, optional
Ligating clip appliers (e.g., Hemoclip appliers), short and medium, optional
Bipolar electrosurgical forceps and cord, optional

Supplies

Basin set
Blades, (2) #15
Needle magnet or counter
Electrosurgical pencil (with needle tip) and cord, optional
Pediatric **nonlatex** suprapubic catheter (e.g., 8Fr), tubing, and urimeter/urometer, as necessary
Ureteral stents, optional
Normal saline irrigation, warm
Syringe, 60 ml (for accurate irrigation measurement), optional
Suction tubing, polyethylene, or other substitute for latex
Dissectors (e.g., peanuts, Kittners), optional
Umbilical tapes, 1/4″ (for retraction), optional; **vessel loops are not used when latex precautions are observed**
Ligating clips (e.g., Hemoclips,), small and medium

Suture to approximate the pubic rami (e.g., #2 nylon)
Pediatric **nonlatex** urinary catheter (e.g., 6 to 8Fr), tubing, and urimeter/urometer
Petrolatum gauze; light pressure genital dressing (for males)

Special Notes

- Apply **Special Notes** from ***Omphalocele Repair***, p. 1008, as applicable.
- **N.B. Reminder:** *For this procedure, the circulator should consult with the surgeon and the anesthesia provider to assure that all possible measures are taken to maintain the infant's body temperature.*

Pediatric Umbilical Herniorrhaphy

Definition

Repair of an abdominal wall defect at the umbilicus through which viscera or fatty tissues protrude.

Discussion

Umbilical hernia occurs when there is incomplete closure of the umbilical ring at the fascial level. Skin coverage is intact. Although noted at birth or early infancy, particularly if small, a significant number of these defects may close in time without treatment. Unless there is a large defect (greater than 2 cm) or symptoms such as pain present, or for cosmetic reasons, surgery may be delayed until 18 months of age (or even until age 4 to or 5). Incarceration and strangulation of the contents of the hernia (e.g., bowel) are emergencies that require immediate surgery. During the surgery, the umbilicus is preserved rather than excised to maintain body image.

Procedure

Pediatric umbilical herniorrhaphy is performed using general anesthesia; however, the anesthesia provider or surgeon may also administer local anesthetics for pain relief immediately postoperatively. Usually an infraumbilical hemicircumferential incision is made. The sac is dissected free and the fascial rim of the defect exposed. The dome of the sac is transected and can be left attached to the undersurface of the umbilical skin. The sac is closed (excess sac is excised) and is replaced intra-abdominally. The fascial anterior rectus sheath defect is closed by any of several simple or overlapping layer techniques. The umbilical skin or retained dome of the sac is sutured to the fascia to recreate the umbilical indentation. The skin incision is closed; fine absorbable sutures may be used.

Preparation of the Patient

The **Preparation of the Patient** is the same as for ***Congenital Diaphragmatic Hernia,*** p. 1003, except that a Foley catheter is not placed. Note that a pediatric electrosurgical dispersive pad is applied for this procedure as well.

Skin Preparation

Using warm prep solutions only, begin at the umbilicus; extend the prep from the axillae to just above the knees (including the genitalia) and down to the table at the sides. Extra care is taken to prep the inguinoscrotal or inguinolabial area well.

Draping

Folded towels and a pediatric laparotomy sheet

Equipment

Radiant heat lamps
Coverings for the head and the extremities
Mattress/pad (e.g., K-Thermia pad) is placed on the table or a warming blanket (e.g., Bair Hugger) may be placed over the child; **do not use both at same time.** Not all warming measures may be employed, e.g., coverings for extremities, as these procedures are usually delayed until the child is at least 18 months old
Padded board to support extremity (IV line placement), optional
Padded extremity restraints, as needed
ESU, monopolar or bipolar
Suction, optional

Instrumentation

Pediatric minor procedures tray
Bipolar electrosurgical forceps and cord, optional

Supplies

Basin set
Electrosurgical pencil (with needle tip) and cord, optional
Blades, (2) #15
Needle magnet or counter
Suction tubing, available
Dissectors (e.g., peanut or kittners), optional

Special Notes

- Apply **Special Notes** from the ***Pediatric Omphalocele***, p. 1008, as applicable.

- **N.B.** An incarcerated or strangulated hernia requires emergency surgery; the surgery should be prepared for accordingly, p. 1014. Additional measures for the child's safety in an emergent situation are performed (e.g., an IV cut-down is inserted, EKG/ECG with pediatric leads are placed, Foley catheter with urimeter/urometer may be placed, IV antibiotic therapy is instituted, and the abdomen may be irrigated with an antibiotic solution, etc.).
- All implemented emergency care measures are documented in the **Perioperative Record.** The time the measure is implemented and the names of the persons who performed the measure are documented; record keeping is vital for patient safety in continuity of care and for medicolegal reasons.
- *The scrub person should be prepared with swabs for culture and sensitivity of the peritoneal fluid if the hernia was incarcerated.*
- *The circulator should prepare the requisition for routine culture and sensitivity of the peritoneal fluid, stating that the hernia was incarcerated on the requisition form.*

Pediatric Inguinal Herniorrhaphy

Definition

Repair of a hernia in which a musculofascial defect containing intraperitoneal viscera presents in the inguinal region.

Discussion

Most pediatric inguinal hernias are indirect; correction is accomplished by high ligation of the patent processus vaginalis (sac) without repair of the inguinal floor. Repair of the transversalis muscle fascia and inguinal canal floor may be done as indicated. In the male, the herniation may be evident in the scrotum; care is taken to avoid injury to the spermatic cord structures. A hydrocele or undescended testis may be associated with the hernia and is corrected at the same time. In females, the hernia presents in the labium majus; ovary and fallopian tubes may be encountered within the hernial sac. These hernias are repaired when the diagnosis is made; if incarceration occurs, it is an emergency. The surgeon may explore the opposite side of the abdomen, even if no evidence of contralateral hernia is present preoperatively.

Open or laparoscopic approaches may be used. Recurrence is somewhat higher and general anesthesia is usually required for the laparoscopic technique, but potential damage to spermatic cord structures (vessels and vas deferens) is minimal.

Procedure

Inguinal Herniorrhaphy, Open Approach is described. A transverse incision is made. The external oblique aponeurosis is exposed and incised. The ilioinguinal nerve is avoided. The contents of the inguinal canal are explored and the sac identified. High ligation is performed with nonabsorbable suture; the sac is transected. If a hydrocele is present, the sac is delivered into the wound and opened, exposing the testis; a portion of the hydrocele sac is usually excised. The external oblique aponeurosis is closed, and the skin is closed using a subcuticular suture. In the female, if a sliding component is present (i.e., if part of the sac wall is broad ligament or mesentery), the sac is transected and ligated, including the round ligament, as close to the sliding portion as possible. Transversalis fascia is closed over the defect prior to closure of the external oblique aponeurosis. A contralateral exploration may be done in addition to the repair, as applicable.

A variation of the open technique may be done by inserting a laparoscope into the opened processus vaginalis for visualization of the contralateral side, thus avoiding an unnecessary contralateral incision. The skin is closed.

Inguinal Herniorrhaphy, Laparoscopic Approach is described. The table may be positioned in the Trendelenburg position. After institution of general anesthesia, pneumoperitoneum is established. Three ports are placed: 5-mm ports in the umbilical position for the laparoscope (0°, 30°, or 70°) and 3- or 5-mm ports in the pararectal areas for instrumentation. The hernia is identified, and the contents of the sac are replaced intraperitoneally. The internal inguinal ring is closed in the female child and repaired for the male child with nonabsorbable sutures; the sac is usually not amputated. The contralateral side is visualized; if the internal opening is greater than 2 mm, closure is performed in the female child and repaired in the male child using the same ports and instrumentation. The incisions are closed.

Preparation of the Patient

The room temperature is adjusted 1 hour prior to the arrival of the child. Measures are applied to maintain the child's body temperature at normothermia (e.g., coverings for the head and the extremities may be applied, a mattress/pad may be placed on the table or a forced-air warming blanket (e.g., Bair Hugger) may be used to cover the child, according to the weight/size/age of the patient. The head and foot sections of the table may be removed. When the patient is an infant or small child, he/she may be placed in a mummy-like wrap until completely anesthetized. Following induction of general anesthesia, the child is placed in supine position. An IV is inserted into a forearm, and the extremity is secured to a padded board. The other extremities are restrained using nonconstricting padded restraints placed after the child is anesthetized. All bony prominences and areas vulnerable to skin and neurovascular trauma or pressure are padded. A pediatric electrosurgical dispersive pad is placed.

Skin Preparation

Using warm prep solutions only, prep the entire abdomen. Begin at the inguinal area on the affected side; extend the prep from nipples to midthighs and down to the table at the sides.

Draping

Folded towels and a pediatric transverse sheet

For **Equipment, Instrumentation, Supplies, and Special Notes,** see **Pediatric Umbilical Herniorrhaphy,** p. 1014.

Supplies, Add

Penrose drain 1/4″″ (for retraction)

For laparoscopic approach, see ***Pediatric Laparoscopy,*** p. 1027 for **Preparation of Patient, Equipment, Instrumentation, Supplies,** and **Special Notes,** as applicable.

Repair of Congenital Atresia of the Esophagus

Definition

Restoration of esophageal continuity and repair of a tracheoesophageal fistula, when present.

Discussion

Several types of anomalies in **congenital atresia of the esophagus** may be seen. In all patients there is a lack of a patent esophagus in continuity with the stomach. The stomach may or may not contain air by virtue of the connection with the trachea.

Types of **congenital atresia of the esophagus** include:

1. The upper esophagus ends blindly and the lower esophagus communicates with the trachea; air distends the stomach (the most common)
2. The upper and lower esophagus may exhibit muscular continuity, but without luminal continuity.
3. The upper esophagus may end blindly, with the lower esophagus extending above the diaphragm for a variable distance but not communicating with the trachea; here the stomach is empty.

Diagnosis is made by the neonate's inability to take oral fluids without regurgitation and aspiration; it is confirmed by x-ray studies.

A Replogle catheter may be inserted into the proximal esophageal pouch to aspirate mucus and secretions. Antibiotics are administered, and dehydration is corrected employing IV therapy. Additional anomalies including those of the cardiovascular and gastrointestinal systems may be encountered.

When air is not present in the stomach, a gastrostomy (see ***Pediatric Gastrostomy***, p. 1035) is performed and tube feedings are begun. Cervical esophagostomy for drainage of secretions may be done when the proximal and distal segments are unlikely to be directly connected. In addition, a limited "sham" feeding may be instituted to help the infant develop swallowing reflexes. When the proximal and distal segments are separated but do not demonstrate adequate length, upper-pouch bougienage can be done twice daily for 6 to 12 weeks prior to direct reconstruction. Definitive reconstruction can be performed in a single-stage procedure (including the closure of the tracheoesophageal fistula), or it may be done in stages.

Final restoration may be delayed (even for as long as 2 years). A colonic segment interposition, the stomach mobilized into the thorax, or a gastric tube (either isoperistaltic or antiperistaltic) may be employed to restore esophageal continuity. Each modality has advantages and disadvantages with respect to regurgitation and the difficulty and potential complications of the respective procedures.

When the air-filled stomach compromises respiration and there is reflux of gastric contents into the trachea, gastrostomy is performed immediately and definitive surgery is delayed. When the stomach is only moderately distended, definitive single-stage correction may be done, employing a transpleural or extrapleural approach.

Improved treatment may include minimal-access procedures such as ***thoracoscopy*** (with and without robotic assistance), p. 1081, tissue engineering for esophageal replacement, and in-utero intervention.

Procedure

A Transpleural Approach to Repair of Congenital Atresia of the Esophagus with Tracheoesophageal Fistula and Discontinuous Esophageal Segments is described. A right posterolateral incision is made over the fifth rib. The pleural cavity is entered in the fourth intercostal space and a Finochietto retractor (infant-sized) is placed; the azygous vein is divided. Care is taken to avoid injury to the vagus nerve trunks, the recurrent laryngeal nerves, and the trachea. The mediastinal pleura is incised, and the lower esophagus is exposed and mobilized, taking care not to compromise the blood supply. The tracheoesophageal fistula is transected and closed with fine nonabsorbable sutures, or staples are employed (leaving a small cuff of esophagus in order not to compromise the tracheal lumen). The integrity of the tracheal closure is tested for air leaks by filling the chest with saline. Extra length to the esophageal segments may be achieved with circular or spiral myotomies.

Esophageal continuity is established by any of several one- or two-layer techniques, depending on the diameter and muscular wall thickness of the upper and lower segments (using absorbable interrupted sutures or stapling device). A small-gauge feeding tube may be passed transnasally into the esophagus across the anastomotic site into the stomach for post-operative feeding (placed prior to closure of the anterior anastomotic layer). The connective tissues around the divided azygous vein may be used to reinforce the anastomosis, as is the mediastinal pleura. A chest tube is placed, the chest is closed, and a chest x-ray may be taken.

Preparation of the Patient

The room temperature is adjusted prior to the arrival of the child. The head and foot sections of the table may be removed. Measures are applied to maintain the child's body temperature at normothermia [e.g., coverings for the head and the extremities may be applied, radiant heat lamps may be positioned over the table, a warming blanket (e.g., Bair Hugger) may be placed over the child]. **Do not place a mattress pad on the table, as it interferes with x-rays and fluoroscopy.** The infant may be placed in a mummy-like wrap until completely anesthetized. Following induction of general anesthesia with endotracheal intubation, an IV cutdown is inserted, secured to a padded board. A hyperalimentation line may be inserted. A Foley catheter is inserted into the patient's bladder, connected to a urimeter/urometer. A small roll may be placed just below the axilla to decrease pressure on the brachial plexus. The right arm is positioned across the chest and secured with a nonconstricting padded restraint. The left leg (lower) is bent and the right leg is extended over the left with a small pillow placed between the legs. The position may be stabilized with 2-inch-wide nonallergic tape placed across the top of the shoulder and across the iliac crest, secured to the underside of the table. The feet are padded, positioned, and supported as necessary to maintain good body alignment. The position is checked for the padding of all bony prominences and areas vulnerable to skin and neurovascular trauma or pressure. A pediatric electrosurgical dispersive pad is placed.

Skin Preparation

Using warm prep solutions only, begin at the mid-chest, at the level of the fifth rib; extend the prep from the shoulder to the iliac crest and down to the table anteriorly and posteriorly.

Draping

Folded towels, sterile, plastic adhesive drape (optional), and pediatric laparotomy or transverse sheet

Equipment

Radiant heat lamps, optional
Forced-air warming blanket (e.g., Bair Hugger)
Do not place warming mattress pad (e.g., K-Thermia pad) as it interferes with x-ray or fluoroscopy
Covering for the head (e.g., tube stockinette and plastic wrap), optional
Covering for extremities (e.g., bias stockinette or Kerlix and plastic wrap), optional
Padded board to support the extremity (IV placement)
Padded extremity restraints, as needed
Small sandbag, small pillow, and padding, as necessary
EKG/ECG monitor and pediatric leads
ESU, bipolar or monopolar
Suction
Scales, metric, to weigh sponges
Fluoroscopy or x-ray cassette (x-ray department)

Instrumentation

IV cutdown tray and supplies
Hyperalimentation tray and supplies
Pediatric major procedures tray
Pediatric thoracotomy tray
Pediatric gastrointestinal tray (available)
Small bone cutter and graduated bougies (e.g., Maloney)
Ligating clip appliers (e.g., Hemoclip appliers), short and medium
Beaver knife handle, optional
ESU, bipolar or monopolar

Supplies

Nasogastric catheter to anesthesia provider
Argyle Repulogle suction catheter, optional
Pediatric Foley catheter tray with urimeter/urometer (for accurate measurement of urine), optional
Cutdown and hyperalimentation trays and supplies
Basin set
Sterile, plastic adhesive drape (optional)
Blades, (2) #15
Beaver blade (ask regarding size), optional
Suction tubing
Needle magnet or counter
Electrosurgical pencil (with needle tip) and cord
Syringe (60-ml) to measure irrigation, optional
Ligating clips (e.g., Hemoclips,), small and medium

Automatic disposable stapling devices with staple cartridge, e.g., EEA®, GIA®, optional
Bone wax, optional
Infant chest sealed underwater drainage unit (e.g., Pleurevac)
Chest tube (e.g., #10 Argyle) and straight or Y connector
Small feeding tube

Special Notes

- Apply **Special Notes** from ***Omphalocele Repair***, p. 1008, as applicable.
- **N. B. Reminder:** *The room must be heated (see p. 983) and radiant heat lamps must be waiting over the OR table to fulfill minimum heating requirements.* The circulator should consult the surgeon and the anesthesia provider to assure that all possible measures are taken to maintain the infant's body temperature at normothermia.
- **N.B.** The circulator should determine if fluoroscopy (image intensifier) or portable x-ray is to be used and prepare the OR table accordingly. **A warming mattress/pad *cannot* be used in conjunction with any type of x-ray.**
- When an x-ray is taken or the image intensifier is used, everyone in the room should observe x-ray precautions by wearing a lead apron or by stepping out of the room.
- When staying in the room when the image intensifier is used or when x-rays are taken, the scrub person and all persons scrubbed should don a lead apron before scrubbing.
- **N.B. Reminder:** *The circulator should determine if an intravenous cutdown and a hyperalimentation line are to be inserted following induction of anesthesia.* Prior to the child's entry to the room, the circulator should obtain the equipment and supplies to perform theses procedures.
- **N.B. Reminder:** *The circulator must confirm that blood or blood products, as ordered, have been typed and screened (or cross-matched) before bringing the patient into the room.* The availability of the blood or blood products is confirmed during "***time out***."
- **N.B. Reminder:** *The circulator assists the anesthesia provider by comparing identifiers to ascertain that the blood or blood product is available in the correct unit for the correctly identified patient.*

- The circulator documents any reaction or the lack of a reaction to blood or blood products administered in the **Perioperative Record,** p. 12.
- The circulator weighs used sponges as soon as possible to reduce "evaporation factor" to help determine blood loss replacement.
- The scrub person measures irrigation fluids accurately to help determine fluid loss replacement.
- The circulator should anticipate advising x-ray personnel that an x-ray may be necessary prior to the patient's departure from the OR.
- **N.B.** When transferring the patient, the closed drainage system is kept below chest level to prevent fluid from entering the lungs.
- **N.B. Reminder:** When the patient is transported to the PACU, the circulator should anticipate providing all possible measures to maintain the patient's body temperature such as normothermia, e.g., using an isolette and keeping the head and extremity coverings on the infant.

Insertion of a Pediatric Central Venous Catheter

Definition

The introduction of Silastic tubing into the subclavian, internal jugular, or femoral vein to administer parenteral nutrition or chemotherapy, to monitor hemodynamics, and to replace fluids and blood.

Discussion

In the pediatric patient, a **central venous catheter** may be inserted on an acute basis for hemodynamic monitoring and for rapid replacement of fluids and blood or for ongoing access for purposes of parenteral nutrition or the administration of chemotherapy or any other drug. The main advantage of this technique is to spare the patient frequent venepunctures and to decrease the likelihood of inducing phlebitis if more peripheral veins are used. The internal jugular vein may be accessed via the external jugular or facial veins and the subclavian directly or via the median cubital or cephalic veins.

In addition to the sites noted above, in the newborn, umbilical or saphenous veins may be used; in older children, the femoral vein can be used if other sites are no longer available. Several types of Silastic catheters are available. When long-term venous access is anticipated, subcutaneous access ports (Port-A-Cath™, Infuse-A-Port™, or Medi-Port™) can be placed to avoid an externalized line.

Procedure

Insertion of a Central Venous Catheter is described. A small incision is made over the external jugular vein in the lateral neck. The catheter is passed into the incised vein (confirmed by the aspiration of blood) traversing the internal jugular vein to a predetermined length in order to be in the superior vena cava. The external jugular vein is ligated proximally and distally about the catheter. A blunt tunneling instrument is employed to tunnel subcutaneously from the incision to the anterior chest lateral to the sternum. The catheter exits through the tunnel and is sutured to the skin. The position of the catheter is confirmed by x-ray or fluoroscopy. The fluid-primed catheter is immediately connected by heparin lock, or three-way stopcock to fluid-primed intravenous tubing. The venotomy is secured and the initial incision is closed. Antimicrobial ointment may be applied around to the exit site. A dressing is placed.

Preparation of the Patient

The room temperature is adjusted prior to the child's arrival. The head and foot sections of the OR table may be removed. To help maintain the patient's body temperature, radiant heat lamps may be positioned over the table, and the patient's head and extremities may be covered (depending on the weight/size/age of the child patient) and a forced-air warming blanket may be used to cover the patient. General anesthesia is employed (most often); the child is placed in supine position with the neck gently extended by placing a small roll under the shoulders to extend the neck, optimizing exposure. The extremities are restrained using nonconstricting padded restraints placed after the child is anesthetized. All bony prominences and areas vulnerable to skin and neurovascular trauma or pressure are padded. A pediatric electrosurgical dispersive pad is placed.

Skin Preparation

Using warm prep solutions only, begin at the supraclavicular area; extend the prep from the infra-auricular border to the umbilicus (including the right shoulder if the catheter is to exit the anterior thorax), down to the table on the right side, and well beyond the midline on the left side. If the catheter is to exit from the epigastrium, extend the prep to the pubic symphysis distally. A lap pad may be placed at the right side of the neck to avoid pooling of the prep solution. Care should be taken in removing the pad ***not*** to contaminate the prepped surgical field.

Draping

Folded towels and a sheet with a small fenestration

Equipment

Overhead radiant heat lamps
Forced-air warming blanket (e.g., Bair Hugger), optional
Warming mattress pad is not used, as x-ray or fluoroscopy is employed
Small roll (placed under the shoulders), optional
Covering for the head (e.g., tube stockinette cap), optional
Covering for extremities (e.g., bias stockinette and plastic wrap), optional
The warming measures listed may be employed, as necessary, depending on the age and weight of the patient
Padded extremity restraints
ESU (monopolar)
Fluoroscopy or x-ray cassette (x-ray department)

Instrumentation

Pediatric major procedures tray
Bulldog (vascular) clamps, assorted, small
Tunneling instrument

Supplies

Basin set
Blades, (1) #15 and (1) #11
Needle magnet or counter
Electrosurgical pencil (with needle tip) and cord
Medicine cups, labels, and marking pen
Local anesthetic (e.g., lidocaine/Xylocaine 1%, control syringe, and #25 needle) for local immediate postoperative pain relief
Graduate pitcher, heparin, and syringe for heparin solution (optional)
Silastic catheter and introducer (e.g., Broviac)
Radio-opaque dye (e.g., Hypaque™, half strength) and syringe, optional
IV tubing and IV solution (e.g., 10% dextrose)
Heparin lock or three-way stopcock
Antimicrobial ointment (ask regarding type) and a transparent dressing, optional
Telfa (optional) and dressing sponges

Special Notes

- Apply **Special Notes** measures from the ***Pediatric Tracheostomy***, p. 992, as applicable.
- The circulator should determine if fluoroscopy (image intensifier) or portable x-ray is to be used and prepare the OR table

accordingly. ***A warming mattress/pad cannot be used in conjunction with any type of x-ray.***

- All medications, dyes, etc., on the sterile field must be labeled according to type and strength to avoid medication error. All medication containers should be kept in the room until the completion of the procedure. Follow all safety precautions to avoid medication errors; see p. 30.
- If Hypaque is used to confirm the placement of the catheter, it is diluted to half strength.
- The circulator should consult the x-ray department regarding confirmation that x-rays or fluoroscopy will be needed. The circulator should notify the x-ray department in advance of the procedure. During ***"time out,"*** confirmation regarding x-ray personnel and the necessary x-ray equipment are present.
- When an x-ray is taken or the image intensifier is used, x-ray precautions are observed by wearing a lead apron or by stepping out of the room.
- When the scrub person (or anyone scrubbed) is staying in the room when x-rays are taken or when the image intensifier is used, he or she should don a lead apron before scrubbing.
- The circulator should prepare the IV tubing by running the IV solution through the tubing until there are no air bubbles in the line to avoid cerebrovascular accident caused by air embolus, e.g., if the child has a patient foramen ovale.
- Extra care is taken by all to avoid infection of the child's wound.

Pediatric Laparoscopy

Definition

The introduction of an endoscope through the abdominal wall to visualize the peritoneal cavity and/or the preperitoneal and retroperitoneal spaces.

Discussion

Pediatric Minimal Access Surgery (MAS) is described. Once practiced with limited application in the pediatric population, pediatric minimal-access procedures (laparoscopic, endoscopic, and thorascopic) are being performed with increasing frequency.

Reasons for previous limited application of this approach included the following:

1. Physical space for the introduction of the instruments is more limited than in the adult.

2. Limited number of smaller sized laparoscopic instrumentation available.
3. Cost of additional instrumentation, equipment, and supplies for the pediatric patient.

Note: An overriding principle of any MAS is that the procedure must be promptly converted to an open procedure when the endoscopic approach is deemed unfeasible or when the patient's safety is compromised.

Pediatric laparoscopy is indicated for diagnosis and treatment of pediatric conditions and diseases, including the following: gastroesophageal reflux (fundoplication); evaluation of the spleen, liver, and lymph nodes in hematologic entities such as spherocytosis, idiopathic thrombocytopenic purpura, etc. (biopsy, splenectomy); sickle-cell disease with cholelithiasis (cholecystectomy); and acute appendicitis (appendectomy).

Another indication for laparoscopy in the pediatric patient is the identification of a contralateral patent processus vaginalis in inguinal herniorrhaphy. A scope is inserted intraperitoneally through the hernia sac on the ipsilateral side. Similarly, the inguinal area may be explored for a nonpalpable intra-abdominal testis; the testis can be mobilized for later replacement into the scrotum, or if the testis is abnormal, it can be excised. Assistance in mobilizing the colon can be achieved laparoscopically in a pull-through procedure for ***Hirschsprung's disease*** (p. 1054).

Laparoscopic diagnostic evaluation of tumors, including retroperitoneal node biopsy, etc., may be performed.

As in the adult, numerous other procedures involving intra-abdominal organs may be performed via laparoscopic approach, or they may be combined with a "limited" open technique, such as **"laparoscopic-assisted" surgery**. Pneumoperitoneum may be established with a Verres needle or by direct puncture under direct vision utilizing a limited cutdown. During needle insertion, the abdominal wall may be pulled up manually, (employing hemostats, tissue hooks, stay sutures, etc.). Prior to the needle insertion, the surgeon may ensure that the child's bladder is empty by utilizing the Credé maneuver. When a tissue specimen is obtained, an endoscopic specimen pouch may be employed to retrieve the specimen.

Procedure

Pediatric Laparoscopy is described. An insufflation needle (e.g., Verres needle with sheath) is inserted, angled towards the pelvis, and gently pushed until it penetrates the peritoneum. The surgeon ascertains that the position of the needle is correct; the needle is removed, leaving the sheath in place. The surgeon attaches Silastic tubing to the sheath. (Following draping, the scrub person will have passed off the other end of the Silastic tubing to the circulator who attached the tubing to the CO_2 source.) Pneumoperitoneum is established with warmed CO_2. A peri-umbilical port is established for the scope; two lateral ports are established for instrumentation.

The initial incision is made a little larger to accommodate the trocar. The trocar is introduced (the tip automatically retracts as the peritoneum is pierced). The trocar is removed; the sheath (now an established port) is secured to the abdominal wall with incorporated screw threads; stay sutures may be used to further secure the port. A laparoscope is inserted through the port (the CO_2 line was previously attached to the sheath to maintain the pneumoperitoneum). The laparoscope may contain a camera (computer chip at its distal end) that provides an image directly onto the monitor(s). Additional ports are placed under visual control, using the telescopic property of the laparoscope.

Preparation of the Patient

The room is heated one hour prior to the arrival of the patient. The head and foot sections of the table may be removed. Warming measures are employed to maintain the pediatric patient's body temperature, and a warming mattress/pad may be placed on the table, or a forced-air warming blanket placed to cover the child. Radiant heat lamps may be positioned over the table, the child's head may be covered with a tube stockinette cap, and the extremities may be covered with bias stockinette or Kerlix and plastic wrap. Gastric contents are emptied by nasogastric tube prior to the induction of anesthesia. Following the administration of general anesthesia via endotracheal intubation, the child is placed in supine position and an IV line is inserted. The child's extremities are restrained using nonconstricting padded restraints, placed after the child is anesthetized. All bony prominences and areas vulnerable to skin and neurovascular trauma or pressure are padded. A pediatric electrosurgical dispersive pad is placed for grounding the patient. The circulator should consult the surgeon regarding emptying the patient's bladder.

Skin Preparation

Using warm prep solution only, clean the umbilicus meticulously. Begin the prep over the right upper abdomen; extend the prep from the axillae to the pubic symphysis and down to the table at the sides.

Draping

Folded towels and a pediatric laparotomy sheet

Equipment

The warming measures listed may be employed, as necessary, depending on the age/weight/size of the child

Overhead radiant heating lamps
Covering for the head (e.g., tube stockinette cap) and covering for extremities (e.g., bias stockinette or Kerlix and plastic wrap), optional
Forced-air warming blanket (Bair Hugger) or warming mattress/pad (K-Thermia pad); **do not use both at the same time**
Padded extremity restraints
Padded board to support extremity with IV, optional
ESU (monopolar)
Suction
Endoscopy cart (where available)
Insufflation device, CO_2
Fiber-optic light source, e.g., Xenon™ 300 W
Monitor(s)
VCR
CD burner
Camera console

Instrumentation

Pediatric minor procedures tray
Pediatric major procedures tray (if laparoscopy converted to open procedure), available
Specific instruments are the same or similar to those used for adult laparoscopy (appropriately smaller): Verres needle, trocars with sleeves, reducers, fiber-optic pediatric laparoscope, and power cord
Endoscopic instrumentation: dissectors, graspers, scissors (blunt and sharp), electrosurgical suction-irrigator, dissectors (including electrosurgical hook dissector and/or monopolar Maryland dissector), scissors (blunt and sharp), graspers (atraumatic, blunt, and heavy), and measuring device (ruler or marked dissector)
Fan retractor (older child)
Camera may be separate, and it attaches to the scope with a coupler or there may be a camera (chip) in the distal end of the scope
Fiber-optic pediatric laparoscope, scope sizes: 2.7 mm with 0° angled lens, 2.7 mm with 30° angled lens, and/or 5.0 mm with 0° angled lens and/or 5 mm with 30° angled lens

Supplies

Pediatric-sized nasogastric tube (to anesthesia provider)
Basin set
Blades, (1) #15
Electrosurgical pencicord
Suction tubing

Needle magnet or counter
Silastic tubing (for CO_2 insufflation)
Fog reduction agent, e.g., FRED™, ELVIS™, optional
Local anesthetic (e.g., lidocaine/Xylocaine 1%), control syringe, and #25 needle for immediate postoperative pain relief at incision sites, optional
TiGold (ligating endoscopic clip applier with nondisposable handle and cartridge or entire unit is disposable with 14 clips in cartridge) small and medium, optional
ENDOLOOP (extracorporeal and intracorporeal ligating suture device with loop sutures and introducer sleeve), disposable, single use, optional
ENDO STITCH® (suture with swaged-on needle), disposable, single use, optional
ENDOKNOT (suture with swaged-on needle and sleeve), disposable, single use, optional
Endoscopic specimen pouch, e.g., Endopouch™, Endosac™, ENDOBAG™, LAP-BAG™, or LAPSAC™, disposable, single use, optional
HandPort®, GelPort™ (laparoscopic-assisted hand port), disposable, single use, optional

Special Notes

- Apply **Special Notes** from ***Abdominal Laparoscopy,*** p. 134, and measures from **Pediatric General Information**, p. 978, as applicable.
- **N.B. Reminder:** *The circulator is responsible for having adequate levels of CO_2 in the tank (cylinder) prior to bringing the patient into the room.* If CO_2 is low, the cylinder should be changed before the procedure begins.
- **N.B. Reminder:** The circulator connects the CO_2 tubing to the insufflator and adjusts the insufflator pressure level. For the pediatric patient, a beginning low flow rate of CO_2 (such as 1 to 1.5 l/min) to effect a pressure of 5 mm Hg is used; later, the flow rate may be adjusted to 8 mm (pressure) for brief periods, as directed by the surgeon.
- **N.B. Reminder:** *As CO_2 can be easily absorbed through the peritoneum, there can be serious consequences for the pediatric patient when it is employed.* By using low pressure and warm humidified gas during insufflation, in addition to careful monitoring, complications such as hypothermia may be avoided.

- The scrub person should be aware that sutures may be placed to secure the trocars, or trocars with screw threads are used (that prevent dislodgement).
- The circulator and scrub person should be aware that extracorporeal and intracorporeal suturing devices should be included in the needle count.
- **Reminder:** Local anesthetic (e.g., lidocaine/Xylocaine 1%) may be injected into the incision sites to the pediatric patient for local immediate postoperative pain relief. For the pediatric patient, the local anesthetic is injected into the incision sites at the time the incisions are made when the surgery takes a short amount of time; local anesthetic is injected at the end of the surgery when the surgery takes longer.
- **N.B. Reminder:** *Injected lidocaine/Xylocaine 1% can be toxic when too much is administered.* The surgeon should be cautious regarding the amount of lidocaine being administered, and he/she, the anesthesia provider, and the circulator should observe the child for signs of lidocaine toxicity, such as arrhythmia, seizures, erythema, bruising, edema, or any allergic-type response in the child, following lidocaine administration.
- **N.B. Reminder:** The rigid telescopes can be autoclaved; the flexible telescopes cannot be autoclaved. **Following manufacturer's directions precisely for sterilization of laparoscopic instruments and telescopes is mandatory.**
- The circulator should position the monitor(s) after the patient is on the table. When the surgery begins, the circulator needs to recheck the position of the monitors to ensure that the surgeon and those assisting can view them easily.
- **Reminder:** Following draping, the scrub person should pass off the end of the CO_2 Silastic insufflation tubing, the fiberoptic light cord (cable), suction tubing, and electrosurgical cord to the circulator. The circulator may connect these items after the team is in position (to avoid tripping over the cords). When determining if laparoscopic equipment is working, the circulator should first check to see that the equipment cords are plugged in.
- For the removal or reduction of fog on the lens of a telescope prior to laparoscopic viewing, a special fog-reduction agent (e.g., FRED, ELVIS) may be used. During intra-abdominal use of the telescope, the surgeon may wipe the lens over moist intra-abdominal tissue to clear the fog, or a lens warmer may be used.

- *All fiber-optic instrumentation and light cables must be handled with great care to avoid breaking the tiny fiber-optic light fibers.* The fiber-optic cables may not be bent or folded.
- **Note:** *The manufacturer has determined whether the particular telescope is autoclavable;* **directions for sterilization of the telescopes should be followed precisely.** Flexible telescopes may be sterilized using ethylene oxide, peracetic acid, or hydrogen peroxide gas plasma; see p. 44.
- **Reminder:** Steris 20™ (peracetic acid) solution system (the most frequently employed) may be used to sterilize laparoscopic instruments and telescopes. The instrument or telescope must be completely submerged for 12 minutes at 50° to 55°C for sterilization requirements to be met; see p. 43.
- **N.B.** *Instrumentation for open surgery should always be available in the room for immediate use should the laparoscopy surgery require conversion to an open laparotomy procedure.*

Pyloromyotomy for Congenital Hypertrophic Pyloric Stenosis

Definition

The hypertrophied muscles of the pylorus are incised to relieve pyloric obstruction.

Discussion

Congenital hypertrophic pyloric stenosis usually becomes evident a few weeks after birth with progressive episodes of vomiting caused by pyloric muscular hypertrophy that creates a mechanical obstruction. The muscle mass ("olive") can often be palpated transabdominally. Ultrasound or a thin solution of barium contrast medium may be necessary to confirm the diagnosis. A **Ramstedt-Fredet pyloromyotomy** is the procedure of choice. The pyloric muscle is divided, leaving the mucosa (and submucosa) intact, relieving the condition. Other modalities, such as transendoscopic balloon dilatation, are successful in some cases, but they can result in rupture of the pylorus.

Pyloromyotomy may be performed laparoscopically.

Procedure

Open Approach (Ramstedt-Fredet Procedure) to Pyloromyotomy is described.

A high right rectus-splitting incision (or a transverse or oblique incision) is made over the liver. (More recently, a supraumbilical incision is becoming increasingly utilized.) The peritoneum is incised, and the pylorus is delivered into the wound. The pylorus is incised longitudinally, anteriorly from the pyloric vein and pyloroduodenal junction, proximally over the extent of the hypertrophic muscle. Using a pyloric spreading forceps, all remaining circular muscle fibers are separated down to the level of the submucosa. (Any laceration of the gastric or duodenal mucosa is immediately repaired.) After hemostasis is obtained, the wound is closed in layers.

Laparoscopic Approach to Pyloromyotomy is described. A periumbilical port is established for the scope, and two lateral ports are established for instrumentation; see Pediatric Laparoscopy, p. 1025. An endoscopic Babcock (or similar) forceps stabilizes either the duodenal or gastric tissue just distal or proximal to the hypertrophied muscle; a retractable arthroscopic knife blade is drawn away from the stabilizing forceps to incise the hypertrophied muscle. An endoscopic spreading forceps is used to dissect the remaining fibers, taking care not to perforate the submucosa and mucosa. Hemostasis is secured, the instruments are withdrawn, and the port incisions are closed.

Preparation of the Patient

The room temperature is adjusted one hour prior to the patient's arrival. The head and foot sections of the table may be removed. Measures to help maintain the patient's body temperature at normothermia are employed, such as covering the patient's head and extremities, placing radiant heat lamps over the table, placing a warming mattress/pad on the table, or covering the patient with a forced-air warming blanket (***both measures are not employed at the same time to avoid burning the patient***), depending on the size/weight/age of the child. Any gastric contents are emptied by nasogastric tube prior to the induction of anesthesia. General anesthesia is administered via endotracheal intubation, and the child is placed in supine position. An IV line is inserted, and the extremities are restrained using nonconstricting padded restraints, placed after the child is anesthetized. All bony prominences and areas vulnerable to skin and neurovascular trauma or pressure are padded. A pediatric electrosurgical dispersive pad is placed.

Skin Preparation

Using warm prep solutions only, begin over the right upper abdomen; extend the prep from the axillae to the pubic symphysis and down to the table at the sides.

Draping

Folded towels and a pediatric laparotomy sheet

Equipment

Overhead radiant heat lamps
Forced-air warming blanket (Bair Hugger) or warming mattress/pad (K-Thermia pad); **do not use both at the same time**
Covering for the head (e.g., tube stockinette cap), optional
Covering for extremities (e.g., bias stockinette and plastic wrap), depending on the size/age/weight of the child, optional

The warming measures listed above are for infants and small children, although hypothermia is an ever-present concern for all patients.

Padded extremity restraints, optional
EKG/ECG monitor and pediatric leads
ESU, monopolar
Suction

Laparoscopic, Add:
Monitor(s)
Endoscopy cart (where available)
Insufflation device (CO_2)
Fiber-optic light source, e.g., Xenon 300 W
VCR
Camera console
CD burner
Printer

Instrumentation

Pediatric major procedures tray
Pediatric gastrointestinal procedures tray
Pyloric spreader
Ligating clip appliers, e.g., Hemoclip appliers (short, medium), optional

Laparoscopic
Pediatric minor procedures tray
Pediatric major procedures tray (available in room for possible conversion)
Pediatric fiber-optic laparoscopes and power cords (e.g., 2 × 7 mm with 0° angled lens and 30° angled lens, and/or 5.0 mm with 0° angled lens and 30° angled lens), depending on the size of the child and surgeon's preference
Camera and coupler or laparoscope with camera chip contained in the distal end of the scope
Pediatric-sized instrumentation is similar to that used for adult laparoscopy, e.g., Verres needle, trocars with sleeves, electrosurgical suction-irrigator, fiber-optic light cable (cord), reducers,

scissors (blunt and sharp), dissectors (3) (e.g., 1 heavy, 1 blunt, 1 hook), electrosurgical dissector, graspers (e.g., 1 atraumatic intestinal, 1 blunt, 1 heavy), knife handle, and fan retractor, optional

Ligating clip applier (short) and clips (small, medium), e.g., TiGold

Supplies

Pediatric-sized nasogastric tube (to anesthesia provider)
Basin set
Blades, (2) #15
Electrosurgical pencil, needle tip, and cord
Needle magnet or counter
Suction tubing
Dissectors (e.g., peanuts, Kittners)
Ligating clips, e.g., Hemoclips (small and medium), optional

Laparoscopic, Add

Silastic tubing (for insufflation)
Fog reduction agent, e.g., FRED, ELVIS
Arthroscopic knife blade
Electrosurgical cord for electrosurgical instruments
Xylocaine/lidocaine/1%, local anesthetic (for immediate postoperative pain relief) and control syringe, with #25 needle, optional
Medicine cups, marking pen, and labels
TiGold, ligating endoscopic clip applier (short) and clip cartridge with 14 clips (small and medium)
ENDOLOOP, ENDO SUTURE (without needlc), ligature or loop sutures, disposable, single use, optional
ENDO STITCH (extracorporeal and intracorporeal suturing device with introducer sleeve, and suture with swaged-on needle), disposable, single use, optional
ENDOKNOT (suture with swaged-on needle and sleeve), disposable, single use, optional

Special Notes

- Apply **Special Notes** from the ***Pediatric Umbilical Herniorrhaphy***, p. 1014, as applicable.
- For the laparoscopic approach to **Pyloromyotomy**, apply **Special Notes** from ***Pediatric Laparoscopy***, p. 1029, as applicable.
- **Reminder:** *The circulator is responsible for having adequate levels of CO_2 in the tank (cylinder) prior to bringing the*

patient into the room. If CO_2 is low, the cylinder should be changed before the procedure begins.

- **N.B.** The circulator should connect the CO_2 insufflator tubing and adjust the insufflator pressure level. For pediatric patient, use a beginning low flow rate of CO_2 (such as 1 to 1.5 l/min) to effect a pressure of 5 mm Hg; later the flow rate may be adjusted to 8 mm (pressure) for brief periods, as directed by the surgeon.
- **Reminder:** *Local anesthetic (e.g., lidocaine/Xylocaine 1%) may be injected into the incision sites for immediate local postoperative pain relief.* For the pediatric patient, the local anesthetic is injected into the incisional sites at the time the incisions are made when the surgery takes a short amount of time; the local anesthetic is injected at the end of the surgery when the surgery is lengthy.
- **Reminder:** *Use safety precautions to identify, label, and dispense medications or solutions and to avoid medication errors; see p. 30.* It is mandatory that all medications and solutions on the sterile field be labeled by name and strength. The medication bottle is retained in the room until the procedure has concluded.
- **N.B. Reminder:** *Xylocaine/lidocaine 1%, a local anesthetic, can be toxic when too much is injected.* The surgeon should be cautious regarding the amount of lidocaine being administered. The surgeon, the anesthesia provider, and the circulator should observe the child for signs of toxicity, arrhythmias, seizure, such as erythema, bruising, or edema when lidocaine is administered.
- **Reminder:** *Laparoscopic (nondisposable) instruments can usually be flash-sterilized (autoclaved); rigid telescopes can usually be flash-sterilized.* Flexible telescopes cannot be autoclaved; they should be sterilized using ethylene oxide, peracetic acid, or gas-plasma hydrogen peroxide (see sterilization techniques, p. 44). ***Follow manufacturer's directions explicitly for sterilization of laparosopic instruments and telescopes.***
- **N.B.** *When laparoscopic pyloromyotomy is performed, instrumentation for immediate conversion to open laparotomy should always be available in the room.*

Pediatric Gastrostomy

Definition

Establishment of an artificial opening into the stomach, exiting onto the skin of the abdominal wall.

Discussion

Pediatric gastrostomy is most frequently performed to permit liquid feedings; it may also be done to permit gastric drainage or retrograde dilation of an esophageal stricture. Some of the techniques for performing a pediatric feeding gastrostomy include the open Stamm, percutaneous endoscopic, open Janeway, and laparoscopic gastrostomy. Gastrostomy can be an independent procedure or performed in conjunction with other abdominal surgeries.

Several percutaneous techniques have been developed. These rely on distention of the stomach with guidance and assistance employing a flexible pediatric gastroscope; they may also be done employing fluoroscopy or ultrasound control. ***(When fluoroscopy is employed, a warming mattress/pad is not placed on the table.)*** Numerous technical maneuvers (Russell, Sachs-Vine, Gauderer-Ponskey) may be utililzed depending on whether the gastrostomy tube is "pushed" or "pulled" into position. Similarly, there are many commercially prepared gastrostomy kits (C.R. Bard, Wilson Cook Medical, etc.), as well as a variety of anchoring devices [e.g., T-anchors (fasteners) and tube replacements (e.g., Bard Button® and MIC-KEY® balloon cannulas)].

For children, the open approach employing the traditional Stamm technique, once the standard, is being replaced by the laparoscopic U-stitch technique. A mini laparoscope (1.6 mm) has been used to verify the visceral site for introduction of instrumentation for the percutaneous procedures. Although the Stamm technique and percutaneous procedures are still performed by some surgeons, the laparoscopic technique seems safer and more versatile.

Procedure

The Stamm (Open) Procedure for Gastrostomy is described. A short left upper-quadrant transverse or vertical incision is made (avoiding proximity to the costal margin). The greater curvature of the stomach is identified. Two concentric purse-string sutures are placed in the stomach; a stab wound is made in the center of the purse strings, and a gastrostomy catheter is inserted. The purse-string sutures are then tightened and tied to secure the tube. The tube is brought out through a stab wound lateral to the incision. The stomach is sutured to the peritoneum about the stab wound. The tube is sutured to the skin. The wound is closed.

As an Alternative to an Open Surgical Procedure, Percutaneous Endoscopic Gastrostomy (PEG), is described. It may be performed in the radiology department special procedure suite or, if necessary, for critically ill patients, at the patient's bedside, as well as in the OR. A well-lubricated flexible fiber-optic gastroscope is passed into the stomach; the stomach is distended with air. The lighted tip of the scope is impacted on the gastric wall that is then positioned to be directly under the parietal peritoneum, displacing the liver edge and colon. X-ray or ultrasound may be employed to confirm the position of the gastric wall onto the parietal abdominal wall. Additionally, finger pressure is exerted over the glow of the scope tip; the endoscopist should see an indentation on the gastric wall. If not, interposition of other viscera (e.g., colon) is presumed and the site of percutaneous puncture is altered. (When the patient is awake, local anesthesia is injected at the site of the intended gastrostomy.) A second operator passes a trocar through a percutaneous stab wound, aiming at the transilluminated gastroscope tip. Following a guide wire and dilators that enlarge the puncture tract, the gastrostomy tube is passed via the abdominal wall into the stomach, where it is seized and its intragastric position confirmed. Various catheters are used, including balloon and loop tips to prevent dislodgement. Tissue anchors (T-anchors) may be placed percutaneously to secure the gastric wall to the parietal abdominal wall about the catheter entry site. The catheter is secured to the skin around the stab wound. As an adjunct to this procedure, a laparoscope can be inserted via an umbilical port to assure by direct vision that the gastric puncture maneuver avoids any adjacent organs (such as the colon).

Laparoscopic gastrostomy is another modality for gastrostomy tube insertion in the pediatric patient. A periumbilical port is established for the laparoscope (3 mm). Two additional ports are established for instrumentation. The site of the gastrostomy is identified and stabilized with grasping forceps. Two concentric purse-string sutures are placed around the intended puncture site. A puncture wound is then made into the stomach (scissors, electrosurgically, etc.), any secretions are aspirated, and the gastrostomy tube (e.g., Foley catheter) is passed via an abdominal stab wound under laparoscopic visual guidance and into the gastric puncture site and the sutures tied after the catheter balloon is inflated. Additional sutures affix the gastric wall to the parietal peritoneum around the entry site of the tube. Pneumoperitoneum is released and the incisions are closed.

Laparoscopic Gastrostomy Employing the U-stitch Technique is described. Following the establishment of pneumoperitoneum, a 3-mm trocar is inserted. The anterior wall of the stomach is grasped. The pneumoperitoneum is slightly deflated. A large curved needle is passed through the abdominal wall, hooking a segment of the anterior wall of the stomach on needlepoint. The needle is rotated and passed back through the abdominal wall. Two adjacent large "bite" sutures are made in the gastric wall, forming a square and stabilizing a segment of the anterior gastric wall. The stomach is insufflated with air. A needle introducer is passed through the abdominal wall and the stomach inside the U-sutures. A guide wire is passed through the needle introducer; the tract over the guide wire is dilated. A gastrostomy tube (with a balloon tip) is introduced over the wire via a stab wound made in the abdominal wall passing through the stomach between the two previously placed "U" sutures. The balloon is inflated. The sutures draw the gastric wall onto the parietal peritoneum and are tied over bolsters or buttons on the skin.

For **Preparation of the Patient, Skin Preparation, and Draping,** see *Pediatric Pyloromyotomy,* pp. 1032–1033.

Equipment

Overhead radiant heat lamps, optional
Forced-air warming blanket (Bair Hugger), optional
Covering for the head (e.g., tube stockinette cap), optional
Covering for extremities (e.g., bias stockinette and plastic wrap), optional
(The warming measures listed above may be employed, as necessary, depending on the age/weight/size of the patient)
Padded extremity restraints
ESU, monopolar (open procedure or laparoscopic)
Suction

Percutaneous Endoscopic, Add

Monitor(s)
Fiber-optic light source, e.g., Xenon 300 W
VCR
CD burner
X-ray or Fluoroscopy (x-ray department)

Laparoscopic, Add

Endoscopy cart
Monitor(s)
Insufflation device (e.g., CO_2)
Fiber-optic light source, e.g., Xenon 300 W
VCR
CD burner
Camera console

Instrumentation

Pediatric minor procedures tray (open procedure and laparoscopic)
Ligating clip applier, e.g., Hemoclip applier, (short and medium) for open and laparoscopic procedures
Pediatric major procedures tray (available in room for possible conversion)

Percutaneous Endoscopic, Add

Guide wires and dilators
Flexible fiber-optic pediatric gastroscope and cord

Laparoscopic, Add

Guide wires and dilators

Fiber-optic pediatric laparoscope, (depending on the size of the child and surgeon's preference) and power cord

Camera may be separate; it attaches to the scope with a coupler or the laparoscope may have a camera (chip) at the distal end of the scope

Pediatric scope sizes: 2.7 mm with 0° angled lens, 2.7 mm with 30° angled lens, 5.0 mm with 0° angled lens, and/or 5 mm with 30° angled lens

Specific instruments are similar to those used for adult laparoscopy, but appropriately smaller: Verres needle, trocars with sleeves, and reducers

Endoscopic instrumentation: dissectors, graspers, scissors (blunt and sharp), electrosurgical suction-irrigator, dissectors (including electrosurgical hook dissector and/or monopolar Maryland dissector), scissors (blunt and sharp), graspers (atraumatic, blunt, and heavy), and measuring device (ruler or marked dissector)

Fan retractor (older child)

Electrosurgical cord for electrosurgical instruments, e.g , electrosurgical suction-irrigator

Supplies

Pediatric-sized nasogastric tube (to anesthesia provider)

Basin set

Electrosurgical pencil with needle tip and cord

Suction tubing

Needle magnet or counter

Blades, (2) #15 and (1) #11

Gastrostomy catheter (e.g., Pezzer, Malecot, or Foley) and catheter plug

Tissue anchors (T-anchors/fasteners), optional

Ligating clips (e.g., Hemoclips), small and medium, optional

Percutaneous Endoscopic, Add

Lubricant, water-soluble

Gastrostomy kit [e.g., percutaneous endoscopic gastrostomy (PEG) kit], optional

Guide wire and a variety of balloon and loop-tipped catheters, optional

Laparoscopic, Add

Medicine cups, labels, and marking pen

Xylocaine/lidocaine 1%, local anesthetic, control syringe, and #25 needle for immediate local postoperative pain relief, optional

Silastic tubing (for insufflation)

Electrosurgical cord for electrosurgical instruments, e.g., electrosurgical suction-irrigator
Fog reduction agent, e.g., FRED, ELVIS, optional
TiGold, ligating endoscopic clip applier (short) and clip cartridge with 14 clips (small, medium)
ENDO SUTURE (e.g., ENDOLOOP, SURGITIE) suture ligature or loop suture for ties (both without needles)
ENDO STITCH suturing device for extracorporeal and intracorporeal stitches with introducer sleeve (with swaged-on needle)
ENDOKNOT or SUTURE ASSISTANT, suturing device, knot-sliding instrument (with swaged-on needle), optional

Special Notes

- Apply **Special Notes** from ***Pediatric Pyloromyotomy,*** (open or laparoscopic) p. 1034, for the laparoscopic approach, as applicable.
- The circulator should determine if fluoroscopy (image intensifier) or portable x-ray is to be used and prepare the OR table accordingly. A warming mattress/pad **cannot** be used in conjunction with any type of x-ray.
- When **PEG** is performed, the circulator should determine if the surgeon or the surgeon's assistant will perform the gastroscopy or if an additional endoscopist (e.g., gastroenterologist) will be required. In the latter, the circulator makes certain that the endoscopist has been notified and is available. Additionally, the circulator makes certain that the gastroscopic instrumentation is available, as well as the gastrointestinal laboratory personnel, as necessary, according to the policy of the facility.
- For **PEG**, the circulator should contact x-ray personnel regarding the need for intraoperative x-rays or fluoroscopy.
- **Reminder:** When an x-ray is taken or the image intensifier is used, x-ray precautions should be observed by wearing a lead apron or by stepping out of the room.
- **N.B. Reminder:** The scrub person, or anyone scrubbed, staying in the room when x-rays are taken or when the image intensifier is used should don a lead apron *before* scrubbing.
- **Reminder:** For the laparoscopic approach, the circulator connects the CO_2 insufflator tubing to the CO_2 insufflator and adjusts the insufflator pressure level. For the pediatric patient, use a beginning low flow rate of CO_2 (such as 1 to 1.5 l/min) to effect a pressure of 5 mm Hg; later the flow rate may be adjusted to 8 mm (pressure) for brief periods, as directed by the surgeon.

- The circulator should check with the surgeon regarding the type and size of the gastrostomy catheter wanted. A catheter plug is required to avoid contamination of the peritoneal cavity and the sterile field.
- The scrub person must keep soiled instruments (those that come in contact with the gastrointestinal tract) isolated in a basin to avoid contamination of the peritoneal cavity.

Pediatric Hepatic Portoenterostomy/ Kasai Procedure

Definition

Anastomosis of the jejunum to the porta hepatis to relieve biliary ductal atresia.

Discussion

Congenital biliary ductal atresia is the most common surgically correctible cause of jaundice in the newborn. Several presentations involving or sparing the main hepatic, the common hepatic, and common bile ducts, as well as the gallbladder and cystic duct, are seen. In addition to comprehensive evaluation in general, a percutaneous liver biopsy and/or cholangiogram may be performed preoperatively (or intraoperatively) When the hepatic ducts are atretic at the porta hepatis, these fibrous cords are excised to expose the liver parenchyma with microbiliary ducts to which a limb of jejunum (e.g., a conduit) is anastomosed (known also as the **Kasai procedure**).

The surgery should be performed prior to 3 months of age to avoid severe liver problems (cirrhosis, portal hypertension, enzyme changes, etc.). Even with successful surgery, most patients will ultimately require liver transplantation for long-term survival.

Procedure

Pediatric Hepatic Portoenterostomy is described. With the patient in supine position, a right subcostal incision is made, and the abdomen explored for other anomalies: If the gall bladder itself is not atretic, a cholangiogram is performed via a catheter placed within the fundus, using appropriately diluted dye. If the proximal and distal major ducts are patent, a liver biopsy is done and the procedure abandoned. When these ducts (and/or the gallbladder) are obliterated, the incision is extended across the midline. The distal common duct is ligated and the hepatic ducts are excised under "frozen section control" to expose bile-draining microducts at the porta hepatis. Care is taken to avoid injury to the hepatic arteries and portal vein, as well as distorting the inferior vena cava, during the mobilization of the liver after transecting the various hepatic ligaments. The proximal jejunum is divided (approximately 10 to 12 cm distal to the ligament of Treitz). The distal section is passed via the transverse mesocolon and anastomosed to the porta hepatis (end to end or end to side). The proximal section is anastomosed to the jejunum approximately 30 to 35 cm distal to the initial division in Roux-en-Y configuration.

Midway in the conduit, an intussuscepted nipple valve may be created (sutured or stapled) to prevent reflux. A liver biopsy is performed, drains are placed about the porta hepatis, and the abdomen is closed. The jejunal conduit is generally no longer exteriorized as a doublebarreled stoma.

Preparation of the Patient

The head and foot sections of the OR table may be removed. Measures are instituted to help retain body heat (depending on the size of the child patient) to maintain normothermia, as radiant heat lamps may be positioned over the table and a forced-air warming blanket may be placed over the patient. The head may be covered with a tube stockinette cap and the extremities may be covered with bias stockinette or Kerlix and plastic wrap. EKG/ECG monitor is employed and pediatric leads are placed. Following induction of general anesthesia, the child is placed in supine position. A Foley catheter is inserted into the bladder with the tubing connected to a urine collection device (e.g., urimeter/urometer) for accurate urine measurement. An IV line is inserted into an extremity (usually a forearm), and the extremity is secured to a padded board. The extremities are restrained using nonconstricting padded restraints, placed after the child is anesthetized. All bony prominences and areas vulnerable to skin and neurovascular trauma or pressure are padded. A pediatric electrosurgical dispersive pad is placed.

Skin Preparation

Using warm prep solution only, begin at the right upper abdomen for a subcostal incision; extend the prep from the axillae to the pubic symphysis and down to the table at the sides.

Draping

Folded towels and a pediatric laparotomy sheet

Equipment

Overhead radiant heat lamps, optional
Forced-air warming blanket (Bair Hugger), optional
Covering for the head (e.g., tube stockinette cap), optional
Covering for the extremities (e.g., bias stockinette and plastic wrap), optional

Padded extremity restraints
EKG/ECG monitor and pediatric leads
ESU, monopolar
Suction
Scales, metric to weigh sponges
Fluoroscopy or x-ray cassette (x-ray department)

Instrumentation

Pediatric major procedures tray
Pediatric gastrointestinal procedures tray
Ligating clip appliers (e.g., Hemoclip appliers), small and medium
Biliary tract procedures tray, p. 1098, when cholangiogram performed
Liver biopsy needle, optional

Supplies

Pediatric-sized nasogastric tube (to anesthesia provider)
Pediatric Foley catheter tray and Urimeter/Urometer
Basin set
Electrosurgical pencil (with needle tip) and cord
Blades, (2) #15 and (1) #11
Needle magnet or counter
Suction tubing
Dissector sponges (e.g., peanuts, Kittners), optional
Vessel loops or 1/4″ umbilical tape
Gastrostomy catheter and plug (e.g., Pezzer, Malecot, or Foley) and PEG kit, T anchors, etc.

For Cholangiogram

Radio-opaque dye, e.g., Hypaque, Renografin 60™ diluted to half strength (labeled as such), or Visipaque™
Small basins (2) for saline and dye
Sterile marking pen and labels (to label radio-opaque dye, saline basins, and syringes)
Control syringes (2)
Polyethylene pediatric cystoscopy tubing, Silastic tubing (or surgeon's preference), and three-way stopcock
Ligating clips, e.g., Hemoclips, small, medium, optional
Liver sutures (special, if liver biopsy done), optional
Intestinal stapler (for Roux-en-Y), e.g., GIA, EEA, optional
Drains, e.g., Jackson-Pratt™ or Hemovac, optional

Special Notes

- Apply **Special Notes** from ***Omphalocele Repair***, p. 1008, as applicable.

- **Reminder:** *The room is heated (see p. 983), and radiant heat lamps are waiting over the OR table to fulfill minimum heating requirements.* The circulator should consult with the surgeon and the anesthesia provider to ensure that all possible measures are taken to maintain the infant's body temperature.
- **N.B. Reminder:** *The circulator should determine if an intravenous cutdown and/or hyperalimentation line are to be done following induction of anesthesia.* Prior to the child's entry to the room, the circulator should obtain the equipment and supplies to perform theses procedures.
- **N.B. Reminder:** *The circulator must confirm that blood or blood products, as ordered, have been typed and screened (or cross-matched) before the patient is brought into the room.* This should be reconfirmed during "***time-out***."
- The circulator should ascertain if cholangiogram is to be done or if fluoroscopy (image intensifier) or portable x-ray is to be used and prepare the OR table accordingly. A warming mattress/pad ***cannot*** be used in conjunction with any type x-ray.
- The circulator should contact the x-ray department regarding need for x-rays or fluoroscopy intraoperatively before the patient is brought into the room. This information should be confirmed during "***time-out***."
- When an x-ray is taken or the image intensifier is used, x-ray precautions are observed by wearing a lead apron or by stepping out of the room.
- The scrub person (or anyone scrubbed) staying in the room when x-rays are taken or when the image intensifier is used should don a lead apron *before* scrubbing.
- When x-rays are taken, the scrub person should cover the surgical field with a sterile towel to protect the sterile field from contamination of the surgical site. This is done to protect the patient from infection.
- **Reminder:** *The circulator assists the anesthesia provider to compare identifiers to ascertain that the correct blood or blood product is available for the correctly identified patient.* He/she documents the reaction or lack of reaction to the blood (or blood products) in the **Perioperative Record,** p. 12.
- The circulator weighs used sponges immediately to reduce "evaporation factor" to help determine fluid loss.
- The scrub person measures irrigation fluids accurately to help determine fluid loss p. 987.

- The scrub person should keep all instruments used on the gallbladder or instruments that come in contact with bile isolated in a basin to avoid contamination of the peritoneal cavity.
- **N.B.** During surgery, a liver biopsy needle should be available as a liver biopsy should be performed before the abdomen is closed. If a biopsy is taken, special liver sutures may be requested. The circulator needs to have the liver sutures available in the room; he/she should prepare requisitions for the liver biopsy.
- **Reminder:** The patient may be transported (in an isolette to help maintain the pediatric patient's body temperature, avoiding hypothermia) to a pediatric intensive care unit or a PACU by the circulator and the anesthesia provider.

Relief of (Pediatric) Intestinal Obstruction

Definition

Reestablishment of intestinal continuity in any number of conditions that present with blockage of the intestinal tract.

Discussion

Obstruction in the gastrointestinal tract of newborn becomes apparent shortly after birth with symptoms of emesis, abdominal distention, and failure to pass flatus and meconium. Urgent treatment is often mandatory. The conditions that may be responsible for the obstruction are numerous, including intussusception, esophageal atresia, atresia and stenosis of duodenum, small bowel, and colon, annular pancreas, hypertrophic pyloric stenosis, imperforate anus, congenital malrotation, volvulus, congenital bands, infarction, meconium ileus, aganglionic megacolon, internal hernias, strangulated hernias, and infection. Treatment depends on the diagnosis; during the course of surgery, the abdomen is explored for additional abnormalities or anomalies.

Relief of pediatric intestinal obstruction may be performed laparoscopically; see **Pyloromyotomy for Congenital Hypertrophic Pyloric Stenosis,** p. 1031.

Intestinal obstructive symptoms may also be seen in otherwise unrelated conditions, such as cerebral injury, with persistent emesis, and in pulmonary infections.

Procedure

Relief of Obstruction of the Duodenum is described. A paramedian or transverse incision is made in the upper abdomen. The abdomen is explored for abnormalities; the site of the obstruction is identified. Bypass, rather than resection of the obstructed duodenal segment (usually second portion), is performed. An antecolic duodenojejunostomy is usually the procedure of choice. A loop of proximal jejunum is brought anterior to the transverse colon to the side of the distended proximal duodenum. A side-to-side anastomosis is fashioned in one or two layers according to the size of the small jejunal lumen and the surgeon's preference. The abdomen is closed in layers.

Preparation of the Patient

The room temperature is adjusted one hour prior to the child patient's arrival. The head and foot sections of the OR table may be removed. Radiant heat lamps may be positioned over the OR table to help maintain the patient's body temperature. EKG/ECG is employed and pediatric leads are placed. Following induction of general anesthesia, the child is placed in supine position. A Foley catheter is inserted into the bladder; the tubing is connected to a urine collection device (e.g., urimeter/urometer) for accurate urine measurement. Prior to positioning, the head may be covered with a tube stockinette cap and the extremitities may be covered with bias stockinette or Kerlix and plastic wrap to help retain body heat (depending on the age, weight, and size of the child patient). An IV line is inserted into one extremity (usually a forearm), and the extremity is secured on a padded board. The extremities are restrained using nonconstricting padded restraints placed after the child is anesthetized. All bony prominences and areas vulnerable to skin and neurovascular trauma or pressure are padded. A pediatric electrosurgical dispersive pad is placed.

Skin Preparation

Using warm preparation solution only, begin at the right upper abdomen for paramedian or transverse incision; extend the prep from the axillae to the pubic symphysis and down to the table at the sides.

Draping

Folded towels and a pediatric laparotomy sheet

Equipment

Overhead radiant heat lamps, optional
Warming blanket (Bair Hugger) or mattress/pad (K-Thermia pad); **do not use both at the same time**
Covering for the head (e.g., tube stockinette cap), optional
Covering for extremities (e.g., bias stockinette and plastic wrap), optional
The warming measures listed may be employed, as necessary, depending on the age, weight, and size of the patient
Padded extremity restraints

EKG/ECG monitor and pediatric leads
ESU, monopolar
Suction
Scales, metric to weigh sponges

Instrumentation

Pediatric major procedures tray
Pediatric gastrointestinal procedures tray
Pediatric Balfour retractor
Ligating clip applier, (e.g., Hemoclip applier) short

Supplies

Pediatric-sized nasogastric tube (to anesthesia provider)
Foley catheter tray and urimeter/urometer
Basin set
Electrosurgical pencil (with needle tip) and cord
Blades, (2) #15
Needle magnet or counter
Suction tubing
Dissectors (e.g., peanut, Kittners), optional
Ligating clips, e.g., Hemoclips, small and medium, optional
Disposable automatic stapling unit with staples, e.g., GIA, ILA, EEA, optional

Special Notes

- Apply **Special Notes** from ***Pyloromyotomy for Congenital Hypertrophic Pyloric Stenosis,*** p. 1034, and ***Pediatric Laparoscopy***, p. 1029, as applicable.
- **N.B. Reminder:** *The circulator should determine if an intravenous cutdown and/or hyperalimentation line are to be done following induction of anesthesia.* Prior to the child's entry to the room, the circulator should obtain the equipment and supplies to perform theses procedures.
- **N.B. Reminder:** *The circulator must confirm that blood or blood products, as ordered, have been typed and screened (or cross-matched) before the patient is brought into the room.* This is reconfirmed during "***time-out***."
- **Reminder:** *The circulator assists the anesthesia provider to compare identifiers to ascertain that the correct blood or blood product is for the correctly identified patient; this is a safety measure that should be documented.*

- The scrub person measures irrigation fluids accurately to help determine fluid loss. The circulator weighs used sponges immediately to reduce "evaporation factor" to help determine fluid loss.
- The scrub person should keep all instruments that come in contact with the gastrointestinal tract isolated in a basin to avoid contamination of the peritoneal cavity and possible infection in the patient when the instruments are reused.

Reduction of Pediatric Intussusception

Definition

Correction of a condition in which there is an invagination of a segment of the intestine into an adjacent segment.

Discussion

Intussusception, typically seen in the older male infant, is characterized by sudden episodes of severe abdominal pain, emesis, and subsequent passage of bloody mucus stools (like "red currant jelly"). The infant seems to feel well shortly thereafter. Additional bouts often follow; ultimately, intestinal obstruction becomes evident. The most common site of intussusception is about the ileocecal valve, in which the terminal ileum (intussusceptum) becomes invaginated into the cecum (intussuscipiens). If not reduced, either spontaneously or by the hydrostatic pressure of an air or barium enema examination (70 to 80 mg Hg; not to exceed 120 mg Hg), gangrene will ensue. When the patient is stable, more than one attempt at hydrostatic enema reduction may be tried prior to performing surgery. Even if reduction is accomplished, any suspicion of bowel wall compromise or perforation necessitates immediate surgery. At surgery, incidental appendectomy is done; cecopexy is not done.

The laparoscopic approach may be used; however, as diminished tactile sensation is inherent in this modality, gentle reduction may not be possible and conversion to an open procedure may be required. If initially the laparoscopic approach is selected, depending on the anatomical presentation, usual techniques for pediatric laparoscopy and possible bowel resection apply.

Procedure

Reduction of Pediatric Intussusception is described. A low midline incision is employed (right lower quadrant Jalaguier-Buck, right transverse supraumbilical, and upper midline incisions are also utilized). The intussusception is manually reduced using a "milking" technique rather than forcibly pulling on the involved viscera. If there is resistance to reduction or compromised bowel is encountered, a resection is done with primary anastomosis, or the ends of the bowel are brought out as stomas through separate incisions and anastomosis is later performed as a secondary procedure. The abdomen is closed.

Preparation of the Patient

The room temperature is adjusted one hour prior to the child's entry. The head and foot sections of the OR table may be removed. Radiant heat lamps may be positioned over the operating table to help maintain body temperature. EKG/ECG monitor is employed and pediatric leads are placed. Following induction of general anesthesia, the child is placed in supine position. A Foley catheter may be inserted into the bladder (optional); when used, the tubing is connected to a urine collection device (e.g., urimeter/urometer) for accurate urine measurement. Prior to positioning, the head may be covered with a tube stockinette cap and the extremities may be covered with bias stockinette or Kerlix and plastic wrap to help retain body heat (depending on the age, weight, and size of the child patient). Then an IV line is inserted into one extremity (usually a forearm) and the extremity is secured on a padded board. The extremities are restrained using non-constricting padded restraints placed after the child is anesthetized. All bony prominences and areas vulnerable to skin and neurovascular trauma or pressure are padded. A pediatric electrosurgical dispersive pad is placed.

The anesthesia provider usually places a nasogastric tube. Intravenous antibiotic therapy is usually begun.

Skin Preparation

Using warm preparation solutions only, begin at the low midline; extend from the nipples to the upper thighs and down to the table at the sides.

Draping

Folded towels and a pediatric laparotomy sheet

Equipment

Overhead radiant heat lamps

Warming blanket (Bair Hugger) or mattress/pad (K-Thermia pad); **do not use both at the same time**

Covering for the head (e.g., tube stockinette cap), optional

Covering for extremities (e.g., bias stockinette and plastic wrap), optional

The warming measures listed may be employed, as necessary, depending on the age, weight, and size of the patient

Padded extremity restraints
EKG/ECG monitor and pediatric leads
ESU, monopolar
Suction

Instrumentation

Pediatric major procedures tray
Pediatric gastrointestinal procedures tray
Ligating clip applier (e.g., Hemoclip), short and medium

Supplies

Pediatric-sized nasogastric tube (to anesthesia provider)
Foley catheter tray and urimeter/urometer, optional
Indelible marking pen, optional
Basin set
Electrosurgical pencil (with needle tip) and cord
Blades, (3) #15
Needle magnet or counter
Suction tubing
Dissectors (e.g., peanut, Kittners), optional
Ligating clips, (e.g., Hemoclips,), small and medium, optional
Vessel loops or umbilical tapes, 1/4″
Disposable automatic stapling unit with staples, e.g., GIA, ILA, EEA, optional

Special Notes

- Apply **Special Notes** from ***Relief of Pediatric Intestinal Obstruction***, p. 1047, as applicable. For the laparoscopic approach, see ***Pediatric Laparoscopy,*** p. 1025, as applicable.
- **Reminder:** *The room must be heated (see p. 983), overhead radiant heat lamps must be waiting, and a warming mattress/pad (e.g., K-Thermia pad) must be on the table to fulfill minimum heating requirements.* The circulator should consult the surgeon and the anesthesia provider to assure that all possible measures are taken to maintain the infant's body temperature.
- **Reminder:** *The circulator should determine whether an intravenous cutdown and/or hyperalimentation line are to be done following induction of anesthesia.* Prior to the child's entry to the room, the circulator should obtain the equipment and supplies to perform theses procedures.
- When a bowel resection is performed, the scrub person should isolate soiled instruments (e.g., those that come in contact with the gastrointestinal tract) in a basin.

- **Reminder:** *For the laparoscopic approach, the circulator should connect the CO_2 insufflator tubing and adjust the insufflator pressure level.* Use a beginning low flow rate of CO_2 (such as 1 to 1.5 liters/min) to effect a pressure of 5 mm Hg; later the flow rate may be adjusted to 8 mm (pressure) for brief periods, as directed by the surgeon.
- **Reminder:** *The circulator must confirm that blood or blood products, as ordered, have been typed and screened (or cross-matched) prior to bringing the patient into the room.* This is reconfirmed during "***time-out.***"

Pediatric Colostomy

Definition

Creation of an opening into the colon that is exteriorized onto the anterior abdominal wall as a stoma.

Discussion

Colostomy is performed to bypass an obstructed colonic segment distally or for diversion of the fecal stream to minimize contamination because of perforation or infection and to "protect" a distal anastomosis by eliminating passage of the fecal stream across it. Additionally, colostomy may be performed as a preliminary procedure prior to correction of involved distal colonic or rectal problems, such as severe presentation of aganglionic megacolon or imperforate anus (see high lesion, p. 1061).

Several types of colostomy may be created; transverse and sigmoid are the most common. Most pediatric colostomies are temporary, but they may be permanent when the rectum is congenitally absent or unable to be reconstructed or in cases of neurological and neoplastic processes, etc. Colostomy may be performed as an independent procedure or in conjunction with other abdominal surgery. The appropriate site is determined preoperatively with x-ray studies modified by intraoperative findings. **Colostomy** may be done as an emergency procedure. ***Children with high "ostomy output" must be watched for electrolyte imbalance and dehydration.***

As this type of surgery often connotes a social stigma (unfortunately), the patient (depending on the age) and the parents will need psychological support to accept the results of the surgery; the circulator may convey measures of comfort by empathizing and using warm gestures such as touch. Both the child (depending on the age) and the parents will require counseling from the surgeon, an enterostomal therapist, and/or RN specialist to be sure the family understands how to care for the patient with a stoma. With information, preparation, and guidance provided, the patient and his/her family may be able to reduce their anxiety. Preoperatively and again postoperatively, the family should be given information regarding a local support "ostomy" group.

Laparoscopic approach may be used to mobilize the colon prior to creation of the stoma(s); for the approach, see **Pediatric Laparoscopy,** p. 1025.

Procedure

Creation of Colostomy is described. For an obstructive process or congenital absence of the distal sigmoid colon or rectum, a sigmoid or descending colon colostomy is made. The potential stoma site(s) are marked. An oblique incision is made in the left lower abdomen, and the muscles are either separated (as in gridiron incision) or divided. The abdomen is explored to identify any associated abnormalities or obstructive bands. The colon may be brought out as a loop over a rod or bridge to prevent retraction, or it can be divided and the proximal end brought out through the incision or through an adjacent limited incision as an end-colostomy. The distal end may be closed and returned intraperitoneally unless the distal colon or rectum is completely obstructed, in which situation a mucous fistula is made (the stoma made at a site away from the functioning proximal stoma).

In either situation, the colon and mesentery are sutured to ensuing layers of abdominal wall to prevent prolapse or herniation. The stoma wall is matured with sutures through the full thickness of the stoma to the skin. Tension on the stomal limb is avoided in order to prevent retraction or circulatory compromise and allowance is made for an increasing thickness of the abdominal wall with growth and improved postoperative nutrition. The main incision is closed and covered with a towel to avoid undue contamination. The sequence of closure of the wound and final preparation of the stoma varies according to the preference of the surgeon. At the completion of the procedure, a colostomy pouch is applied to the stoma (and a separate dressing or pouch to the mucous fistula, if present).

For **Preparation of the Patient, Draping, Equipment,** and **Instrumentation,** see ***Relief of Pediatric Intestinal Obstruction,*** p. 1046.

Skin Preparation

Using warm preparation solutions only, begin at the lower left abdomen; extend the prep from the nipples to the upper thighs and down to the table at the sides.

Supplies

Pediatric-sized nasogastric tube (to anesthesia provider)
Foley catheter tray and urimeter/urometer, optional

Basin set
Blades, (3) #15
Electrosurgical pencil (with needle tip)
Vessel loops or umbilical tapes, 1/4″, optional
Dissectors (e.g., peanut, Kittners), optional
Suction tubing, optional
Drain, e.g., Hemovac or Jackson-Pratt
Vaseline® gauze (neonates and infants), optional
Glass rod, tubing, and colostomy pouch (e.g., Karaya Seal®), optional
Plastic bridge and loop colostomy set (e.g., Hollister®), older children, optional

Special Notes

- Apply **Special Notes** from ***Relief of Pediatric Intestinal Obstruction***, p. 1047, as applicable.
- The perioperative practitioner in the preoperative area should provide emotional support to the parents, family, and the child, as this procedure is emotionally laden with inappropriate social taboos. He/she should take every opportunity to provide emotional reassurance and factual information to the parent(s), family, and the child (if he or she is old enough to understand).
- **Reminder:** *Soiled instruments (e.g., those that come in contact with the gastrointestinal tract) are isolated in a basin to avoid contamination of the peritoneal cavity by preventing their inadvertent reuse.*
- **N.B.** At the conclusion of the procedure, the stomas of neonates and infants may be covered with Vaseline gauze or a stoma appliance; older children require a one-piece stoma appliance that can be cut to fit around the stoma.
- **Reminder:** The patient is usually transported to PACU by the circulator and the anesthesia provider. The circulator provides the necessary measures required to maintain the pediatric patient's body temperature and avoid hypothermia, such as using warmed blankets during the transportation of the child.
- On the nursing unit, an enterostomal therapist may have the opportunity to demonstrate to the parents the correct way to place a colostomy bag securely. He/she should emphasize to the parent the importance of using a bag that fits the stoma to prevent leaks that could lead to embarressment for the patient due to odor and stains. On a more serious note, a poorly fitting appliance may lead to complications such, as skin irritation, excoriation, and infection.

- When time permits, the perioperative practitioner in the PACU should ascertain if the parents have been given adequate information to initiate contact with an enterostomal therapist or RN specialist.

Pediatric Colorectal Resection for Aganglionic Megacolon (Hirschsprung's Disease)

Definition

Removal of the aganglionic portion of the colon and rectum with the anastomosis of the proximal normal colon to the distal rectum or anus.

Discussion

In pediatric patients with aganglionic megacolon, the section of colon that is resected can include a short segment of rectum and/or colon or, less often, the entire colon. The section represents a functional obstruction caused by a lack of ganglion cells in the muscular layer (Auerbach or myenteric plexus and Meissner or submucosal plexus). Because the distal segment is unable to relax, it does not permit the passage of feces. The problem may be recognized soon after birth or in later infancy (or if the absence of ganglion cells is partial, diagnosis may be delayed until adulthood). Males are affected more than females. Additional congenital abnormalities (such as *Down syndrome* and cardiac malformations) may be present. A purely genetic cause for this entity has been investigated but not established. *Constipation* with abdominal distention, growth failure, anemia, and episodes of paradoxical diarrhea occur. *Necrotizing enterocolitis* can develop in the neonate and is often fatal if not treated promptly. Reestablishing normal fluid and electrolyte balance, preventing bowel overdistension (with possible perforation), and management of ensuing complications, such as sepsis, must be achieved. Thus, medical treatment includes hydration, nasogastric decompression, and antibiotics.

Barium enema examination and rectal muscle biopsy (full-thickness biopsy) under anesthesia or a suction biopsy may be performed without anesthesia, the latter of which may not provide adequate tissue for evaluation) to demonstrate absence of ganglion cells are diagnostic. Immunohistochemical studies that note the absence of "pick-up" of special stain for certain nervous system proteins in aganglionic muscle, the stains for presence of acetylcholine esterase, and other laboratory studies help to confirm or negate the diagnosis when, on routine staining, nonganglionic cells may give impression of a false or equivocal presence of ganglion cells. Colostomy (see ***Pediatric Colostomy***, p. 1051) is indicated in newborns and children who are either ill or not responsive to measures to alleviate constipation and abdominal distention. The site of the colostomy must be proximal to the aganglionic segment, as confirmed by histologic examination (employing frozen section examination). When the infant has regained good health and weight of 13.5 kg (30 pounds), or even until late childhood, surgical correction is undertaken. The aganglionic segment is resected, and the proximal colon is anastomosed to the distal rectum or anus.

The Swenson "Pull-through" Procedure (most often employed) to Treat Aganglionic Megacolon is described. The ***Duhamel procedure,*** in which the distal rectum is not excised but allowed to form a common lumen with a segment of normal proximal colon brought anterior to the rectum by crushing the adjacent bowel walls with gastrointestinal clamps or a GIA or similar stapler, may be employed. In the ***Soave procedure***, the distal rectum is preserved but denuded of mucosa, forming a sleeve through which a normal colonic segment is passed to the anus with local anastomosis. These latter procedures (and modifications thereof to clear) avoid dissection in the pelvis, sparing possible injury to genital nerves, but do not necessarily give better results than the Swenson procedure or its several modifications. For an "ultra-short" aganglionic segment, ano-rectal myomectomy is done.

Additionally, in selected cases, a perineal approach such as for ***perineal rectosigmoidectomy*** (see pp. 272–273) may be employed to eliminate intra-abdominal dissection.

A laparoscopic approach can be used to determine the transitional level of the aganglionic colon, to mobilize the colon and rectum, to pass the proximal bowel, and to prolapse the rectal remnant. Prior to establishing pneumoperitoneum, the surgeon may employ the Credé maneuver to ensure that the patient's (catheterized) bladder is empty. Three ports in the upper abdomen and one port in the right lower quadrant are established. To establish pneumoperitonieum, see ***Pediatric Laparoscopy***, p. 1025.

When there is uncontrolled bleeding or if there is trauma to another intra-abdominal organ, the surgery is converted to an open procedure.

Procedure

Pediatric Colorectal Resection for Aganglionic Megacolon (Hirshchsprung's Disease) using the Swenson Procedure is described. A left paramedian incision is made. The sigmoid colon is mobilized and superior hemorrhoidal vessels are divided, taking care not to injure the ureters and vasa deferens. Frozen section of colon muscle biopsies may be done at the level of the division of the bowel to make certain of the presence of ganglia. The pelvis is entered, the lateral rectal ligaments are cut, and the rectum is further mobilized, staying close to the bowel to avoid injury to the autonomic nerves. If a colostomy had not been done, after confirmation of the level of resection, the distal agangliotic colon and proximal rectum are stapled closed and removed. When a colostomy is present, after being separated from the abdominal wall, it is stapled closed and the proximal colon mobilized to permit tension-free passage to the depths of the pelvis.

An operator from below (perineal field) may dilate the anal canal and then evert the rectal stump. A ring clamp or long Babcock forceps is inserted transanally, and a segment of the dissected proximal healthy colon is seized from within; with counter pressure from the pelvis, the colon is "pulled through" the anus. The coats of the everted very distal rectum just proximal to the dentate margin are circumferentially incised amputating the remaining aganglionionic segment. The distal end of the proximal pulled-through colonic segment (including the closed stapled margin) is excised and the retained segment sutured (or stapled) in a single or double layer to the remaining rectal remnant and the anastomosis completed. The anastomosis is then inverted, replacing it within the anal canal. The abdominal incision is closed.

Preparation of the Patient

The head and foot sections of the OR table may be removed. A warming blanket may be placed on the OR table, and radiant heat lamps are positioned over the table to help maintain body temperature. EKG/ECG monitor is employed and pediatric leads are placed. Prior to positioning, the head may be covered with a tube stockinette cap and the extremities may be covered with bias stockinette or Kerlix and plastic wrap to help retain body heat (depending on the weight, size, and age of the child patient). After the child is anesthetized, an IV is inserted into an extremity (usually a forearm) and the extremity is secured to a padded board; padded nonconstricting restraints are placed on the upper extremities. Intravenous antibiotic therapy is usually begun. The child is placed in a modified lithotomy position (or the surgeon's modification of the same) to provide access to the lower abdomen and perineum. A folded towel (or towel-covered plastic IV bag) is placed under the buttocks. The legs may be held in position using pediatric stirrups or abdominal dressing pads and adhesive tape; care is taken to avoid direct skin contact with the tape and to maintain good body alignment. The circulator should consult the surgeon regarding insertion of a Foley catheter (at which time to be done and by whom); the tubing is connected to a urine collection device (e.g., urimeter/urometer) for accurate urine measurement. Irrigation of the rectum may be done with a small rectal tube and warm saline or lactated Ringer's solution (**not water**) prior to skin preparation. All bony prominences and areas vulnerable to skin and neurovascular trauma or pressure are padded. A pediatric electrosurgical dispersive pad is placed. The anesthesia provider inserts a nasogastric tube.

Skin Preparation

Combined Approach. Using warm prep solutions only, begin just left of the midline for a left paramedian incision; extend the prep from the nipples to the knees and down to the table at the sides. Prep the inner thighs, genitalia, exposed buttocks, perineum, and anus (in that order), discarding each sponge after prepping the anus.

Separate Approaches: Perineal. Begin at the pubic symphysis; extend the prep to include the inner thighs, genitalia, exposed buttocks, perineum, and anus (discarding each sponge after prepping anus).

Abdominal. Begin just left of the midline for a left paramedian incision; extend the prep from the nipples to the midthighs and down to the table at the sides. If a colostomy is present, it is protected with a separate sponge soaked in prep solution.

Draping

The patient may be draped all at once for the combined abdominal and perineal approaches, or the patient may be prepped and redraped for the perineal approach.

For Combined Approach. A drape sheet is tucked under the patient's buttocks. The abdomen and perineal area are draped with folded towels. Towels may be secured by using a sterile, plastic adhesive drape, staples, or sutures. A pediatric laparotomy sheet covers the field. A colostomy stoma is covered with an adherent plastic film (e.g., SteriDrape).

For Perineal Approach. The abdominal wound is covered. The patient is prepped and redraped. A portion of a pediatric laparatomy sheet may be cut (in the perineal area). A drape sheet is tucked under the patient's buttocks; the perineum is draped with folded towels and a pediatric laparotomy sheet.

Abdominal Approach. After the perineal portion is completed, for closure, the abdomen may undergo limited local reprepping and is redraped with folded towels and a pediatric laparotomy sheet. Gowns, gloves, and the instruments are changed.

Equipment

- Overhead radiant heat lamps
- Warming blanket (Bair Hugger) or mattress/pad (K-Thermia pad); **do not use both at the same time**
- Covering for the head (e.g., tube stockinette cap), optional
- Covering for extremities (e.g., bias stockinette and plastic wrap), optional
- Padded extremity restraints

EKG/ECG monitor and pediatric leads
ESU, monopolar
Pediatric stirrups or ABD pads and adhesive tape (modified lithotomy position)
Suction
Scales, metric to weigh sponges
Mayo stand (additional) and/or back table for perineal approach

Instrumentation

Abdominal Approach
Pediatric major procedures tray
Pediatric gastrointestinal procedures tray
Pediatric Balfour retractor (if larger than 3¾″ size retractor on tray is required)
Ligating clip appliers, e.g., Hemoclip appliers (short and medium)
Hegar dilators
Automatic small, disposable stapling device (e.g., GIA), optional
Ruler (or measurements marked on knife handle or marking pen may be used)

Perineal Approach
Pediatric major procedures tray

Supplies

Pediatric-sized nasogastric tube (to anesthesia provider)
Bulb syringe, warm normal saline, and small basin (for rectal irrigation), optional
Foley catheter tray and urimeter/urometer
Basin set
Sterile marking pen, optional
Blades,(1) #10, and (4) #15
Electrosurgical pencil (with needle tip) and cord
Vessel loops or umbilical tapes, ¼″, optional
Dissectors (e.g., peanut, Kittners), optional
Suction tubing
Ligating clips, (e.g., Hemoclips), small and medium, optional
Drain, e.g., Hemovac or Jackson-Pratt, optional

Special Notes

- Apply **Special Notes** from ***Relief of Pediatric Intestinal Obstruction***, p. 1047, as applicable. For the laparoscopic approach, apply measures from ***Pediatric Laparoscopy***, p. 1025, as applicable.

- **Reminder:** The room must be heated (see p. 983), overhead radiant heat lamps must be waiting, and a warming mattress/pad (e.g., K-Thermia pad) must be on the table to fulfill minimum heating requirements. The circulator should consult the surgeon and the anesthesia provider to assure that all possible measures are taken to maintain the infant's body temperature.
- **Reminder:** The circulator should determine if an intravenous cutdown and/or hyperalimentation line are to be done following induction of anesthesia. Prior to the child's entry to the room, the circulator should obtain the equipment and supplies to perform these procedures.
- **Reminder:** The circulator must confirm that blood or blood products, as ordered, have been typed and screened (or cross-matched). This should be done before the patient is brought into the room; it is confirmed during "*time-out*."
- The circulator should bring the correctly identified x-ray study films into the room for the correctly identified patient.
- The circulator should consult the surgeon regarding the need for warm saline irrigation of the colon.
- The scrub person should check the temperature of the irrigation fluid prior to its administration to avoid burn injury to the rectal mucosa and to avoid systemic injury by hypothermia.
- The circulator should exercise great care to avoid perforation of the rectum (during colonic irrigation) to avoid the risk of sepsis and tissue injury.
- **N.B.** The circulator should consult the surgeon regarding the approach (combined or separate abdominal and perineal), the position, and the insertion of a Foley catheter (at which time to be done and by whom).
- In positioning the patient, if pediatric stirrups are not available, do not allow the adhesive tape (used in positioning) to come in direct contact with the skin to avoid injury. Protect the skin with tincture of benzoin if the tape must touch the skin.
- If stirrups are used, prevent the risk of positioning injury with stirrups that are padded and positioned correctly, avoiding skin and neurovascular pressure or trauma.
- **N.B.** ***As there are two separate surgical fields, the circulator and the scrub person should exercise particular care to avoid confusion when counting sponges, needles and sharps, and instruments.***

- **N.B.** The scrub person should be prepared for multiple bowel tissue biopsies; each specimen sent for frozen section may be placed on Telfa (or similar pad) and labeled (with marking pen) to avoid identification error.
- **N.B.** The circulator must consult the surgeon for the exact location and the tissue type (e.g., bowel mucosa or muscular layer of the bowel wall) to identify the tissue type from which a biopsy is taken; this information should be written clearly on the pathology requisition.
- **Reminder:** When a bowel resection is performed, the scrub person should isolate soiled instruments (e.g., those that come in contact with the colon) in a basin to avoid sepsis injury.
- "Clean" closure of the abdomen requires regowning, regloving, redraping, and "new" instruments (e.g., Pediatric major procedures tray) are used to avoid the risk of infection.
- **Reminder:** For the laparoscopic approach, the circulator should connect the CO_2 insufflator tubing and adjust the insufflator pressure level. Use a beginning low flow rate of CO_2 (such as 1 to 1.5 l/min) to effect a pressure of 5 mm Hg; later the flow rate may be adjusted to 8 mm (pressure) for brief periods, as directed by the surgeon. To prepare for the laparoscopic approach, see ***Pediatric Laparoscopy***, p. 1025.
- **Reminder:** The circulator assists the anesthesia provider to compare identifiers to ascertain that the correct blood or blood product has been obtained for the correctly identified patient to avoid error.
- The circulator weighs used sponges immediately to reduce "evaporation factor" to help determine fluid loss replacement.
- The scrub person measures irrigation fluids accurately to help determine fluid loss replacement.
- **Reminder:** The patient is usually transported to the PACU by the circulator and the anesthesia provider. The circulator provides the necessary measures required to maintain the pediatric patient's body temperature and avoid hypothermia, such as using an isolette or, when a crib is used, warmed blankets during the transportation of the child.
- **Reminder:** In addition to the orders given to the perioperative practitioner by the anesthesia provider, the circulator gives an intraoperative report regarding the patient care that was implemented and the desired patient outcomes achieved for patient safety regarding continuity of care and for medicolegal reasons.

- **N.B.** When the child does not pass a stool on the nursing unit postoperatively in due time, the child's rectum needs to be irrigated. ***Only the surgeon should irrigate the child's rectum at this critical time.***

Repair of Imperforate Anus

Definition

Establishment of colorectal continuity where there is an absence of an anal opening.

Discussion

There have been multiple classifications of **imperforate anus**. Currently, these anomalies are regarded as "low" or "high." The level of the low lesions present at or inferior to the levator muscle complex; these include a membranous barrier at the anal opening, simple stricture, perineal cutaneous fistulae, labial fistulae, ectopic placement of the anus, etc. The lesions are usually treated locally, often 24 hours after birth without colostomy. The level of high lesions includes the agenesis of the anorectum, rectourethral and rectovesical fistulae (male), rectovestibular and rectovaginal fistulae (female), and cloaca formation. Also, in presentations where there is no fistula, there may be a discontinuity of the colon and rectum at different levels (and other intestinal malformations). These lesions are treated initially with colostomy and with definitive correction later on. Frequently, other anomalies occur in these infants, e.g., in the urinary tract, spine (including tethered cord, sacral agenesis, etc.), or duodenum (atresia, see p. 1045), or they may present as tracheoesophageal fistula (p. 1017), etc. X-ray, magnetic resonance imaging (MRI), and ultrasound examinations may be performed to delineate the array of lesions. Some of the anorectal presentations can be surgically corrected but may not result in a functional ability to control defecation; later sphincter corrective surgery may apply in selected cases. In all of the patients who undergo correction of imperforate anus, careful attention to bowel management and dilatation of the newly formed anus is necessary.

Primary diagnosis relies on the absence of a normally situated anus (including a "flattened" perineum) or local fistulae (as noted above), and after 16 to 24 hours to allow air to enter the gastrointestinal tract, a cross table lateral prone position x-ray may be taken to note the position of the terminal bowel or its absence. When the air pattern is 1 to 1.5 cm from the expected anal opening, the lesion is regarded as "low"; if >1 to 1.5 cm, the lesion is regarded as "high."

High lesions require colostomy to permit passage of stool or to bypass any distal fistulae. A divided descending colostomy is preferred. The distal limb is irrigated, and water-soluble contrast studies (colostographic examinations) are performed to delineate the anatomical pathology in the intestinal and urinary tracts, as applicable, to plan for later repair (usually at age 3 months).

The low lesions are repaired according to presentation. A membrane may be incised and the anal canal repaired (if needed); a simple stricture is serially dilated. The various fistulae are repaired by **posterior sagittal anorectoplasty (PSARP)** or other local surgery. After colostomy, the local rectal correction is done by PSARP combined with intraperitoneal surgery, according to the defects encountered. In all cases, prolonged medical management is required postoperatively. The key to success requires management of constipation proactively. The patient is monitored regularly, and laxatives and dietary management are begun at the first sign of constipation.

There are four classes/types of imperforate anus:

I. Stenosis at the anus or distal rectum
II. Membranous barrier at the anus
III. Rectum ending in a blind pouch above the perineum
IV. Anus and distal rectum ending in a blind pouch proximally, and the more proximal rectum ending in a blind pouch above the distal segment

Type I may be treated by dilation (with colostomy if fecal drainage is impaired); ultimately, if stricture persists, a plastic procedure will be necessary.

In *Type II,* a simple anal membrane needs only to be incised and dilated. The mucosa can be sutured to the skin.

Type III is often associated with various fistulae (including rectovesical, rectourethral, rectovaginal, and rectoperineal) that may allow the passage of the fecal stream by way of the genitourinary tract. Correction of these conditions depends on their presentation. Type III, with its variety of fistulae, is initially treated by colostomy, especially if other abnormalities are present and the infant is in otherwise ill health or premature. Definitive repair can be performed after 3 months of age.

Type IV (rare) is treated first by preliminary colostomy with secondary definitive repair performed several months later by direct anastomosis, or "pull-through," procedure (see ***Pediatric Colonic Resection***, p. 1055).

Imperforate anus may be treated by a laparoscopic-assisted procedure using a 30° laparoscope. Preoperative decompression of the colon is mandatory.

Postoperative complications include edema and urinary retention. Long-term issues and concerns include incontinence, constipation, neurogenic bladder, stricture of neoanus, prolapse of neoanus, and perineal rash.

Procedure

The Standard Procedure for Repair of Imperforate Anus, Posterior Sagittal Anorectalplasty (PSARP), is described. Note that the procedure described is applicable for low and high lesions. Antibiotics are given, a Foley catheter is placed, and the patient is placed in the prone position. A percutaneous electrode from a nerve stimulator (e.g., Pena®) is used to locate the anal dimple. The nerve stimulator is used for short-term sacral nerve stimulation of sacral reflexes that regulate rectal sensitivity and contractility and anal motility.

For low lesions, a midline incision is made from the sacrococcygeal level to the anal site. The external sphincter mechanism is divided and tagged for later repair. The rectum and local fistula are exposed; the rectum may be incised to divide and close the fistula in layers. Absorbable suture is employed for urinary tract structures (such as urethra). The rectum is repaired and tapered (excising a wedge prior to repair to enable passage of the mobilized rectum into its anatomical position) and placed within the center of the delineated sphincter muscular structures; it exits through an incision at the determined site of the anus. The wound is repaired and the distal rectum (any excess amputated) is secured to the anal skin; a perineal anoplasty is performed. A drain is usually not placed.

For high lesions, via a left paramedian incision (or other comparable access), intraperitoneal surgery is employed to divide any fistula accessible above the pelvic floor (e.g., vaginal) and mobilizes the colon (or rectum) for tension-free passage to the perineum. Any collection of stool is irrigated out via the established colostomy; care is taken to protect the wound from contamination. Election to restore continuity of the colostomy is made (or may be done subsequently). The abdominal wound is closed.

The patient is then turned prone to permit **PSARP**; any low fistula is corrected and the proximal mobilized bowel is placed in its correct intrasphincteric position to create the anal opening, as described above. The intraperitoneal portion of the procedure may be performed laparoscopically. To prepare for the laparoscopic approach, see **Pediatric Laparoscopy,** p. 1025.

In the male type III procedure without fistula, the procedure is done by the *perineal approach* only when x-ray confirms the blind pouch is less than 1.5 cm from the anal dimple. A catheter (8 or 10Fr) is passed into the bladder, and a nerve stimulator is used to determine the location of the anal sphincter. A small vertical incision is made within the anal dimple. The rectal pouch is dissected free from surrounding structures so that it can be brought to skin level without tension. The bowel is opened and meconium aspirated. The full thickness of the rectal wall is sutured to the (perianal) skin.

When the rectal pouch is greater than 1.5 cm above the sphincter, a combined abdominoperineal approach is used. The bladder is catheterized with the patient in modified lithotomy position. (This permits simultaneous access to the abdomen and perineum.) An incision is made within the anal dimple as above, and the sphincter is dilated. A left lower oblique or a left paramedial abdominal incision is made. The sigmoid colon and rectum are mobilized, taking care not to injure the ureters. Meconium is aspirated from the distal portion of the colon with a large-bore needle, and the puncture site sutured closed. Dissection continues until the rectum can reach the perineal floor without tension. Care is taken to preserve vascular arcades. The end of the bowel is passed through a tunnel within the levator muscles, made via the perineal incision. The pelvic peritoneum is closed. The abdominal wound is closed. The full thickness of the rectum is sutured to the skin passed through the sphincter as above.

Preparation of the Patient

The room temperature is adjusted one hour prior to the child's arrival. The head and foot sections of the OR table may be removed. Some surgeons prefer to place the infant on the OR table sideways. A warming blanket may be placed on the OR table and radiant heat lamps may be positioned over the OR table to help maintain the patient's body temperature. EKG/ECG monitor and pediatric leads are placed. Prior to positioning, the head may be covered with a tube stockinette cap and the extremities may be covered with bias stockinette or Kerlix and plastic wrap to help retain body heat (depending on the weight, size, and age of the child patient). After the child is anesthetized, an IV is inserted into an extremity (usually a forearm) and the extremity is secured to a padded board; padded nonconstricting restraints are placed on the upper extremities. Intravenous antibiotic therapy is usually begun prior to induction of anesthesia (if IV line established). Positioning is done according to the particlar variant of the presentation; if abdomen and perineum are to be accessed, the child is placed in a modified lithotomy position (or the surgeon's modification of same) to provide said access to the lower abdomen and perineum simultaneously. A folded towel (or towel-covered plastic IV bag) is placed under the buttocks. The legs may be held in position using pediatric stirrups or abdominal dressing pads (ABDs) and adhesive tape; care is taken to avoid skin contact with the tape and to maintain good body alignment. The circulator should consult the surgeon regarding insertion of a Foley catheter (at which time to be done and by whom); the tubing is connected to a urine collection device (e.g., urimeter/urometer) for accurate urine measurement. Irrigation of the rectum may be done with warm saline prior to skin preparation. All bony prominences and areas vulnerable to skin and neurovascular trauma or pressure are padded. A pediatric electrosurgical dispersive pad is placed. A nasogastric tube is inserted by the anesthesia provider. (The patient is turned to prone position for the PSARP portion of the surgery.)

Skin Preparation

Some surgeons prefer to have the prep extend from the nipples to the toes.

Combined Approach. Using warm prep solutions only, begin just left of the midline for a left paramedian incision; extend the prep from the nipples to the knees and down to the table at the sides. Prep the inner thighs, genitalia, exposed buttocks, perineum, and anus (in that order), discarding each sponge after prepping the anus.

Separate Approaches: Abdominal. Begin just left of the midline for a left paramedian incision; extend the prep from the nipples to the midthighs and down to the table at the sides.

Perineal. Begin at the pubic symphysis; extend the prep to include the inner thighs, genitalia, exposed buttocks, perineum, and anus (discarding each sponge after prepping anus).

PSARP. See pilonidal cystectomy (p. 273).

Draping

Combined Approach. A drape sheet is tucked under the patient's buttocks. The abdomen and perineal area are draped with folded towels. Towels may be secured using a sterile, plastic adhesive drape (e.g., SteriDrape), staples, or sutures. A portion of a pediatric laparatomy sheet may be cut (in the perineal area).

Abdominal Approach. The abdominal aspect of the surgery is performed and the wound is covered. Closure performed after the completion of the perineal phase is done after limited reprepping, fresh draping, and unused instruments (e.g., Pediatric minor procedures tray).

Perineal Approach. The patient is prepped and redraped as above. A pediatric laparotomy sheet covers the field.

PSARP. See pilonidal cystectomy (p. 273).

Equipment

Overhead radiant heat lamps
Warming blanket (Bair Hugger) or mattress/pad (K-Thermia pad); **do not use both at the same time**

Covering for the head (e.g., tube stockinette and plastic wrap), optional
Covering for extremities (e.g., bias stockinette and plastic wrap), optional
Padded board to support extremity with IV line, optional
Padded nonconstricting extremity restraints
EKG/ECG monitor and pediatric leads
ESU, monopolar
Suction
ABD pads and adhesive tape for positioning (modified lithotomy), available
Suction
Scales, metric to weigh sponges
Mayo stand (additional) and/or back table for perineal approach
Sacral nerve stimulator unit, e.g., Pena

Instrumentation

For an Extensive Procedure

Pediatric major procedures tray (pediatric Balfour retractor and brain/ribbon/malleable retractors on tray)
Ligating clip appliers, e.g., Hemoclip appliers (short and medium)
Hegar dilators, probes (small), if requested
Automatic stapling device (disposable), optional
Ruler (or measurements marked on knife handle or marking pen may be used), optional
Sacral nerve stimulator cord with electrodes (e.g., Pena)

For a Limited Procedure

Pediatric major procedures tray
Pediatric gastrointestinal procedures tray
Hegar dilators, probes

Supplies

Pediatric-sized nasogastric tube (to anesthesia provider)
Bulb syringe and lubricant (for rectal irrigation), optional
Foley catheter tray and urimeter/urometer, optional
Basin set
Sterile marking pen, optional
Blades,(1) #10, (4) #15
Needle magnet or counter
Electrosurgical pencil (with needle tip) and cord
Vessel loops or umbilical tapes, 1/4″, optional
Dissectors (e.g., peanut, Kittners), optional
Suction tubing

Ligating clips, e.g., Hemoclips (small and medium)
Drain, e.g., Hemovac or Jackson-Pratt, optional

Special Notes

- Apply **Special Notes** from **Pediatric Colorectal Resection for Aganglionic Megacolon (Hirshchsprung's Disease),** p. 1058, as applicable.
- **Reminder:** The room must be heated (see p. 983), overhead radiant heat lamps must be waiting, and a warming mattress/pad (e.g., K-Thermia pad) must be on the table to fulfill minimum heating requirements. The circulator should consult with the surgeon and the anesthesia provider to assure that all possible measures are taken to maintain the infant's body temperature.
- **N.B.** The circulator should consult the surgeon regarding the extent of the skin prep, as the surgeon may request that the infant be prepped from nipples to toes.
- **N.B.** The circulator should ascertain whether a sacral nerve stimulator (e.g., Pena) is needed. He/she brings the sacral nerve stimulator (in good repair) into the room. It is used to locate the anal dimple, prior to the patient's arrival in the room. This information should be confirmed during "***time-out.***"
- **Reminder:** Following the surgery, the patient may be transported (in an isolette to help maintain the pediatric patient's body temperature and to avoid hypothermia en route) to a pediatric intensive care unit or a PACU by the circulator and the anesthesia provider.
- **Reminder:** In addition to the orders given to the perioperative practitioner by the anesthesia provider, the circulator gives a full intraoperative report, including the patient care that was implemented, and the patient outcomes achieved for patient safety regarding continuity of care and for medicolegal reasons.

Pediatric Laparoscopic Appendectomy

Definition

Excision of the appendix through a laparoscope.

Discussion

Indications for **pediatric laparoscopic appendectomy** are similar to the standard approach, but laparoscopy should not be attempted when the disease has reached an advanced stage or when peritonitis is present. An additional benefit of the laparoscopic approach is the ability to identify other causes of the acute abdomen, such as ovarian pathology, congenital abnormalities (e.g., *Meckel's diverticulum*), and numerous abdominal infections. When the laparoscopic approach is employed, prior to pneumoperitoneum, the surgeon ensures that the patient's bladder is empty; the surgeon may employ the Crede maneuver, if necessary.

Many pediatric surgeons prefer (in the smaller child and the thin male) to perform an open procedure regardless, as the abdominal portal incisions may be longer than the standard incision.

Procedure

Pediatric Laparoscopic Appendectomy is described. Following the establishment of pneumoperitoneum, a periumbilical port is established for the scope and two lateral ports are established for instrumentation; see ***Pediatric Laparoscopy***, p. 1025. If early appendicitis is identified, two additional portals are established at the right anterior axillary line and in the left lower quadrant. The Trendelenburg position used to establish pneumoperitoneum is maintained. The appendix is placed in traction using suture (e.g., the ENDOLOOP) or atraumatic grasping forceps. The mesoappendix is either clipped (e.g., with TiGold clips) or, during a laparoscopic-assisted approach, stapled (using smallest disposable endoscopic automatic stapler). The appendix is ligated in the same manner and amputated.

The specimen is delivered; an endoscopic specimen bag may be used to retrieve the specimen. If the appendix is perforated or covered by purulent exudate, the use of a specimen bag is mandatory (to avoid further contamination). The abdomen may be irrigated and a drain placed, as indicated. If additional pathology (e.g., **Mekel's diverticulum,** p. 230) is encountered during a laparoscopic-assisted approach, and peritoneal contamination is minimal, the diverticulum can be resected with the smallest endoscopic intestinal stapler. The portals are removed and the incisions closed.

For **Preparation of the Patient, Skin Preparation, Draping, Equipment,** and **Supplies,** see ***Pediatric Laparoscopy,*** p. 1025, as applicable.

Special Notes

- Apply **Special Notes** from ***Pediatric Laparoscopy,*** p. 1029, as applicable.
- **Reminder:** Before the patient is brought into the room, the circulator and the scrub person must familiarize themselves with the instrumentation used in laparoscopy and the equipment on the laparoscopy cart. (Learning about laoparoscopy should have been done previously in an inservice meeting.)

- **N.B. Reminder:** The circulator should connect the CO_2 insufflator tubing and adjust the insufflator pressure level. For the pediatric patient, use a beginning low flow rate of CO_2 (such as 1 to 1.5 l/min) to effect a pressure of 5 mm Hg; later the flow rate may be adjusted to 8 mm (pressure) for brief periods, as directed by the surgeon.
- **N.B.** As CO_2 can be easily absorbed through the peritoneum, there can be serious consequences to the pediatric patient when it is employed. By using low pressure and warm humidified CO_2 gas during insufflation, in addition to careful monitoring, complications such as hypothermia may be avoided.
- **N.B. Reminder:** Injected lidocaine/Xylocaine 1% can be toxic when too much is administered (at incisional sites). The surgeon should be cautious regarding the amount of lidocaine being administered; the child is observed for signs of lidocaine toxicity (e.g., erythema, bruising, edema, arrhythmias, seizures, or any allergic-type response in the child following lidocaine administration).
- ***Following the manufacturer's directions precisely for sterilization of laparosopic instruments and telescopes is mandatory.***
- **Reminder:** The circulator should position the monitor(s) after the patient is on the table. When the surgery begins, the circulator needs to recheck position of monitors to ensure that the surgeon and those assisting can view them easily.
- **Reminder:** Following draping, the scrub person should pass off the end of the CO_2 Silastic insufflation tubing, the fiberoptic light cord (cable), suction tubing, and electrosurgical cord to the circulator. The circulator may connect these items after the team is in position (to avoid tripping over the cords).
- **Reminder:** Following the surgery, the patient may be transported in an isolette (to help maintain the pediatric patient's body temperature at normothermia and to avoid hypothermia) en route to a pediatric intensive care unit or a PACU by the circulator and the anesthesia provider.
- **Reminder:** In addition to the orders given to the perioperative practitioner by the anesthesia provider, the circulator gives an intraoperative report of the patient's status, the patient care measures that were implemented, and the patient outcomes achieved for patient safety regarding continuity of care and for medicolegal reasons.

Pediatric Laparoscopic Fundoplication/ Nissen Procedure

Definition

Endoscopic wrapping of the gastric fundus about the cardia to correct esophageal reflux.

Discussion

Pediatric Laparoscopic Fundoplication/Nissen Procedure, a minimal-access procedure (MAS), has become the standard of care in children with gastroesophageal reflux disease (GERD). Indications for the Nissen procedure include respiratory compromise (obstructive apnea and aspiration pneumonia), neurological impairment, failure to thrive, esophagitis, and esophageal stricture. An inadequate anti-reflux barrier may be the cause.

This procedure may be performed as a reoperative procedure if the first attempt at fundoplication failed.

The benefits of MAS for the pediatric patient are similar to those for the adult patient:

1. Smaller incisions
2. Reduced analgesic requirements
3. Shortened length of stay
4. Faster return to normal level of activity

The laparoscopic approach is particularly beneficial in children with chronic cough (e.g., cystic fibrosis) regarding postoperative pain that is minimized with easier pulmonary toilet.

Complications include perforation of the esophagus or the stomach. When there is a perforation, it may be repaired laparoscopically, or immediate conversion to an open procedure may be indicated.

Procedure

Pediatric Laparoscopic Fundoplication/Nissen Procedure is described. The anesthesia provider passes a dilator into the esophagus; the dilator should be passed prior to creating the pneumoperitoneum. After pneumoperitoneum is established, four portals are placed: umbilical, mid-upper rectus, and left and right paraumbilical. A laparoscope with a 30° angled lens is used. The triangular ligament of the liver is incised, and the phrenicoesophageal ligament is divided. The esophagus is dissected, protecting the vagus nerves. The crura are dissected, and the dilator is removed. The gastric fundus is mobilized, dividing short gastric vessels, as necessary. A Nissen wrap (or partial wrap) is accomplished with two or three nonabsorbable sutures (sometimes reinforced by staples or two layers of suture). The fundus can then be stapled to the right crus.

If a **gastrostomy,** p. 1035, is indicated, the stomach is inflated with carbon dioxide through a nasogastric tube. Four T anchors are inserted into the stomach percutaneously with a special slotted needle, and a catheter (e.g., Foley) is passed into the center of the square of fasteners. The "T anchors" are tied over stents at the skin level.

If gastric emptying is a problem, ***pyloromyotomy***, p. 1031, or ***pyloroplasty,*** p. 205, may be performed, laparoscopically mobilizing the pylorus, which may be delivered onto the abdominal wall through an enlarged port, and the definitive procedure performed. The pneumoperitoneum is released, and the ports are closed in the routine manner.

For **Preparation of the Patient, Skin Preparation,** and **Draping see Pediatric Laparoscopy,** p. 1025.

Equipment

Overhead radiant heat lamps, optional
Warming blanket (Bair Hugger) or mattress/pad (K-Thermia pad); **do not use both at the same time**
Covering for the head (e.g., tube stockinette and plastic wrap), optional
Covering for extremities (e.g., bias stockinette and plastic wrap), optional
The warming measures listed may be employed, as necessary, depending on the age, weight, and size of the patient
Padded extremity restraints
Padded board to support the extremity for IV line, optional
Padded armboards (if patient is school age or older)
EKG/ECG monitor and pediatric leads
ESU, monopolar
Suction
Monitor(s)
Insufflation device (CO_2)
Fiber-optic light source, e.g., Xenon 300 W
VCR
Camera console
Printer
CD burner

Instrumentation

Pediatric minor procedures tray
Pediatric major procedures tray (available)
Esophageal dilators (e.g., Hurst or Maloney) to the anesthesia provider
Pediatric laparoscopes (2.7 mm × 30° angled lens and/or 5.0 mm × 30° angled lens), and light cord with built-in camera

Size of the laparoscope depends on the size of the child and the surgeon's preference

Pediatric-sized instrumentation (in a range of sizes) is similar, but smaller than that used for adult laparoscopy: Verres needle, trocars with sleeves, 2.7 and 5.0 mm × 230 mm scope, electrosurgical suction-irrigators, fiber-optic light cables (cords), reducers, dissectors, electrosurgical hook dissector, scissors (blunt and sharp), graspers (atraumatic, blunt, and heavy), ruler (or measuring device), and Maryland dissector

Older child fan retractor, extracorporeal and intracorporeal suturing device with introducer sleeve, ligature or loop sutures, knot-sliding instrument, e.g., TiGold

Supplies

Pediatric-sized nasogastric tube (to anesthesia provider)
Basin set
Blades, (1) #15 and (1) #12, optional
Electrosurgical cord
Suction tubing
Needle magnet or counter
Silastic tubing (for CO_2 insufflation)
Fog reduction agent, e.g., FRED, ELVIS, optional
Local anesthetic (e.g., lidocaine/Xylocaine 1%), control syringe, and #25 needle for local immediate postoperative pain relief, optional
Gastrostomy catheter (of choice), catheter plug, T-anchors, bolsters, and stents (for percutaneous insertion of gastrostomy catheter), optional
Tissue anchors (T-anchors), e.g., Moss, optional
Ligating endoscopic clip applier (short) and clips (small, medium), TiGold

Special Notes

- Apply **Special Notes** from the ***Pediatric Laparoscopy***, p. 1029, as applicable.
- Before the patient is brought into the room, the circulator and the scrub person must refamiliarize themselves, as necessary, with the instrumentation used in laparoscopy and the equipment on the laparoscopy cart. Learning about laparoscopy, instrumentation, etc. should be done previously in an inservice meeting.
- **Reminder: *Following manufacturer's directions precisely is mandatory for sterilization of laparoscopic instruments and telescopes.***

- **N.B.** The circulator must be certain that the anesthesia provider is in possession of the surgeon's choice of dilators (e.g., Maloney) prior to starting the surgery; this should be confirmed during "time-out."
- The anesthesia provider may be requested to pass the dilator into the esophagus down to the cardiac junction prior to establishing the pneumoperitoneum. Intraoperatively, he/she may be asked to move the dilator in and out of the junction, prior to its dissection, at the direction of the surgeon. ***Great care is taken not to perforate the esophagus or the stomach.***
- **Reminder:** The circulator is responsible for having adequate levels of CO_2 in the tank (cylinder) prior to bringing the patient into the room. If CO_2 is low, the cylinder should be changed before the procedure begins.
- **N.B. Reminder:** The circulator should connect the CO_2 insufflator tubing and adjust the insufflator pressure level. For the pediatric patient, use a beginning low flow rate of CO_2 (such as 1 to 1.5 l/min) to effect a pressure of 5 mm Hg; later the flow rate may be adjusted to 8 mm (pressure) for brief periods, as directed by the surgeon.
- **N.B.** As CO_2 can be easily absorbed through the peritoneum, there can be serious consequences to the pediatric patient when it is employed. By using low pressure and warm humidified gas during insufflation, in addition to careful monitoring, complications such as hypothermia may be avoided.
- **N.B. Reminder:** Local anesthetic (e.g., lidocaine/Xylocaine 1%) may be injected into the incision sites for local immediate postoperative pain relief when the surgery takes a short amount of time; when the surgery takes longer, local anesthetic is injected at the end of the surgery.
- **N.B. Reminder:** Injected lidocaine/Xylocaine 1% can be toxic when too much is administered. The surgeon must be cautious regarding the amount of lidocaine being administered. The child should be observed for signs of lidocaine toxicity, such as erythema, bruising, edema, arrhythmias, seizures, or any allergic-type response in the child following lidocaine administration.
- The circulator should consult the surgeon regarding an indication for *gastrostomy*, p. 1035; the surgeon's choice of gastrostomy tube (and plug) should be in the room.
- **N.B. Reminder:** Instrumentation and supplies for an open procedure should always be in the room for immediate use,

should the laparoscopic surgery require conversion to an open laparotomy procedure.

- **Reminder:** Following the surgery, the patient may be transported via isolette to help maintain the pediatric patient's body temperature and to avoid hypothermia en route to a pediatric intensive care unit or a PACU by the circulator and the anesthesia provider.
- **Reminder:** In addition to the report (including vital signs) and orders given to the perioperative practitioner by the anesthesia provider, the circulator gives a full intraoperative report, including patient care that was implemented, and the patient outcomes achieved for patient safety regarding continuity of care and for medicolegal reasons.

Excision of Wilms' Tumor

Definition

Excision of a malignant tumor arising in renal embryonal tissue.

Discussion

Wilms' tumor, a nephroblastoma, the most common of childhood intra-abdominal tumors, is usually found in young children prior to age 4 and rarely in neonates or adults. The tumor presents as a flank mass, sometimes with abdominal pain, hematuria, and hypertension, depending on its extension into the renal parenchyma. Multiple studies can reveal its size, bilaterality, extension into the kidney, intravascular extension into the renal vein, inferior vena cava, hepatic veins, or right atrium, and whether there are pulmonary and liver metastases. The approach to treatment begins with nephrectomy (p. 412), followed by chemotherapy with or without postoperative radiotherapy. Recent chemotherapy regimens have been effective but are usually reserved for postoperative treatment unless the tumor is extensive or bilateral.

At the initial surgery, when venous extension is suspect, cardiopulmonary bypass (p. 514) is performed to excise intra-atrial tumor, if present; if liver metastases are found, local hepatic excision is performed. Isolated pulmonary metastases can be excised at a formal thoracotomy later on. The ipsilateral adrenal gland is removed unless the lesion is well confined to the lower pole of the kidney. Bilateral lesions may be treated, providing half of a kidney can be preserved. A second-look procedure may be utilized after a course of chemotherapy for further extirpation of residual tumor. Despite its ominous presentation, surgery and chemotherapy (and radiation therapy) can lead to better than 50% survival, even with metastatic disease.

Procedure

Excision of Wilms' Tumor is described. The patient is supine with a folded towel placed under the affected flank. Multiple vascular lines and monitoring channels are established (and means for cardiopulmonary bypass when significant venous extension is suspect). A bilateral transverse supraumbilical incision is made. The opposite kidney, liver, diaphragm, and adjacent organs are explored for evidence of tumor; lymph nodes are sampled and sites marked with clips for directing postoperative radiation therapy, if needed. Adjacent organs are mobilized to expose the renal pedicle. The renal, gonadal, and adrenal veins are divided (noting the anatomical differences between left and right sides of these vessels). Renal vein tumor extension is determined and treated even to the right atrium under bypass, as necessary. The renal and adrenal arteries are divided and the tumor mass dissected from surrounding structures.

Intimately adherent portions of colon, diaphragm, liver, etc., may be part of an en bloc resection with extension of the incision into the thorax, as needed. Care is taken to avoid tumor "spillage." The ureter is divided close to the bladder and the kidney; adrenal (when same cannot be spared) and tumor mass are removed. After usual completion of hemostasis, irrigation, placement of additional clips to mark the extent of the tumor, etc., the wound is closed.

Preparation of the Patient

The room temperature is adjusted prior to the child's arrival. The head and foot sections of the OR table may be removed. Radiant heat lamps may be positioned over the table to help maintain body temperature. EKG/ECG monitor is employed using pediatric leads. Following induction of general anesthesia, the child is placed in supine position with a folded towel or a small roll placed under the flank on the same side as the lesion; however, depending on tumor distribution, another position (e.g., lateral) may be necessary. A Foley catheter may be inserted into the bladder; the tubing is connected to a urine collection device (e.g., urimeter/urometer) for accurate urine measurement. Prior to positioning, the head may be covered with a tube stockinette cap and the extremities may be covered with bias stockinette or Kerlix and plastic wrap to help retain body heat (depending on the size and age of the child patient). An IV is inserted (into a forearm), additional lines are placed (e.g., an arterial and a central venous pressure), and the extremities may be secured on padded boards. The extremities are restrained using nonconstricting padded restraints placed after the child is anesthetized. All bony prominences and areas vulnerable to skin and neurovascular trauma or pressure are padded. A pediatric electrosurgical dispersive pad is placed.

See ***cardiopulmonary bypass (CPB)*** (p. 514) if this approach is employed when the tumor involves the right atrium.

Skin Preparation

Using warm prep solutions only, prep the entire abdomen and the thorax. For a suprasternal transverse incision, begin the prep on same side as the tumor; extend the prep from the axillae to the pubic symphysis and down to the table at the sides.

Draping

Folded towels and a pediatric laparotomy sheet

Equipment

Radiant heat lamps, optional

Warming blanket (e.g., Bair Hugger) or mattress/pad (e.g., K-Thermia pad); **do not use both at same time**

Covering for the head (e.g., tube stockinette and plastic wrap), optional

Covering for extremities (e.g., bias stockinette or Kerlix and plastic wrap), optional

Note: The above warming measures may be employed, as requested by the surgeon; however, as this tumor is not usually seen in the neonate, the covering for head and extremities is not used.

Padded boards (e.g., to support upper extremities) when an IV and arterial and central venous pressure lines are placed, optional, or padded armboards may be used (depending on the size of the patient), optional

EKG/ECG monitor and pediatric leads (anesthesia provider)

Suction

Scales, metric to weigh sponges

Instrumentation

Pediatric major procedures tray

Pediatric gastrointestinal procedures tray

Cardiac procedures trays (available)

Vascular procedures tray (available)

Ligating clip appliers (e.g., Hemoclip appliers), short and medium

Supplies

Nasogastric tube (to anesthesia provider)

Supplies for IV, arterial, and central venous lines, (include warmer unit), optional

Pediatric Foley catheter tray and urimeter/urometer

Basin set

Blades, (2) #15
Needle magnet or counter
Electrosurgical pencil (with needle tip) and cord
Syringe, 60 ml (for accurate irrigation measurement), optional
Suction tubing
Dissectors (e.g., peanuts, kittners), optional
Vessel loops or umbilical tapes, 1/4″ (for retraction), optional
Ligating clips (e.g., Hemoclips), small and medium

Special Notes

- Apply **Special Notes** from ***Repair of Diaphragmatic Hernia,*** p. 1005, as applicable.
- **Reminder:** The room must be heated (see p. 983), overhead radiant heat lamps must be waiting, and a warming mattress/pad (e.g., K-Thermia pad) must be on the table to fulfill minimum heating requirements. The circulator should consult the surgeon and the anesthesia provider regarding all possible measures to be taken to maintain the infant's body temperature.
- **N.B. Reminder:** The circulator should determine if an intravenous cutdown and/or hyperalimentation line are to be inserted following induction of anesthesia. Prior to the child's entry to the room, the circulator should obtain the equipment and supplies to perform these procedures.
- **N.B. Reminder:** The circulator must confirm that blood or blood products, as ordered, have been typed and screened (or cross-matched) before bringing the patient into the room. Orders for ordering blood and or blood products are confirmed during "***time-out***."
- **Reminder:** The circulator assists the anesthesia provider to compare identifiers to ascertain that the correct blood or blood product unit is there for the correctly identified patient.
- The circulator documents any reaction or the lack of reaction to blood or blood products that are administered in the **Perioperative Record,** p. 12.
- **N.B. Reminder:** Sponges should be weighed as soon as possible to avoid the evaporation factor. To weigh sponges, see **Pediatric General Information**, p. 978.
- **N.B. Reminder:** The scrub person tests the temperature of irrigation fluid before use.
- The scrub person measures the total volume of irrigation solution accurately as it is administered.

- **Reminder:** The circulator and the scrub person must ensure that all fluids (e.g., IV, prep, and irrigation) that come in contact with the patient are warmed to body temperature.
- The scrub person measures irrigation fluids accurately to help determine fluid loss.
- The scrub person may want to receive the large specimen in a basin (for easy handling).
- **Reminder:** The patient is transported to the PACU by the circulator and the anesthesia provider. The circulator provides the measures required to maintain the pediatric patient's body temperature such as using an issolette or warmed blankets in the crib during the transportation of the child.
- **Reminder:** In addition to the orders given to the perioperative practitioner by the anesthesia provider, the circulator gives an intraoperative report of the patient's status, the patient care measures that were implemented, and the patient outcomes achieved for patient safety in continuity of care and for medicolegal reasons.

Excision of Sacrococcygeal Teratoma

Definition

Removal of a neoplastic mass of the sacrococcygeal region.

Discussion

A *sacrococcygeal tumor* of pluri-potential tissues (from more than one germ layer) is usually benign but may contain malignant cells or later develop into a malignancy. *Teratomas* may be derived from cells in the testes in males and the ovaries in females. It presents in a variety of sizes (usually a large mass) and degrees of symmetry. Extensions from the sacrococcygeal area may be found in the pelvis, abdomen, or spinal canal.

Sacrococcygeal teratomas may be diagnosed through ultrasound testing in utero. When associated with fetal hydrops and high output cardiac failure, in utero surgery may be necessary. Whereas this entity is grossly apparent and is successfully treated in the neonatal period, lesser presentations may not be evident until later childhood or in the adult (noted as a small mass or draining sinus that has become malignant). If the tumor is malignant, adjunctive therapy in addition to surgical excision can be offered, but often with less than favorable outcome.

Procedure

Excision of Sacrococcygeal Teratoma is described. With the patient in the prone position, a hemicircumferential incision is made about the superior aspect of the tumor mass. The tumor is excised en bloc, including the coccyx; care is taken to avoid injury to the rectum. To reduce chances of recurrence, the coccyx must be excised with the tumor. As an additional abdominal incision is needed to excise pelvic or intra-abdominal extensions when present, the patient may need to be turned to the supine position for that portion of the surgery. A drain may be placed, and the wound(s) are closed.

Preparation of the Patient

The room temperature is adjusted one hour pror to the child's arrival. The head and foot sections of the table may be removed. A warming mattress/pad may be placed on the table and radiant heat lamps may be positioned over the table to help maintain the patient's body temperature. EKG/ECG monitor and pediatric leads are placed. A Foley catheter may be inserted into the bladder; the tubing is connected to a urine collection device (e.g., urimeter/urometer) for accurate urine measurement. Prior to positioning, the head may be covered with a tube stockinette cap and the extremities may be covered with bias stockinette or Kerlix and plastic wrap to help retain body heat (depending on the weight, size, and age of the child patient). An IV is inserted into a forearm, and for large tumors, additional lines are placed (e.g., an arterial and a central venous pressure). All lines are placed after the child is anesthetized. Following induction of general anesthesia, the airway (endotracheal tube) is secured and the patient turned over to the prone position (at the direction of the anesthesia provider). In the prone position, the face is placed downward on a padded donut (to protect the face), or the head is turned to either side on a donut or pillow and the ear is well padded. The hips are positioned over the middle break of the table to permit flexion. Small chest rolls are placed under the thorax and abdomen to facilitate respiration. A small pillow is placed in front of the knees, and a small roll is placed in front of the toes to prevent nerve damage. Adhesive tape is secured from across the thighs to the underside of the table to stabilize the position (after checking the chart for patient allergy to latex products); the skin under the tape should be protected with an ABD pad. Care is taken to be certain that the tape is not in contact with the skin and that it does not constrict blood flow. Tincture of benzoin is painted on the areas where the tape will be placed to protect the skin. The arms are extended and the hands are positioned on padded boards, with the forearms pronated. All bony prominences and areas vulnerable to skin and neurovascular trauma or pressure are padded. A pediatric electrosurgical dispersive pad is placed.

If an additional abdominal incision is needed to excise pelvic or intra-abdominal tumor extensions, the patient may need to be turned to the supine position for that portion of the surgery. ***The patient is turned only when the anesthesia provider indicates that he/she is ready to move the patient.*** The patient may be turned *only* at the direction of the anesthesia provider; care must be taken not to dislodge IV lines, the urinary catheter, etc.

Skin Preparation

A sterile, plastic adhesive drape may be placed to drape the anus out of the field. Begin at the midline of the back; extend the prep from the level of the axillae to the midthighs and down to the table at the sides.

If patient is turned to supine position, begin at the midline; extend the prep from the axillae to the top of the thighs and down to the table at the sides.

Draping

Folded towels and a pediatric laparotomy sheet

If patient is turned to supine position, redraping using folded towels and a pediatric laparotomy sheet are necessary

Equipment

Overhead radiant heat lamps, optional
Warming mattress/pad (e.g., K-Thermia pad), optional
Covering for the head (e.g., tube stockinette cap)
Covering for extremities (e.g., bias stockinette and plastic wrap), depending on the infant's size, age, and weight, optional
Small donut, pillows, padding, and rolls for positioning (prone)
Adhesive tape, 3″, and an ABD pad placed under the tape to protet the skin (for prone position), available
Padded boards to support upper extremities, optional
Padded nonconstricting upper-extremity restraints, optional
EKG/ECG monitor and pediatric leads
Monopolar ESU
Suction
Suction (with special trap for accurate blood loss measurement), optional
Scales, metric (gram) to weigh sponges
Sacral nerve stimulator unit, e.g., Pena, optional

Instrumentation

Pediatric major procedures tray
Pediatric gastrointestinal procedures tray, available
Vascular procedures tray, available

Ligating clip appliers, e.g., Hemoclip appliers, (short and medium)
Sacral nerve stimulator with electrodes and cord (e.g., Pena), optional
If patient is turned from prone to supine position, an additional pediatric major procedures instrument tray is needed

Supplies

Supplies for IV, arterial, and central venous lines, including warmer unit, optional
Pediatric Foley catheter tray and device for accurate measurement of urine (urimeter/urometer)
Basin set
Blades, (2) #15
Needle magnet or counter
Electrosurgical pencil (with needle tip) and cord
Syringe, 60 ml (for accurate irrigation measurement), optional
Suction tubing
Dissectors (e.g., peanuts, Kittners), optional
Vessel loops or umbilical tapes, 1/4″ (for retraction), optional
Ligating clips (e.g., Hemoclips), small and medium, optional
Scales, metric (2), optional
Drain (e.g., Hemovac or Jackson-Pratt), optional

Special Notes

- Apply **Special Notes** from ***Excision of Wilms' Tumor***, p. 1077, as applicable.
- **Reminder:** The room may be heated (see p. 983), and radiant heat lamps may be waiting over the table to fulfill minimum heating requirements. The circulator should consult the surgeon and the anesthesia provider to ensure that all possible measures are taken to maintain the infant's body temperature.
- **N.B.** The scrub person should anticipate that the patient will be turned from the prone to the supine position; additional drapes, equipment, instruments, and supplies will be necessary. The patient will be prepped and redraped, and a new tray of instruments is required.

Pediatric Thoracoscopy

Definition

Endoscopic visualization of the lungs and the pleural space.

Discussion

Pediatric Thoracoscopy is performed in the OR by a pediatric surgeon experienced in thoracic surgery or a pulmonologist. Most often, a flexible fiber-optic thoracoscope is employed. The pediatric patient receives general anesthesia or titrated IV sedation administered by an anesthesia provider, with local anesthesia injected by the surgeon at the incisional site for a limited procedure (diagnostic). Thoracoscopy affords the surgeon direct visualization of the thoracic cavity for the identification and biopsy of solitary peripheral lesions, evaluation of lung diseases, assessment of the resectability of masses, lysis of empyema cavity in the early stages, and identification of mediastinal masses. Thoracoscopy is considered the optimal technique for the management of many thoracic disorders in children, pulmonary biopsies in the immunosuppressed child, biopsy of pulmonary masses associated with malignancy, excision of mediastinal masses, and lobectomy. Other indications for pediatric thoracoscopy include blebectomy and excision of intrathoracic masses, including bronchogenic cysts.

Prior to thoracoscopic biopsy, x-ray studies, computed tomography (CT) scan, or MRI is indicated; their findings help to localize a lesion and determine optimal patient positioning for surgery. Most often the lateral position is employed for lung biopsy and modified supine position is indicated for mediastinal lesions. If biopsy specimens are sent for frozen section, the ports are not removed until diagnosis is confirmed.

Potential problems inherent in thoracoscopy are the inability to palpate lesions and the potential development of recurrent disease at the trocar sites.

Pediatric thoracoscopy is contraindicated for larger lesions, small children (less than 6 months old), established pleural dense adhesions, and patients on whom mechanical ventilation must be maintained.

It should be noted that a limited biopsy through a small opening incision is efficient and less costly, especially when diffuse disease is present. Postoperative recovery is faster, the patient returns to normal activities sooner, and usually few complications result.

Pediatric thoracoscopy may be performed as a video-assisted thorascopic surgery (VATS) and as a robotic VATS.

Procedure

Pediatric Thoracoscopy is described. General anesthesia is employed. With the patient positioned in a lateral or modified supine position, single-lung ventilation is performed with a double-lumen endotracheal tube on the contralateral side. Unless the patient is unable to tolerate same, the anesthesia provider induces collapse of the ipsilateral lung (creating pneumothorax); three or four ports are established, and 3- and 5-mm instruments are utilized. Using a 5-mm trocar for simple biopsies, a cup biopsy forceps is used. (Note that direct leaks are rare following biopsies.) For more involved procedures, selective intubation is necessary for single lung ventilation of the contralateral lung. On occasion, a Fogarty catheter can be placed to obstruct the ipsilateral bronchus. Using low pressure CO_2 insufflation, 4 to 6 mm, can further assist in collapsing the operative side (in which case, insufflation supplies must be used).

Portal placement and position of the patient depend on preoperative localization of the lesion (e.g., if the lesion is posterior, lean the patient forward). The initial portal is made in the fifth or sixth intercostal space on the midaxillary line. After exploration, other ports are placed accordingly. Endoscopic staplers are helpful in sealing the wound edges following excision of tissues (e.g., lung); note, however, that in small patients, an endoscopic gastrointestinal stapler must be introduced as far from the operative site as possible to allow 5-mm clearance to operate the instrument. Certain lesions, such as a posterior mediastinal neuroblastoma, can be excised employing electrosurgery or a laser. A large specimen can be morcellated in a specimen bag to facilitate its extraction. After lysis of empyema cavities prior to the fibrothorax stage, urokinase (an enzyme) may be instilled into the pleural space. Bleeding is controlled with electrosurgery, laser, ultrasonic shears, or endoscopic sutures. Re-expansion of the lung may also be effective in controlling bleeding.

A chest tube is usually not employed postoperatively unless the patient requires assisted ventilation. The use of endoscopic staplers across divided lung tissue permits removal of the chest tube prior to the patient leaving the operating room (i.e., negligible air leak).

Preparation of the Patient

The room temperature is adjusted prior to the arrival of the child. The head and foot sections of the OR table may be removed. Radiant heat lamps may be positioned over the table, a warming mattress/pad may be placed on the table, or a forced-air warming blanket may be placed over the patient to help maintain body temperature (both devices are not used at the same time to avoid burning the patient). EKG/ECG monitor and pediatric leads are placed. Following induction of general anesthesia, the child is placed in a modified supine position or lateral position (affected side up). In the modified supine position, a folded towel or a small roll is placed under the flank on the same side as the lesion; for the lateral position, see p. 26. Prior to positioning, the head may be covered with a tube stockinette cap and the extremities may be covered with bias stockinette or Kerlix and plastic wrap to help retain body heat (depending on the weight and age of the child patient). An IV is inserted into a forearm, and the forearm may be secured on a padded board. The extremities are restrained using nonconstricting padded restraints, placed after the child is anesthetized. All bony prominences and areas vulnerable to skin and neurovascular trauma or pressure are padded. A pediatric electrosurgical dispersive pad is placed.

Skin Preparation

Using only warm prep solutions, begin at the level of the fourth costal interspace on the operative side; extend the prep from the shoulders to the pubic symphysis and down to the table at the sides.

Draping

Folded towels and a pediatric laparotomy sheet

Equipment

Radiant heat lamps, optional
Forced-air warming blanket (e.g., Bair Hugger) or warming mattress/pad (e.g., K-Thermia pad); **do not use both at same time**
Covering for the head (e.g., tube stockinette cap), optional
Covering for extremities (e.g., bias stockinette or Kerlix and plastic wrap), optional
Padded board to support the upper extremity for an IV, or padded armboards (on the child school-aged or older), optional
EKG/ECG monitor and pediatric leads (anesthesia provider)
Suction
ESU, monopolar
Laser (e.g., Nd:YAG), optional
Ligasure® Vessel Sealing Generator, optional
Scales, metric (gram) to weigh sponges, optional
Monitor(s)
Fiber-optic light source, e.g., Xenon 300 W
VCR
Printer
CD burner
Camera console

Instrumentation

Pediatric minor procedures tray
Pediatric major procedures tray (available)
Pediatric thoracoscope (telescope) and light cord; thorascope may have built-in camera or the camera may be a separate unit attached by a coupler
Pediatric laparoscopic instrumentation (in a range of sizes) is similar or the same as that used for adult laparoscopy, except it is smaller: trocars with sleeves 2.7 and 5.0 mm × 230 mm, electrosurgical suction-irrigators, fiber-optic light cables (cords), reducers, [see dissectors, electrosurgical hook dissector, scissors (blunt and sharp), graspers (e.g., atraumatic, Babcock), sponge-holding forceps, ruler (or other measuring device], Maryland dissector, morcellator, and fan retractor

Ligating endoscopic clip applier (short) and clips (small and medium), e.g., TiGold, optional
Endoscopic or endovascular linear stapler stapler, optional
Laser hand piece, fiber tip and cord, optional
Ligasure handpiece (reusable), cord, and snap-in electrode, optional
Cavitational Ultrasonic Aspirator (CUSA) generator with foot pedals, optional, or
Cavitron generator, ultrasonic hand piece and instrument (dissector, shears, aspiration tip, etc.) and cord, generator

Supplies

Pediatric-sized nasogastric or orogastric tube (to anesthesia provider)
Basin set
Normal saline irrigation (warm) and 2 bulb syringes, optional
Blades,(1) #10 and (2) #15
Needle magnet or counter
Electrosurgical cord for electrosurgical instruments
Suction tubing
ENDO SUTURE (suture ligature or loop sutures (e.g., ENDOLOOP, SURGITIE) both without needles
ENDO STITCH, extracorporeal and intracorporeal suturing device with introducer sleeve (e.g., with swaged-on needle)
ENDOKNOT or SUTURE ASSISTANT, ligature or loop sutures, with knot-sliding instrument (both with swaged-on needle)
Endoscopic specimen pouch, e.g., Endopouch, Endosac, ENDOBAG, LAP-BAG, or LAPSAC, endoscopic specimen pouch, optional
Endoscopic or endovascular staples, optional
Medicine cups, labels, and marking pen, optional

Medications

Xylocaine/lidocaine 1%, local anesthetic, control syringe, and #25 needle for local immediate postoperative pain relief, optional

Urokinase, enzyme used following debridement, for adhesiolysis (100,000 to 200,000 units of urokinase is added to 30 ml of normal saline), optional, Chest drainage unit, underwater seal (e.g., Pleurovac™) and drainage tube(s) (e.g., Argyle), and straight or Y connector, optional

Special Notes

- Apply **Special Notes** from ***Pediatric Laparoscopy***, p. 1029, as applicable.

- **Reminder:** The scrub person should be aware that sutures may be placed to secure the trocars or that trocars with screw threads that prevent dislodgement are used.
- **Reminder:** Local anesthetic (e.g., lidocaine/Xylocaine 1%) may be injected into the incision sites for local immediate postoperative pain relief. For the pediatric patient, the local anesthetic is injected into the incision sites at the time the incisions are made when the surgery takes a short amount of time; local anesthetic is injected at the end of the surgery when the surgery takes longer.
- The circulator may be requested to prepare the Urokinase (an enzyme used following debridement); to debride the pleural cavity, 100,000 to 200,000 units of Urokinase is introduced into 30 ml of normal saline.
- **N.B. Reminder:** Injected lidocaine/Xylocaine 1% can be toxic when too much is administered. The surgeon is cautious regarding the amount of lidocaine being administered. The child is observed for signs of lidocaine toxicity, such as erythema, bruising, edema, arrhythmia, seizures, or any allergic type response in the child following lidocaine administration.
- The circulator should position the monitor(s) after the patient is on the table. When the surgery begins, the circulator needs to recheck position of the monitors to ensure that the surgeon and those assisting can view them easily.
- Following draping, the scrub person should pass off the fiber-optic light cord (cable), suction tubing, and electrosurgical cord to the circulator. The circulator may connect these items after the team is in position (to avoid tripping over the cords).
- **Reminder:** All fiber-optic instrumentation and light cables must be handled with great care to avoid breaking the tiny fiber-optic light fibers. The fiber-optic cables may not be bent or folded.
- **Note:** The manufacturer has determined whether the particular telescope is autoclavable; directions for sterilization of the telescopes should be followed precisely. Telescopes may be sterilized using ethylene oxide, peracetic acid, or hydrogen peroxide gas plasma; see p. 44.
- Steris 20 (peracetic acid) solution system (the most frequently employed) may be used to sterilize telescopic instruments and telescopes. The instrument or telescope must be completely submerged for 12 minutes at 50° to 55°C for sterilization requirements to be met, see p. 43.

- **N.B.** Instrumentation should always be available in the room for immediate use, should the thoracoscopic surgery require conversion to an open thoracotomy procedure.
- **Reminder:** The patient is usually transported to the PACU by the circulator and the anesthesia provider. Necessary measures are required to maintain the pediatric patient's body temperature, such as using an isolette or warmed blankets in the crib during the transportation of the child.
- **Reminder:** In addition to the orders given to the perioperative practitioner by the anesthesia provider, the circulator gives an intraoperative report regarding the patient's status, the patient care that was implemented, and the desired patient outcomes achieved related to patient safety in continuity of care and for medicolegal reasons.

Pediatric Laparoscopic Splenectomy

Definition

The endoscopic excision of the spleen.

Discussion

Primary indications for **pediatric laparoscopic splenectomy** are hematological. The decision to perform a splenectomy depends on the severity and the prognosis of the disease or condition causing the hypersplenism. Performing the procedure is restricted, as there are concerns regarding exposure of patients to a lifelong risk of overwhelming infections (due to loss of immunologic function of the spleen). Hypersplenism is almost always associated with splenomegaly. *Splenomegaly* may be caused by *cirrhosis of the liver, leukemia, lymphomas (both Hodgkin's and non-Hodgkin's), primary cancer of the spleen, hereditary spherocytosis* (a hematological disorder in which red blood cells are destroyed in the spleen) may present at any age, including the newborn; splenectomy is delayed until at least age 5 or 6. *Idiopathic thrombocytopenia* (characterized by destruction of platelets). Another indication for which splenectomy is done is trauma. Whenever possible, **splenorrhaphy** or **partial splenectomy** is performed in cases of trauma. Some children who have had a splenectomy are placed on antibiotics until the age of 16 prophylactically; these children are then given a booster dose of pneumococcal vaccine every 5 to 10 years. The risk of a child dying from an infection is highest in the first 2 years following surgery. A search for accessory spleens is done, and, if identified, they are excised.

If ***cholecystectomy*** (p. 148) is likewise indicated, ***laparoscopic cholecystectomy*** (p. 153) is similar to that performed in the adult (except that smaller instruments are used). ***Intraoperative cholangiogram*** to identify the small biliary ductal structures is done through the gallbladder or cystic duct. Colonic preparation is usually done.

Prior to starting the procedure, the patient's bladder should be empty. If the anticipated surgery will be brief, the surgeon may avoid a Foley catheterization by applying the *Credé's maneuver* to empty the child's bladder; for longer procedures or for procedures where significant blood loss is expected, a Foley catheter may be ordered. The anesthesia provider usually inserts a nasogastric or orogastric tube to ensure that the patient's stomach is empty. Often, antibiotics are administered prophylactically.

Contraindications for **pediatric laparoscopic splenectomy** include uncorrected coagulopathy, hemodynamic instability or shock, and diffuse, dense adhesions that preclude safe access.

Procedure

Pediatric Laparoscopic Splenectomy is described. With the patient in modified supine position, an infraumbilical incision is employed; the trocar is inserted under direct vision, and pneumoperitoneum is established. Sutures may be used to secure the port. The laparoscope is inserted, and three or four portals in the midline or left of the midline are placed. The short gastric vessels are divided. The splenocolic ligament is divided, employing electrosurgery or an endoscopic linear stapler; attachments to the diaphragm and perinephric tissues are divided. The remaining short gastric vessels are also divided. The endovascular linear stapler is placed across the splenic hilum, avoiding the tail of the pancreas. The specimen is delivered in a specimen-retrieval bag with morcellation of the spleen, as necessary. Accessory spleens, if present, are excised. Hemostasis is achieved. The pneumoperitoneum is released, and the ports are closed.

Preparation of the Patient

The room temperature is adjusted prior to the child's arrival. The head and foot sections of the table may be removed. Radiant heat lamps may be positioned over the table to help maintain body temperature. EKG/ECG monitor is employed with pediatric leads. A forced-air warming blanket or a warming mattress/pad may be used. Following induction of general anesthesia, the child is placed in a modified supine position or lateral position. In the modified supine position, a folded towel or a small roll is placed under the flank on the same side as the lesion; for the lateral position, see p. 26. Prior to positioning, the head may be covered with a tube stockinette cap and the extremities may be covered with bias stockinette or Kerlix and plastic wrap to help retain body heat (depending on the size and age of the child patient). An IV line is inserted into a forearm and secured on padded boards. The extremities are restrained using nonconstricting padded restraints, placed after the child is anesthetized. A Foley catheter may be inserted in the patient's bladder, and the tubing is attached to a urimeter/urometer. All bony prominences and areas vulnerable to skin and neurovascular trauma or pressure are padded. A pediatric electrosurgical dispersive pad is placed to ground the electrosurgical instruments.

Skin Preparation

Using only warm prep solutions, the umbilicus is meticulously cleaned. Begin at the umbilicus; extend the prep from the axillae to the pubic symphysis and down to the table at the sides.

Draping

Folded towels and a pediatric laparotomy sheet

Equipment

Radiant heat lamps, optional
Forced-air warming blanket (e.g., Bair Hugger) or mattress/pad (e.g., K-Thermia pad); **do not use both at same time**
Covering for the head (e.g., tube stockinette cap), optional
Covering for extremities (e.g., bias stockinette or Kerlix and plastic wrap), optional
Padded board to support the upper extremity for an IV line, padded armboards (may be used for school-aged children), optional
EKG/ECG monitor and pediatric leads (to anesthesia provider)
Suction
ESU, monopolar
Insufflation device (CO_2)
Fiber-optic light source, e.g., Xenon 300 W
VCR
Laser (e.g., Nd:YAG), optional
CUSA Generator with foot pedals, (e.g., Cavitron), optional

Instrumentation

Pediatric minor procedures tray
Pediatric major procedures tray (available for conversion)
Laparoscopes, 5 mm × 0° angle lens and 5 mm × 30° angle lens, with camera chip and cord or separate camera attached with coupler
Laparoscopes, from 1.7 to 4 mm in diameter with viewing angles from 0° to 70° (available)
Pediatric-sized instrumentation (in a range of sizes) is similar or the same as that used for adult laparoscopy: Verres needle, trocars

with sleeves, electrosurgical suction irrigators, fiber-optic light cables, reducers, and dissectors (e.g., reusable), monopolar electrosurgical Maryland dissector and electrosurgical hook dissector, scissors (blunt and sharp), graspers (atraumatic, e.g., Babcock), ruler (measuring device), needle holders, and fan retractor

Ultrasonic irrigation/aspiration hand piece, (e.g., Cavitron), optional

Supplies

Pediatric-sized nasogastric or orogastric tube (to anesthesia provider)
Foley catheter and urimeter/urometer
Basin set
Normal saline irrigation, warm, and 2 bulb syringes, optional
Blades,(1) #10 and (2) #15
Needle magnet or counter
Electrosurgical cord (for electrosurgical instruments)
Silastic tubing (for CO_2 insufflation)
Suction tubing
ENDO SUTURE (without needle), suture ligature, or loop sutures (e.g., ENDOLOOP, SURGITIE)
ENDO STITCH (with swaged-on needle), extracorporeal and intracorporeal suturing device with introducer sleeve
ENDOKNOT or SUTURE ASSISTANT, knot-sliding instrument (both with swaged-on needle)
Endoscopic specimen pouch, e.g., Endopouch, Endosac, ENDOBAG, LAP-BAG, or LAPSAC, optional
Ligating endoscopic clip applier (short) and clips (small, medium), e.g., TiGold
Endoscopic or endovascular linear stapler with staples, optional
Medicine cup, labels, and marking pen, optional
Local anesthetic (e.g., lidocaine/Xylocaine 1%), control syringe, and #25 needle for local immediate postoperative pain relief, optional

Special Notes

- Apply **Special Notes** from ***Laparoscopic Fundoplication (Nissen Procedure)***, p. 1072, as applicable.

PART 5 Instrument Trays

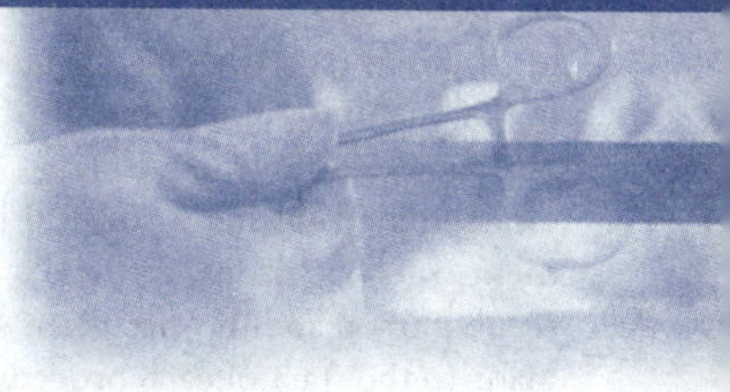

Introduction

The most important aspect of surgical instrumentation is related to the function of the instrument. Many instruments are multipurposed or can be used to perform similar tasks in varying specialties. There may be a difference of opinion as to which instruments should be specifically selected, though surgeons the world over frequently choose the same or similar instruments when performing a particular surgery. In this guide, the instrument trays have been organized to represent those instruments classically selected for use in a particular specialty, allowing for substitutions by individuals and institutions. Universally, availability and cost containment influence the ultimate selections.

The ever-increasing number and variety of surgical instruments is influenced by the development of technological advances in innovative procedures and surgical approaches. Many traditionally-used instruments have been discarded or modified. Some instruments are known by more than one name or by various colloquial names even within the same institution. The composition of the trays appearing in this guide, therefore, will be familiar to most readers, although they may not reflect precisely what might be encountered at their own hospital or surgical institution.

The following trays are based on surgical specialties or frequently-performed specific surgical procedures. To simplify the listings of the trays' components, certain liberties have been taken to avoid excessive terminology and subsections. Therefore, the category of "Forceps" refers only to "thumb" forceps. The category of "Clamps" includes the many types of forceps, including hemostatic, biopsy, and grasping forceps; towel clips; and needle holders. The "Miscellaneous" subheading is an all-inclusive category for instruments that do not fit under any of the main categories. The sizes of most instruments have been included to aid in their identification.

Each surgical facility has its own written policies and procedures that serve as a guideline for individual practice. Following the accepted standard practice established by the Association of periOperative Nurses (AORN) regarding the counting of instruments, all objects that are potentially subject to inadvertent inclusion within a wound must be counted (see Chapter 2, p. 39). That refers not only to the counting of each instrument but also to the counting of components, separate or removable parts (e.g., parts of a refractor, assembled and disassembled during a surgical procedure), or portions of an instrument, such as blades, screws, washers, nuts, tips of suctions, etc. The scrub person and the circulator should perform the instrument counts prior to the start of each procedure and, subsequently, prior to closure of a body cavity or a deep or large wound and again prior to the closure of the skin. The scrub person and the circulator count concurrently (aloud) all instruments (and parts thereof, as applicable) on the sterile field as the scrub person touches each item. The circulator immediately records the number (count) of each type of instrument, as the recording of the count is the circulator's legal responsibility. If there is any uncertainty regarding the counting of any instrument(s), the counting of that type of instrument(s) is repeated. See counting procedure, Chapter 2, p. 39.

Usually, personnel in the central supply department prepare instrument sets/trays with predetermined numbers and types of each instrument in the tray, according to the discretion of the surgical department. Counting is expedited when an initialled document accompanies each tray indicating the number and type of instrument(s) and the name of the person who assembled the tray, with a notation regarding any missing instrument. When used, this protocol facilitates the counting of instruments and avoids searching for missing instruments not included on the tray.

CHAPTER 32

General Surgery Instrument Trays

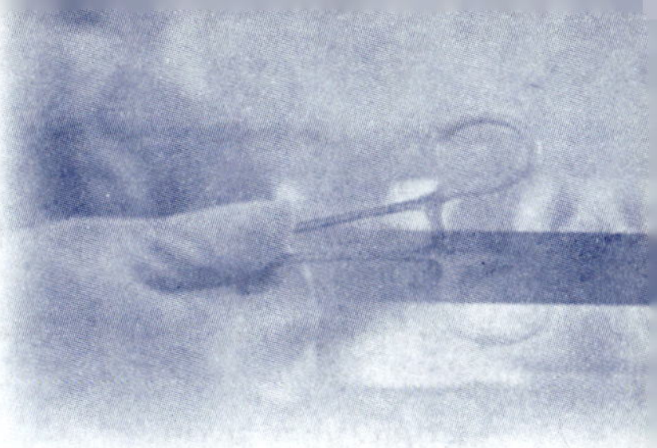

Major Procedures Tray

Retractors

- 2 Ribbon/malleable, (1) 1 1/2″ and (1) 2 1/2″
- 3 Richardson (1 small, 1 medium, 1 large)
- 2 Goelet, 7 1/2″
- 2 Army-Navy/USA, 8 5/16″
- 3 Deaver (1 narrow, 1 medium, 1 wide)
- 2 Harrington, (1) 1 1/2″ and (1) 2 1/2″

Forceps

- 2 Tissue smooth/plain/dressing (without teeth), (1) 6″ and (1) 10″
- 3 Tissue with teeth, (2) 6″ and (1) 10″
- 2 Russian, (1) 7″ and (1) 10″
- 4 DeBakey, (2) 7 3/4″ and (2) 9″
- 2 Ferris Smith, 7″
- 1 Adson, smooth/plain/without teeth, 4 3/4″
- 2 Adson with teeth, 4 3/4″

Scissors

- 2 Straight Mayo, 6 1/4″
- 1 Curved Mayo, 6 1/4″
- 1 Metzenbaum, 7″
- 1 Wire cutter

Clamps

- 8 Towel clip, nonpiercing, (4) 3 1/2″ and (4) 5″
- 8 Towel clip, piercing, (4) 3 1/2″ and (4) 5″
- 18 Curved Crile, 6 1/2″
- 6 Straight Crile, 6 1/2″
- 12 Curved Pean/Mayo Pean, (6) 7″ and (6) 8″
- 8 Straight Kocher/Ochsner, (4) 6 1/4″ and (4) 8″
- 6 Allis, 6″
- 4 Babcock, 6″
- 4 Tonsil/Schnidt, 7 1/4″
- 2 Right-angle/Mixter, (1) 7 1/4″ fine and (1) 9″

8 Needle holder, (2) Mayo Hegar (heavy), 6″; (2) Ryder, 6″; (2) Crile Wood, 7 1/2″; and (2) Crile Wood, 9″
4 Sponge (ring) forceps (Foerster), 10″

Suction Tubes or Tips

1 Poole/Pool (suction tube and sleeve; 2 pieces), 8 1/4″
1 Yankauer, (suction tube and tip; 2 pieces), 10 3/8″

Miscellaneous

3 Knife handles, (2) #3 and (1) #7
1 Probe, malleable
1 Grooved director

Optional

Balfour self-retaining retractor (with 2 central blades, regular and deep, and 2 pairs fenestrated side blades, regular and deep)
Bookwalter™ self-retaining retractor set (with a variety of parts, as segmented half circles, screws, oval ring, straight extensions, ratchet mechanisms, horizontal bars, post couplings, and a variety of assorted blades)
Martin's arm (fixed table retractor with 3 joints)

Basic/Minor Procedures Tray

Retractors

2 Goelet, 7 1/2″
2 Army-Navy/USA, 8 1/2″
1 Weitlaner, sharp, 6 1/2″
1 Ribbon/malleable/Ochsner malleable, 1″ wide
1 Deaver, narrow, 1″ wide
1 Richardson, small blade, 7/8″
2 Rakes, sharp (4 prong), 8″
2 Senn sharp, 6″

Forceps

2 Tissue/smooth/plain/dressing/fingers, without teeth, (1) 6″ and (1) 10″
4 Tissue with teeth, (2) 6″ and (2) 10″
1 Adson without teeth, 4 3/4″
2 Adson with teeth, 4 3/4″
1 Russian, 7″
2 DeBakey, 6″

Scissors

1 Curved Mayo, 6 1/4″
2 Straight Mayo, 6 1/4″
3 Metzenbaum, (1) 5 1/4″; (1) 6″; and (1) 7″
1 Stevens tenotomy, 4 1/2″
1 Curved Iris, 4″
1 Straight Iris, 4″

Clamps

8 Towel clip, piercing, (4) 3 1/2″ and (4) 5″
8 Towel clip, nonpiercing, (4) 3 1/2″ and (4) 5 1/2″
12 Curved mosquito, 5″
2 Straight mosquito, 5″
12 Curved Crile, 6 1/2″
2 Straight Crile, 6 1/2″
2 Babcock, 6″
4 Allis, 6″
4 Straight Kocher/Ochsner, 6 1/4″
2 Webster needle holder, 4 1/2″
4 Needle holder, (2) Mayo Hager (heavy), 6″ and (2) Ryder (fine), 7″
2 Forester sponge forceps, 7″

Suction Tubes or Tips

1 Yankauer (suction tube and tip; 2 pieces) 10 3/8″
1 Frazier, #10

Miscellaneous

3 Knife handles; (2) #3 and (1) #7
1 Probe, malleable
1 Grooved director
2 Medicine cups

Limited Procedures Tray

Retractors

2 Joseph skin hooks, single, 6″
2 Senn, sharp, 6″

Forceps

2 Tissue with teeth, 6″
1 Adson without teeth, 4 3/4″
2 Adson with teeth, 4 3/4″
1 Adson-Brown, 5″

Scissors

1 Straight Mayo, $6^1/_4''$
2 Metzenbaum, (1) $5^1/_4''$ and (1) $6''$
1 Stevens tenotomy, $4^1/_2''$
1 Curved iris, $4''$
1 Straight iris, $4''$

Clamps

4 Curved Crile, $6^1/_2''$
2 Straight Crile, $6^1/_2''$
4 Curved mosquito, $5''$
2 Straight mosquito, $5''$
2 Needle holder, $6''$
8 Towel clip, piercing, (4) $3^1/_2''$ and (4) $5''$
8 Towel clip, nonpiercing, (4) $3^1/_2''$ and (4) $5''$

Suction Tubes or Tips

1 Frazier, #10

Miscellaneous

2 Knife handles, #3
2 Medicine cups

Thyroid Tray

Retractors

2 Senn, sharp, $6''$
2 Lahey, $8''$
2 Greene, $8^1/_2''$
2 Cushing vein, $9''$
4 Gelpi, $4^1/_2''$, $5^1/_2''$, $7^1/_2''$, and $10^1/_2''$
1 Weitlaner, sharp, $5^1/_2''$
1 Adson, $4^3/_4''$
1 Mahorner
2 Joseph single skin hooks, $6^1/_4''$
2 Joseph double skin hooks, $6^1/_4''$

Forceps

1 Tissue without teeth, $6''$
2 Tissue with teeth, $6''$
2 Cushing without teeth, $7''$
2 Cushing with teeth, fine, $7''$
2 Adson with teeth, $4^3/_4''$

2 Adson without teeth, 4 3/4″
2 DeBakey, 6″

Scissors
2 Straight Mayo, (1) 5 1/4″ and (1) 6 1/4″
1 Straight Metzenbaum, 5 1/4″
2 Metzenbaum, (1) 5 1/4″ and (1) 7″
1 Straight Iris, 4
1 Curved Iris, 4

Clamps
6 Curved mosquito, 5″
6 Straight mosquito, 5″
8 Curved Crile, 6 1/2″
2 Curved Pean/Mayo Pean, 7″
6 Allis, 6″
2 Babcock, 6″
2 Tonsil/Schnidt, 7 1/4″
2 Right-angle, Mixter (fine), 6 1/4″
2 Right-angle, Mixter, 6 1/4″
2 Straight Kocher/Oschner, 6″
4 Lahey, 6″
2 Webster needle holder, 4 1/2″
2 Needle holder, 6″
8 Towel clip, piercing, (4) 3 1/2″ and (4) 5″
8 Towel clip, nonpiercing, (4) 3 1/2″ and (4) 5″

Suction, Suction Tubes or Tips
1 Frazier #8
1 Andrews (suction tube and tip; 2 pieces), 9 1/2″
1 Adnoid suction, (suction tube and tip; 2 pieces), 7 1/4″

Miscellaneous
3 Knife handles, (2) #3 and (1) #7

Long Instruments Tray

Forceps
1 Tissue smooth/plain/fingers without teeth, 10″
1 Tissue with teeth, 10″
2 DeBakey, (1) 9 1/2″ and (1) 12″

Scissors
2 Metzenbaum, (1) 9″ and (1) 10″

Clamps

4 Collier needle holders, 10½″
2 Right-angle/Mixter, 11″
2 Tonsil/Schnidt, 10″
2 Tonsil/Bridge, 11″
4 Pean/Mayo Pean, 12″
4 Allis, 10″
2 Babcock, 10″
2 Kocher/Ochsner, 10″
2 Needle holder, 10″

Miscellaneous

1 Knife handle, #3L, 8″

Biliary Tract Procedures Tray

Forceps

2 DeBakey, (1) 9½″ and (1) 12″
4 Randall stone forceps (¼ curved length through 1 full curved length)

Clamps

2 Borge cystic duct clamp, (1) 4Fr and (1) 6Fr
2 Long tonsil/Schnidt, 10″
2 Long right angle/Mixter, 10″

Scissors

1 Metzenbaum scissors, 9″
1 Potts scissors, 45° angle, 9″

Scoops

3 Ferguson gallstone scoops (1 small, 1 medium, 1 large)

Miscellaneous

9 Bakes common duct dilators, sizes 3 to 11
1 Knife handle, #3L, 8
1 Spoon
1 Medicine cup
1 Probe, malleable, 15, 18, or 20Fr
1 Alcock conical catheter adaptor, 18 to 25Fr
1 Ochsner gallbladder trocar, 12 Fr

Choledochoscopy Tray ("Open" Procedure)

Scope

1 Choledochoscope, fiber-optic, rigid, or flexible, with sheath, adaptor, and cord
1 Camera, coupler, and cord, or built-in camera chip

Extras

1 Instrument guide
1 Stone crusher
1 Stone-retrieval basket
1 Stopcock
1 Rubber washer
2 Rubber caps

Laparoscopic Cholecystectomy

(Many of the following instruments are available as disposable)

Verres needle with stylet, medium and long
Silastic tubing with Luer-Lok tip (male)
Trocars (e.g., 5 mm, 10 mm, 12 mm, and Hasson)
Cannulas (sleeves, sheathes, or ports) and obturators
Reducer caps, port caps, nipples, 2 each
Smoke evacuator

Scopes

Laparoscope(s), fiber-optic (operating telescope) with camera chip, and cord(s) or camera is separate and a coupler is used

Endoscopic Instrumentation

2 Babcock forceps
4 Scissors or endoshears, insulated (curved, hook, straight, and micro)
Electrosurgical Metzenbaum
Curved and straight Maryland dissector
Right angle dissector
Microdissector
Kelly clamp
Multifire ligating clip applier (assorted sizes)
Fan retractor
2 Grasping forceps
1 Large-toothed grasping forceps
2 Dissecting forceps, insulated (right angle, J tip, or hook)
Electrosurgical dissector

Irrigator-aspirator
Olsen cholangiogram clamp
Dormia stone-retrieval basket

Many of the items listed as supplies in this text are disposable instruments

ENDO STITCH® (suture with swaged-on needle), disposable, single use, optional
ENDOKNOT (suture with swaged-on needle and sleeve), disposable, single use, optional
ENDOBAG (specimen retrieval pouch), disposable, single use, optional
Fogarty catheters, assorted sizes, to aid in stone retrieval (by stone dislodgement), available

Laparoscopic Choledochoscopy

Choledocoscope, flexible fiber-optic (operating flexible scope with small working channel) and cord
1 Stone-retrieval basket

Special Notes

- A ureteroscope may be substituted for a choledochoscope.
- Ultrasound wand or laser fiber (may be requested).

Basic Rigid Sigmoidoscopy Tray

1 Anoscope (e.g., Hirschmann, medium)
1 Standard rigid sigmoidoscope (steel) with obturator, or 1 disposable rigid sigmoidoscope (plastic) with obturator, and fiber-optic light cord
1 Illuminator head unit (reusable), for disposable scope only
1 Insufflation bulb and tubing

Special Notes

- Standard rigid sigmoidoscope is 25 cm (long) × 19 mm (diameter). Disposable rigid plastic sigmoidoscope is 25 cm (long) × 18 mm (diameter); disposable scopes are usually preferred over the metal scopes.
- Other rigid sigmoidoscopes may be requested, e.g., 11-, 15-, or 27-mm diameter.

Gastrointestinal Procedures Tray

Forceps

2 DeBakey forceps, 9 1/2″, 12″

Scissors

2 Metzenbaum scissors, 9″,10″

Clamps

4 Long Pean/Mayo Pean, 10″
4 Long Babcock, 10″
4 Long straight Kocher/Ochsner, 9″
4 Long Allis, 10″

Special Notes

- A variety of additional pairs of noncrushing clamps may be used on the bowel, straight or right angle, such as:

  4 Glassman intestinal clamps: 2 angled, 2 straight, 9″ with 2″ jaws

  2 DeBakey vascular clamps, obtuse 60° angle, 12″

  2 DeBakey aortic aneurysm clamps, 12″
- A variety of disposable stapling devices may be used instead to "clamp, cut, and staple" the bowel, such as GIA, EEA, ILA, or TA.

Ano-Rectal Procedures Tray

Retractors

1 Parks or 1 Pratt rectal speculum (with 1 set screw)
3 Sawyer (1 small blade 3/4″, 1 medium blade 1 1/8″, 1 large blade 1 1/2″)

Forceps

1 Tissue plain/smooth (without teeth), 6″
2 Tissue (with teeth), 6″
1 Adson-Brown tissue forceps, 4 3/4″

Scissors

1 Straight Mayo, 6 1/4″
1 Curved Mayo, 6 1/4″
1 Metzenbaum, 7″

Clamps

6 Curved Crile, 6 1/2″
6 Allis, 6″

8 Towel clip, piercing, (4) 3 1/2″ and (4) 5″
8 Towel clip, nonpiercing, (4) 3 1/2″ and (4) 5″
4 Pennington, 5 1/2″
2 Mayo Hager needle holders, 6″

Suction Tubes or Tips

1 Yankauer suction (suction tube and tip; 2 pieces) 10 3/8″

Miscellaneous

2 Knife handles, #3
1 Probe, malleable
1 Grooved director
1 Crypt hook

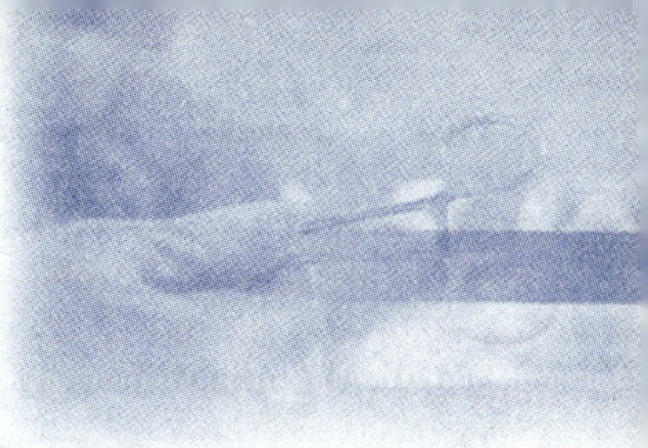

CHAPTER 33
Gynecologic and Obstetric Trays

Dilatation and Curettage (D&C) Tray

Retractors
1 Auvard vaginal speculum, weighted

Forceps
1 Tissue without teeth, 10″
1 Tissue with teeth, 10″

Scissors
1 Straight Mayo, 6 1/4″

Clamps
1 Straight Crile, 5 1/2″
2 Towel clips, piercing, 5 1/2″
2 Towel clips, nonpiercing, 5 1/2″
1 Needle holder, 8″

Tenaculums
1 Schroeder, single-toothed, 9 1/2″
1 Schroeder, double-toothed, 9 1/2″
1 Jacobs, 8 1/4″

Dilators
8 Hegar (#3 to #4 through #17 to #18)
1 Goodell, 13″

Curettes
3 Sims, sharp (1 small, 1 medium, 1 large)
1 Heaney endometrial, 9 1/2″
1 Kevorkian, sharp, 13″
1 Thomas blunt, medium, 11″

Miscellaneous
1 Biopsy punch
1 Randall stone forceps (1/4 curved length), 9 1/4″
1 Bozeman packing forceps, 10″

2 Sponge forceps, (1) straight and (1) curved, 10″
1 Uterine sound, 10 1/2″

Cervical Conization Tray

Additional Trays
D&C Tray

Retractors
2 Heaney, 8 1/2″

Forceps
1 Tissue without teeth, 10″
2 Tissue with teeth, (1) 5 1/2″ and (1) 10″

Scissors
1 Straight Mayo, 6 1/4″
1 Curved Mayo, 6 1/4″
1 Metzenbaum, 7″

Clamps
6 Curved Crile, 5 1/2″
2 Straight Kocher, 6 1/4″
6 Allis, 6″
2 Towel clips, 5 1/2″
1 Needle holder, 7″

Miscellaneous
2 Knife handles, (1) #3 and (1) #7

Hysteroscopy Tray

Additional Trays
D&C Tray

Limited Procedures Tray

Extras
Cervical cannula
Rubber caps, nipples (fine, glass, and medium)
Universal stopcock
Gynecological bridge
Hamou Hysteromat II tubing and tip
Essure device kit, optional

Scopes

Flexible fiber-optic hysteroscope, diagnostic, 0° angle lens, 15° angle lens, 30° angle lens, and panoview × 25 mm, with sheath and cord
Operating fiber-optic rigid hysteroscope, 10° and 45°, and cord
Continuous-flow sheath and rotating continuous-flow sheath (for operating)
Iglesias resectoscope and cord
Camera, coupler, and cord or built-in camera chip

Endoscopic

Probes
Electrosurgical suction-irrigator-aspirator dissector
Cannulas
Electrosurgical scissors
2 Babcock forceps
Electrosurgical biopsy forceps
Graspers
Intrauterine device grasper
Gynecologic and micro scissors
Electrosurgical tips
Loops
Cup forceps (assorted)
Alligator forceps
Punch forceps
Kleppinger bipolar forceps

Pelvic Laparoscopy Tray

Additional Trays

Limited Procedures Tray

D&C Tray

Retractors

Uterine retractors and uterine manipulator

Extras

Verres needle (disposable, if available)
Trocars, obturators, and sheathes (5 mm, 10 or 11 mm, 12 mm, or Hasson)
Reducers, nipples, and connectors

Scopes

Fiber-optic rigid laparoscope, 30° angle lens, and sheath, camera chip, and cord; 0° scope, optional
Camera and coupler (if not included in scope)

Endoscopic

2 Babcock forceps,
3 Scissors (curved, hook, straight)
Right-angle dissector
Curved DeBakey dissector
Graspers (straight and curved)
Kelly clamps
Multifire ligating clip applier
Dissecting forceps
Straight, right-angle, and hook irrigation-suction-electrosurgical dissectors
Beaver knife handle
Irrigator-aspirator
Aspiration needles
Biopsy forceps
Fimbrial grasper
Pancake grasper
Kleppinger bipolar forceps
Alligator forceps
Loop ligation sutures, e.g., Endoloop™ (with introducer sleeve), disposable

Optional

Argon beam coagulator, electrode and cord, optional
Hydrodissector hand piece with cannula and cord

Vaginal Hysterectomy Tray

Retractors

1 Auvard vaginal speculum, weighted
1 Glenner, weighted, 10 1/2″ with blade 5″ × 1″
1 Deaver, narrow
2 Jackson, short, 6 3/4″ × 8 1/2″
2 Heaney, 1″ × 6 1/2″

Forceps

3 Tissue without teeth, (1) 6″; (1) 8 1/2″; and (1) 10″
3 Tissue with teeth, (1) 6″; (1) 8 1/2″; and (1) 10″
1 Russian, 7″

Scissors

1 Curved Mayo, 6 1/2″
2 Straight Mayo, 6 1/2″
2 Metzenbaum, 7″ and 9″

Clamps

8 Straight Crile, $5^1/_2''$
8 Curved Crile, $5^1/_2''$
4 Allis, 6″
8 Allis Adair, $6^1/_2''$
6 Curved Pean, $6^1/_4''$
12 Straight Kocher (Ochsner), (8) $6^1/_4''$ and (4) 8″
4 Curved Kocher (Ochsner), 8″
4 Heaney, straight, $8^1/_4''$
4 Heaney, curved, $8^1/_4''$
4 Heaney Balentine, $8^1/_2''$
2 Babcock, 10″
2 Tonsils, $7^1/_4''$
2 Lahey, 8″
4 Foerster sponge forceps, 10″
4 Needle holder, (2) 6″ and (2) 7″
2 Heaney needle holder, $8^1/_2''$
4 Towel clip, piercing, $5^1/_2''$
2 Towel clip, nonpiercing, $5^1/_2''$

Suctions

1 Yankauer, 10″
1 Poole, $8^1/_4''$

Tenaculums

1 Schroeder single-toothed, $9^1/_2''$
1 Schroeder double-toothed, $9^1/_2''$
1 Jacobs, $8^1/_4''$

Miscellaneous

1 Bozeman packing/dressing forceps, $10^1/_2''$
1 Uterine sound, $13^1/_2''$
3 Knife handles, (1) #3; (1) #3L 10″; and (1) #7

Abdominal Hysterectomy Tray

Additional Trays

Major Procedures Tray

Retractors

O'Sullivan O'Connor with 3 blades

Forceps

1 Tissue with teeth, 10″

Scissors

1 Curved Mayo, 6 1/4″
1 Curved Jorgenson, 9″

Clamps

2 Lahey, 8″
5 Heaney, 8 1/4″
6 Long straight Kocher/Ochsner, 8″
6 Long, curved Kocher/Ochsner, 8″
4 Heaney Balentine, 8 1/2″
2 Long Babcocks, 9″
1 Somer, 9″
6 Curved Phaneuf, 8 1/4″
6 Long Allis, 10″
2 Heaney needle holders, 8 1/2″

Tenacula

1 Jacobs, 8 1/2″
1 Schroeder single-toothed, 9 1/2″
1 Schroeder double-toothed, 9 1/2″

Miscellaneous

1 Knife handle, #3L

Laparoscopic Hysterectomy

Additional Trays

Limited Procedures Tray
D&C Tray
Vaginal Hysterectomy Tray (for Laparoscopic-Assisted)

Retractors, Vaginal

Uterine manipulator, e.g., Kronner Manipujector or Valtchev uterine mobilizer, with multiple tips

Scopes

Fiber-optic rigid laparoscope, 0° angle lens, with sheath, camera chip, and cord
Camera and coupler (if not contained in scope)

Endoscopic

Electrosurgical suction-irrigator-dissector
Electrosurgical scissors
Multifire clip appliers with medium and large clips

Babcock forceps
Scissors (blunt and sharp)
Serrated-edged macro-morcellator (SEMM) with drill tip and cord

Special Notes

- Loop ligation sutures, e.g., Endoloop (with introducer sleeve, intracorporeal available for ties), disposable, optional
- Endopouch™, disposable
- Endoport™ (laparoscopic-assisted), disposable, optional

Laparoscopic Tubal Sterilization

Additional Trays

Limited Procedures Tray
D&C Tray

Extras

Verres needle (disposable), available
Trocar, sheath, and obturator (5 mm, 10 or 11 mm, 12 mm, or Hasson)
Reducers and connectors
Hamou Hysteromat II tubing and tip

Scopes

Fiber-optic laparoscope, 30° angle lens or 0°angle lens, with sheath, camera chip, and cord or camera (separate), cord, and coupler

Endoscopic

Electrosurgical dissector
2 Babcock forceps
Scissors (blunt, fine, and sharp)
Electrosurgical suction-irrigator
Multifire ligating clip applier with clips
Kleppinger bipolar forceps and cord
3 Graspers (with teeth, without teeth, and fine)

Clips or Banding

Hulka or Hulka-Clemens (plastic clip with stainless-steel hinge and gold-plated spring), small or medium, and applicator
Field sheath clip or Filschie clip (titanium clip with silicone rubber lining) and applicator
Silicone banding

Optional

Laser (CO_2 or KTP) hand piece with fiber tip and cord
Argon beam coagulator hand piece with electrode and cord

Cesarean Section Tray

Retractors

2 Richardson (1 small, 1 medium)
1 Deaver, extra wide, 3″
2 Goelet, 7 1/2″
1 DeLee universal, 9 1/2″

Forceps

2 Tissue with teeth, 6″
2 Adson with teeth, 4 3/4″
1 Russian, 7″

Scissors

2 Straight Mayo, 6 1/4″
1 Curved Mayo, 6 1/4″
1 Metzenbaum, 7″
1 Umbilical, 4″
1 Lister bandage, 3 1/2″, 4 1/2″, 5 1/2″, 7 1/2″, 8″

Clamps

4 Towel clips, piercing, 5 1/2″
4 Towel clips, nonpiercing, 5 1/2″
12 Curved Crile, 5 1/2″
4 Straight Crile, 5 1/2″
2 Babcock, 6″
6 Allis, 6″
6 Straight Kocher, 6 1/4″
6 Pean/Mayo Pean, 6 1/4″
4 Foerster sponge forceps, 7″
4 Pennington, 7 1/2″
4 Needle holder, (2) 7″ and (2) 8″

Suction Tubes or Tips

1 Poole (suction and sheath; 2 pieces), 8 1/4″
1 Yankauer, 10″

Miscellaneous

3 Knife handles, (2) #3 and (1) #4
1 Somer uterine elevator, 9″
1 Simpson obstetrical delivery forceps, 12″

CHAPTER 34
Genitourinary Trays

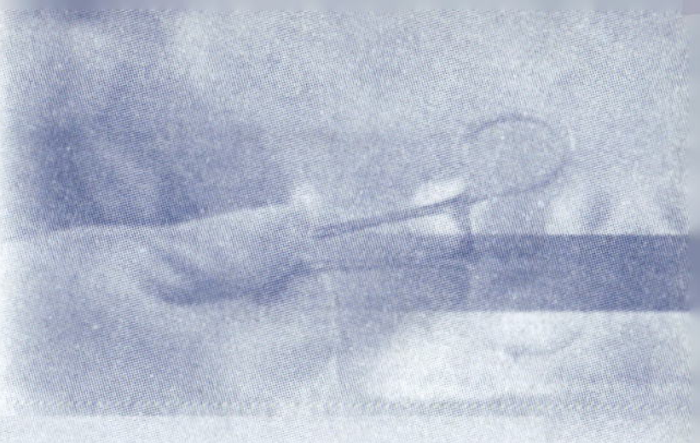

Hypospadias Tray

Additional Trays
Vasectomy Tray

Forceps
2 Castroviejo, 0.3-mm tip
1 Bishop Harmon, 1 × 2 T, 0.6 mm
1 Bipolar, straight

Scissors
1 Wescott, 4 1/4″

Miscellaneous
1 Castroviejo needle holder, straight, 5″
1 Castroviejo caliper
1 Beaver knife handle

Vasectomy Tray

Retractors
2 Joseph skin hook, 6″
2 Senn, sharp, 6″

Forceps
1 Tissue without teeth, 6″
1 Tissue with teeth, 6″
1 Adson with teeth, 4 3/4″

Scissors
1 Metzenbaum, 5 1/4″
1 Straight Mayo, 6 1/4″

Clamps
2 Curved Crile, 5 1/2″
2 Curved mosquito, 5 1/4″
2 Allis, 6″
2 Towel clips, piercing, 5″
2 Towel clips, nonpiercing, 5″
1 Needle holder, 6″

Miscellaneous

1 Knife handle, #3

Vasovasostomy Tray

Additional Trays

Vasectomy Tray

Forceps

2 Jeweler, bipolar
1 Tying, straight, 4″
6 Nerve holding (2, 2.5, 3, 4, 5, and 6 mm)
2 Tissue, straight, 6″

Scissors

1 Adventitia, straight
1 Castroviejo, micro, 4″

Clamps

2 Vasoepididymostomy approximator for anastomosis, (1) end-to-side and (1) end-to-end
Microspike™ (microvascular) approximator clamp
2 Micro vas clamps

Miscellaneous

2 Vessel dilators (10° angulated tip, 0.2 mm)
1 Dennis blade holder, 4 1/2″
2 Needle holders, smooth

Cystoscopy Tray

Forceps

3 Biopsy

Scissors

1 Straight Mayo, 6 1/4″

Clamps

1 Towel clip, piercing, 3 1/2″
2 Towel clip, nonpiercing, 3 1/2″
2 Pean/Mayo Pean, 6 1/4″
2 Crile, (1) straight and (1) curved, 5 1/2″

Scopes and Extras

Bridges (double-catheterizing) cystoscope
Alberrán (double-catheterizing) cystoscope

Operating (Alberrán) cystoscope
Obturator (light) cord/cable and 2 short telescope bridges
1 Cystourethroscope, rigid, (e.g., 30° angle lens, 70° angle lens, and 0° angle lens)
Telescope
1 Stationary catheter deflector mechanism with 2 instrument channels
Obturator (for each cystoscope)
1 Double-catheterizing fin
Working element (biopsy forceps)
Bugbee electrode
Electrosurgical cord
1 Biopsy forceps
1 cystourethroscope sheath
Obturator
Visual obturator
Bridge (telescope adapting)
Urethrotome (e.g., Otis) with 2 blades and cord
1 Iglesias resectoscope with sheath (insulated)
Obturator
2 urethrotome blades and cord

Optional

1 Hendrickson-Bigelow lithotrite
1 Camera and cable/cord

Miscellaneous

1 Drainage pan or receptor kit
Sterile screen unless cystoscopy drape used (sterile screen incorporated)
1 Cone-shaped syringe (female)
1 Acorn adaptor on disposable syringe (male)
1 Cunningham penile clamp
1 Water connector
1 Collar
8 Plastic adaptors or nipples
2 Glass syringes, (1) 10 ml, (1) 20 ml
2 Medicine cups
1 Ellik evacuator
5 Van Buren urethral bougies or sounds, 8 to 16Fr (male)

Special Notes

- **Cystoscopy** utilizes a cone-shaped syringe (female), acorn adaptor on disposable syringe (male) penile clamp, 2 medicine cups, 10- and 20-ml glass syringes, a rigid cystourethroscope (e.g., 30°, 70°, and/or 0° sheath), obturator, visual obturator, short bridge, water connector, Luer-Lok stopcock, nipples, cord, calibrated container, and test tubes with screw tops.

- The additional instruments are chosen according to the procedure to be performed, e.g., urethral dilation, bladder biopsy, ureteral catheterizations, lysis of urethral stricture, etc.

Prostatectomy Instrument Trays

Abdominal and Perineal Additional Trays

Major Procedures Tray
Long Instruments Tray

Retractors

1 Judd-Masson, total opening, 5″

Clamps

6 Allis, 10″
6 Babcock, 10″
4 Lahey, 8″
1 Stratte needle holder, 9″
2 Heaney needle holder, 8 1/2″

Forceps

Prostatic lobe

Scissors

1 Metzenbaum, 9″
1 Jorgenson, 9″

Miscellaneous

1 Prostatic enucleator
8 Ligating clip appliers, e.g., Hemoclip™ appliers (e.g., 4 regular length, 2 medium, 2 large or 4 long, 2 medium, and 2 large)
1 Boomerang suture passer
Otis prostatic urethral sounds

For Suprapubic, Add
Lowsley tractors, straight and curved
Jacobsen bladder retractor (3 or 4 blades)

For Retropubic, Add
Millin-Bacon retropubic prostatic bladder retractor (2 side blades, 1 center blade), crossbar, 18 1/2″

For Perineal, Add

Retractors

Retractors Lateral, anterior, bifurcated

Denis-Browne perineal self-retaining and/or Turner-Warrick bladder neck spreader

Roux, 6″

Young, bulb, 8 1/2″, bifid, 8″

For Transurethral Resection of the Prostate, Add

Scopes

Brown-Berger rigid fiber-optic cystoscope

McCarthy panendoscope or Wappler cystourethroscope

Lateral and foroblique fiber-optic telescopes (interchangeable with all sheaths) and (power) cords

Iglesias, Nesbit, Baumrucher, and Stern-McCarthy resectoscopes (resecting sheath, insulated resecting sheath), Timberlake obturator, deflecting obturator, Bakelite® oculars, working element, electrodes (sharp, ball, loop and roller ball electrodes) and cord

Miscellaneous

Sterile screen unless cystoscopy drape used (sterile screen incorporated)

Stopcock, hemostat, and catheter nipples

Penile clamp (used following local anesthetic instillation in males)

Urethral sounds, 8 to 40Fr

Otis urethrotome

Bridge (e.g., short, Alberrán)

For Bladder Fulguration, Add

Scopes

McCarthy, Nesbit, Iglesias bipolar resectoscopes with sheath, obturator, and cutting loops

Foroblique and lateral telescopes and (fiber-optic light) cords with rotating contact

Miscellaneous

Urethral dilators

Van Buren or Otis urethral sounds, 8 to 16Fr

Hemostat and stopcock

Toomey syringe

Ellik evacuator

Bridge, 1, Alberrán, short

1 Double-catheterizing bridge

Rubber tips, electrosurgical cord, 30-ml glass syringe

Laparoscopic Approach

Additional Trays

Limited Procedures Tray

Extras

Verres needle (disposable, when available)
Trocars, obturators, and sheathes (5, 10, 11, or 12 mm)
Connectors and reducers
Endopouch™ (disposable)

Scopes

Fiber-optic laparoscopes, 30° with sheath, built-in camera, and cord (type most often used), and 0° scope, and cord, optional

Endoscopic

2 Babcock forceps
Scissors (curved, hook, straight)
Electrosurgical Metzenbaum scissors
Right angle dissector
Kelly clamps
Straight, right angle, and hook electrosurgical suction-irrigators-dissectors
Forceps (fine, blunt, bipolar)
Locking grasping forceps
Suture loop (e.g., Endoloop™) with intracorporeal introducer sleeve, Beaver knife handle
Ligating clip applier with clips
Suturing device with curved needle

Miscellaneous

Rectal bougie
Urethral sounds

Robotic

DaVinci robot 4 articulated arms with seven degrees of freedom and 90° articulation
Aesop robotic arm, voice-activated and magnetically connected, holds laparoscope with camera chip

Special Note

- In the laparoscopic prostatectomy, the flexible fiber-optic cystoscope is employed for patients unable to tolerate the lithotomy position.

Kidney, Ureter, Bladder Tray

Additional Trays

Major Procedures Tray
Long Instruments Tray

Retractors

1 Judd-Masson, total opening, 5″
2 Cushing vein, 9″
5 Gil-Vernet renal sinus, 91/2″ × 9, 11, 13, 15, 18 mm

Clamps

4 Babcock, 9″
2 Herrick kidney pedicle, 91/2″
2 Walther kidney pedicle, 93/4″
1 Kaufman kidney clamp, 16″
1 Mayo ureter isolation forceps9″
2 Hendren ureteral, 8″
2 Pean vessel, 10″
2 Mayo-Guyon pedicle, 91/4″
2 Millin Campbell ureteral forceps, 91/2″

Forceps

4 Randall Stone (1/4 curved length through 1 full curved length)
1 Singley fenestrated tissue, 93/4″

Scissors

1 Metzenbaum, 9″, 11″
1 Nelson, 9″
1 Potts 45°, 8″
1 Jorgenson, 81/2″

Suction Tubes or Tips

1 Andrews-Pynchon (suction tube and tip; 2 pieces), 91/2″

Miscellaneous

1 Gluck rib cutter, 8″
2 Alexander's periosteotome, 6″ and 8″
2 Doyen rib strippers, right 7″ and left 7″
2 Doyen costal elevator (1 medium, 1 large)
2 Greenwald dilators, (1) 24Fr and (1) 28Fr

CHAPTER 35
Thoracic Instrument Trays

Bronchoscopy Instrument Trays

Rigid Bronchoscopy

Rigid bronchoscope(s), child sizes 3 to 5 mm × 15 to 30 cm and adult sizes 5 mm to 9 mm × 25 to 40 cm with fiber-optic light carrier(s) and fiber-optic cord(s)
Endotracheal adaptor (for bronchoscope)
Electrosurgical suction cannula(s), range 3 to 5 mm × 20 to 60 cm
Electrosurgical cord(s)/cable(s)
Cytology brush
2 Bronchoscopy sponge carriers
Biopsy forceps, e.g., Takahashi handle (nondisposable) with 1 curved and 5 straight cannulas, (disposable)
Nagashima universal forceps tips, variety
Hot (electrosurgical) biopsy forceps
Grasping forceps (Jackson serrated, side grasping, fenestrated)
Clerf-Arrowsmith safety-pin closer
Gordon bead grasper

Flexible Bronchoscopy

Flexible fiber-optic bronchoscopes, (outer diameter, 3.7 to 6.0 mm; inner channel, 1.3 to 2.8 mm; length, 55 to 70 cm), light carrier, and cord
Flexible video camera (e.g., camera chip) in fiber-optic bronchoscope and cord
Camera and coupler (if not contained in scope)
Endotracheal adaptor
Cytology brush
Electrosurgical suction/aspiration cannula, tubing, electrosurgical
Biopsy forceps, variety of tips
1 Alignment wrench

Miscellaneous

Foreign body retrieval snares and baskets
Laser hand piece and fiber tip

Mediastinoscopy Tray

Retractors

2 Senn, sharp, 6″
2 Army-Navy/USA, 8$^5/_{16}$
2 Carlens introducer
1 Weitlaner, blunt, 5½″

Forceps

1 Tissue with teeth, 6″
1 Adson with teeth, 4″
1 DeBakey, 6″

Scissors

1 Straight Mayo, 6¼″
1 Metzenbaum, 7″

Clamps

1 Straight Crile, 5½″
4 Curved Crile, 5½″
4 Towel clips, piercing, 5″
2 Towel clips, nonpiercing, 5″
2 Ryder needle holders, fine, 6″

Suction Tubes or Tips

1 Frazier #10
2 Electrosurgical suctions with cord and tubing

Scopes

1 Rigid fiber-optic Carlens mediastinoscope, 13 cm and 17 cm with introducer, fiber-optic light carrier, and cord

Miscellaneous

3 Biopsy forceps (up, down, straight)
1 Circular biopsy forceps
1 Grasping forceps
1 Jackson forceps
1 Electrosurgical cord
2 Stamey needles (aspiration needles)
1 Knife handle, #3

1 Aspirating tube
1 Syringe, Luer Lok, 5 ml

Thoracoscopy or Video-Assisted Thoracic Surgery Tray

Additional Trays

Major Procedures Tray (available)
Thoracotomy Tray (available)
Vascular Procedures Tray (available)

Retractors

1 Modified small Finochietto rib (long blades) or infant Finochietto rib spreader, blades 5.4 cm, length 10.2 cm
1 Weitlaner, blunt and sharp, 11 cm and 16 cm

Extras

Trocars (Thoracoports), (2) 5 mm, (2) 10.5 mm, (1) 12 mm, and (1) 15 mm (disposable), single use, optional
Reducers

Scopes

1 Fiber-optic rigid thoracoscope 0° angle lens, 30° angle lens, and 30° angle lens, rotating, with cord
1 Fiber-optic flexible videothoracoscope with camera chip and cord
Camera, coupler, and cord (if not contained in scope)

Endoscopic

Electrosurgical suction, tubing, and cord, or electrosurgical irrigator-aspirator (orthopedic type)
Fan, vein, and/or Naticoke retractor
Graspers (Allis, Babcock, tonsil, right-angle, modified ring, Duval, and Pennington), dissectors, and scissors
Harper clamp and suture loop (e.g., Endoloop™) with intracorporeal introducer sleeve
Thoracoscopy biopsy forceps or mediastinoscopy biopsy forceps (preferred)
DeBakey forceps
Long curettes
Ligating clip applier with clip cartridge
Stapler, 30 and 60 mm × 2, 2.5, 3.5, and 4.8 mm, e.g., gastrointestinal anastomosis or transverse anastomosis articulated, rotating

Miscellaneous

Argon beam coagulator (ABC) 80 W hand piece with electrode, optional

ABC Bend-a-Beam® malleable hand piece with electrode (disposable), optional

Laser (15 W Nd:YAG) hand piece with fiber, optional

Special Note

- A gastroscope may be substituted for a thoracoscope.

Thoracotomy Tray

Additional Trays

Major Instruments Tray

Long Instruments Tray

Retractors

1 Finochietto rib (with 6 blades), adult size, total opening 10″

1 Finochietto rib (with 4 blades), child size, total opening 6″

Forceps

1 Russian, 10″

6 DeBakey, (2) 6″, (2) 8″, and (2) 9½″

Scissors

1 Long Metzenbaum, 11″

1 Nelson, 8″

Clamps

2 Duval-Crile lung, 19.7 cm with tip 1.3 cm

4 Long right-angle/Mixter, (1) 9″ and (1) 11″

2 Long tonsil/Schnidt, 10″

4 Babcock, 10″

1 Crile Wood needle holder, fine, 10½″

Rib Elevators

2 Doyen elevator and raspatory (stripper), 1 left, 7″ and 1 right, 7″

1 Matson stripper and elevator, 8⅝″

2 Alexander costal periosteotomes, 6″ and 8″

2 Langenbeck periosteal elevator, narrow, ¼″ × 8″ and wide, 11/16″ × 7½″

1 Alexander rib raspatory, double-ended, 8½″

Rib Shears

1 Bethune, 14″
2 Gluck, 8″
1 Sauerbruck double-action rongeur, 10½″
1 Stille, 10″

Miscellaneous

2 Bailey rib approximator (contractor), 6¾″ and 7¾″
1 Lebsche knife, 10″
1 Bone mallet

Pacemaker Tray

Retractors

2 Senn, blunt, 6″
2 Weitlaner, sharp, 5½″ and 7½″
2 Rake, blunt (4 prong), 7″
2 Army-Navy/USA, 8 5/16″

Forceps

1 Tissue without teeth, 6″
1 Tissue with teeth, 6″
1 Adson without teeth, 4¾″
2 Adson with teeth, 4¾″
2 DeBakey, 6″

Scissors

1 Metzenbaum, 7″
1 Straight Mayo, 6¼″
1 Stevens tenotomy, 4½″
1 Curved iris, 4″
1 Straight iris, 4″
1 Potts with 45° angle tip, 5½″

Clamps

2 Right-angle, 8″
2 Tonsil (Schnidt), 7¼″
8 Curved Crile, 5½″
6 Curved mosquito, 5¼″
2 DeBakey, multipurpose, 6″, (1) 30° and (1) 60°
1 Mayo-Hegar needle holder, heavy, 6″
1 Ryder needle holder, fine, 6″

4 Towel clip, piercing, 5″
2 Towel clip, nonpiercing, 5″
2 Forester sponge forceps, 10″

Suction Tubes or Tips

1 Frazier, #10
1 Andrews, $9^1/_2$″

Miscellaneous

2 Knife handles, #3
1 Medicine cup
1 Crawford-Cooley tunneling instrument, 18″
2 Modified ring forceps (limited thoracotomy)

CHAPTER 36
Cardiovascular Procedures Instrument Trays

Abdominal and Thoracic Vascular Procedures Tray

Additional Trays

Major Procedures Tray
Long Instruments Tray
Thoracotomy Tray, optional

Retractors

2 Harrington, 12½″ with 2½″ blades
Balfour self-retaining retractor set (with 2 central blades, regular and deep, and 2 pairs of fenestrated side blades, regular and deep)
Bookwalter, large, self-retaining retractor set

Forceps

1 Tissue/plain/smooth/dressing (without teeth), 6″
2 Tissue with teeth, 6″
2 Russian, 7″, 10″
1 Adson without teeth, 4¾″
2 Adson with teeth, 4¾″
1 Adson-Brown, 5″
6 DeBakey, (2) 6″, (2) 8″, and (2) 9½″
2 Gerald forceps, smooth, 7″

Scissors

2 Potts-Smith, (1) 7¼″ × 25° angle tip and (1) 7½″ × 45° angle tip
1 Long Metzenbaum, 9″

Clamps

4 Bridge/tonsil, curved, 11″
2 DeBakey-Mixter/right-angle, 11″
8 Ligating clip appliers, medium and long, with 2 small and 2 medium clip cartridges

Vascular Clamps

2 DeBakey multipurpose, (1) 9¾″ and (1) 12″
1 DeBakey curved aorta aneurysm, 11¼″

5 DeBakey tangential occlusion clamps (7½″, 9¾″, 10″, 10¼″, 10½″)
1 Hufnagel ascending aorta
2 Angled DeBakey, 60° × 9⅝″ and 90° × 10″
4 Satinsky, 10¾″
1 DeBakey Aorta, 10½″
1 Medium curved Crawford auricle, 9¼″
1 Glover coarctation, straight, 8¾″
1 Glover coarctation, angled, 8¾″
1 Glover patent ductus, straight, 8″
1 Glover patent ductus, angled, 8″
1 Straight Glover, 6¾″
2 Curved Glovers, (1) 6¾″ and (1) 8¼″
1 Cooley multipurpose, angled, 6¼″
2 Cooley multipurpose, straight, 7″
1 Curved Cooley, pediatric, 6¾″
6 Cardiovascular needle holders, (2) 7″, (2) 8″, and (2) 9″
6 DeBakey needle holders, (2) 7¾″, (2) 9½″, and (2) 12″
4 Glover bulldog, 2″, 2 straight and 2 curved
4 DeBakey cross-action bulldog, 2½″, 2 straight, 2 curved
4 Johns Hopkins bulldog (mini), 1½″, 2 straight, 2 curved
Ligating clips

Miscellaneous

Doppler probe and cord, optional
Venting needle, 18 gauge

Arteriovenous (A-V) and Carotid Artery (CA) Shunt Instrument Tray

Additional Trays

Limited Procedures Tray

Retractors

2 Senn, blunt, 6″
2 Rake, blunt (4 prong), 7″
2 Cushing vein, 8″
1 Weitlaner, straight, blunt, 5″
1 Weitlaner, curved, blunt, 5″
2 Alm, blunt, 3⅞″ and 4″

Forceps

1 Tissue without teeth, 5½″
2 Adson, 1 without teeth, 1 with teeth, 4¾″

1 Adson, without teeth, 4¾
2 DeBakey, 6″
2 Gerald, with teeth and without teeth, 7″

Scissors

1 Straight Mayo, 6¼″
2 Metzenbaum, 5″, 1 curved, 1 straight
2 Castroviejo, 1 straight, 3½″, 1 curved, 3¾″
2 Potts, 1 short, 7½″ and 1 long blade, 9″

Clamps

2 Right-angle (Mixter), 5¼″, 7″
2 Needle holders, 5½″

Vascular Clamps

2 DeBakey multipurpose, 5½″
4 DeBakey cross-action bulldog, 1¼″, 2 straight, 2 curved, 2½″, 2 straight, 2 curved
4 Glover bulldog, 2″, 2 straight, 2 curved
4 Johns Hopkins bulldog (mini), 1½″, 2 straight, 2 curved
2 Sponge forceps, 7″
2 Shunt clamps
2 Vascular needle holders, 7″
4 Towel clips, piercing, 3½″ and 5″
2 Towel clips, nonpiercing, 3½″ and 5″

Suction Tubes or Tips

1 Frazier, #8
1 Yankauer, 8″

Miscellaneous

1 Probe, malleable (A-V)
2 Shunt connectors (A-V)
1 Curette (A-V)
1 Freer elevator (A-V)
2 Olive-tip heparin needles (A-V)
Shunt PTFE cannulas (A-V)
Doppler probe and cord, optional
Rumel tourniquet, optional (C-A)
High-speed drill, e.g., Hall oscillating with endarterectomy valvutome

Microscopic

Micro tissue forceps (with teeth)
Curved smooth forceps (2), 6″

Harms curved tying forceps, 9 cm, straight and curved
Dujovny micro-dissector, 4¼″
Castroviejo needle holder, 4¾″, optional

Peripheral Vascular Procedures Tray

Retractors

2 Army-Navy/(USA), 8½″
2 Goelet, 7½″
2 Senn, blunt, 6″
2 Rake, blunt (4 prong), 8½″
2 Cushing vein, 9″
1 Weitlaner, straight, blunt, 5″
1 Weitlaner, curved, blunt, 5″
1 Gelpi, 4½″, 5½″, 7½″, 10½″

Forceps

1 Tissue without teeth, 6″
2 Tissue with teeth, 6″
1 Russian, 6″
1 Adson without teeth, 4¾″
2 Adson with teeth, 4¾″
1 Adson-Brown
2 DeBakey, 6″
2 Micro

Scissors

2 Straight Mayo, 6¼″
2 Curved Metzenbaum, (1) 5″ and (1) 7″
1 Straight Metzenbaum, 5″
2 Potts-Smith, 7¼″, 25°, 7½″, 45°

Clamps

6 Straight mosquito, 5¼″, 2 fine, 4 regular
6 Curved mosquito, 5¼″, 2 fine, 4 regular
12 Crile, 6 straight, 5½″, 6 curved, 5½″
4 Curved Pean, 6¼″
2 Tonsil (Schnidt), 7½″
5 Right angle (Mixter), (2) 5¼″, (2) 7″ fine, and (1) long jaw
10 Towel clips, piercing, 3½″
2 Towel clips, nonpiercing, 5″
4 Ryder needle holders, (2) 5″ and (2) 7½″
1 Castroviejo needle holder, 5⅛″

Vascular Clamps

2 DeBakey multipurpose, 5½″
4 Glover bulldog, 2″, 2 straight, 2 curved
8 DeBakey cross-action bulldog, 1¼″, 2 straight, 2 curved, 2½″, 2 straight, 2 curved
4 Johns Hopkins bulldog (mini), 1½″, 2 straight, 2 curved
2 Carotid shunt tube clamps, smooth
2 Carotid micro shunt tube clamps, smooth

Suction Tubes or Tips

Cell Saver® suction tube
1 Andrews, 9½″
1 Yankauer, 10⅜

Miscellaneous

1 Probe (malleable)
2 Knife handles, #3
2 Micro dissectors, 4¼″
1 Doppler probe
1 Valvutome, e.g., Mills, optional

Cardiac Procedures Instrument Trays

Open Heart Basic Instrument Tray

Retractors

1 Sternal retractor with attachments (some disposable)
1 Loc Ness™ epicardial tissue stabilizer with articulated arm, optional
2 Himmelstein sternal retractor (with hinged arms), optional
2 Inge lamina spreader, 1 small, 6″ and 1 large, 10″
1 Ribbon (malleable), narrow

Forceps

4 Tissue with teeth, 5½″
1 Tissue without teeth, 5½″
2 Cushing vein forceps, 1 with teeth, 1 without teeth
2 Adson with teeth, 4¾″
1 Adson without teeth, 4¾″
2 Russian, 6″, 10″
10 DeBakey, (1) 7¾″, (8) 9½″, and (1) 12″

Scissors

2 Straight Mayo, 6¼″
1 Curved Mayo, 6¼″
3 Metzenbaum, 7″, 8″, 9″
3 Potts, (1) 25°, (1) 45°, and (1) 60°
2 Tenotomy, 3½″ and 4½″
1 Cooley, 7¼″
1 Wire cutter, 4½″

Clamps

12 Mosquito, 5¼″, 6 curved, 6 straight
2 Jacobson mosquito, 5″ and 7″
8 Curved Crile, 5½″
6 Straight Crile, 6½″
2 Curved Pean, 6¼″
2 Herrick kidney, 9½″
2 Straight Kocher (Ochsner), 8″
2 Mixter (right-angle), 8″
2 Tonsil (Schnidt), 7½″

Vascular Clamps

3 Derra (1 small, 1 medium, 1 large)
2 DeBakey coarctation, 8½″
2 Crawford aortic aneurysm, 9½″
2 DeBakey tangential occlusion, (1) 9¾″ and (1) 10″
2 Satinsky, 9½″
1 DeBakey patent ductus, straight, 7½″
1 DeBakey patent ductus, angular, 7½″
8 Vascular needle holders
2 Sternal needle holders, 7″
2 Sponge forceps, 10″
18 Towel clips, piercing, 5½″
6 Towel clips, nonpiercing
1 Wire holder-twister, 7″

Suction Tubes or Tips

2 Yankauer, 8″, 10″
1 Cell Saver (Harmonics®) suction tube

Miscellaneous

5 Knife handles, (2) #3, (2) #7, and (1) #3L
2 Beaver knife handles, 4″
1 Lebsche sternal knife, 10″
1 Mallet
2 Awls
Oscillating saw, sternal, e.g., Sarns, Hall

1 Toomey adaptor
3 Olive-tipped heparin needles
1 Pliers, needle nose, 6½″
6 DeBakey bulldog clamps, 2 curved, 2 straight
3 Partial-occlusion tube clamps
6 Tubes, occluding
Line tubing holder
Phrenic nerve pad
Ligating clip appliers, e.g., Hemoclip® appliers (various lengths with clip cartridges small, medium, large)
Epicardial pacemaker leads
Internal defibrillator paddles

Optional

Sternal saw, oscillating, e.g., Sarns™, Stryker®
Laser hand piece and tip, e.g., CO_2 or holmium:YAG
Harmonic scalpel® and ultrasonic tips

For Valves, Add

1 Atrial valve retractor
1 Sculptor annuloplasty ring retractor (mitral valve repair)
1 Chordae tendinae retractor
4 Richardson retractors, (2) 9½″ with ¾″ × 1″ blade and (2) 9½″ with 1″ × 1¼″ blade
2 Cardiac suction tips
4 Allis clamps, (2) 6″ and (2) 10″
4 Babcock clamps, 10″
3 Cardiac curettes, 000 to 0
1 Freer elevator, 8″
1 Smithwick hook, 8¼″
2 Graham blunt nerve hooks, 6½″
1 Dental mirror, sizes 1 to 6
2 Pituitary rongeurs, 6″, 7″, 8″ with jaw bite 1½ mm and 2 mm

For Coronary Artery Bypass Graft (CABG), Add

1 Shaw internal mammary artery retractor
1 Internal mammary artery scissors
9 Coronary artery probes (vessel dilators) (1, 1.25, 1.5, 1.75, 2, 2.25, 2.5, 2.75, 3 mm)
1 Parsonette retractor
1 Ribbon retractor, small
1 Aortic punch set (3.0 to 3.6, 4.0 to 4.4, 4.8 to 5.2, 5.6 to 6.3)
3 Castroviejo needle holders (1 straight, 1 curved, 1 long)
2 Gerald forceps, 7″
1 Ruler or caliper

1 Titanium bipolar bayonet forceps, fine, 8¾″
2 DeBakey forceps, fine, 7¾″ and 9½
2 Selmaning forceps, fine, 6″

CABG Leg Tray, Add

2 Goulet, 7½″
2 Greene, 8¾″
1 Richardson, small
2 Army-Navy/(USA)
2 Cushing vein, 9″
2 Senn, sharp, 6″
2 Rake (3 prong), sharp, 7¾″
4 Rake (4 prong), 2 sharp, 2 dull, 8″
2 Adson or 2 Weitlaner (medium), self-retaining, straight, 5½″
2 Beaver blade holders
6 Long Kocher (Ochsner) clamps, 9″
1 Valvutome, e.g., Mills
1 Endarterectomy knife
4 DeBakey cross-action bulldog, 2½″, 2 straight, 2 curved
2 Selman short, fine ring forceps, 6″
4 Vascular needle holders
5 Heparin tips, (3) 18 gauge and (2) 23 gauge
6 Towel clips, piercing, 3½″
6 Towel clips, piercing (baby), 3½″

Special Note

- For "off-pump" minimally invasive and endoscopic instrumentation and robotic systems, refer to Chapter 22, Cardiac Surgery, p. 512.

CHAPTER 37

Orthopedic Instruments Trays

Minor Orthopedic Procedures Tray

Retractors

2 Joseph skin hooks, 6″
2 Senn (sharp), 6″
2 Volkmann rake, 2 prong, 8″
2 Weitlaner, sharp, 5½″

Forceps

1 Tissue without teeth, 5½″
1 Tissue with teeth, 5½″
1 Adson without teeth, 4¾″
2 Adson with teeth, 4¾″
1 Adson-Brown, 5″

Scissors

2 Straight Mayo, 6¼″
3 Metzenbaum, (1) 5¼″, (1) 6″, and (1) 7″
1 Stevens tenotomy, 4½″
2 Iris, 4″, (1) curved and (1) straight
1 Wire cutter, 5″
1 Liston bone cutter, 5½″

Clamps

4 Curved mosquito, 5¼″
2 Straight mosquito, 5¼″
4 Curved Crile, 5½″
2 Straight Crile, 5½″
2 Allis, 6″, straight
6 Kocher (Ochsner), (4) 6″ and (2) 10″
2 Needle holders, 6″
1 Scissors needle holder, Olsen Hegar 5½″, 6½″, 7½″
1 Webster needle holder, 5″
8 Towel clips, piercing, (4) 3½″ and (4) 5½″
8 Towel clips, nonpiercing, (4) 3½″ and (4) 5½″

Suction Tubes or Tips

1 Frazier #10

Miscellaneous

2 Knife handles, #3
1 Small rasp, 7″
1 Zaufal-Jansen small double-action rongeur, 6¼″
1 Ruskin small double-action bone cutter, 6″
1 Small mallet, 7¼″ or 7½″
1 Mc Ewen small chisel, 7½″ × ¾″
1 Freer elevator dissector, 8″
1 Malis short blunt nerve hook, 7″
1 Straight Key elevator, ½″ blade
1 Curved Key elevator, ¼″ blade
3 Curettes, 000 to 0
1 Ruler, 6″
2 Tendon passers, e.g., Bunnel malleable, small, 18.5 cm with 5 cm diameter, and large 23 cm with 5 cm diameter
5 Osteotomes, (3) straight 4, 6, and 8 mm, (1) angled 6 mm, and (1) curved 8 mm
Bone tamps, 6″, 2 to 10 mm diameter
1 Awl, 6¼″

Basic Orthopedic Procedures Tray

Retractors

2 Rake (4 prong), sharp, 8″
2 Rake (6 prong), sharp, 6″
2 Weitlaner, sharp, 4″ and 6½″
2 Army-Navy/USA, 8 5/16″

Forceps

2 Tissue with teeth, 5½″
2 Adson with teeth, 4¾″

Scissors

2 Straight Mayo, 6½″
1 Curved Mayo, 6¼″
2 Metzenbaum, (1) 6″ and (1) 7″
1 Bandage, 8″
1 Wire cutter, 5″ × 0.7 mm, 6″ × 1.1 mm, or 7″ 1.6 mm
1 Pin cutter, 9½″ × 3.2 mm

Clamps

2 Curved Pean, 6¼″
2 Kocher-Lovelace, 6″

5 Curved Crile, 5½″
2 Needle holders, 7″
8 Towel clips, piercing, (4) small, 3½″ and (4) large, 5″
8 Towel clips, nonpiercing, (4) small, 3½″ and (4) large, 5″
1 Foerster sponge forceps, 9½″

Suction Tubes or Tips

1 Yankauer, 10⅜″

Miscellaneous

3 Knife handles, (2) #3, (1) #7
2 Pliers, (1 regular, 1 needle nose)
2 Screwdrivers, (1 Phillips, 1 blade)
1 Mallet, 7¼″ or 7½″, head 1½″, 1 and 2 pounds
1 Ruler and/or caliper, 6″
1 Depth gauge, 6½″
3 Guide wires
1 Drill bit, 7/64″
3 Wire passers, (small, medium, large)
1 Rasp, 7″
1 Hand drill with chuck, 11″, up to 3.2 mm diameter
3 Liston bone cutters, 6″, 7½″, 8⅜″
2 Langenbeck periosteal elevators, 1 narrow, ¼″ × 8″ 1 wide, 11/16″ × 7½″
1 Periosteal elevator, Joseph, 7½″
1 Joker, Cushing, "little joker" elevator, 15.2 cm
1 Freer dissector, 8″
6 Curettes, #0 to #5
1 Blunt nerve hook, 7¼″
1 Gigli saw with 2 handles, 20″ wire saw
6 Osteotomes, 7″, 3 straight, 10, 20, and 25 cm, 3 curved, 5, and 10 mm

Bone-Holding Instruments Tray

2 Lane retractors, 12½″
3 Lowman clamps, 4¾″, 7¼″, or 8″
5 Verbrugge forceps (1 large, 1 medium, 1 small, 2 very small)
2 Lewin bone clamps, 7″
2 Bishop clamps

Knee Arthrotomy Tray

Additional trays
Basic Orthopedic Procedures Instrument Tray

Retractors
6 Grey
1 Blount, 8¾″
2 Doane, 57 mm × 69.8 deep and 63 mm × 76.2 deep

Scissors
1 Cartilage, 6″ smooth or 8″ serrated

Clamps
1 Cartilage (modified Martin), 7½″
2 Lahey, 8″

Miscellaneous
1 Semi-lunar cartilage knife
3 Smilie cartilage knives, 6¾″ (1 right, 1 left, 1 neutral)
1 Meniscotome
1 Beaver knife handle, 10″
1 O'Donahue suture passer
1 Adson blunt hook, 8″

Hip Instruments Tray

Retractors
2 Goelet, 7½″
2 Bennett, large, 10″ with 2½″ blade
2 Hibbs, 9½″ blade, 1″ × 3″
2 Dingman bone hooks
2 Weitlaner, sharp, 8″
2 Femoral neck
1 Hip skid
2 Israel, 8″, 3- or 4-prong
2 Meyerding, blade, small 2″ deep × ⅝″ wide and large 3″ × 1″
4 Cobra, pointed, blunt smooth, blunt serrated, long 14″
2 Hohmann, 10 mm and 18 mm
1 Bone hook (e.g., T-handled)

Scissors

3 Mayo, 2 straight, 1 curved, 6¼″
1 Metzenbaum, 7½″
1 Stille-Liston bone cutter, 10¾″

Forceps

2 Tissue with teeth, 6″
1 Russian, 7″
1 Cushing forceps, 7″
2 Adson with teeth, 4¾″

Clamps

4 Curved Crile, 6½″
2 Straight Crile″, 6½″
2 Peans, 7″
2 Tonsils, 7¼″
2 Allis, 6″
4 Kocher (Ochsner), 8″
2 Crile-Wood needle holder, 6″
8 Towel clips, piercing, (4) small, 3½″ and (4) large, 5″
8 Towel clips, nonpiercing, (4) small, 3½″ and (4) large, 5″

Suction Tubes or Tips

2 Yankauer, suction tube and tip; 2 pieces, 10⅜″, 12″
2 Adson with finger valve controls and stylets, 15Fr × 8″, 11Fr × 6″

Miscellaneous

6 Knife handles, (2) #3, (1) #3L, (2) #4, (1) #7
1 Acetabular knife
1 Bone chip impactor/bone tamp
1 Hex screw
2 Long, large bone curettes, 25 cm large and small
1 Corkscrew head remover, 12.7 diameter, 194 mm
1 Freer elevator, 8″
2 Langenbeck periosteal elevators, 1 wide, 11⁄16″ × 7½″, 1 narrow, ¼″ × 8″, 1 wide
1 Duckbill rongeur, 229 mm with cup 3 × 10 mm
1 Straight double-action rongeur, Stille multiple action, straight, 9″
1 Rongeur, large, straight, 7″-Luer
1 Rasp, large, flat, 10½″
1 Scott-McCracken elevator,
2 Key elevators, ¾″, ½″
1 Bone mallet, heavy, 8″

1 Pliers, heavy, 216 mm
4 Osteotomes, e.g., (2) straight 3/4″, 1″, and 2 curved 1/4″, 1″
Large bone curettes, straight and angled, graduated sizes, Innomed®, 10½″
1 Moore hollow chisel, according to prosthesis chosen
1 Prosthesis driver, according to prosthesis chosen
1 Femoral head extractor
1 Metal ruler, caliper, and/or measuring gauge, 6″
1 Cement gun, optional
1 Cement applying restrictor, optional

Total Hip Systems Instrument Tray

The following instruments are representative of the many that may be required according to the specific brand of total hip replacement prosthesis. Each hip system has its own system specific instrumentation that must be used to assure the accurate implantation of the prosthetic components. Refer to specific instrumentation companies such as DePuy; Smith and Nephew; Zimmer; and Howmedica.

Additional Trays

Open Hip Instruments Tray

Retractors

1 Charnley retractor
2 Posterior inferior, 1 left, 1 right
2 Anterior, 1 left, 1 right
1 Superior retractor
1 Femoral retractor

Miscellaneous

T-handle coupling adaptor (for femoral reamers)
Rod for central placement (of femoral prosthesis)
Reamers, tapered, selected
Trial broach for femur
Femoral head extractor
Set femoral stem trials
Impactor (nylon, polyethylene, or similar head)
Femoral stem inserter with distractor device
Neck-cutting guide
Acetabular reamer handle
Acetabular drill guide handle
Acetabular cup positioner
Acetabular pusher (cup impactor with alignment rod)

Trial broach for acetabular cup
Set acetabular cup trials
Acetabular curettes, small, medium, large
Acetabular cup retainer
Measuring gauge
Extractor, brand specific
Extractor with 2 hooks and spare hook
Bone cement block inserter rod

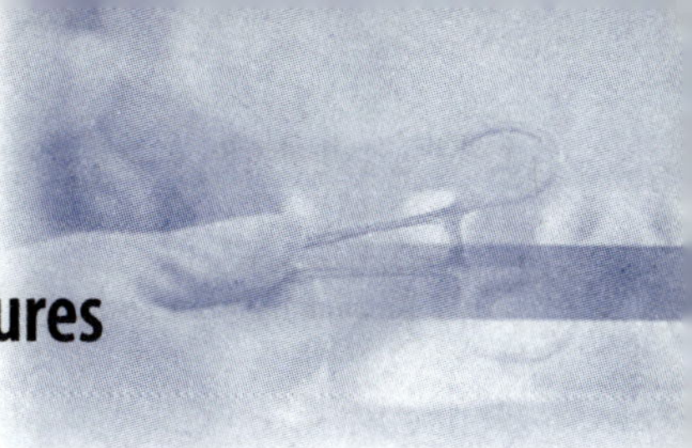

CHAPTER 38
Neurosurgical Procedures Instrument Trays

Craniotomy Tray

Additional Trays

Kerrison Rongeurs and Pituitary Forceps Tray

Retractors

2 Army-Navy/(USA), 8½″
1 Jansen mastoid, self-retaining, 4″ or 4½″
2 Weitlaner self-retaining, straight, (1) 5½″, (1) 6½″
1 Weitlaner, self-retaining, curved, 6½″
2 Adson cerebellar self-retaining (1) straight, 7½″ and (1) curved, heavy, 7″
8 Davis malleable brain spatulas, double-ended (¼″ to 1¼″)
2 Malis nerve hooks, 1 sharp, 7¼″ 1 blunt, 7¼″
2 Love nerve root, straight blade 7⅝″ × ½″
2 Hoen dura separators, (1) 45°, (1) 90°
2 Dura hooks, 8″
3 Cushing subtemporal decompression, 6¾″, 7¾″, and 11″
1 BUDDE-Halo self-retaining retractor system with flexible arms, multiple attachments
1 BUDDE-Halo radiolucent self-retaining retractor system with flexible arms, multiple attachments
1 Greenberg Universal retractor system with malleable blades, various bar and arm lengths, and attachments
1 Leyla-Yasargil self-retaining retractor with 2 flexible arms
1 Fiber-optic rhinoplasty retractor and cord (craniofacial)

Forceps

3 Tissue with teeth, (2) 5½″ and (1)10″
2 Adson with teeth, 4¾″
1 Adson without teeth, 4¾″
4 Cushing with teeth, (2) 7″ and (2) 8″
2 Cushing without teeth, 8″
1 Watchmaker
2 Adson hypophyseal bayonet, 9″
2 Tumor bayonet cup, 8″
3 Gerald, 7″, 1 with teeth and 2 without teeth

2 DeBakey, 6″
1 Bipolar bayonet and cord (e.g., Malis, SilverGlide)

Rongeurs

2 Kerrison up-bite, 40°, 6″ and 7½″
1 Kerrison straight, 40° × 6″
1 Kerrison up-bite, 40° × 8″
1 Leksell double-action (heavy), 9½″
1 Ruskin double-action, slightly curved (fine), 6″ with 2 to 3 mm jaws
1 Decker alligator, serrated, 6″ × 1.4 mm jaw

Scissors

2 Straight Mayo, 6¼″
1 Curved Mayo, 6¼″
2 Metzenbaum, (1) 5½″ and (1) 7″
2 Potts 7¼″, (1) straight and (1) 25° angled
1 Wire cutter

Clamps

6 Curved Mosquito, 5″
2 Straight Mosquito, 5″
8 Curved Crile, 5½″
2 Straight Criles, 5½″
2 Curved Pean, 6¼″
2 Tonsil (Schnidt), 7½″
2 Right angles (Mixter), 8″
4 Allis, (2) short, 6″, and (2) long, 7¼″
4 Kocher (Ochsner), (2) 6″ and (2) 8″
36 Dandy hemostatic scalp clamps, serrated, 5½″ (add 10 rubber bands) or
2 Raney or Michel scalp clip appliers with clip cartridges, or 2 Raney scalp clip appliers with LeRoy-Raney clip applier, 6¼″ disposable clips, or ACRA-CUT®, Caspar, or ScalpFix® system with gun and scalp clips
2 Webster needle holders, fine, 5″
2 Adson dura needle holders, 7¼″
2 Crile needle holders, 5¼″
2 Crile-Wood needle holders, 6″
4 Towel clips, piercing, 5″
2 Towel clips, nonpiercing, 5″
Sponge (ring) forceps (Foerster), 10″

Suction Tubes or Tips

4 Frazier with stylets, #7, #9, #10, #12
1 Bucy-Frazier electrosurgical suction tip, 10Fr × 5″

Drills and Saws

2 Gigli saw handles, pair with 2 blades and 1 saw guide (e.g., Bailey), standard 12″ and long 20″
Hand drill, e.g., Hudson brace with key and 1 set drill bits, burrs, and perforator (Raney or Hudson), or Craniotome (high-power micro drill) with modular attachment, compression ring, cranio-blade, skull perforator, skull perforator guard, cranio-blade (disposable), dura guard (fixed or swiveling), such as UHT Stryker™ micro drill with Duraguard® and integrated irrigation
Hall Surgairtome™, or ACRA-CUT Smart Drill Perforator (cordless, battery powered) with bone pad remover, or Medtronic Midas Rex™ Legend® pneumatic drills, also with saw attachment or
Triton® micro drill
MicroAire™ self-contained power micro drill (cordless, battery powered)
Micro power saws with cord, blade, chuck, key, and attachments, e.g., Stryker CORE® micro sagittal saw with Duraguard and integrated irrigation pump
MicroAire pneumatic-powered (nitrogen) micro saw

Miscellaneous

Prongs for skull clamp (e.g., Yasargil, Gardner, Mayfield, etc.)
1 Basin (tiny)
4 Medicine cups
1 Anspah® neurosurgical sponge tray (pattie plate)
4 Knife handles, (1) #3, (2) #7, (1) Beaver
2 Langenbeck periosteal elevators, 7½″ and 8″
1 Key periosteal elevator, 7½″
2 Freer elevators, 8″
1 Cushing "Little Joker" periosteal elevator, 6″
2 Woodson dental probes, double-ended, 7″
1 Hoen dura separator, 6½″
5 Penfield dissectors, #1 to #5
1 Straight pituitary forceps, 7″ with 1.5 to 2 mm bite
1 Angled pituitary forceps, up-bite, 6″ with 1.5 to 2 mm bite
3 Blunt ventricular needles with stylets, (1) #11, (1) #14, (1) #16

1 Campbell sharp ventricular needle with stylet, 4″
4 Syringes, Luer lok (control), 10 ml
2 Olive-tip heparin needles
2 Brain spoons
3 Pituitary spoons (1 small, 1 medium, 1 large)
1 McKissack fine-needle driver
4 Ligating clip appliers, e.g., Hemoclip® or Weck® clip applier®, 2 short, 2 medium

Microsurgical (Titanium Instruments)

Microscopic or microendoscopic (robotic, optional)

Micro forceps, micro bayonet forceps, micro scissors (curved, straight), Beaver knife handle, micro needle holders (curved, straight), diamond microknife, micro curettes (curved, straight, angled), micro suction tips, micro hooks (90°, semi-sharp, blunt), bipolar bayonet forceps and cord, micro dissectors (small, medium, large, straight), micro elevators (variety of straight and curved), assorted aneurysm clips and clip appliers (e.g., Heifetz, Yasargil, Sundt-Kees, Mayfield, Keer, Olivecrona, Surgita)

Endoscopic (Ebonized)

Hopkins rigid endoscope (0°, 30°, 70°, and 120°), 2.7 mm, 20 cm with sheath (6.5- or 4.0-mm "mini"), camera and optical bridge, surgical tips attached to telescope, electrosurgical suction-irrigator and coaxial cable, laser fiber and hand piece, 1-mm scissors, 1-mm pituitary forceps, 1-mm grasping forceps, and endoscopic ligating clip appliers (Ligaclips®)

Transsphenoidal Stereotactic Instruments Limited Procedures Tray

Microsurgical (titanium) instruments, e.g., 3 nasal specula (1 long, 1 short, 1 oro-nasal), bayonet smooth dressing forceps, blunt Senn retractors, small blunt rakes, Cottle elevator-freer, transsphenoidal micro curettes (angled, assorted), micro dissectors (angled up and down), enucleators, micro bayonet bipolar forceps, micro bayonet 3-prong fork, micro bayonet knife handle, micro bayonet needle holders, micro hooks, micro suction, and micro dissectors

Optional

When a laser, e.g., Ho:YAG, Nd:YAG, KTP, Argon, or CO_2 is employed, endoscopic micro instruments are used, as follows:

CO_2 laser beam with microsurgical approach, with fiber-optic camera, camera-coupling micromanipulator
Instruments with Rhoton, black anodized, or other nonreflective covering (e.g., micro dissectors, micro elevators, micro hooks, micro needles, micro bayonet forceps, micro tying forceps, micro curettes, micro needle holders, etc.)
Cavitational UltraSound Aspirator (CUSA)

Kerrison Rongeurs and Pituitary Forceps Tray

Kerrison Laminectomy Rongeurs

2 Angled, 40° up-bite, 6″, (1) 3 mm, (1) 5 mm
2 Angled, 90° up-bite, 7½″, (1) 3 mm, (1) 5 mm
2 Angled, 90° down-bite, 6″, (1) 3 mm, (1) 5 mm
2 Angled, 90° down-bite, 7½″, (1) 3 mm, (1) 5 mm

Intervertebral Disc Rongeur

2 Straight (Ferris Smith or Sterling), 7″, (1) 2 × 10 mm cup, (1) 4 × 10 mm cup
2 Angled, up-bite (Ferris Smith or Sterling), 7″, (1) 2 × 10 mm cup, (1) 4 × 10 mm cup
2 Angled, down-bite (Ferris Smith or Sterling), 7″, (1) 2 × 10 mm cup, (1) 4 × 10 mm cup

Clamps

1 Ligamentum flavum forceps

Laminectomy Tray

Additional Trays

Kerrison Rongeurs and Pituitary Forceps Tray

Retractors

2 Army-Navy/(USA), 8 5/16″
2 Goelet, 7½″
4 Weitlaner self-retaining, 6½″, 2 blunt, 2 sharp
2 Gelpi self-retaining, 7″
2 Beckman-Adson self-retaining (sharp), 12″
2 Meyerding, small, 9½″, with blade, (1) 5/8″ × 2″, (1) 1″ × 3″
4 Taylor, (2) 1¼″ × 3, (2) 2¼″ × 4″
1 Downing self-retaining with 6 blades (2 small, 2 medium, 2 large)

1 Laminar or vertebral spreader and wrench each, 1 large, 1 small
1 Dura self-retaining with 3 malleable blades
2 Scoville, racheted with hinged arms, blades, 1″ to 3½″, 1 straight, 1 angled
2 D'Errico angled nerve root, 9″ with blade ¼″
6 Love nerve root, 2 straight, 2 angled 45°, 2 angled 90°
2 Cushing dura hooks, 5½″
2 Graham nerve hooks, 7″

Forceps

2 Tissue with teeth, 6″
2 Adson with teeth, 4¼″
2 Cushing without teeth, 7″ or 8″
2 Cushing with teeth, 7″ or 8″
2 Cushing, 4¾″ura, fine
3 Hardy bayonet without teeth, 8¼″
1 Bipolar bayonet forceps and cord (e.g., Malis, SilverGlide)

Scissors

1 Straight Mayo, 6¼″
1 Curved Mayo, 6¼″
1 Metzenbaum, 7″
1 Potts, 25° angle, 7½″

Rongeurs

1 Leksell double-action rongeur, 9½″
1 Stille-Luer double-action rongeur (gooseneck), 8½″ or 9½″

Clamps

6 Curved mosquito, 5¼″
18 Curved Crile, 5½″
2 Curved Pean, 6¼″
2 Kocher (Ochsner), 6¼″
2 Kocher-Lovelace, fine short jaws, 6″
4 Needle holders, (2) 6″, (2) 7″
4 Towel clips, piercing, 3½″
2 Towel clips, nonpiercing, 3½″
2 Sponge forceps (Foerster), 10″

Suction Tubes or Tips

3 Frazier, 7Fr, 9Fr, 11Fr
1 Adson, 12Fr

Drills

High-power micro drill with cord, chuck, drill-sleeve, drill bits, burrs, and drill guard, e.g., UHT Stryker micro drill with Duraguard and integrated irrigation or Hall Surgairtome or self-contained (battery)

MicroAire

Miscellaneous

5 Knife handles, (2) #3, (2) #7, (1) Long Beaver
1 Cordotomy knife (e.g., Bucy or Humby)
1 Anspah neurosurgical sponge tray (pattie plate)
1 Probe, malleable, 12 1/2 cm to 16 cm
1 Grooved director, 12 1/2 cm to 16 cm
1 Blunt nerve hook (Hoen), 8 1/4″ with hook 1/4″ deep
1 Ruler, 6″
2 Jokers, 6″
2 Penfield dissectors, double-ended, 7″ and 11 1/2″
2 Freer dissectors, 8″
3 Cobb elevators 1 small, 1 medium, 1 large .
2 Key elevators, (1) 3/4″ and (1) 1″
1 Electrosurgical unit spatula blade
1 Langenbeck periosteal elevator, 11/16″
1 Freer chisel, curved, 7 1/2″
1 Mallet
2 Medicine cups
4 Long curettes, 0 to 3
2 Ring curettes, 1 small, 1 medium
4 Ligating clip appliers, e.g., Hemoclip, or Weck clip applier, 2 short, 2 medium

Micro Instruments

Williams micro-lumbar disectomy self-retaining retractor with deep blades, 4 sizes, in pairs

Williams micro-lumbar disectomy forceps, 1 mm × 5 1/2″

Williams micro-lumbar disectomy suction retractor (nerve root), 6″

Micro forceps, 3 mm, micro needle holders (straight and curved), micro scissors (straight and curved), micro tying forceps

Micro biopolar forceps (straight and bayonet)

Laser Micro Instruments (Rhoton for Laser Safety)

Curettes, dissectors, elevators, alligator forceps, bayonet forceps, forceps, dura forceps, tumor forceps, hooks (blunt and sharp), needle holders (straight and bayonet), scissors (straight and bayonet)

Iliac Bone Graft

Limited Procedures Tray

Taylor or Richardson retractors, blades, 4″ deep and 3″

Bone gouge (medium), bone impactor, and mallet, or Hudson brace (drill), 10½″

Cloward drill shaft, dowel cutter (with removable nut), and dowel bone graft cutters, drill tips

Cloward bone graft impactor and mallet or electric Midas Rex Legend Bone Mill

Cloward punch

Anterior Fusion

Cloward self-retaining retractor with 4 blades, 2 short, 2 long

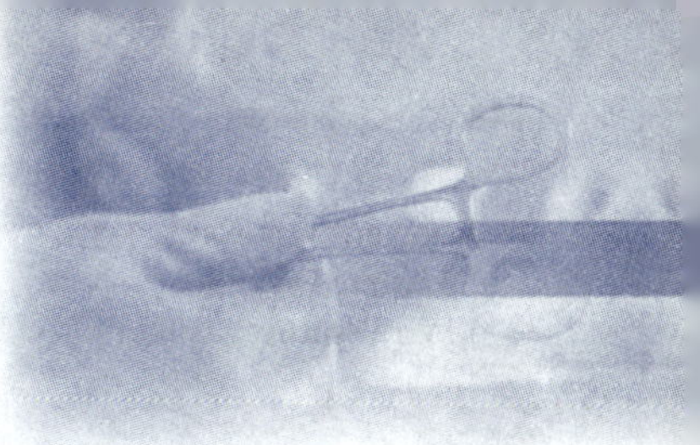

CHAPTER 39 Plastic Surgery Instrument Trays

Basic Plastic Procedures Tray

Retractors

- 2 Joseph skin hooks, single, 6″
- 2 Guthrie skin hooks, double, 5″
- 1 Graham nerve hook, 7″
- 2 Army-Navy/ USA, 8 5/16″
- 2 Senn, blunt, 6″
- 2 Cushing vein, 9″
- 2 Rake (four prong), blunt, 8″
- 2 Cherry, S-shaped, double-ended, ⅜″ and ½″
- 5 Malleable (Ribbon) brain, (1) ¼″, (1) ½″, (1) ⅜″, (1) ¾″, (1) 1″
- 1 Gilles zygoma hook, 7″ or 1 Dingman bone hook, 7″
- 2 Richardson, small
- 1 Deaver, medium
- 2 ALM, blunt, (1) 2¾″ and (1) 3″ deeper blades
- 2 Weitlaner, 1 sharp, 4½″ and 6¾″ and 1 blunt, 4½″ and 6¾″

Forceps

- 2 Tissue with teeth, 6″
- 1 Tissue without teeth, 6″
- 2 Cushing with teeth, 7″
- 1 Cushing without teeth, 7″
- 1 Cushing bayonet forceps, 7″
- 2 Adson with teeth, 4¾″
- 1 Adson without teeth, 4¾″
- 1 Adson-Brown, 5″
- 2 Jansen bayonet dressing, 6½
- 2 DeBakey, 6″
- 1 Bipolar bayonet with cord

Scissors

- 1 Straight Mayo, 6¾″
- 2 Metzenbaum, curved, fine tip, (1) 5¾″ and (1) 7″
- 1 Metzenbaum, straight, blunt tip, 5¾″
- 2 Iris, 1 curved, 1 straight, 4¾″

1 Stevens tenotomy, 4½″
1 Littler, 4¾″
1 Wire (suture) scissors

Clamps

4 Mosquito, curved, fine tip, 5″
6 Mosquito, 5¾″, 4 curved, 2 straight
6 Crile, 5½″, 4 curved, 2 straight
2 Pean, baby (delicate), 5⅛″
2 Pean, curved, 6″
2 Allis, 6″
2 Babcock, 6″
2 Kocher, 6″
1 Castroviejo micro needle holder, 5⅛″
2 Webster needle holder, 4½″
2 Crile needle holders, 5⅛″
2 Johnson needle holders, 6″
2 Crile-Wood needle holder, fine, 7″
8 Towel clips, piercing, (4) 3½″ and (4) 5″
8 Towel clips, nonpiercing, (4) 3½″ and (4) 5″
4 Sponge forceps (Foerster or Ballenger), straight, 7″ and 7½″

Suction Tubes or Tips

4 Frazier (with finger control and stylet), (1) 5Fr, (1) 7Fr, (1) 9Fr, (1) 11Fr
1 Andrews with tip (2 pieces), 9½″

Miscellaneous

4 Knife handles, calibrated, (2) #3, (1) #7, (1) Beaver
1 Probe, malleable
1 Ruler and/or 1 caliper
1 Freer elevator, 7½″
1 Joseph periosteal elevator, 6½″
2 Medicine cups

Optional Additional Plastic Instruments or Equipment Grouped According to Use

Skin Grafting Instruments

Oscillating knife (Humby, Blair), Weck blade, or Brown, Reese, Padgett-Hood, or Zimmer air dermatome electric handheld oscillating dermatome with blade (disposable) and cord

Padgett or Zimmer skin graft mesher, or Intregra® Brennen non-crushing skin mesher and Meshgraft® skin expander, Derma Carrier (used with meshing device)

Dermabrasion

Dermabrader and cord (e.g., Stryker®), wire brush, and sanding cylinder

Cleft Lip or Cleft Palate

Lip clamp
High power micro drill, with drill bits (fine), and cord or unit may be battery powered (self-contained)
Dingman mouth gag with 3 blades (1) 25 mm wide × 5.6 cm length, (2) 27 mm × 5.9 cm, and (3) 30 mm × 7.2 cm
2 Salyer palate hooks, 17.5 cm 2 prongs, 7″, and 12.5 cm 1 prong, 5″
4 Wang palate elevators, 18 cm, 1 left, 1 right, 1 angled left, and 1 angled right or
3 Blair palate elevators, 1 L-shape, 19.7 cm, blunt tip, 1 right angle, 19.7 cm semi-sharp tip, and 1 curved blunt tip, 20.3 cm
2 Salyer palate retractors, 1 large, 15 mm, 18 cm, 7″, and 1 small, 10 mm, 18 cm, 7″
Latrobe soft-palate retractor, 5 1/2″
Foman lower-lateral scissors, 5″
2 Logan's lip traction bow, small and large with spread 2.8 cm to 3.5 cm

Nasal Fracture (see Nasal Procedures Tray, p. 1156)

Add

Cottle chisel-osteotome, 4 mm

Mandibular Fracture

Closed

2 Bite blocks or mouth props, 1 adult, 1 child
1 Yankauer (suction and tip; 2 pieces), 10 3/8″
2 Weder tongue depressors, (1) large, 3.5 cm wide and (1) small, 2.8 cm
1 Needle-nose pliers and wire cutter, 6.5″
1 Obwegeser wire twister, 13.5 cm
2 Mayo-Haney needle holders (heavy), 6″
Arch bars, latex bands, or stainless-steel wire

Open

Cloward bone-grafting instruments

2 Cloward bone punches, 1 square 9″ × 13 mm and 1 plain 9 3/8″
4 Cloward bone punches with 40°, 3 mm × 7″, 5 mm × 7″, 3 mm × 8″, 5 mm × 8″
1 Cloward bone-graft double-ended impactor, 11/14 mm ends
1 Cloward drill shaft with 4 drill tips, 10, 12, 14, 16 mm
6 Cloward dowel cutters with center pins, 12 to 18 mm
1 Cloward dowel handle, cone tip with spring
2 Weder tongue depressors (1) large, 3.5 cm wide and (1) small, 2.8 cm
2 Lewin bone-holding clamps
2 Gilles bone hooks, 6.5″ and 7.5″
High-speed micro power drill (e.g., Mini Stryker or Hall II®), cord, micro bits, tap, and drill guide
Depth gauge, 6 1/2″
Nerve stimulator (e.g., Concept, Pulsatron® II)

Special Note

- **N.B.** *Any time the jaws are wired, a disposable wire cutter must be available in case of emergency.* For both closed and open reduction of mandibular fracture, disposable wire cutter may be taped to the head of the bed; ***the disposable wire cutter must accompany patient in case of emergency.***
- For any procedure on the face in which nerve damage might result, it is wise to set up a nerve stimulator. The unit (e.g., Concept or Pulsatron II), faces the anesthesia provider for monitoring.

Facial Fractures

Kerrison rongeurs, assorted
3 Carroll jaw bone hooks, 7″ long with hook lengths, 5/16″, 7/16″, 11/16″
2 Gilles zygomatic bone hook
2 Gilles bone and zygoma hook, retractors, 6.5″ and 7.5″
High-speed micro power drill (e.g., Mini Stryker or Hall II), bits, tap, drill guide, and cord
Depth gauge, 6.5″
Nerve stimulator (e.g., Concept)

Rhinoplasty and Nasal Procedures (see Nasal Procedures Instrument Tray, p. 1156)

Rhytidectomy

Basic Plastic Procedures Tray
2 Deaver retractors, narrow, 1″

Bipolar bayonet forceps
1 Gorney or 1 Castanares facelift scissors

Otoplasty

Small rasp, bayonet shank, 9″
1 Langenbeck periosteal elevator, narrow, 8″
Hand drill and fine drill points, 5½″
Microinstruments: Von Graefe muscle hook, jewelers' forceps (2), micro elevator, microdissector, micro electrosurgical suction, diamond knife, Castroviejo-Vannas scissors, Castroviejo needle holder without lock, Castroviejo needle holder with lock
ALM self-retaining retractor, 2¾″ or 3″

Vascular and Nerve Procedures

Nerve stimulator (e.g., Concept)
Microinstruments: Von Graefe muscle hook, jewelers' forceps (2), micro elevator, microdissector, micro electrosurgical suction, diamond knife, Castroviejo-Vannas scissors, Castroviejo needle holder without lock, Castroviejo needle holder with lock

Breast Reduction

Freeman areola marker, sizes 18 to 52 mm blades
Fiber-optic lighted retractor with sleeve, blades, and cord, 70 × 25 mm to 220 × 27 mm
Hopkins rigid endoscope and cord
Endoscopic: electrosurgical suction-irrigator and endoscopic instruments
CO_2 laser hand piece and cord (Rhoton instruments for laser safety)
Harmonic Scalpel® hand piece with scissors or blade tip and cord
Liposuction hand piece with blunt suction cannulas, e.g., Tulip BioMed™ handpiece with micro cannulas
High-pressure tumescent fluid infusion pump (e.g., Cabot)

Breast Augmentation

Fiber-optic lighted retractor, 70 × 25 mm to 220 × 27 mm blades, and cord (optional)

Transaxillary and Transumbilical

Johnson endotube, pocket expander, inflatable trial prosthesis
Hopkins rigid endoscope with sleeve, cord, electrosurgical suction-irrigator and cord, camera

Liposuction

Fiber-optic retractor, blades, and cord
Blunt suction cannulas and/or Mercedes-tip cannulas
Ultrasound hand piece and probe, e.g., Misonix™ unit, LySonix™, Mentor Contour™
High-pressure tumescent fluid infusion pump (e.g., Cabot)

CHAPTER 40
Otorhinolaryngologic (ENT) Instrument Trays

Ear Procedures Instrument Tray

Retractors

2 Joseph skin hook, 6″
2 Senn-Kanavel or House double-ended, dull prongs, 6″
2 Army-Navy/(USA), 8 5/16″
1 Wullstein-Weitlaner, 13 cm, 3 × 3 blunt prongs
1 Miltex Jansen mastoid, 4 1/4″, 3 × 3 blunt prongs
1 Shea articulated speculum holder (with assorted specula), 11 13/16″ × 30 cm

Forceps

2 Adson with teeth, 4 3/4″
1 Adson-Brown, 5″
1 Bayonet, short (Jansen), 6″

Scissors

1 Straight Mayo, 6 1/4″
2 Metzenbaum, (1) 5 1/4″ and (1) 7″
1 Strabismus, 10 cm
3 House-Bellucci alligator, 1 small, 6 cm and 9 cm

Clamps

8 Mosquito, 5 1/4″, (4) straight, (4) curved
4 Crile, 5 1/2″, 2 curved, 2 straight
2 Curved Pean, 6 1/4″
2 Allis, 6″
2 Webster needle holders, 5″
8 Towel clips, piercing, (4) 3 1/2″ and (4) 5 1/2″
2 Towel clips, nonpiercing, (4) 3 1/2″ and (4) 5 1/2″
1 Sponge forceps, straight (Ballenger), 7″

Suction Tubes or Tips

2 Frazier (with finger control and stylets), (1) 7Fr, (1) 9Fr
3 Baron, (1) 3Fr, (1) 5Fr, (1) 7Fr
3 House suction-irrigator, (1) 3Fr, (1) 5Fr, (1) 7Fr
4 Rosen, 3 3/8″, 14Fr, 16Fr, 18Fr, 22Fr

Miscellaneous

1 Knife handle, #3
1 Ruler, 6″
1 House elevator
6 Endaural specula, 1 to 6
1 speculum
1 House-Dieter malleus nipper, 14 cm
3 Cup forceps, 1 small, 1 medium, 1 large
2 Alligator forceps, 1 small, 1 large
3 Hartman forceps, jaws, 6 cm, 5⅝″ total length
2 Mastoid gouges, (1) 2 mm and (1) 4 mm
2 House stapes curettes (double-ended), 6¼″
3 Mastoid curettes, 000 to 0
1 House Gelfoam pressure forceps, 6″
1 House Teflon® block

Delicate Middle-Ear Sharp Instruments (In Protective Rack in Preselected Set)

1 Ring curette
2 Wax curette, (1) #1 and (1) #2
1 Double-ended J curette
1 Duckbill knife-elevator
1 Right-angle elevator
1 Oval curette
1 Excavator
1 Heavy needle
2 Picks, angled, (1) 45° and (1) 90°
1 Austin pick, 25° angle
1 Rosen (House-Rosen) needle
1 Paparella straight needle
1 Curved needle
1 Attic dissector
2 House picks, (1) 1 mm and (1) 3 mm
2 Whirlybird, 1 left, 1 right
1 Strut caliper
1 Straight chisel
1 Canal knife
1 Sickle knife (House)
1 Incal stapedial knife
1 Drum scraper
1 Oval window rasp
1 Hough hoe
2 Footplate hooks
1 House alligator crimper forceps (for prosthesis)

Optional

Medtronic Universal handle and instruments, or Kavanaugh universal hand stabilizer® and instruments, e.g.; straight vertical scissors, 3-mm blade; straight serrated alligator forceps, 4-mm blades; 1-mm round straight cup forceps; 1-mm round angled-up cup forceps; 1-mm round curved right cup forceps; 1-mm round curved left cup forceps; McGee crimper, 3.5 mm; House crimper, 3.5 mm; Gruppe crimper, 3.5 mm

Micro Instruments Tray

Micro fiber-optic light and cord, micro electrosurgical suction and cord, micro curettes, micro alligator forceps, measuring gauge, attic hook, House strut hook, House oval window hook, Schucknecht roller knife

Endoscopic Instruments Tray

Rigid fiber-optic endoscopes, 0° and 30°, with cords (robotic voice directed, optional)

Ports available for camera with coupler and laser (Ebonized or Rhoton instrumentation for laser safety)

Micro instrumentation similar to the middle-ear sharp instruments, e.g., Rosen needle, micro dissector, micro elevators, micro suctions with side opening for varying the amount of suction, micro curettes, micro alligator forceps, Austin strut caliper and measuring gauge, attic hook, House strut hook, House oval window hook, Schucknecht roller knife, prosthesis footplate hooks, and McGee crimper

High-Speed Power Micro Drill

Micro Stryker® with chuck, key, micro drill bits, micro burrs, guards, and cord, etc., or Visao® high-speed otologic drill with irrigation, micro drill bits, micro burrs and extended burr guard, tubing, and cord

CO_2, KTP, or Er:YAG Laser and Rhoton micro instruments (for laser safety)

Myringotomy Instruments Tray

Additional Trays

Ear Procedures Tray

Retractors

1 Shea speculum holder (articulated), n/a or 1 Universal speculum holder (articulated)

3 Oval aural specula, (1 small, 1 medium, 1 large)
4 Boucheron round aural specula, metal (assorted sizes)

Forceps

1 Bayonet, 5½″

Scissors

1 Straight iris, 4″

Suction Tubes or Tips

3 Frazier (with finger control and stylets), (1) 3Fr, (1) 5Fr, (1) 7Fr
1 Baron, 5Fr

Miscellaneous

1 Long metal applicator
1 Medicine cup
2 Wire ear curettes, 1 small, 1 medium
1 Sexton ear knife, straight, 7″ or 1 myringotomy knife, double edged, disposable, or 1 Sexton ear knife reverse swivel handle, 7½″ or 1 Storz folding handle myringotomy knife 7½″
1 Noyes serrated alligator forceps, 5½″
1 Noyes smooth alligator forceps, upbite, 5½″
1 Rosen needle, blunt, 6½″

Nasal Procedures Instrument Tray

Retractors

2 Joseph skin hooks, 2 single, 6″
2 Guthrie double skin hooks, 5″
2 Killian nasal specula, (1) 3″ and (1) 2″
1 Cottle nasal speculum, narrow, 5¼″
1 Cushing bivalve speculum
2 Aufricht nasal specula, 1 long, 1 short
1 Cottle guide and retractor, 8″
1 Nerve hook, Graham, 7″

Forceps

2 Jansen bayonet dressing, coated (serrated tips), 8¼″ or 2 Cushing bayonet, 7″, 1 without teeth, 1 with teeth
1 Brown bayonet, 7¼″
1 Adson Brown, with teeth, 4¾″

Scissors

2 Fomon, 5¼, 1 dorsal angular, and 1 lower lateral, full curve

4 Knapp, iris, 4″, curved blunt, straight blunt, curved sharp, and straight sharp
1 Cottle spring, straight, 19 cm
1 Cottle dorsal spring, 17 cm
1 Knight nasal, angled on side, 6¾″
1 Becker septum, serrated, $7^3/_{32}$″

Clamp

2 Jacobson bayonet needle holders, smooth, spring, 8½″
2 Johnson needle holders, 5″
1 Cottle columella, 11 cm, jaws 11 mm
4 Towel clips, piercing, (2) 3½″ and (2) 5″
2 Towel clips, nonpiercing, (2) 3½″ and (2) 5″

Suction Tip

1 Antrum, grasping, curved down, 10 cm
3 Frasier (with finger control and stylets), (1) 3Fr, (1) 5Fr, and (1) 7Fr
1 Andrews with tip, suction tube + tip; 2 pieces, 22 cm

Miscellaneous

1 Basin, small
2 Long metal applicators
1 Asch septal forceps, 9″
1 Takahashi nasal forceps, 120 mm, cups, 2 × 10 mm
1 Ferris-Smith fragment forceps, 7″
1 Jansen-Middleton forceps, 8″
3 Knight polyp forceps, (1 small, 1 medium, 1 large)
1 Cartilage knife
1 Cottle knife, 5.5″
2 Joseph knives, 1 sharp, 1 blunt
1 Joseph button-end knife
1 McKenty knife
1 Ballenger swivel knife, 7½″ long and 3 to 5 mm blade
1 Freer septum knife
1 Freer elevator, 7½″
1 Joseph periosteal elevator, 6½″
1 Gilles elevator
1 Septal displacer
1 Septal cutting scissors, Caplan, 8″
1 Septal straightener
1 Rubin nasal cartilage crushing forceps or morselizer, 8″
1 Kazanjian nasal hump forceps
1 Double-action nasal rongeur

3 Kerrison rongeurs, up-bite, (1) 2 mm, (1) 4 mm, and (1) 6 mm
1 Reamer
4 Nasal rasps, 1 Lewis, 1 Maltz, 2 Aufricht, large and small
2 Nasal saws, 1 right, 1 left
1 Cottle mallet, flat
1 Rubin nasofrontal osteotome, 7″
2 Converse chisels, guarded, 1 right curved, 1 left curved
1 Parks lateral osteotome chisel
1 Ballenger chisel
2 Gouges, (1) 2 mm and (1) 4 mm
2 Osteotomes, (1) 2 mm and (1) 4 mm
1 Antrum trocar and stylet

Optional

Fiber-optic nasal retractor and cord
Fiber-optic sinuscope
Nasal polypectomy instruments
1 Faulkner antrum curette, double-ended
6 Nasal antrum curettes, angled (Coakley), assorted
1 Bruening bayonet nasal snare (with disposable wires)
1 Jansen-Middleton septum forceps
1 Knight polyp and turbinate forceps

Tonsillectomy and Adenoidectomy Instruments Tray

Retractors

1 Fulton mouth gag
1 McIvor mouth gag (fits all), with 3 McIvor tongue blades, 1 large, 1 medium, 1 small
2 Jennings mouth gags, adult, (1) 4½″ and (1) 6″
1 Jennings mouth gag, child, 4″
1 Boyle Davis mouth gag and tongue blade
1 Love uvula
1 Hurd dissector and pillar retractor

Scissors

1 Metzenbaum, 7″
1 Straight Mayo, 6¼″
1 Dean, angled, 6¾″

Clamps

4 Tonsil (Schnidt), 7½″
2 Allis, 6″

2 Allis, curved, long, 10″
1 Straight sponge forceps (Foerster), 10″
2 Curved sponge forceps (Ballenger), 7″
1 Needle holder, 7″
2 Towel clips, piercing, 3½″
2 Towel clips, nonpiercing, 3½″

Suction Tubes or Tips

1 Yankauer and tip (2 pieces), 10⅜″
1 Andrews-Pynchon and tip (2 pieces), 8½″
1 Adenoid
1 Electrosurgical suction

Miscellaneous

2 Medicine cups
1 Knife handle, #7
1 Beck-Schenck or Tydings tonsil snare with wire (plus 3 extra wires)
1 Adenoid punch
1 Fisher tonsil knife
3 Barnhill adenoid curettes, (1) #1, (1) #2, (1) #3
3 La Force adenotomes, 1 small, 1 medium, 1 large
1 Bipolar electrosurgical unit bayonet forceps, or 1 bipolar diathermy forceps, or 1 thermal welding forceps (Starion®)

Optional

Bifrazier Bipolar Coagulating Suction®
Harmonic Scalpel®
Laser (CO_2 or KTP)
Monopolar radio-frequency ablation
Bipolar radio-frequency coblation
Microdebrider (rotary shaver with continuous irrigation-suction)
1 SLT Contact Laser Technology System® with direct-contact probe and scalpel, tip and fiber (disposable and reusable)

Tracheostomy Instruments Tray

Retractors

2 Army-Navy/(USA), 8 5/16″
2 Senn, blunt, 6″

Forceps

1 Tissue with teeth, 6″
1 Adson with teeth, 4¾″

Scissors

2 Mayo, 6¼″, 1 straight, 1 curved
1 Metzenbaum, 7″

Clamps

4 Curved mosquito, 5¼″
4 Curved Crile, 5½″
2 Allis, 6″
1 Needle holder, 6″
4 Towel clips, piercing, 3½″
2 Towel clips, nonpiercing, 3½″
2 Sponge forceps, short (Foerster)

Suction Tubes or Tips

1 Yankauer (suction tube and tip; 2 pieces), 10⅜″
1 Andrews (suction tube with tip; 2 pieces), 9½″
1 Frazier #10 with stylet

Miscellaneous

2 Knife handles, #3
2 Knife blades (in wrapper), (1) #11, (1) #15
1 Syringe, 5 ml, Luer lok control
2 Needles, (1) 1″, 20 gauge and (1) 25 gauge
1 Tracheostomy dilator
1 Tracheostomy hook
1 Tracheal punch
1 Stoma spreader
1 Tracheostomy tube and obturator, plus 1 extra tracheostomy tube (kept with patient)
1 Flexible guide wire, 1.32 mm
10 Sponges, 4 × 4
1 Prep solution cup

Optional

In the Operating Room. Bronchoscopic: guided percutaneous tracheostomy employing direct bronchoscope or bronchoscopic video imaging

At Bedside Percutaneous Dilatational Tracheostomy (PDT) Kit. 22-gauge needle and Luer lok syringe; short-punch dilator (11Fr); 1.32-mm guidewire; 8Fr guiding catheter; dilators (18Fr, 21Fr, 28Fr, 32Fr, 36Fr, and 38Fr); Shiley tracheostomy tube (8 double cannula)

Fiber-optic bronchoscope (optional)

Guidewire Dilating Forceps (GWDF) Kit. 14-gauge needle and Luer lok syringe; guidewire (J tip Seldinger); scalpel, #11 or #15; Kelly forceps; Shiley tracheostomy tube (8 double cannula and curved obturator); Fiber-optic bronchoscope (optional)

Rapitrach Kit. 12-gauge needle and Luer lok syringe; short guidewire; scalpel, #11 or #15; Rapitrach PCT dilator; Portex 8 mm (standard tracheostomy tube with curved obturator)

Fiber-optic bronchoscope (optional)

CHAPTER 41
Ophthalmic Procedures Trays

Basic Eye Procedures Tray

Retractors

1 Eye speculum (Lancaster, Barraquer) 3″ length, opens to 20 mm aperture

Scissors

1 Stevens, blunt, 4½″
1 Iris, curved, 4¾″
1 Stevens, tenotomy, curved, blunt, 4½″
1 Suture, 6¼″

Clamps

3 Halsted mosquito, 5″, 2 straight, 1 curved
1 Castroviejo standard needle holder, straight with lock, 4¾″
2 Serrefine clamps, straight, 1½″
4 Towel clips, piercing, (2) 3½″ and (2) 5″
4 Towel clips, nonpiercing, (2) 3½″ and (2) 5″

Miscellaneous

1 Irrigating tip, #21
1 Knife handle, #9
6 Medicine cups
Needles, 2 Hypodermic, (1) 23 gauge × 1″, (1) 25 gauge × ⅝″; 4 Retrobulbar, (2) 23 gauge, (2) 25 gauge
7 Syringes, Luer lok, (2) 5 ml and (5) 2 ml
1 Eye pad
2 Eye shields, 1 metal, 1 plastic

Special Notes

- **N.B.** *To avoid medication errors, labeling syringes, and medicine cups is mandatory.* The scrub person uses a skin marking pen and paper labels that have been steam sterilized.
- When steam-sterilizing (autoclaving) eye pads, leave them in their original wrapper (unopened) and place in the instrument tray prior to autoclaving.

Basic Eye Procedures Microscope Tray

Retractors

1 Eye speculum, Kratz-Berraquer, Castroviejo, or Lancaster, (Lancaster 8 cm length, 15 mm blade length, 35 spread)
1 Barraquer speculum, 3″, open, 20 mm
2 Desmarres lid retractors, (1) 5½″ × 12 mm and (1) 5½″ × 14 mm
1 Jameson muscle hook, small 5″ length, 9 mm × 1.3 mm blade
1 Stevens tenotomy hook, 5″
1 Green muscle hook, 5⅛″
1 Gass retinal detachment hook, 5⅗″

Forceps

2 Extra fine, 4″, serrated, 1 straight and 1 half-curved
1 Castroviejo W-H fixation, 0.3 mm tip
2 Castroviejo W-H suture, (1) 0.12 mm and (1) 0.5 mm tips
1 Troutman Barraquer, 0.12 mm tip
1 Jameson muscle, adult, left and right, 5″
1 McPherson or Kelman-McPherson suture, straight, 3½″
1 Bishop-Harmon, 1 × 2 teeth, 0.7 mm, 3⅜″ length
1 Lester fixation, 1 × 2 teeth, 3¾″ length
1 McCullough utility, serrated, 4″
4 Towel clips, piercing, (2) 3⅛″ and (2) 5″
4 Towel clips, nonpiercing, (2) 3⅛″ and (2) 5″

Scissors

1 Suture, 6¼″
1 Dolphin-nose Stevens, 3½ to 4½″
2 Carb-edge iris, 4½″, 1 straight, 1 curved
1 Barraquer-Dewecker iris, 5.5 cm
1 Westcott tenotomy, curved slightly right, 10.5 cm
1 Wescott stitch, curved slightly left, 10.5 cm

Clamps

5 Halsted mosquito, 5¼″, 2 straight and 3 curved
2 Serrefine clamps, straight, 1½″
1 Barraquer needle holder, curved with lock, 4¾″
1 Castroviejo standard needle holder, straight with lock, 4¾″
4 Towel clips, piercing, 3½″
2 Towel clips, nonpiercing, 3½″

Miscellaneous

1 Knife handle, #9
1 Knife handle #3KS, round, 4″
1 Jarit steel rule, 6″
1 Castroviejo caliper, straight, 3½″
1 Castroviejo blade breaker and holder, 5.5 cm
1 Scleral twist hook, 4¼″, right
6 Medicine cups
5 Syringes, Luer lok, (2) 5 ml, (3) 2 ml
2 Air injection cannulas, (1) 27 gauge and (1) 30 gauge

Basic Eye Muscle Procedures Tray

Retractors

1 Maumenee-Park speculum, solid, 8 cm
1 Barraquer speculum, wire, 1.3″ or 1.6″
3 Demarres lid, 5½″, (1) 12 mm, (1) 14 mm, and (1) 16 mm
1 Agrikola lacrimal sac (self-retaining), 4.5 cm
2 Stevens tenotomy hook, 13cm
2 Jameson muscle hooks, 1 small 5″ and 1 large 5¼″
3 Von Grafe strabismus hook, 5½″, 1 small, 1 medium, and 1 large

Forceps

1 McCullough utility forceps, serrated, 4″
1 Troutman-Barraquer forceps, 0.12 mm, tip
2 Jameson muscle, adult, 5″, 1 left and 1 right
2 Berens muscle, child, 9.8 cm, 1 left and 1 right
1 Jameson recession, 9.8 cm, 1 left and 1 right
3 Bishop-Harmon, 1 heavy, 3.5″, tip 0.3 mm, 1 fine, 3.5″, tip 0.5m, and 1 serrated, 3.5″, tip 0.3m
1 McPherson cornea, angled, 3½″
1 Lister fixation 8.5 cm
2 Castroviejo W-H suturing, (1) 0.12 mm, (1) 0.5 mm
1 Castroviejo W-H fixation, 0.3 mm

Scissors

1 Wescott tenotomy, straight, 4½″
1 Wescott stitch, curved, 4¼″
1 Wescott tenotomy, curved right, 4½″, or 1 Stevens tenotomy, curved right, 4½″
1 Carb-edge iris, 4½″
1 Suture (Troutman) 10 cm

Clamps

2 Halstead mosquito, curved, 5¼″
2 Serrefine clamp, straight, 1½″
1 Kalt eye needle holder, 12.5 cm, 14 cm
1 Castroviejo needle holder, standard straight with lock, 4¾″
1 Barraquer needle holder, curved without lock, 4¾″
4 Towel clips, piercing, (2) 3½″ and (2) 5″
4 Towel clips, nonpiercing, (2) 3⅛″ and (2) 5″

Miscellaneous

1 Knife handle, #9
1 Caliper, straight (Castroviejo), 3½″
1 Jarit steel rule, 6″

Eyelid and Conjunctival Procedures Tray

Retractors

2 Senn, 6″
4 Skin hooks, 6″ (2) single prong and (2) double-prong
1 Eye speculum (e.g., Barraquer, Lancaster), 3″ open 20 mm
1 Knapp lacrimal sac, 5½″
5 Desmarres lid, 14 cm length, (2) #1 13 mm, (1) #2 13 mm, and (2) #3 15mm
2 von Graefe muscle hooks, 14.4 cm length (1) #1 0.7 × 1 mm blade and (1) #3 10 × 1.5 mm blade
1 Chalazion clamp (Desmarres), 3¾″

Forceps

2 Fixation (e.g., Lester), 3¾″
2 Bishop-Harmon suturing, 3.5″, tip 0.3mm and 0.7mm
1 Castroviejo W-H suturing, 0.5 mm
2 Conjunctival, 1 with teeth, 1 serrated
1 Dressing, fine, serrated, 10 cm
1 Tying (e.g., Castroviejo), 11 cm
1 Lid (Green), 10 cm × 5 mm
1 Lambert chalazion, 3½″
1 Desmarres chalazion, medium, 3¾″
1 Entropion (Snellen), 35 mm × 9.5 cm, left and right
1 Jarit micro stitch, curved, 4″

Scissors

1 Westcott or Stevens tenotomy, 4⅛″
1 Vannas iridocapsulotomy, curved, 7.5 cm

1 McPherson vannas micro, 3″
1 Jarit micro stitch, curved, 4″

Clamps

2 Halstead mosquito, curved, 3½″
1 Jaeger lid plate, 4½″
1 Kalt needle holder, 12½ cm
1 Castroviejo needle holder, standard curved with lock, 5½″
4 Towel clips, piercing, (2) 3½″ and (2) 5″
4 Towel clips, nonpiercing, (2) 3½″ and (2) 5″

Miscellaneous

1 Knife handle, #9
1 3KS knife handle, round, 4″
1 Corneal knife (Gill), 4 mm blade
1 Beaver knife handle, 4″
1 Castroviejo caliper, straight, 3½″
3 Chalazion curettes, Meyerhoffer, (1) 1½″, (1) 2″, and (1) 2½″

Dacryocystorhinostomy Tray

Retractors

1 Maumenee-Park speculum, fenestrated blade, 8 cm
1 Knapp, 5″
2 Lacrimal sac, 4 prong (Knapp, Stevenson), 4 mm wide, 14 cm long
1 Lacrimal sac, self-retaining (Agrikola), 4.5 cm
3 Killian nasal speculum with set screw, 12½ cm length, with blades, (1) short, 6.5 cm, (1) medium, 7.5 cm, (1) long, 9 cm

Forceps

2 Bayonet, 7¼″
2 Jewelers bipolar forceps, straight, 10 cm and curved 11 cm
1 Extra-fine serrated, straight, 4″
1 Bishop-Harmon, 1 × 2 teeth, 0.7 mm, 8.6 cm
2 Castroviejo W-H suturing, 0.12 mm (1), and 0.5 mm (1)
1 McCullough utility forceps, serrated, 4″

Scissors

2 Carb-edge iris, 4½″, 1 curved and 1 straight
1 Stevens tenotomy, curved, 4⅛″
1 Westcott, straight, 4¼″
1 Westcott stitch, curved, 4¼″
1 Metzenbaum scissors, straight, 5″

Clamps

4 Halstead mosquito, 5″, 2 curved and 2 straight
2 Lid everters (Berens)
2 Webster needle holders, 12.5 cm
1 Castroviejo needle holder, standard straight with lock, $5\frac{1}{8}$″
4 Towel clips, piercing, (2) $3\frac{1}{2}$″ and (2) 5″
2 Towel clips, nonpiercing, (2) $3\frac{1}{2}$″ and (2) 5″

Suction Tubes or Tips

2 Frazier (with finger control and stylets), (1) #5 and (1) #7

Miscellaneous

1 Lacrimal trephine (Arruga)
1 Joseph periosteal elevator, curved and straight, $6\frac{1}{2}$″
1 Freer elevator, double ended, $7\frac{1}{2}$″
1 Key elevator, $\frac{1}{8}$″ wide × $6\frac{3}{4}$″ long
2 Lacrimal chisels, (1) 2 mm and (1) 4 mm
2 Lacrimal gouges, (1) 2 mm and (1) 4 mm
2 Lacrimal osteotomes, (1) 2 mm and (1) 4 mm
1 Mallet, small
2 Kerrison rongeurs, (1) 2 mm and (1) 4 mm
1 Lempert rongeur, delicate, curved, $7\frac{1}{2}$″
1 Takahashi straight nasal forcep, 5″
2 Blakesley nasal cutting forceps, 5″, (1) straight and (1) curved
1 Worst "pigtail" probe, 9.5 cm
6 Lacrimal probes (0000 to 000 to sizes 7 to 8)
3 Wilder lacrimal dilators, 4″ length, 1 short, 1 medium, and 1 fine tapers
1 Ruedemann lacrimal duct dilator
2 Jarit lacrimal duct cannulas, 1 straight and 1 curved, bulbous tip
1 Air-injection cannula, 27 gauge

Globe and Orbit Procedures Tray

Retractors

1 Eye speculum (Guyton-Park, Lancaster, 31 mm)
1 Schepens orbital, $5\frac{3}{4}$″
1 Lacrimal sac (Fink)
4 von Graefe muscle hook, 14 cm length, (2) #17 mm blade and (2) #3 10 mm blade
1 Jameson muscle hook, large, $5\frac{1}{4}$″
1 Converse alar, double-ended, 4″

Forceps

1 Extra-fine serrated, straight, 4″
2 Bishop-Harmon with 1 × 2 teeth 0.7 mm, 3½″ length
2 Lister fixation, 4¼″
2 Suturing (Castroviejo), 4″
2 Recession (Jameson) 3¾″, right and left

Scissors

1 Suture (Stevens)
2 Wescott, 4½″ 1 left, 1 right
2 Stevens tenotomy, 4⅛″, 1 straight, 1 curved
1 Enucleation, strong curve, 5

Clamps

4 Halstead mosquito, 5¼″, 2 curved, 2 straight
1 Crile, straight, 5½″
1 Right angle (Mixter), 6¼″
2 Tonsil (Schnidt), 7¼″
2 Needle holders, Barraquer 5⅛″, with lock and without lock
4 Towel clips, piercing, (2) 3½″ and (2) 5″
2 Towel clips, nonpiercing, (2) 3½″ and (2) 5″

Miscellaneous

1 Castroviejo blade breaker and holder, 5½″
1 Arruga orbital/elevator, 5¾″
1 Freer periosteal elevator, double ended, 6″
1 Cottle septum elevator, double ended, 9″
1 Bone cutter
1 Lacrimal sac chisel, 4mm × 6″
1 Mallet, small
2 Kerrison mastoid rongeurs, 1 up 40° × 6″ and 1 down 40° × 6″
1 Rongeur, single-action (Lempert), 7½″
1 Castroviejo enucleation snare
2 Evisceration spoons, Bunge, 1 large, 12 mm and 1 small, 8 mm
1 Wells enucleation spoon, 6″
1 Sphere introducer

Corneal Procedures Tray

Retractors

1 Maumenee-Park speculum, solid, 3¼″
1 Eye speculum, Lancaster, 3¼″
2 Muscle hook (Green, O'Connor, Jameson, von Graefe)
1 Sinskey reverse hook, blunt

Forceps

2 Bishop-Harmon, 8.6 cm length, 1 × 2 teeth, 0.7 mm and 0.3 mm
1 Castroviejo Colibri, 4¼″
2 Cohan corneal utility (Colibri style)
2 Castroviejo W-H suturing, (1) 0.12 mm and (1) 0.3 mm
2 Polack double corneal, 0.1 mm and 1.2 mm
1 McPherson suture, straight, 3½″
1 McPherson cornea, 3″
1 Charlie (coapts at distal tip)

Scissors

1 Curved suture, Gradle, 3¾″
2 Troutman-Castroviejo, mini, 1 right, 1 left
1 Castroviejo cornea BLT, curved
2 Castroviejo, mini, 1 right blade, 1 left blade
2 Katzin mini cornea, 1 right, 1 left
1 Straight iris (Barraquer-DeWecker)
1 Wescott tenotomy, right, 4½″
1 Wescott stitch, curved, 4¼″
1 Gills-Welch Vannas, 3⅜″

Clamps

5 Halstead mosquito, curved, 5″
1 Serrefine clamp, straight, 1½″
1 Barraquer needle holder, curved, with lock, 4¾″
2 Straight micro needle holder (Castroviejo, Barraquer)
1 Anis needle holder, with lock, 4¾″
4 Towel clips, piercing, (2) 3½″ and (2) 5″
4 Towel clips, nonpiercing, (2) 3½″ and (2) 5″

Miscellaneous

2 Trephine handles (Weck)
3 Trephine blades, (1) 7.5 mm, (1) 8.0 mm, and (1) 8.5 mm
1 Base plate with corneal Teflon® block
1 Iris spatula, Wecker, 30 × 2 mm
1 Paton spatula
1 Castroviejo or Wheeler cyclo spatula, silver, 5¼″
1 Castroviejo caliper, straight, 3¼″
1 Corneal knife (Gill), 4¾″
1 Paufique graft knife, angled, 4¾″
1 Corneal dissector (Troutman)
2 Corneal markers, Galand 3.0 mm to 8.0 mm
2 Air injection cannulas, (1) 27 gauge, (1) 30 gauge

Cataract Extraction and Lens Procedure Tray

Additional Trays

Basic Eye Microscope Procedures Tray
Specific Lens Procedure Tray and IOL Lens Implant

Retractors

- 2 Barraquer eye speculums, 1 child size, (open, 14 mm) 1 adult size, (open 20 mm)
- 1 Kuglen iris hook manipulator
- 1 Iris hook, blunt (Bonn), 4⅞″
- 1 Iris hook, IOL (Sinskey), 4¾″
- 1 Muscle hook (von Graefe or Green); von Graefe #1 14.4 cm length, 0.7 × 1 mm blade
- 1 Lens hook (Fenzl)
- 1 Micro lens hook (Sinskey)

Forceps

- 1 Bishop Harmon 1 × 2 T, 0.6 mm
- 1 Troutman, Troutman-Barrequer superior rectus, 0.3 mm
- 1 Castroviejo colibri, 4¼″
- 1 Curved iris (von Graefe)
- 1 Capsulotomy (Arruga), 4″
- 1 Serrefine, straight, 1½″
- 1 Bonn, 0.12 mm
- 1 Lens holding (Shepard or Clayman)
- 1 Straight tying (McPherson, Kelman-McPherson)
- 1 Curved tying (McPherson or Harms)
- 2 Suturing, Castroviejo, (1) 0.12 mm and (1) 0.5 mm
- 4 Towel clips, piercing, (2) 3½″ and (2) 5″
- 4 Towel clips, nonpiercing, (2) 3½″ and (2) 5″

Scissors

- 1 Tenotomy (Wescott) 4½″
- 1 Wescott stitch, curved, 4¼″
- 1 Straight iris (Barraquer-DeWecker), 5.5 cm
- 1 Vannas, Gills-Welsh capsulotomy, 3⅜″
- 1 Iridotocapsulotomy
- 1 Castroviejo cornea BLT, curved
- 2 Corneal Troutman, 1 left, 1 right, or 2 Castroviejo mini, 1 left, 1 right , 4″ length, 6 mm blade

Clamps

1 Serrefine clamp, straight, 1½″
1 Castroviejo needle holder with lock, standard straight
1 Barraquer needle holder without lock, curved, 4¾″
4 Towel clips, piercing, (2) 3½″ and (2) 5″
4 Towel clips, nonpiercing, (2) 3½″ and (2) 5″

Miscellaneous

1 Beaver knife handle, selected
1 Knife handle, #3 KS, round, 4″
1 Castroviejo blade breaker, 5½″
1 Jeweler's bipolar forceps, straight, 4″
1 Clayman guide 45D, 4½″
1 Lens loop (Gills-Welsh or New Orleans), 5″
1 Lens manipulator (Kugler)
1 Lens folder (2 parts)
1 Phacoemulsification tray, with I/A unit (e.g., McIntyre infusion set with connector and coaxial irrigation-aspiration system, Cavitron Phaco Emulsifier unit with AVIT ultrasonic hand piece with irrigation cystotome; Infiniti™ FMS ultrasound hand piece; Infiniti FMS Aqualase™ Liquefaction hand piece with polymer Aqualase tip and [disposable] micro smooth infusion-irrigation sleeve; Infiniti FMS Neosonix™ hand piece with linear ultrasonic motion with oscillatory sonic motion)
1 Olive-tip irrigator
1 Crescent knife
1 Corneal knife (Gill)
1 Kelman cystotome knife, 22 gauge, curved, 60°
1 Castroviejo caliper, straight, 3½″
1 Iris spatula (Wheeler)
1 Castroviejo cyclodialysis spatula or synechia spatula, 5½″
1 Hydrodissector hand piece and cannula (e.g., Santer)
1 Irrigating vectis loop, ½″
4 Syringes, Luer lok, (2) 5 ml and (2) 2 ml
2 Air or Healon injection cannulas, (1) 27 gauge and (1) 30 gauge

Glaucoma Procedures Tray

Retractors

1 Eye speculum (Barraquer, Lancaster)
1 Iris hook (Bonn)

Forceps

1 Corneal (Colibri, 0.12 mm)
1 Suturing (Castroviejo, 0.12 mm), 4″
1 Bonn, 0.1 mm
2 Suturing (Bishop-Harmon), 8.6 cm length 1 heavy 0.7 mm teeth, 1 fine, 0.3 mm teeth

Scissors

1 Westcott (blunt-tipped), 10.5 cm
1 Suture (Troutman)
1 Iris (Barraquer-DeWecker)
1 Strabismus (Knapp)
1 Iridocapsulotomy (Vannas)
1 Tenotomy (Westcott), 10.5 cm

Clamps

1 Kalt needle holder, 5¼″
1 Barraquer needle holder (curved, nonlocking), ¾″
4 Towel clips, piercing, (2) 3½″ and (2) 5″
4 Towel clips, nonpiercing, (2) 3½″ and (2) 5″

Miscellaneous

1 Beaver knife handle (selected)
1 Corneal knife (Gill)
1 Blade breaker (Castroviejo, Barraquer), 5½″
1 Tonometer (Schiotz), with 5.5, 7.5, 10, and 15 gram weights
1 Corneal dissector (Troutman)
1 Corneoscleral punch (Rumex)
2 Harms Trabeculotome, 1 right, 1 left
1 Kozlova glaucoma cutting board
1 Kozlova glaucoma polisher
1 Kozlova trabeculectomy flap marker
1 Kozlova glaucoma marker, 45°, angled blades, 4.00 mm
1 Castroviejo caliper, 3¼″
3 Castroviejo cyclodialysis spatula, (1) 5¼″, with blade 10 mm × 0.5 mm, (1) 0.75 mm, (1) 1 mm
1 Glaucoma draining device with introducing forceps (Titanium)
1 Kozlova glaucoma probe
1 Iris spatula (Wheeler)
1 Irrigating tip, #27
1 Air-injection cannula, 27 gauge

Basic Eye Procedures Microscope Tray

Retractors

1 Eye speculum (Barraquer, Lancaster)
5 Desmarres lids, (2) #1, (1) #2, (2) #3
2 Muscle hooks
1 Kuglen iris hook and lens manipulator

Forceps

2 Castroviejo suturing, (1) 0.12 mm and (1) 0.5 mm
1 Bishop-Harmon suturing, 8.6 cm
1 Fixation (Lester, von Graefe)
1 Corneal (Colibri 0.12 mm)
2 McPherson tying, 1 curved, 1 straight
2 Straight suture tying (Castroviejo)

Scissors

1 Suture (Troutman)
2 Castroviejo corneal, blunt tip, 1 left, 1 right, 10.1 cm length, 7 mm blade
2 Carb-edge iris, $4^1/_2''$, 1 curved, 1 straight
1 Suture iris (Barraquer-DeWecker)
1 Iridocapsulotomy (Vannas)
1 Intraocular vitrectomy scissors

Clamps

1 Barraquer needle holder, nonlocking, 110 mm length × 9 mm
2 Needle holders (Troutman-Barraquer), length 114 mm, smooth jaw 6 mm
4 Towel clips, piercing, (2) $3^1/_2''$ and (2) 5″
4 Towel clips, nonpiercing, (2) $3^1/_2''$ and (2) 5″

Miscellaneous

1 Knife handle, #9
1 Beaver knife handle (selected)
1 Iris spatula (Barraquer, Wheeler), e.g., Barraquer, 9.5 cm overall length, (1) 0.5 mm × 13 mm blade length or (1) 0.25 mm × 13 mm blade length
1 Corneal knife, Gill, flat, serrated handle, curved, (1) 3.5 mm × 121 mm or straight, (1) 3.5 mm × 121 mm

Retinal Procedures Tray

Retractors

1 Eye speculum (Weiner, Lancaster, or Guyton-Park), e.g., Guyton-Park, length 83 mm, (1) fenestrated blade, 14 mm with 48 mm blade spread or (1) solid blade 14 mm with 48 mm blade spread
1 Muscle hook, small, (von Graefe #1 or Jameson), e.g., Jameson, length 124 mm, with hook 9 mm × 1.3 mm
1 Stevens tenotomy hook, length 117 mm with hook 5 mm × 1 mm
1 Retinal detachment hook (Gass)
1 Des Marres lid, Size 2, 140-mm-length, 15-mm-wide blade
1 Arruga
1 Schepens

Forceps

1 Extra-fine serrated, straight, 4″
1 Bishop-Harmon 1 × 2 teeth, 0.5 mm, 8.6 cm length
1 Jewelers bipolar forceps, straight, 4″
1 Jameson muscle (recession), adult, angled left, 117 mm length, with (6) 1 mm teeth
1 Troutman-Barraquer, 0.12 mm
3 Castroviejo W-H, (1) 0.12 mm, (1) 0.3 mm, and (1) 0.5 mm
1 Watzke sleeve spread, 4½″
2 Suturing (Bishop-Harmon), 8.6 cm length 1 heavy 0.7 mm teeth, 1 fine, 0.3 mm teeth
1 McPherson suturing, straight, 3½″
1 McPherson cornea, angled, 3½″
2 Tying (McCollough, Alabama)
1 Fixation (Elshnig, von Graefe, or Lester), 3¾″

Scissors

2 Carb-edge iris, 4½″, 1 curved, 1 straight
1 Wescott tenotomy, 4½″, right
1 Stevens tenotomy, curved, 4⅛″
1 Wescott stitch, curved, 4¼″
1 McClure iris, angled, 4¼″
2 Stevens suturing, 1 straight, 1 curved

Clamps

5 Halstead mosquito, curved, 5¼″
1 Serrefine forceps, straight, 1½″

1 Castroviejo needle holder, standard straight with lock, $4^3/_4''$
1 Anis needle holder, curved with lock, $4^3/_4''$
1 Barraquer needle holder, Titanium, standard or with lock handle, 110 mm length × 9 mm
1 Kalt needle holder, $5^1/_4''$
4 Towel clips, piercing, $3^1/_2''$
2 Towel clips, nonpiercing, $3^1/_2''$

Miscellaneous

2 Beaver knife handles (selected)
1 Gill corneal knife, flat, serrated handle, curved, (1) 3.5 mm × 121 mm or straight, (1) 3.5 mm × 121 mm
1 Knife handle, #9
1 3KS knife handle, round, 4″
1 Tonometer (Schiotz), with 5.5, 7.5, 10, and 15 gram weights
1 Castroviejo blade breaker, $5^1/_2''$
1 Castroviejo caliper, straight, $3^1/_4''$
1 Scleral depressor (Schepens), thimble style, length 43 mm × 8 mm wide
3 Diathermy tips
2 Retinal probe, 1 straight, 1 curved
1 Retinal probe sleeve
2 Air injection cannulas, (1) 27 gauge and (1) 30 gauge

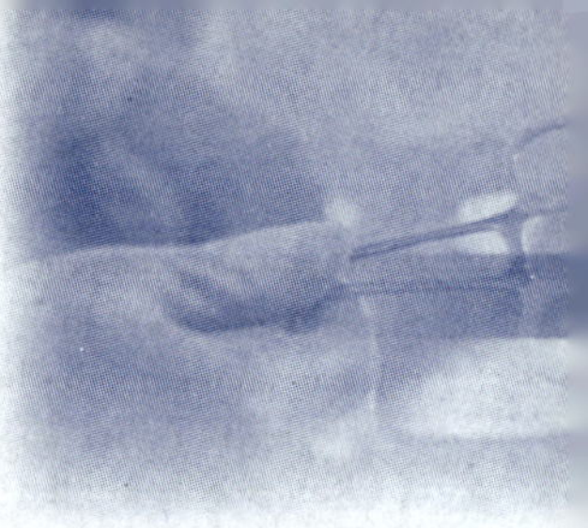

CHAPTER 42
Dental Instrument Trays

Dental Instruments for Extractions Tray

Additional Trays

Limited Procedures Trays
Tracheostomy Tray and various-sized tracheostomy tubes, available

Retractors

2 Senn, sharp, 6″
2 Joseph skin hook, sharp, 6″
1 Minnesota, large 15.5 cm
2 Jennings mouth gags, adult, (1) 4½″ and (1) 6″
1 Jennings mouth gag, child, 4″
3 McIvor tongue blades, 1 large #4, 1 medium #3, and 1 small #2.5
2 Weder tongue depressors, 1 large, 3.5 cm wide and 1 small, 2.8 cm wide
2 Toe-in retractors

Forceps

1 Bayonet, smooth, 7¼″
1 Cotton forceps or pliers, 11½″ to 12″, 14″to 14½″
1 Mandibular reduction
3 Dingman holding, 7″
1 Young tongue, 6¼″
1 Extracting (assorted sizes and configurations)

Scissors

1 Suture, 6¼″
1 Gingival (gum), e.g., Goldman Fox, 10.5–3.5 cm
1 Wire cutter and twister
1 Arch bar cutter

Clamps

4 Halstead mosquito, 5″, 2 curved and 2 straight
2 Allis, 6″
1 Wyman crown gripper and crown remover
2 Mayo-Haney needle holders
2 Towel clips, piercing, 3½″ and 5″
2 Towel clips, nonpiercing, 3½″ and 5″

Suction Tubes or Tips

1 Yankauer (suction tube and tip; 2 pieces), $10^3/_8''$
2 Frazier suction, straight (with fingertip control and stylets), 1 small (7Fr), 1 large (10Fr)
1 Frazier suction, curved, large

Miscellaneous

1 Bite block
1 Suture holder
1 Suture scissor, $6^1/_4''$
1 Bard-Parker scalpel, #3
1 Medicine cup
1 Disposable control syringe and needle (25 or 27 gauge), or 1 VibraJect® with shield
1 Dyna Surg irrigation-aspiration (I/A) hand piece (with 2 tubing clips, irrigation needle)
1 Periodontal probe
1 Periodontal knife
2 Periosteal elevators, 1 Seldin, 1 Joseph
1 Molt periosteal elevator, #9
1 Freer elevator, 9″
1 Explorer, 1 elevator, 1 excavator (assorted)
1 Set assorted picks (set of 5 or 7)
1 Scaler, Jacquette
2 Bone files
3 Curettes
1 Gracey curette
1 Lucas curette
1 Back-action hoe scaler
2 Kerrison rongeur, 6″, 3 mm tip, up and down biting
1 Depth gauge, marked with a scale (8–15 cm depth, 2.8–3.5 mm diameter)
1 Ruler, 6″
1 Gardner mallet
1 Gardner chisel
2 pliers, 1 wire bending, 1 needle nose
2 Thomas spatulas, 1 wax, 1 cement
1 Hollenback wax carver
1 Friedman Rongeur
1 Sharpening stone
2 Awls, 1 mandibular, 1 zygomatic
1 Dental mirror and handle (e.g., cone and stem)
Arch bars (cut to appropriate sizes)

Latex bands or retention bolsters
1 Coil stainless steel wire, 25 or 26 gauge
High-speed power dental drill hand piece, diamond drills and burrs, cord (with foot pedal)
Dental implant (prosthesis) with specific instrument system

Dental Restoration with Implant

Additional Trays

Add to Dental Instruments for Extractions Tray

Minor Orthopedic Procedures Tray
Tracheostomy Tray with tracheostomy tubes

Miscellaneous

Dyna Surg I or Dyna Surg II (Intl Dental) irrigation system with 3 hand pieces
Rotex® or Radiosurg®
High-speed fiber-optic dental drill with 3 hand pieces: HS Canister, Push Button, or Quick disconnect
Low-speed dental drill, Merus electric irrigation latch, and 3 contra-angle hand pieces
Cover screw/healing cap
Dental implant (prosthesis) with specific instrument system
Arch bar application

Instruments

Bite block
Yankauer and Frazier suction tips
Bayonet forceps
Weider tongue depressors (large and small)
Freer septal elevator
Probe
Wire cutter
Wire twister
Mayo-Heaney needle holders
Ruler (or calipers)
Needlenose pliers
Suture scissors

Temporomandibular Joint (TMJ) Procedures Instrument Tray

Add to Dental Instruments for Extractions Tray

Nasal Procedures Tray, available

Minor Orthopedic Procedures Tray
Tracheostomy Tray and tracheostomy tubes, available

Miscellaneous

1 Dingman mouth gag set
2 Sets osteotomes (curved, straight)
2 Sets chisels (curved, straight)
1 Bone clamp
High-speed dental reciprocating sagittal saw, blades, and cord
Diamond-coated cortical screws
1 Phillips screwdriver
Maxillofacial fixation plating system and instrumentation
TMJ implant (prosthesis) with specific instrument system

Orthognathic/Maxillofacial Procedures Instrument Tray

Add to Dental Instruments for Extractions Tray

Additional Trays
Nasal Procedures Tray,
Minor Orthopedic Procedures Tray, available
Tracheostomy Tray and various-sized tracheostomy tubes, available

Miscellaneous

High-speed dental reciprocating sagittal saw hand piece, blades, cord
Diamond-coated cortical screws
2 Sets osteotomes (curved, straight)
2 Sets chisels (curved, straight), 3–7 mm width, $5\frac{1}{2}$–$6\frac{3}{4}$″ length
1 Bone clamp
Maxillofacial fixation plating system and instrumentation
Distractor system
Alloplastic chin implant (prosthesis) and instrument system

Special Notes

- *For all instrument trays, include a wire cutter in addition to the one on the* ***Dental Extraction Instruments Tray.*** A disposable wire cutter must **always** accompany the patient (in whom jaws have been wired) in case of emergency (e.g., choking). Tape a disposable wire cutter to the top of the gurney.

CHAPTER 43

Pediatric Instrument Trays

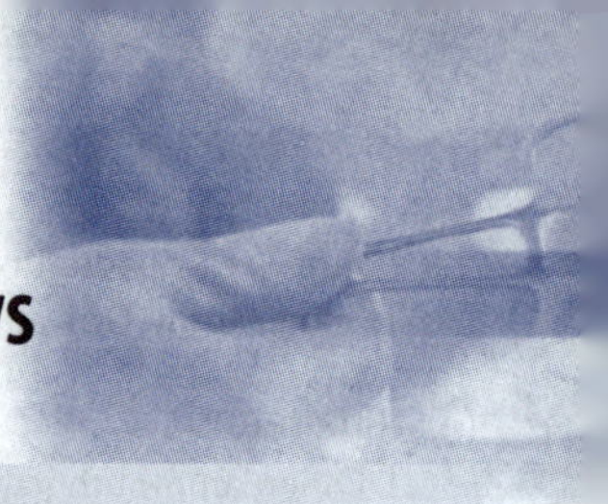

Pediatric Major Procedures Tray

Retractors

2 Senn, blunt, 6″
4 Gans, (2) #1 and (2) #2
2 Cushing vein, 9″
5 Malleable brain (spatulas), (1) ¼″, (1) ½″, (1) ¾″, (1) 1″
2 Deaver, small
2 Richardson, (1) ½″ × 1″, (1) 1″ × 1″
1 Heiss self-retaining, 4″
1 Balfour, infant with bladder blade (total opening, 3¾″ with 2.5 cm blades)

Forceps

1 Tissue with teeth, 6″
1 Wells tissue, 6″
2 Adson without teeth, 4¾″
2 Adson with teeth, 4¾″
1 Cushing without teeth, 7″
1 Cushing with teeth, 7″
4 DeBakey, fine, (2) 6″ and (2) 7¾″

Scissors

2 Straight Mayo, 6¼″
1 Curved Mayo, 5½″
3 Metzenbaum, curved, (1) 5¼″, fine tip, (1) 6″, and (1) 7″
1 Metzenbaum, straight, 6″
2 Potts, 25° angle, 5¼″ and 7″
1 Stevens tenotomy, 4½″
2 Iris, 1 curved, 1 straight, 4¾″

Clamps

16 Mosquito, 5¼″, 4 straight, 12 curved
10 Crile, 5½″, 4 straight, 6 curved
2 Pean, baby (delicate), 5⅛″
2 Pean, curved, 6″
4 Babcock, 5¾″
4 Allis, fine, (2) 5¾″ and (2) 6″
8 Kocher, 5½″, (4) straight (4) curved

2 Kocher-Lovelace, fine
2 Tonsil (Schnidt), 7½″
4 Right-angle, (2) 5½″ and (2) 7½″
1 Ruler, 6″
2 Webster needle holders, 4½″
2 Crile needle holders, 5⅛″
4 Towel clips, piercing, (2) 3½″ and (2) 5″
4 Towel clips, nonpiercing, (2) 3½″ and (2) 5″
4 Sponge forceps (Foerster), 7″

Suction Tubes or Tips

1 Poole with sheath (2 pieces), 9¼″
1 Andrews with tip (2 pieces), 9½″
1 Frazier (with finger control and stylet), 7Fr

Miscellaneous

5 Knife handles, (2) #3, (1) #7, (1) #9, and (1) Beaver
1 Ballinger elevator, 8¼″, blade ¼″
1 Elevator dissector
1 Elevator probe
1 Ruler, 6″

Pediatric Minor Procedures Tray

Retractors

2 Senn, blunt, 6″
2 Gans, #1

Forceps

2 Tissue without teeth, 6″
2 Adson without teeth, 4¾″
2 Adson with teeth, 4¾″
2 DeBakey, 6″

Scissors

2 Straight Mayo, 6¼″
2 Metzenbaum, curved, fine tip, (1) 5½″ and (1) 6″
1 Straight Metzenbaum, 5¼″
1 Stevens tenotomy, 4½″
2 Iris, 1 curved, 1 straight, 4″

Clamps

8 Mosquito, 5¼″, 2 straight and 6 curved
8 Crile, 5½″, 2 straight and 6 curved

2 Tonsil (Schnidt), 7½″
2 Right-angle, 5½″
2 Babcock, baby, 5½″
2 Webster needle holder, 4½″
4 Towel clips, piercing, (2) 3½″ and (2) 5″
4 Towel clips, nonpiercing, (2) 3½″ and (2) 5″

Miscellaneous

1 Medicine cup
3 Knife handles, (2) #3 and (1) #7

Pediatric Gastrointestinal Procedures Tray

Additional Trays

Pediatric Major Procedures Tray

Clamps

2 DeBakey peripheral vascular, straight, 7½″
2 DeBakey, 60°, multipurpose, 8½″
2 Pean, straight, 6″

Forceps

2 DeBakey, extra-delicate tissue, 7¾″ S

Special Note

- For **Pediatric Laparoscopic/Endoscopic Instruments,** refer to the specific procedure.
- Automatic (disposable) stapling devices with staples, e.g., end-to-end anastamosis (EEA) should be available in the room.
- During pediatric gastrointestinal surgery, ligating clip appliers, e.g., Hemoclip™ appliers, and assorted-size clip appliers with clip cartridge, small, medium, medium large, and large clips should be available in the room.
- For pediatric laparoscopic and endoscopic surgeries, Multi-Fire™ Endo clips, Endo Stitch (or similar), should be available in the room.

Pediatric Thoracotomy Tray

Retractors

2 Finochietto rib, infant size, total opening, (1) 2 ½″ and (1) 3½″
1 Finochietto rib (4 blades), child size, total opening, 6″

Miscellaneous

1 Freer elevator
2 Langenbeck periosteal elevators, (1) 1/4″ and (1) 11/16″
1 Beyer double-action rongeur, 7″
1 Bailey rib contractor, 6 3/4″

Special Notes

- **Pediatric Thoracotomy** is avoided whenever the surgery can be accomplished thoracoscopically. A **Pediatric Thoracotomy Tray** must always be available in the room in case the **thoracoscopy** must be converted to an **open thoracotomy**. Ligating clip appliers, e.g., Weck or Hemoclip appliers, assorted-size clip appliers with clip cartridge, small and medium clips; large clips, to be available in the room.
- Automatic small, disposable, stapling devices with staples, e.g., gastrointestinal anastomosis (GIA™), end-to-end anastomosis EEA™) should be available in the room.
- For **Pediatric Thoracoscopic Instruments,** refer to Instrumentation within **Pediatric Thoracoscopy**, p. 1081.

Bibliography

Chapter 1 Perioperative Care of the Patient

Adams, James D. Herbal Drug Interactions. USC School of Pharmacy. Personal Communication (lecture, Medical Center of Tarzana, Nov 3, 2003), JAdams@hsc.usc.edu

Beyea, Suzanne C. Patient Identification: A Crucial Aspect of Patient Safety. AORN J, Sept 2003, 78:478

Clavreul, Genvievève M. Being the Patient Advocate: What Does It Really Mean? Working Nurse, Sept 13–Oct 4, 2004, pp. 6–10

Fortunato, Nancymarie. Berry & Kohn's Operating Room Technique, ed IX. Mosby, 2000

Fortunato, Nancymarie. Berry & Kohn's Operating Room Technique, ed IX. Chapter Two: Foundations of Patient Perioperative Care. Mosby, 2000

Newhouse, Robin P., et al. Perioperative Nurses and Patient Outcomes: Mortality, Complications, and Length of Stay. AORN J, 2005, 81:508–526

Nicoll, Leslie H. Patient Advocacy. Advance for Nurses, July 11, 2005, vol 12, no 11

Nurses Push Protocol. AORN Connections: Special Edition, Sept 2004, pp. 14–15

Patient Partners and Advocates. Nursing Spectrum. Nurse Week, 2005. Specialty Guide for the Perioperative Nurse, pp. 14–16

Perioperative and Intraoperative Records Format and West Hills Hospital, West Hills, California. 2002 Northridge Hospital Medical Center, Northridge, California

Post Anesthesia Care Unit (PACU) Guidelines: 2001, West Hills Hospital, West Hills, California

Rothrock, Jane C. Alexander's Care of the Patient in Surgery, ed XII. Supplementary Information Incorporating AORN Standards, Practice Guidelines, and Recommendations for Perioperative Care of the Patient in Surgery, Both Nursing and Technical. Mosby, 2003

Rothrock, Jane C. Concepts Basic to Perioperative Nursing. Alexander's Care of the Patient in Surgery, ed XII. Mosby, 2003, p. 1–39

Rutherford, Colleen J. Differentiating Surgical Instruments. F.A. Davis, 2005

Tighe, Shirley M. Instrumentation for the Operating Room, ed VI. Mosby, 2003

Surgical Consent and Sterilization Consent Formats:

2004 California Healthcare Association, Health and Safety Code Section 1690

2001 Department of Health Services, State of California Health and Welfare Agency

2001 West Hills Hospital, West Hills, California
2005 Encino-Tarzana Regional Medical Center, Tarzana, California

Surgical Preoperative Assessment and Checklist Formats:

1999 UCLA Medical Center, Los Angeles, California
2001 West Hills Hospital, West Hills, California
2002 Encino-Tarzana Regional Medical Center, Tarzana, California

Anesthesia Record Format:

2001 West Hills Hospital, West Hills, California
2001 Encino-Tarzana Regional Medical Center, Tarzana, California
Caruthers, Bob, et al. Surgical Technology for the Surgical Technologist, Delmar, 2001

Chapter 2 Protection of the Patient in Surgery/Patient Safety

AORN Correct Site Surgery Tool Kit. AORN supplied to members
AORN Guidance Statement. Safe Medication Practices in Perioperative Practice Settings, Mar 2002
Artificial Nails Should Not Be Worn. Standards, Recommended Practices, and Guidelines With Official AORN Statements. AORN, Inc, Denver, 2003
Berk, Beth. Taking Off the Gloves. Nurse Week, January 13, 2003, p. 12–13
Chyna, Julie. Time Out! Advocates: Nursing Spectrum. Nurse Week, 2005, p. 62–65, Specialty Guide: Perioperative Nurse
Clavreul, Geneviève M. Universal Precautions. Working Nurse, Aug 2, 2004
Collaborative Instrumentation Standards; Fire Protection Standards; Sterilizers; Medical Gas Fittings; Borrowing Instruments. Association for the Advancement of Medical Instrumentation (AAMI) Standards for Instrument Care, www.redorbit.com/news/health/288898/collaborative_instrumentation_standards_fire_protection_standards_sterilizers_medical_gas_fittings/?source=r_health_
Comparison of Correct Site Processes, AORN Connections. June 2003, vol 1, no 6, p. 12–13
Correct Site Surgery. AORN Connections. Dec 2003, vol 1, no 13, p. 1–4
Correct Site Surgery. AORN Connections. Apr 2004, vol 4, no 2, p. 1
Croteau, Rick. JCAHO Protocol to Eliminate Wrong-Site, Wrong-Procedure, Wrong Patient Surgery. Personal Communication, Dec 5, 2003, Medscape Medical News

Domrose, Cathryn. Senior Surgery Outcomes Improving for Elderly Patients. Nurse Week, Oct 24, 2004, vol 18, no 22, p. 10–11

Dunn, Deborah. Incident Reports: Their Purpose and Scope. AORN J, July 2003, 78:46

Dunn, Deborah. Reprocessing Single-Use Devices. AORN J, May 2002, 75:989

Evacuation of Laser Plume. Healthcare Epidemiology Policies and Procedures. University of Texas Medical Branch (UTMB), Revised 2003, pp. 1–3

Fire Safety in the OR. Reprint from Bulletin of American College of Surgeons. Aug 1997, vol 82, no 8

Fortunato, Nancymarie. Surgical Positions. Berry & Kohn's Operating Room Technique, ed IX. Mosby, 2000, p. 491–499

Hand Cleaning Policies (Related to Hand Hygiene, Surgical Scrub, Artificial Nails, etc.). Tenet California Health System Memorandum, Dec 8, 2003

JCAHO Sets Patient Safety Goals for '05. Nurse Week, Aug 9, 2004

Joint Commission Releases 2005 Safety Goals. AORN Connections, pp. 1, 8–9

Joint Commission Resources. Patient Safety Special Report, 2005. Joint Commission National Patient Safety Goal: Practice Strategies and Helpful Solutions for Meeting these Goals

Lafreniere, Rogier, et al. Preparation of the Operating Room. ACS Surgery Principles and Practice, 2003. Medscape, updated 10/14/03, www.medscape.com/view article462684

Larkin, Brenda. The Ins and Outs of Body Piercing. AORN J, Feb 2004, 79:333

Lopes, Rosimeire. A Review of Latex Sensitivity Related to the Use of Latex Gloves in Hospitals. AORN J, July 2004, 80:64

Lorenz, JM. Developing Patient Education Materials. Advance for Nurses, 1:15–17, 2004

Low-Temperature Gas Plasma: A New Sterilization Technology. Dupont, www.tyvek.com/na/medical pack/english/techinfo/95-1ste.html

Low-Temperature Hydrogen Peroxide Gas Plasma Sterilization. The Sterrad System, www.communicore.com/downloads/approd.txt

Low-Temperature Oxidative Sterilization Methods for Sterilizing Medical Devices. Nov 2001, www.p2pays.org/ref/20/19926/p2_opportunity_handbook/12_3.html

Macilquham, Michael. Identifying Lost Surgical Needles Using Radiographic Techniques. AORN J, July 2003, 78:73

Module Virtual Reality Surgical Suite Module 2004. US Department of Labor, Occupational Safety & Health Administration, www.osha.gov/SLTC/etools/hospital/surgical/surgical.html

Paulson, Daryl S. Efficacy of Preoperative Antimicrobial Skin Preparation on Biofilm Bacteria. AORN J, 2005, 81:492–500

Paulson, Daryl S. Hand Scrub Products: Performance Requirements vs. Clinical Relevance. AORN J, 2004, 80:225

Perioperative Disaster Preparedness Resource Manual. AORN, Inc, Denver, 2003
Positioning Guidelines, 2000–2006. University Hospitals of Cleveland Department of Anesthesia, www.uhcaneanesthesia.com
Preparation of the Operating Room. ACS Surgery Principles and Practice, 2003, WebMD, Inc
Preventing Venous Thromboembolism. OR Insider, Nov 2005, pp. 24–26
Recommended Practices for Electrosurgery. AORN J, Mar 2005, 81:616–638
Reyes, Suzanne C. Counting Instruments and Sponges. AORN J, Aug 2003, 78:290
Rothrock, Jane C. Surgical Positions. Alexander's Care of the Patient in Surgery, ed XII. Mosby, 2003, p. 176–179, 181–184
Rusynko, B. and Perry-Ewald, J. Keeping Patients Safe: Procedure and Site Verification and Pre-Procedural Pause. AORN J, 2004, 79:787
Schultz, Alyce. Predicting and Preventing Pressure Ulcers in Surgical Patients. AORN J, May 2005, 81:986
Smart PACU. Innovation for the Medical Environment. ConMed Integrated Systems. 2004, www.conmedis.com/products/smartpacu.html
Surgical Positions. Dorland's Medical Dictionary, ed XXVIII. Saunders, pp. 1338
Surgical Positions. Taber's Cyclopedic Medical Dictionary, ed XX. F.A. Davis, 2001, p. 1736–1737
The Risk of the Rings. Nursing Spectrum. Nurse Week, Specialty ed, Spring 2004
The Three R's (Right Site, Right Procedure, Right Patient). Nurse Week, July 26, 2004
Two AORN Groups Address Safety Issues. AORN Connections. July 2004, p. 12
Watters, James, et al. The Elderly Surgical Patient. 2004, www.acssurgery.com/abstract/acs/acs0801.htm
2006 Position Statements (Regarding Safety Issues). AORN Connections Practice Issues Special Edition. Feb 2006, vol 4, no 2

Chapter 3 Safety Measures for Operating Room Personnel

AORN Guidance Statement: Safe Medication Practices in Perioperative Settings. AORN J, Mar 2004, vol 79, no 3, p. 674
AORN Takes a Stand on Practice Issues. AORN Connections, Mar 2005, vol 3, no 3
Cuming, Richard. Reducing the Hazards of Exposure of Cornstarch Glove Powder. AORN J, Aug 2002, 76:288
Evacuation of Laser Plume. Healthcare Epidemiology Policies and Procedures. University of Texas Medical Branch (UTMB), Online Documentation, Revised 2003
Goulette, Candy. Safety First. Advance for Nurses, Oct 14, 2004, vol 1, no 7, pp. 22–24
Habel, Maureen. Document It Right. Nurse Week, Jan 13, 2003, p. 20–22

High Tech Helpers: Changing the Lives of Patients and Nurses. Nurse Week, Specialty Guide Perioperative Nurse, 2005, p. 22–24

Hughes, Karen J. Backing Up Nurses (Strategies to Reduce Injuries). Advance for Nurses, Southern California, vol 3, no 8, p. 35–36

Icon, Erica. Relax, Your Job Depends on It. Working Nurse, Sept 13–Oct 4, 2004, p. 20–21

Icon, Erica. Overtime: Knowing When to Say When. Working Nurse, Oct 4–Oct 25, 2004, p. 32–35

JCAHO Requirement. Joint Commission Resources: Emergency Management Standards-EC.1.4 and EC.2.9.1, Jan 1, 2003

Latex Allergy: Perioperative Aspects. Department of Anesthesia University Hospital of Cleveland, www.uuhcanesthesia.com/guidelines/latex/

McCarthy, Patricia M. and Gaucher, Kenneth A. Fire in the OR! A Plan for Safety. AORN J, Mar 2004, 79:588–600

Nunnelee, Jance. Needlesticks (suppl). What You Must Know. RN Professional Journal, Nov 2005, vol 68, no 11, p. 32–36

Nurse's Assistant® OR Control System. ConMed Integrated Systems, 2004, www.conmedis.com/products/na.html

Preventing Surgical Fires. AORN Connections, Sept 2003

Salmon, Liane. Fire in the OR: Prevention and Preparedness. AORN J, July 2004, 80:42–44

Sawicki, Jack. Protection From Chemical and Biological Warfare. GEOMET® Technologies, LLC, Surgical Services Management (publication of AORN). Sept 1999, www.aorn.org/ssm/

Smart OR™ Nurse's Station. ConMed Integrated Systems, 2004, www.conmeds.com/products/ns.html

Specialty Guide Perioperative Nurse, www.NAPPSI.org

Wide. Hazards Module. U.S. Department of Labor. Occupational Safety & Health Administration Health Care, p. 1–10, www.osha.gov/SLTC/etools/hospital/hazards/hazards.html

Wilder, Jan. High Tech Helpers: Eliminating Suture Needlesticks Through Primary Prevention. Nursing Spectrum. Nurse Week, 2005, p. 32–35

Chapter 4 Anesthesia Modalities

Backman, Steven, et al. Perioperative Considerations for Anesthesia, www.acssurgery.com/abstract/acs/acs0103.htm

Coby, Lisa R. New Reusable Laryngeal Mask. Mar 29, 2006, www.ambuusa.com/ambuus/final.nsf/(docshortname)/uswebsitemain8c4fe3f9dmain

Dantrium® (dantrolene sodium). Proctor & Gamble Pharmaceuticals, 2006, www.pgpharmaceuticals.com

Emergency Therapy for Malignant Hyperthermia (wall chart), revised 1999. Malignant Hyperthermia Association of the U.S. (MHAUS), www.mhaus.org

Fortunato, Nancymarie. General Anesthesia: Techniques and Agents. Berry & Kohn's Operating Room Technique, ed IX. Mosby, 2000, p. 397–421

Hommertvheim, Ruth and Steinke, Elaine. Malignant Hyperthermia: The Perioperative Nurse's Role. AORN J, 81:83, pp. 151–164

Kleinman, Wayne. Anesthesia Modalities, Anesthetic Agents, and Ancillary Use of Pharmacologic Agents. Personal Communication, 2005

Litman, Ronald S. and Rosenberg, Henry. Malignant Hyperthermia: Update on Susceptibility Testing. JAMA, 2005, 293:2918–2924

Litman, Ronald S., et al. Malignant Hyperthermia (Critical Review). Medscape Critical Care, Oct 2004

Malignant Hyperthermia, www.mhaus.org

Miller, Ronald (ed). Anesthesia, ed VI, vol 1 (multiple citations). Elsevier, Churchill Livingstone Division of Harcourt Brace, 2003

Neuromonitoring Guides: Anesthesia Reduces Awareness During Surgery. Medscape Article 479507 from Lancet, 2004, 363:1747, 1757–1763

Rothrock, Jane C. Anesthesia. Alexander's Care of the Patient in Surgery, ed XII. Mosby, 2003, p. 219–250

Chapter 5 General Anesthesia

ASA Practice Parameters, Guidelines, Statements. Department of Anesthesia, University Hospital of Cleveland, www.uhcanesthesia.com/guidelines/

Kleinman, Wayne. General Anesthesia Considerations. Personal Communication, 2005

Miller, Ronald (ed). Anesthesia, ed VI, vol 1 (multiple citations). Elsevier, Churchill Livingstone Division of Harcourt Brace, 2003

Propofol Administration. AORN Online: Clinical Issues. Nov 2004

Rothrock, Jane C. General Anesthesia. Alexander's Care of the Patient in Surgery, ed XII. Mosby, 2003, p. 230–239

Chapter 6 Conduction Anesthesia

Consideration for Policy Guidelines for Registered Nurses Engaged in the Administration of Sedation and Analgesia Adopted by AANA Board of Directors. June 1996, Revised June 2003

Fortunato, Nancymarie. Local and Regional Anesthesia. Berry & Kohn's Operating Room Technique, ed IX. Mosby, 2000, p. 423–438

Kleinman, Wayne. Methods of Conduction Anesthesia. Personal Communication, 2005

Kosta, Michael. Administration of Conscious Sedation/Analgesia. Nursing Spectrum, Perioperative Specialty Edition, 2004, www.nursingspectrum

Rothrock, Jane C. Regional (Conduction) Anesthesia. Alexander's Care of the Patient in Surgery, ed XII. Mosby, 2003, p. 239–246

Chapter 7 Laser Technology

Anderson, Karen. Safe Use of Lasers in the OR: What Perioperative Nurses Should Know. AORN J, Jan 2004, 79:171–187

Ball, Kay. Lasers: The Perioperative Challenge, ed III. Mosby, 1995

Guidelines for Laser Safety and Hazard Assessment (OSHA). Jan 5, 2001, www.osha.gov/pls/oshaweb/owadisp.show_document?p_table=directives&p_id=1705

Laser Surgery and Laser Safety Precautions. Alexander's Care of the Patient in Surgery, ed XII. Mosby, 2003, p. 78–86

Medical Lasers. Shore Laser Center, Oct 25, 2004, www.shorelaser.com/aboutlasersmed.htm

Ngyuen, Ann. Photodynamic Therapy With Porfimer Sodium (Photofrin™) Laser, www.meniscus.com/web/publications/hl/arth_151.html

Photodynamic (Laser) Therapy. Mar 2000 (revised), www.cancer.org/docroot/cr1/content/cri_2_6xphotodynamictherapy.asp?sitearea=cri.view

Standards of Perioperative Clinical Practice in Laser Medicine and Surgery, www.aslms.org/health/standards_perioperative.html

Troust, D, et al. Surgical Laser Properties and Their Tissue Interaction. Mosby Year Book, 1992, p. 131–162

U.S. Department of Labor Guidelines for Laser Safety and Hazard Assessment. Safe Use of Lasers in Health Care Facilities. z136.3–2005, Jan 5, 2005, www.osha.gov/pls/oshaweb/owadisp.show_document?p_table=directives&p_id=1705

Chapter 8 Endoscopy: A Minimal Access Approach

Ball, Kay. Endoscopic Surgery. Mosby, 1997, p. 33, 46, 86–99, 111, 146

Bragg, K, et al. Trends in Minimally Invasive Surgery. AORN J, Dec 2005, 82:1005–1020

Darzi, Ara. Recent Advances in Minimal Access Surgery. British Medical Journal, 2002, 324:31–34, www.bmj.com/czi/content/ful/324/7328/31

Levitt, Marc A and Singh, Kirpal. Minimal Access Surgery. eMedicine, Mar 28, 2006, www.emedicine.com/ped/topic2977.htm

Chapter 9 Robotics

Aesop Surgical Systems® (Robotic), http:www.computermotion.com/aesop.html

Anvari, Mehran, et al. Establishment of the World's First Telerobotic Remote Surgery Service. Annals of Surgery, 2005, 241:460

DaVinci Surgical Systems® (Robotic). Intuitive Surgical, www.intuitivesurgical.com/products/indexaspx

Domrose, Cathryn. Working Smart: Advances in OR Technology. Nursing Spectrum. Nurse Week, Mar 8, 2004, www.Nurseweek.com/NEWS/FEATURE/04–03/OR.asp

Hermes Intelligent Operating Room®, www.trueforce.com/medical_robotics/medical_robotics_companies_hermes.htm

Kaul, Sanjeev. Laparoscopic and Robotic Radical Prostectomy. eMedicine, Feb 28, 2005, www.emedicine.com/med/topic3723.htm

Lanfranco, Anthony, et al. Robotic Surgery. Annals of Surgery, 2004, 239:14

Reger, T. B. and Janhke, M. E. Robotic Cardiac Surgery. AORN J, 2003, 77:182

Robotic Cardiac Surgery. Department of Cardiothoracic Surgery, USC, http://www.cts.usc.edu/rsi-cardiacsurgery.html

Robotics and Technology. Wikipedia, Nov 2006, http://en.wikipedia.org/wiki/robotic_surgery

Robotics: The Future of Minimally Invasive Heart Surgery, www.biomed.brown.edu/courses/b1108/b1108_2002_groups/heart_surgery/robotics.html

Talamini, Mark A. and Hanly, Eric J. Technology in the Operating Suite. JAMA, Feb 16, 2005, vol 293, no 7

Zeus Surgical Systems® (Robotic), http:www.computermotion.com/zeus.html

Chapter 10 Microsurgery

AROSurgical™ Microsurgery Product Line. Handheld microinstrument sets, Bear single-use micro vessel clamps, sterile suture, nonsterile suture, www.arosurgical.com/index.ctm?cfid=114488&cftoken=42656870

Gilbert, Bruce. Microsurgical Equipment and Instrumentation, www.brucegilbertmd.com/publications/chapters/BRGmicro.html

Microsurgery. Encyclopedia of Surgery: A Guide for Patients and Caregivers. 2006, www.surgeryencyclopedia.com/la-pa/microsurgery.html

Microsurgery. Campbell's Operative Orthopedics, ed X. Mosby, 2003, p. 3288–3317

Williams, Keith D and Park, Ashley L. Lower Back Pain and Disorders of the Intervertebral Discs (Microdiscectomy). Campbell's Operative Orthopedics, ed X. Mosby, 2003, p. 1982–2013

Chapter 11 Harmonic Scalpel and Plasma Scalpel

Harmonic Scalpel®. Gateway Products Information and Ultrasonic Cutting and Coagulation Devices. Johnson & Johnson, 2001–2006, Ethicon Endo-surgery, Inc, www.harmonicscalpel.com

Harmonic Scalpel®. Intermedix International Experts, Inc, www.armonic-scalpelrepaircenter.com/harmonic.html

Link, W. J. A Plasma Scalpel: Comparison of Tissue Damage and Wound Healing With Electrosurgical and Steel Scalpels. Arch Surg, Apr 1976, 111(4):392–397, www.ncbi.nlm.nih.gov/entrez/query.fcgi?cmd=retrieve&db=pubmed&list_uids=1259576&

Minimally Invasive Techniques Gradually Gain Ground in Ear, Nose, and Throat Surgery. Virtual Medical Worlds Monthly. Dec 15, 1998

Siperstein, Allan E., et al. Use of Harmonic Scalpel® vs Conventional Knot Tying for Vessel Ligation in Thyroid Surgery. Arch Surg, 2002, 1337:137–142

Chapter 12 Argon Beam Coagulator

Application of Argon Beam Coagulation in Plastic Surgery. Perspectives in Plastic Surgery, 1991, 5:91–98

Argon Beam Coagulator®. Conmed® Argon Beam Technology System 7500®

Marino, Ignazio RA. New Option for Patients Facing Liver Resection Surgery. 2006 Plasma Surgical Limited, www.plasmasurgical.com/article–Marino.htm

Chapter 13 Radiofrequency Ablation

Cronin, Colleen. Radiofrequency Catheter Ablation for Atrial Fibrillation. eMedicine, http://healthinfo/cedars-sinai-edu/library/healthguide/en-us/illness/topic.asp?hwid-H159948

Greenberg, Mark L. and Chandrakanton, Arvind. Radiofrequency Catheter Ablation. eMedicine, Aug 26, 2006, www.com/med/topic2957.htm

Radiofrequency Catheter Ablation (RFA). Society of Interventional Radiology, www.sirweb.org/patpub/radiofrequencyablation.shtml#4

Williams, Jason. Radiofrequency Ablation: A Minimally Invasive Technique for Treating Cancer, www.cancerlynx.com/rfa.html

Chapter 14 Integumentary and Minimally Invasive Surgery

Larson, Shawn D., et al. Vascular Access: Surgical Perspective. eMedicine, updated Oct 20, 2006, www.emedicine.com/ped/topic3050.htm

Scott-Conner, Carol E. H. and Radebold, Klaus. Lipomas. eMedicine, updated Apr 17, 2006, www.emedicine.com/med/topic 2720.htmøp

Veys, Nic, et al. Percutaneous Dialysis Catheters vs Surgical Placement. Oxford Journals, 2002, www.ndt.oxfordjournals.org/cgi/content/full/17/2/210

Chapter 15 Breast Surgery

Barclay, Laura. Outcomes Comparable in Skin-Sparing Mastectomy, Modified Radical Procedures. Medscape from WebMD, Jul 3, 2003, www.medscape.com/viewarticle/458204?mpid=15685

D'Amours, Amy. Lymph Node Biopsy and Lymphoscientigraphy. Surgical Technologist Jan 2003, 35:7–15

Harlow, Seth, et al. Lymphatic Mapping and Sentinel Node Biopsy. American College of Surgery: Principles and Practice, Medscape, Jan 30, 2005, www.medscape.com/viewarticle/498442?src-mp

Kellar, Stephanie. Sentinel Lymph Node Biopsy for Breast Cancer. AORN J, Aug 2001, 74:197

Sardi, Armando, et al. The Benefit of Using Two Techniques for Sentinel Node Mapping in Breast Cancer. The American Surgeon, 2002, 68:24

Tuttle, Todd, et al. Subareolar of Tc^{99} Facilitates Sentinel Lymph Node Identification. Annals of Surgical Oncology 2002, 9:77–81

Veitz, Alice. Breast Cancer and Genetic Testing. Advance for Nurses, 7/25/05, vol 2, no 12

Chapter 16 Abdominal Extraintestinal Surgery

Ballantyne, Garth H. (ed). Atlas of Laparocopic Surgery. WB Saunders, May 5, 2000

Cook® Surgical. Nathanson Liver Retractors, www.cookgroup.com/cook_surgical/features/nlrs.html

Erickson, Richard A. Pancreatic Cancer. eMedicine, Dec 15, 2005, www.emedicine.com/med/topic1712.htm

Extracorporeal Shock Wave Lithotripsy of Gallstones. Shackelford's Surgery of the Alimentary Tract. Saunders, 1996, p. 240–241

Keefe, Sandy. Cell Salvaging. Advance for Nurses, May 30, 2005, vol 2, no 8

Lingvay, Ildik and Aung, K. Amebic Hepatic Abscess. eMedicine, Nov 2004, www.emedicine.com/med/topic2662.htm

Mulagha, E. and From, H. J.. Extracorporeal Shock Wave Lithotripsy of Gallstones Revisited: Current Status and Future Promises. J Gastroenterology Hepatology, 2000, 15:239

Nathanson Liver Retractors (Cook® Surgical), www.cookgroup.com/cook_surgical/features/nlrs.html

Nyhus, Lloyd, et al. Liver Surgery, Mastery of Surgery, ed III. Little, Brown and Co, 1997, p. 1080–1082

Pankaj, Chaturved and Chamberlain, Ronald S. Carcinoma of the Ampulla Vater. eMedicine, Sept 2005, www.emedicine.com/topic2676.htm

Pofahl, Walter E. and Di Palma, Jack A. Acalculous Cholecystopathy. eMedicine, 1, Nov 15, 2005, www.emedicine.com/med/topic347.htm#section~treatment

Radiofrequency Catheter Ablation (Liver Metastases), www.sirweb.org/patpub/radiofrequencyablation.html

Rau, J., et al. Jet-Cutting Supported by High Frequency Current: New Technique for Hepatic Surgery. World J Surgery, 1997, 2:254

Sawyer, Micheal H. and Telian, Simon. Pseudocyst, Pancreatic. eMedicine, Sept 20, 2002, www.emedicine.com/radio/topic576.htm

Wolf Corp. Laparoscopic Equipment and Instruments. 2004, www.richardwolfusa.com/generalsurgery/

Chapter 17 Gastrointestinal Surgery

A Comparison of Laparoscopically Assisted and Open Colectomy for Colon Cancer. Clinical Outcomes of Surgical Therapy Study Group. New England Journal of Medicine, May 13, 2004, 350:20

Barrow, Cynthia. Roux-en-Y Gastric Bypass for Morbid Obesity. AORN J, 2002, 76:593

Biliopancreatic Diversion With Duodenal Switch. Reviewed Oct 9, 2003 by Rhoads, C.S., 2005, Kaiser Permanente

Brolin, Robert E. Bariatric Surgery and Long-Term Control of Morbid Obesity. JAMA, 12/11/02, 288:2793–2796

Colorectal Aganglionosis. Handbook of Colon and Rectal Surgery. Lippincott, Williams & Wilkins, 2002, p. 285–286

Davies, Roger, et al. Percutaneous Jejunostomy Using CT Fluoroscopy. Am J Radiol, 2001, 176:808–810

DeMaria, Eric J. Bariatric Procedures. ACS Surgery: Principals & Practice, WebMD, 2005, www.Medscape.com

Ethicon Endo-Surgery, Inc. Endo Cutters: Linear and Circular Cutters and Staplers, www.ethiconendo.com/surgical.jsp

Graling, Paula and Elariny, Hazem. Perioperative Care of the Patient With Morbid Obesity. AORN, 77:802–819

Harbe, Karla. Adjustable Band Obesity Surgery Successful in Out Patients. Medscape Medical News, reviewed by Vogin, Gary D, May 17, 2004, www.medscape.com/view article/477744_print

Hulka, Fabian H. and Reich, Harry. Laparoscopy, ed III. Saunders, 1997

Hurst, Roger D. and Michelassi, Fabrizio. Fulminant Ulcerative Colitis. WebMD, 2005, www.acssurgery.com/abstracts/acs/acs0513.htm

Introducer Gun for T Anchors. Moss™ Tubes, www.mosstubesinc.com/tdiagram.html

Laparoscopy. Autoclavable Laparoscopes and Components. Innovative Endoscopic Components, Inc, Endoscopy.MD, 2004

Mulsow, J, et al. Sentinel Lymph Node Mapping in Colorectal Cancer. Br J Surg, 2003, 90:659–667

Nyhus, Lloyd, et al. Anal Neo-Sphincter Procedures. Mastery of Surgery, ed III. Little, Brown and Co, 1997, p. 1585

Nyhus, Lloyd, et al. Bariatric Surgical Procedures. Mastery of Surgery, ed III. Little, Brown and Co, 1997, p. 983–990

Nyhus, Lloyd, et al. Ileal Pouch With Ileoanal Anastomosis. Mastery of Surgery, ed III. Little, Brown, and Co, 1997, p. 1449–1453

Oelschlager, Brandt. Surgical Management of Achalasia. Medscape, General Medicine, Dec 15, 2003, 5(4)

Payer, Marilyn, et al. Panniculectomy: An Option for People Who Are Morbidly Obese. AORN, 2003, 77:782–794

Roux-en-Y. Gastric Bypass Surgery. Gastric Bypass Surgery Center, 2002–2004, www.obesitysurgerycenter.com

Saunders, V. (ed). Laparoscopic Jejunostomy. Shackelford's Surgery of the Alimentary Tract, 2002, p. 250–251

Schwartz, Lewis, et al. Atlas of Laparoscopic Surgery. Current Medicine, Philadelphia, 1996

Stein, Patricia. Ulcerative Colitis: Diagnosis and Surgical Treatment. AORN J, 2004, 80:242

Surgisis® AFP™ Anal Fistula Plug Overview (Cook Surgical®). Cook Biotechnology, 2003, www.cooksis.com/products/surgis_afp/index.html

Todd, Steven, et al. Outpatient Laparoscopic Nissen Fundoplication. AORN J, 2002, 75:956

U.S. Surgical Corporation (USSC). Auto Suture® (Endo Stitch) Single Use, www.autosuture.com/imageserver.aspx?contentid=3231&contenttype=application/pdf

Wolf Corp. Laparoscopic GI and GYN Surgery Instruments. 2004, www.richardwolfusa.com/generalsurgery/

Zuidema, G. and Yeo, C. Laparoscopic Partial (Guarner) Fundoplication. Minimally Invasive Esophageal Procedures. ACS Surgery Principles and Procedures, WebMD, 2005, p. 250–251

Zuidema, G. and Yeo, C. Surgery of the Alimentary Tract, ed V. 2002

Chapter 18 Gynecologic and Obstetric Surgery

A New Choice: The Essure Method. Nurse Week, May 17, 2004, p. 9–12

Bristow, Robert E. Secondary Cytoreductive Surgery for Isolated Nodal Recurrence of Ovarian Cancer. Annals of Surgical Oncology, 11(7):639

de Candolle, G. and de Jolinière, Bouquet J. Management of Tubal Infertility. Geneva Foundation for Medical Education and Research, www.gfmer.ch/books/reproductive_health/tubal_infertility.html

Ectopic Pregnancy. Operative Gynecology, ed II. WB Saunders, 2001, p. 655–665

Essure. Mayo Clinic, www.mayoclinic.com/invoke.cfm?objectid=264df9-ffbf-4c69-b0ac30778b

Farrell, S. A., et al. Tension Free Vaginal Tape (TVT) Procedure. J Obstet Gynaecol Can, 2003, 25(8):692–694, 695–668

Hill, D. Ashley. Hysteroscopy: Issues and Procedures in Women's Health. OBGYN.net, http://home.mpinet.net/dahmd

Introducing the Essure™ Procedure (booklet). Conceptus®, Inc, San Carlos, CA, www.essure.cm and www.conceptus.com

League, Diane D. Endometrial Ablation as an Alternative to Hysterectomy. AORN J, 2003, 77:321

Ngoh, Nkele Ndeki. Management of Tubal Obstruction. 8/13/03, www.gfmer.ch/presentations_en/management_tubal_obstruction.htm

Olympus©. Hysteroscope. Essure Instrumentation, www.olympusamerica.com/gy

Radical Vulvectomy. Operative Gynecology, ed II. WB Saunders, 2001, p. 237–259

Schrecengost, Ann. Ovarian Mass Benign or Malignant. AORN J, Nov 2002, vol 76, p. 789, 792–802, 805–806

Sepilian, Vicken and Wood, Ellen. Ectopic Pregnancy. eMedicine, Oct 10, 2005, www.emedicine.com/med/topic3212.htm

Uterine Myomectomy. Operative Gynecology, ed II. WB Saunders, 2001, p. 517–521

Wolf Corp. Laparoscopic GI and GYN Surgery Instruments. 2004, www.richardwolfusa.com/generalsurgery/

Chapter 19 Genitourinary Surgery

Bickert, D. and Frickel, D. Laparoscopic Radical Prostatectomy. AORN, 2002, 82:760

Chambers, Ann. Transurethral Resection Syndrome: It Does Not Have To Be a Mystery. AORN J, 2002, 75:156

Cystoscopy. Autoclavable Cystoscopes and Components. Innovative Endoscopic Components, Inc, Endoscopy. MD, 2004

Dyer, Raymond et al. Percutaneous Nephrostomy With Extensions of the Technique. Radiographics, 2002, 22:503

Extracorporeal Shockwave Lithotripsy. Dornier Compact Delta II Manual. 2005, www.emedicine.com/med/topic3024.htm

Feste, J. Laparoscopic Retropubic Colposuspension: The Burch Procedure. OB/GYN News, Jan 1, 2000, www.OB.GYN.net

Grasso, Michael, et al. Intracorporeal Lithotripsy. eMedicine, Sept 2004, updated May 17, 2006 www.emedicine.com/med/topic3034.htm

Gynecare (TVT) Procedure, Tension Free Vaginal Tape. Support for Incontinence International Urology. IUGA Abstract #116, Oct 2003, www.gynecare.com

Hautmann, Stefan. Nephrostomy. eMedicine, updated Jan 31, 2006, www.emedicine.com/med/topic3040.htm

Herr, H. W., et al. Cancer of the Bladder. Principals and Practice of Oncology, ed VI. Lippincott, Williams & Wilkins, 2001, p. 1396

Herr, H. W., et al. Ileal Conduit. Principles and Practice of Oncology, ed VI. Lippincott, Williams & Wilkins, 2000, p. 1396

Jarred, David F. Urothelial Tumors of the Renal Pelvis and Ureters. eMedicine, updated Aug 4, 2006, www.emedicine.com/med/topic3088.htm

Kaul, Sanjeev. Laparoscopic and Robotic Radical Prostectomy. eMedicine, Feb 28, 2005, www.emedicine.com/med/topic3723.htm

Laparoscopic Radical Cystectomy With Ileal Conduit Diversion. Urological Reports. 2005, 6:93

Laparoscopic Varicocelectomy. Laparoscopy Hospital, 2001, www.laparoscopyhospital.com/laparoscopic_varicocelectomy.htm

Lee, David I. and Landman, Jaime. Novel Approach to Minimizing Trocar Sites During Challenging Hand-Assisted Laparoscopic Surgery. Utilizing the Gelport®: Trans-Gel Instrument Insertion and Utilization. J Endourology, Mar 2003, vol 17, no 2

Leslie, Stephen W. Transuretheral Resection of the Prostate. eMedicine 05, updated Oct 3, 2006, www.emedicine.com/med/topic3071.htm

Orchiectomy, www.health.enotes.com/surgery_encyclopedia/orchiectomy

Papanikolaou, Frank and Notz, Laurence. Orchiectomy, Radical. eMedicine, Feb 2, 2006, www.emedcine.com/med/topic3063.htm

Rothrock, Jane C. Percutaneous Nephrostomy. Alexander's Care of the Patient in Surgery, ed XII. Mosby, 2003, p. 606

Rothrock, Jane C. Urethroplasty. Alexander's Care of the Patient in Surgery, ed XII. Mosby, 2003, p. 544–545

Sabanegh, E. Vasovasostomy and Vasoepididymostomy. eMedicine, Oct 18, 2006, emedicine.com/med/topic3090.htm

Sabiston, David C. and Lyerly, H. Kim. Essentials of Surgery (multiple citations). WB Saunders, 2002

Sajadi, Kamran. Artificial Urinary Sphincter. eMedicine, July 1970, www.emedicine.com/med/topic3019.htm

Santucci, Richard A and Knopick, Christopher. Penile Prosthesis Implantation. eMedicine, updated Mar 8, 2006, www.emedicine.com/med/topic3047.htm

Santucci, Richard A. Radical Nephrectomy. eMedicine, updated Aug 24, 2005, www.emedicine.com/med/topic3062.htm

Steidle, Chris. Penile Prostheses (Implants). eMedicine, updated Sept 2003, www.SeekingWellness.com/MenSexuality/penimpl.htm

Terris, Martha K. Pyelolithotomy. eMedicine, updated June 12, 2006, www.emedicine.com/med/topic3060.htm

Urethroplasty. Campbell's Urology, ed VIII. WB Saunders, 2002, p. 3915

Chapter 20 Thoracic Surgery

Acton, Robert D. and Saltzman, Daniel. Surgical Corrective Treatment for Pectus Excavatum and Pectus Carinatum. University of Minnesota, Sept 29, 2004, www.pectusdeformity.com

Allen, Gloria. Thoracoscopic Sympathectomy for Palmer Hyperhydrosis. AORN J, 2001, 74:178

Flores, Raja M., et al. VATS. American College of Surgeons: Surgery Principles and Practice. WebMD, Mar 2005, www.acssurgery.com/acsonline/pdf/acs50407.pdf

Hebra, Andre. Pectus Excavatum. eMedicine, updated Jul 24, 2006, www.emedicine.com/ped/topic2558.htm#Section~treatment

Instrumentation, Equipment, and Devices used in Thoracic Open and Endoscopic Surgery. Kelleher Medical, Inc, Richmond, VA, www.Kellmed@kellerhermedical.com

Kaseda, Shizuka. Better Pulmonary Function and Prognosis With Video-Assisted Thoracic Surgery. Annals Thoracic Surg, 2000, 70:1644–1646

Livesay, JJ. Surgical Experience in Descending Thoracic Aneurysmectomy With and Without Adjuncts to Avoid Ischemia. Annals Thoracic Surg, 39:37–46

Lorenz® Pectus Bar for the Nuss Procedure. BIOMET® Lorenz Surgical Headquarters, Jacksonville, Florida

Surgical Treatment for Pectus Excavatum. UK Pectus Excavatum and Pectus Carinatum Information Site, www.pectus.org/surgical.htm

Chapter 21 Vascular Surgery

Aortic Stent Grafts, www.medscape.com/newarticle/503004_6

Arko, Frank, et al. Repair of Infra-Renal Abdominal Aortic Aneurysms, www.acssurgery.com/abstracts/acs/acs0505.htm

Arterial Thromboembolectomy. Rutherford Vascular Surgery, ed V. WB Saunders, 2000, p. 822–835

Bergan, John and Pascarella, Luigi. Varicose Vein Surgery. Rutherford Vascular Surgery, ed V. WB Saunders, 2000, p. 822–835

Bergan, John and Pascarella, Luigi. Varicose Vein Surgery. 2004, www.acssurgery.com/abstracts/acs/acs0513.htm

Criado, Frank J. Access Strategies for Carotid Artery Intervention. J Invasive Cardiol, 2000, 12(1):61–69

Cundy, JoAnn. Carotid Artery Stenosis and Endarterectomy. AORN J, 2002, 75:309

Dong, Charles, et al. Intraoperative Spinal Cord Monitoring During Descending Thoracic and Thoracoabdominal Aneurysm Surgery. Annals of Thoracic Surgery, 2002, 74:1873–1876

Eskandari, Mark. Aortoilliac Reconstruction. June 2003, www.medscape.com/viewarticle/457766?mpid=15685.html

Hall, Susan. Endovascular Repair of Abdominal Aortic Aneurysms. AORN J, 2003, 77:630

Hanni, Cary. Modern Treatment of Abdominal Aortic Aneurysm (Endoscopic). Deceptive Pain Conference, 2000. Discover Magazine, Jan 2001

Kinney, T. B., et al. Stent Grafts for Abdominal and Thoracic Aortic Disease. Aortic Stent Grafts. Applied Radiology, vol 34, no 10, www.medscape.com/viewarticle/503004–6

Livesay, J. J. Surgical Experience in Descending Thoracic Aneurysmectomy With and Without Adjuncts to Avoid Ischemia. Ann Thorac Surg, 39:37–46

Madani, M. M. and Jameson, S. W. Pulmonary Thromboendarterectomy: Cardiac Surgery in the Adult. Cohn, L.H. and Edmunds, L.H. Jr, eds. New York: McGraw-Hill, 2003, p. 1205–1228

Moore, Wesley. Carotid Artery Procedures. 2003, www.medscape.com/viewarticle/457757.htm

Pearce, William. The Evolution of Varicose Vein Treatment. Sept 2003, www.medscape.com/view article/461016.htm

Sullivan, Timothy. Carotid Angioplasty and Stenting, www.acssurgery.com/abstracts/acs/acs0521.htm

Tani, D., et al. Fluorescence Detection of Arteriosclerotic Arteries (Paper). Intra-Balloon Angioscope. Tokyo Medical University, Tokyo, Japan

Chapter 22 Cardiac Surgery

Aortic Aneurysms and Dissections. Student Handout. Cardiothoracic Surgery Service LAC+USC Medical Center

Aortic Valve Bypass, www.umm.edu/heart/avb.html

Berul, Charles. Pacemaker Therapy. eMedicine, May 5, 2006, www.emedicine.com/ped/topic2711.htm

Bhimji, Shabir. Transmyocardial Laser Revascularization. eMedicine, June 8, 2006, www.emedicine.com3575.htm

Chikwe, J., et al. Surgical Management of Aortic Valve Disease. Posted Jan 30, 2004 http://www.medscape. com/viewarticle/466235_1

Cohn, L. H. and Edmunds L. H. Jr., eds. Cardiac Surgery in the Adult. New York: McGraw-Hill, 2003, p. 581–607

Combined Minimally Invasive Heart Bypass Surgery and Stented Angioplasty, www.umm.edu/heart/hybrid.htm

Cremer, Jochen T., et al. Minimally Invasive Coronary Artery on the Beating Heart. Ann Thorac Surg, 2000, 69:1787–1791

Genessee® BioMedical, Inc. Instrumentation for Cardiac Valves and Cardiac Stabilizers

Green, Beverly. Maze III Surgical Procedure. AORN, 2002, 76:133

Greenberg, S., et al. Trimethoprim-Sulfamethoxazole Induces Reversible Hyperkalemia. Ann Intern Med, 1993, 119:291–295

Gregoric, Igor, et al. Off-Pump Coronary Artery Bypass Grafting and Transmyocardial Laser Revascularization via a Left Thoracotomy. Tex Heart Inst J, 2003, 30:13–18

Huang, J. K. C., et al. The Bair Hugger Patient Warming System in Prolonged Vascular Surgery: An Infection Risk? Posted Aug 20, 2003. Crit Care 2003, 7(3):r13-r16, www.medscape.com/viewarticle/459057_print

Hybrid Procedure: Combined Minimally Invasive Heart Bypass Surgery and Stented Angioplasty, www.umm.edu/heart/hybrid.html

Implantable Left Ventricular Assist Devices, www.medscape.com/viewarticle/4625593

Keefe, Sandy. Cell Salvaging. Advance for Nurses, May 30, 2005, 3:17–19

Lipscomb, K. J., et al. Implantation of a Cardioverter Defibrillator Under Local Anesthesia. Heart Online, 1998, 79:253–255, www.heart.bmj.com/cgi/content/full/79/3/253

MAZE Procedure, www.umm.edu/heart/maze.html

Minimally Invasive Aortic Valve Surgery Incision Options, www.umm.edu/heart/aortic_valve.html

Minimally Invasive Coronary Bypass Surgery, www.umm.edu/heart/cabg.html

Ninami, H., et al. Partial Median Sternotomy as a Minimal Access for Off-Pump Coronary Artery Bypass Grafting: Feasibility of the Lower-End Sternal Splitting Approach. Ann Thorac Surg, 2001, 72:1041–1045

Pacifico, Antonio, et al. Long Term Follow-Up of Cardioverter-Defibrillator Implanted Under Conscious Sedation in Prepectoral Subfascial Position. 1997, www.circ.ahajournals.org/cgi/content/full/95/4/946

Petrou, Mario. Implantable Left Ventricular Assist Devices. Br J Cardiol, 2003, 10(5):aic78-aic81, posted 01/05/04

Ramchandani, Majesh. Off Pump Coronary Bypass Surgery. Feb 2005, www.drramchandani.com/surgery/coronary/offpump.asp

Reger, TB and Janhke, ME. Robotic Cardiac Surgery. AORN J, 77:182, 2003

Ross Procedure, www.umm.edu/heart/threevalvereplace.html

Sample, Susan. Left Ventricular Assist Devices. RN Professional Journal, Nov 2005, vol 68, no 11, p. 46–51

Seguin, J. R., et al. Aortic Valve Repair With Fibrin Glue for Type A Acute Aortic Dissection. Ann Thorac Surg, 2001, 72:510–514

Subramanian, V.A., et al. Robotic Assisted Multivessel Minimally Invasive Direct Coronary Artery Bypass With Port-Access Stabilization and Cardiac Positioning: Paving the Way for Outpatient Coronary Surgery? Ann Thorac Surg, 2005, 79:1590–1596

Tapson, Victor F. Massive Pulmonary Embolism. Sep 10, 1999, www.cambi.bjmu.edu.cn/update/critical%20care/emboli/massive%20pulmonary%20embolism.htm

Trans-Myocardial Revascularization, www.umm.edu/heart/tmr.html

"Transmyocardial Revascularization" or "Laser Heart Surgery." J Thorac Cardiovasc Surg, 2000, 120:1104–1111

Transmyocardial Revascularization, www.umm.edu/heart/tmr.html

Tremper, Roberta. Intra-Aortic Balloon Pump Therapy. AORN J, July 2006, 84:34–44

Videoscopic Minimally Invasive Mitral Valve Repair, www.umm.edu/heart/mitral_min.html

Woo, Y. J. and Gardner, TJ. Myocardial Revascularization With Cardiopulmonary Bypass. Updated Sep 28, 2005

Zeiner, Andrea, et al. Hypothermia to Improve Neurological Outcome After Cardiac Arrest. Stroke, 2000, 31:86.

Zimmerman, Lani. Comparison of Recovery Patterns for Patients Undergoing Coronary Artery Bypass Grafting and Minimally Invasive Direct Coronary Artery Bypass in the Early Discharge Period. Progress in Cardiovascular Nursing, Sep 30, 2002, vol 20, no 2

Chapter 23 Orthopedic Surgery

Arthroscopic Hip Surgery. AORN J, Feb 2006, 82:976–1000

Bach, Bernard and Boonos, Cynthia. Anterior Cruciate Reconstruction. AORN J, Aug 2001, 74:152

Belkin, Nathan L. Laminar Airflow and Surgical Wound Infections. AORN J, Aug 1998

Betz, Randal. Thoracoscopic Anterior Instrumentation for Scoliosis, www.spineuniverse.com/displayarticle.php/article504.html

Biomet® Orthopedic Instruments and Prostheses

Branson, Jill and Goldstein, Wayne. Primary Total Hip Arthroplasty. AORN J, Dec 2003, 78:947

Cemented and Cementless Knee Replacement. American Academy of Orthopedic Surgeons, www.orthoinfo.aaos.org/fact/printer_page.cfm?topcategory=knee&thread_id=281

Coblation in Brief, www.ArthroCare.com/our_technology/ot_coblation_explained.htm

DeOrio, James. Claw Toe, www.eMedicine.com/orthoped/topic51.htm

Drake, Cynthia, et al. Revision Total Hip Arthroplasty. AORN J, Sept 2002, 76:414

Fortunato, Nancymarie. Microsurgical Technique and Equipment. Berry & Kohn's Operating Room Technique, ed IX. Mosby, 2000, p. 333–342, 764–766

Geissler, William and Walsh, John. Wrist Arthroscopy. eMedicine, updated Feb 15, 2005

Haddad, S. L. Total Ankle Arthroplasty: Orthopedic Technology Review. Mar/Apr 2003, vol 5 no 2

Hips and Knees, www.njrcentre.org.uk/documents/reports/part2.pf

Hohler, Sharon. Minimally Invasive Hip Arthroplasty. AORN J, June 2004, 79:1244

Instrumentation Systems for Scoliosis Surgery, www.scoliosis.org/old/instrusu.html

Johnson, Don. Arthroscopic Rotator Cuff Repair: Advancing a New Gold Standard. Campbell's Operative Orthopedics, ed X, Mosby, 2003, p. 3260–3265

Johnson, Don. Update on Minimally Invasive Hip and Knee Arthroplasty. Campbell's Operative Orthopedics, ed X. Mosby, 2003, p. 2458–2467

Knee Implants. American Academy of Orthopedic Surgeons, www.orthoinfo.aaos.org/fact/printer_page.cfm?topcategory=knee&thread_id=279

Knee Surgery, www.eMedicine.com/orthoped/topic347.htm

Lin, J. S. H., et al. Use of Reconstruction Nails to Manage Ipsilateral Displaced Femoral Neck/Shaft Fractures: Assessment of a New Approach. J Orthopedic Surg, 2002, 10:185–93, www.josonline.org/abstracts/v10n2/185.html

Marcus, Randall E. Diagnosis and Treatment of Forearm Fractures. Medscape, 15th Annual Vail Orthopaedics Symposium, Jan 2001

Microsurgical Technique. Campbell's Operative Orthopedics, ed X. Mosby, 2003, p. 3287

Multilok® Hand Operating Table, www.osiosi.com/handsurgery.cfm

Picetti, George. Idiopathic Scoliosis: Discectomy, www.spineuniverse.com/displayarticle.php/article475.html

Picetti, George. Idiopathic Scoliosis: Surgical Setup and Equipment, www.spineuniverse.com/displayarticle.php/article473.html

Pilney, J. Arthroscopy in the Diagnosis and Therapy of Wrist Disorders. Acta Chir Orthop Tramatol Chech, 2004, 71:106–109

Repair of Achilles Tendon. Campbell's Operative Orthopedics, ed X. Mosby, 2003, p. 24, 58–67

Richardson, Michael L. Orthopedic Hardware. 2000, www.rad.washington.edu:8080/mskbook/orthopedichardware

Rothrock, Jane C. Microsurgical Replantation. Alexander's Care of the Patient in Surgery, ed XII. Mosby, 2003, p. 1038–1041

Rothrock, Jane C. Shoulder Arthroplasty. Alexander's Care of the Patient in Surgery, ed XII. Mosby, 2003, p. 909–912

Schmidt, Andrew H. Shoulder Arthroplasty. Campbell's Operative Orthopedics, ed X. Mosby, 2003, p. 3260–3265

Schmidt, Andrew H. Shoulder Arthroplasty. Medscape, 15th Annual Vail Orthopaedics Symposium, Jan 2001

Schramm, Carol A., et al. Triple Arthrodesis. AORN J, July1996, 64:31–52

Scoliosis Surgery, www.spine-health.com/topics/cd/scoliosis/scoliosis04.html

Scoliosis Treatment Options, Mar 1, 2002, updated Dec 27, 2005, www.isoliosis.com/stripcontent.php?parent_file=/treatment-surgical.html

Shea, Kevin P. Shoulder Replacement. Medscape, June 2000

Surgical Treatment of Idiopathic Scoliosis, www.thaispinecenter.com/scoliosis.htm

Swank, M. L. and Lehnert, I. E.. Orthopedic Roles in the OR for Assisted Total Knee Arthroplasty. AORN J, Oct 2005, 82:631

Taljanovic, M. S., et al. Knee Arthroplasty and Prosthesis, www.radialgraphics.rsnajn/s.org/cg1/content/full/23/5/1295

Trail, Ian. Metacarpophalangeal, Wrist, and Elbow Arthroplasty, www.medscape.com/viewarticle/42502

Transposition of the Ulnar Nerve. Campbell's Operative Orthopedics, ed X. Mosby, 2003, p. 3260–3265

Wrist Arthroscopy and Arthroplasty. Orthopaedic Institute Medical Staff. American Orthopedic Association, edited Jan 2003

Yian, Edward and Karunakar, Madhav. Distal Humerus Fractures. Hand and Upper Extremity Specialties. Orthopedic Surgery. eMedicine, www.emedicine.com/orthoped/topic145.htm

Chapter 24 Neurologic Surgery

Akizuki, T. A. Distraction for Osteogenesis. Neurosurg Focus, 2000, 9(3):2000

An, Howard and Juarez, Christen. Artificial Disc Replacement, 2004, www.spineuniverse.com/displayarticle.php/article1671ml

Artificial Disc Replacement Surgery. Depuy Spine, www.charitedisc.com/charitedev/domestic/patients/treatment_artificialdisc.asp

Bajnoczy, Susan. Artificial Disc Replacement: Evolutionary Treatment for Degenerative Disc Disease. AORN J, 2005, 82(2):192, 195–202, 205–206

Balloon Kyphoplasty. 2004–2006, www.kyphon.com/media.cfm

Balloons for Bones (Kyphoplasty) and KyphX® Inflatable Bone Tamps. Georgia Orthopedics and Spine Medicine Clinic (Spinal Division), 2004, www.swgspine.com/balloons_for_bones.com.htm

Brady, Sharon and Jackson, Sarah. Anterior Lumbar Interbody Fusion: Advances in Spinal Fusion Technology. AORN J, 2005, 82:817

Cedars-Sinai Outpatient Cancer Center. Stereotactic Radiosurgery. 9/27/05, www.cedars-sinai.edu/pf

Cherry, Cecile. Anterior Cervical Discectomy and Fusion for Cervical Disc Disease. AORN J, 2002, 76:996

Dickman, C. and Mican, C. Multilevel Anterior Thoracic Disectomies and Anterior Interbody Fusion Using Microsurgical Thoracic Approach, www.AANS.ORG/education/ Journal/neurological/Nov99/7-5-2.html

Emergency Craniotomy, www.uscneurosurgery.com/infonet/ecrani/setup.htm

Endoscopic Hypophysectomy, www.bhj.org/journal/1999_4104oct99/sp_686.htm

Fully Endoscopic Removal of Acoustic Neuromas. 2005, www.skullbaseinstitute.com/acoustic_neuroma/acoustic_neuroma.htm

Gokaslan, Z. L., et al. Intraoperative Monitoring of Spinal Cord Function Using Motor Evoked Potentials via Transcutaneous Epidural Electrode During Anterior Cervical Spinal Surgery. J Spinal Disorders, 1997, 10:29

Grant, G. A. Failure of Autologous Bone-Assisted Cranioplasty Following Decompressive Craniectomy in Children and Adolescents. AORN J, Aug 2005, 82:192–205

Intracranial Endoscopy, Endoscope-Assisted Microsurgery, Intraventricular Tumors, Stereotactic Biopsy, www.aans.org/education/journal/neurosurgical/apr99/6-4.asp?showmenu=false&s

Intraoperative Spinal Cord Monitoring, www.bku.bk/ortho/ortho/cspine/10m.htm

Kanan, Angela and Gasson, Beth. Brain Tumor Resections Guided by MRI. AORN J, 2003, 77:590

Legatt, Alan and Soliman, Emad. Somatosensory Evoked Potentials. eMedicine, May 2006, www.emedicine.com/neuro/topic640.htm

Mejia, M. Experiences With Intraoperative MRI System in Neurosurgery. AORN J, 2004, 80:432

McAfee, Paul C. Spinal Disc Replacement with the Charité Artificial Disc. Updated Mar 30, 2005, www.spine-health.com/research/discupdate03.html

Microdiscetomy. Youman's Neurological Surgery, ed IV. WB Saunders, 1996, p. 2369–2370, 2382–2388

Neurosurgery for Variety of Neurological Conditions. Hyman-Newman Institute for Neurology and Neurosurgery, www.neurosurgery.org/index.html

Nucleotome: Automated Percutaneous Lumbar Discectomy, www.clarus-medical.com/nucleotome.htm

OWL Universal RF Lesion Generator and Monitors System. Diros Technology, Inc., 2005, www.dirostech.com/urf1.html

Parthiban J. K., et al. Custom Cranioplasty Using Rapid Prototyping Technology. Neurol India [serial online], 2004 [cited 2/4/06], 52:520, http://www.neurologyindia.com/article.asp?issn=0028-3886;year=2004;volume=52;issue=4;spage=520;epage=520;aulast=Parthiban

Rediscovery of Neuroendoscopy. 2005, www.medscape.com/viewarticle/520939_2

Russell, Laurie. Intraoperative MRI Safety. AORN J, March 2003, 77:590

Schroeder, Henry WS and Gaab, Michael R. Intracranial Endoscopy. Neurosurgical Focus J, 1999, 6(4), Article 1, www.aans.org/education/journal/apr99/6-4-1.asp?showmenu=false&show print=false

Sealants (Duraseal©) to Prevent Leakage of CSF from Dural Suture, www.medscape.com/viewarticle/503292?src=DDD

Strayer, Andrea. Lumbar Spine: Common Pathologies and Interventions. J Neuroscience Nursing, 2005, 37(4):181–193, www.Medscape.com/viewarticle/512033_1

Three Minimally Invasive Endoscopic Approaches to Craniopharyngiomas. Skull Base Institute Text Navigation, 2005, www.skullbaseinstitute.com/craniopharyngioma/index.htm

Total Disc Replacement: A New Alternative to Spinal Fusion Surgery, www.medcompare.com/spotlight.asp?spotlight10=119

Total Disc Replacement (Artificial). Georgia Orthopedics and Spine Medicine Clinic (Spinal Division), 2004, www.swgspine.com/new_page_1.htm

Treatment Options for Pituitary Tumors at Mayo Clinic, www.mayoclinic.org/pitutary-tumors/treatment.html?wt.mc_id=1&wt.mc_n=os

Vertebroplasty and Kyphoplasty: Percutaneous Injection Procedures for Vertebral Fracture. 2004, www.pmrehab.com/kyphop.htm

Chapter 25 Plastic Surgery

A Prospective Study of Orbital Fracture Sequelae After Change of Surgical Routines. J Oral Maxillofacial Surg, 2003, 61:1375

Bonilla, Arturo J. Microtia. eMedicine, Mar 30, 2006, www.emedicine.com/ped/topic3003.htm

Bradford, C. R. and Prince, M. E. Oral Cavity Procedures. ACS Surgery Principles and Practices. Oct 12, 2004, www.medscape.com/viewarticle/491045

Chang, Edward W. Chin Augmentation. Medline Plus Encyclopedia, updated Nov 10, 2005

Clark, C. P. Breast Augmentation, Endoscopic-Assisted. eMedicine, Apr 24, 2003

Duod-Galli, Susan K., and Miller, Phillip J. Chin Implants. eMedicine, Aug 9, 2006, www.emedicine.com/ent/topic628.htm#top

Glenn, Lyle W. Breast Reduction, Superior Pedicle. eMedicine, Jan 27, 2005

Grossman, John A. Liposuction, Thigh and Knee. eMedicine, 12/7/04

Hua, Xi, et al. Repair of Hard Cleft Palate With Absorbable Membranes Made by Poly-DL-Lactic Acid: A Feasibility Study [in Chinese]. Medscape, 2004, 22(2):132–134

Hypospadiac or Intact Foreskin Graft for Syndactyly Repair. Medscape Newsletters. J South Orthop Assoc, 2000, 9:81–90

Lee, Steve, et al. Dupuytren's Contracture. eMedicine Specialties: Hand and Upper Extremity. June 6, 2003, www.emedicine.com/orthoped/topic81.html

Meronk, Frank. Lower Blepharoplasty Eyelid Surgery. Blepharoplasty Information Service, 2002–2006, www.drmeronk.com/insidersguide/18.html

Meronk, Frank. Upper Blepharoplasty Eyelid Surgery. Blepharoplasty Information Service, 2002–2006, www.drmeronk.com/insidersguide/18.html

Merritt, Linda. Physical Assessment of the Infant With a Cleft Lip and/or Palate. Advances in Neonatal Care, 2005, 5(3):125–134

Nyhus, Lloyd, et al. Common Facial Injuries. Mastery of Surgery, ed III. Little, Brown, and Co, 1997, p. 456

Osteomed®. Oral and Maxillofacial Instrumentation and Prostheses

Padgett Dermatome Integra®. June 2005, www.padgettinst.com/products/?product=17

Payer, Marilyn, et al. Panniculectomy: An Option for People Who Are Morbidly Obese. AORN, 2003, 77:782–794

Peltier, Jacques. Mandible Fractures. Grand Rounds Presentation, University of Texas Medical Branch, May 26, 2004

Rettinger G. and O'Connell M. The Nasal Base in Cleft Lip Rhinoplasty. Facial Plast Surg, 2002, 18(3):165–178

Revis, Don R. Dupuytren's Contracture. eMedicine, 1/6/06, www.eMedicine.com/med/topic592.htm

Revis, Don R., et al. Skin Grafts. eMedicine, Nov 2003, www.emedicine.com/plastic/topic392.htm

Sandberg, Debra, et al. Neonatal Cleft Lip and Cleft Palate Repair. AORN J, 2002, 75:490, www.aorn.org/journal/homestudy/mar2a.pdf

Scalfani, Anthony P. and Ranaudo, Jeffrey. Otoplasty. eMedicine, Aug 29, 2006, www.emedicine.com/ent/topic110.htm#section~treatment

Segal, Zachary, et al. Facial Trauma, Zygomatic Complex Fractures. eMedicine, July 13, 2004

Shelton, Ron and Rokhsar, Cameron R. Tumescent Liposuction. eMedicine, Sep 1, 2006, www.emedicine.com/derm/topic526.htm

Thornton, James F. Breast Reduction, Lejour (Technique). eMedicine, Dec 2, 2003

Chapter 26 Neck Surgery

Carling, T. and Udelsman, R. Parathyroid Surgery in Familial Hyperparathyroid Disorders. J Intern Med 2005, 257(1):27–37

Chheda, Hemant. SPECT Scanning of Parathyroid Tumor. Endocrine Web and Norman Endocrine Clinic, 1997–2002, www.endocrineweb.com/SPECT.html

Ghorayeb, Bechara Y. Intraoperative Recurrent Laryngeal Nerve Monitoring for Thyroid and Parathyroid Surgery. Otolaryngology Houston, www.ghorayeb.com/recurrentlaryngealnervemonitoring.html

Ghorayeb, Bechara Y. Parathyroid Sestamibi & Minimal Parathyroidectomy. Otolaryngology Houston, Oct 31, 2006

Hyperparathyroid Surgery, www.rush.edu/rumc/page-1099611533367.html

March, Abe. Radical Neck Dissection. eMedicine, Nov 2005

Norman, James. Minimally Invasive Parathyroid Surgery. June 2005, www.endocrineweb.com/MIRP.html

Norman, James. Parathyroid Sestamibi & Minimal Parathyroidectomy. Endocrine Web, June 2005

Santacroce, Luigi. Thyroidectomy, Papillary Carcinoma. eMedicine, July 22, 2005, www.emedicine.com/med/topic2464.htm

Sharma, Pramod K. Thyroid Cancer. eMedicine, June 29, 2006, www.eMedicine.com/ent/topic646.htm

Smith, Jonathan C. and Johnson, Jonas T. Neck, Cysts. eMedicine, Aug 24, 2005. www.emedicine.com/ent/topic238.htm

Smith, Jonathan. Thyroglossal Duct Cyst. eMedicine, www.emedicine.com/ent/topic283.htm

Sutherland, Michael and Peyton, B. Zenker's Diverticula. eMedicine, Jan 15, 2006, www.entcolumbia.org/divert.htm

Uvulopalatophyaryngoplasty. Ballenger's Otorhinolaryngology Head and Neck Surgery, ed XVI. 2003, p. 1045

Valledes, J, et al. Re: Use of Hi-Lo Endotracheal Tube: Continuous Aspiration of Subglottic Secretions in Preventing Ventilator-Associated Pneumonia (VAP). Annals of Internal Medicine 1995, 122(3): 179–186

Werning, John. Modified Radical Neck Dissection, eMedicine, August 2004, www.emedicine.com/ent/topic748.htm

Wright G. M. Video-Assisted Thoracoscopic Thymectomy (VATS) for Myasthenia Gravis. Int Med J, 2002, 32(8):367–371, www.medscape.com/medline/abstract/12162392

Chapter 27 Otorhinolaryngological Surgery

Ankit, M. and Vaughn, Winston C. Surgical Treatment of Sinusitis, Maxillary, Chronic. eMedicine, May 19, 2005, www.emedicine.com/ent/topic339.htm

Chahin, Fadi and Kaufman, Matthew K. Salivary Gland Tumors, Minor, Benign. eMedicine, UCLA Medical Center, Nov 10, 2005, www.emedicine.com/ent/topic2790.htm

Cochlear Implant. Ballenger's Otorhinolaryngology Head and Neck Surgery, ed XVI. BC Decker, Inc, 2003, p. 476

Cochlear Implants. JAMA, 2004, 291:2398

Cochlear Implants. National Institute on Deafness and Other Communication Disorders. Updated Oct 5, 2006, www.nidcd.nih.gov/health/hearing/coch.asp

Colin, S. and Duval, S. Surgical Treatment of Sleep Apnea. AORN, 2005, 82:371

Devan, P. P. and Donaldson, John D. Mastoiditis, Middle Ear. eMedicine Journal, Oct 6, 2006, www.emedicine.ent/topic740.htm

Drake, Amelia and Carr, Michele M. Tonsillectomy. eMedicine, June 15, 2005, www.emedicine.com/ent/topic315.htm

Endoscopic Electrosurgical Adnoidectomy. Journal of Otolaryngology, 2004, 33:82–87

ENT Endoscopy Instrumentation. Endoscopy. MD, 2004, http://www.endoscopy.md/earnose.html

Ghorayeb, Bechara Y. Otosclerosis and Stapedectomy. Otolaryngology Houston, 3/19/06

Gidley, Paul. Mastoidectomy. Medical Center Ear Nose and Throat Associates of Houston, PA. Sep 11, 2003, updated Mar 31, 2004, http//:www.mcenta.com/for%20%20and%20hearing/mastoidectomy.htm

Gosselin, Benoit J. Malignant Tumors of the Mobile Tongue. eMedicine, May 5, 2006, www.emedicine.com/ent/topic256.htm

Guerrissi, J. Endoscopic Excision of Submandibular Gland by Intraoral Approach. Journal of Craniofacial Surgery, 2001, 12:299–303

Howard, Matthew L. Middle Ear, Tympanic Membrane Perforations. eMedicine Journal, Mar 22, 2006, www.emedicine.com/ent/topic206.htm

Jackson, Lance. Minimally Invasive Otological Surgery (Personal Communication). University School of Medicine, St. Louis, MO, Sept 8, 2003

Kluge, David. Tonsil: A Review of Methods and Adjunctive Therapy. Nov 3, 2005, www.siumed.edu/surgery/otol/ppts/11-03-05_entgr_tonsillectomy.ppt

Lango, Miriam N, et al. Neck Dissection. ACS Surgery Principles and Practice. WebMD, July 2004, www.acssurgery.com/abstracts/acs/acs0206.htm

Laser Myringotomy Policy Statement. American Academy of Otolaryngology. Head and Neck Surgery. Mar 4, 2001

Lee, Dennis and Krishna, Priya. Acute Frontal Sinusitis, Surgical Treatment. eMedicine, 11/07/05, www.emedicine.com/ent/topic342.htm

Lindman, Jonathan P and Morgan, Charles E. Tracheosteomy. eMedicine, Oct 27, 2006, www.emedicine.com/ent/topic356.htm#section~treatment

McClay, John E. Nasal Polyps. eMedicine, Apr 20, 2006, www.emedicine.com/ped/topic1550.htm

Megerian, Cliff A and Murray, Gail S. Cochlear Implants, Surgical Technique. eMedicine, May 24, 2006, www.emedicine.com/ent/topic425.htm

Patel, Ankit M. and Vaughn, W. C. Sinusitis, Maxillary, Chronic, Surgical Treatment. eMedicine, May 19, 2005, www.emedicine.com/ent/topic339.htm

Patel, Ankit M., et al. Functional Endoscopic Sinus Surgery. eMedicine, 10/31/05, www.emedicine.com/ent/topic758.htm

Rothrock, Jane C. Frontal Sinus Trephination. Alexander's Care of the Patient in Surgery, ed XII. Mosby, 2003, p. 775–776

Rothrock, Jane C. Intranasal Antrostomy. Alexander's Care of the Patient in Surgery, ed XII. Mosby, 2003, p. 777

Scully, Crispian. Cancers of the Oral Mucosa. eMedicine, Sep 15, 2006, www.emedicine.com/derm/topic565.htm

Shabana, Yousef, et al. Laser Stapedotomy. Journal of Laryngology and Otology, 1999, 113:413–416

Shah, Nishit J. Functional Endoscopic Sinus Surgery. Bombay Hospital Journal, October 1999, vol 41, no 4, www.indegene.com/ent/featart/indentfeatart7.html

Shin, J. J. and Hartnick C. J. Pediatric Endoscopic Transnasal Adnoid Ablation. Annals of Otorhinolaryngology, 2003, p. 511–514, www.medscape.com/medline/abstract/12834118?querytext=endoscopic%20adnoidectomy

Singer, D. Anatomical and Surgical Approach to Submandibular Resection. Plastic and Reconstructive Surgery, Sept 2003, 112:1150–1154

Strong, E. Bradley. Fractures of the Frontal Sinus. eMedicine, Jun 28, 2006, www.emedicine.com/ent/topic419.htm

Terris, David J. Conservation Laryngeal Surgery, Subtotal Laryngectomy. eMedicine, Aug 19, 2004, www.emedicine.com/ent/topic569.htm

Total Laryngectomy. MD Anderson Cancer Center, University of Texas Patient Information, 2006, http://www.mdanderson.org/departments/headandneck/display.cfm?id=eff107f2-87df-11d4-b10b00508b603a14&method=displayfull&pn=dc30f0bf-7545-11d4-aec300508bdcce3a

Uvulopalatopharyngoplasty. Alexander's Care of the Patient in Surgery, ed XII. Mosby, 2003, p. 803–804

Uvulopalatopharygoplasty. Ballenger's Otorhinolaryngology Head and Neck Surgery, ed XVI. 2003, p. 1045

Uvulopalatopharyngoplasty. Surgical Technology for the Surgical Technologist. 2001, p. 517–522

Watson, Deborah and Rivkin, Alexander. Septoplasty. eMedicine, Mar 31, 2006, www.emedicine.com/ent/topic128.htm

Weber, Rainer, et al. Success of Stenting in Endonasal Frontal Sinus Surgery. ENT J, Dec 2000, www.entjournal.com/archives_fr.htm?id=2008&md=search

Weisskopf, Peter A. and Anurag, Jain. Middle Ear, Chronic Suppurative Otitis, Surgical Treatment. eMedicine from WebMD, June 15, 2006, www.emedicine.com/ent/topic215.htm#top

Chapter 28 Ophthalmic Surgery

Acutome.com. 2004, Eye Surgery Equipment, Instruments, and Products, www.accutome.com/

Alvarenga, L. S. Fibrin Glue in Pterigium Surgery. Br J Ophth 2005, 89:392

Ayyala, Ramesh S and Hong, Chian. Glaucoma Drainage Devices. eMedicine, Oct 31, 2005

Bashour, Mounir. Eyelid Reconstruction, Lower Eyelid. eMedicine, Feb 24, 2006, www.emedicine.com/plastic/topic10.htm

Bashour, Mounir. Eyelid Reconstruction, Upper Eyelid. eMedicine, Feb 24, 2006, www.emedicine.com/plastic/topic11.htm

Belkin, M., et al. Management of Non-Magnetic Intraocular Bodies. Archives of Ophthalmology, Jan 2001, 97:106

Bashour, Mounir. Myopia, Radial Keratotomy. eMedicine, June 2005, www.emedicine.com/oph/topic669.htm

Bashour, Mounir. Nasolacrimal Duct Congenital Anomalies. eMedicine, June 10, 2005, www.emedicine.com/oph/topic392.htm

Belkin, Mounir, et al. Management of Non-magnetic Foreign Bodies: A New Approach With the Use of Diagnostic X-ray and Spectrometry. Archives of Ophthalmology, 2001, 97:106

Burns, Frank. Eyelid Diseases and Surgery, www.frankburnsmd.com/faq/eyelid_diseases_surgery.htm#top

Cataract Surgery. Wikipedia, http://www.en.wikipedia.org/cataract_surgery

Chen, Amy Y. Facial Reanimation of the Chronically Paralyzed Face. eMedicine, 9/28/94, www.bcm.edu/oto/grand/92994.html

Cohen, A. J. Blepharotosis Repair. Review of Ophthalmology, Aug 2003, 10:08

Dacryocystorhinostomy (Pawar Implant). Intracystic Implant (P05)-G Surgiwear, Ltd, www.allproducts.com/surgiwear/p05.html

DeBacker, Christopher and Dryden, Robert M. Entropion. eMedicine, Aug 5, 2005, updated Nov 10, 2006, www.emedicine.com/oph/topic212.htm

Descemets Stripping Automated Endothelial Keratoplasty (DSAEK), New Corneal Transplantation Technique Offers Fewer Risks (Descements Stripping Automated Endothelial Keratoplasty), www.musc.edu/catalyst/archive/2006/co3-10new.html

Douglas, Raymond S. Retinal Detachment Repair (Scleral Buckling). UCLA Medical Center, Apr 8, 2005, www.umm.edu/enc/05/article/002960.htm

Duong, Hon-vu and Copeland, Robert. Basal Cell Carcinoma, Eyelid. eMedicine, Mar 2006, updated Mar 10, 2006, www.emedicine.com/oph/topic199.htm

EyeMDLink.com. Dacryocystorhinostomy for Tearing. www.eyemdlink.com/eyeprocedure.asp?eyeprocedureid=32

Fernandes, Valentine S. Dacryocystorhinostomy. eMedicine, last updated May 5, 2005, www.emedicine/ent/topic452.htm

Fischer, Jerome P and Trattler, William. Pterygium. eMedicine, Dec 12, 2005

Foster, Stephen C. and Ocampo, Vicente Victor D. Esotropia, Infantile. eMedicine, Aug 4, 2005, www.emedicine.com/oph/topic328.htm

Freund, K. Vitrectomy, eMedicine, Nov 2004, updated Jan 11, 2005, www.vrmny.com/vitrectomy.htm

Fulcher, J., et al. Nasolacrimal Intubation in Adults. British Journal of Ophthalmology, 1998, 82:1039–1041

Glaucoma Tool (The EYEPASS Procedure). December 2004, www.noorvision.com/weblog/archives/2005/01/index.html

Glynn-Milley, Catheryn. Outlook Positive for Today's Cataract Patients. Nurse Week, Ape 25, 2005, p. 17–18

Goosey, John. Laser Vision Correction, www.johngoosey.com/about DSAEK.asp

Hays, James and Thornton, Spencer. Astigmatic Keratotomy. eMedicine, Mar 14, 2006, www.emedicine.com/oph/topic654.htm

Hertle, Richard W. Understanding and Treatment of Infantile Nystagmus Syndrome, www.nystagmus.org/doc/conf2005/hertle_ann.pdf

Ing, Edsel. Ectropion. eMedicine, May 1, 2005, www.emedicine.com/oph/topic211.htm

International Eye Foundation. Eye Instruments and Eye Procedures Instrument Trays, www.sightreachsurgical.com

Jordan, David R and Klapper, Stephen R. Anophthalmic Orbital Implants: Current Concepts and Controversies. Medline, Jan 3, 2006

Jordan, D. The Anophthalmic Patient (Eviseration of the Eye, Orbital implants, and Reconstructive Procedures). 2004, www.ocularist.org/surgical.html

Kuhn, Ferenc and Wong, David T. Intraocular Foreign Bodies. eMedicine, October 2004, updated Aug 3, 2006, www.emedicine.com/oph/topic648.htm

Lasik, www.lasereyecenter.com/ggl/proc_lasik.php

Lasik vs PRK, www.lasik1.com/lasikvsprk.html

Lehmann, Robert P. Aqualase for Refractive Lens Exchange. Cataract and Refractive Surgery. Nov/Dec 2005

Manners, T., et al. Trabeculectomy With Mitomycin C in the Treatment of Post-Traumatic Angle Recession Glaucoma. British Journal of Ophthalmology, 2001, 85:159

Naradzay, Jerome FX and Santen, Salley. Chalazion. eMedicine, Specialties Emergency Medicine Ophthalmology, last updated May 2, 2006

Phakic IOLs, www.lasereyecenter.com/ggl/proc_phakic.php

Pterygium Surgery, www.harvardeye.com/procedures/pterigium.html

Radial and Astigmatic Keratotomy, www.vision-institute.com /techniques/ radial.html

Reddy, Madhusulany Y, et al. Silicon Implant Dacryocystorhinostomy. Asian J Ophthalmology, 2005, 7(2):34–37, www.seagig.org/toc/v7n2p34.pdf

Repair of Retinal Detachment/Scleral Buckling, www.health.enotes.com/ surgery-encyclopedia/scleral buckling

Rumex® International Microsurgical Ophthalmic Instruments. Micro Incision Cataract Surgery, Thermo Cut® Diamond Knives, Limbal Relaxing Incision Instruments, Intra Lasik instruments, Acqua® Choppers, Lasek Instruments, www.rumex.net/pdf/abc_index.pdf

Surevision® Eye Centers, St. Louis, MO. Ophthalmic procedures instrument trays. Jul 31, 2006, www.surevision.us/index

University of Maryland Medical Center. Apr 2005, www.umcm.edu/ medical-terms/06084.htm

Wilson, R. Trabeculectomy. eMedicine, 2005, www.wills-glaucoma.org/ trab.htm

Wong, D. and Giavendoni, L. A Simple "Lasso" Technique for Intraocular Foreign Bodies. Ophthalmic Surgery and Lasers, 1999, 30:63

Yepez, J., et al. Modified Self-Sealing Sclerotomy for Drainage of Subretinal Fluid During Scleral Buckling Surgery. British Journal of Ophthalmology, 2004, 88:589

Yo, Christopher and Agawal, Soma. Lasik, Future Advances. eMedicine, Apr 13, 2006, www.emedicine.com/oph/topic759.htm

Chapter 29 Dental Surgery

Ash® Instruments, Inc. Dental Specialty Instruments

Atraumatic Ridge Expansion and Implied Site Prepared With Motorized Bone Expanders. Practice of Procedural Aesthetics Journal, 2001, 18:17–22

Baur, Dale A. and Helman, Joseph. Distraction Osteogenesis of the Mandible. eMedicine, June 2005, www.emedicine.com/ent/topic765.htm

Burstein, F., et al. The Use of Hydroxyappatite Cement in Craniofacial Reconstruction. Emory University and San Diego Children's Hospital, 2003, www.ehoa.org/menus/documents/ourservices/d921r9089.pdf

Christensen. TMJ Implant System Co-Cr-Mo Glenoid Fossa Eminence Prosthesis. BIOMET© Lorenz Surgical Headquarters, Jacksonville, FL

Clinical Implication Dentistry and Related Research. PubMed, 2005, 7:209–220

Hu-Friedy® instrumentation for dental specialties

Immediate and Early Replacement Implications and Restorations. Implant Dentistry, June 2006, 33:262–264, 266–268

Manganello-Souza, L. C. and Mariani, P. B. Temporomandibular Joint Ankylosis. Intl J Oral Maxillofacial Surgery, 203, 32:24

Park, J., et al. Surgical Management of Advanced Degeneration Arthritis of TMJ With Metal fos-em Hemijoint Replacement Prosthesis: 8 Year Retro Pilot Study.

Patel, Pravin K., et al. Craniofacial Orthognathic Surgery. eMedicine, June 28, 2006, www.emedicine.com/plastic/topic177.htm

Piehl, Joel Dental Implantation Surgery Personal Communication 2006

Sullivan, R. Implant Dentistry and the Concept of Osseointegration, 2001

Temporomandibular Joint Arthroscopy and Surgery. Surgical Technology for the Surgical Technologist, ed II. Del Mar, 2004, p. 681

TenHulzen, D. Temporomandibular Joint Surgery, www.Drtenhulzen.com/procedures/tmj.html

Chapter 30 Radiation Therapy/ Radiotherapy Procedures

Breast Brachytherapy, www.brachytherapy.c/breast-brachy.html

Bucci, Kara M., et al. Advances in Radiation Therapy. Cancer Journal for Clinicians, 2005, 55:117, www.oralcancerfoundation.org/facts/pdf/radiation-types.pdf-2431k

Clinica Universitaria New Technique in Brachytherapy for Treatment of the Lung. www.basqueresearch.com/berria

Demanes, Jeffrey D. Gynecologic Brachytherapy. California Endocurie Therapy Cancer Center, 2006, www.cetmc.com/gynecologic.html

Dickler, A, et al. The MammoSite® Breast Brachytherapy Applicator. Brachytherapy, 2005, 4:130

Domanovic, Mary Ann, et al. Using Intraoperative Radiation Therapy: A Case Study. AORN, 2003, 77:412, www.aorn.org/journal/2003/febtoc.htm

Duffy, Frederick J and Rossi, Rene M. Head and Neck Cancer: Radiation. eMedicine, 3/26/06, www.com/plastic/topic374.htm

Fortunato, Nancymarie. Radiation Safety. Berry and Kohn's Operating Room Technique, ed IX. 2000, Mosby, p. 388

Grimm, Peter. Prostate Seed Implantation. Prostate Cancer Research Institute, Nov 2003, www.prostate-cancer.org/education/localdis/grimm_seed_implantation.html

Internal Radiation Therapy. Cedars-Sinai Outpatient Cancer Center, www.csmc.edu/3156.html

Intraoperative Radiation Therapy at Mayo Clinic. Nov 8, 2005, www.mayoclinic.org/intraoperative-radiation

Intensity Modulated Radiation Therapy. Cedars-Sinai Outpatient Cancer Center, www.csmc.edu/3153.html

McCammon, Robert J. Radiation Therapy in Gynecology. eMedicine, June 22, 2006, www.emedicine.com/med/topic3307.htm

Ozohan, Mary L. Radiation Therapy. Personal Communication, 2006

Padmanabhan, T. K. Radiotherapy in the CNS: Neurosurgery on the Web. Amirtha Institute of Medical Sciences, Cochin, India, www.Thamburaj.com/radiotherapy.htm

Rothenberger, David A. and Ricciardi, Rocco. Procedures for Rectal Cancer: Introduction. Medscape General Surgery, June 2006, www.medscape.com/viewarticle533583.rss

Syed A. M. N., et al. High-Dose-Rate Brachytherapy in the Treatment of Carcinoma of the Prostate. Cancer Control, 2001, 8:511

Tannehill, Scott. High Dose Rate Brachytherapy Guide. Cancer Center, University of Wisconsin Department of Human Oncology. May 22, 2006, www.humonc.wisc.edu/pts/brachytherapy/cervical/#content

Theodorescu, Don and Krupski, Tracey L. Prostate Cancer: Brachytherapy (Radioactive Seed Implantation Therapy). eMedicine, Mar 10, 2005, www.emedicine.com/med/topic3147.htm

Chapter 31 Pediatric Surgery

Albanese, Craig T. Perils and Pitfalls During Laparoscopic Repair of High Imperforate Anus. Society of Gastrointestinal Endoscopic Surgeons. SAGES Postgraduate Course IV: April 19, 2001, St Louis, MO

Beals, Daniel. Imperforate Anus. eMedicine, June 14, 2004

Becmeur, Francois, et al. Sept 2004, www.websurg.com/ref/expert_Francois_Becmeur_France-625.htm

Cendron, Marc and Wajsman, Zev. Wilms' Tumor. eMedicine, June 29, 2006

Chahine, Alfred, et al. Intussusception. eMedicine, April 2006, www.emedicine.com/ped/topi1208.htm

Congenital Diaphragmatic Hernia. Texas Pediatric Surgical Associates, www.pedisurg.com/pteduc/congenital_diaphragmatic_hernia.htm

Congenital Dislocation of the Hip. Alexander's Care of the Patient in Surgery, ed XII. 2003, p. 1255

Congenital Dislocation of the Hip. Campbell's Operative Orthopedics, ed X. Mosby, 2003, pp. 1079–1123

de Jongee, Rogier C. J., et al. Central Venous Catheter Use in the Pediatric Patient. PCCM, 2005, 6:329–339

Dillon, Peter. Congenital Pediatric Colorectal Disorders. American Society of Colon and Rectal Surgeons, 2003, www.fascrs.org/displaycommon.cfm?an=1&subarticlenbr=116

Excision of Wilm's Tumor. Mastery of Surgery, ed III. Little, Brown and Co, 1997, p. 1685

Georgeson, Keith E. Laparoscopic Gastrostomy. Society of Gastrointestinal Endoscopic Surgeons. SAGES Postgraduate Course IV. April 19, 2001, St Louis, MO

Glasser, James. Omphalocele and Gastroschisis. eMedicine, June 8, 2006, www.emedicine.com/ped/topic1642.htm

Haijai, M. Hirschsprung's Disease: Revisited. J Postgrad Med, 2000, 46: 52–54

Hebra, Andre. Pediatric Hernias. eMedicine, May 30, 2006, www.emedicine.com/ped/topic2559.htm

Hepatic Portoenterostomy. Mastery of Surgery, ed III. Little, Brown and Co, 1997, p. 1159–1162

Jona, Juda Z. Laparoscopy for Hirschsprung's Disease. Society of Gastrointestinal Endoscopic Surgeons. SAGES Postgraduate Course IV: April 19, 2001, St Louis, MO

Larson, Shawn D., et al. Pediatric Vascular Access. eMedicine, Nov 2004, updated Oct 20, 2006

Lee, Steven, et al. Hirschprung's Disease. eMedicine, Mar 2006, www.emedicine.com/ped/topic1016.htm

Levitt, Marc A. and Pena, Alberto. Imperforate Anus: Surgical Perspective. eMedicine, Apr 24, 2006

Levitt, Marc A. and Singh, Kirpal. Minimal Access Procedures. eMedicine, Mar 28, 2006, www.emedicine.com/ped/topic2977.htm

Lewis, Nicola and Glick, Philip. Diaphragmatic Hernias. eMedicine, May 22, 2006, www.emedicine.com/ped/topic2937.htm

Lobe, Thom E. Pediatric Laparoscopy: General Considerations. 1996, www.sages.org/primarycare/chapter36.html

Lobe, Thom E. Pediatric Laparoscopy General Considerations. 2005, www.sages.org/primarycare/chapter#content.html

Mickes, R. K, et al. Congenital Anomalies of the Esophagus. eMedicine, May 3, 2006, www.emedicine.com/ped/topic2934.htm

Minkes, Robert K., et al. Stomas of the Small and Large Intestine. eMedicine, Oct 2006, www.emedicine.com/ped/topic2994.htm

Molmenti, Hebe. Omphalocele Repair. Medline Plus Medical Encyclopedia, Oct 25, 2004, www.nlm.nih.gov/medlineplus/encyclopedia/presentation/1000033_1.htm

Mooney, David P. Emergency Vascular Access Procedures. American College of Surgeons Committee on Trauma, Sept 1999

Nazer, Hisham, et al. Pyloric Stenosis, Hypertrophic. eMedicine, July 20, 2006

Oak, Sanjay, et al. Minimal Access Surgery in Children: 5 Years Institutional Experience. Journal of Minimal Access Surgery, July 7, 2005, vol 1, no 3, 121–128

Oak, Sanjay, et al. Laparoscopic Surgery of Inguinal Hernia in Children. Indian Journal of Surgery, 2004, 66:70

Pediatric Anesthesiology, www.anesthesiawisc.edu/med3/peds/pedshandout.html

Pediatric Urology. Campbell's Urology, ed VIII. 2002, p. 2136–2196

Romino, Stacy, et al. Parental Presence During Anesthesia Induction in Children. AORN J, 2005, 81:779–792

Rothrock, Jane C. Hepatic Portoenterostomy (Kasai Procedure). Alexander's Care of the Patient in Surgery, ed XII. 2003, p. 1237

Rothrock, Jane C. Pediatric Anesthesia. Alexander's Care of the Patient in Surgery, ed XII. Mosby, 2003, p. 1216–1219

Steinhorn, Robin H. Congenital Diaphragmatic Hernia. eMedicine, May 2004, www.eMedicine.com/ped/topic2603.htm

The First Decade's Experience With Laparoscopic Nissen Fundoplication. J Ped Surg, 2005, 40:142–147

Tran, Cecelia. Considerations in Pediatric Tracheostomy. Baylor College of Medicine, Jan 20, 2005, www.bcm/edu/oto.grand/91202005.htm

Vaizey, CJ, et al. Effects of Short Term Sacral Nerve Stimulation on Anal and Rectal Function in Patients With Anal Incontinence. Gut, 1999, 44:407–412

Warner, B. and Sexton, M. Umbilical Hernia in Children. Quest Diagnostics, Feb 15, 2006, www.bcbswny.com/kbase/topicmini/th17785/treatment.htm

Wise, Barbara V. Nursing Care of the Pediatric General Surgical Patient. Aspen Publishers, 2000

Wulkan, Mark L. Pitfalls of Laparoscopic Fundoplication. Society of Gastrointestinal Endoscopic Surgeons. SAGES Postgraduate Course IV: April 19, 2001, St Louis, MO

Yerkes, Elizabeth B. and Rink, Richard C. Exstrophy and Epispadias. eMedicine, May 18, 2006, www.emedicine.com/ped/topic704.htm

Zamack, Sherry M. Laparoscopic vs Endoscopic Gastrostomy: A New Gold Standard. J Ped Surg, 2005, 40:859–862

Zamakhshery, M., et al. Laparoscopic vs Percutaneous Endoscopic Gastrostomy Insertion: A New Pediatric Standard? J Pediatr Surg, 2005, 40(5):859–862

Chapter 32 Through Chapter 43, Instrument Trays

The surgical inventory in health-care facilities are procured utilizing a number of sources and resources in each specialty. The format of this text precludes the extensive citation of individual surgical instruments, equipment, and supply companies, domestic and international, many of which offer excellent but similar products. The reader is reminded, however, that, when applicable, certain proprietary products have been suggested within the text to perform the particular procedure; the inclusion of those brands hopefully clarifies the type of items needed.

Index

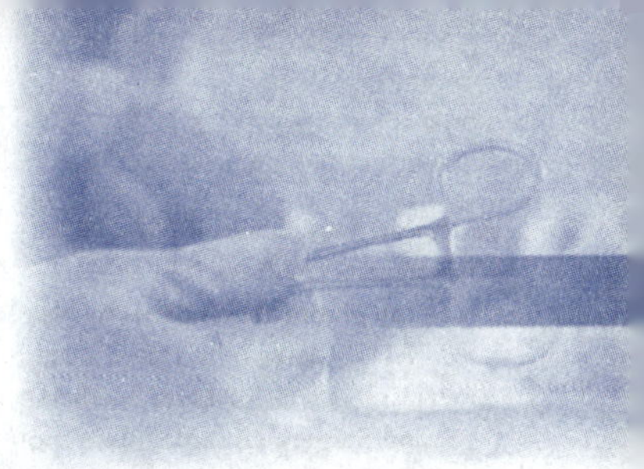

A

B

C

D

E

G

H

I

M

P

S